CHAPMAN'S ORTHOPAEDIC SURGERY

CHAPMAN'S ORTHOPAEDIC SURGERY

Third Edition

VOLUME 4

Edited by

MICHAEL W. CHAPMAN, M.D.

Professor Emeritus and David Linn Chair of Orthopaedic Surgery
University of California Davis
Sacramento, California

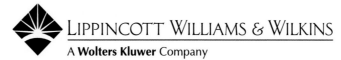

LIPPINCOTT WILLIAMS & WILKINS
A **Wolters Kluwer** Company

Philadelphia • Baltimore • New York • London
Buenos Aires • Hong Kong • Sydney • Tokyo

Acquisitions Editor: Anne Schuldiner Patterson
Developmental Editor: Maureen Iannuzzi
Production Editor: Penny Bice
Manufacturing Manager: Tim Reynolds
Cover Designer: Diana Andrews
Compositor: Maryland Composition
Printer: Courier Westford

© 2001 by LIPPINCOTT WILLIAMS & WILKINS
530 Walnut Street
Philadelphia, PA 19106 USA
LWW.com

Printed in the USA

Library of Congress Cataloging-in-Publication Data

Chapman's orthopaedic surgery/edited by Michael W. Chapman.—3rd ed.
    p. ; cm.
  Rev. ed. of: Operative orthopaedics. 2nd ed. c1993.
  Includes bibliographical references and index.
  ISBN 0-7817-1487-7
    1. Orthopedic surgery. I. Title: Orthopaedic surgery. II. Chapman, Michael W. III. Operative orthopaedics.
  [DNLM: 1. Orthopedic Procedures. WE 168 C466 2000]
  RD731 .O64 2000
  617.4'7—dc21   00-057610

10 9 8 7 6 5 4 3 2 1

To

Our teachers on whose shoulders the contributors to the third edition and I stand.
Our patients who inspired us to write this book so that they will receive the finest of care.
Our students, residents, fellows, and colleagues whose questions and guidance provided the guideposts
for the text.

And

To my wife, Elizabeth (Betty) Casady Chapman, whose patience and support endures,
and to my parents, William P. and Ethel B. Chapman, whose skills in parenting induced the discipline
necessary to take on the monumental task of writing and editing this book.

Michael W. Chapman, M.D.

CONTENTS

VOLUME 2

SECTION III
THE HAND
Robert M. Szabo

VOLUME 3

SECTION IV
SPORTS MEDICINE (CONTINUED)
Richard A. Marder

SECTION EDITORS

MICHAEL W. CHAPMAN, M.D.
Professor Emeritus and David Linn Chair of Orthopaedic
  Surgery
University of California Davis
Sacramento, California

JOSEPH M. LANE, M.D.
Professor of Orthopaedic Surgery
Weill Medical College of Cornell University
Orthopaedic Attendant
Hospital for Special Surgery
New York, New York

ROGER A. MANN, M.D.
Orthopaedic Surgeon
Summit Hospital
The Surgery Center
Oakland, California
San Leandro Hospital
San Leandro, California

RICHARD A. MARDER, M.D.
Professor
Department of Orthopaedic Surgery
University of California Davis
Sacramento, California

ROBERT F. McLAIN, M.D.
Director, Spine Research
Department of Orthopaedics
The Cleveland Clinic Foundation
Cleveland, Ohio

GEORGE T. RAB, M.D.
Professor
Department of Orthopaedic Surgery
University of California Davis
Sacramento, California

ROBERT M. SZABO, M.D., M.P.H.
Professor and Chief
Hand, Microvascular, and Upper Extremity Surgery
Department of Orthopaedics and Plastic Surgery
University of California Davis
Sacramento, California

KELLY G. VINCE, M.D., FRCS(C)
Associate Professor
University of Southern California
Los Angeles, California

CONTRIBUTING AUTHORS

Louis M. Adler, M.D.
Longmeadow, Massachusetts

Behrooz A. Akbarnia, M.D.
Clinical Professor
Department of Orthopaedics
University of California San Diego
Medical Director
San Diego Center for Spinal Disorders
San Diego, California

Edward Akelman, M.D.
Professor and Vice-Chair
Orthopedics
Brown University
Surgeon-in-Charge
Division of Hand Surgery
Rhode Island Hospital
Providence, Rhode Island

David A. Alessandro, M.D.
Massachusetts General Hospital
Boston, Massachusetts

Howard S. An, M.D.
The Morton International Professor of
Orthopaedic Surgery
Department of Orthopaedic Surgery
Rush Medical College
Director of Rush Spine Center
Rush-Presbyterian-St. Luke's Medical Center
Chicago, Illinois

Reynaldo L. Aponte, PA-C
Physician Assistant
Division of Plastic, Reconstructive,
Maxillofacial and Oral Surgery
Duke University Medical Center
Durham, North Carolina

James Aronson, M.D.
Chief of Pediatric Orthopaedic Surgery
Arkansas Children's Hospital
Professor
Department of Orthopaedic Surgery
University of Arkansas for Medical Sciences
Little Rock, Arkansas

Edward A. Athanasian, M.D.
Assistant Attending Surgeon
Hospital for Special Surgery
Assistant Professor
Cornell University Medical College
New York, New York

Bernard R. Bach, Jr., M.D.
Professor, Department of Orthopaedics
Rush Medical Center
Director, Sports Medicine Section
Rush-Presbyterian-St. Luke's Medical Center
Chicago, Illinois

Roland J. Barr, M.D.
Southern Orthopaedics Associates
Southern Illinois Healthcare
Carbondale, Illinois

Gordon R. Bell, M.D.
Vice-Chairman, Department of Orthopaedic
Surgery
Head, Section of Spinal Surgery
Cleveland Clinic Foundation
Cleveland, Ohio

Daniel R. Benson, M.D.
Professor, Dept. of Orthopaedic Surgery
Chief, Spine Service
Dept. of Orthopaedic Surgery
University of California Davis
Sacramento, California

Richard Berger, M.D., Ph.D.
Associate Professor
Departments of Orthopedic Surgery and
Anatomy
Mayo Clinic/Mayo Foundation
Rochester, Minnesota

Robert M. Bernstein, MD
Assistant Chief of Staff
Department of Pediatric Orthopedics
Shriners Hospitals for Children
Associate Clinical Professor
Department of Orthopaedic Surgery
UCLA School of Medicine
Los Angeles, California

Daniel J. Berry, M.D.
Consultant
Department of Orthopaedics
Mayo Clinic
Associate Professor of Orthopaedic Surgery
Mayo Medical School
Rochester, Minnesota

Bruce Beynnon, M.D.
University of Vermont Medical School
Department of Orthopaedics
Burlington, Vermont

Leslie J. Bisson, M.D.
Northtowns Orthopedics, P.C.
E. Amherst, New York

William F. Blair, M.D.
Steindler Orthopaedic Clinic
Iowa City, Iowa

Walther H. O. Bohne, M.D.
Director, Children's Foot Service
Co-Director Adult Foot Service
Hospital for Special Surgery
New York, New York

Lawrence B. Bone, M.D.
Director of Musculoskeletal Trauma
Department of Orthopaedics
Erie County Medical Center
Associate Professor
State University of New York at Buffalo
Buffalo, New York

F. William Bora, Jr., M.D.
Penn Medicine at Radnor
Chief, Department of Hand Surgery
Hospital of the U. of Pennyslvania
Professor
Dept. of Orthopaedic Surgery
University of Pennsylvania
Philadelphia, Pennsylvania

Mathias Bostrom, M.D.
Hospital for Special Surgery
New York, New York

Michael J. Botte, M.D.
Head, Section of Neuromuscular
Reconstructive Surgery & Rehabilitation
Division of Orthopaedic Surgery
Scripps Clinic and Research Foundation
La Jolla, California
Clinical Professor
Department of Orthopaedic Surgery
University of California School of Medicine
San Diego, California

J. Richard Bowen, M.D.
Chairman, Department of Orthopaedics
DuPont Hospital for Children
Wilmington, Delaware

David J. Bozentka, M.D.
Assistant Professor
Department of Orthopaedic Surgery
Hospital of the University of Pennsylvania
Penn Hand Specialists
Philadelphia, Pennsylvania

David S. Bradford, M.D.
University of California Medical Center
San Francisco, California

Paul W. Brand, M.D., M.B.B.S. (Lond.),
FRCS (Eng.)
Clinical Professor Emeritus
University of Washington
Seattle, Washington

Timothy J. Bray, M.D.
Associate
Reno Orthopaedic Clinic
Associate Clinical Professor
Dept. of Orthopaedic Surgery
University of California Davis Medical
Center
Sacramento, California

Nigel S. Broughton, FRCSEd, FRCS, FRACS
Consultant Orthopaedic Surgeon
Frankston Hospital
Victoria, Australia

Dennis W. Burke, M.D.
Department of Orthopaedic Surgery
Massachusetts General Hospital
Harvard Medical School
Boston, Massachusetts

Jesse Butler, M.D.
Adjunct Instructor
Department of Physical Medicine
Northwestern University
Attending
Department of Orthopaedic Surgery
Our Lady of Resurrection Spine Center
Chicago, Illinois

Jason H. Calhoun, M.D., FACS
Professor and Chairman
Department of Orthopaedics &
Rehabilitation
The University of Texas Medical Branch
Galveston, Texas

Michelle Gerwin Carlson, M.D.
Attending Hand Surgeon
Department of Orthopaedics
The Hospital for Special Surgery
Assistant Professor
Dept. of Surgery (Orthopaedics)
Cornell University Medical College
New York, New York

Charles Carroll IV, M.D.
Attending Staff
Department of Orthopedic Surgery
Northwestern Memorial
Assistant Professor of Clinical Orthopedic
Surgery
Northwestern University Medical School
Chicago, Illinois

Mark Casillas, M.D.
Clinical Instructor of Orthopaedics
University of Texas Health Sciences Center
in San Antonio
San Antonio, Texas

Michael W. Chapman, M.D.
Professor and David Linn Chair of
Orthopaedic Surgery
Department of Orthopaedic Surgery
University of California Davis
Sacramento, California

Larry K. Chidgey, M.D.
Department of Orthopaedics &
Rehabilitation
University of Florida
Gainesville, Florida

Loretta B. Chou, M.D.
Assistant Professor
Department of Functional Restoration
(Orthopaedic Surgery)
Stanford University School of Medicine
UCSF Stanford Health Care
Stanford, California

William G. Clancy, Jr., M.D.
American Sports Medicine Institute
Staff Orthopaedic Surgeon
Clinical Professor of Orthopaedic Surgery
Alabama Sports Medicine & Orthopaedic
Center
University of Alabama/Birmingham
Birmingham, Alabama

Charles R. Clark, M.D.
Professor of Orthopaedic Surgery
Professor of Biomedical Engineering
University of Iowa, College of Medicine &
College of Engineering
Staff Physician
Department of Orthopaedic Surgery
University of Iowa Health Center
Iowa City, Iowa

Charles N. Cornell, M.D.
Hospital for Special Surgery
New York, New York

Michael J. Coughlin, M.D.
Oregon Health Sciences University
Portland, Oregon
Treasure Valley Hospital
Boise, Idaho

David B. Coward, M.D.
Clinical Assistant Professor
Dept. of Orthopaedic Surgery
University of California Davis
Senior Staff
Dept. of Orthopaedic Surgery
Sutter Medical Center
Sacramento, California

Edward V. Craig, M.D.
Attending Orthopaedic Surgeon
The Hospital for Special Surgery
Department of Surgery
New York-Presbyterian Hospital
New York, New York

Gordon Derman, M.D.
Attending Surgeon
Plastic and Reconstructive Surgery
Rush Presbyterian St. Luke's Medical Center
Assistant Professor
Dept. of Plastic Surgery
Rush Medical College
Chicago, Illinois

James H. Dobyns, M.D.
Division of Hand Surgery
Department of Orthopaedic Surgery
Mayo Clinic
Rochester, Minnesota

Xavier A. Duralde, M.D.
Attending Physician
Peachtree Orthopaedic Clinic
Piedmont Hospital
Clinical Instructor
Department of Orthopaedics
Emory University
Atlanta, Georgia

Sridhar M. Durbhakula, M.D.
Research Fellow
Orthopaedic Surgeon
Albany Medical Center
Albany, New York

Kenneth A. Egol, M.D.
Department of Orthopaedic Surgery
Carolinas Medical Center
Charlotte, North Carolina

Jan Paul Ertl, M.D.
Kaiser-Permanente Hospital
Sacramento, California

John L. Esterhai, Jr., M.D.
Associate Professor of Orthopaedic Surgery
Department of Orthopaedics
Hospital of the University of Pennsylvania
Philadelphia, Pennsylvania

Peter J. Evans, M.D., Ph.D., FRCSC
Assistant Professor
Department of Orthopaedic Surgery and
Rehabilitation
Johns Hopkins University School of
Medicine
Baltimore, Maryland

Richard D. Ferkel, M.D.
Attending Surgeon & Director of Fellowship
Southern California Orthopedic Institute
Clinical Instructor
Dept. of Orthopedic Surgery
UCLA
Center for Health Sciences
Los Angeles, California

James D. Ferrari, M.D.
Director Sports Medicine
Department of Orthopaedic Surgery
Denver Health Medical Center
Assistant Professor
Department of Orthopaedic Surgery
University of Colorado Health Science
Center
Denver, Colorado

Linda Ferris, MB/BS, BSc (med), FRACS
Wakefield Orthopaedic Clinic
Adelaide, Australia

Christopher G. Finkemeier, M.D.
Assistant Professor
Department of Orthopaedic Surgery
University of California Davis
Sacramento, California

Evan Flatow, M.D.
Professor
Mt. Sinai Medical Center
New York, New York

William F. Flynn, Jr., M.D.
St. Mary's Hospital
Waterbury, Connecticut

Deborah A. Frassica, M.D.
Johns Hopkins Radiation Oncology at
Greenspring Station
Assistant Professor of Radiation Oncology
Department of Oncology
Johns Hopkins University
Baltimore, Maryland

Frank J. Frassica, M.D.
Professor of Orthopaedic Surgery and
Oncology
Department of Orthopaedic Surgery
Johns Hopkins University
Baltimore, Maryland

Alan E. Freeland, M.D.
Professor & Director of Hand Surgery
Service
Department of Orthopaedic Surgery
University of Mississippi Medical Center
Jackson, Mississippi

Dennis L. Fung, M.D.
Department of Anesthesiology
University of California Davis
Sacramento, California

Robert W. Gaines, Jr., M.D.
Professor/Spine Surgeon
Department of Orthopaedic Surgery
University of Missouri Hospital & Clinics
University of Missouri
Health Sciences Center, M-562
Columbia, Missouri

Dina Hulsizer Galvin, M.D.
Instructor, Orthopaedics
Department of Orthopaedics
Brown University School of Medicine
Providence, Rhode Island

Kevin L. Garvin, M.D.
Professor
Department of Orthopaedic Surgery
University of Nebraska Medical Center
Omaha, Nebraska

Mark C. Gebhardt, M.D.
Associate Orthopaedic Surgeon
Department of Orthopaedic Surgery
Children's Hospital
Associate Professor of Orthopaedic Surgery
Department of Orthopaedics
Harvard Medical School
Boston, Massachusetts

Richard H. Gelberman, M.D.
Department of Orthopaedic Surgery
Barnes Hospital
St. Louis, Missouri

Claude Gelinas, M.D.
Southwest Spine Center
Albuquerque, New Mexico

M. Eric Gershwin, M.D.
Division Chief of Rheumatology/Allergy
Davis, California

Paramjeet S. Gill, M.D., FRCSC
Assistant Clinical Professor, Division of
Orthopaedic Surgery
University of California, San Francisco
School of Medicine
University Medical Center
Fresno, California

Steven Gitelis, M.D.
Professor
Dept. of Orthopaedic Surgery
Rush Medical College
Associate Chairman
Dept. of Orthopaedic Surgery
Rush-Presbyterian-St. Luke's Medical Center
Chicago, Illinois

Ronald E. Glousman, M.D.
Partner, Vice-President
Kerlan-Jobe Orthopaedic Clinic
Clinical Associate Professor
Dept. of Orthopaedic Surgery
University of Southern California
Los Angeles, California

Michael J. Goebel, M.D.
Blue Ridge Bone and Joint
Orthopaedic Surgeon
Department of Surgery
Mission/St. Joseph's Health System
Asheville, North Carolina

Vijay K. Goel, M.D.
Department of Biomedical Engineering
University of Iowa
Iowa City, Iowa

**Stuart B. Goodman, M.D., Ph.D., FRCSC,
FACS**
Chief of Orthopaedic Surgery
Stanford University Medical Center
Stanford, California

John S. Gould, M.D.
Orthopaedic Surgeon
Alabama Sports Medicine and Orthopaedic
Center
Health South Medical Center
Clinical Professor of Orthopaedic Surgery
University of Virginia
Birmingham, Alabama

James A. Goulet, M.D.
University of Michigan Hospital
Ann Arbor, Michigan

Steven M. Green, M.D.
Associate Chief Hand Surgery
Dept. of Orthopaedic Surgery
Hospital for Joint Diseases
Assoc. Clinical Professor
Dept. of Orthopaedic Surgery
Mt. Sinai Medical School
New York University
New York, New York

Stuart A. Green, M.D.
Clinical Professor
Dept. of Othopaedic Surgery
University of California Irvine
Orange, California

William L. Green, M.D.
Dept. of Orthopaedics
California Pacific Medical Center
Clinical Professor
Dept. of Orthopaedic Surgery
University of California San Francisco
San Francisco, California

Adam Greenspan, M.D., FACR
Department of Radiology
University of California Davis
Sacramento, California

Letha Y. Griffin, M.D.
Staff
Peachtree Orthopaedic Clinic
Team Physician
Georgia State University
Atlanta, Georgia

Paul P. Griffin, M.D.
Greenville Memorial Hospital
Professor Emeritus
Department of Orthopaedic Education
Medical University of South Carolina
Greenville, South Carolina

Munish C. Gupta, M.D.
Assistant Professor
Department of Orthopaedic Surgery
University of California Davis
Sacramento, California

David J. Hak, M.D.
Assistant Professor
Department of Surgery
University of Michigan Hospital
Ann Arbor, Michigan

Mark N. Halikis, M.D.
Chief, Hand Surgery Service
Long Beach Veterans' Affairs Medical
Center
Assistant Clinical Professor
Dept. of Orthopaedic Surgery
University of California Irvine
Orange, California

Robert A. Hart, M.D., MA
Assistant Professor
Chief, Division of Spine Surgery
Department of Orthopaedic Surgery
Oregon Health Sciences University School of
Medicine
Portland, Oregon

Eric A. Heiden, M.D.
Assistant Professor
Department of Orthopaedic Surgery
University of California Davis
Faculty
Department of Orthopaedics
University of California Davis Medical
Center
Sacramento, California

Karen D. Heiden, M.D.
Department of Orthopaedic Surgery
University of California Davis Medical
Center
Sacramento, California

Lior Heller, M.D.
Fellow in Wound Healing and Plastic
Surgery
Division of Plastic, Reconstructive,
Maxillofacial and Oral Surgery
Duke University Medical Center
Durham, North Carolina

Harry N. Herkowitz, M.D.
Chairman
Dept. of Orthopaedic Surgery
William Beaumont Hospital
Royal Oak, Michigan

John A. Herring, M.D.
Chief of Staff
Department of Orthopaedics
Texas Scottish Rite Hospital for Children
Professor
Department of Orthopedic Surgery
University of Texas Southwestern Medical
School
Dallas, Texas

Anne Hollister, M.D.
Department of Orthopaedic Surgery
Louisiana State University Medical Center
Shreveport, Louisiana

Serena S. Hu, M.D.
Associate Professor
Department of Orthopedic Surgery
University of California San Francisco
Spine Specialist
Department of Orthopedics
Moffett Long Hospitals
San Francisco, California

Michelle A. James, M.D.
Assistant Chief
Department of Orthopaedic Surgery
Shriners Hospital for Children, Northern
California
Associate Clinical Professor
University of California Davis
Sacramento, California

Louis G. Jenis, M.D.
Staff Surgeon
Department of Orthopaedic Surgery
New England Baptist Hospital
Clinical Instructor in Orthopaedic Surgery
Tufts University School of Medicine
Boston, Massachusetts

Robert J. Johnson, M.D.
University of Vermont
Department of Orthopaedics &
Rehabilitation
Attending Orthopaedist
Fletcher Allen Health Care
Burlington, Vermont

Deryk G. Jones, M.D.
Assistant Professor
Department of Orthopaedic Surgery
Tulane University School of Medicine
Staff
Tulane University Medical Center
New Orleans, Louisiana

Michael A. Joyce, CP
The Joyce Center
Manhasset, New York

Jesse B. Jupiter, M.D.
Director, Orthopaedic Hand Service
Massachusetts General Hospital
Professor, Orthopaedic Surgery
Harvard Medical School
Boston, Massachusetts

James C. Karageannes, M.D.
Blue Ridge Bone & Joint
Adult Reconstruction Surgery Fellow
Hospital for Special Surgery
New York, New York

Lori A. Karol, M.D.
Staff Orthopaedist
Department of Orthopaedics
Texas Scottish Rite Hospital
Associate Professor
Department of Orthopaedic Surgery
University of Texas
Southwestern Medical Center
Dallas, Texas

Carol K. Kasper, M.D.
Emeritus Professor of Medicine
Department of Medicine
University of Southern California
Emeritus Director
Hemophilia Center
Orthopaedic Hospital
Los Angeles, California

Barry M. Katzman, M.D.
Orthopaedic Care & Surgery
Department of Orthopaedics
University of Pennsylvania
Philadelphia, Pennsylvania

Mary Ann E. Keenan, M.D.
Director, Neuro-Orthopaedics Program
Department of Orthopaedic Surgery
Albert Einstein Medical Center
Professor
Department of Orthopaedic Surgery
Temple University School of Medicine
Philadelphia, Pennsylvania

Howard A. King, M.D.
St. Luke's Regional Medical Center
Boise, Idaho

Graham J. W. King, M.D., MSc, FRCSC
Chief, Orthopaedic Surgery
Department of Surgery
St. Joseph's Health Center
Associate Professor
Department of Surgery
University of Western Ontario
London, Ontario
Canada

L. Andrew Koman, M.D.
Professor
Department of Orthopaedic Surgery
Division of Surgical Sciences
Wake Forest University School of Medicine
Winston-Salem, North Carolina

Kenneth J. Koval, M.D.
Chief, Orthopaedic Fracture Service
Hospital for Joint Diseases
Associate Professor
Dept. of Orthopaedics
NYU School of Medicine
New York, New York

Thomas E. Kuivila, M.D.
Attending Surgeon
Department of Orthopaedic Surgery
Section of Pediatric Orthopaedics
The Cleveland Clinic Foundation
Cleveland, Ohio

Ashkan Lahiji, M.D.
Department of Orthopaedic Surgery
Hospital University of Pennsylvania
Philadelphia, Pennsylvania

Joseph M. Lane, M.D.
Hospital for Special Surgery
Chief
Metabolic Bone Disease Service
Professor of Orthopaedic Surgery
Weill Medical College of Cornell University
New York, New York

William C. Lauerman, M.D.
Chief, Division of Spine Surgery
Georgetown University Medical Center
Associate Professor
Dept. of Orthopaedic Surgery
Georgetown University
Washington, D.C.

Donald H. Lee, M.D.
Associate Professor/Hand Fellowship
Director
Division of Orthopaedic Surgery
University of Alabama at Birmingham
Birmingham, Alabama

Guy Alan Lee, M.D.
Department of Orthopaedic Surgery
Albert Einstein Medical Center
Moss Rehab Hospital
Philadelphia, Pennsylvania

Robert D. Leffert, M.D.
Massachusetts General Hospital
Boston, Massachusetts

Michael T. LeGeyt, M.D.
Instructor, Orthopaedics
Department of Orthopaedics
Brown University School of Medicine
Providence, Rhode Island

Ross K. Leighton, M.D., FRCSC, FACS, BSc
Associate Professor
Department of Surgery
Dalhousie University
Halifax, Nova Scotia
Canada

Robert H. Leland, M.D.
Assistant Professor
Chief of Foot and Ankle Surgery
Department of Orthopaedic Surgery
Wayne State University School of Medicine
Hutzel Hospital
Department of Orthopaedics
Detroit, Michigan

L. Scott Levin, M.D.
Associate Professor of Plastic and
Orthopaedic Surgery
Chief—Division of Plastic, Reconstructive,
Maxillofacial and Oral Surgery
Duke University Medical Center
Durham, North Carolina

Alan M. Levine, M.D.
Director
Alvin & Lois Lapidus Cancer Institute
Sinai Hospital of Baltimore
Clinical Professor of Othopaedic Surgery
Department of Surgery
University of Maryland
Baltimore, Maryland

George Lian, M.D.
Assistant Clinical Professor
Department of Orthopaedic Surgery
University of California Davis School of
Medicine
Sacramento, California

Isador Lieberman, BSc, M.D., FRCS
Orthopaedic & Spinal Surgeon
Department of Orthopaedics
The Cleveland Clinic Foundation
Cleveland, Ohio

Steven A. Lietman, M.D.
Assistant Professor of Orthopaedic Surgery
Department of Orthopaedic Surgery
Johns Hopkins University
Baltimore, Maryland

Terry R. Light, M.D.
Dr. William M. Scholl Professor and Chair
Department of Orthopaedic Surgery and
Rehabilitation
Loyola University Chicago
Stritch School of Medicine
Chief
Department of Orthopaedic Surgery &
Rehabilitation
Foster McLean Loyola Medical Center
Maywood, Illinois

Judith C. Lin, M.D.
Staff Hematologist, Hemophilia Center
Orthopaedic Hospital
Los Angeles, California

Paul R. Lipscomb, M.D.
Professor Emeritus of Orthopaedics
School of Medicine
University of California Davis
Sacramento, California

Randall T. Loder, M.D.
Chief of Staff
Shriners Hospital for Children
Clinical Professor
Dept. of Orthopaedics
University of Minnesota
Minneapolis, Minnesota

Laurence J. Logan, M.D.
Director, Hemophilia Treatment Center
Department of Vascular Medicine
Orthopaedic Hospital
Clinical Associate Professor
Department of Medicine (Hematology)
University of Southern California
Los Angeles, California

John D. Lubahn, M.D., FACS
Hand Microsurgery & Reconstructive
Orthopaedics
Chairman, Department of Orthopaedic
Surgery
Hamot Medical Center
Erie, Pennsylvania

James V. Luck, Jr., M.D.
Chief of Orthopaedics
Hemophilia Center, Orthopaedic Hospital
Los Angeles, California
Executive Vice Chairman
UCLA-Orthopaedic Hospital
Department of Orthopaedics
University of California at Los Angeles
Los Angeles, California

William G. Mackenzie, M.D.
Assistant Professor
Jefferson Medical College
Wilmington, Delaware

Jon T. Mader, M.D.
Section Chief, Surgical Infectious Diseases
Department of Internal Medicine
Adjunct Professor of Orthopaedic Surgery
University of Texas Medical Branch
Galveston, Texas

Martin Malawer, M.D.
Washington Cancer Institute
Washington, D.C.
George Washington University School of
Medicine
Washington, D.C.

Martin G. Mankey, M.D.
Clinical Instructor, Department of
Orthopaedics
University of Washington
Seattle, Washington

Jeffrey A. Mann, M.D.
Oakland, California

Roger A. Mann, M.D.
Orthopaedic Surgeon
San Leandro Hospital
Summit Hospital
The Surgery Center
San Leandro, California

Mark W. Manoso, M.D.
Department of Orthopaedic Surgery
Johns Hopkins Hospital
Johns Hopkins University School of
Medicine
Baltimore, Maryland

Paul R. Manske, M.D.
Professor of Orthopaedic Surgery
Washington University
St. Louis, Missouri

Richard A. Marder, M.D.
Professor
Department of Orthopaedic Surgery
University of California Davis
Sacramento, California

Guido Marra, M.D.
Instructor
Loyola University Medical Center
Loyola University of Chicago
Maywood, Illinois

Robert G. Marx, M.D.
Hospital for Special Surgery
New York, New York

Jeffrey W. Mast, M.D.
Professor Orthopaedic Surgery
Department of Orthopaedic Surgery
Wayne State University School of Medicine
Detroit, Michigan

Joel M. Matta, M.D.
University of Southern California School of
Medicine
Los Angeles, California

Jack K. Mayfield, M.D., M.S.
Adjunct Professor
Department of Materials, Chemical and
Bioengineering
Arizona State University
and Phoenix Spine Center
St. Luke's Hospital Center
Phoenix, Arizona

Paul C. McAfee, M.D.
Chief of Spinal Surgery
Dept. of Orthopaedic Surgery
St. Joseph's Hospital
Associate Professor
Dept. of Orthopaedic Surgery
Johns Hopkins School of Medicine
Johns Hopkins Hospital
Baltimore, Maryland

Edward F. McCarthy, M.D.
Director of Bone Pathology
Department of Pathology
Johns Hopkins Hospital
Associate Professor of Orthopaedics and
Oncology
Department of Pathology & Orthopaedic
Surgery
Johns Hopkins University
Baltimore, Maryland

Patrick J. McDaid, M.D.
Department of Orthopaedic Surgery
Albert Einstein Medical Center
Moss Rehab Hospital
Philadelphia, Pennsylvania

Douglas J. McDonald, M.D.
Professor
Department of Orthopaedic Surgery
Washington University School of Medicine
St. Louis, Missouri

Steven J. McGrath, M.D.
Southern California Orthopedic Institute
Van Nuys, California

Theresa M. McKillip, PA-C
University of Nebraska Medical Center
Department of Orthopaedic Surgery
Omaha, Nebraska

Robert F. McLain, M.D.
Director, Spine Research
Department of Orthopaedics
The Cleveland Clinic Foundation
Cleveland, Ohio

Dana C. Mears, M.D., Ph.D.
Professor and Chief
Division of Orthopaedic Surgery
The Albany Medical College
Albany, New York

John P. Meehan, M.D.
Assistant Professor
General Orthopaedics
University of California Davis
Department of Orthopaedics
Sacramento, California

Malcom B. Menalaus, M.D., FRCS, FRACS
Chief Orthopaedic Surgeon, Emeritus
Royal Children's Hospital
Melbourne, Australia

Alan C. Merchant, M.D., MS
Clinical Professor, Orthopaedic Surgery
Stanford University School of Medicine
Stanford, California
Staff Surgeon, Department of Orthopedic
Surgery
El Camino Hospital
Mountain View, California

R. Scott Meyer, M.D.
Assistant Clinical Professor
Department of Orthopaedics
University of California San Diego
Department of Orthopaedics
UCSD Medical Center
San Diego, California

Kimberly K. Mezera, M.D.
Assistant Professor
Department of Orthopaedic Surgery
Hand, Wrist, Elbow, Shoulder &
Microvascular Surgery
Southwestern Medical School
Dallas, Texas

John D. Miles, M.D.
Spine Surgeon
Columbia Spine Center
Columbia, Missouri

Gary A. Miller, M.D.
Associate Professor
Washington University School of Medicine
St. Louis Veterans Affairs Medical Center
Orthopaedic Surgery
St. Louis, Missouri

Hanno Millesi, M.D.
Professor Emeritus of Plastic Surgery
University of Vienna Medical School
Medical Director Vienna Private Hospital
Director Ludwig-Boltzmann Institute for
Experimental Plastic Surgery
Vienna, Austria

Joseph C. Milne, M.D.
Fort Worth Bone and Joint Clinic
Fort Worth, Texas

Roby D. Mize, M.D.
Clinical Associate Professor
Orthopaedic Surgery
University of Texas Southwestern Medical
School
Orthopaedic Staff Member
Orthopaedic Surgery
Presbyterian Medical Center of Dallas
Dallas, Texas

Mark S. Mizel, M.D.
Associate Professor
University of Miami
Miami, Florida

Michael A. Mont, M.D.
Associate Professor
Department of Orthopaedic Surgery
Johns Hopkins University School of
Medicine
Baltimore, Maryland

Matthew A. Mormino, M.D.
Assistant Professor
University of Nebraska Medical Center
Department of Orthopaedic Surgery
Omaha, Nebraska

Carol D. Morris, M.D., MS
Department of Orthopaedic Surgery
Memorial Sloan-Kettering Cancer Center
New York, New York

Vincent S. Mosca, M.D.
Children's Hospital and Regional Medical
Center
Seattle, Washington

Colin I. Moseley, M.D.
Shriner's Hospital
Los Angeles, California

Scott J. Mubarak, M.D.
Director of Orthopaedic Program
Children's Hospital
Clinical Professor
Department of Orthopaedics
University of California San Diego
San Diego, California

Robert J. Neviaser, M.D.
Professor and Chairman
Department of Orthopedic Surgery
George Washington University
Washington, D.C.

Beth G. Nicholson, OTR, CHT
Alabama Sports Medicine and Orthopaedic
Center
Birmingham, Alabama

Hugh O'Flynn, M.D.
Beverly Hospital
Beverly, Massachusetts

Steven A. Olson, M.D.
Associate Professor
Chief, Orthopaedic Trauma
University of California Davis Medical
Center
Department of Orthopaedic Surgery
Sacramento, California

George E. Omer, Jr., M.D., MS
Professor and Chairman Emeritus
Department of Orthopaedics and
Rehabilitation
The University of New Mexico Health
Sciences Center
Albuquerque, New Mexico

William L. Oppenheim, M.D.
Professor and Head
Division of Pediatric Orthopaedics
UCLA School of Medicine
Consultant, Shriners' Hospital
UCLA Medical Center
Los Angeles, California

A. Lee Osterman, M.D.
Professor of Orthopaedics and Hand Surgery
Philadelphia Hand Center
King of Prussia, Pennsylvania

Dror Paley, M.D.
Kerman Hospital
Baltimore, Maryland

Carl F. Palumbo, M.D.
Department of Orthopaedic Surgery
University of California Davis Medical
Center
Sacramento, California

Wayne G. Paprosky, M.D., FACS
Associate Professor
Department of Orthopaedic Surgery
Rush Medical College
Chicago, Illinois
Attending Orthopaedic Surgeon
Central DuPage Hospital
Winfield, Illinois

Michael J. Patzakis, M.D.
Professor and Chairman
The Vincent and Julia Meyer Chair
Department of Orthopaedic Surgery
USC Medical School
Los Angeles, California

Terrance D. Peabody, M.D.
University of Chicago Hospitals and Clinics
Department of Surgery
Section of Orthopaedic Surgery and
Rehabilitation Medicine
Chicago, Illinois

Clayton A. Peimer, M.D.
Professor of Orthopaedic Surgery and Chief
of Hand Surgery
Hand Center of Western New York
Buffalo, New York

Jacquelin Perry, M.D., D.Sc. (Hon)
Professor Emeritus of Orthopaedics
Professor Emeritus of Biokinesiology and
Physical Therapy
University of Southern California
Rancho Los Amigos Medical Center
Downey, California

Martin A. Posner, M.D.
Clinical Professor of Orthopaedics
New York University School of Medicine
Chief of Hand Services:
HJD—New York University Department of
Orthopaedic Surgery
Lenox Hill Hospital
New York, New York

Patricia A. Post, M.D.
Department of Orthopaedics and
Rehabilitation
Vanderbilt University
Nashville, Tennessee

Mark E. Pruzansky, M.D.
Assistant Professor of Clinical Orthopaedic
Surgery
Mt. Sinai School of Medicine
New York, New York

Beth A. Purdy, M.D.
Children's Rehabilitative Services,
Orthopedic/Hand Surgery
Hand Surgery Associates
Phoenix, Arizona

Christian M. Puttlitz, Ph.D.
Post-Doctoral Research Fellow
Orthopaedic Bioengineering Laboratory
Department of Orthopaedic Surgery
University of California San Francisco
San Francisco, California

George T. Rab, M.D.
Professor
Department of Orthopaedic Surgery
University of California Davis
Sacramento, California

Kamshad Raiszadeh, M.D.
Clinical Instructor
Department of Orthopedics
University of California—San Diego School
of Medicine
San Diego Center for Spinal Disorders
San Diego, California

John R. Raskind, M.D.
Assistant Clinical Professor
Department of Orthopaedic Surgery
University of California Davis
Sacramento, California

Lawrence A. Rinsky, M.D.
Stanford University Medical Center
Stanford, California

Charles A. Rockwood, Jr., M.D.
Department of Orthopaedics
University of Texas Health Science Center
San Antonio, Texas

Juan J. Rodrigo, M.D.
Professor
Department of Orthopaedic Surgery
University of California Davis
Sacramento, California

Patricia G. Rossbach, RN
Amputee Coalition of America
Knoxville, Tennessee

David S. Ruch, M.D.
Assistant Professor
Department of Orthopaedic Surgery
Division of Surgical Sciences
Wake Forest University School of Medicine
Winston-Salem, North Carolina

Peter B. Salamon, M.D.
Department of Orthopaedic Surgery
University of California Davis
Sacramento, California

Richard F. Santore, M.D.
Department of Orthopaedic Surgery
University of California San Diego
Sharp Memorial Hospital
San Diego, California

Michael F. Schafer, M.D.
Ryerson Professor and Chairman
Department of Orthopaedic Surgery
Northwestern University Medical School
Chicago, Illinois

Eric Schaffer, CP
The Joyce Center
Manhasset, New York

David J. Schurman, M.D.
Stanford Medical Center
Stanford, California

Yoshio Setoguchi, M.D.
Clinical Professor
Department of Pediatrics
UCLA School of Medicine
Shriner's Hospital of Los Angeles
Los Angeles, California

Gary Shapiro, M.D.
Hospital for Special Surgery
New York, New York

Franklin H. Sim, M.D.
Professor of Orthopaedic Surgery
Mayo Clinic
Rochester, Minnesota

Edward H. Simmons, M.D.
Buffalo, New York

Michael A. Simon, M.D.
Department of Surgery
Section of Orthopaedic Surgery and
Rehabilitation Medicine
University of Chicago Hospitals and Clinics
Chicago, Illinois

Robert R. Slater, Jr., M.D.
Assistant Professor
Department of Orthopaedic Surgery
Sacramento, California

Beth Paterson Smith, Ph.D.
Assistant Professor
Department of Orthopaedic Surgery
Division of Surgical Sciences
Wake Forest University School of Medicine
Winston-Salem, North Carolina

Dan M. Spengler, M.D.
Vanderbilt University Medical Center
Department of Orthopaedics
Nashville, Tennessee

Paul D. Sponseller, M.D.
Associate Professor
Chief, Pediatric Orthopaedics
Johns Hopkins Hospital School of Medicine
Baltimore, Maryland

Lynn T. Staheli, M.D.
Director, Department of Orthopaedics,
CHMC
Professor, Department of Orthopaedics
University of Washington
Children's Hospital and Regional Center
Seattle, Washington

Deborah F. Stanitski, M.D., FRCSC
Professor
Pediatric Orthopaedics/Scoliosis/Limb
Deformity
Department of Orthopaedic Surgery
Medical University of South Carolina
Orthopaedic Services
Charleston, South Carolina

David R. Steinberg, M.D.
Assistant Professor of Orthopaedic Surgery
University of Pennsylvania
Philadelphia, Pennsylvania

Marvin E. Steinberg, M.D.
Professor and Vice Chairman
Department of Orthopaedic Surgery
University of Pennsylvania School of
Medicine
Philadelphia, Pennsylvania

Peter J. Stern, M.D.
Norman S. & Elizabeth CA. Hill Professor
Chairman, Department of Orthopaedic
Surgery
Department of Orthopaedic Surgery
University of Cincinnati College of Medicine
Cincinnati, Ohio

Thomas R. Stevenson, M.D.
Division of Plastic Surgery
University of California Davis
Sacramento, California

Marc F. Swiontkowski, M.D.
Professor and Chair, Department of
Orthopaedic Surgery
University of Minnesota Medical School
Minneapolis, Minnesota

Robert M. Szabo, M.D., M.P.H.
Professor and Chief
Hand, Microvascular and Upper Extremity
Surgery
Department of Orthopaedics and Plastic
Surgery
University of California Davis
Sacramento, California

Julio Taleisnik, M.D.
Department of Orthopaedic Surgery
University of California Irvine
Orange, California

J. Charles Taylor, M.D.
Memphis, Tennessee

Kevin Tetsworth, M.D.
Maryland Center for Limb Lengthening and
Reconstruction
University of Maryland
Baltimore, Maryland

James S. Thompson, M.D.
Hand and Upper Limb Reonstructive
Surgeon
Carolina Hand Surgery Associates
Mission-St. Joseph's Health System
Carolina Hand Surgery Associates
Asheville, North Carolina

George H. Thompson, M.D.
Professor, Orthopaedic Surgery and
Pediatrics
Director, Division of Pediatric Orthopaedics
Rainbow Babies and Children's Hospital
Case Western Reserve University
Cleveland, Ohio

Laura A. Timmerman, M.D.
Associate Clinical Professor
Orthopaedic Surgery
University of California Davis
Team Physician,
University of California Berkeley
Private Practice, Walnut Creek
Walnut Creek, California

Kenneth B. Trauner, M.D.
Department of Orthopaedic Surgery
University of California Davis
Sacramento, California

Eeric Truumees, M.D.
Spinal Surgery Fellow, William Beaumont
Hospital
Troy, Michigan

James R. Urbaniak, M.D.
Professor of Orthopaedic Surgery
Chief, Division of Orthopaedic Surgery
Vice Chairman, Department of Surgery
Duke University School of Medicine
Duke University Medical Center
Durham, North Carolina

Kelly G. Vince, M.D., FRCS(C)
Associate Professor
University of Southern California
Los Angeles, California

Kent A. Vincent, M.D.
Staff Surgeon, Shriners Hospital for
Children, Portland
Department of Orthopaedics, Oregon Health
Sciences University
Portland, Oregon

Peter Walker, Ph.D.
Institute of Orthopaedics
Director, Division Biomedical Engineering
University College London
Brockley Hill
Royal National Orthopaedic Hospital
United Kingdom

Jon J.P. Warner, M.D.
Chief, The Harvard Shoulder Service
Associate Professor
Partners Department of Orthopaedics
Harvard Medical School
Massachusetts General Hospital
Boston, Massachusetts

Robert G. Watkins, M.D.
Los Angeles, California

Hugh G. Watts, M.D.
Shriners' Hospital
Department of Orthopaedics
Clinical Professor
UCLA School of Medicine
Los Angeles, California

Kristy L. Weber
University of Texas
M.D. Andersen Cancer Center
Houston, Texas

Andrew J. Weiland, M.D.
Hospital for Special Surgery
New York, New York

Arnold-Peter C. Weiss, M.D.
Professor of Orthopaedics
Brown University School of Medicine
Providence, Rhode Island

James F. Wenz, M.D.
Assistant Professor of Orthopaedic Surgery
Department of Orthopaedic Surgery
Johns Hopkins University
Baltimore, Maryland

Thomas P. Whetzel, M.D.
Division of Plastic Surgery
University of California Davis
Sacramento, California

Sam W. Wiesel, M.D.
Professor and Chairman
Department of Orthopaedic Surgery
Georgetown University Hospital
Washington, D.C.

Robert L. Wilson, M.D.
Hand Surgery Consultant
Phoenix Orthopedic Program
Maricopa Medical Center
Associate in Surgery
University of Arizona
Tucson, Arizona

Russell E. Windsor, M.D.
Hospital for Special Surgery
New York, New York

Michael A. Wirth, M.D.
Department of Orthopaedics
San Antonio, Texas

Jennifer Moriatis Wolf, M.D.
Resident
Department of Orthopaedics
Brown University School of Medicine
Rhode Island Hospital
Providence, Rhode Island

Kevin P. Yakuboff, M.D.
Associate Professor of Surgery
Division of Plastic, Reconstructive & Hand
Surgery
Attending Burn Surgeon
Shriners Burns Institute
University of Cincinnati
Cincinnati, Ohio

Ken Yamaguchi, M.D.
Assistant Professor, Orthopaedic Surgery
Washington University School of Medicine
Barnes Jewish Hospital
St. Louis, Missouri

Francis Young-In Lee, M.D.
Assistant Professor
Department of Orthopaedic Surgery
Columbia-Presbyterian Medical Center
College of Physicians & Surgeons of
Columbia University
New York, New York

Thomas A. Zdeblick, M.D.
Professor and Chair
Orthopaedic Surgery
University of Wisconsin
Madison, Wisconsin

PREFACE TO THE THIRD EDITION

The third edition of *Operative Orthopaedics* has been retitled *Orthopaedic Surgery* to better reflect its content. While the book is predominantly concerned with operative orthopaedics, it also provides a review of general principles and the nonoperative care of musculoskeletal disorders. This book has been written primarily for the practicing orthopaedic surgeon who needs a comprehensive reference text on orthopaedic surgery to meet the demands of his or her practice in the twenty-first century. It is also an ideal textbook for the orthopaedic resident that will be useful from the first year of training on into practice after graduation. Due to the breadth of the field of orthopaedic surgery, busy orthopaedic surgeons often encounter conditions that they see only infrequently or are required to perform operations that they don't often do. There is a need for a resource that can be pulled off the shelf or brought up on the computer as a CD-ROM that efficiently answers a diagnostic problem or provides a "brush up" on an operative procedure. The section editors and I have designed this book to be useful not only to the practicing general orthopaedic surgeon but also to subspecialists in orthopaedic surgery who need a comprehensive reference book that provides cutting edge information from highly respected colleagues in their subspecialty.

To meet this need, we have substantially reorganized the third edition to provide a more logical sequence of chapters and identified major sections in each chapter with icons. Additionally, we have placed emphasis on providing "information at a glance" using numerous figures, tables, and algorithms. Color has been added to make it easier to identify important information and to enhance the clarity of the illustrations. A select group of illustrators was used to provide consistency in the art. Important information in the body of the text has been highlighted. For instance, the surgical techniques are presented in an easy to read style that uses blue squares to designate each significant step in the procedure. Careful page layout keeps descriptions of surgical techniques in close proximity to relevant illustrations, making it easier for the reader to follow the steps of the procedures. Finally, the new organization of the text is particularly suited for use on the computer, making the associated CD-ROM very accessible and user friendly.

The table of contents and the detailed chapter outlines provided at the beginning of each chapter make it easier for readers to find the material covering the subject or operative procedure they seek. The comprehensive index will be very helpful to readers as well. In addition, throughout the text we provide frequent cross-referencing to other chapters.

As all surgeons know, there are many hints and tricks that master surgeons have learned to ensure the success of their procedures, to help them avoid pitfalls, and to minimize the risk of complications. These are presented in hints and tricks boxes scattered throughout the text. The authors describe pitfalls and how to avoid complications in a separate section, and provide their personal perspective at appropriate points in each chapter.

The 180 chapters in the third edition are organized to provide a tightly focused discussion on the topics of concern. This also allows topical organization of the references, which are now annotated with symbols to designate the article as a historical classic (*), a basic science article relevant to the clinical topic (!), an article on clinical results or outcomes (+), or a review article (#).

For the more than 300 contributing authors, the seven section editors and me, this revision has been an enormous task. Aside from some portions of the basic principles chapters, the book has been essentially rewritten. Orthopaedic surgery and musculoskeletal medicine continue to advance at an astounding rate in diagnostic techniques, nonoperative treatments, and surgical procedures. Each author describes operative procedures and techniques that, in their own personal experience and on the basis of the best evidence available, have proven to be the most reliable. Surgical procedures and techniques of purely historical interest are mentioned only in passing.

Section I, edited by Michael W. Chapman, has nine chapters covering the basic principles underlying the practice of orthopaedic surgery including surgical approaches, imaging modalities, preoperative planning and perioperative management, orthopaedic anesthesia and postoperative pain management, as well as chapters on instrumentation, implants, bone grafting, and soft-tissue management. Chapter 4 on imaging includes expanded coverage of MRI, and Chapter 9 on bone grafting includes an expanded discussion of bone graft substitutes and growth factors.

Section II, also edited by Michael W. Chapman, contains 23 chapters on the management of fractures and dislocations. The section opens with an extensive discussion of closed treatment (Chapter 10) and the following four chapters cover the basic principles of fixation, treatment of open fractures, compartment syndromes, and management of polytrauma. Chapters 15 through 25 address the diagnosis and surgical treatment of fractures and dislocations on an anatomical basis. Chapters 27 through 32 are organized on an anatomical basis and focus on the diagnosis and treatment of nonunions and malunions. Chapter 32 is an extensive chapter, broken down into individual sections with multiple authors addressing the complex topic of application of Ilizarov techniques to the management of fractures, nonunions, malunions, limb-length discrepancy, and bone loss.

Section III, edited by Robert M. Szabo, has 43 chapters which provide the most comprehensive coverage of hand, upper extremity, and microvascular surgery available in a general orthopaedic textbook today. Chapters 33 to 36 address management of vascular disorders and microvascular surgery. The principles of hand surgery and surgical approaches are covered in Chapter 37. Chapters 38 through 49 cover hand and upper extremity trauma including both bone and soft-tissue injuries. The remainder of this section covers the entire field of hand and upper extremity surgery. Arthroscopic surgery of the wrist is covered in this section (Chapter 75), rather than in the sports medicine section.

Section IV, edited by Richard A. Marder, presents sports medicine and in 23 chapters thoroughly covers the surgery of athletic injuries. A new chapter on adolescent sports injuries (Chapter 97) and an entire chapter on the use of lasers in orthopaedic surgery (Chapter 98) have been added.

Section V, edited by Kelly G. Vince, covers joint reconstruction in 11 chapters. Chapter 99 addresses the management of arthritis. Chapter 100 provides the knowledge about design, manufacture, and materials of prosthetic implants that is necessary to perform modern total joint arthroplasty. Chapters 101 through 109 are organized on an anatomical basis and discuss primary and revision arthroplasty of each of the major joints. A discussion of arthrodesis is included in each of the chapters on revision arthroplasty. Chapter 104 on osteotomies about the hip has been substantially expanded due to the recent success of periacetabular osteotomies and other osteotomies about the hip.

Section VI, edited by Roger A. Mann, in 10 chapters covers the important issues in the care of disorders of the foot and ankle. (Fractures of the ankle are covered in Section II on trauma.)

In Section VII, edited by Joseph M. Lane, neoplastic, infectious, neurologic, and other skeletal disorders are covered in 17 chapters (120 through 136). This section opens with three chapters on the principles of amputations and prosthetics. Chapters 126 through 130 focus on orthopaedic oncology and Chapters 132 through 135 discuss the treatment of orthopaedic infection. The remaining chapters address specific problems such as treatment of stroke (Chapter 123), heterotopic ossification and Charcot neuroarthropathy (Chapter 124), osteonecrosis (Chapter 125), metabolic bone disease (Chapter 131), and management of hemophilic arthropathy (Chapter 136).

Section VIII, edited by Robert F. McLain, in 27 chapters (137 through 163), presents an exhaustive coverage of spinal disorders and surgery. The section opens with the general principles of spinal instrumentation (Chapter 137) and surgical approaches to the spine (Chapter 138). Chapters 139 through 142 address the treatment of fractures and dislocations of the spine, and Chapters 143 through 149 address the treatment of degenerative disorders of the spine. Tumors and infection are covered in Chapters 150 through 152 and inflammatory arthritis of the spine in Chapters 153 and 154. Scoliosis and deformity surgery are covered in Chapters 155 through 163.

Section IX, edited by George T. Rab, covers pediatric disorders in 17 chapters (164 through 180). Pediatric orthopaedics is an enormous field covered in detail in separate textbooks. It is addressed in these seventeen chapters in sufficient detail that the general orthopaedic surgeon will find excellent coverage of the most frequently encountered pediatric disorders and surgical procedures.

Based on my experience as the chair of the Department of Orthopaedic Surgery at the University of California Davis and Director of Resident Education from 1979 to 2000, I highly recommend this text for residents and fellows training in orthopaedic surgery and other specialties involving musculoskeletal care, as well as for paraprofessionals treating musculoskeletal disorders. Medical students and residents in their first two years of training will receive a solid background in orthopaedic surgery and musculoskeletal medicine by reading Section I on basic principles as well as the principles chapters in each section

(Chapters 10–14, 26, 37, 76, 83, 84, 99, 100, 116, 120–122, 126, 132, 137, 138, 145, 156 and 164). In the last three years of residency training, through fellowship, and on into the active practice of surgery, *Chapman's Orthopaedic Surgery* will help provide the solid, comprehensive base in clinical orthopaedic surgery required to pass board certification and to achieve a high level of confidence as a practitioner.

A CD-ROM is now included with this book and therefore deserves comment. This enhanced CD-ROM has an advanced search engine that lets a user search for information in many different ways from full-text, to tables, figures, references, and annotations. The hypertext links allow you to move through the document without losing your place. The bookmarking feature lets you return to frequently used text with ease. The zoom feature lets you examine any figure in detail, and the slide show feature allows you to use illustrations for review or lectures. The print feature lets you output relevant material for use in your office with patients or paraprofessionals. The editing feature lets you add your own annotations. Equally as important, the CD-ROM gives you access to an expanded source of references and other materials through access to PUBMED and other Internet resources with just a click of your mouse. The CD-ROM not only provides value added information but also allows you to gain access to *Chapman's Orthopaedic Surgery* and more by simply carrying the disc with you and popping it into your laptop or a computer wherever you are. Please visit our website at LWW.com/chapman as this evolving website will provide useful supplemental material.

Michael W. Chapman, M.D.
Editor
Professor Emeritus and David Linn Chair of
Orthopaedic Surgery
University of California Davis, Sacramento, California

PREFACE TO THE FIRST EDITION

Over the last 30 years surgical intervention has been increasingly accepted by the orthopaedic community as the preferred procedure for a growing number of orthopaedic conditions. There are a number of reasons for this: increased high-energy trauma in patient populations; improvements in antibiotics; innovations in design of orthopaedic implants; the rapid development of sophisticated and powerful instrumentation, especially in arthroscopy and radiology; and the change in philosophy that increasingly recognizes the value of early mobilization. With this growing preference for surgical intervention has come a continuously improving prognosis for a variety of orthopaedic conditions.

The expansion and diversification of orthopaedic surgical procedures, however, also demands an ever greater technical expertise from the orthopaedic surgeon. Many of the several thousand procedures current in orthopaedic surgery are difficult and complex, and their success or failure depends very much on the orthopaedic surgeon's mastery of the subtleties of technique.

This book has been developed to meet the need for a text that stresses the technical details that the orthopaedic surgeon must know to perform these intricate surgical procedures well. The emphasis throughout is on the details essential to rapid, smooth, complication-free surgery. Each contributor has written a tightly focused chapter, in which he describes his preferred method of performing specific operations—including hints and 'fine points' that have proven of value in his own experience. A particularly important feature of each chapter is the discussion of how to avoid pitfalls and manage complications.

The table of contents, index, and detailed outline of headings at the beginning of each chapter should facilitate rapid and easy location of any procedure. Because no book can describe in detail every orthopaedic surgical procedure, alternative methods to those discussed in the text are noted and cited in the comprehensive reference lists appearing at the end of each chapter. Historical aspects, reviews of the literature, and compilations of results are mentioned only in passing, although necessary data are provided to justify the recommendation of the specific procedures described.

The text has been organized with the aim of making it as useful as possible to the practicing orthopaedic surgeon. The many operative procedures included are arranged partly according to anatomic region, partly according to surgical modality, and partly according to type of injury or disease—depending on the context in which a particular procedure is most likely to be considered by the orthopaedic surgeon. The eight chapters in Section I, Surgical Principles and Techniques, provide a unifying overview of the general principles important to successful surgery—particularly preoperative planning, a neglected topic that is critical to success. Each of the fourteen major sections of the text that follow begins with several chapters on general principles that introduce the chapters on specific operations. The technical expertise and experience represented in these chapters is the foundation of this book.

ACKNOWLEDGMENTS

It takes many skilled and dedicated people to write and publish a textbook of this magnitude. First and foremost are our more than 300 contributing authors who are practicing orthopaedic surgeons who have taken valuable time from their families, patients, and their own leisure interests to set down their expertise and experience for the benefit of their colleagues and students. I cannot thank them enough for their extraordinary contributions. The section editors, without whose superb knowledge of their subspecialties this book could not have been written, were essential in establishing the table of contents and chapter outlines, recruiting and working with the authors, and assuring that the content is current, accurate, and clinically and scientifically valid.

The organization, writing, and publishing of the third edition have required more than three years. In that period of time a number of Lippincott Williams & Wilkins staff working on the book have moved on to other opportunities. I thank them for their contributions but most importantly I wish to thank the key staff who have seen the text through to its completion.

Kathey Alexander, Executive Vice President, Professional Medical Publishing, at Lippincott Williams & Wilkins was instrumental in executing the third edition. Her depth of experience in medical publishing, sage advice, and assistance in recruiting contributing authors was essential and greatly appreciated. It has been a pleasure working with Anne Schuldiner Patterson, Vice President and Publisher for Lippincott Williams & Wilkins, who has been responsible for the publication of this text. Maureen Iannuzzi, Developmental Editor, expertly edited the manuscript, ensured the proper flow of the manuscript in the editing process, and patiently and doggedly worked with the contributing authors, illustrators, section editors, and me to get the text into production on a timely basis. Her contributions were invaluable. I gratefully acknowledge the contributions of Sandra Rush, Sarah Fitz-Hugh, and Mary Patton-Nelson, who did developmental line editing, and Gina Read, who did word processing. Our illustrators did a wonderful job of providing upgraded and uniform art throughout the text. In particular I would like to thank Theodore G. Huff at Theodore Huff and Associates, George Barile at Accurate Art Inc., and Richard Fritzler with Design Pointe Communications. The production staff at Lippincott Williams & Wilkins did a terrific job of putting the book together, particularly Penny Bice, Tim Prairie, and Tim Reynolds. An important addition to the text is the enhanced CD-ROM for which the development editor was Lisa Consoli.

I gratefully thank the many secretaries and staff who supported the contributing authors. It is they who put up with our demands to meet deadlines and have tirelessly placed our thoughts on the typewritten page, in particular my administrative assistants Norma Sigerseth and Shannon Ackerman.

Most importantly, I thank my wife, Elizabeth (Betty) Casady Chapman, whose patience and skill at keeping our busy lives functioning allowed me to make the major time commitment that was required to produce this book.

Michael W. Chapman, M.D.

SECTION VIII

THE SPINE

SECTION EDITOR

Robert F. McLain

CHAPTER 137

BIOMECHANICS OF SPINAL INSTRUMENTATION

Christian M. Puttlitz, Vijay K. Goel, and Robert F. McLain

The spine is a mechanical entity. Its most important function is to protect the spinal cord from damage while allowing physiologic motions at each vertebral level. Many times, especially in disease states or in the case of trauma, vertebral motion may produce impingement on the spinal canal, resulting in elevated pressure on the spinal cord. Some spinal disorders may reduce mechanical stability, resulting in abnormal motion, pain, or deformity in the face of normal loads and activity. The primary goal of surgical intervention is to relieve extraneous spinal pressure, reduce the patient's pain, and obtain correct spinal alignment.

Obtaining a solid fusion of the affected levels is often the long-term goal of surgery. It is commonly achieved by open reduction and bone grafting, with the postoperative reduction maintained by fixation implants. Each stage in treatment has an associated biomechanical implication that cannot be overlooked.

NORMAL MOTION

The normal motion of the spine is determined by the spinal structures, particularly the facet joints and intervertebral disc. The spine exhibits two types of motion: in-plane and "coupled" motion. Coupled motion is defined as movement that is out of the plane of the applied loads. The orientation of the facet joints primarily determines the magnitude of in-plane and coupled motion.

Range-of-motion (ROM) characteristics are determined partially by the intervertebral disc and ligaments. Hyperextension, for instance, is limited by the anterior longitudinal ligaments and the anterior portion of the annulus fibrosis (16). Flexion is limited primarily by the posterior ligamentous complex and capsules of the facet joints. The degree of lateral bending is usually checked by the capsular ligaments and facet joints. Axial rotation is regulated by the intervertebral discs including Luschka's

C. M. Puttlitz: Research Fellow, Departments of Biomedical Engineering and Orthopaedic Surgery, University of Iowa, Iowa City, Iowa, 52242.

V. K. Goel: Professor, Department of Biomedical Engineering; Professor, Department of Orthopaedic Surgery; Co-Director, Iowa Spine Research Center, University of Iowa, Iowa City, Iowa, 52242.

R. F. McLain: Director of Spine Research, Department of Orthopaedic Surgery, The Cleveland Clinic Foundation, Cleveland, Ohio, 44195.

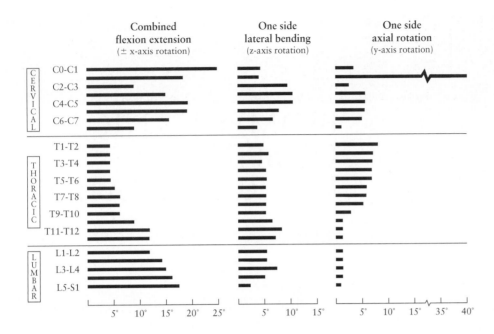

Figure 137.1. Mapping of the normal ranges of motion in combined flexion and extension, lateral bending, and axial rotation as a function of spinal position. Note that these values should not be regarded as absolute and that considerable variation exists within the population. (From White AA, Panjabi MM. *Clinical Biomechanics of the Spine,* 2nd ed. Philadelphia: J.B. Lippincott Co., 1990:107, with permission.)

joints (cervical spine), facet joints, and capsular, interspinous, and supraspinous ligaments. It has been demonstrated that 90% resistance to axial rotation in the lumbar spine is provided by the facet joints and intervertebral discs; the ligaments are responsible for the remaining 10% (10).

The upper cervical region, the occipitoatlantoaxial complex (C0–C1–C2), is the most mobile area of the spine (Fig. 137.1). Both the occipitoatlantal and atlantoaxial levels allow greater than 20° of flexion and extension. Also, the C1–C2 facets and the atlantodental articulation allow for 40° to 50° of axial rotation to each side. The lower cervical spine (C3–C7) exhibits more lateral bending than the occipitoatlantoaxial complex. Sagittal plane and axial rotation diminish from the C4–C5 level and below.

Because of its articulation with the rib cage, the thoracic region is the least mobile portion of the spine. The upper thoracic spine allows significant axial rotation (approximately 10°), but below T8–T9, the major motion of the thoracic spine is in flexion and extension. The lumbar spine permits a significant degree of flexion and extension across all levels. There is a sharp increase in the amount of lateral bending exhibited by the L3–L4 level, with a corresponding decrease at the L2–L3 and L4–L5 motion segments. Axial rotation in the lumbar spine is limited by the vertical orientation of the facet joints.

INSTABILITY

Measurement of spinal stability (or instability) is integral to the diagnosis and treatment of the lumbar spine. Insta-

bility of the spine can be a result of a purely mechanical disorder or a disorder of another origin.

Incorrect judgments of spinal stability can lead to unnecessary surgery in some cases or inadequate treatment in others. Unrecognized and untreated instability exposes the patient to an increased risk of neurologic injury, pain, and in the upper cervical spine, mortality. White and Panjabi (54) define clinical instability as "the loss of the ability of the spine under physiologic loads to maintain its pattern of displacement so that there is no initial or additional neurological deficit, no major deformity, and no incapacitating pain." The key phrase within this definition, for the purpose of understanding stability, is "to maintain its pattern of displacement." Trauma, degeneration, and certain clinical procedures can severely alter the spine's normal pattern of displacement and lead to instability.

A checklist based on clinical and radiographic criteria has been developed to help the physician determine the degree of instability; see Table 137.1. (43) Radiographs of the spine are taken, whereupon the physician assigns a certain number of points depending on range of motion and condition of spinal elements. According to this system, a total of five points or more indicates a clinically unstable spine.

Sagittal plane displacement greater than 4.5 mm or 15% of the anteroposterior diameter of the vertebral body or relative angulation greater than 22° denotes potential instability (45,50). Also, relative sagittal rotation greater than 15% at L1–L2, L2–L3, and L3–L4; greater than 20° at L4–L5; or greater than 25° at L5–S1 represents an abnormal range of motion and potential instability (54). The presence of a neurologic deficit is also diagnostic of spinal stability.

*Table 137.1. Checklist for the diagnosis of clinical instability of the lumbar spine**

Element	Point value
Anterior elements destroyed or unable to function	2
Posterior elements destroyed or unable to function	2
Radiographic criteria	4
Flexion-extension radiographs	
Sagittal plane translation >4.5 mm or 15%†	2
Sagittal plane rotation	
>15° at L1–L2, L2–L3, and L3–L4	2
>20° at L4–L5	2
>25° at L5–S1	2
Resting radiographs	
Sagittal plane displacement >4.5 mm or 15%†	2
Relative sagittal plane angulation >22°	2
Cauda equina damage	3
Dangerous loading anticipated	1

* A total of five points or greater indicates clinical instability of the spine. (Adapted from White AA, Panjabi, MM. *Clinical Biomechanics of the Spine*, Philadelphia: J.B. Lippincott Co., 1990, with permission.
† Of the anteroposterior diameter.

A theory that has gained some popularity in assessing spinal instability involves the idea of quantifying the "neutral zone" (43). Within the neutral zone, there is minimal resistance to intervertebral motion; minor changes in load result in considerable shifts in position. A patient in pain may reveal an increase in the neutral zone, allowing motion to occur beyond the pain-free zone under physiologic loads, while showing no change in the spine's overall range of motion. In contrast, when the spine is stabilized, pain may decrease because of a decrease in the range of the neutral zone as well as the overall range of motion.

At present, clinicians can quantify the degree of instability within the lumbar spine through the use of magnetic resonance imaging (MRI), computed tomography (CT) scans, and radiographs, which can indicate the spine's range of motion. (Take care to identify whether the data are based on active or passive range of motion, because there is a difference between the two.) Many recent studies have also postulated that a measurement of the time course of motion within the spine may be as important as range of motion in determining degrees of instability (34,40).

These studies suggest that both velocity and acceleration of movement give key insight into the patient's condition. Slow motion could indicate a patient's lack of confidence or pain. Jerky movements may be indicative of a lack of fine motor control. Some studies suggest that the dynamics behind the movement of the spine are subject to a great amount of variability depending on neuromuscular coordination, motivation, skill, physiologic strength and flexibility, and metabolic support (24).

How much each one of these factors contributes to the speed at which the patient moves is unknown. No conclusive evidence has indicated that velocity measurements are more sensitive to impairment than ROM measurements. The large amount of variability found in studies that examine movement velocity for diagnostic purposes has limited the clinical usefulness of such measurements. Therefore, a dynamic analysis of the spine should be used as a supplement to static radiographs for the determination of spinal instability; flexion and extension x-ray studies are the most widely used studies for this purpose.

Spinal instability can be the direct result of trauma, degeneration, tumor, infection, muscle dysfunction, surgical intervention, or any combination thereof. Damage to any portion of the functional spinal unit (vertebra-disc-vertebra assembly) can lead to instability. The most important spinal elements contributing to instability are the intervertebral disc, facet joints, and the perispinal ligaments. It is often necessary to dissect some or all of these components during spinal surgery. Just exposing the spine can damage fine nerves that contribute to muscle function and coordination (38,44). Nerve damage can upset the normal distribution and transmission of loading, leading to further instability. Thus, it is necessary to describe the biomechanical effects due to partial or complete spinal element removal. The three most common procedures involving spinal element resection are laminectomy, facetectomy, and partial or complete removal of the intervertebral disc.

Laminectomy involves partial or complete removal of the posterior vertebral arch to decompress the neural elements, cord and nerve r ts. Partial laminectomy does not necessarily result in inst. ility. Cadaver experiments show that partial laminectomy has a greater effect on the amount of flexion and axial rotation (approximately a 15% to 20% increase) than lateral bending (less than a 5% increase) (23). Controversy exists as to whether fusion is necessary following laminectomy procedures. Degenerative spondylolisthesis cohort studies suggest that laminectomy with fusion results in a decrease in pain, with increased stability. However, follow-up studies on patients who had laminectomies for spinal stenosis showed no difference in outcome whether or not a coincident fusion procedure was performed. It appears that an indication for fusion depends more on the evidence of pre-existing instability than on the decompression itself.

The geometry of the posterior facets is important in determining the relative amount of motion at each spinal level. In particular, the facets serve to resist axial rotation and extension motion. Farfan et al. (10) demonstrated that, in the lumbar region, the facets alone resist approximately 50% of the torsional loads experienced by the spine.

It would seem intuitive that partial or complete removal of these vertebral elements would result in an unstable spine. In fact, however, partial unilateral or bilateral facetectomy at one level results in greater motion but may not produce instability (23). Complete facetectomy (unilateral or bilateral) increased motion by 78% in extension, 63% in flexion, 15% in lateral bending, and 126% in axial rotation as compared with the intact controls, confirming that the degree of instability can be directly correlated with amount of facet removal.

Intervertebral disc disorders can produce instability. The intervertebral disc can degenerate, becoming dehydrated and fissured, resulting in nonphysiologic loading (18). The nucleus pulposus can evidence fibrous tissue formation, leading to nonhomogeneous stresses within the disc. The intervertebral disc, which may protrude or herniate, causing nerve root compression, has been implicated as common source of low back pain ("discogenic pain"). Thus, many surgical interventions involve removing part or all of an intervertebral disc, as do interbody fusion techniques.

Partial removal of the disc can lead to iatrogenic instability. It has also been shown that discectomy with minimal removal of the lamina does not produce instability. In fact, complete discectomy (partial laminectomy, partial facetectomy, partial annulus removal, and complete nucleotomy) results in an 80% increase in flexion, an increase of 60% in extension, a 38% increase in lateral bending, and a 62% increase in axial rotation (14). Post-discectomy back pain may be associated with more extensive disc removal at the time of surgery.

FUSION AND INSTRUMENTATION

Spinal stabilization and fusion procedures have been used to treat ailments ranging from fractures and tumors to spondylolisthesis and disc degeneration. Eliminating motion between the affected segments increases the likelihood of fusion and may reduce the degree of pain the patient experiences (41,53). Properly applied, spinal instrumentation maintains alignment and shares spinal loads until a solid, consolidated fusion is achieved.

As instrumentation procedures have become increasingly popular (9,30), the number of available fixation systems has grown. With few exceptions, these systems are used in combination with bone-grafting procedures and may be augmented by external bracing systems.

Most often, spinal instrumentation systems are described in terms of where the hardware is attached: anterior, posterior, or interbody.

- The "anterior" devices such as anterior plates and screw systems usually are classified as those systems that are designed to attach to the anterior or anterolateral aspect of the vertebral body. Typically, the plate or rod construct is transfixed to the involved vertebral segments by screws that pierce one or both cortices as well as gain purchase in the cancellous bone of the vertebral body.
- "Posterior" systems are affixed to the elements situated posterior to the vertebral body, the spinous processes, pedicles, facets, or laminae. These instrumentation systems use laminar hooks, pedicle screw systems, facet screws and wiring techniques.
- Finally, interbody fusion systems promote fusion between the vertebral bodies by the incorporation of a device or graft that spans the disc space. Although allograft and autograft spacers are routinely used in combination with other anterior or posterior instrumentation, a variety of "stand-alone" devices are now available and approved for implantation. Usually, the interbody systems are further classified by the surgical approach used during device implantation. The comingling of system and approach has given rise to such contemporary terminology as anterior lumbar interbody fusion (ALIF), transforaminal lumbar interbody fusion (TLIF), and posterior lumbar interbody fusion (PLIF) procedures.

POSTERIOR DEVICES

The earliest form of spinal fusion was developed using the posterior fusion technique. The concept originated using the midline fusion technique wherein the graft material spanned adjacent spinous processes and lamellae (Fig. 137.2A). This technique is biomechanically disadvantageous. The graft material is situated far from the center of rotation and experiences tensile forces when the spine is put in flexion, both factors that may induce excessive motion and cause the graft to migrate before it can incorporate and consolidate. The measured stress increases as the distance from the center of rotation increases; thus, grafts placed at this distance may result in a nonunion due to resorption or material failure. In addition, tensile loads experienced by the graft also may cause it to fail because bone is inherently more stable in compression than in tension. The clinical outcome is delayed union or nonunion.

These mechanical disadvantages were manifested in the relatively high pseudoarthrosis rate with early posterior fusion techniques. The most commonly employed contemporary method of fusion, the posterolateral fusion technique (Fig. 137.2B), addresses many of these flaws. The posterolateral technique involves fusion of the transverse

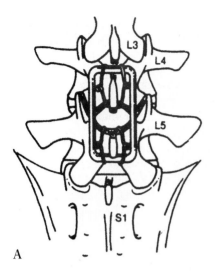 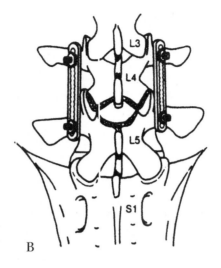

A   B

Figure 137.2. Schema depicting two types of posterior fusion devices. **A:** The Luque Loop application is a midline procedure that uses wiring to achieve fixation to the spine. **B:** The posterolateral application of Steffee plates involves pedicle screw fixation (From Goel VK, Lim TH, Gwon J, et al. Biomechanics of Fusion. In: Andersson GBJ, NcNeill TW, eds. *Lumbar Spinal Stenosis.* Chicago: Mosby–Year Book, 1996:403, with permission.)

processes and the facet joints of adjacent vertebrae. The intertransverse fusion allows placement of the graft in closer proximity to the center of vertebral rotation than the midline fusion, thus reducing the tensile loads experienced by the graft and decreasing the risk of graft migration.

Both factors increase the probability of obtaining a solid fusion. Although aggressive removal of the facet cartilage does reduce the inherent stability of the motion segment, the increased surface area for fusion and close apposition of the facet joint surfaces facilitates the rate of fusion. Internal fixation using wiring, pedicle screw fixation, and hooks usually reduces the risk of graft displacement by decreasing displacement and the loads through the graft during the healing process.

Posterior implant systems have evolved from simple distraction devices, using hooks to force the laminae apart and straighten the spine. Sublaminar wires were the first implant used to provide "segmental" fixation, attaching the rod to the spine at multiple points along the length of the construct. They are still used in deformity surgery, but because they do not provide axial stability, they are a poor choice for stabilizing fractures or bone loss due to tumors. Sublaminar wires have greater leverage in directly pulling the displaced element to the correcting rod than the distraction systems could safely generate, but they cannot prevent these elements from sliding down the rod should adjacent levels collapse.

Contemporary segmental systems use a variety of hooks to attach to multiple points along the construct, and they offer a means of locking the hook to the rod at any given point to maintain axial distraction or compression forces after implantation. Pedicle screws, large fixation screws implanted through the lamina and pedicle into the vertebral body, allow segmental fixation even in areas where the laminae have been removed. Pedicle screws are

the only devices available that provide fixation to all three vertebral columns. When used in combination with sublaminar wires and pedicle screws, contemporary posterior instrumentation systems are highly versatile and effective devices.

Pedicle screw systems in particular continue to gain use. These systems provide a high degree of construct stability as well as afford good fixation to the spine. Because pedicle screws are inserted into the vertebral body, these posterior devices can directly manipulate the intervertebral space. Pedicle screws also allow one to apply distraction, compression, lordosis, rotation, and anterolisthesis or retrolisthesis forces selectively. They are the most important factor that provides torsional stiffness in thoracolumbar spinal constructs. Pedicle screw systems provide a means to treat thoracolumbar instability after burst fracture or resection of a spinal tumor. However, they must be augmented with anterior column support to avoid exposing the screws to excessive cantilever loads that might cause bending failure or breakage.

As the indications for the use of pedicle screw systems have increased, additional modifications have become essential to increase their effectiveness and compensate for the shortcomings of the system for a given indication. For example, studies reported a high rate of screw failure when first-generation screws were used to treat thoracolumbar burst fractures (39). Implant failure, by either acute bending failure (postyield deformation) or acute fracture, was seen in young patients with axial instability due to trauma. Screw failure contributed to loss of alignment and fixation. Loosening, toggling, or backing out of the screw owing to failure of bone may occur, early or late, in older patients with weak, osteoporotic bone.

Fatigue failure, occurring after the bony healing period, often results in asymptomatic screw breakage and is usually not a problem clinically. To reduce screw-bone interface problems, augmentation of thoracolumbar constructs with offset laminar hooks has been recommended (51). Laminar hooks help decrease the load transmitted between the bone and pedicle screws, thereby protecting the screws and the bone. Injection of bone cement in the hole before insertion of the screw has also been suggested to increase the bone–screw interface strength, but this approach has limited effectiveness in severely osteoporotic patients and introduces some very real, if uncommon, risks.

Clinical failure in pedicle screws occurs two ways—by loosening and fixation failure and by acute or subacute bending failure or breakage. Loosening occurs as repetitive loading persists beyond the tolerance of the bone, which is usually due to delayed union or excessive activity. The screw is exposed to a combination of cantilever bending and axial pullout loads. Cantilever bending loads may also exceed the yield point of the screws, resulting in acute bending failure and breakage. Even in the degenerated and collapsed disc, axial loads impart small cyclic displacements that generate significant cantilever loads and bending moments. These are most pronounced around the screw hub, inside the pedicle. When the pedicle screws are forced to bear most or all of the anterior column's axial loads, as in burst fracture or tumor reconstruction, excessive bending moments predictably lead to screw failure and progressive kyphosis.

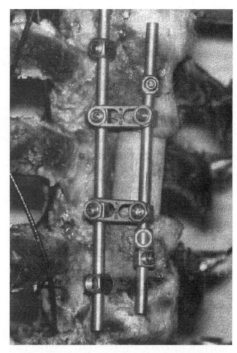

Figure 137.3. An example of an anterior instrumentation device (applied to a cadaveric specimen). This device (ALC dynamized system, AcroMed, Inc., Cleveland, OH) uses screws driven into the vertebral body with bars spanning between the screws. These devices are commonly used in conjunction with vertebrectomy procedures.

ANTERIOR DEVICES

The advantage of the anterior approach to the spine is that it gives direct access to the area of disease, which is frequently the disc or vertebral body. The anterior approach allows the surgeon to decompress the neural structures, resect the disease, reduce deformity, and stabilize the injured segment. Fusion anteriorly has the mechanical advantage of being in closer proximity to the vertebral center of rotation, thus reducing the stresses on the graft and hardware, as well as being placed in compression.

Anterior reconstructions directly oppose the greatest forces acting on the thoracic and thoracolumbar spine—the anterior compressive forces generated by gravity, posture, activity, and muscular contraction. Unopposed, these forces lead to progressive and disabling kyphosis. Whereas posterior systems depend on long lever arms and cantilever forces to resist kyphotic collapse, anterior struts are loaded in nearly pure compression, the cortical bone's strongest aspect. Anterior instrumentation need only share the compressive load and resist translation and torsion to be effective.

Biomechanical animal studies (59) have demonstrated the efficacy of obtaining a solid fusion when anterior instrumentation is used. These studies also indicate that fusion mass consolidation is greater when anterior instrumentation is used, resulting in higher torsional stiffness of

the fused levels. Most anterior fixation systems use screws placed into the vertebral body with rods or plates, or both (Fig. 137.3). The weak link in these constructs is most often the bone–screw interface, or fatigue failure of the implant occurs due to nonunion.

Although rigidity of the implant seems to be the most important feature associated with immediate postoperative stability, the higher stiffness fixation systems can, in time, impart progressively deleterious effects. "Stress shielding" is a phenomenon that occurs with both anterior and posterior devices when a relatively stiff implant bears a disproportionately large amount of physiologic loads compared with the host bone. The biologic response of the bone to the reduction in load is resorption of the bone around the implant.

Stress shielding of the graft and surrounding bone by the implant can lead to progressive angular deformities and loss of fixation of the implant to the bone owing to weakening or resorption of the bone around the implant, which leads to migration of the implant in the bone. More rigid fixation, however, has been associated with greater degrees of immediate postoperative stability. Thus, the dilemma is that although higher implant rigidity is needed in the immediate postoperative period, it may contribute to stress shielding as time proceeds.

The clinical importance of stress shielding in any given construct remains unclear. Additionally, the controlled subsidence of the graft into the vertebral endplate may be a contributing factor to successful fusion, which stiffer implants may impair. At the extreme, resorption of the graft adjacent to a rigid implant may convert a "load-sharing" device to a "load-bearing" device, leading predictably to implant failure.

To overcome these perceived deficiencies, several new devices of more flexible design have come on the market (48). The flexible devices theoretically permit more load-bearing through the interbody bone graft. They may not, however, provide the same degree of immediate stability until fusion occurs. In newer implants the rigidity of the device decreases as a function of time, providing a rigid construct for the initial healing phase and thereafter permitting larger loads through the fusion site because of a gradual decrease in the rigidity of the device (20). The newer anterior as well as posterior "dynamized" systems seek to allow a preset degree of axial subsidence due to graft resorption and settling, thereby allowing temporal load-sharing as graft consolidation proceeds (28). These devices are quite new, however, and are still in evaluation and thus not accepted for general use.

INTERBODY FUSION DEVICES

Total disc removal alone or in combination with other surgical procedures invariably leads to a loss of disc height and an unstable segment. Both allografts and autologous bone grafts have been used as interbody spacers. Autogenous bone grafts have the disadvantage of donor site morbidity, and both autografts and allografts are subject to dislodgement when used anteriorly, resulting in loss of alignment.

The use of disc space inserts fabricated from synthetic materials has gained popularity. These inserts may be implanted through an anterior or posterior approach.

Interbody cages composed of titanium or carbon fiber mesh promote fusion by imparting immediate postoperative stability, promoting fusion through the incorporation of bone chips packed inside the cage (29). Anterior procedures used to implant cages usually require extensive removal of the anterior portion of the annulus fibrosis and anterior longitudinal ligament. The strength of the construct relies in part on distraction, which produces tension in the remaining annulus (11).

Posterior interbody fusion procedures require removal of various posterior elements. Iatrogenic or acquired (spondylolytic) posterior column instability frequently requires posterior fixation. Combined anterior or posterior interbody fusion and posterior instrumentation and fusion in the lumbar spine usually requires partial or complete facetectomy, removal of the pars interarticularis, and partial or complete discectomy. These constructs require a significant amount of load-bearing by the graft (and cage) construct and posterior hardware to resist translation and torsion forces (47).

BIOMECHANICAL EVALUATION OF INSTRUMENTATION AND DEVICE FAILURE

The development of various spinal devices has come, in large part, from a desire on the part of surgeons to improve success rates. The operative assumption is that better instrumentation will produce better surgical results, whether success is defined in terms of fusion rate, correction of deformity, pain relief, or hardware survival. Thus, it is no surprise that the engineering community, in concert with surgeons, is constantly evaluating the mechanical performance of spinal instrumentation.

Over the years, a vast number of biomechanical studies have appeared in peer-reviewed journals publishing data on a multitude of clinically relevant mechanical parameters, collected using an equally large and diverse number of *in vitro* and *in vivo* testing methods. The literature can be loosely divided into several distinct categories that outline the stepwise evolution that typically occurs in the design and development of spinal implants and subsequent release for clinical use (1,2,13,46). The majority of data deal with three mechanical parameters: construct stiffness, load to failure, and fatigue load (7,12,26,29,42,55,59,60).

Stiffness is the ratio of the applied load to the resultant displacement. The failure load defines the maximum load that can be applied to the construct before component or fixation failure occurs. Fatigue load is usually defined as the number of loading cycles, at physiologic loading levels, that can be applied to a given system before hardware or fixation failure.

The goal of most instrumentation systems is to minimize motion between the affected levels; thus knowledge of the construct stiffnesses in flexion, extension, lateral bending, and axial rotation is requisite for a complete understanding of a particular hardware system. Load-to-failure studies reveal how the implant is likely to behave when it is first applied. Fatigue studies give insight into the likelihood and type of failures to be expected when the system is exposed to normal loads over time. Several important categories of biomechanical testing modalities illustrate the nature and value of data obtained from each study type.

1. *Interconnection testing* of spinal instrumentation systems has become increasingly more common, owing to the complexity of contemporary designs. This type of testing seeks to characterize mechanically the slip and failure properties of the various interfaces within

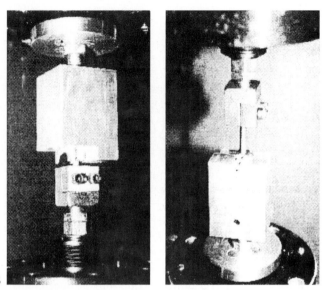

A,B

Figure 137.4. Interconnection testing seeks to characterize mechanically the interfaces within an assembled device. Pictured are two examples: testing of the hook–rod interface (**A**) and the screw–rod interface (**B**).

the device (Fig. 137.4). Interconnection testing performed for pedicle screw and rod systems can assess the failure load needed to produce appreciable slip at the screw-rod junction.

Because these tests are standardized as to configuration and loading, comparisons between various studies can be made. Figure 137.5, for example, shows the loads needed to produce failure slip under both axial and rotational forces for many contemporary lumbar designs (21).

2. *Plastic vertebrae (simulated corpectomy) models* are tests that mimic the performance of fixation devices under the worst possible clinical scenario, which is where an anterior gap is produced by vertebrectomy. Tests using plastic models standardize the bone-screw interface and, thus, highlight the performance of the assembled device as distinguished from the bone-screw interface. The devices are mounted onto molded plastic vertebral components (Fig. 137.6) (8,48) and subjected to axial compression, compression-flexion bending, and torsional modes, loading either statically or cyclically (fatigue testing).

Results show that most devices fail at up to 50% less load, when fatigue tested to 5 million cycles, as compared to the loads they can withstand when loaded statically (22). Failure always seems to occur at points of stress concentration, such as attachment of the rod to the screw, at threads in the rod, at the junction of the cross-links, and in the longitudinal members. These failure patterns are supported by pedicle-screw loading studies.

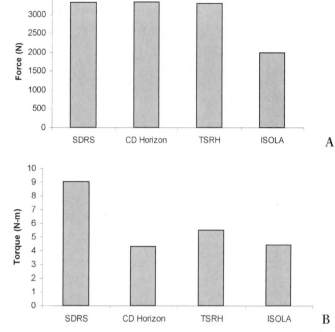

A

B

Figure 137.5. Data from interconnection testing for both (**A**) axial load and (**B**) axial rotation. The four systems tested were the Surgical Dynamics Rodding System (SDRS), Cotrel-Dubousett Horizon (CD-Horizon), Texas Scottish Rite Hospital (TSRH), and ISOLA system.

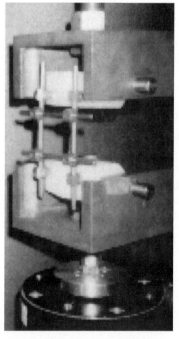

Figure 137.6. Instrumentation testing using the plastic vertebrae model. The construct is assembled with the two plastic blocks representing the vertebral bodies. The assembly depicted here is being subjected to a combined loading of flexion and compression.

One such study (56) demonstrated that the maximum stresses are seen near the hub of the screw and decay nonlinearly to zero at the screw tip. Additionally, the stress concentrations introduced by the geometry of the screw hub–shaft junction increased the stresses experienced by the screw such that the screw would be at risk of fatigue failure. Biomechanical studies using analog models have shown that even small changes in screw orientation or insertion technique can affect screw bending moments (35–37). Thus, it seems that with the development of more versatile pedicle screw systems, the clinical ease for implanting the devices may improve but may introduce additional stress concentration sites. This type of testing clearly shows the need for coordination between implant design engineers and clinicians to ensure that the likely locations of failure will be the least problematic.

Tests of the compression strength of cortical and cancellous bone dowels and cortical femoral rings, inserted between plastic blocks having matching geometry and loaded in axial compression using a servohydraulic testing machine, have shown that fresh human cancellous bone fails at an average load of 863 N, whereas cortical bone dowel strength may exceed 24,000 N (4).

3. *The strength of the bone–implant interface* is as important as the strength of the implant in preventing failure. Axial pullout tests, which evaluate the fixation characteristics of different screw types (31), have led to optimization of screw placement (6) and thread design, producing instrumentation systems that are less likely to fail clinically owing to fixation failure. Use of offset hooks has been suggested as a supplement to pedicle screw fixation. Yerby et al. (57) demonstrated that hook augmentation to screw fixation decreased the bending moment experienced by pedicle screws by approximately 30%, leading to reduced screw migration during *in situ* contouring of the rods.

The strength of pedicle screw fixation can be augmented by filling the screw holes with hydroxyapatite grouting material. This method can increase screw purchase in situations in which the bone quality is diminished.

In an animal study, Spivak et al. (49) used hydroxyapatite as a grouting material for posterior screw placement. They showed that grouting significantly improved screw pullout strength 6 weeks following implantation. Histologic analysis showed that this was most likely due to new bone formation within the grout material around the screw.

In an acute pullout study, Yerby et al. (58) performed similar testing to determine the potential improvement in fixation provided by hydroxyapatite augmentation for revision pedicle screws. They simu-lated revision by pulling out 6.0 mm screws and replacing them with 7.0 mm screws. The results showed that hydroxyapatite augmentation increased the pullout strength by 325%. They also showed that 7.0 mm screws that pulled out could be salvaged by augmention with hydroxyapatite.

Pullout studies have also been used to study the parameters governing cage migration and extrusion in the immediate postoperative period. Brantigan and Steffee (5) reported that an average force of 342 N was required to dislodge their fiber cage, whereas a force of 122 N was required to extract rectangular PLIF bone plugs. Bagby and Kuslich (3) determined that a mean force of 569 N was needed to dislodge the BAK interbody fusion cage, compared with a mean force of 271 N for corticocancellous bone dowels.

4. *Cadaveric construct testing* (Fig. 137.7) provides important information about the effectiveness of a device in reducing intervertebral motion across the affected and adjacent segments during quasiphysiologic loading.

For example, a cadaver study (28) was used to compare the load-deformation characteristics of three different anterior devices: the Synthesis Anterior Thora-

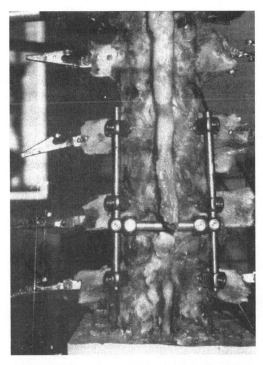

Figure 137.7. Cadaver construct testing is an important evaluation in the testing protocol. In this example, a pedicle screw system is applied to the lumbar spine and pure moments are applied to the superiormost vertebra. The motion of each lumbar vertebra is tracked to determine the hardware's effectiveness in reducing motion at the affected and adjacent levels.

columbar Locking Plate (ATLP, Synthes, Paoli, PA), the AcroMed Smooth Rod Kaneda System (SRK, Acro-Med Corp., Cleveland, OH), and Z-Plate (Sofamor-Danek, Inc.). Loads of 0 to 6 Nm were applied in increments of 1.5 Nm to thoracolumbar spine segments from T9–L3. Following destabilization by L-1 corpectomy and removal of the adjoining discs, a wood dowel was placed between the T-12 and L-2 vertebral bodies to simulate the presence of an interbody bone graft to restore bony alignment and height.

Results showed that the SRK device provides greater stiffness than the ATLP, although neither is different from the intact spine (Fig. 137.8A). The Kaneda rod system provided the highest degree of immediate stability, which should provide the best chance of fusion. The stiffness of the construct obtained with the SRK and ATPL systems were equivalent to the intact spine. The SRK and Z-Plate systems withstood best fatigue loading in 5,000 cycles of flexion and extension (Fig. 137.8B). The data show that the SRK and Z-Plate system will maintain their structural integrity in the face of repeated physiologic loading, thus reducing the chance of failure. Most important, the stability of construct using existing anterior devices can, at best, only approach that of the intact spine.

In flexion and extension, rigid posterior devices provide a 70% reduction in motion across the L4–L5 level, compared with the intact spine. Similar results were obtained for three different systems which were loaded in lateral bending and axial rotation as well (27).

Pedicle screw systems are effective, at least initially, in stabilizing the motion segment, irrespective of screw size, implant shape, or other variables. This finding is not surprising in that stainless steel and titanium implants are many orders of magnitude stiffer than the bony and ligamentous components of an intact spine. As a result, slight variations in the shapes and sizes of pedicle screw devices are not likely to affect the stability of constructs to any significant degree.

Flexible restraints have been tried. The Graf system is an extreme example of a flexible posterior system, in which bilateral polyester tension bands span the vertebral pedicle screws (51). After laminectomy, this system restored axial rotation to normal stiffness levels. It also significantly decreased the range of motion in flexion and extension and lateral bending. Flexible systems have not proven successful in restoring stability to a severely destabilized spinal segment such as after partial or total discectomy.

The major concern with dynamized systems is whether they can impart initial rigidity comparable to that of traditional systems using plates, bars, and screws. Hitchon et al. (28) evaluated the stiffness properties of one such anterior dynamized system, the An-

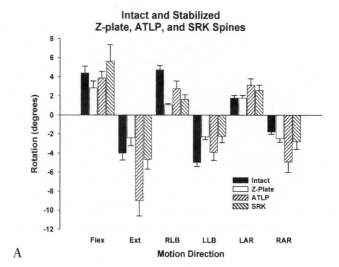

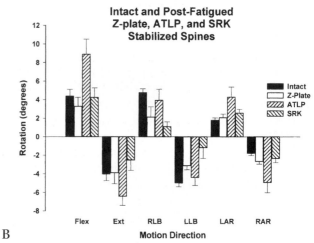

Figure 137.8. Rotational data of the intact spine and the spine stabilized using three devices: the Synthesis Anterior Thoracolumbar Locking Plate (ATLP, Synthes, Palo, PA), the AcroMed Smooth Rod Kaneda System (SRK, AcroMed Corp., Cleveland, OH), and Z-Plate (Sofamor-Danek, Inc.). **A:** Following stabilization, a significant difference was observed between the ATLP and both the SRK and Z-Plate in extension. **B:** After cyclic testing, the SRK was found to provide significantly more stability to the segment, as compared with the ATLP device, in flexion, extension, lateral bending, and right axial rotation. The Z-Plate was significantly more stable as well in flexion, extension, and axial rotation.

terolateral Controlled Compression (ALC) device (AcroMed, Cleveland, OH). The implant can be applied as a dynamized device (ALC) or can be attached rigidly (ALCR). Both applications produced the same degree of stiffness in flexion, extension, lateral bending, and axial rotation (Table 137.2). There seems to be no loss of immediate stability using the implant as a dynamized device, which may reduce long-term, deleterious effects due to stress shielding.

Table 137.2. Angular Rotations (Degrees)

	Flex.	Ext.	RLB	LLB	RAR	LAR
Intact	5.7 ± 1.1	−5.1 ± 0.8	8.8 ± 1.0	−12.2 ± 2.2	1.3 ± 0.3	−1.5 ± 0.3
ALC	3.2 ± 1.0	−3.0 ± 0.7	1.2 ± 0.3	−1.6 ± 0.2	5.1 ± 1.3	−8.4 ± 3.6
ALCR	2.0 ± 0.6	−2.1 ± 0.5	0.6 ± 0.1	−0.8 ± 0.1	2.9 ± 0.6	−2.7 ± 0.4

Angular rotation data in flexion (Flex.), extension (Ext.), right lateral bending (RLB), left lateral bending (LLB), right axial rotation (RAR), and left axial rotation (LAR) for the dynamized (ALC) and rigid (ALCR) Anterolateral Controlled Compression device. Each loading case represents 6.0 Nm of pure load applied to the L1 of the L1–L6 calf spines. The data indicate that the dynamized device (ALC) was able to reduce significantly the motion seen in the intact case and closely approximate the motion reduction obtained with the rigid device (ALCR).

In a similar study (48), this group compared the Segmental Spine Correction System (SSCS), which is a pedicle hinged screw-rod system (Osteotech, Inc. Eatontown, NJ), with its equivalent rigid screw system. The hinged screw allows 15° of movement, at which point the hinge mechanism engages the screw shaft; it then behaves like a rigid screw. The researchers showed a 65% reduction of motion in flexion and extension and 90% reduction in lateral bending across the destabilized segment for both devices when compared with the intact spine.

Interbody fusion cages have also been mechanically evaluated using cadaver models (42,52). Nibu et al. (42) studied the stabilizing effect of implantation of the BAK (Spine Tech Inc., Minneapolis, MN) interbody fusion device in human lumbrosacral specimens (L5–S1). They found that range of motion was reduced by 46% in flexion, 66% in lateral bending, and 40% in axial rotation after implantation of the device as compared with the intact spine. However, extension range of motion increased by 14% after implantation of the device owing to the anterior approach, which required cutting the anterior longitudinal ligament and the anterior annulus, which compromises the stability in extension.

5. *Analytic modeling* (15,19), such as finite element (FE) analysis, is a valuable tool for determining how implant and intraosseous loading patterns change with varying parameters of the device design. FE modeling can also help predict bone remodeling in response to the implant; therefore, it helps in evaluating stress shielding. Goel et al. (13) have generated osteoligamentous one-segment (L3–L4) and two-segment (L3–L5) FE models of the intact lumbar spine. Using the L3–L4 model, they simulated bilateral fusion using unilateral and bilateral plating, and measured the magnitude and position of internal stresses in bone, ligament, and the

implants. They normalized their data to an intact model. Bilateral plating models showed significantly reduced stresses in cancellous bone. In a simulated consolidated fusion mass, there was unloading of the cancellous bone, even after simulated removal of the device. This model predicts that removal of the fixation would not alleviate stress-shielding–induced osteopenia, which may be due to the fusion mass itself.

Models of unilateral plating revealed higher initial trabecular bone stresses than were seen with bilateral plating. However, the degree of initial stability was reduced. Thus, the best appears to be a fixation system that allows the bone to bear greater load as fusion proceeds, which would offer higher initial stability and yet minimize the problem of long-term stress-shielding–induced bone resorption.

FE modeling (17) of newer dynamic fixation systems shows that the load through the bone graft increases 10% compared with the rigid systems. Thus, it seems that the competing criteria can, in some part, be simultaneously satisfied with these dynamized devices.

FE modeling coupled with adaptive bone remodeling algorithms has been used to predict temporal changes that may be associated with interbody fusion devices. Grosland et al. (25) studied the BAK device (Fig. 137.9) and showed that implantation of this interbody fusion device results in hypertrophy of bone directly overlying and underlying the implant, whereas lateral atrophy occurs due to the stress-shielding effects associated with the relatively high stiffness of the implant. The model also predicts that bone would be stimulated to grow into and around the larger holes in the implant, resulting in sound fixation of the device.

The value of FE modeling is that mapping of the stresses and strains in bone, ligaments, and instrumentation can be obtained in a relatively inexpensive and

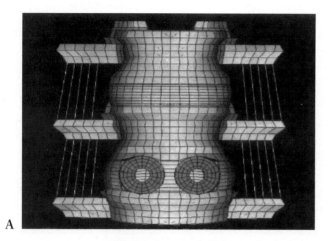

A

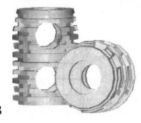

B

Figure 137.9. Finite element (FE) modeling has proved to be an invaluable tool for determining the changes in load sharing associated with device implementation. The schematic depicts the implantation of an interbody fusion device into a three-vertebrae FE model. This model has been used to characterize not only the loading changes that will occur immediately in the postoperative period but also as consolidation of the graft proceeds.

time-efficient manner. In addition, it yields important predictive data concerning temporal changes in bone in response to implantation of a device. It also facilitates quick assessment of the relative advantages and disadvantages of design iterations. Actual mechanical testing of constructs is still necessary, from time to time, to validate theoretical assumptions and confirm FE predictions.

6. *Animal studies* provide real-time *in vivo* data concerning the performance and associated biologic response to an implant. Temporal changes in both the host biologic tissue and associated instrumentation can be assessed with selective intermittent sacrificing of the animals.

The usefulness of these tests is best illustrated by the animal studies performed by McAfee et al. (32, 33). They investigated the effects of instrumentation on fusion consolidation and peri-implant bone density in 63 canines. The data confirmed a higher probability of achieving fusion when instrumentation was used. Mechanical testing of the fusion sites after sacrifice (and removal of all metal components) revealed that fusions achieved with instrumentation were more rigid

than those that occurred without instrumentation. There was, however, an inverse correlation between volumetric density of bone and rigidity of the implant, implying that utilization of the implant resulted in an osteoporotic effect owing to stress shielding. These findings could not have been predicted by the FE models available at the time.

The findings of animal models must be evaluated in terms of their inherent limitations. Most animal studies involve quadrupeds; thus, the loading imposed on the spinal instrumentation may not represent the loading that it would experience in patients.

For example, in the study mentioned earlier, McAfee et al. used a complete corpectomy model, with the device spanning the vertebrectomy space. In patients, one would expect a degenerated disc or interbody bone graft between the vertebral bodies. Hence, in the experimental model, the device assumed 100% of the load in contrast to the load-sharing capabilities for which it was designed.

The greatest value of animal studies is to provide bioengineers and clinicians with data as to how the osseous and soft tissues adapt to the altered loading environment produced by instrumentation. They also demonstrate the impact of normal and altered biology on the healing process.

The biomechanical evaluation of spinal fusion and stability has produced a large knowledge base that has allowed for the design, development, and implementation of progressively more sophisticated devices. The preceding methods are used to demonstrate the safety and potential effectiveness of instrumentation. Of course, the ultimate measure of efficacy of any system is based on well-designed and selected studies.

AUTHORS' PERSPECTIVE

The human disc, facets, and the ligaments of a spinal segment work in unison to transmit loads and permit motion. If the degenerative process, trauma, or any other factor affects an anatomic component, changes in loading and motion patterns result. Modern imaging techniques and clinical observations have adequately delineated morphologic changes in certain spinal structures that may precede degeneration of the spine. A surgeon combines this information with his or her experience to assess instability and the need for surgery, especially when conservative treatment options fail to produce satisfactory results.

The choice of technique, whether anterior, posterior, or interbody, and fixation system must be approached from a biomechanical perspective. The biomechanical data available can make the choice a more informed one. On a short-term basis, rigid fixation devices (both anterior and posterior) are capable of imparting stability to an injured or unstable segment. The degree of stability imparted, at least in the physiologic range of motion, does not vary significantly with the screw size, implant shape, or other variables.

The rigidity of the construct and the ability of a spinal fixation device to share a load with the maturing fusion mass are essential for fusion to occur. If the load transferred through the fusion mass is increased without sacrificing the rigidity of the construct, a more favorable environment for fusion may be created. Finally, although a host of experimental methods have enabled researchers to evaluate initial device performance and failure characteristics, the true measure of a device's effectiveness can be assessed only through properly designed clinical outcome studies.

REFERENCES

Each reference is categorized according to the following scheme: *, classic article; #, review article; !, basic research article; and +, clinical results/outcome study.

! 1. Ashman RB. Mechanical Testing of Spinal Implants. *Seminars in Spine Surgery* 1993;5:73.

! 2. Ashman RB, Birch JG, Bone LB, et al. Mechanical Testing of Spinal Implementation. *Clin Orthop* 1988;227: 113.

+ 3. Bagby GW, Kuslich SD. Arthrodesis of the Lumbar Spine Utilizing a Rigid Housing Containing Bone Graft—the BAK Interbody Fusion Method. In: Thalgott JS, Aebi, eds. *Manual of Internal Fixation of the Spine.* Philadelphia: Lippincott-Raven Publishers, 1996:156.

! 4. Brantigan JW, Cunningham BW, Warden K, et al. Compression Strength of Donor Bone for Posterior Lumbar Interbody Fusion. *Spine* 1993;18:1213.

! 5. Brantigan JW, Steffee A, Geiger J. A Carbon Fiber Implant to Aid Interbody Lumbar Fusion: Mechanical Testing. *Spine* 1991;16:S277.

! 6. Carlson GD, Abitbol JJ, Anderson DR, et al. Screw Fixation in the Human Sacrum—an In Vitro Study of the Biomechanics of Fixation. *Spine* 1992;17:S196.

! 7. Chang KW, Dewei Z, McAfee PC, et al. A Comparative Biomechanical Study of Spinal Fixation Using the Combination Spinal Rod-plate and Transpedicular Screw Fixation System. *J Spinal Disord* 1989;1:257.

! 8. Clausen JD, Goel VK, Sairyo K, Pfeiffer M. A Protocol to Evaluate Semi-rigid Pedicle Screw Systems. *J Biomech Eng* 1997;119:364.

+ 9. Davis H. Increasing Rates of Cervical and Lumbar Spine Surgery in the United States, 1979–1990. *Spine* 1994; 19:1117.

+ 10. Farfan HF, Gracovetsky S. The Nature of Instability. *Spine* 1984;9:714.

+ 11. Fraser RD. Interbody, Posterior, and Combined Lumbar Fusions. *Spine* 1995;20:167S.

! 12. Glazer PA, Colliou O, Klisch SM, et al. Biomechanical Analysis of Multilevel Fixation Methods in the Lumbar Spine. *Spine* 1997;22:171.

13. Goel VK, Gilbertson LG. Basic Science of Spinal Instrumentation. *Clin Orthop* 1997;335:10.

! 14. Goel VK, Goyal S, Clark C, et al. Kinematics of the whole lumbar spine. *Spine* 1985;10:543.

! 15. Goel VK, Grosland NM, Grobler LJ, Griffith SL. Adaptive Internal Bone Remodeling of the Vertebral Body Following an Anterior Interbody Fusion—a Computer Simulation. The 24th Annual Meeting of the International Society for the Study of the Lumbar Spine, Singapore. 1997.

! 16. Goel VK, Grosland NM, Scifert JL. Biomechanics of the Lumbar Disc. *Journal of Musculoskeletal Research* 1997;1:81.

! 17. Goel VK, Konz RJ, Chang H-T, et al. Hinged-dynamic Posterior Device Permits Greater Loads on the Graft and Similar Stability as Compared to Its Equivalent Rigid Device—a Three-dimensional Finite Element Assessment. Submitted for publication, 1999.

! 18. Goel VK, Lim TH. Mechanics of Spondylolisthesis. *Seminars in Spine Surgery* 1989;1:95.

! 19. Goel VK, Lim TH, Gilbertson LG, Weinstein JN. Clinically Relevant Finite Element Models of a Ligamentous Lumbar Motion Segment. *Seminars in Spine Surgery* 1993;5:26.

! 20. Goel VK, Lim TH, Gwon J, et al. Effects of Rigidity of an Internal Fixation Device: A Comprehensive Biomechanical Investigation. *Spine* 1991;16:S155.

! 21. Goel VK, Scifert JL, Grosland NM. Evaluation of Surgical Dynamics Rodding System (SDRS) Using ASTM Standard Methodologies. (Personal Communication), 1998.

! 22. Goel VK, Winterbottom JM, Weinstein JN. A Method for the Fatigue Testing of Pedicle Screw Fixation Devices. *J Biomechanics* 1994;27:1383.

+ 23. Goel VK, Woodhouse J, Hitchon PW. Stability Considerations for the Lumbar Spine. In press, 1998.

! 24. Gomez T, Beach G, Cooke C, et al. Normative Database for Trunk Range of Motion, Strength, Velocity, and Endurance with the Isostation B-200 Lumbar Dynometer. *Spine* 1991;16:15.

! 25. Grosland NM, Goel VK, Grobler LJ, Griffith SL. Adaptive Internal Bone Remodeling of the Vertebral Body Following an Anterior Interbody Fusion—a Computer Simulation. 24th Annual Meeting of the International Society for the Study of the Lumbar Spine, Singapore, 1997.

! 26. Gurr KR, McAfee PC, Shih CM. Biomechanical Analysis of Anterior and Posterior Instrumentation Systems after Corpectomy. *J Bone Joint Surg* 1988;70-A:1182.

! 27. Gwon JK, Chen J, Lim TH, et al. In Vitro Comparative Biomechanical Analysis of Transpedicular Screw Instrumentations in the Lumbar Region of the Human Spine. *J Spinal Disord* 1991;4:437.

! 28. Hitchon PW, Goel VK, Serhan H, et al. Biomechanical Studies on a Dynamized Anterior Thoracolumbar Implant. *Spine* 2000;25:306.

+ 29. Hoshijima K, Nightingale RW, Yu JR, et al. Strength

and Stability of Posterior Lumbar Interbody Fusion—Comparison of Titanium Fiber Mesh Implant and Tricortical Bone Graft. *Spine* 1997;22:1181.

+ 30. Katz JN. Lumbar Spinal Fusion—Surgical Rates, Costs and Complications. *Spine* 1995;20:78S.

! 31. Lieberman IH, Khazim R, Woodside T. Anterior Vertebral Body Screw Pullout Testing. A Comparison of Zielke, Kaneda, Universal Spine System, and Universal Spine System with Pullout-resistant Nut. *Spine* 1998;23:908.

+ 32. McAfee PC, Farey ID, Sutterlin CE, et al. Device-related Osteoporosis with Spinal Instrumentation. *Spine* 1989;14:919.

! 33. McAfee PC, Farey ID, Sutterlin CE, et al. The Effect of Spinal Implant Rigidity on Vertebral Bone Density: A Canine Model. *Spine* 1991;16:S190.

+ 34. McGregor AH, McCarthy ID, Hughes SFP. Motion Characteristics of the Lumbar Spine in the Normal Population. *Spine* 1995;20:2421.

! 35. McKinley TO, McLain RF, Yerby SA, et al. The Effect of Pedicle Morphometry on Pedicle Screw Loading in Unstable Burst Fractures: A Synthetic Model. *Spine* 1997;22:246.

! 36. McKinley TO, McLain RF, Yerby SA, et al. Effects of Pedicle Screw Insertion Techniques on Pedicle Screw Bending Moments: A Biomechanical Analysis. *Spine* 1999;24:18.

! 37. McLain RF, McKinley T, Sarigul-Klijn N, et al. The effects of Cancellous Bone Quality on Pedicle Screw Loading in Axial Instability: A Synthetic Model. *Spine* 1997;22:1454.

! 38. McLain RF, Pickar JG. Mechanoreceptor Endings in Human Thoracic and Lumbar Facet Joints. *Spine* 1998;23:168.

+ 39. McLain RF, Sparling E, Benson DR. Early Failure of Short-segment Pedicle Instrumentation for Thoracolumbar Fracture. *J Bone Joint Surg* 1993;75A:162.

! 40. Menezes AP, Davies KE, Hulkins DWL, Jayson MIV. Measurement of the Time Course of Bending of the Back in the Sagittal Plane. *Eur Spine J* 1995;4:24.

! 41. Nagel DA, Edwards WT, Schneider E. Biomechanics of Spinal Fixation and Fusion. *Spine* 1991;16:S151.

! 42. Nibu K, Panjabi MM, Oxland T, Cholewicki J. Multidirectional Stabilizing Potential of Bak Interbody Spinal Fusion System for Anterior Surgery. *J Spinal Disord* 1997;10:357.

43. Panjabi MM. Low Back Pain and Spinal Stability. In: Weinstein GS, ed. *Low Back Pain: A Scientific and Clinical Overview.* San Diego: American Academy of Orthopaedic Surgeons, 1996.

! 44. Pickar JG, McLain RF. Responses of Mechanosensitive Afferents to Manipulation of the Lumbar Facet in the Cat. *Spine* 1995;20:2379.

! 45. Posner I, White AA, Edwards WT, Hayes WC. A Biomechanical Analysis of the Clinical Stability of the Lumbar and Lumbosacral Spine. *Spine* 1982;7:374.

! 46. Puttlitz CM, Goel VK, Pope MH. Biomechanical Testing Sequelae Relevant to Spinal Instrumentation. *Orthop Clin North Am* 1998;29:571.

! 47. Rapoff AJ, Ghanayem AJ, Zdeblick TA. Biomechanical Comparison of Posterior Lumbar Interbody Fusion Cages. *Spine* 1997;22:2375.

! 48. Scifert JL, Sairyo K, Goel VK, et al. Stability Analysis of an Enhanced Load Sharing Posterior Fixation Device and Its Equivalent Conventional Device in a Calf Model. *Spine* 1999;24:2206.

+ 49. Spivak JM, Neuwirth MG, Labiak JL, et al. Hydroxyapatite Enhancement of Posterior Spinal Instrumentation Fixation. *Spine* 1994;19:955.

+ 50. Stagnara P, DeMauroy JC, Dran G, et al. Reciprocal Angulation of Vertebral Bodies in a Sagittal Plane: Approach to References for the Evaluation of Kyphosis and Lordosis. *Spine* 1982;7:335.

! 51. Strauss PJ, Novotny JE, Wilder DG, et al. Multidirectional Stability of the Graf System. *Spine* 1994;19:965.

! 52. Tencer AF, Hampton D, Eddy S. Biomechanical Properties of Threaded Inserts for Lumbar Interbody Spinal Fusion. *Spine* 1995;20:2408.

53. Traynelis VC, Goel VK, Gilbertson LG. Biomechanics of the Throracolumbar Spine. In: Sonntag MAAV, ed. *Principles of Spinal Surgery.* New York: McGraw-Hill, 1995:85.

54. White AA, Panjabi MM. *Clinical Biomechanics of the Spine,* 2nd ed. Philadelphia: J.B. Lippincott Co., 1990.

! 55. Wittenberg RH, Shea M, Edwards WT, et al. A Biomechanical Study of the Fatigue Characteristics of Thoracolumbar Fixation Implants in a Calf Spine Model. *Spine* 1992;17:S121.

! 56. Yerby SA, Ehteshami JR, McLain RF. Loading of Pedicle Screws within the Vertebra. *J Biomechanics* 1997;30:951.

! 57. Yerby SA, Ehteshami JR, McLain RF. Offset Laminar Hooks Decrease Bending Moments of Pedicle Screws during In Situ Contouring. *Spine* 1998;23:276.

! 58. Yerby SA, Toh E, McLain RF. Revision of Failed Pedicle Screws Using Hydroxyapatite Cement. *Spine* 1998;23:1657.

+ 59. Zdeblick TA, Shirado O, McAfee PC, et al. Anterior Spinal Fixation after Lumbar Corpectomy. *J Bone Joing Surg* 1991;73-A:527.

! 60. Zdeblick TA, Warden KE, Zou D, et al. Anterior Spinal Fixators—a Biomechanical In Vitro Study. *Spine* 1993;18:513.

CHAPTER 138

SURGICAL APPROACHES TO THE SPINE

Robert G. Watkins

As late as 1980, spinal surgeons, and therefore spinal patients, were severely limited in the options available to them for surgical treatment. The source of this limitation was a combination of technology and the experience in surgical approaches. Very few spinal surgeons had the ability to approach every aspect of the spine with the optimal exposure. Spinal access surgeons were few and far between. The microscopic and endoscopic approaches that protect normal tissue and speed recovery were scarcely available to unavailable. The evolution of spinal surgery now allows the surgeon to approach their pathology so as to optimize the resection of a pathologic lesion and reconstruct the spine to optimal biomechanical advantage. Perfecting the approach is the first step to perfecting the surgery and a major step in protecting the patient.

R. G. Watkins: Los Angeles, California, 90033.

THE CERVICAL AND THORACIC SPINE

POSTERIOR APPROACH TO C1–C2

- For the posterior cervical exposure of any level, position the patient's head in the self-retaining neurosurgical head fixation device that is attached to the surgical table. Attach the drapes to the patient's neck with stay sutures. Neck flexion will increase exposure, but flexion is limited by the type of pathologic process present, usually to a neutral, slightly flexed position. In the presence of spinal instability, confirm the position of the spine with radiographs.

- Incise the skin and subcutaneous tissue in the midline to the fascia, and obtain hemostasis with rapid application of hemostats and electrocautery. Insert self-retaining retractors.

- Deepen the incision with the cautery knife, staying within the thin white median raphe; avoid cutting muscle tissue. The medial raphe of the cervical spine is a

3633

tortuous structure that does not follow a straight path. Open the median raphe to the spinous processes of C-2 and C-3, the occiput, or any level needed. In children, expose no spinal levels unnecessarily to avoid spontaneous fusion at adjacent levels, including the occiput.

- With a #15 blade or cutting cautery, expose the bulbous bifid tips of the spinous processes. The ligamentous attachments to C-2 are very prominent. The large spinous process of C-7 and T-1 can be identified. Identify any spina bifida of the cervical spine on preoperative radiographs and be aware of these areas at surgery. Insert the Cobb elevator, first facing up to elevate the tip of the spinous process subperiosteally, then facing down to complete the subperiosteal elevation from medial to lateral for a width of approximately 1 inch (2.5 cm) at each level. At levels below C-2, identify the medial edge of the facet joint at the base of the lamina and pack each level as it is exposed. When necessary, expose the occiput with elevators. Insert the self-retaining retractors to expose the base of the skull and the dorsal spine of C-2. The area in between will contain the ring of C-1. This is often very deep compared with the spinous process of C-2.

- Maintaining firm lateral retraction of the wound, identify the posterior tubercle of C-1 longitudinally in the midline by probing with a sharp Cobb elevator. Begin the subperiosteal dissection to expose the bone.

- Often the C-1 ring is very thin, and direct pressure can fracture it or cause the instrument to slip off the ring and penetrate the atlantooccipital membrane. Elevation on this ring can be very dangerous if there is subluxation with constriction of the posterior dura under this ring. The dura may be vulnerable on both the superior and inferior edges of the ring of C-1.

- At the level of C-1, dissect laterally only approximately 1.5 cm. The second cervical ganglion is an important landmark on the ring of C-1 laterally; it lies approximately 1.5 cm laterally on the lamina of C-1 in the area of the groove for the vertebral artery. Carefully identify the most medial aspect of the groove for the vertebral artery and vein on the superior border of the C-1 ring. The bluish color of the vein is visualized first. By seeing the initial ridge or the vein, damage to the artery can be avoided. There is seldom any indication for dissection lateral to the groove of the vertebral artery on C-1. The vertebral artery and vein are vulnerable in the groove; in addition, as the artery passes from the foramen transversarium of C-2 to that of C-1, it is in close proximity laterally and posteriorly to the joint (29) (Figs. 138.1 and 138.2).

- The vertebral artery enters the foramen transversarium at the sixth vertebra and progresses cephalad. It exits through the foramen transversarium of C-1 and progresses posteriorly as well as medially in the groove of

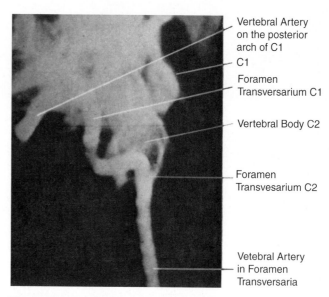

Vertebral Artery on the posterior arch of C1
C1
Foramen Transversarium C1
Vertebral Body C2
Foramen Transvesarium C2
Vetebral Artery in Foramen Transversaria

Figure 138.1.   The course of the vertebral artery is from the foramen transversarium of C-1 posteriorly in the region of the C1–C2 articulation through the transversarium of C-1, then posteromedially to the posterior rim of C-1.

the superior border of C-1 toward the midline, then turns cephalad along the spinal cord to enter the foramen magnum. The vertebral artery can be damaged by penetrating the atlanto-occipital membrane off the superior border of the ring of C-1 more lateral than the usually safe 1.5 cm from the midline.

- Following exposure of the ring of C-1 and exposure to bone of the posterior occiput, different operative procedures require exposure of the dura under the edge of the foramen magnum (17,25,26). Never attempt to decompress the posterior fossa under the edge of the foramen magnum without sufficient visualization of the area cephalad to the foramen. This is best accomplished by placing two burr holes just off the midline of each side of the skull (Fig. 138.3). The caudal extent of the holes is usually determined by the angle of the drill on the skull as limited by the patient's shoulders.

- In the posterior approach to the foramen magnum, first place burr holes in the occiput above the foramen magnum. Two parasagittal holes allow removal of bone from the dura with a Harrison-type rongeur. Careful dissection medially from the burr holes provides protection from the often significant fragile venous sinus, and dissection caudally approaches the foramen magnum. After removal of the occiput including the bony rim of the foramen magnum, which is a sharp-lipped structure projecting directly anterior in the transverse plane, the fibrous attachment of the inner periosteum of the skull to the dura at the rim of the foramen magnum is encountered. When a transverse venous sinus in this area

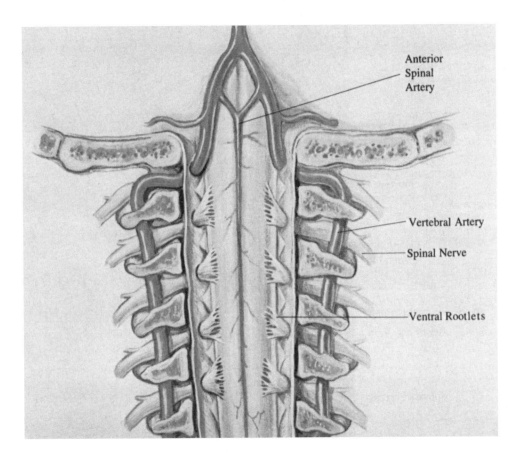

Figure 138.2. The anterior view without vertebral bodies emphasizes the formation of the anterior spinal artery. There are numerous variations in this formation, ranging from a unilateral vertebral artery contribution to no contribution.

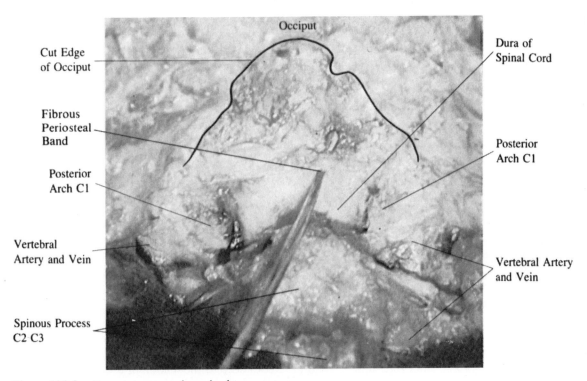

Figure 138.3. Posterior approach to the foramen magnum.

is torn, bleeding can be significant. Attachment to the dura in this area produces a dural leak unless the area is carefully dissected.

- Penetrate to the inner periosteum and the bone edge with a small dissector. Expand the hole caudally to the foramen with rongeurs. The edge itself curves under and projects anteriorly. The periosteum of the skull at this point is often conjoined with the dura of the spinal cord. There is a median venous sinus in the midline, and the fascial attachment of the periosteum of the skull to the dura often contains a transverse sinus as well.
- Passing instruments under the edge of the foramen can produce dangerous bleeding in the posterior fossa with no means of control. Therefore, resect the bone down to this edge from above.
- For a more lateral approach to the C1–C2 facet joint, the vertebral artery between C-1 and C-2 must be identified. In rotatory dislocations of C1–C2, the artery is stretched tightly across the joint on the side that C-1 is anterior to C-2, and it is easily damaged (29).
- For nerve root exposure below C-2, identify the junction of the lamina and the inferior facet. Then identify the junction of the interlaminar area and the facet joint. Expanding these areas with a burr or a micro-Kerrison rongeur allows entry into the intervertebral foramen and exposure of the nerve root.

TRANSORAL APPROACH TO C1–C2

For preoperative preparation, take oral and nasal cultures of the patient in case problems develop later (1). Use standard prophylactic antibiotics because no special antibiotic coverage for normal oral flora is needed. I do not use preoperative antiseptic gargles or tetracycline (7).

Always perform a tracheostomy, using a short-cuffed tube.

- Position the patient supine with the head slightly flexed on occipital pads, or put the head into a halo. A more upright position can be used with certain precautions.
- The Boyle-Davis or McIver ear, nose, and throat (ENT) retractor allows depression of the tongue and self-retaining retraction of the mouth. The lips and teeth should be adequately padded.
- Incise the soft palate with a curvilinear incision around the uvula, and retract the cut edges with stay sutures to the lateral walls of the oropharynx or to an especially bent, blunt-tipped Gelpi retractor (7,14). Prep the oropharynx with povidone-iodine (Betadine) solution and reculture it.
- Enhanced hemostasis by injecting the posterior pharyngeal tissue with a solution of 5% lidocaine and 1:500,000 epinephrine.

- After palpation and radiographic confirmation of the ring of C-1, make a vertical incision from approximately 1 cm cephalad to the tip of the odontoid to 2 cm distal to the anterior tubercle of C-1. Incise the four layers (posterior pharyngeal mucosa, superior constrictor muscle of the pharynx, the prevertebral fascia, and the anterior longitudinal ligaments) directly to the bone.
- Bluntly dissect the soft tissue off the body of C-2 below the odontoid and off the anterior tubercle of C-1.
- *Caution: The longus colli muscle inserts on the anterior tubercle of C-1, and sharp dissection may be needed to remove it. Venous bleeding may arise from the recesses just lateral to the base of the odontoid.*
- When necessary, the lateral masses of C1–C2 can be exposed by bluntly dissecting the bone both transversely and vertically.
- *Caution: Avoid plunging lateral to the facet joints. To avoid damage to the internal carotid, do not pass a stay suture too deeply into the lateral pharyngeal wall.*
- Remember, this is a deep wound, requiring long instruments with fine tips. Most operations done with this exposure require use of the microscope for lighting and magnification.
- After the bony work is completed and good hemostasis is obtained, close the posterior pharynx in a single layer with interrupted absorbable sutures.

ANTEROLATERAL APPROACHES TO C-1, C-2, AND C-3

- Position the patient supine with the appropriate support for the cervical spine mentioned earlier. For two levels of pathology, it is a transverse incision, one finger-breadth medial to the medial border of the sternocleidomastoid. Open layers in a fashion similar to that used with the standard cervical approaches.
- For higher anterior approaches to C-1, C-2, and C-3, identify the superior thyroid artery and vein. The superior thyroid artery arises from the external carotid artery at approximately the level of the hyoid bone. It crosses through the carotid triangle, arches deep to the strap muscles, and enters the lateral superior aspect of the thyroid gland. Retract the superior thyroid artery and vein inferiorly.
- Identify and retract the hypoglossal nerve. The hypoglossal nerve is found passing from lateral to medial superficial to the external carotid, lingual, and facial arteries (Fig. 138.4). It exits the skull in close proximity to the vagus nerve and courses beneath the internal carotid artery and internal jugular vein, becoming superficial at the angle of the mandible. After the usual point of identification of the hypoglossal nerve over the arteries, it passes deep to the tendon of the digastric muscle and stylohyoid muscle for distribution to the muscles

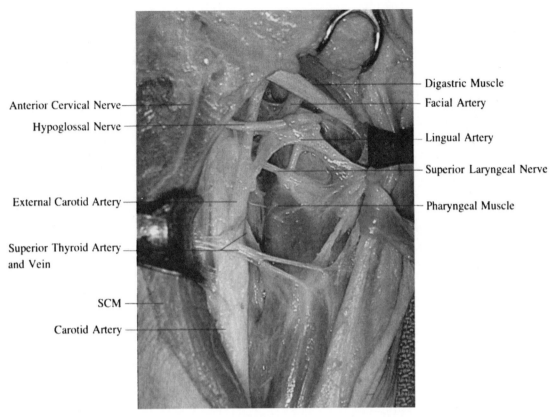

Anterior Cervical Nerve

Hypoglossal Nerve

External Carotid Artery

Superior Thyroid Artery
and Vein

SCM

Carotid Artery

Digastric Muscle

Facial Artery

Lingual Artery

Superior Laryngeal Nerve

Pharyngeal Muscle

Figure 138.4. Dissected anatomy of the carotid triangle and area just below emphasizes the importance of identification of the hypoglossal nerve before ligation of the arterial structures in this area. The most common approach is cephalad to the superior thyroid artery and caudad to the digastric muscle. SCM, sternocleidomastoid.

of the tongue. Retract the hypoglossal nerve cephalad; usually, the superior thyroid artery and vein are retracted caudad.

- Be certain of the identification of the hypoglossal nerve before ligating any structure. It is a superficial structure, first coursing vertically and parallel to the carotid sheath, then horizontally, crossing medially over the carotid and its branches.
- Identify the lingual artery, which arises from the external carotid. From the level of the hyoid, it crosses under the digastric and stylohyoid muscles in its ascent to the oral pharynx.
- Identify and ligate the facial artery. The facial artery next leaves the external carotid artery, coursing under the ramus to the mandible within the carotid triangle. It passes deep into the digastric muscle and enters the face at the anterior edge of the mastoid after crossing on the submandibular gland.
- Identify the digastric muscle. This muscle is easily retracted cephalad with the hypoglossal nerve. When necessary, divide the stylofascial band running from the stylohyoid process to the posterior pharynx.

- Difficulties may be encountered with the superior laryngeal nerve, both external and internal branches, and the pharyngeal branches of the vagus nerve. These nerves should be identified and retracted, but they frequently suffer from the retraction. Continue to use finger palpation to identify the spine and the carotid artery.
- Retract the carotid sheath and the ligated stumps of the lingual and facial arteries laterally, and retract the musculovisceral column medially with deep right-angle, hand-held blunt retractors.
- With a Kittner dissector, make a careful, blunt dissection at this point, to identify the prevertebral fascia.
- Elevate the fibers of the longus colli muscle and fascia off the vertebral body in a lateral and cephalad direction. Insert the sharp claw blades of the Cloward retractor under the longus colli. The smooth-tipped blades can be used if firm fixation cannot be obtained under the longus colli (3). Deep hand-held retractors are also quite effective (Fig. 138.5).

The external investing fascia forms the anterior and posterior sheaths of the sternocleidomastoid muscle and

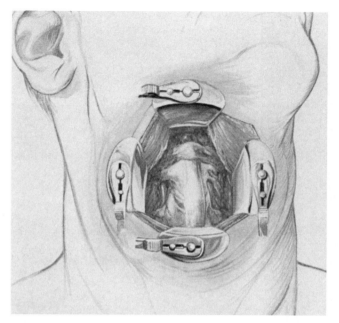

Figure 138.5. The spine is exposed with deep retractor blades.

the fascial covering of the visceral structures of the neck (10). This investing layer of cervical fascia is attached inferiorly to the acromion, clavicle, and manubrium of the sternum in an outer and inner layer superiorly to the hyoid bone, posteriorly to the mandible and mastoid processes, and superior to the nuchal line. The interval between the two laminae of the external investing fascia is called the suprasternal space, or the space of Burns. This space, which contains the anterior jugular veins and sternal head of the sternocleidomastoid, is referred to as the cul-de-sac of Bruger. Communication between the anterior and external jugular veins is channeled through this inner laminar area.

The middle cervical fascia attaches to the carotid sheath and joins the external investing fascia at the posterior border of the sternocleidomastoid muscle. Inferiorly, the middle cervical fascia attaches to the posterior surface of the sternum, as do the muscles that they cover. It is the middle cervical fascia that attaches to the clavicle and forms the loop for the inferior belly of the omohyoid muscle.

The prevertebral fascia is continuous with the endothoracic fascia caudally, and laterally it covers the levator scapulae and splenius muscles. It extends posteriorly to attach to the spinous processes of the vertebrae. In the neck and throughout the spinal column, it covers the longus colli and capitus muscles and is secured to the tips of the transverse processes.

The origin of the anterior scalene muscle rises from the anterior tubercles of the transverse processes of C-3, C-4, C-5, and C-6. It inserts into the scalene tubercle on the inner border of the first rib and into the ridge on the cranial surface of the rib ventral to the subclavian groove. The scalenus medius originates from the posterior tubercle of the transverse processes of the last six cervical vertebrae and inserts into the first rib.

The scalenus medius is a muscular reinforcement of Sibson's fascia. These fascial connections and the scalenus minimus connect the transverse processes of the seventh cervical vertebra to the first rib. Sibson's fascia, as a portion of the prevertebral fascia, becomes continuous with the endothoracic fascia on the inner surface of the first rib. Extending medially between the anterior scalene muscle and the spine is the all-important retropharyngeal fascial cleft. This is the space beneath the visceral structures, superficial to the prevertebral fascia; it is in this space that retraction and work on the anterior portion of the spine takes place.

ANTEROMEDIAL APPROACH TO THE MIDCERVICAL SPINE

■ Position Gardner-Wells tongs or headhalter traction for cervical traction. Position the head in slight extension and rotation to the right. Contour a small, curved sand bag under the neck to support the spine. Drape off the entire neck with adhesive towel drapes. Select the level of the skin incision. Superficial landmarks are used to determine the appropriate placement of the skin incision over the appropriate level of the spine. For approaches to C-1, C-2, and C-3, start the incision midline extended to the lateral border of the carotid sheath, one fingerbreadth below the angle of the madible. For approaches to C2–C3 start the incision at the midline and extend it to the lateral border of the sternocleidomastoid at the level of the cephalad margin of the thyroid cartilage. For C4–C5, start the incision at the midline and extend it to the medial border of the sternocleidomastoid at the level half way between the cricoid cartilage and the superior border of the tyroid cartilage. For C5–C6, start the incision at the midline on the cephalad margin of the cricoid cartilage and extend it to the medial border of the sternocleidomastoid. For C6–C7, start the incision at the midline of the caudal margin of the cricoid cartilage and extend it to the medial border of the sternocleidomastoid. For C7–T1, start the incision at the midline; extend it just lateral of the medial border of the sternocleidomastoid, halfway between the cricoid cartilage and the clavicle. We prefer the midline starting point, because retraction of the medial muscular visceral column is the strongest structure requiring retraction. Having the skin open to the midline eases that retraction. The self-retaining retractor is

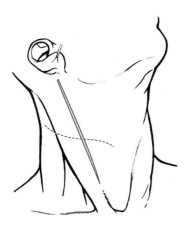

Figure 138.6. The more cosmetically suitable transverse incision is made at the appropriate level and should allow exposure of up to two discs and three vertebrae. A vertical incision can be used for an even greater exposure.

placed in the midline. Having the skin open to the midline aids in that retraction.

- After making a transverse skin incision at the appropriate level (Fig. 138.6), dissect through the subcutaneous tissue to the platysma muscle. Elevate the platysma muscle with Adson forceps, and open it carefully, in the line of the fibers, when possible. Beware of damage to veins and the sternocleidomastoid muscle (2,21). Insert a spring retractor.
- Open the superficial cervical fascia and identify the medial border of the sternocleidomastoid muscle (25). The first key to successful exposure is adequate identification of the medial border of the sternocleidomastoid so that it may be retracted laterally (23) (Fig. 138.7). With identification of this medial border, bluntly develop the interval between the sternocleidomastoid muscle and the sternohyoid muscles. Retract the posterior cutaneous nerves. Bluntly dissect the soft tissue and spread it vertically in this interval.
- Retract the sternocleidomastoid laterally and the strap musculature medially with angled retractors. Identify the middle cervical fascia. The omohyoid muscle crosses from proximal medial to lateral distal through the middle cervical fascia at C6–C7. Retract the omohyoid; when necessary, divide it and later repair it in its midportion.
- After retracting the sternocleidomastoid muscle laterally and the strap musculature medially, identify the arteriovenous structures of the middle cervical fascial layer (Fig. 138.8). Palpate the carotid pulse. Open the midline cervical fascia medial to the carotid artery. Ligate and tie the medial thyroid vein. Retract cephalad

the superior thyroid artery and retract caudad the inferior thyroid artery to expose the midcervical spine.

- Spread the middle cervical fascia just medial to the carotid sheath (23), with finger dissection spreading vertically and horizontally (3). Identify the inconstant middle thyroid vein crossing at approximately C-5, and ligate and divide it when needed. Identify the spine with finger palpation of the anterior surface of the vertebral body. Insert a blunt, nonlipped Cloward hand-held retractor into the wound directly down to the spine. Hold the retractor on the right longus colli. Beware of entering the tracheoesophageal groove (and thereby damaging the recurrent laryngeal nerve with the retractor tip) (19).
- Distally retract the inferior thyroid artery and vein at the C6–C7 level, and proximally retract the superior thyroid artery and vein with the superior laryngeal nerve at C3–C4.
- Do not mistake the transverse process for the anterior surface of the vertebral body because an incision deep in this area will damage the longus colli, the sympathetic chain, and possibly the vertebral artery. An incision into the longus colli produces bleeding.
- Palpate a disc in the midline of the spine and open the prevertebral fascia with a small dissector longitudinally until the disc can be identified. If the finger dissects directly to the spine and the retractor is then inserted, the esophagus cannot be seen. The empty esophagus is only a soft, flat ribbon-like structure simulating the musculature over the anterior portion of the spine. Always use either an esophageal stethoscope or a nasotracheal tube to identify the esophagus.
- Insert a needle into a disc for lateral radiographic confirmation of the level.
- Retract the esophagus, trachea, and anterior strap muscles medially and the carotid sheath and sternocleidomastoid muscle laterally.
- Incise the prevertebral tissue in the midline on the disc. Use a bipolar coagulator along the medial edge of the longus colli as needed. Using sharp periosteal elevators, fashion a flap of muscle under which the retractor can be inserted laterally from the midline. Insert the clawed blades of the Cloward deep self-retaining retractor under the longus colli on both sides of the spine. To expose the desired disc, use the blunt-tipped Cloward retractor vertically (3).
- Insert the clawed retractor first. Hold it down on the spine while inserting the near retractor. The Cloward curved periosteal elevator can lift up the flap for insertion of the blade retractor.
- After hemostasis has been achieved, close the deep wound by removing the retractors. Use subcuticular skin closure, and always use a closed suction wound drainage system.

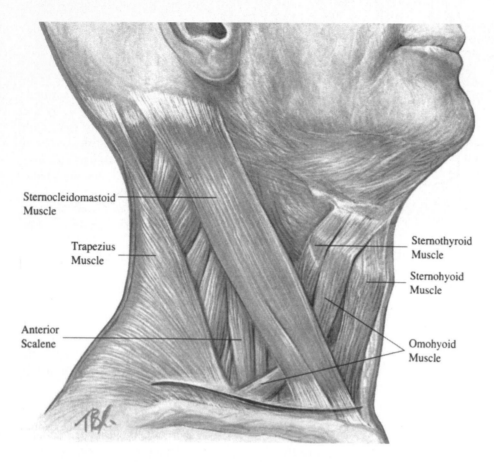

Figure 138.7. The key to the dissection at this point is to identify the medial border of the sternocleidomastoid muscle. With lateral retraction of the sternocleidomastoid, the interval between this muscle and the medial strap msucles is delineated.

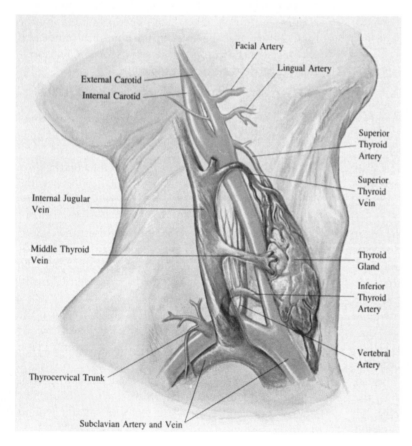

Figure 138.8. Arteriovenous structures of the middle cervical fascial layer.

SUPRACLAVICULAR APPROACH

- Place the patient in the supine position with the neck slightly hyperextended and rotated away from the side of the approach. Use an inflatable cervical pillow for support; a small roll under the shoulder often helps to extend the neck.
- *Caution: Location of the thoracic duct and recurrent laryngeal nerve becomes even more important at this level. Approaches from the left for C6–T2 are directly in the vicinity of the thoracic duct. Identify the thoracic duct when possible and protect it. A large fatty meal the day before surgery will help. If the thoracic duct is inadvertently divided, double ligate both ends well. The approach to the right definitely requires identification and protection of the recurrent laryngeal nerve. I recommend the left supraclavicular approach to avoid risk to the recurrent laryngeal nerve.*
- Make a transverse incision approximately one fingerbreadth above the clavicle from the midline to the posterior border of the sternocleidomastoid muscle. After the skin and subcutaneous tissue are divided and small skin self-retaining retractors are placed, incise the playtsma muscle in the line of the incision. As in the higher approaches, identification of the medial border of the sternocleidomastoid muscle is imperative.
- In addition, identify and define the anterior and posterior borders of the sternocleidomastoid muscle. The external jugular vein, although somewhat variable, is usually directly in the operative field, and the anterior jugular vein is positioned more medially. Divide it, if necessary.
- Incise the external investing fascia. Pass a probe or finger laterally from the medial border of the sternocleidomastoid to clear off the venous structures underneath the clavicular head of the sternocleidomastoid.
- Divide the sternocleidomastoid laterally to medially 1 inch from its insertion, watching for the internal jugular vein (12). If required for visualization, remove the sternal head of the sternocleidomastoid muscle in the same fashion. Eventual reattachment depends on suturing the fascial covering of the muscle.
- Retract the divided sternocleidomastoid in a cephalad-caudad direction with self-retaining blunt retractors. The floor of the incision, at this point, consists of the middle cervical fascia, which contains the omohyoid and the sternohyoid muscles.
- Enter the middle cervical fascia lateral to the carotid sheath. Bluntly dissect to the surface of the anterior scalene muscle. The superficial surfaces of the anterior scalene are composed of the outer layer of prevertebral fascia, which is the third and deepest of the fascial layers dealt with in this approach. Lying on the surface of the anterior scalene muscle is the phrenic nerve. The phrenic nerve crosses from lateral to medial, and cephalad to caudad. Retract the phrenic nerve medially after freeing it from the surface of the anterior scalene muscle. Identify the large internal jugular vein medially and feel for the carotid pulse. Although retraction of the carotid sheath is possible laterally, attempt to retract the internal jugular vein and carotid sheath medially (24). Retract the phrenic nerve to obtain good visualization of the anterior scalene, which is between the phrenic nerve and the middle scalene. The brachial plexus and suprascapular nerves are more superficial at the lateral border of the anterior scalene.
- Delineate the medial and lateral borders of the anterior scalene muscle. The fascia on the deep surface of the anterior scalene is Sibson's fascia, a continuation of the prevertebral fascia that encloses this muscle. The apex of the parietal pleura and lung form the undersurface of Sibson's fascia.
- Retract the anterior scalene laterally. Now carry out blunt dissection medially under the retracted carotid sheath. Stay on the prevertebral fascia of the spine.
- If more exposure is needed, carefully approach under the anterior scalene without violating the major portions of Sibson's fascia, and divide the anterior scalene muscle. The scalene can be retracted cephalad to caudad with self-retaining blunt retractors. Sibson's fascia now makes up the floor of the wound; the large internal jugular vein and the carotid sheath are located medially; the apex of the lung is beneath Sibson's fascia in the floor of the wound; and laterally, the brachial plexus courses superficial to the scalenus medius. The proximal portion of the anterior scalenus muscle may be dissected from the anterior tubercle of the transverse processes to allow greater exposure of the spine or brachial plexus (22).
- Incise Sibson's fascia at the transverse processes and bluntly retract it inferiorly. This retracts the pleura of the lung, which is usually at the T-1 level. Mobilize the recurrent laryngeal nerve medially with the carotid sheath and medial visceral column. Expose the spine by opening the fascia in the midline over the body. The transverse processes and rib heads can be exposed (18).
- Dissect to the second and third rib heads. This produces a rather lateral exposure of the spine. From the rib heads, dissect medially to enter the retropharyngeal fascial cleft on the anterior surface of the spine without having to dissect the longus colli muscle. Identify the vertebral artery entering the spine at C-6. The subclavian vein courses on the floor of the wound.
- If the approach is done from the left, the junction of the internal jugular veins and the subclavian veins will contain the thoracic duct. Identify the thoracic duct. In case of damage, double ligate it proximally and distally. Chylothorax can be prevented with proper ligation.

Often, a more judicious approach involves blunt dissection, progressing cephalad to caudad, as has been described for the transverse processes of C-5, C-6, and C-7, to the rib head of the first rib down on the spine. This will sweep most of these structures cephalad to caudad. The danger, of course, lies in cutting restraining structures that cross the field. The sympathetic chain (stellate ganglion at C-7) lies on the rib heads in a lateral position. Avoid damage by dissecting more medially.

THIRD RIB RESECTION IN THE TRANSTHORACIC APPROACH

Third rib resection is used for the transthoracic approach to the T1–T4 area. Resection of the third rib allows greater spreading of the intercostal area than does second rib resection (13). The cephalad extension of the exposure is enhanced with kyphosis deformity of the cervicothoracic junction area. The second rib can be removed if the operative exposure is inadequate.

- Place the patient in the lateral decubitus position, with the left side up. Prep and drape the entire left upper extremity in a sterile manner (Fig. 138.9).
- Incise the skin and subcutaneous tissue from the lateral paraspinous area at T-2, along the medial caudal border of the scapula, under the axilla to the costal cartilage of the third rib.
- Carefully divide each subsequent muscle layer down to the level of the rib, sectioning portions of the trapezius, latissimus dorsi, rhomboid major, and serratus posterior as needed. Careful dissection with electrocautery

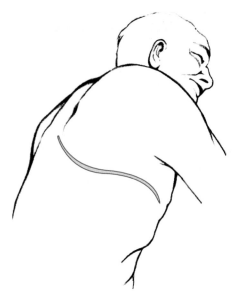

Figure 138.9.   Skin incision for third rib resection for the transthoracic approach.

and meticulous cauterization of each muscle bleeding point allows exposure to the outer periosteum of the third rib with a minimal amount of bleeding. As the muscle layers are divided, retract the scapula cephalad and medially to tense the muscle tissue for easier cutting. Palpate the chest wall cephalad for identification of the third rib. Remember that the first rib is situated inside the second; this is important for reaching the correct rib level (Fig. 138.10).

- Dissect the external periosteum off the third rib with periosteal elevators. Excise the third rib from the angle

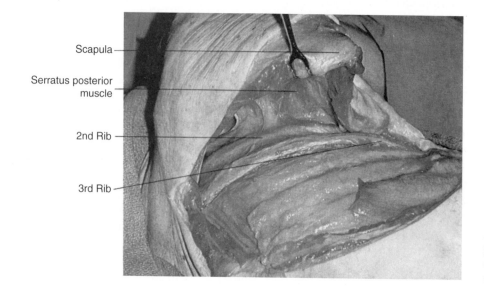

Scapula

Serratus posterior muscle

2nd Rib

3rd Rib

Figure 138.10.   Elevation of the scapula aids in the division of the muscles attached to the scapula and allows visualization of the third rib.

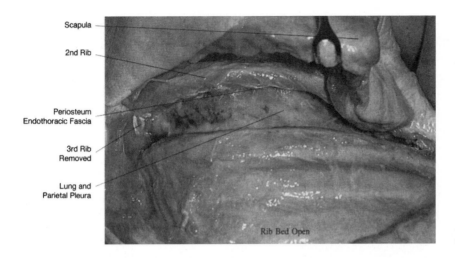

Figure 138.11. Excise the third rib from the angle of the rib to the costal cartilage.

of the rib to the costal cartilage. Open the rib bed as in the standard thoracotomy approach (Fig. 138.11). The rib bed consists of periosteum, endothoracic fascia, and parietal pleura. Incise the parietal pleura, carefully avoiding damage to the underlying lung. Pick up the inner periosteum of the rib bed with Adson forceps and open the rib bed with scissor tips or fine dissection with a knife blade. To avoid lung and pleural adhesions just under the rib, complete the opening of the rib bed with semiclosed scissors, using a finger to clear lung from the undersurface.

■ Use the Feochetti rib spreader to open the intercostal area. Deflate or retract the lung with a spatula-type retractor (Fig. 138.12).

■ Identify the aorta, spine, ribs, parietal pleura, and veins under the parietal pleura in the wound. The highest intercostal vein is usually seen.

■ Use an Adson forceps and Metzenbaum scissors to open the parietal pleura delicately over the costovertebral articulations.

■ Identify the prominent soft or white tissue of the intervertebral disc. This is a relatively avascular, safer plane for dissection than the surface of the vertebral body. Make an intraoperative radiograph to verify the level.

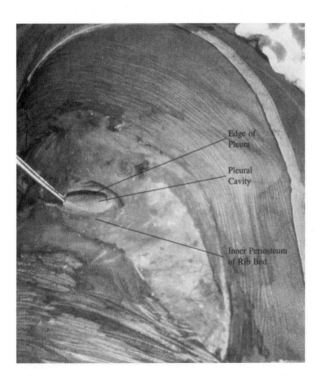

Figure 138.12. With the rib bed open, place the Feochetti rib-separating retractor and retract the lung with a spatula lung retractor.

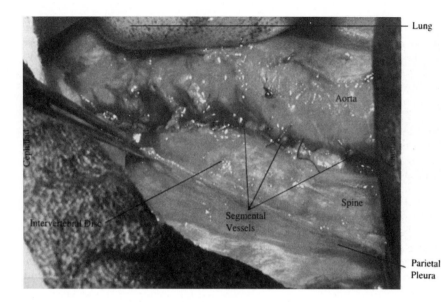

Figure 138.13. After the parietal pleura is opened, bluntly dissect its edges off the spine with a "peanut" or sponge. The parietal pleura may be sutured back laterally with stay sutures when necessary for continued retraction.

- Dissect each intercostal vessel, tying and ligating it over the vertebral body. Bluntly dissect the soft tissue from the vertebral body (Fig. 138.13).
- Fully expand the lung and visualize in all areas before closure. Close the parietal pleura over the spine whenever possible. Place the chest tube through a separate aperture, preferably in the ninth intercostal space. Protect the lung during closure. Close the chest with the rib approximator. Close the rib bed with interrupted permanent braided Dacron sutures. The chest tube can usually be removed within 48 to 72 hours, depending on drainage and expansion of the lung.

THORACOTOMY APPROACH

The standard thoracotomy approach is used for safe exposure of vertebral levels T-2 to L-2. Rib selection depends on the location and extent of the pathologic process. Anatomic variations at the cervicothoracic and thoracolumbar junction dictate the rib to be taken. Choose the rib to be resected for a certain vertebral level by one of two methods:

1. When the pathology dictates a direct anterior approach to the vertebral column (e.g., kyphotic tuberculous abscess), choose the rib directly horizontal to the vertebral level at the midaxillary line in an anteroposterior chest radiograph. The rib removed must be cephalad to the lesion to give adequate proximal exposure of the lesion (13).
2. When direct access to the spinal canal is needed at one disc (e.g., ninth rib to the T8–T9 disc), use a left approach because it is much easier to deal with the aorta and the segmental vessels from the left side. For

patients with a large abscess in the right chest or in other circumstances that dictate a right thoracic approach, be prepared to mobilize the vena cava and associated veins from that side.

- Place the patient on the bean bag. Use a double-branched endotracheal tube into the right and left mainstem bronchi to allow selective collapse of the left lung. Center the midthorax of the patient over the break in the table. Pad the dependent axilla, and pad and protect the left arm. Stabilize the pelvis with a strap to the table. Place a pillow between the legs, and pad all the bony prominences. Flex the table to allow better exposure.
- Open the skin and subcutaneous tissue from the lateral border of the paraspinous musculature to the sternocostal junction over the rib to be resected. Inject the incision with 1:500,000 epinephrine. Place the thoracotomy incision slightly tangential to the rib to be resected, allowing easier resection of more than one rib if necessary.
- After inserting the self-retaining retractors, extend the wound with the electrocautery down through the muscle layers to the thorax. When necessary for full exposure, the latissimus dorsi, trapezius, and rhomboid major and minor muscles can be sectioned.
- After the chest wall is exposed, count the ribs from the twelfth up to the appropriate rib or from the first rib downward. The first rib appears to be inside the second when one is palpating from this angle, and it is often difficult to find. Each rib articulates with the superior portion of the body in the area of the disc space of the level above. Therefore, the twelfth rib inserts closer to the T11–T12 intervertebral disc space. Confirm identification of the rib with a radiograph.

- Expose the outer periosteum of the rib with the electrocautery and cut directly to the bone through the periosteum from the angle of the rib to the costal cartilage. Elevate the periosteum off the outer rib surface. Use the curved-tip rib elevator to strip the superior and inferior borders of the rib, maintaining an intact elevated periosteum. Elevate the inner periosteum of the undersurface of the rib with the Doyen elevator.
- *Caution: Avoid damaging the intercostal vessels that course on the inferior surface of the rib. Elevate the periosteum of the rib by cutting with the elevator directly on bone. Avoid plunges that might inadvertently enter the pleura.*
- With the intact periosteum freed from the rib, cut the rib with the rib cutter as far posteriorly as necessary between the costotransverse joint and the angle of the rib and anteriorly at the costal junction. Remove the rib and save it for bone graft. Lightly wax the bone on the end of the rib after rasping to make sure there are no ragged edges. Tie a sponge on the tip of the stump to protect the surgeon during the procedure.
- Pick up the inner periosteum of the rib bed with Adson forceps and open the rib bed with scissor tips. Avoid lung and pleural adhesions. Complete the opening of the rib bed with a semiclosed scissors after using a finger to clear lung from the undersurface. When pleural adhesions exist, first attempt to dissect the adhesions bluntly with the finger or sponge stick. If necessary, sharply dissect dense adhesions and ligate vascular structures.
- Retract the lung medially with a spatula lung retractor or deflate it. Retraction of the lung should be removed at least every 20 minutes to allow adequate expansion of the lung and to prevent postoperative atelectasis. Insert the Feochetti separator in the rib resection defect, with moist lap sponges over the edges. Expand the Feochetti separator to allow adequate visualization inside the thoracic cavity. Flexion of the table may be of benefit.
- The anatomy of the spine at this point is obscured by the reflection of the parietal pleura as it covers the soft-tissue structures over the spinal column. Elevate the parietal pleura with Adson forceps and open it with Metzenbaum scissors. Extend the opening of the parietal pleura cephalad and caudad on the spine by cutting over a peon dissected under the pleura. The presence of a large paravertebral abscess at this point means only that the abscess should be exposed just as the spine would be. When an abscess is present, cut its outer wall longitudinally and approach the spine through the abscess.
- The disc is the more prominent, softer, white structure of the spine. The discs are relatively avascular and a much safer area for dissection. An intercostal vein and artery cross the midportion of each vertebral body.
- Bluntly dissect the edges of the parietal pleura off the spine with a Kittner dissector or sponge. Elevate the pleura on the discs and lift it off the vessels on the vertebral body. Dissection begun over the disc is less likely to cause bleeding. Make a radiograph at this point to verify the level. After the parietal pleura is opened, it may be sutured back on itself laterally with two stay sutures.
- Separate, sever, and ligate each of the intercostal vessels over the vertebral body. If a large paravertebral abscess is present, the arteries enter the abscess. Take care to avoid clamping segmental arteries too close to the aorta so as to lose the tie or too close to the intervertebral foramen. Tie arteries and veins separately or together, depending on their size. Pass a right-angled clamp under the vessels, and use a braided 2-0 suture in a free tie to tie off first the medial and then the lateral exposed vessels; use vascular clamps in a similar fashion.
- *Caution: Take care to dissect adequately under the vessels. A common mistake is to have both ligature sutures in the same place under the vessel and not have adequate room for cutting between them. Handle every segmental vessel in the area of where bony work will be done in this manner. Paralysis due to ligation of a segmental artery on the vertebral body has not been a problem (13).*
- *Caution: Do not dissect into the intervertebral foramen.*
- Bluntly expose the outer surface of the spine after division of the segmental vessels. When bone and disc exposure is needed, cut with the cautery directly to bone. Use the periosteal elevator to dissect the annulus off the disc and the periosteum off the bone medially and laterally, exposing the entire disc and vertebral column. The tendency is not to dissect the soft tissue laterally enough off the spine. The rib head articulates with the cephalad half of its appropriate vertebral body and the disc space above. Access to the posterior disc and spinal column can be gained by resecting the rib head (Fig. 138.14). Removal of the head of the rib and its articulation allows excellent exposure of the posterolateral aspect of the intervertebral disc. After the rib head and disc are removed, identify the intercostal nerve, dural sac, posterior vertebral body wall, and spinal canal. The costal vertebral articulation is a major stabilizing structure in the thoracic spine. Identifying the left pedicle in a left-sided approach helps locate the spinal canal for orientation. The vertebral body can be completely exposed by resecting the disc above and below to identify the posterior body wall and spinal canal and dissected laterally to identify the pedicle and spinal canal.
- Visualize the lung fully expanded in all areas before closure. Close the parietal pleura over the spine whenever possible. Place the chest tube through a separate aperture, preferably in the ninth intercostal space. Protect the lung during closure. Close the chest with the rib approximator. Close the rib bed with interrupted

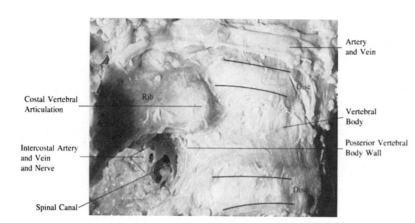

Costal Vertebral
Articulation

Rib

Artery
and Vein

Disc

Vertebral
Body

Posterior Vertebral
Body Wall

Intercostal Artery
and Vein
and Nerve

Disc

Spinal Canal

Figure 138.14. The rib articulates with the cephalad half of its appropriate numbered vertebral body and with the disc space above. Therefore, the tenth rib articulates at T9–T10.

permanent braided Dacron sutures. The chest tube connects to the water seal. With the lung re-expanded, the chest tube can usually be removed within 48 to 72 hours, depending on drainage and expansion of the lung.

THE THORACOLUMBAR JUNCTION

The rules for resecting the best rib for exposure of the thoracolumbar junction are much the same as in the rest of the thoracic spine. Hodgson and Rau (13,14) recommend a ninth rib resection for T10–L1. Dwyer et al. (6) recommend a tenth rib resection with the standard thoracolumbar approach for the T10–L1 area. For exposure of the T12–L1 area, Perry (19) recommends a tenth rib resection. Ideally, choosing the rib in the midaxillary line opposite the lesion or the apex of a curve allows adequate proximal exposure for working "down" or caudad on the lesion.

Transthoracic resection of the ninth rib is usually best for maximum exposure of T11–T12. A tenth rib thoracoabdominal approach is preferred for exposure of the T12–L1 area. Both techniques involve detaching the diaphragm at its circumference. A twelfth rib approach is used in cases in which less exposure is needed or when it is imperative that the diaphragm not be taken down. A twelfth rib extrapleural retroperitoneal approach is recommended for exposure of L1–L2.

The approach through the eleventh rib, a more demanding approach with less expansive exposure, is the highest practical, extrapleural, retroperitoneal anterior approach for the exposure of the T10–L2 area. It is ideally used in severely ill patients in whom avoiding opening the pleural cavity and cutting the diaphragm is an advantage. Another alternative for limited extrapleural exposure with low morbidity is the posterior costotransversectomy approach. The vertebral body and spinal canal can be ex-

posed by following the twelfth subcostal nerve to T12–L1. Unless at least two levels are exposed with the approach, the visualization necessary to perform total discectomy, vertebrectomy, and strut grafting is extremely poor compared with the anterior approach.

A third approach that may be used in special situations is the tenth rib thoracolumbar approach for long exposures of the thoracic and lumbar spine. This approach allows proximal and distal extension for multilevel operations and optimum exposure for bony work.

TENTH RIB THORACOABDOMINAL APPROACH

■ Place the patient in the lateral decubitus position. Make the approach from the convexity of the scoliosis or from the left side, when possible (Fig. 138.15). A left-sided approach is preferred because of ease of mobilization of the aorta compared with the vena cava and because splenic retraction is easier than hepatic reconstruction. Open the skin and subcutaneous tissue from the lateral

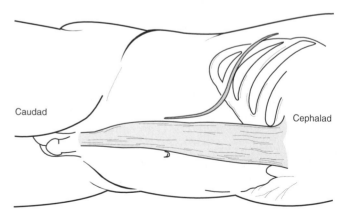

Caudad

Cephalad

Figure 138.15. Skin incision for a tenth rib thoracoabdominal approach.

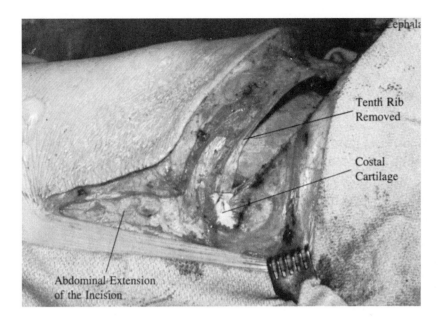

Figure 138.16. With the rib removed, carefully delineate the costal cartilage.

border of the paraspinous musculature over the tenth rib to the junction of the tenth rib and costal cartilage (20). Curve the incision anteriorly from the tip of the tenth rib to the lateral rectus sheath and distally down the edge of the sheath as far as necessary for exposure. Use electrocautery to slowly extend the incision through each muscle layer while an assistant aggressively picks up bleeders with two Adson forceps.

■ Open the superficial periosteum of the tenth rib to the costal cartilage. Use the sharp, curved periosteal elevator to remove the superficial and deep periosteum off the rib. Take care to avoid the neurovascular bundle on the inferior surface of the rib. Cut posteriorly at the angle of the rib, and cut at the junction of the rib and costal cartilage. Remove the rib. On opening the pleural space, retract the lung and fully open the rib bed with scissors (Fig. 138.16). At this point, the intrapleural cavity is opened and the retroperitoneal cavity is still closed.

■ Split the costal cartilage with a knife along its length. Open the undersurface of the costal cartilage and retract the two tags of cartilage (5,6,20) (Fig. 138.17).

■ Identify the peritoneum and retroperitoneal space by blunt dissection under the retracted split tips of the costal cartilage. The guide to the retroperitoneal space is the light areolar tissue of the retroperitoneal fat (Fig. 138.18).

■ Bluntly dissect the peritoneum off the inferior surface of the diaphragm (Fig. 138.19). The peritoneum is swept, using a sponge, first from the undersurface of the diaphragm, then from the transversalis fascia, and finally from the abdominal wall.

■ After the peritoneum is retracted, carefully open the abdominal musculature (the external oblique, the internal oblique, and the transversus abdominis) one layer at a time, with complete hemostasis. At this point the chest and retroperitoneal space are open and the diaphragm is the intervening structure in the wound.

■ Incise the diaphragm from inside the chest with clear visualization under the diaphragm in the retroperitoneal space. Extend the incision in the diaphragm circumferentially, 1 inch from its peripheral attachment to the chest wall (28). Use marker clips throughout the take-down of the diaphragm to allow accurate reapproximation.

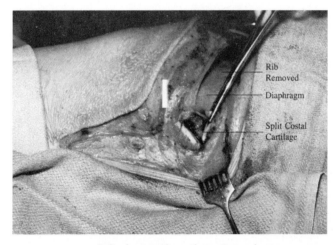

Figure 138.17. Split the costal cartilage. Open the most superficial layer of soft tissue under the costal cartilage enough to allow retraction of the cartilage tips.

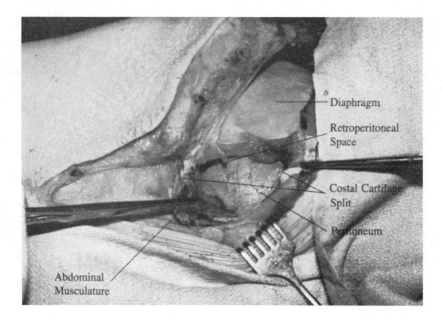

Figure 138.18. Retract the split tips of costal cartilage. Identify the insertion of the diaphragm into the cephalad cartilage tip and the insertion of the abdominal musculature into the caudad cartilage tip.

■ For work on T2–L1, resect the diaphragm to the spine. Cut the crus of the diaphragm and elevate it off the spinal column. Use protected Deaver retractors to retract the peritoneal sac anteriorly. Identify the psoas muscle with its most cephalad attachment to the transverse process of L, and protect the muscle because the lumbosacra plexus is under it. With a large rib retractor, such as the Feochetti, open the tenth rib incision in the chest. The spine will be visualized from approximately T-6 as far distally in the lumbar spine as necessary. In the lumbar spine, remove the crus of the diaphragm and the attachments of the psoas muscle, if needed, for proper visualization of the spine. In the thoracic spine,

the parietal pleura is opened as in a standard thoracotomy approach. Tie and ligate the intercostal artery and vein to allow mobilization of the major vascular trunks. If it is identified as in the operative area, the thoracic duct, which usually crosses right to left around T4–T5, is tied off. Avoid the sympathetic plexus. After the intercostal vessels are removed, cut directly to the spine. Dissection is carried out on the spine, and soft tissue is removed laterally.

■ The key to closure is the reapproximation of the costal cartilage. After the diaphragm is resutured with multiple interrupted sutures and the split cartilage is reapproximated, insert the chest tube in the eighth intercos-

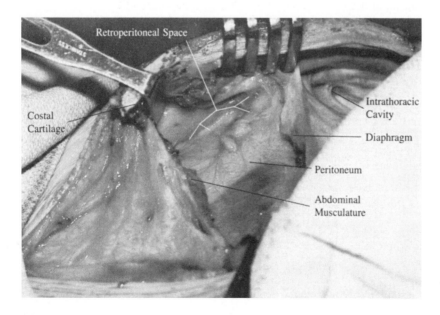

Figure 138.19. Bluntly dissect the periosteum off the inferior surface of the diaphragm.

tal space and pass it posterosuperiorly. Attached to the cephalad half of the costal cartilage is the insertion of the diaphragm and the interthoracic fascia. Inserting into the distal split of costal cartilage is the transverse abdominal fascia and attachment for the abdominal musculature. With the costal cartilage reapproximated, the layers of the abdominal musculature are better defined. Close each layer of the abdominal wall separately when possible, and close the chest as in a standard thoracotomy.

THE LUMBOSACRAL SPINE

PARARECTUS INCISION FOR L2–S1

- Position the patient supine on the table with the lower lumbar spine at the level of the kidney rests.
- Make a lower abdominal pararectus incision through the skin and subcutaneous tissue. The most immediate layers are those of the external oblique with its transition into the linea semilunaris, which leads to the fascia of the rectus sheath. The linea semilunaris is composed of the aponeurosis of the three layers of the abdominal musculature and their fascia.
- Incise the fibers of the external oblique, the internal oblique, and the small thin layer of transversus abdominis muscles laterally to the semilunaris in line with the skin incision.
- Identify the transversalis fascia, which is the internal investing fascial layer of the abdominal cavity. Dissect the outer surface of the transversalis fascia to the edge of the rectus sheath. The transversalis fascia splits at this point to form the lamina of the rectus sheath. The posterior lamina of the rectus sheath forms the endoabdominal fascia in this area.
- Carefully incise the transversalis fascia laterally to the linea semilunaris, and identify the peritoneum through the incision.
- Begin the incision in line with the skin incision. Dissect the peritoneum with a sponge or gloved hand off the undersurface of the transversalis fascia. Open the abdominal wall after the peritoneum has been identified and cleared.
- Bluntly dissect the peritoneum from the lateral abdominal wall, progressing posteriorly. Identify the psoas muscle, as in any retroperitoneal approach to the spine. Retract the peritoneum off the left iliac artery and vein by use of the surgeon's hand, a padded deaver retractor, or sponge sticks. Sweep the peritoneum with the ureter from left to right, and expose the left common iliac artery and vein. Insert Freebody pins or special retractors.
- Palpate and identify the intervertebral disc. Remember that this is a relatively avascular area. With any approach to the L4–S1 area, identify the left iliolumbar

vein and ligate it when necessary. Dissection within the bifurcation of the aorta should be blunt and as avascular as possible. Remember, the left common iliac vein lies in the bifurcation over the L4–S1 disc. The variation in inferior vena cava and lumbar veins often dictates the exact approach from this point.
- Bluntly retract and protect the hypogastric plexus.
- Allowing the peritoneal sac to fall into place, close the muscle layers with a running suture. The transversus abdominis and the internal oblique may be closed together.

ANTERIOR RETROPERITONEAL FLANK APPROACH TO L2–L5

For the retroperitoneal exposure of the lumbar spine, an anterior pararectus vertical incision, a J-shaped renal incision, or a horizontal lateral abdominal incision can be used (Fig. 138.20). I prefer the horizontal oblique incision.

- Place the patient in the supine position over the kidney rests. For patients with a large abdominal pannus, the left lateral decubitus position can be used. In the lateral position, too much hip flexion at this point will limit the operative exposure anteriorly.
- Start the incision equidistant between the lowest rib and the superior iliac crest in the midaxillary line, and extend it approximately to the edge of the rectus sheath. The level of the incision varies according to the level of the spine approached: L5–S1 is in the lower half of the distance between umbilicus and symphysis, L4–5 is in the upper half, L3–4 is at the umbilicus, and L2–3 is above the umbilicus. The length of the incision can vary according to the surgeon's experience, the exposure needed, and the operation to be done.
- Muscle relaxation allows greater mobility to the ab-

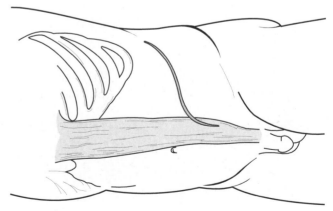

Figure 138.20. For retroperitoneal exposure of the lumbar spine, an anterior pararectus vertical incision, a J-shaped renal incision, or a horizontal lateral abdominal incision can be used.

dominal wall and decreases the contractility of the muscle as it is incised. First, open the muscle layers as laterally as possible because they are thicker here and there is less chance of penetrating the peritoneum. The muscle layers thin out, and the layers of the fascia become almost joined medially. The peritoneum is very superficial. Inadvertent penetration of the peritoneum is most likely just lateral to the rectus sheath. Dissect through the external oblique and the internal oblique muscle. Inferior to the internal oblique is the transversus abdominis. Use care in inserting self-retaining retractors into the muscle layers so as not to damage the peritoneum. Often, the transversus abdominis muscle is a very thin or absent muscle layer. Bluntly spread this thin muscle in line with its fibers to expose the transversalis fascia.

■ Open the transversalis fascia in the lateral portion of the wound (Fig. 138.21). Lift the transversalis fascia with Adson forceps and carefully open it with blunt scissors. The retroperitoneal fat allows room to enter the extraperitoneal space.

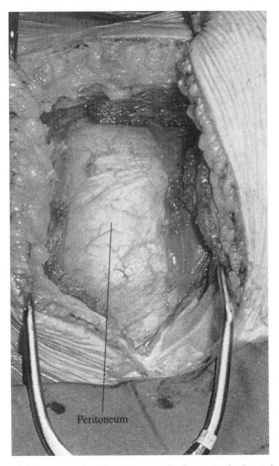

Figure 138.21. Open the transversalis fascia in the lateral portion of the wound. Lift it with Adson forceps and carefully open it with blunt scissors.

■ Enter the retroperitoneal space laterally. Identify the peritoneum and the fat of the peritoneal space. Remove the peritoneum from the remaining transversalis fascia with blunt dissection. Extend the incision after the peritoneum has been safely removed. The sheath may be incised for added exposure. Torn peritoneum should be repaired promptly (19).

■ Identification of the psoas muscle is the key to the retroperitoneal approach. Pass your hand directly to the psoas. Avoid opening the retropsoas space, which is a blind pouch. The genitofemoral nerve can be identified on the psoas. The spine is immediately medial to the psoas and can be partially obscured by it. Palpate and identify the psoas muscle, the intervertebral disc, the aorta, and the vertebral body. The paravertebral sympathetic chain lies medial to the psoas muscle. The ureter will be reflected medially with the undersurface of the peritoneum. If a retroperitoneal abscess is well developed, open it and dissect inside the abscess to the spine.

■ The key at this point is to identify the raised, white, softer disc by direct palpation with the finger, as opposed to the lower, concave vertebral body, where the lumbar vessels are found. The discs are the hills, and the vertebral bodies are the valleys. The vessels are in the valleys.

■ Once the lumbar disc can be identified, insert a blunt elevator or padded small retractor to sweep the soft tissue from left to right across the disc space. The lumbar veins are a horizontal tether. Variations in formation of the inferior vena cava and lumbar veins are the rule rather than the exception (11). The most important of these veins is the iliolumbar vein, which crosses the body of L-5 from right to left and ascends in the left paraspinous area (13). This vessel is a direct tether to the left-to-right retraction of the aorta off the spine and is very vulnerable to avulsion.

■ For operations on the L4–L5 disc space, identify the iliolumbar vein early in the dissection (Fig. 138.22). Ligate it after clamping the vein with angled tonsil clamps and passing two or three ligatures around the vein. These ligatures should not be tied too close to the vena cava because a sidewall injury can occur. Transect the vein after securing the permanent ties. Greater mobilization of the vena cava and venous structures, left to right, is thereby obtained. The iliolumbar vein consistently requires ligation.

■ Lumbar veins of varying sizes at various positions are always present. Some may be directly posterior to the vena cava and of quite large diameter. Dissection on the anterior spine consists of gentle stretching and pulling of the structures, blunt dissection, direct pressure over many small bleeding areas with a sponge, and a minimum of electrocautery. The paraspinous sympathetic plexus between the spine and the psoas muscle varies in size and number of fibers. Branches course between the preaortic and paraspinous chains. Preserve paraspinous sympathetic fibers that do not impede dissection.

■ Dissect with the fingertip and blunt elevators all the vascular structures from left to right to give adequate visualization of the end plate of the vertebral body above the disc (27).

■ Use malleable Deaver-type retractors or blade spike retractors around the disc space. Alternatively, prepare four Freebody Steinmann pin retractors with rubber sleeves and mount them in a Steinmann pin holder (9). For any sharp stay-retractor that is driven into the body, stabilize the pin on the finger and engage the tip into the vertebral body under direct vision. The assistant taps the pin into the body while the surgeon maintains control of the pin. Avoid the tendency for the pin to enter the disc space by directing the tip of the pin horizontal to the disc space. Allow a sufficient distance from the endplate to allow work on the disc space without dislodging the pin. Place the superior and inferior right-sided pins before placing the left-sided pins.

■ Expose the annulus of the disc (Fig. 138.23). There should have been minimal sharp dissection and cautery in this area. Now prepare the disc for the operative procedure. The vena cava and iliac artery and vein are held by the retractors.

■ Special curved or malleable retractors can be used between the stay retractors for protection of the vena cava.

■ Extract the retractors with the same amount of care as when they were inserted. The sheath and a finger must

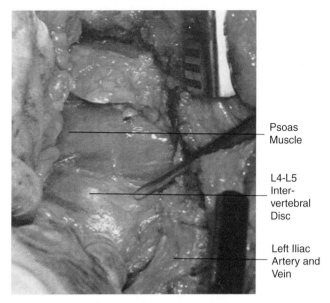

Figure 138.23. Expose the annulus of the disc.

Psoas Muscle

L4-L5 Inter-vertebral Disc

Left Iliac Artery and Vein

guard the tip; otherwise the vena cava will be torn as the sharp tip passes the vessel that is tented around it.

■ Remember:

1. When making the incision, follow the skin guidelines for optimum spine exposure.
2. Achieve careful hemostasis in the muscle layers.
3. Incise the transversus abdominus muscle layer and the transversalis fascia in the lateral portion of the wound.
4. Beware of thinning muscle layers and the peritoneum's superficial position medially near the rectus sheath.
5. Pass directly to the psoas muscle.
6. Identify the raised, soft, white disc.
7. Identify, ligate, and divide the iliolumbar vein.
8. Sweep prevertebral tissue left to right across the disc.
9. Insert the Steinmann pin after placing it directly on bone with the fingertip.

■ Retract the Steinmann pin, again with the fingertip preventing the tip of the pin from damaging the left iliac artery.

RETROPERITONEAL EXPOSURE OF L5–S1

■ Palpate the spine with a finger and find a disc for orientation. Usually, it is the L4–L5 disc. With identification of the L4–L5 disc, palpate the pulse of the left common iliac artery and the aortic bifurcation. The bifurcation of the aorta is critical in determining the exact approach

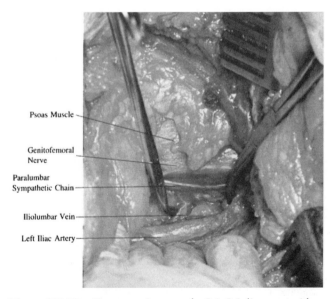

Psoas Muscle

Genitofemoral Nerve

Paralumbar Sympathetic Chain

Iliolumbar Vein

Left Iliac Artery

Figure 138.22. For operations on the L4–L5 disc space, identify the iliolumbar vein early in the dissection.

from this point. The usual bifurcation at the L4–L5 disc level was present in 69% of anatomic dissections performed by Harmon (11), but great variation exists.

■ Palpate the left common iliac artery and pass over it medially to the L5–S1 disc. By placement of the finger and a subsequent blunt retractor such as a sponge-covered elevator, develop a plane just to the right of the left common iliac artery.

■ The left iliac vein lies within the aortic bifurcation. It often courses directly on the surface of the L5–S1 disc and may be flattened against the disc or L-5 body, with its venous character obscured. Mobilize it to the left and cephalad with the left iliac artery.

■ The middle sacral artery and veins are present in the bifurcation. The key to handling these structures is blunt dissection just to the right of the left common iliac artery, sweeping from left to right the prevertebral tissue, including the middle sacral vessels and superior hypogastric plexus, off the lumbosacral disc. Occasionally, the middle sacral vessels are of formidable size, but seldom do they have to be ligated (4).

■ An additional structure in the bifurcation is the superior hypogastric sympathetic plexus.

■ The thoracolumbar sympathetic chain extends down anterior to the aorta and vertebral bodies in the retroperitoneal space as the preaortic sympathetic plexus. At approximately the L3–L4 level, the inferior hypogastric plexus extends to L4–S1 as the superior hypogastric plexus (Fig. 138.24). The structure of the superior hypogastric plexus varies considerably because the preponderance of the superior hypogastric plexus fibers is usually closer to the left iliac artery as they arch over the L5–S1 disc in the bifurcation of the aorta (Fig.

138.25) (16). There may be multiple strands or one predominant large simple nerve trunk. The superior hypogastric plexus contains the sympathetic function for the urogenital system. The S1–S4 nerve roots that contribute to the pelvic splenic nerves provide parasympathetic function for the urogenital system. The pudendal nerve covers somatic function from S-1, S-2, S-3, and S-4.

■ Ejaculation is predominantly a sympathetic function, whereas through control of the vasculature of the penis, erection is predominantly a parasympathetic function. Retrograde ejaculation and sterility result from disruption to the sympathetic plexus. The main effect of damage to the superior hypogastric plexus is improper closing of the bladder neck, with resultant retrograde ejaculation, although the sympathetic fibers also have some effect on the motility of the vas deferens, which is important in the transportation of the spermatozoa from the epididymis to the seminal vesicle (15).

■ The prognosis for recovery from retrograde ejaculation is good (8). Sperm can be obtained in refractory cases by bladder aspiration techniques. Damage to the superior hypogastric plexus should not produce impotence or failure of erection. Avoid damaging the hypogastric plexus by doing the following (4):

1. For the transperitoneal midline approach, carefully open the posterior peritoneum and bluntly dissect the prevertebral tissue from left to right (9).
2. Visualize and retract the prevertebral tissues by opening the posterior peritoneum higher over the bifurcation and then extending the opening down over the sacral promontory (4,8,9,15).

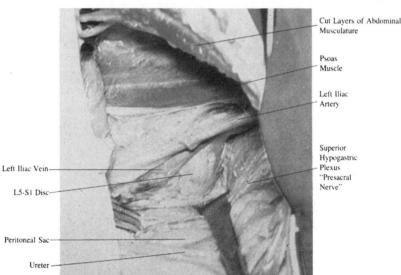

Figure 138.24. Sweep the prevertebral tissue bluntly off the front of the L5–S1 disc. The superior hypogastric plexus may be a diffuse plexiform nerve formation that is retracted with the other tissue, or it can be a discrete well-defined presacral nerve.

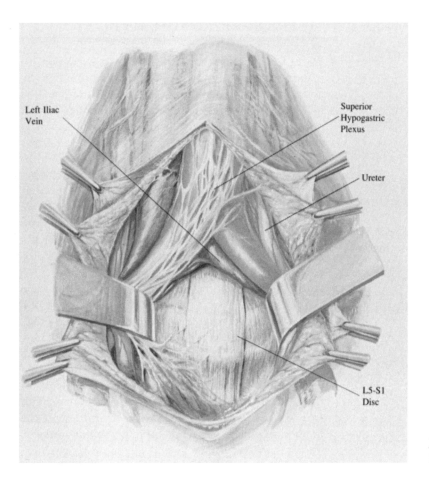

Left Iliac
Vein

Superior
Hypogastric
Plexus

Ureter

L5-S1
Disc

Figure 138.25. The superior hypogastric plexus is within the bifurcation of the aorta.

3. Remove the prevertebral tissue from the L5–S1 disc with blunt dissection, retraction, and spreading.
4. Attempt to retract the middle sacral artery and vein without electrocautery by spreading and blunt dissection. Use vascular clips or tie ligation when this vessel is of considerable size.
5. Until the annulus of the disc is clearly exposed, make no transverse scalpel cuts on the front of the L5–S1 disc.
6. Do not use electrocautery within the aortic bifurcation.

■ The key to avoid damaging the superior hypogastric plexus is to avoid transverse cuts on the face of the disc until all the prevertebral tissue has been elevated from the annulus and to avoid electrocautery on the surface of the L5–S1 disc. Small bleeding points are encountered when doing this dissection, but they are usually easily controlled by direct finger pressure or packing with hemostatic gauze. Usually, the left iliac artery and vein will be retracted to the left, but it may require retraction to the right on occasion.
■ Locate and ligate the iliolumbar vein before any mobilization of the left iliac artery to the right.

■ Always obtain radiographic confirmation of the level. It can be done easily by inserting a #22-gauge spinal needle and taking a radiograph. Because the L5–S1 disc and the sacrum are often angled very horizontally, the body of L-5 can be mistaken for the sacrum.
■ Insert appropriate Freebody Steinmann pin stay-retractors, blade-point retractors, or hand-held retractors.

TRANSPERITONEAL EXPOSURE OF L5–S1

■ For the transperitoneal exposure, use either a vertical midline incision or a transverse "smile" incision. The "smile" is better cosmetically and gives excellent exposure, but it requires transection of the rectus abdominus sheath. Identify and open the rectus sheath, and transect the rectus abdominus muscle. The posterior rectus sheath, the abdominal fascia, and the peritoneum are conjoined in this area. Carefully open the posterior rectus sheath and abdominal fascia to the peritoneum.
■ Pick up the peritoneum. Open the length of the wound carefully, avoiding damage to the bowel. Identify the

posterior peritoneum over the sacral promontory after packing off the bowel.

- Palpate the aorta and both iliac vessels through the posterior peritoneum. Feel the softer texture of the L5–S1 disc.
- Inject the retroperitoneal space with saline to achieve separation of the peritoneum from the vascular structures.
- Pick up the peritoneum with Adson forceps; handle it delicately.
- Avoid use of the electrocautery anterior to L5–S1 to prevent damage to the superior hypogastric plexus, despite the fact that there is bleeding in this area. The left common iliac vein often lies as a flat, white, bloodless ribbon across the L5–S1 disc within the aortic bifurcation.
- After the left common iliac artery and left common iliac vein are identified, use blunt dissection to the right of the left iliac artery and hypogastric plexus and soft tissue, moving from left to right (Fig. 138.26).
- Bluntly dissect the middle sacral artery and vein from left to right without sacrifice at this point. Longitudinal blunt dissection allows better mobilization of these vascular structures. When bleeding is encountered, use direct finger and sponge pressure for a short time, followed by blunt dissection. Control hemorrhage with packing and pressure. Divide and tie the middle sacral artery and vein, if necessary.

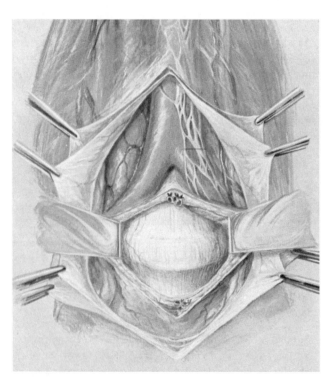

Figure 138.26. Exposure of the L5–S1 disc. See text for a description of the technique.

POSTERIOR APPROACH TO L1–S1

- Position the patient to allow full chest excursion, to maintain the neck in a safe position, and to allow the abdomen to hang completely free of pressure. Flex the hips and knees enough to relieve nerve root tension but not so much as to obstruct arterial flow to the legs or to produce any abdominal pressure. I prefer the Andrews frame.
- Obtain a skin marker radiograph by inserting two #20-gauge spinal needles perpendicular to the skin approximately three fingerbreadths lateral to the spine. Using the alignment of the needles, put the skin incision in the midline over the disc space. Paraspinous needles allow a more accurate skin incision than a spinous process marker.
- Use a skin marking pencil to draw a vertical, midline skin incision relative to the two needles over the disc space. Make a dermal skin incision only. The average length is 3.2 cm for a one-level microscopic discectomy, longer for a more extensive decompression. Inject 25 to 50 ml 1:500,000 epinephrine through the dermal incision into the subcuticular tissue and directly down to the lamina into the paraspinous muscle mass. Cut with a scalpel directly to the fascial layer. Preserve the lumbodorsal fascial attachments to the spinous process, the interspinous ligament, and the supraspinous ligaments by making a paraspinous fascial incision that can be sutured at closure without tension. This is preferable to removing all soft-tissue fascial attachments from the spinous process, unless a total laminectomy is to be done, in which the fascia is totally removed from the spinous process and lamina with the electrocautery.
- The lumbodorsal fascia is critical for stability of the spine. Maintaining the fascial attachments to the spine is important and should be done when possible. The abdominal, trunk, and gluteal muscles contract and tense the lumbodorsal fascia; the fascia attachment to the spine allows these muscles to stabilize the spine.
- Make an incision into the lumbodorsal fascia just lateral to the bulbous tips of the spinous processes. Lengthen the fascial incision. Insert a Cobb elevator, with the tip turned upward, onto the spinous process just under its bulbous tip, and start the subperiosteal dissection. Then turn the elevator bevel down. Dissect, identify by touch the cephalad and then the caudad lamina, and clear the interlaminar area. Take care not to cut through the outer cortex of the lamina. Sweep the superficial soft tissue off the interlaminar area laterally out to the facet joint capsule. Do not damage the capsule. Protect the facet joint capsule. Remember that the two laminae and their interlaminar areas are the only areas that need be exposed for an operation on one intervertebral disc.

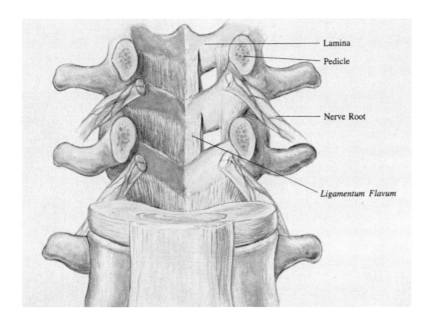

Figure 138.27. This underview of the posterior elements from the intervertebral canal demonstrates the ligamentum flavum and its insertion on the lamina.

■ Following exposure of the intralaminar area, place a Williams self-retaining retractor with the blade retracting laterally over the facet joint capsule with the pointed tip placed medially. For larger, bilateral exposures, I use the Wiltse retractors with both sides exposed similarly.

■ The superficial ligamentum flavum blends laterally into the facet joint capsule. Incise the superficial ligamentum flavum with the #15 blade or electrocautery laterally or at the junction of the superficial ligamentum flavum and the facet joint capsule. Use a curet to elevate the superficial ligamentum flavum from the deep ligament moving from lateral to medial. Remove the superficial ligament with a pituitary rongeur. The vertical striations of the yellow deep ligamentum flavum can be seen in the depths of the interlaminar area. Use an angled curet to clear under the caudal edge of the cephalad lamina and a straight curet to define the ligamentum flavum attachment to the caudad lamina (Fig. 138.27). Expose the deep portion of the ligamentum flavum's vertical striations.

■ Several factors concerning the anatomy of the ligamentum flavum are important:
  ■ It has a deep and superficial portion.
  ■ It blends with the facet joint capsule laterally.
  ■ It inserts over the caudal 50% of the undersurface of the cephalad lamina.
  ■ It inserts on the cephalad edge of the caudad lamina.
  ■ Its undersurface is the ideal dural covering.
  ■ It has a vertical, parasagittal orientation deep in the lateral recess under the superior facet that may contribute to lateral recess stenosis.
  ■ It is the main stabilizing ligament of the posterior column, and preservation of as much of it as possible will benefit spine stability at that motion segment.
  ■ It is the soft-tissue roof of the intervertebral foramina.

LAMINOTOMY

■ Perform as much of the lateral wall resection and laminectomy as possible before opening the ligamentum flavum. Estimate the size of the interlaminar area that will be needed for correcting the pathologic process. A portion of the caudad edge of the cephalad lamina can be removed if it is believed that exploration of the spinal canal will require greater cephalad exposure. The walls of the interlaminar area may be the area to be removed. Progressing from dorsal to ventral, the lateral wall of the interlaminar area is composed of the facet joint capsule, the inferior facet, the intra-articular space of the facet joint, the superior facet, the deep capsule and ligamentum flavum, the nerve root, the blood vessels, and the floor of the canal. The preoperative CT scan should determine the amount of lateral recess stenosis and how much of a medial facetectomy is needed. Remove as much bone as necessary. For a standard L5–S1 discectomy, I seldom remove any bone. At L3–L4, a centimeter of cephalad lamina is often removed. Evaluate the CT scan for cephalad migration of a disc fragment that would require the removal of more lamina. To allow a more lateral approach to a larger extruded disc fragment, remove a small portion of the medial facet. More extensive exposure may be required depending on the pathology.

- For a discectomy, make an incision with a #15 blade into the deep portion of the ligamentum flavum, approximately 50% of the width of the interlaminar area. Incise the ligamentum flavum by feathering the knife blade, allowing one to see the edge of the knife cutting into the ligamentum flavum. Make the incision by long cuts into the ligamentum flavum reaching from lamina to lamina with careful observation for any sign of the white undersurface of the ligamentum flavum, followed by the bluish hue of the dura. Once the undersurface is reached, use the handle of the knife or a Penfield 4 elevator to open the last few underlayers of the ligamentum flavum. Use the Penfield 4 elevator to separate the entire length of the ligamentum flavum. Under the ligamentum flavum is usually a layer of epidural fat over the dura, but with a large space-occupying lesion in the canal, the dura may be immediately adjacent to the undersurface of the ligamentum flavum. Pass the Penfield 4 elevator under the lateral leaf of the ligamentum flavum, and retract the dura medially away from the lateral leaf of the ligamentum flavum. A cottonoid can be placed under the lateral leaf of the ligamentum flavum. With a Kerrison rongeur angled 40° in the dominant hand and the Penfield 4 elevator in the other hand, pass the Kerrison rongeur under the lateral ligamentum flavum and remove the lateral ligamentum flavum.

- The epidural fat, the dura, the nerve root, and the longitudinal blood vessels in the lateral recess can usually be identified after the lateral half of the ligamentum flavum is removed. The deep portion of the ligamentum flavum runs vertically in the lateral recess and attaches to the facet joint capsule. Position the cottonoid or Penfield 4 elevator between this portion of the ligament and the underlying nerve root. This stage of entering the canal is often an anxious one because of fear of bleeding and damaging the nerve root. The more delicate the approach, the less bone that is cut, and the less vigorous the removal of the lateral ligamentum flavum, the less bleeding there will be. Magnification is of tremendous value in identifying vessels and allowing safe, accurate retraction and bipolar coagulation, if needed. Removal of fat causes bleeding and later scarring. Bleeding often starts when exposing the disc or nerve root. When lateral exposure is obtained out to the pedicle, the longitudinal vessels lateral to the root can be identified and cauterized with the bipolar cautery. Cottonoids placed laterally at the cephalad and caudad extremes of the exposure can collapse the vessels and allow work in the area between the cottonoids.

- A transverse or horizontal vascular supply exits each intervertebral foramen. The most consistent vascular leash is found just caudad to the nerve root exiting in the caudal portion of the intervertebral foramen at the cephalad portion of the disc. For large exposures, when the dural sac needs to be retracted to the midline, identify and coagulate the vascular leash with a bipolar cautery. Minimize the use of electrocautery because the more that is used, the more scarring there will be. The use of cottonoids, Surgicel, and thrombin-soaked Gelfoam retards bleeding. I prefer not to leave Gelfoam and Surgicel packing in the spinal canal. Cottonoids remove epidural fat and should be used judiciously.

- The surgeon needs to know where the disc and root are without undue exploration. The key to intracanal anatomy is the pedicle (Fig. 138.28). The pedicle is deep to the caudad third of the inferior facet. After the ligamentum flavum is removed, palpate into the canal with a nerve hook or dental tool. Often, the pedicle is lateral

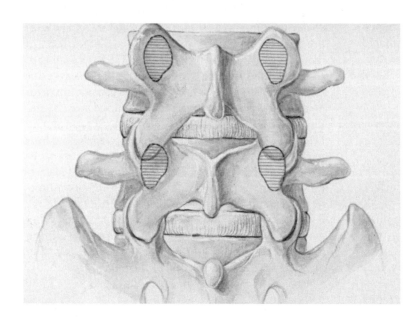

Figure 138.28. The pedicle is the key to the intracanal anatomy. Identification of the pedicle will lead to the location of the disc and nerve root.

under an overhanging roof of superior facet. In fact, the superior facet may be mistaken for the pedicle. To remove the roof of the lateral recess and to relieve lateral recess stenosis, remove the facet joint with the Kerrison rongeur medially to the parasagittal plane of the medial border of the pedicle.

- Knowing the location of the pedicle tells you the following:
  - The disc space is less than 1 cm cephalad to the pedicle. It often appears to be immediately cephalad adjacent to the pedicle.
  - The intervertebral foramen above the pedicle is for the exiting nerve root and the intervertebral foramen below the pedicle is the foramen for the transversing nerve root.
  - Dorsal and immediately cephalad to the pedicle is the superior facet. The superior facet is the roof of the intervertebral foramen for the exiting nerve root.
  - Just medial to the pedicle is the traversing nerve root.
- Extensive probing should not be done in the medial pedicular area because the pedicular plexus will bleed. Remember, at higher lumbar levels, the disc is farther cephalad relative to the interlaminar space. Therefore, the L5–S1 disc is approximately at the level of the interlaminar space between L-5 and S-1. The L2–L3 disc space is well cephalad under the lamina of L-2 rather than at the level of the interlaminar space between L-2 and L-3. The ligamentum flavum covers the interlaminar area.
- Often, it is imperative to expose the disc space. The disc is a raised, white, soft structure that may be covered by epidural fat, veins, and the nerve root. Feel for the disc using the Penfield 4 elevator. It causes little bleeding and allows for palpation of the disc with the tip of the instrument. Reach out laterally and feel for the floor of the canal. Gently retract medially with the Penfield 4 elevator. Feel for obstruction to this medial retraction. Do not retract against a major obstruction. Retract gently, and insert the microsucker retractor. Lift the root up and medial with the nondominant hand; expose the disc with the Penfield 4 elevator in the dominant hand.
- When there is difficulty in finding the disc or retracting the nerve root, several methods have been used to prevent damage to the nerve root. Knowing the location of the pedicle in the canal is probably the most significant way to avoid major damage to the nerve root. Find the pedicle. The transversing nerve root is adjacent medially to the pedicle. Identify the nerve root medial to the pedicle. If the root cannot be retracted because it is tightly against the medial wall of the pedicle, proceed cephalad to a point slightly lateral to the medial wall of the pedicle. The transversing nerve root should not be lateral to the medial wall of the pedicle. Exposing the disc cephalad to the pedicle and lateral to the medial

wall of the pedicle can avoid nerve damage. The nerve root exiting in this intervertebral foramen cephalad to the pedicle will usually be further cephalad, just under the pedicle above. The exiting nerve root runs obliquely across the intervertebral disc laterally in or lateral to the intervertebral foremen. The farther lateral on the intervertebral disc, the more likely the cephalad exiting nerve root is reached. A lateral disc herniation may trap the exiting nerve root in the intervertebral foramen. A conjoined root may totally fill the entire foramen from pedicle to pedicle. An exiting conjoined nerve root limits exposure of the disc. It can usually be identified preoperatively on the myelogram and contrast CT scan. The key to avoiding damage to a conjoined nerve root is recognition. This is facilitated by lateral exposure of the traversing root shoulder.

- For further exposure of the disc, determine the amount of tension in the nerve root. Do not retract the root against a solid obstruction. If it can be retracted easily, retract it medially with the nerve root retractor. If it is tight, it will feel like you are retracting against a solid wall.

There are five common methods of dealing with a tight nerve root:

1. Explore the axilla of the transversing root with the Penfield 4 elevator. The axilla is in the caudal part of the exposure between the root and the dural sac. If a fragment is found, remove it with the nerve hook. Bleeding may be encountered.
2. Obtain more lateral exposure. Be sure you have identified the pedicle and have exposure lateral to the medial wall of the pedicle. The traversing nerve root should not be lateral to the medial wall of the pedicle.
3. Enter the disc space lateral to the root, and try to decompress the disc and pull disc material from under the root through the disc space.
4. Be sure that the root is free cephalad to the disc and that the ligamentum flavum or undersurface of the cephalad lamina is not a factor. Remove enough lamina and ligament cephalad to expose the shoulder of the nerve root.
5. The nerve root may be tethered caudally in the foramen below the pedicle. Remove the roof (the junction of the caudad lamina and the superior facet) over the transversing root as it exits around the pedicle. A foraminotomy of the foramen below may allow better retraction of the root.

- Gently lift and retract the nerve root with a sucker retractor in the nondominant hand and explore the disc area with a nerve hook in the dominant hand. Take great care not to stretch the nerve root. Exploration underneath the dural sac may reveal a large fragment of herniated disc that can be pulled out from under the nerve root with the nerve hook. The lateral exposure allows this fragment of disc to be pulled laterally rather than vertically. Removing the fragment laterally from under the nerve root will decrease the nerve root tension and allow better visibility and protection for the nerve root. Large dilated vessels often decrease in size and not bleed when the fragment is removed, relieving vascular distention.

▪ Expose the annulus with the Penfield 4 elevator. Determine the texture of the annulus, amount of bulge, presence of herniation, or presence of a hole in the annulus, and perform a discectomy.

▪ More exposure is needed for significant spinal stenosis or central, lateral recess or foraminal stenosis.

LAMINECTOMY

▪ When a total laminectomy is needed to expose the dura and nerve roots, remove the fascia entirely from the tip of the spinous process bilaterally. Extend the exposure laterally from the spinous process to the lamina with the Cobb elevators. Carefully protect the facet joint capsule. The exposure may be to the tips of the transverse processes if a fusion is to be done.

▪ *Note:* The most important structure that must be exposed and clearly seen is the pars interarticularis. Identification of the pars is imperative to prevent its transection with subsequent spinal instability. By continually visualizing the pars, removal of the lamina can be done quickly and safely. The bone cutters remove the spinous process. I prefer to use the Midas Rex AM1 (Medix Rex Pneumatic Tools, Inc., Fort Worth, TX) to remove all of the lamina over the ligamentum flavum and down to a 1 mm thin shell over the dura. Alternatively, I use the Luxel rongeur by inserting it under the caudad edge of the cephalad lamina and rotate the instrument cephalad, rolling a bite of lamina off. This allows visualization under the instrument to see a possible inadvertent dura pinch early. Before using the Midas Rex tool, I expose the pars by curetting the caudal tip of the inferior facet. Seeing the articular surface of the superior facet and the pars at each level allows full removal of lamina and medial portion of the facet without danger of cutting the pars. Identify the pedicle as soon as possible to avoid removing too much facet.

▪ To expose the lateral portion of the spinal canal, remember that the lateral wall may protrude significantly into the spinal canal. If the partial medial facetectomy is to be done, use the Midas Rex AM1 or AM3, the Kerrison rongeur, the Cloward chisel, or the Pheasant discotome. Starting medially on the lamina, cut the caudal portion of the lamina and continue laterally onto the inferior facet. The amount of inferior facet removed

varies according to the pathology. If the chisel is used, insert it to remove the appropriate amount of the medial portion of the inferior facet and twist the chisel, removing the bone medially. This allows visualization of the facet join space and the superior facet. The shiny cartilaginous floor is the superior facet. The ligamentum flavum inserts on the superior facet. The nerve root may be under this superior facet.

▪ The ligamentum should be opened at this point by one of numerous methods. Use the curet to detach the lateral ligamentum flavum from the edge of the superior facet. Position the Penfield 4 elevator, Penfield 3 elevator, or the cottonoid under the superior facet to protect the nerve. Use the Kerrison rongeur to remove the medial portion of the superior facet and the most lateral ligamentum flavum. The chisel is quite safe on the inferior facet because the superior facet provides a guard from possibly injuring the nerve root. With skill and experience, the superior facet likewise can be removed with a chisel by cutting over the pedicle with the Penfield elevator, protecting the nerve. With lateral recess stenosis, remove the medial facet to the parasagittal level of the medial wall of the pedicle.

▪ I prefer to use the Midas Rex bone cutter because it causes less splintering. Cut the lamina down centrally with the AM1. With the AM3, extend the bone removal laterally over the ligamentum flavum and foramen.

▪ After the lamina is burred down to a thin layer over the dura and totally off the ligamentum flavum, open the ligament with a Penfield 3 elevator and clasp it with a ligamentum flavum clamp. Pass a cottonoid between the ligament and the dura. Remove the major portion of the ligament with a large, straight curet from the opposite side of the table. The most lateral ligament is removed by undercutting with the angled kerrison chisel from across the table. Position the cottonoid and have the assistant remove the ligamentum flavum with a 45° Kerrison rongeur from the other side of the table. Remove the medial edge of the superior facet with the lateral-most ligamentum flavum. The assistant on the opposite side of the table also can position this cottonoid very effectively using the sucker and the bayonet. Use the 90° Kerrison rongeur to remove this lateral portion of the ligamentum flavum.

▪ The ligamentum flavum can be detached with a curet from its caudad and lateral attachments, and a curved osteotome can be used to free the cephalad attachment of the ligamentum flavum from the undersurface of the cephalad lamina. Use a nerve hook to pull the detached cephalad edge of the ligamentum flavum into the intralaminar area. Use a straight curet to detach the caudad edge of the ligamentum flavum from the edge of the caudad lamina and an angled curet to detach the lateral ligamentum flavum. With this detaching method, the ligamentum flavum can be retracted intact with a medial attachment to the ligamentum flavum from the opposite side, allowing access to the spinal canal without excision of the ligamentum flavum. Although the ligamentum flavum, being elastic, will shrink from its original attachment, it will still provide an excellent dural covering when reapproximated on closing. There is some danger in detaching this ligamentum flavum in the lateral recess because of the nerve root. Be careful over the "critical angle," which is the junction of the base of the superior facet and the caudad lamina, because the nerve root exits under this angle.

FORAMINOTOMY

- The key to a safe, effective foraminotomy is to expand the intervertebral foramen without damaging the pars interarticularis or the facet joint. A foraminotomy begins after removal of the lateral recess, identification of the pedicle, and identification of the pars interarticularis. The medial caudal aspect of the pedicle is the beginning of the intervertebral foramen. The pars forms part of the bony roof of the intervertebral foramen. The root exits around the pedicle, and it is the roof over that root as it exits that must be expanded first. I use the Midas Rex AM3 or M8 to an arc over the root, leaving a thin shell of bone over the root and plenty of the facet undersurface. Then insert the Kerrison rongeur on the root and remove the bone touching the nerve and any ligamentum flavum attached to it. Probe the foramen until it is clear. I use gallbladder probes up to 5 mm in diameter or a Woodson probe. Often, the tip of the superior facet compresses the nerve root from below. I routinely remove the cephalad tip of the superior facet with the Cloward chisel. The curved Kerrison rongeur removes more of the roof of the foramen laterally. Protect the pars. A portion of its undersurface can be carefully expanded to open the intervertebral foramen.

- Uncinate ventral spurs may arise from the caudal vertebral body, caudal to the pedicle, at the edge of the disc space below; they are seen on CT foraminal reconstructions. The root can be tented over the spur and tethered laterally by foraminal ligaments. Removing the roof is not enough to relieve this nerve root tension. The spur under the root should be removed. Although these spurs can be removed from cephalad to caudad by putting a chisel under the root, they are more easily approached from the level below. Remember, these spurs are under the annulus of the disc below and covered with soft tissue, making removal with a chisel more difficult. Putting a knife under the nerve root is dangerous.

- Expose the disc below. Working from caudad to cephalad, identify the exiting root. Open the disc with a knife laterally. Use the chisel and curet to burrow under the spur and then the endplate of the vertebra. Hollow out a space. Insert an angled curet between the root and the annulus-covered spur, and knock the spur into the hole. Leave it in the hole or remove it. It is safer to remove it after the root tension is relieved.

- The foraminotomy can be performed from the "outside in." Move to a paraspinous position through the same incision. Identify the superior facet and transverse processes above and below the pars. Several tacks can be taken from this point. One is to remove the intertransverse ligament, identify the nerve, and follow it back into the canal, removing any obstructions for a foraminotomy. I prefer to expose the caudal surface of the pedicle above, using the pars and transverse process as guides. Identify the nerve there and expand the intervertebral foramen. If there is a foraminal herniated nucleus pulposus, expose the cephalad surface of the pedicle below, and work cephalad to identify the disc, the nerve, and the herniation.

- After the discectomy, the delicacy of the approach will determine how much fat is left covering the nerve root. Supplement this procedure with a free fat graft taken from the layer above the fascia in the caudal portion of the wound. When fat is not available, I use Depo-Medrol–soaked Gelfoam.

- After closing any dead space left by the fat graft, close the fascia with interrupted 0 Vicryl. When midline fascial structures have been removed from the spinous process, reattach them. The layers above the fascia are closed with multiple layers of interrupted 2-0 Vicryl. Close the subcutaneous fat in at least two layers, tacking each layer to the lower layer. I usually drain both the subfascial and suprafascial layers. Close the subcutaneous layer immediately adjacent to the subcuticular layer. Close the skin with subcuticular sutures, benzoin, and Steristrips. Retract and cut off the sutures after the Steristrips are applied.

LATERAL APPROACH TO THE DISC

- Position the patient on a standard operating frame.
- Use skin-marking needles to identify the pedicles of the involved segment with a lateral radiograph. For L4–L5, align the needle markers over the pedicle at L-4 and the pedicle at L-5. Make the incision one fingerbreadth lateral to the spinous process, spanning between the pedicles of the involved segment (Fig. 138.29).
- Carry the incision through the skin and subcutaneous tissue. Open the fascia enough to admit an index finger that dissects down in a muscle-splitting dissection to the cephalad transverse processes. Use a Penfield 1 instrument or a small Cobb elevator to identify the transverse processes, but do not carry out vigorous muscle dissection at this point. Use your finger to palpate medi-

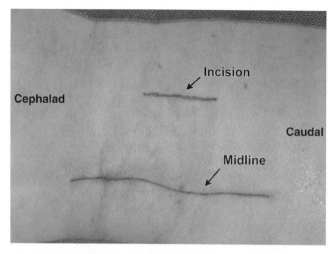

Figure 138.29. Make the incision one fingerbreadth lateral to the spinous process, spanning between the pedicles of the involved segment.

ally on the cephalad-transverse process to the area of the pars interarticularis, just cephalad to the facet joint. Rest the Penfield 1 on the more cephalad transverse process and position the McCulloch blade-spike retractor by placing the blade laterally against the soft tissue, then placing the spike medially just dorsal to the pars interarticularis. Do not hook it under the pars interarticularis.

■ By opening the retractor, visualize the transverse process. Obtain a lateral radiograph with a needle on the transverse process to confirm levels.
■ Use the Bovie and curet to dissect the soft tissue off

the pars interarticularis and the base of the transverse process.

■ It is important to see the bone of the pars interarticularis. Too often, the dissection is carried out too far laterally. The transverse process is cleared off, but the actual location of the pedicle is more medial, and too much time is wasted in a more lateral position. Identify the pars and follow the bone of the transverse process back to the dorsal surface of the pedicle. At this point, there are times when a portion of the cephalad facet joint, or cephalad lateral portion of the inferior facet, has to be removed with Kerrison rongeur to provide proper exposure of the intertransverse area. For better exposure, laterally retract the muscle off the intertransverse ligament and hold it with the lateral blade retractor (Fig. 138.30).

■ Using a straight and an angled curet, detach the intertransverse ligament from the cephalad-transverse process, the dorsal surface of the pedicle, and the lateral surface of the pars interarticularis. Identify this ligament, hook it with a blunt nerve hook, pull it laterally, and free it up with the small Kerrison rongeur under direct visualization.

■ *Caution: Sometimes, distinguishing the ligament from the nerve is not easy. Proceed carefully.*

■ Identify the nerve as it exits around and just caudal to the cephalad pedicle (Fig. 138.31).

■ Use the Penfield 4 elevator to palpate gently cephalad to the nerve, starting at the medial wall of the pedicle and progressing laterally. Beware of bleeding in this area.

■ Identify the caudal aspect of the nerve and use the microsucker retractor to retract the nerve cephalad. Using

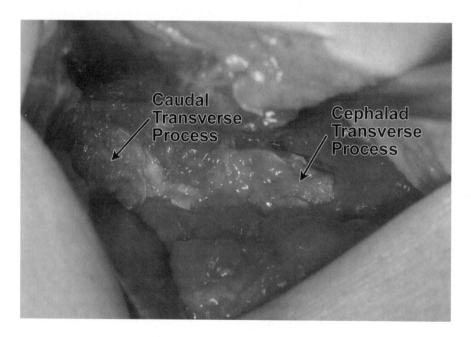

Figure 138.30. For better exposure of the intertransverse area, laterally retract the muscle of the intertransverse ligament. (Note: The illustration depicts a larger field of visualization than actually performed.) After opening the fascia, use finger dissection to clear the transverse process. Insert the retractor.

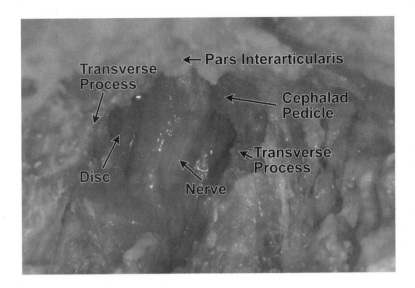

Figure 138.31. Identify the cephalad transverse process, then expose the part interarticularis medially. Detach the intertransverse ligament. Identify the pedicle, then the nerve exiting just caudal to the pedicle. The disc is caudal to the nerve.

the Penfield 4 elevator, identify the disc caudal to the nerve. Be aware that the dorsal ganglion of the nerve may feel like a disc fragment under the nerve. Carefully identify the nerve and the disc (Fig. 138.31). Follow the nerve laterally to insure removal of any lateral disc fragments.

▪ Remember:
  ▪ Identify the cephalad transverse process.
  ▪ Identify the pars interarticularis to stay medially.
  ▪ The pedicle is the key landmark.
  ▪ Laterally retract the intertransverse ligament.

REFERENCES

Each reference is categorized according to the following scheme: *, classic article; #, review article; !, basic research article; and +, clinical results/outcome study.

+ 1. Apuzzo MJ, Weiss MH, Hyden JS. Transoral Exposure of the Atlanto-Axial Joint. *J Neurosurg* 1978;3:201.

+ 2. Bailey RW, Bagley CD. Stabilization of the Cervical Spine by Anterior Fusion. *J Bone Joint Surg Am* 1960; 42:565.

+ 3. Cloward R. *Ruptured Cervical Intervertebral Discs. Codman Signature Series 4.* Codman and Shurtleff, 1974.

+ 4. Duncan HMM, Jonck LM. The Presacral Plexus in Anterior Lumbar Fusion of the Lumbar Spine. *S Afr J Surg* 1965;3:93.

+ 5. Dwyer AF. Experience of Anterior Correction of Scoliosis. *Clin Orthop* 1973;93:192.

+ 6. Dwyer AF, Newton NC, Sherwood AA. An Anterior Approach to Scoliosis. *Clin Orthop* 1969;62:192.

+ 7. Fang HSY, Ong BG. Direct Anterior Approach to the Upper Cervical Spine. *J Bone Joint Surg* 1962;44-A: 1588.

+ 8. Flynn JC, Hoque A. Anterior Fusion of the Lumbar Spine. *J Bone Joint Surg* 1979;61-A:1143.

+ 9. Freebody D, Bedall R, Taylor RD. Anterior Transperitoneal Lumbar Fusion. *J Bone Joint Surg* 1971;53-B:617.

10. Goss CM, ed. *Gray's Anatomy of the Human Body*, 29th ed. Philadelphia: Lea & Febiger, 1973.

+ 11. Harmon PH. Anterior Extraperitoneal Lumbar Disc Excision and Vertebral Bone Fusion. *Clin Orthop* 1963; 16:169.

12. Henry AK. *Extensive Exposure.* Baltimore, Williams & Wilkins, 1959.

13. Hodgson AR, Rau ACM. Anterior Surgical Approaches to the Spinal Column. In: Apley AG, ed. *Recent Advances in Orthopedics.* Baltimore, Williams & Wilkins, 1964:326.

+ 14. Hodgson AR, Rau ACM. Anterior Approach to the Spinal Column. *Recent Advances in Orthopaedics IX* 1969;9:289.

+ 15. Johnson RM, McGuire EJ. Urogenital Complications of Anterior Approaches to the Lumbar Spine. *Clin Orthop* 1981;154:114.

+ 16. LaBate JS. The Surgical Anatomy of the Superior Hypogastric Plexus-Presacral Nerve. *Surg Gynecol Obstet* 1938;67:199.

17. Logue V. Compressive Lesions at the Foramen Magnum. In: Ruge D, Wiltse L, eds. *Spinal Disorders: Diagnosis and Treatment.* Philadelphia, Lea & Febiger, 1977:249.

+ 18. Nanson EM. The Anterior Approach to Upper Dorsal Sympathectomy. *Surg Gynecol Obstet* 1957;104:118.

19. Perry J. Surgical Approaches to the Spine. In: Pierce D, Nichols V, eds. *The Total Care of Spinal Cord Injuries.* Boston: Little, Brown & Co., 1977:53.

+ 20. Riceborough EJ. The Anterior Approach to the Spine for Correction of the Axial Skeleton. *Clin Orthop* 1973;93: 207.

+ 21. Riley L. Surgical Approaches to the Cervical Spine. *Clin Orthop* 1973;91:16.

+ 22. Riley L. Surgical Approaches to the Anterior Structures of the Cervical Spine. *Clin Orthop* 1973;91:10.

\# 23. Robinson RA. *The Craft of Surgery,* 2nd ed. Boston: Little, Brown & Co., 1971.

\# 24. Robinson RA. Approaches to the Cervical Spine C1-T1. In: Schmidek HH, Sweet WH, eds. *Current Techniques in Operative Neurosurgery.* New York: Grune & Stratton, 1978.

\# 25. Robinson RA, Southwick WO. Surgical Approaches to the Cervical Spine. *Instr Course Lect* 1960;17:299.

\# 26. Rothman R. *The Spine,* Vol I. Philadelphia: W.B. Saunders, 1975.

+ 27. Royal ND. A New Operative Procedure in the Treatment of Spastic Paralysis and Its Experimental Basis. *Med J Anat* 1924;77:30.

+ 28. Scott R. Innervation of the Diaphragm and Its Practical Aspects in Surgery. *Thorax* 1965;20:357.

\# 29. Watkins RG, O'Brien JP. *Anatomy of the Cervical Spine (Sound/Slide Program).* Atlanta, American Academy of Orthopaedic Surgeons, 1980.

## CHAPTER 139

UPPER CERVICAL SPINE FRACTURES AND INSTABILITY

Claude Gelinas and Alan M. Levine

INTRODUCTION

Upper cervical spine fractures include a wide spectrum of injuries whose patterns differ from those of injuries in the lower cervical, thoracic, and lumbar spine because of the unique anatomic configuration of the vertebral elements of the craniocervicum (45,57). The craniocervicum includes the base of the skull, the atlas, and axis, and is unique both in its bony as well as ligamentous structure. A variety of conditions can lead to upper cervical spine instability (infections, tumors, spondylosis, and congenital abnormalities), but the most common cause is direct trauma. Although upper cervical fractures occur as a result of mechanisms of injury that are similar to those causing other spine fractures (i.e., motor vehicle accidents, falls, diving, or direct trauma), they are nevertheless unique for

several reasons. First, in autopsy series (2,13,17), many injuries to the upper cervical spine resulted in trauma to the brain stem and thus immediate death. In addition, in those patients surviving their initial trauma, the incidence of neurologic injury as a direct result of fractures and dislocations in the craniocervicum is proportionately less than the incidence in other areas of the cervical spine because of the relatively large area available for the spinal cord within the spinal canal. Again, because of the unique relationship of this spinal region to the skull, most fractures in the upper cervical spine result from a force applied through the skull, with resultant excessive motion of the head and upper cervical spine, creating the injury pattern. Although the fractures in the upper cervical spine may be survivable, some of these patients succumb as a result of associated severe head injury. In fact, many of the neurologic deficit patterns are a result not of the injuries to the spine but of direct head injuries. To understand the nature of these injuries and to be able to apply the most appropriate treatment methodologies, the physician must first thoroughly appreciate the anatomic considerations of the

C. Gelinas: Southwest Spine Center, Albuquerque, NM.
A. M. Levine: Director, Alvin and Lois Lapidus Cancer Institute, Professor of Orthopaedic Surgery and Oncology, Sinai Hospital of Baltimore, Baltimore, Maryland, 21215.

craniocervicum and then fully understand the mechanism associated with each injury pattern. Appreciation of the significance of the injury in relation to the immediate and subsequent potential instability is important in preventing both undertreatment and overtreatment of injuries in this location. It also may alert the physician to potential pitfalls in treatment modalities that may apply to the various injury types.

REGIONAL ANATOMY

The term "craniocervicum" is generally applied to the area at the base of the skull, the atlas, and the axis. The area is unique because it is the junction between the skull and the cervical spine, and is characterized by extreme mobility (37). It is unique also because of the size, shape, and location of the joints that allow motion between the occiput and the atlas or the atlas and the axis. At the lower end of the craniocervicum (C2–C3), there is a transition in the size, shape, and location of the joints, transitioning to the more usual pattern seen in the lower cervical spine. Forces applied to the craniocervicum may result in injuries having far different patterns and resultant instabilities than those seen in the lower cervical spine.

The occipitocervical articulations lie anterolaterally with reference to the spinal canal in that area. Those joints are made up of convex-shaped lateral masses adjacent to the foramen magnum that articulate with the concave lateral masses of the atlas. The joints are trapezoidally shaped and are somewhat wider medially than laterally. In children, these joints are less concave and flatter, and therefore, they restrict motion to a less significant degree than they do in adults. Therefore, children have more mobility and are more predisposed to injury at this level (5). The normal range of motion at the occipitocervical junction is 21° of extension (which is in part limited by the occiput abutting on the posterior arc of the atlas) (89), 3° of flexion, 7° of rotation, and 5° of lateral bending (64).

The atlas is unique in that it has no distinct body, an element present in the remainder of the vertebrae of the cervical spine. Embryologically, the vertebral body of C-1 is absorbed into the formation of the dens process of C-2; therefore, the atlas has two lateral masses connected by an anterior and a posterior arch. The anterior arch is thicker and shorter than the posterior arch. The posterior arch has a tubercle in its posterior midportion and two relatively flatter areas just posterior to the lateral masses, over which the vertebral artery runs after it exits from the foramen in C-2. The shape of the lateral masses is important because it helps one understand how injuries to C-1 occur. The articular surfaces for C1–C2 and also occiput–C1 are concave, with that of the atlantoaxial joint being somewhat flatter than that of the occipitocervical joint. The resultant shape of the C-1 lateral mass is

that it is thinner medially than laterally; thus, when axial loading forces are applied across the craniocervicum, there is a resultant force that serves to displace the lateral masses of C-1 in a lateral direction.

The axis is also unique in its relationship to the atlas because the atlantoaxial joint has two different sets of articulations. The first is the articulation of the slightly convex inferior articular process of the atlas with a slightly convex superior articular process of the atlas. Both joints are oriented in the horizontal plane with a medial inclination of approximately 35°. These joints permit rotation, accounting for nearly 50% of the rotation in the cervical spine (69). The odontoid process projects up inside the ring of the axis, forming a second joint with the anterior arch of the atlas. The dens generally is between 14 and 15 mm in height and thus is approximately 40% of the overall height of the axis (74). The overall diameter of the atlas is quite large in relation to the space necessary for the spinal cord (82). Generally, the midsagittal diameter of the cord is one third of the midsagittal diameter of the inner surface of the axis. Actual rotation between the occiput and C-1 is generally approximately 5° to 7°, with more than 8° being pathologic, and at the atlantoaxial joint, the amount of normal rotation is approximately 43°, with more than 50° representing hypermobility and approximately 65° of rotation required for atlantoaxial dislocation (20,38). At C-2, the isolation of the pedicles of the axis between the atlantoaxial joint anterior to them and the C2–C3 joint posterior to them contributes to the occurrence of fractures at the base of the pedicles. The relative stability of the craniocervicum as a unit isolates the pedicles of C-2, predisposing them to fractures. Finally, the large bifid process of C-2 is an anatomic landmark for physical examination as well as for anatomic dissection.

An understanding of the embryologic and postnatal development of the upper cervical spine is also helpful in further understanding injuries to this area. Although all other cervical vertebrae develop from at least three ossific nuclei, the atlas develops from only two centers of ossification, which usually fuse together between 3 and 5 years of age. Because there is an ossific center in each lateral mass, defects in both the anterior arch and posterior arch can occur. The axis has four centers of ossification, which also tend to fuse together between 3 and 6 years of age, with the exception of the junction between the odontoid process and the body, which may persist up to 11 years of age. The presence of persistent congenital defects in the ring of C-1 or C-2 in the adult and delayed fusion of ossific nuclei in children should not be confused with acute fractures.

The arterial supply to the dens initially comes from both the anterior and posterior ascending arteries from the vertebral arteries that anastomose to create a rich vascular network. The cartilage plate that separates the odontoid from the body of C-2, as previously mentioned, tends to ossify around 7 years of age, preventing direct vascularization from the rich plexus in the vascular body. There is also a zone of ossification at the tip of the dens, which appears between 3 and 6 years of age and can remain open until 12 years of age. Both of these delayed closures can be mistaken as fractures.

The relationship between the bony elements at each level of the craniocervicum is far different from that between the bony components of the lower cervical spine. The major difference is that there is no disc between occiput and C-1 or between C-1 and C-2 because there is no vertebral body at C-1. Therefore, without the stability provided by the intervertebral discs, the ligamentous integrity of the craniocervicum is provided by a structure quite different from that in the lower cervical spine. The central point of ligamentous stability in the upper cervical spine is the odontoid process. Affixed to it are several ligaments, which provide resistance to translation, flexion, extension, and rotation. The *transverse ligament* is fixed at the tubercle on the lateral mass at one side of the atlas and traverses just posterior to the odontoid process to attach to the tubercle of the contralateral lateral mass. It secures the anterior surface of the dens in close proximity to the posterior facet of the anterior arch of the atlas. The transverse ligament provides stability in flexion between the atlas and the axis, and also prevents anterior translation of the atlas on the axis (29). The *alar ligaments* attach to the tip of the dens (Fig. 139.1). They actually arise from the medial aspect of the occipital condyles and insert along the tip of the odontoid. They function to prevent anterior translation at C1–C2 as well as to restrict rotation and lateral bending at that level (22,23). The *apical ligament* arises from the rim of the foramen magnum and inserts more centrally than the alar ligaments into the tip of the dens. Finally, the *accessory ligaments* arise from the lateral masses of C-2 and insert into the base of the dens. These three types of ligaments—the alar, apical, and accessory ligaments—act as important secondary restraints to C1–C2 translation, especially in the event of failure of the transverse ligament (29).

The transverse ligament may become incompetent through two different mechanisms of injury. First, a severe flexion force between C-1 and C-2 may result in failure of the transverse ligament by impingement on the dens process, and this may also result in failure of the alar, apical, and accessory ligaments. In contrast, the transverse ligament can fail in tension with axial loading applied across C1–C2, resulting in failure of the accessory ligaments and transverse ligaments, but because of the direction of attachment, the alar and apical ligaments remain intact. Additional stability to this complex is imparted by the joint capsules, especially the C1–C2 capsules (16). These capsules function to limit rotation and, to a lesser degree, translation at the C1–C2 level. Posterior to the

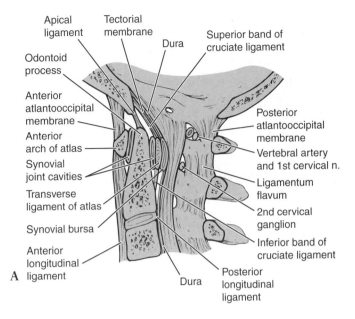

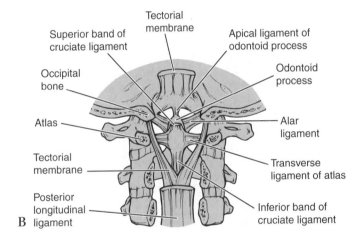

Figure 139.1. **A:** A midsagittal section through the craniocervical junction. This figure shows the appropriate relationship of the basion or anterior aspect of the foramen magnum to the ring of C-1 and the odontoid process, and nicely illustrates the ligaments at the occipitocervical junction. **B:** A coronal section demonstrating the ligaments at the craniocervical junction. Note especially the alar ligaments and the tectorial membrane. (Redrawn from Martel W. The Occipito-atlantoaxial Joints in Rheumatoid Arthritis and Ankylosing Spondylitis. *AJR* 1961; 86:223, with permission.)

central ligamentous complex is the pectoral ligament. This is an attenuation of the interspinous ligament, which is a direct restraint to flexion. The final ligamentous component in the upper cervical spine is the continuation of the anterior longitudinal ligament. This, again, is somewhat attenuated, although it provides restraint to extension in the upper cervical spine.

The final anatomic element with a critical role in treating injuries of the craniocervicum is the vascular anatomy (66). There are three elements in the vascular anatomy of concern: the position and course of the vertebral arteries; the plexus of thin-walled vessels lying just posterior to the facet capsule at C1–C2; and the vascular supply surrounding the dens process. The vertebral arteries course upward through the foramen in C-2, then loop over the posterior arch of the atlas approximately 1.5 to 2 cm lateral to the tubercle of the posterior arch. The vertebral artery is vulnerable to injury during surgery in two separate areas. Dissection of the ring of C-1 more than 2 cm lateral from the midline may expose the vertebral artery to trauma. Also, the insertion of atlantoaxial screws exposes the vertebral artery to injury by direct trauma from a drill bit as it traverses the C-2 body. Because the location of the vertebral artery within C-2 varies, determine its position radiographically before screw fixation (65). It is, however, also important to know that because the vertebral arteries are paired structures (with one usually larger and, therefore, dominant over the other in terms of blood supply), injury to a single vertebral artery rarely results in significant neurologic deficit. In addition, as shown by Rauschning, there is a plexus of thin-walled vessels lying superficial to the facet capsule of C1–C2 with exposure of the C1–C2 articulation from a posterior direction. Sharp dissection through the soft tissue superficial to these vessels may result in profuse bleeding; there is less probability of injuring this vascular network by blunt dissection of the soft tissues caudal to rostral along the pedicle of C-2. Although the bleeding may be bothersome during the course of surgery, the consequences of disruption of the venous plexus is not significant.

Although it was originally thought that avascularity was the sole reason for the high rate of nonunion of the dens, it has since been found that in fact there is a significant endosteal and ligamentous blood supply (Fig. 139.2). The combination of the carotid arteries and vertebral arteries supply sufficient blood vessels to the dens process. Even the internal carotid supplies vessels to the dens through arteries that anastomose in a vascular arcade, and the dens may even have a direct blood supply through an ascending pharyngeal artery.

EVALUATION AND MANAGEMENT OF PATIENTS WITH INJURIES TO THE CRANIOCERVICUM

Although it is vital that any patient with potential trauma to the cervical spine be first assessed for adequacy of airway, breathing, and circulation according to the American Trauma Life Support (ATLS) protocols, it is even more vital in patients with injuries to the upper cervical spine. Especially with injuries caused by distraction at the level of occiput–C1 or C1–C2, brain stem contusion is possible, resulting in cessation of spontaneous respiration. Emergent maintenance of airway and respiration may be the key to patient survival. Treat any patient with a head injury who is comatose or obtunded as if an injury is present until it is clearly ruled out. As with other spinal injuries, immobilize the entire spine on a backboard with a rigid collar. The physical examination of patients with upper cervical spine injuries begins with an evaluation of the skull for evidence of head trauma, including scalp or facial lacerations. Localizing signs, such as tenderness and especially the location of trauma to the skull, is helpful in

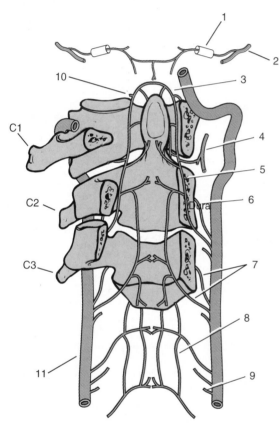

Figure 139.2. The arterial supply to the upper cervical vertebrae and the odontoid process. 1, Hypoglossal canal containing the meningeal artery. 2, Occipital artery. 3, Apical arcade of the odontoid process. 4, Ascending pharyngeal artery giving a collateral branch beneath the anterior arch of the atlas. 5, Posterior ascending artery. 6, Anterior ascending artery. 7, Precentral and postcentral arteries to a typical cervical vertebral body. 8, Anterior spinal plexus. 9, Medullary branch of the vertebral artery. Radicular, prelaminar, and meningeal branches are also found at each level. 10, Collateral to the ascending pharyngeal artery passing rostral to the anterior arch of the atlas. 11, Left vertebral artery. (Redrawn from Parke WW. The Vascular Relations of the Upper Cervical Vertebrae. *Orthop Clin North Am* 1978;9:879, with permission.)

the further evaluation of the patient as well as ultimately determining the mechanism of injury. In the awake, alert patient, palpate the entire spine for areas of localized tenderness or asymmetry.

In the initial neurologic examination, test for muscle function and strength; evaluate sensation with pinprick and light-touch; check the deep tendon reflexes, cranial nerves, and rectal tone and perianal sensation. Physical findings help in ordering proper radiographic evaluation of the patient.

In upper cervical spine injuries, dense incomplete neurologic injuries are rare. The most common neurologic patterns are Brown–Séquard syndrome resulting from rotatory injuries at the occiput–C1 or C1–C2 areas, or flexion injuries with rupture of the transverse ligament. Brain stem injuries with impairment of respiration most commonly occur in occipital–cervical dissociations and often result in sudden death because of lack of respiratory effort. Radicular injuries (aside from injury to the occipital nerve, which can occur with fractures at C-1 resulting in numbness in the posterior aspect of the skull) are infrequent in the craniocervicum. Because of the large area available for the spinal cord, incomplete spinal cord injury as seen in the lower cervical spine is uncommon. Neurologic deficit in patients with this type of injury is usually either severe or trivial. Fractures in patients without a neural deficit or with trivial deficits are usually diagnosed either on routine radiographic screening (especially in the elderly where pain may not be a significant component) or by the presence of pain in the upper cervical spine. Document the complete neurologic examination on a form such as the American Spinal Injury Association (ASIA) Neurologic Assessment form.

The initial radiographic series obtained by most surgeons includes a lateral cervical spine roentgenogram and may also include an anteroposterior (AP) roentgenogram, and for the upper cervical spine, an open mouth view. Correlate the findings on the initial roentgenograms of the upper cervical spine with the initial physical examination to determine whether additional radiographic workup is necessary.

RADIOGRAPHIC EVALUATION

Radiographic evaluation of a patient suspected of having a spinal injury has two separate components. The first is to "clear" the cervical spine. The ultimate goal of this phase of evaluation is to ascertain as definitively as possible whether there is an injury in the cervical spine. The second phase is to define fully the nature of the spine injury once it has been shown to exist.

This evaluation ideally should be broken down into two separate approaches. In patients who are alert, oriented, nonintoxicated, and have no pain or neurologic symptoms, more than a single, lateral radiograph is unnec-

essary. The probability of finding significant injuries is very low in such patients. However, in patients with tenderness of the cervical spine or an altered state of consciousness, or in any polytrauma victim, perform a good quality lateral cervical spine film. An AP as well as an open mouth view may be indicated as part of the initial screening. It is clearly of no additional value to perform a five-view cervical spine radiograph (including two pillar views) unless you are trying to delineate a specific injury further. In patients with negative roentgenograms who are symptomatic and have no neurologic deficit, obtain physician-supervised flexion-extension lateral views in an awake, alert patient to rule out ligamentous instability.

There is also considerable controversy concerning what should contribute final clearance of the cervical spine in an obtunded patient. The opinions range from keeping the patient immobilized until responsive enough to undergo further radiographic evaluation to performing an magnetic resonance imaging (MRI) scan to look for ligamentous disruption. If all radiographs are negative, we prefer to keep the patient immobilized until he or she is responsive enough to cooperate with further testing.

Assess the lateral radiograph in an organized way:

- Assess overall alignment.
- Evaluate each vertebral level (base of the skull, C-1, and C-2) for orientation. If one level is true lateral and the next is oblique, a rotatory abnormality can be inferred.
- Look for translation or kyphosis on the lateral view. Assess routine parameters such as the anterior spinal line, the posterior spinal line, and the spinolaminar line for continuity.
- Identify the line forming the base of the clivus (known as Wachenheim's line) to verify the appropriate glenooccipital relationships. Draw a line along the posterior surface of the clivus and extend it inferiorly; it should intersect or lie tangentially to the posterior cortex of the odontoid.
- The distance between the tip of the clivus (basion) and the odontoid process, the basion–dental interval, should be less than 1.2 cm in adults.
- The Powers' ratio (71) is also useful in assessing possible occipital–cervical dissociation (Fig. 139.3). This is the ratio of the distance between the basion and posterior arch of C-1 to the distance between the posterior margin of the foramen magnum (opisthion) and the anterior arch of C-1. A ratio of greater than 1.0 is abnormal and further imaging with a computed tomography (CT) scan is indicated.
- The lateral roentgenogram also defines the atlanto–dens interval (ADI), which should be 3 mm or less in adults and 5 mm or less in children (32).
- Actual radiographic visualization of dens fractures may be difficult on the lateral roentgenogram. However, the angle of the dens with reference to the vertebral body

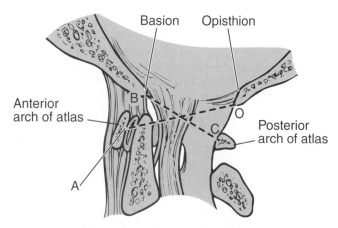

Basion   Opisthion

Anterior
arch of atlas

Posterior
arch of atlas

Figure 139.3. Powers' ratio: if BC/OA is greater than 1, then an anterior occipitoatlantal dislocation exists. Ratios less than 1 are normal except in posterior dislocations, associated fractures of the odontoid process or the ring of the atlas, and congenital anomalies of the foramen magnum. (Redrawn from Jarrett PJ, Whitesides TE Jr. Injuries of the Cervicocranium. In: Browner BD, Jupiter JB, Levine AM, et al, eds. *Skeletal Trauma: Fractures, Dislocations, Ligamentous Injuries,* Vol 1. Philadelphia: W.B. Saunders Co., 1992:668, with permission.)

of C-2 should be evaluated. Angles exceeding 20° should probably be considered abnormal or at least suggestive of a fracture and requiring additional evaluation.

- Fractures of the posterior arch of C-1 are generally visible on the lateral roentgenogram, but significant angulation of the posterior arch may be the only visible sign when the fracture line is in close proximity to the lateral mass of C-1.

Most types of traumatic spondylolisthesis in the axis can be visualized and fully defined on the plain lateral radiograph. Vertical distraction injuries at either occiput–C1 or at C1–C2 are easily visualized on the lateral roentgenogram and are most clearly defined on that study. Finally, the lateral roentgenogram can also be of some value in assessing the retropharyngeal soft-tissue shadow (68,85). The prevertebral soft tissue anterior to C-1 is clearly thicker than that more distal in the cervical spine. An increase in prevertebral soft-tissue shadow may not be present within the first hour or two of injury and is a quite unreliable sign in an uncooperative or screaming or crying patient. Soft-tissue shadows anterior to C-1 of greater than 10 mm in a cooperative patient suggest that there is some anterior column injury causing bleeding into the retropharyngeal space. This finding, in combination with a posterior arch fracture at C-1, would suggest that there is an anterior element injury as well.

The final critical element in evaluating lateral films is to look for contiguous or noncontiguous injuries in the cervical spine (55). Injuries in combination usually have

the same mechanism of injury. The initial lateral roentgenogram may reveal an associated injury in 22% to 50% of patients, depending on the pattern and severity of the upper cervical injury.

The AP view contributes relatively less to the evaluation of the upper cervical spine than it does to the evaluation of the lower cervical spine. However, the posterior elements of C-1 and C-2 can be visualized with this view. One of the more critical features is to assess the orientation of the spinous processes. Loss of alignment of the spinous processes is highly suggestive of a rotatory injury in the upper cervical spine. In addition, an angular deformity on the AP roentgenogram may also be helpful, especially in patients with torticollis, for whom the lateral may be extremely difficult to assess. The AP is also helpful for assessing concurrent injuries in the lower cervical spine.

A well-oriented open mouth view defines the occipital condyles, may show evidence of a fracture of the occipital condyles, and also gives an excellent view of the lateral masses of C-1. Spreading of the lateral masses of C-1 is indicative of a fracture of the anterior arch of C-1, as seen in Jefferson's fractures. The total displacement of the lateral masses can be evaluated (80), providing an indication of rupture of the transverse ligament. The radiographic appearance of a rotatory subluxation at C1–C2 is often defined on the open mouth radiograph with the so-called "wink" sign [overlapping of the inferior edge of the lateral mass of C-1 and the superior edge of the lateral mass of C-2, thus apparently eliminating the joint space (31)]. The odontoid–lateral mass relationship (distance from lateral mass to dens on each side), which sometimes is cited as a pathologic sign, is, in fact, asymmetric in many normal individuals and is of little significance (52,67).

The primary use of CT scans is to enhance the anatomic delineation of fractures that have already been identified. Make the slices at a 1.5 or 2 mm interval to enhance coronal and sagittal reconstructions and three-dimensional reconstructions. In fractures of the atlas, the gantry of the CT scanner must be parallel to the arch of C-1. If care is not taken with the orientation, the views will be difficult to interpret and not add much information to the plain radiographs. At C-1, the CT scan is most helpful in defining the nature of injuries involving the ring. For injuries of the transverse ligament, CT scanning is of help where the disruption of the transverse ligament is with a bony avulsion. In those dens fractures in which the fracture line is not clearly visualized on either the AP or the lateral plain radiographs, but an angular deformity of the dens is noticed, a CT scan with midsagittal reconstructions may define the injury. CT scanning is also helpful for defining dens anatomy before screw fixation (44). It is excellent in defining abnormal C1–C2 relationships, especially in rotatory dislocations and subluxations (21,50,61,63), and as defined by Sonntag and Dickman (79), the CT scan with appropriate reconstruction may also help define the position of the vertebral artery and determine whether placement of an atlantoaxial screw is possible in both sides.

MRI in upper cervical spine injuries is becoming more useful. It has recently been used to allow direct visualization of the transverse ligament, especially in patients with head injuries. The gradient echo MRI pulse sequence is of greatest value (18). Although MRI is helpful in delineating compression injuries to the brain stem and spinal cord in the upper cervical spine, it is of less value than the CT scan in defining bony anatomy. Because the majority of concerns in upper cervical spine trauma are about bony anatomic relationships, the role of MRI remains limited.

EMERGENT IMMOBILIZATION OF THE UPPER CERVICAL SPINE

Patients who have sustained high-velocity vehicular injury, or those who are suspected of having a spine injury, will usually present to the emergency facility immobilized in a collar and on a spine board. Continue this immobilization until the spine has been cleared or until definitive immobilization and treatment can be instituted. Most upper cervical spine injuries in patients without neurologic deficit can be continuously immobilized in a collar until evaluation by CT scan and MRI is completed. Thus, a neurologically intact patient with a posterior arch fracture who is suspected of having a Jefferson fracture may undergo a CT scan using collar immobilization. In contrast, some place patients with transverse ligament rupture and a Brown–Séquard lesion in traction immobilization before initiating any further radiologic studies. It is our preference to keep the patient immobilized in a Philadelphia collar or Miami J collar and not to convert the patient to traction until the workup is completed. This makes transfer into the imaging machinery easier. With transfer in and out of a CT scanner or MRI machine, any traction will generally need to be discontinued several times, with some additional risk to the patient. Furthermore, it is critical with certain injuries, such as traction injuries to the upper cervical spine, that traction not be applied at all. If this mechanism is not recognized, even traction weights as small as 10 lb can cause stretching of the brain stem or cord with additional neurologic injury.

Next, decide what type of traction immobilization to apply once the radiologic examination is completed. The decision depends on two factors: What personnel are available to apply the traction device? What is the goal of applying the device to the patient? It is far simpler and more expeditious in the emergency setting to place Gardner–Well tongs, because this procedure can be done accurately by one person in a very short period of time and with minimal movement of the patient. Placement of a halo ring requires precise positioning of the patient and a surgeon and an assistant to make sure that the ring is applied properly. If the goal is simply to apply a traction

force to either reduce or stabilize an injury before surgery, in which the surgical procedure will give definitive stabilization not requiring postoperative immobilization in a halo vest, Gardner–Wells tong traction is preferred. In contrast, in injuries that require initial reduction by traction and that will either be treated definitively in a halo vest or treated by surgery most likely will require additional postoperative immobilization in a halo vest, initial placement of a halo is appropriate. A third group of patients—those with distraction injuries to the cervical spine, such as occiput–C1 dissociations or type IIA traumatic spondylolisthesis of the axis—will be placed in a halo and then immediately in a halo vest for stabilization. No traction is indicated in either of those injuries but ensuring stability is important.

Decide whether the halo can be placed with the patient in a supine position or whether the erect position is safe, which simplifies the placement. Patients with grossly unstable injuries or multiple injuries cannot tolerate a sitting position, and thus require application in the supine position using a head-positioning apparatus and an open ring halo to allow accurate placement. In those patients who have an isolated upper cervical spine injury, such as a minimally displaced dens fracture, the halo ring can be applied by applying a cervical collar and placing the patient in the sitting position, for placement of the ring and, subsequently, the vest.

Application of Skull Tong Traction

- Apply cervical tongs, such as Gardner–Wells tongs, in the supine position. Cleanse the hair directly above the external auditory meatus of the ear with povidone-iodine (Betadine) solution, but shaving the patient's hair is not necessary.
- Place the sterile pins through the ring and insert at a site directly superior to the external auditory meatus and one fingerbreadth above the pinna. Before application of the tong, inject the area down to the periosteum of the skull with 1% lidocaine, usually with epinephrine (1:100,000).
- Do not incise the skin. Tighten the pins simultaneously and, depending on the manufacturer's recommendations, bring the pressure indicators either to the level of outer surface of the pin or approximately 1 mm beyond.
- The initial traction weight in an adult is generally 10 lb, but before adding any weight, ascertain that the injury will not be made worse by traction.
- Increase the weights incrementally and obtain an appropriate radiograph between each increase to ensure that overdistraction is not occurring.

Although the general formula of 5 lb (2.3 kg) per cervical level above the fracture, with an initial 10 (4.6 kg) to 15 lb (6.8 kg) to overcome the friction of the head on the bed has been suggested, this is often not enough to reduce certain cervical spine injuries. The weight in certain types of traumatic spondylolisthesis as well as Jefferson's fractures will need to be increased to as much as 30 lb (13.6 kg) before an acute injury can be reduced. Between each 5 lb (2.3 kg) increment, however, appropriate radiographic evaluation is critical.

Application of a Halo Vest

Placement of a halo and subsequently a halo vest is more difficult and requires at least two people.

- Before placing the ring, measure the head and torso and size for the halo and vest according to the manufacturer's instructions.
- Place the patient in the supine position or an operating table and use either a mechanical head holder or positioner, or apply the halo with the patient in the sitting position.
- Select the pin sites carefully; four pin sites are adequate in the adult, but more may be needed in the elderly patient with a thin skull or in the child.
- The preferred sites for halo insertion have been determined by a series of radiographic, cadaver, and clinical studies (36): Anteriorly place the pins approximately 1 cm superior to the orbital ridge, below the equator of the skull, and over the lateral two-thirds of the orbit. This will generally avoid the temporalis muscle, the supra-orbital branch of the trochlear nerve, and the frontal sinuses (Fig. 139.4).
- Place the pins as far laterally as possible to minimize prominent scarring. Avoid placement within the temporalis muscle and fossa because it is particularly painful with motion and could cause significant bleeding; in addition, the area has a very thin cortical base, making perforation more common.
- The posterior sites are less critical and are generally placed at 180° on the contralateral side. Any area 2 to 3 cm posterior to the edge of the pinna of the ear is generally satisfactory. Shave the areas so that hair is not trapped as the pin is placed.
- Prepare and anesthetize each pin site by passing the needle for the local anesthetic through the selected hole or from above the halo to the exact contact point on the skin. Infiltrate the skin and deep tissues down to the skull.
- Ask the patient to close his or her eyes, and then make a small vertical incision with a #11 blade, directly in line with the selected screw holes. Some surgeons place the pins without using skin incisions (10). Place the four pins through the halo and screw them into the small incisions. Tighten the pins in a sequential fashion so that the halo is not shifted by overtightening one side before tightening the other.
- Tighten the pins in 2-inch-pound increments to a maximum of 8 inch-pounds in the normal adult skull.

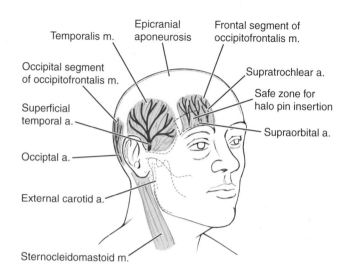

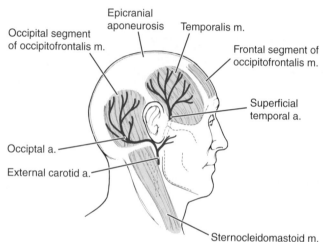

Figure 139.4. The "safe zone" for placement of halo fixator pins. Place the anterior pins anterolaterally, approximately 1 cm above the orbital rim, below the equator of the skull, and cephalad to the lateral two thirds of the orbit. The safe zone avoids the temporalis muscle and fossa laterally, and avoids the supra-orbital and supratrochlear nerves and the frontal sinus medially. (Redrawn from Ballock RT, Botte MJ, Garfin SR. Complications of Halo Immobilization. In: Garfin SR, ed. *Complications of Spine Surgery.* Baltimore: Williams & Wilkins, 1989, with permission.)

Tighten to lower levels when multiple pins are used in either the child or the osteoporotic elderly adult (9). Although 6 inch-pounds were initially used, 8 inch-pounds appears to have a lower rate of complications in terms of loosening and infection (9).

- Once the optimal torque is achieved with a torque screwdriver or a disposable wrench, place lock nuts over the pins and tighten them to prevent backing out of the pins.
- Apply traction through the halo ring using a bale, or

the halo can now be connected to a vest. After applying a halo vest in the supine position, mobilize the patient to an upright position and recheck the halo vest.

■ Now check the reduction of the cervical spine with a radiograph with the patient supine, if applied in the supine position, and then obtain a second radiograph in the upright position to be certain that the reduction does not shift. Obtain another upright roentgenogram 24 hours after the patient is allowed to ambulate, to ensure the maintenance of position. Subsequent adjustments to the halo, in terms of position of the fracture, should be done in the upright position for optimal vest fit.

■ With a torque wrench, retighten all four pins in the halo at 24 hours back to 8 inch-pounds. Teach the patient to cleanse the pin sites daily and to inspect for any problems.

CLASSIFICATION, PATHOLOGY, AND TREATMENT OF UPPER CERVICAL SPINE INJURIES

Bony and ligamentous injuries can be classified in a number of different ways, although it is probably easiest to classify them by level as opposed to any type of mechanistic classification (Table 139.1).

Occipital–Cervical Injuries

Injuries involving the occipital–cervical junction are extremely rare and often are fatal. This group of injuries includes dislocations that can occur with or without occipital condyle fractures, as well as occipital condyle fractures that occur without any subluxation. In addition, there are pure distraction injuries at the occipital–cervical junction. These are the most commonly fatal. These injuries may be overlooked in the acute emergency because they are uncommon and difficult to diagnose on plain roentgenograms. Many of these injuries are found only at autopsy (3). The injuries are commonly associated with other noncontiguous cervical spine fractures and with head injuries. The presence of a high-level neurologic deficit, often with involvement of all four extremities plus abnormal respiratory function, known as "pentaplegia," is a tipoff to injury at the occipital–cervical junction. As a group, these injuries most commonly result from high-speed motor vehicle accidents or are found in pedestrians struck by motor vehicles (3,4,51,53,56,78,86). The cause of death may be due to the associated head injury or sudden loss of voluntary respiratory function because of brain stem injury from the occipital–cervical dissociation (53).

Patients with isolated occipital condyle fractures have a higher rate of survival than occipital–cervical dissociations or dislocations. Patients may present with cranial nerve involvement as well as persistent occipital headaches. The mechanism of injury of all occipital condylar fractures is believed to be either sudden deceleration or direct axial loading on the cranium. Occipital–cervical dislocations can occur as a result of violent hyperextension or distraction forces in which the torso is pinned in position and the distraction force applied to the neck by a force applied beneath the patient's chin. Occipital condyle fractures have been characterized by Anderson and Montesano (4) (Fig. 139.5). A type I fracture (Fig. 139.5A) is a unilateral undisplaced, comminuted fracture of the condyle, usually resulting from axial impact between the skull and the axis. The alar ligament may be disrupted on that side, but the segment is usually stable. A type II fracture (Fig. 139.5B) is a unilateral occipital condyle fracture that is associated with a basilar skull fracture on the same side. The mechanism is generally axial loading with lateral bending, and this injury is generally stable. Type I and II injuries can be treated nonoperatively using a rigid cervical orthosis for 6 to 8 weeks; halo mobilization is not generally required. The type III fracture (Fig. 139.5C) is a unilateral alar ligament avulsion from the occipital condyle. It occurs as a result of extreme lateral bending, rotation, or a combination of the two. This injury, because it has a ligamentous component, may be associated with atlanto-occipital dislocations. Type III fractures may be unstable. Treatment is based on the degree of instability, ranging from collar immobilization, to halo immobilization, to posterior occipital–cervical fusion if associated disruption of the occiput–C1 complex is significant. Perform flexion-extension radiographs at the end of nonoperative management to assess the degree of stability. At that

---

Table 139.1. Classification of Injuries by Cervical Level

• Occiput-cervical injuries
  Occipital
  Condyle fracture
  Occipital-cervical ligamentous injury

• C-1 injuries
  Posterior ring fractures
  Lateral mass fractures
  Jefferson fracture
  Avulsions of the anterior ring

• C1–C2 injuries
  Rotational (atlantoaxial rotatory) instability
  Transverse ligament injuries (with atlantoaxial
    instability)

• C-2 injuries
  Dens fracture
  Traumatic spondylolisthesis
  Extension teardrop fracture

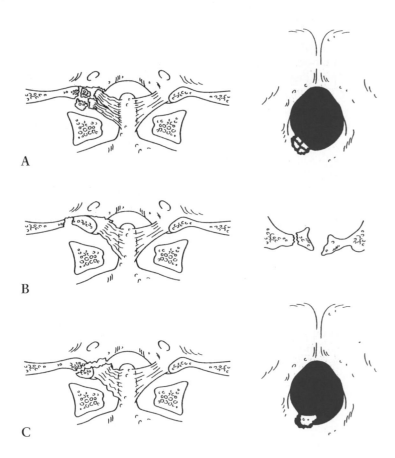

Figure 139.5. The classification of Anderson and Montesano describes three basic types of occipital condyle fractures. **A:** An impaction-type fracture, which is usually the result of an asymmetrical axial load to the head; it may be associated with other lateral mass fractures in the upper cervical spine. **B:** A basilar skull-type occipital condyle fracture. **C:** An avulsion-type occipital condyle fracture, which may be the result of a distraction force applied through the alar and apical ligament complex. (Redrawn from Anderson P, Montesano P. Morphology and Treatment of Occipital Condyle Fractures. *Spine* 1988;13:731, with permission.)

point, abnormal motion can be considered evidence of either nonunion or nonhealing of the ligamentous injuries, which requires treatment with an occipital–cervical fusion. Occipital condyle injuries are commonly unilateral but may be bilateral as well.

Occipital–cervical subluxations and dislocations have been incorporated into a single classification described by Traynelis et al. (86) (Fig. 139.6). Type I injuries are anterior dislocations and generally have the highest survivability. Type II injuries demonstrate vertical displacement, usually from a distraction mechanism: type IIa injuries occur at the occipital–cervical junction, and type IIb injuries occur between the atlas and axis. In some cases, these injuries may be combined injuries. When there is greater than 2 mm of vertical displacement between the occiput and C-1 (IIa), a rupture of the tentorial ligament and alar ligaments must be suspected. At the C1–C2 level (IIb), the joint capsule is usually involved as well as the tentorial membrane and the alar ligaments. Injuries to the transverse ligament can also occur. Type II injuries should not be placed in longitudinal traction. Type III injuries are posterior dislocations and are often fatal, although accompanying fracture of the C-1 arch may increase the chance of survival. Types I and III injuries may be realigned initially using traction, although the degree of ligamentous

disruption is difficult to assess initially. Traction should be used only in type I and type III injuries, with traction restricted to between 2 (0.9 kg) and 5 lb (2.3 kg). Interestingly, gravity itself is usually sufficient to reduce any translation. Increased survival has been reported with traction (26). After closed reduction is achieved, immediately place the patient in a halo vest and obtain a CT scan to identify any fractures. After this assessment, treat only patients with minimal ligamentous destruction and minimal bony disruption definitively in a halo vest for a period of 3 months. At the conclusion of that time, perform flexion-extension roentgenograms to check stability and decide whether a occipital–cervical fusion is necessary based on the degree of residual translation.

Posterior Occipital Fusion   In most cases, however, these are extremely unstable injuries and a posterior occipital–cervical fusion is indicated. Various techniques have been used to achieve an occipital–cervical fusion. The most rigid fixation involves the use of a contoured plate secured with multiple occipital screws and a C1–C2 transarticular screw (24,38,39) (Fig. 139.7). Techniques for occipital–cervical wiring, described by Wertheim and Bohlman (90), require postoperative immobilization in a halo vest, but in their series, all 13 patients developed a

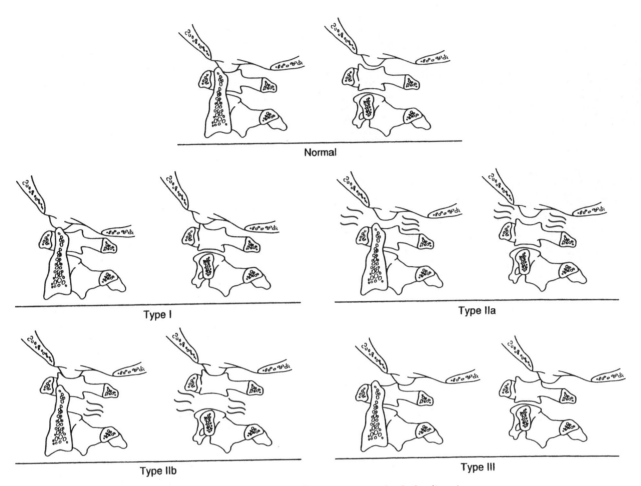

Figure 139.6. The classification of Traynelis and others takes into account both the direction and level of upper cervical dislocation. Type I injuries (antero-occipital–cervical dislocations) are more common than type III, but both are easily missed on routine radiographs. Type II injuries are distraction types, with type IIa occurring predominantly at the occipitoatlantal level and type IIb occurring at the atlantoaxial level. Not accounted for in this classification are double-level distraction injuries, which are uniformly fatal. Type III injuries, which are quite infrequent, are posterior atlantooccipital dislocations. (From Levine AM, Eismont FJ, Garfin SR, Zigler JE. *Spine Trauma.* Philadelphia: W. B. Saunders Co., 1998, with permission.)

solid arthrodesis. Other techniques using corticocancellous struts wired into the skull and beneath the spinous processes of C-1 and C-2 similarly have had high rates of union with minimal loss of fixation in patients treated postoperatively in a halo vest. A contoured occipital–cervical rod has also been described by a number of authors, giving additional stability that is not provided by bone graft alone (73,79). Irrespective of the type of construct, overall fusion rates for occipital–cervical fusions, when properly immobilized postoperatively, are in excess of 90%.

The advantage of occipital–cervical fusion with two plates and screws is that there is no need for halo immobilization.

▪ With the patient in the traction applied at the time of admission, perform an awake fiberoptic intubation. Then turn the patient into the prone position while still awake.

▪ Use a three-pin Mayfield (Ohio Medical Instrument Co., Inc., Cincinnati, OH) or halo modified headrest to secure the head. Induce general anesthesia once appropriate positioning is obtained and the patient's neurologic status is reassessed and found to be unchanged.

▪ Any manipulation of the head is done before inducing general anesthesia. Avoid extreme positions of flexion or extension because the plate fixation is rigid.

▪ Set up fluoroscopy so that AP and lateral images can be easily obtained, preferably simultaneously with two machines.

▪ Before incision, hold a guidewire alongside the neck

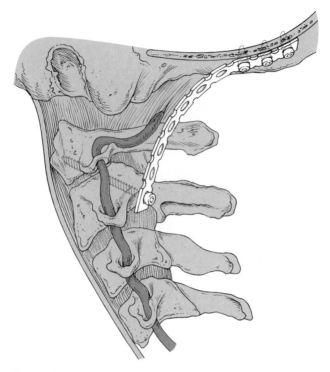

Figure 139.7.   Lateral view of the occipitocervical plating technique using C1–C2 transarticular screws and titanium reconstruction plates with bicortical cranial screws.

and visualize it on a flouroscope to be sure that the C1–C2 transarticular screw can be placed with the patient as positioned. This technique generally cannot be accomplished in patients with an upper thoracic kyphosis or gibbous.

▪ Make a posterior incision from the occipital prominence and extend it to the midcervical spine. Elevate all soft tissue off the bone from the greater occipital prominence to the C2–C3 joint.

▪ Select two plates with appropriate hole spacing and then contour them to fit the occipital–cervical junction, with at least three fixation holes available in the occiput and extending far enough distally to allow a C1–C2 transarticular screw to be placed on each side.

▪ Take care in contouring the occipital portion of the plates so that the terminal end is not prominent and the screw fixation is on the undersurface of the occiput rather than on its most prominent posterior portion.

▪ After templating and drilling the C1–C2 transarticular screw according to the technique described by Magerl and Seemann (Figs. 139.7 and 139.12) (59), select the appropriate-length screw, place the plate into position, and pass the transarticular screw through the plate, tightening it so that the plate lies in the appropriate position against the occiput on one side.

▪ Then place the occipital screws using three bicortical

screws per side. The screws are typically between 6 and 12 mm in length. In older patients, the dura may be adherent to the inner surface of the skull, causing a small cerebrospinal fluid (CSF) leak, but this can be easily stopped by simply placing the screw in the hole.

▪ Then apply the second plate in a similar fashion.

▪ Fashion a corticocancellous graft to lie between the two plates, covering the posterior portion of the occiput, the posterior arch of C-1, and around the spinous process of C-2. Hold this graft in place using heavy suture or wire.

▪ If transarticular screw fixation cannot be achieved because of the patient's position, alternatively, a C-2 pedicle screw can be placed, generally in combination with a C-3 lateral mass screw and a wire or suture placed around the arch of C-1 and tied to the plate on either side.

▪ Immobilize the patient postoperatively in a rigid collar for 12 weeks. While the patient is in the collar, be certain that he does not develop an occipital decubitus either because of the cervical spine trauma resulting in anesthesia in the area of the greater occipital nerve or as a result of the surgical dissection.

Fractures in the Atlas (C-1 Injuries)

Almost 50% of fractures involving the atlas are associated with a second fracture, and approximately 25% of them are associated with noncontiguous second fractures. The two most common types of fractures associated with a fracture of the atlas are fractures of the dens (27,55,58) or type I traumatic spondylolisthesis (55). Because the majority of injury patterns for fractures of the atlas involve widening of the space available for the cord rather than narrowing of the canal area, these injuries are not generally associated with neurologic deficit. If a deficit is present, its etiology may be from another associated or nonassociated spine or head injury. Multiple types of fractures of the C-1 arch have been identified (Fig. 139.8). The initial description of fractures of the C-1 arch was by Jefferson (48,49). He described isolated fractures of the posterior arch as well as multiple fractures of the arch, although his name is most associated with the four-part fracture. Segal et al. (77) have actually identified six different fracture patterns. However, the most common injury type is the posterior arch fracture. This is thought to be the result of a hyperextension-axial loading injury in which the posterior arch is pinched between the occiput and the ring of C-2 (92). These fractures tend to occur at the area just behind the lateral mass where the vertebral artery passes over it. Associated with this hyperextension-axial load mechanism of injury are other fractures that have a similar mechanism, such as posteriorly displaced dens fractures, type I traumatic spondylolisthesis of the axis, and C-2 anterior extension teardrop fractures.

The second most common type of injury, the lateral

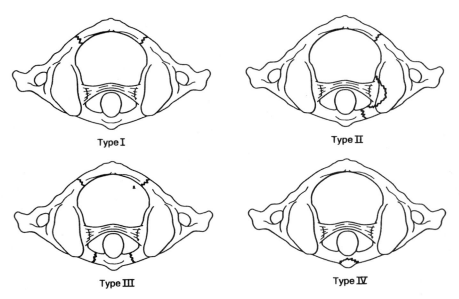

Figure 139.8. Four major types of fractures can occur at the level of the atlas. Type I is the most common and is a posterior arch fracture, which is the result of hyperextension and axial loading. It may be associated with other injuries caused by the same mechanism, such as traumatic spondylolisthesis. Type II, or lateral mass fracture, is the result of axial loading and lateral bending. There is usually a fracture line anterior and posterior to the lateral mass, causing asymmetric spreading. A second fracture line can also be present in the contralateral posterior arch. Type III, or Jefferson's fracture, is a burst fracture resulting from axial loading of C-l. Two to five fracture lines can be present, although most commonly there are four fracture lines: two in the anterior arch and two in the posterior arch. The final category, type IV, is an avulsion fracture of the anterior tubercle of the atlas. (From Levine AM, Eismont FJ, Garfin SR, Zigler JE. *Spine Trauma.* Philadelphia: W. B. Saunders Co., 1998, with permission.)

mass fracture, is generally composed of a fracture anterior to the lateral mass and one posterior to the lateral mass. In some instances, there may also be a fracture through the posterior arch on the contralateral side (42,55). These fractures have the same degree of instability, whether they are two-part or three-part injuries. The mechanism of injury is an axial load with lateral bending. The presence of a second fracture on the contralateral side would suggest at least some slight extension associated with this injury. In addition, the most common fracture occurring in association with this type is a lateral mass fracture in the lower cervical spine, which also has the same mechanism of extension, axial loading, and lateral bending.

The third type of fracture is what has been called the Jefferson fracture, which is a classic bursting injury of the ring of C-1. It has variably been described as having two fractures, one in the anterior arch and one in the posterior arch; or having three fractures, one in the anterior arch and two in the posterior arches; or having four or five fractures, with at least two in the anterior arch and two in the posterior arch. On open mouth radiograph view, this generally shows symmetric displacements of the lateral masses of C-1 (43,48,49,55,77). The injury is believed

to be the result of axial loading applied to the skull. Because the lateral masses of C-1 are wider laterally than medially, they act like a wedge when they are axially loaded, driving the lateral masses laterally and disrupting the ring. Splaying of the lateral masses more than 6.9 mm on an open mouth view may indicate disruption of the transverse ligament (80).

The fourth type of fracture is an avulsion fracture off the inferior portion of the anterior tubercle of C-1, where the longest colli muscle inserts. It is generally the result of hyperextension and, therefore, is an avulsion injury. It is completely stable (83). The final type of injury is a transverse process fracture, which may be either unilateral or bilateral (15).

In general, isolated posterior arch fractures can be treated nonoperatively with 6 to 12 weeks of immobilization in a hard collar. Nonunion is exceedingly rare (55, 77). Patients who have a dens fracture in association with a posterior arch fracture cannot be stabilized by standard C1–C2 wiring techniques. Without the integrity of the posterior arch, either an anterior dens screw or a posterior transarticular C-1 atlantoaxial arthrodesis may be necessary when operative treatment is indicated. Avulsions

from the anterior tubercle and transverse process fractures can be treated symptomatically with simple collar immobilization until pain relief is achieved.

Lateral mass and Jefferson's fractures can be divided into two groups: those that are only minimally to moderately displaced (less than 7 mm total displacement on an open mouth view) and those that are more significantly displaced. Controversy remains concerning the most effective treatment for these injuries. For minimally to moderately displaced fractures, the transverse ligament is intact. Immobilization in a hard collar for less significantly displaced injuries or immobilization in a halo vest for more significantly displaced injuries appears to give adequate long-term results. The most common complications of treating these patients is symptomatic nonunion (77) in those patients who have displaced fragments of the ring that do not unite. If the fragments are symptomatic, they may require arthrodesis. Remember that the halo and vest cannot be expected to reduce the ring fragments, even with traction. Once traction is removed, the original displacement will recur. Thus, placing the patient in traction for several days before immobilizing the patient in a halo vest does not improve the degree of displacement (42,94).

Patients who have had rupture of the transverse ligament and, therefore, more than 7 mm displacement on an open mouth radiographic view can be treated in one of two ways. Although it was initially thought that these patients would have long-term instability without surgical intervention, on the basis of the apparent rupture of the transverse ligament (75), this has turned out not to be the case (51). Thus, if the patient can achieve union of the ring of C-1, the degree of instability, after treatment, is limited. As demonstrated earlier by Fielding (29), this is because only the transverse ligament is ruptured, and the alar, apical, and accessory ligaments as well as the joint capsule are still intact and providing sufficient stability. Thus, the degree of C1–C2 instability is minimal when the ring heals solidly (55). Therefore, patients can be treated with enough longitudinal traction to reduce the splaying of the lateral masses to anatomic position and then held in longitudinal traction until early healing takes place (approximately 6 weeks). Once preliminary healing has occurred, the patient can be mobilized in a halo vest for an additional 6 weeks without risk of loss of reduction.

If, however, the reduction is achieved initially and then the patient is immediately mobilized (within the first week), reduction will be lost. Because of the long hospitalization required, long-term traction is less popular than it was previously. In addition, if the patient cannot be left in a supine position on a Stryker (Stryker Corp., Kalamazoo, MI) frame for long periods of time, operative treatment for significantly displaced fractures may be indicated.

In that case, reduce the ring with axial traction and then perform a C1–C2 transarticular screw fixation (62).

Posterior C1–C2 Arthrodesis, Modified Magerl Technique   The treatment of a widely displaced lateral mass or Jefferson's fracture is the modified Magerl transarticular C1–C2 screw fixation. The technique, however, has to be modified over that originally described by Magerl and Seemann (Fig. 139.9) (59) because a considerable portion of the stability of the technique is with the bone block that is usually placed between the intact posterior arch of C-1 and the spinous process of C-2. Because a Jefferson's fracture has an incompetent C-1 arch, additional stress is placed on the screws, risking early failure of fixation. Therefore, denude the cartilage of the facet joints, and pack bone directly into the posterior aspect of the C1–C2 joint. Also, place graft between the ring of C-1 and C-2, recognizing, however, that its structural integrity is compromised. Postoperatively, additional immobilization may be necessary in the form of a rigid collar or a halo vest, depending on the original degree of instability, the quality of the patient's bone, and the quality of the fixation.

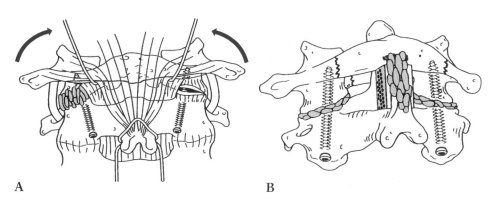

A   **B**

Figure 139.9. An alternative method for the treatment of a widely displaced lateral mass or Jefferson's fracture is the Magerl transarticular C1–C2 screw fixation. See text for details.

- Reduce the fracture with halo traction using about 30 to 35 lb (13.6 to 15.9 kg) of traction to achieve an anatomic reduction, which makes placement of the screws relatively straightforward. Further reduction is not possible once operative stabilization has begun. Use a biplanar fluoroscope imaging.
- The only variation in the standard technique is that the joints are fully exposed (Fig. 139.9*A*) so that the cartilage can be curetted out for fusion, and no fixation of bone graft is possible between the fractured arch of C-1 and the lamina of C-2.
- Graft directly into the facet joints and also do an onlay graft from C-l to C-2 (Fig. 139.9*B*) so that as healing occurs, a solid arthrodesis will also occur. With satisfactory screw fixation, either the halo vest can be continued postoperatively or hard collar can be used.

In patients treated with arthrodesis who attain a satisfactory fusion, long-term results in terms of stability are excellent. In patients with relatively undisplaced lateral mass fractures and Jefferson's fractures treated only in a collar or halo vest, late instability is rare if union is achieved between all fragments (55,77). The motion between C1–C2 however rarely returns to normal. In the Levine and Edwards series (55), up to 80% of patients had some residual neck pain, although none required secondary fusions for neck pain (55). The significant joint incongruity and resultant degenerative changes in fractures that are significantly displaced at the conclusion of treatment will commonly lead to pain and secondary occipital cervical fusion. In one study, nonunions occurred in 17% of patients (77), and nonunion was directly related to the amount of displacement. Patients with a nonunion and displacement of the posterior arch could sustain neural compression on the basis of the displaced fragment, but this is a rare complication.

Atlantoaxial Instability (C1–C2 Injuries)

Atlantoaxial instability may occur secondary to trauma, congenital abnormalities, infection, and arthritis. Traumatic atlantoaxial instability can be of two types. It can be related to flexion instability with anterior translation of the atlas on the axis resulting from rupture of the transverse ligament and disruption of the secondary stabilizers—the alar, apical, and accessory ligaments. The second type of atlantoaxial instability is a rotatory instability, which can be of several different types and be the result of both bony and ligamentous injuries. The transverse ligament is the primary stabilizer, preventing anterior translation of C-1 on C-2, but the alar, apical, and accessory ligaments, as well as the capsular ligaments, offer secondary stabilization. Posterior translation of C-1 on C-2 is prevented by the impingement of the anterior ring of C-1 on the dens. As shown by early work by Fielding et al. (29), a maximum of 3 mm of anterior translation of C-1

on C-2 can occur with an intact transverse ligament in the adult. Within the range of 3 to 5 mm of translation, catastrophic failure occurs, usually within the midsubstance of the ligament rather than at the bony attachments. No correlation has been made between the strength of the transverse ligament and age other than that children tend to be slightly more lax and, therefore, an ADI of 5 mm of translation can be accepted in children as normal. Simple experimental sectioning of the transverse ligament without disruption of the alar, apical, and accessory ligaments results in an ADI of only 5 mm in the adult in the experimental setting (29). In patients with gross instability with an ADI greater than 10 mm, not only does the transverse ligament need to be sectioned but all of the secondary restraints as well.

Most of these injuries are the result of significant trauma to the head, although they may occur in older patients with a simple fall and striking of the occiput. Patients may have varying neurologic involvement, from being neurologically normal with severe neck pain to a transient quadriplegia to a Brown–Séquard–type syndrome. The diagnosis of this injury is generally made on a lateral roentgenogram. If roentgenograms are taken in the supine position, the subluxation may reduce, especially in a patient whose chest is disproportionately large in relation to his or her head, thus placing the patient in extension, as is frequently the case with children. If the patient does not have neurologic deficit and injury is suspected, physician-supervised flexion-extension films in the alert, awake, neurologically intact, cooperative patient may be very helpful in making the diagnosis. In contrast, if the patient has severe neck pain and paraspinous muscle spasm, adequate-quality flexion-extension films may not be attainable. There may not be enough motion in the cervical spine to indicate whether the patient has instability. In that case, several options are available. The patient may be simply immobilized in a hard collar, and when the spasm subsides, adequate flexion-extension films can be obtained. Alternatively, under physician supervision, the amount of spasm in the paraspinous musculature can be reduced by intramuscular injection, allowing flexion-extension roentgenograms to be taken. An MRI may be used to investigate the integrity of the ligamentous complex.

Healing of the transverse ligament, even in the case in which its insufficiency is the result of the avulsion from its insertion on the lateral mass, is uncommon. This is one of the few injuries in the upper cervical spine that routinely requires surgical intervention. There are a variety of techniques to achieve C1–C2 arthrodesis. These are commonly done by posterior arthrodesis because it is infrequent to have a fracture of the posterior arch and a rupture of the transverse ligament from a flexion type injury. C1–C2 fusion, using either a Gallie (35), Brooks (12), or

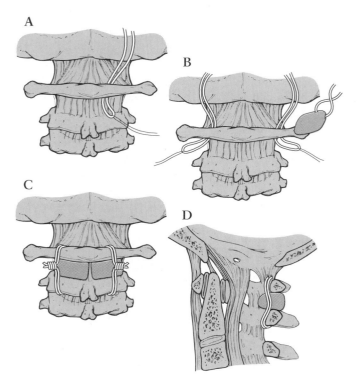

Figure 139.10. Brooks fusion: The occipital nerves emerge through the interlaminar space between the atlas and the axis, the vertebral arteries are more lateral. See text for a description of the surgical technique. (Redrawn from Jarrett JP, Whitesides TE Jr. Injuries of the Cervicocranium. In: Browner BD, Jupiter JB, Levine AM, et al, eds. *Skeletal Trauma: Fractures, Dislocations, and Ligamentous Injuries,* Vol 1. Philadelphia, W. B. Saunders Co., 1992:689, with permission.)

a Magerl (46) C1–C2 transarticular screw fixation, will give satisfactory results in this situation.

Until recently, the most common method for surgical stabilization for C1–C2 was either a Gallie (35) or a Brooks (12) fusion (Fig. 139.10). With any method, significant loss of rotation at the atlantoaxial joint will occur postoperatively because 50% of neck rotation normally occurs at this joint. In fact, because of compensatory motion at other joints, the loss is often less, as reported by Fielding et al. (30). Fielding demonstrated that an average loss of only 13% of rotational motion occurred in patients younger than 20 years of age; a 25% loss occurred in those in the 20-to-40-year-old age group, and a 28% loss occurred in those older than 40 years of age.

Modified Brooks Fusion   In both the Brooks' and Gallie's techniques, wires are passed beneath the arch of C-1, around the spinous process of C-2 in the Gallie technique and sublaminarly beneath the arch of C-2 in the Brooks technique. With the Gallie technique, a corticocancellous bone lock is laid on the arch of C-1 and notched

to fit around the spinous process of C-2. There are a number of different modifications of the Brooks technique, ranging from two wedge-shaped blocks (Fig. 139.10), one on each side, with a single wire around them, to two wires around them, to instances of a single block in the center with wires that pass beneath the laminar at C-1 as well as sublaminar at C-2.

Brooks Fusion   The occipital nerves emerge through the interlaminar space between the atlas and the axis; the vertebral arteries are more lateral.

- Make a midline approach. The arteries and nerves are fairly well protected by the neck muscles. Expose C-1 and C-2.
- On both the right and left, pass sutures under the posterior arch of the atlas (Fig. 139.10A). Then pass the sutures on the lamina of C-2. A twisted wire is then tied to the suture, which is used to guide the wire under the arch of the atlas and the lamina of the atlas (Fig. 139.10B).
- In the Figure 139.10C the wires are now in place and lie anterior to the anterior portion of the atlantoaxial membrane, which was not removed during exposure of the posterior elements of the atlas and axis.
- Harvest either two iliac crest corticocancellous grafts or one larger midline graft and fashion them to fit between the posterior arches of C-1 and C-2. Bevel edges to fit in the interval between the atlas and axis. Hold the graft in place with a towel clip. When they are wired in place, the beveled edges will be in contact with the arch of the atlas and the lamina of the axis.
- Secure the graft or grafts with the wires (Fig. 139.10D)

Several congenital anomalies are associated with atlantoaxial instability. These include Down's, Morquio's, and Klippel–Feil syndromes, as well as occipitalization of the atlas. The incidence of atlantoaxial instability in Down's patients has been reported to be as high as 20%. There is still controversy surrounding the need for prophylactic fusion in these individuals. Most recommend restriction of contact activities in patients with an ADI of less than 7 mm. Prophylactic fusion is recommended for displacement of greater than 7 mm.

Atlantoaxial Rotatory Deformities

Atlantoaxial rotatory deformities have a number of different etiologies including trauma, tumors, and inflammatory conditions (31,54,93). They have been classified anatomically by degree of subluxation (31) and clinically by the duration of symptoms, response to treatment, or their underlying etiology. They are most commonly due to infection or trauma and have been reported in all age groups, with a higher incidence in children (70) and young adults, regardless of the etiology. The typical presentation is a sudden onset of torticollis in which the head is rotated away and tilted anteriorly toward the rotated side with

associated spasm of the sternocleidomastoid muscle. The patients generally have significant neck pain and an inability to rotate the head past neutral. By palpating the posterior wall of the oropharynx, it is possible to feel the difference between the normal and abnormally rotated lateral masses. On the subluxed side, it is possible to appreciate a stepoff from the C-1 lateral mass to the C-2 lateral mass. Any motion produces significant discomfort. In long-standing cases, facial asymmetries may occur. Compensation for the torticollis may occur after some time as a result of counterrotation in the lower cervical spine or atlanto-occipital joint.

The most characteristic finding on the lateral radiograph is an obliquity in the orientation of the posterior arch of C-1 in comparison to the remaining lower spinous processes. A widened ADI may be seen. On the open mouth view, the anteriorly rotated lateral mass can appear wider and closer to the midline than the opposite side. However, the most pathognomonic sign on the open mouth view is the "wink" sign when the inferior edge of the lateral mass of C-1 on the affected side overlaps the lateral mass of C-2, obliterating the joint space. On an AP view the spinous process of C-2 may be rotated away from the side of the anterior displaced lateral mass, known as Sudeck's sign (84). A fixed subluxation can be easily seen on a thin-cut CT scan, which demonstrates the abnormal relationship of C-1 to C-2 (21,33,63). The dimensional reconstructions are also very useful for complete delineation of the injury. For reducible subluxations, a dynamic CT scan in maximal left and right rotation will generally reveal the deformity.

The classification is based on the integrity of the transverse ligament and the direction of the deformity (7,31). A type I deformity indicates an intact transverse ligament and a fixed C1–C2 position within a normal range of rotation. Type II deformities show mild deficiency of the transverse ligament with an ADI of 3 to 5 mm. Mild fixed rotation exceeds the normal motion of the C1–C2 joint. A type III deformity has an ADI greater than 5 mm, and both lateral masses of C-1 are displaced anteriorly, with one side rotated farther than the other. A type IV deformity describes a posterior subluxation of one or both lateral masses. Types III and IV have greater instability with increased neurologic risk, and decreased success with conservative management. Posttraumatic episodes of atlantoaxial deformity have a higher rate of instability and require more aggressive treatment. Rotatory dislocations of traumatic origin may have not only ligamentous disruption but also bony avulsions or fractures from the C-1 joint surfaces, increasing the degree of instability.

With an infectious etiology, treatment is initially geared toward eradicating the organism responsible with intravenous antibiotics. Treatment is then primarily based on the duration of the deformity at presentation. If the deformity has been present for less than 1 week, place the patient in a soft collar and put him on bed rest. If the deformity does not spontaneously reduce, institute halo traction. The weight initially used is based on the age of the patient: 7.7 lbs (3.5 kg) for younger children and up to 13 to 17.6 lb (6 to 8 kg) for adults. The weight may be increased in increments of 1.1 lb to 2.2 lbs (0.5 to 1 kg) every 3 to 4 days until reduction is achieved to a maximum limit of 13.2 lb (6 kg) in children (70) and 19.8 lb (9 kg) in adults. If the deformity has been present for more than 1 week, start halo traction immediately. Continue traction for up to 3 weeks, but if reduction is not accomplished, a surgical stabilization procedure in symptomatic individuals is indicated.

If reduction is achieved, continue immobilization to allow the capsules and ligaments to heal. Wetzel and La Rocca (91) devised a protocol for immobilization based on the type of deformity. They recommend a soft collar for type I, a rigid collar for type II, and a halo for types III and IV for a duration of up to 3 months. After treatment, obtain flexion-extension radiographs to document stability.

Surgical intervention is indicated when there is evidence of significant instability or neurologic deficits, when there is failure to achieve or maintain a reduction in an acute traumatic deformity, or if symptoms persist after conservative treatment. A posterior C1–C2 fusion is recommended. *In situ* fusion is recommended by some, but the passing of sublaminar wires is more difficult because of the narrowed space behind the posterior ring of C-1. Improvement in the cosmetic deformity is usually slow and often occurs through rotation at cephalad and caudal levels, which may become symptomatic in the future. Some surgeons recommend an attempt at open reduction.

Open Reduction

- Pass a sublaminar wire under the posterior arch of C-1 and gently applying traction in order to manually derotate the atlas.
- After reduction is achieved, incorporate the wire into a Gallie or Brooks C1–C2 fusion, or C1–C2 transarticular screw fixation can be done. The C1–C2 transarticular screw fixation is the most stable construction to prevent redisplacement if reduction can be achieved either preoperatively or intraoperatively.
- Screw placement is difficult when residual rotatory deformity exists at the time of screw passage.
- If neurologic deficit is present and reduction cannot be achieved, perform a decompression of the posterior arch of C-1, followed by an occipitocervical fusion.

C-2 Injuries

Fractures of the Odontoid (Dens)   Fractures of the odontoid account for approximately 15% of all cervical spine fractures. Neurologic deficits occur in approximately 25% of patients with fractures and can range from quadriplegia to slight neuralgias. There is a higher mortality rate associated with this fracture in elderly patients. In younger patients, these fractures tend to occur as a result of motor vehicle accidents; in older patients, they tend to result from falls. The mechanism is forceful flexion or extension with an axial load. Flexion results in anterior subluxation, whereas extension results in posterior subluxation.

The classification system for dens fractures was described by Anderson and D'Alonzo (3) (Fig. 139.11). A type I fracture is an avulsion fracture at the tip of the odontoid above the transverse ligament. A type II fracture occurs at the junction of the body and dens, and may be transverse or oblique. A type III fracture extends into the cancellous portion of the body of C-2.

The treatment of type I fractures is a period of immobilization with a soft collar until symptoms resolve. However a type I fracture may be an indication of a distraction injury at C1–C2 and thus may be a grossly unstable injury requiring C1–C2 arthrodesis. Take flexion-extension ra-

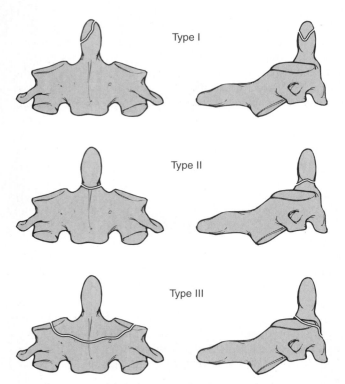

Figure 139.11. Classification of odontoid fractures: Three types of odontoid fractures as seen on AP and lateral radiographs. Type I is an oblique fracture through the upper part of the odontoid process. Type II is a fracture at the junction of the odontoid process with the vertebral body of the second cervical vertebra. Type III is a fracture through the body of the axis. (Redrawn from Anderson LD, D'Alonzo RT. Fractures of the Odontoid Process of the Axis. *J Bone Joint Surg [Am]* 1974;56: 1664, with permission.)

diographs to document stability because some instances of type I fractures are associated with other significant ligamentous injuries that can be grossly unstable. The outcomes are excellent, with few residual symptoms; even persistent nonunion of the avulsion fragment offers no long-term problems.

The treatment of type II fractures is somewhat controversial. The nonunion rate for nonoperative treatment is widely variable (1,3,6,14,40,41,60,88) and ranges up to 75% in some series. It appears to correlate with several factors:

- Posterior displacement (19)
- Initial displacement of greater than 5 mm (41)
- Inability to obtain or maintain an anatomic reduction
- Advanced patient age
- Pre-existing diabetes or rheumatoid arthritis in the injured patient

In these high-risk patients, initial surgical stabilization is recommended. In addition, the inability to achieve a reduction in traction or the inability to maintain a reduction in a halo vest is an indication for surgical stabilization.

Type III fractures have relatively low nonunion and malunion rates (less than 15%) when treated appropriately (14). Nondisplaced type III injuries can be treated in a rigid collar, but displaced injuries usually require halo vest immobilization for 12 weeks. If the fracture line is oblique, it is generally not possible to correct collapse, but angulation can be corrected and maintained to healing. Obtain flexion-extension radiographs at 12 weeks to document stability. Treat failures of halo treatment with a C1–C2 fusion. Loss of initial reduction is also an indication for fusion.

The most common method of treatment for dens fractures is C1–C2 arthrodesis by either the Gallie (35) or Brooks (12) methods, as previously described. The Gallie method is not indicated for posteriorly displaced fractures. Results of treatment of dens fractures uniformly demonstrate an arthrodesis rate of approximately 90% irrespective of the technique used.

When the posterior arch of C-1 is fractured or the dens fragment is so unstable that it translates both anteriorly and posteriorly, a C1–C2 transarticular screw (59) or a direct anterior osteosynthesis of the dens is necessary (Fig. 139.12). This technique provides increased initial stability when compared with wiring techniques but is technically challenging.

Magerl Fusion C1–C2
- Perform an awake fiberoptic intubation and turn the patient prone. Position the patient's head in a Mayfield three-pronged head holder. Verify the neurologic status and initiate general anesthesia.
- Set up fluoroscopy so that both AP and lateral images

can be obtained, preferably simultaneously. Place the patient's neck in as much flexion as possible without displacing the dens. Place a guide wire along the neck and image to verify that the trajectory needed can be obtained.

■ The position of the neck that can be achieved consistent with reduction of the deformity influences exposure. If the neck can be flexed (Fig. 139.12*A1*) and reduction achieved (as is the case with a posteriorly displaced dens fracture), then the drill insertion and instrumentation can usually be done through the primary surgical incision. If the neck cannot be significantly flexed and the position maintained, as is often the case with ruptures of the transverse ligament (Fig. 139.12*A2*), then use a shorter primary incision with the drills and taps passed percutaneously into the primary incision.

■ Make a midline incision from occiput to the C-4 spinous process, exposing the posterior arch of C-1 to the C2–C3 facet joint. Carefully dissect with a Penfield elevator to expose the pedicle of C-2 all the way up to the posterior capsule of the C1–C2 joint. Remove the joint capsule. This dissection is done by elevating carefully along the proximal edge of the lamina of C-2 in a lateral direction until the pedicle is identified. Take care at this point to sweep the soft tissues proximally over the C-1 lateral mass rather than incise them because the greater occipital nerve and a very friable complex of thin-walled venous lakes overlie those structures. Significant bleeding may occur.

■ Clearly dissect the medial aspect of the pedicle (Fig. 139.12*B*). The landmarks for the starting holes for the drill need to be near the medial edge of the facet and inferior margin of the lamina.

■ Hold the soft tissue out of the way by placing a small K-wire below it drilled into the upper edge of the facet (Fig. 139.12*C*).

■ Elevate the ligamentum flavum from under the posterior arch, and pass a sublaminar wire (Fig. 139.12*E*). Gentle traction on the wire may be needed to reduce any residual subluxation. The wire will be used later to secure the bone graft.

■ Drill a guidewire under fluoroscopic visualization, en-

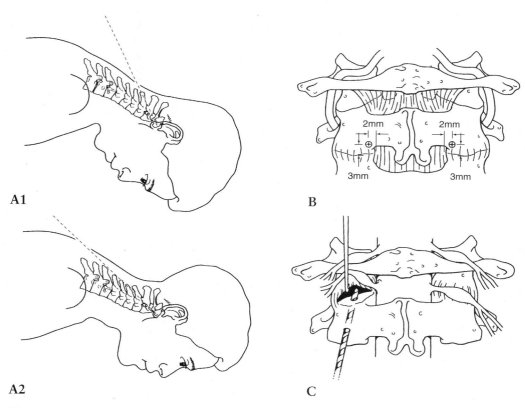

A1

A2

B

C

Figure 139.12. The C1–C2 fusion technique of Magerl. **A1, A2, B to F:** The surgical technique; see text for details. **G:** Lateral view of the completed fixation. [Redrawn from (parts **C** and **G**) the Barrow Neurological Institute, Phoenix, AZ and (parts **A** and **B**, and **D** to **F**) from Levine AM, Eismont FJ, Garfin SR, Zigler JE. *Spine Trauma.* Philadelphia: W. B. Saunders Co., 1998, with permission.] *(continued)*

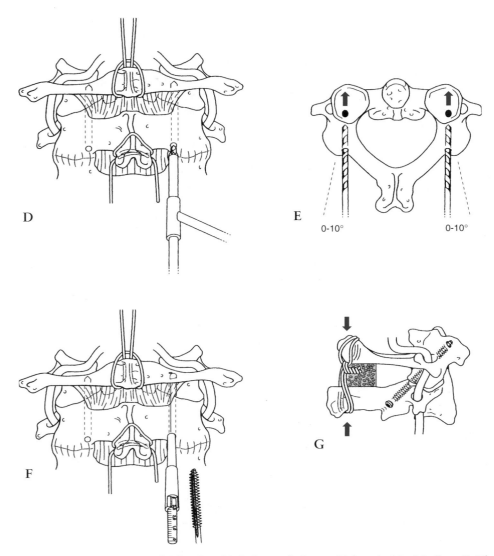

Figure 139.12. *(continued)* The C1–C2 fusion technique of Magerl. **A1, A2, B to F:** The surgical technique; see text for details. **G:** Lateral view of the completed fixation. [Redrawn from (parts **C** and **G**) the Barrow Neurological Institute, Phoenix, AZ and (parts **A** and **B**, and **D** to **F**) from Levine AM, Eismont FJ, Garfin SR, Zigler JE. *Spine Trauma*. Philadelphia: W. B. Saunders Co., 1998, with permission.]

tering the most inferior aspect of the C-2 lamina, 2 to 3 mm lateral to the medial border of the C-2 pedicle.

■ The orientation of the drill should be from the medial starting hole to slightly lateral; do this by direct visualization of the path. It is important to monitor the position on the lateral image carefully so that the drill exits the C-2 lateral mass at its posterior aspect (Fig. 139.12E).

■ Advance the wire slowly toward the posterior rim of the superior facet of C-2, across the joint, and into the middle or posterior third of the inferior articular process of C-1. Advance the wire toward the superior margin of the anterior arch of C-1. A percutaneous ap-

proach through the soft tissues at the C6–C7 level is sometimes necessary to obtain the correct trajectory.

■ Use a cannulated screw system to simplify the remaining steps, but take great care because inadvertent advancement of the guidewire can cause significant injury. This method requires constant imaging.

■ Drill and tap for 3.5 or 4 mm screw and determine the depth (Fig. 139.12F). A 3.5 mm fully threaded screw is most commonly used, with the length varying between 40 and 50 mm, depending on patient size and screw trajectory.

■ Next, harvest a rectangular tricorticocancellous bone

graft and notch it to fit between the decorticated spinous process of C-2 and posterior arch of C-1.

■ Secure it in place with the sublaminar wire previously passed using Gallie technique.

Immobilize the patient postoperatively with a rigid collar for 6 to 8 weeks if no posterior arch fracture is present. If a posterior arch fracture is present or if the fixation is weak, immobilize the patient for 12 weeks in either a halo vest or suboccipital-mandibular immobilization (SOMI)-type brace.

In the interest of preserving as much rotational motion as possible, a direct anterior screw fixation technique has been recommended by some and has shown high union rates, requiring only limited postoperative immobilization (Fig. 139.13) (8,47). The complication rates, however, have been reported to be as high as 20%. The indications include acute type II fractures and very selected type III fractures without much C-2 body involvement. Contraindications include comminuted fractures, associated unstable ring fractures, atypical oblique coronal fractures, irreducible fractures, and nonunion with poor bone quality. It is essential that the fracture be reducible; reducibility must be verified preoperatively with either fluoroscopy or plain radiographs. A small amount of displacement significantly decreases the area available for insertion of the screw. Large amounts of cervicothoracic kyphosis make this procedure technically unfeasible because adequate space must be available for the correct screw trajectory. This procedure is technically difficult in posteriorly displaced fractures because reduction will be lost as extension of the cervical spine as is required to achieve access to C2. The postoperative range of motion has been shown to still be reduced, possibly secondary to adhesions and callus formation.

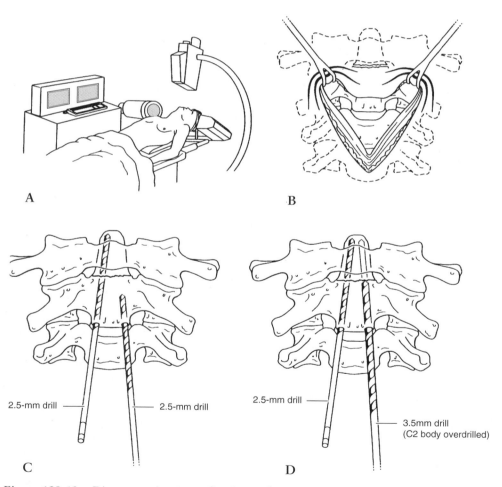

2.5-mm drill — — 2.5-mm drill

2.5-mm drill —

— 3.5mm drill (C2 body overdrilled)

A   B   C   D

Figure 139.13.   Direct anterior screw fixation technique. See text for details. [Part (**A**) redrawn from Grob D, Magerl F. Operative Stabilisirrung bei Frakturen von C1 and C2. *Orthopade* 1987:16; parts (**B** to **I**) redrawn from Muller ME, Allgower M, Schneider R, et al., eds. *Manual of Internal Fixation Techniques Recommended by the AO-ASIF Group*, ed 3. Berlin: Springer-Verlag, 1991:638, with permission.] *(continued)*

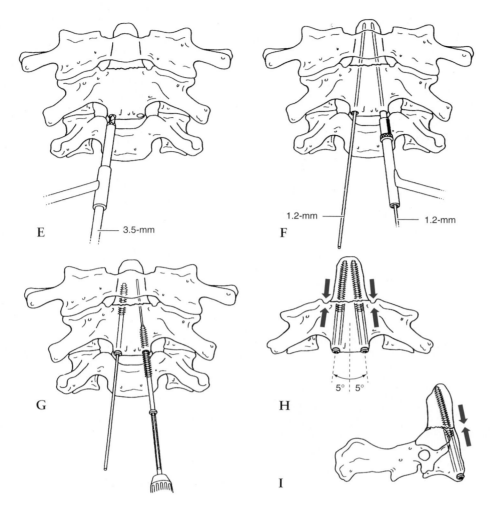

Figure 139.13. *(continued)* Direct anterior screw fixation technique. See text for details. [Part (**A**) redrawn from Grob D, Magerl F. Operative Stabilisirrung bei Frakturen von C1 and C2. *Orthopade* 1987:16; parts (**B** to **I**) redrawn from Muller ME, Allgower M, Schneider R, et al., eds. *Manual of Internal Fixation Techniques Recommended by the AO-ASIF Group,* ed 3. Berlin: Springer-Verlag, 1991:638, with permission.]

Anterior Screw Fixation of the Odontoid

■ Positioning of the patient for anterior dens osteosynthesis is critically important. Place the patient in the supine position with the neck extended so that exposure of the inferior edge of C-2 is possible. Rest the head on a Mayfield horseshoe head support. If fracture reduction is lost (as may happen with posteriorly displaced dens fractures), use less extension until provisional fixation has been achieved. Biplanar image intensification monitoring is essential (Fig. 139.13A). Perform an awake fiberoptic intubation and document the neurologic status. Aid reduction by placing a rolled towel under the neck for anterior displacement and under the head for posterior displacement.

■ Set up fluoroscopy so that satisfactory AP and lateral views can be obtained; simultaneous imaging is preferred.

■ When reduction is obtained, make a standard anterior lateral approach through a transverse incision centering the incision at the C5–C6 level (Fig. 139.13B)

■ Make a retropharyngeal approach, as described by Smith-Robinson (see Chapter 138), at the C5–C6 disc space level and carry the dissection up to the C2–C3 disc space. Make an incision in the anterior longitudinal ligament at the level of the inferior portion of the C-2 body. A one- or two-screw technique can then be used.

■ Starting 3 mm to either side of the midline and on the caudal edge of the body, medially insert a 1.5 mm K-wire to ascertain trajectory and stabilize the fragment (Fig. 139.13C). Insert it across the fracture into the center of the odontoid. Two K-wires can be placed and a cannulated system used, but inadvertent advancement of the wire is a complication; preferably, one wire is removed and replaced at a time with a solid 2.5 mm drill bit advancing to the tip of the dens.

■ Pass the drill bit over the guidewire and advance it under fluoroscopic control. Take care—there have been instances in which the guidewire has been advanced into the spinal cord.

■ Because a lag effect is desired, either a partially threaded screw can be used or one drill bit can be removed and the near fragment overdrilled with a 3.5 mm drill bit (Fig. 139.13D). Tap the near cortex only (Fig. 139.13E to G). Be sure that all threads of this lag screw are across the fracture site.

■ Final screw fixation should have the screw slightly oblique toward the midline and optionally may perforate the cortex of the tip of the dens (Fig. 139.13H and I). Take care to begin the screw on the undersurface and not the anterior surface of the C-2 body to achieve the proper trajectory (Fig. 139.13I).

Studies have shown no significant increase in biomechanical stability with two screws, and anatomic studies have revealed that some odontoids are of inadequate size to accommodate two screws (1,8,28,59). Postoperative immobilization in a Philadelphia collar for 6 weeks is generally sufficient.

Traumatic Spondylolisthesis of the Axis Traumatic spondylolisthesis of the axis is a fracture that occurs through the pars interarticularis usually at its junction with the posterior aspect of the vertebral body. Such fractures are relatively uncommon and the mechanism of injury varies with the fracture type. These usually occur in motor vehicle accidents in which the head strikes the windshield or dashboard. The amount of displacement and angular deformity is related to the amount of rebound occurring from the associated acceleration and deceleration forces. These fractures are generally not associated with significant neurologic deficits because most of the injury patterns expand the canal diameter. As with fractures of the atlas, if a deficit is present, it may be related to a head injury or to some associated injury. Diligently search for associated injuries that can occur in up to 30% of patients with these fractures. Most of the concurrent injuries occur in the adjacent three cervical levels (56).

Several different classification systems have been used to describe traumatic spondylolisthesis of the axis. The systems have been based on either instability criteria (34), mechanism of injury (56), or anatomic or radiologic criteria (25,56,81). The classification most commonly used now is based on four patterns, each of which has both

common radiographic and mechanistic characteristics (Fig. 139.14) (56).

A type I injury has a fracture through the pedicles of C-2, just posterior to the junction of the body and the pedicles. A type I injury (Fig. 139.14A) is either a nondisplaced fracture or minimally displaced, with less than 3 mm of displacement and no angulation. It usually results from an axial load with an associated hyperextension moment. The type IA, or atypical hangman's pattern (81), involves a fracture between the junction of the pedicle and the body of C-2 in which, at least on one side, a portion of the posterior wall breaks off and remains attached to the pedicle. The significance of this pattern is that, if there is any displacement, the cord can be compressed between the ring of C-1 and the retained portion of the posterior wall. The fracture line frequently traverses the foramen for the vertebral artery and may result in intimal damage. A higher incidence of neurologic deficits is associated with this pattern.

The type II injury (Fig. 139.14B) involves displacement and angulation of C-2 on C-3. A type II injury is the result of a hyperextension axial load, which breaks the neural arch, followed by a flexion injury, which results in significant translation. The pattern of the fracture line is similar to that seen with a type I injury.

The type IIA injury (Fig. 139.14C) has only minimal translation of C-2 over C-3 but has severe angulation. The type IIA injury is characterized by minimal translation and significant angulation with widening of the posterior aspect of the disc space. With application of traction, these are the injuries that will demonstrate significant widening of the disc. The mechanism is different in that this type of injury occurs as a result of a flexion distraction force. The fracture line, instead of being vertical at the junction of the pedicle and the body is obliquely through pedicle. Traction may produce distraction, leading to potential neurologic injury.

The type III injury (Fig. 139.14D) is a pars fracture with an associated C2–C3 unilateral or bilateral facet dislocation. The mechanism most probably is initial flexion-distraction, which causes the dislocation, and then extension, which causes the traumatic spondylolisthesis. Reversing the mechanism would not permit the dislocation to occur, because the inferior facet of C-2 would then be detached from the cervicocranium, which serves as the lever for the dislocation. This pattern is associated with a higher incidence of neurologic deficits.

Radiologic evaluation and determination of the traumatic spondylolisthesis can usually be made on a lateral cervical spine roentgenogram. However, because most radiographs of this injury are performed in the supine position, the true nature of the injury may be obscured because any displacement may be reduced in the supine position. Thus, to ensure that the injury is indeed a type I, physician-supervised flexion-extension radiographs are necessary to

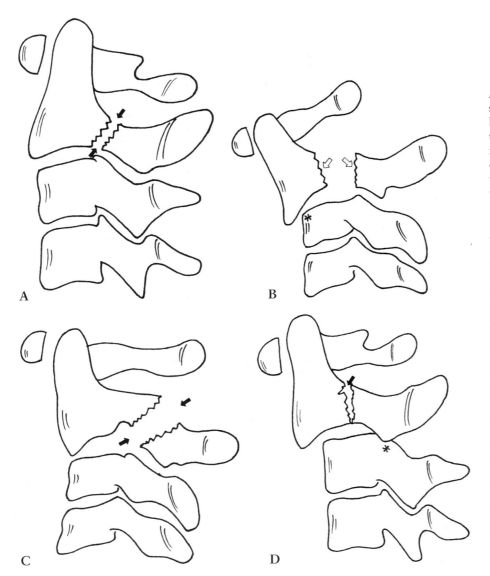

Figure 139.14. Traumatic spondylolisthesis of the axis can be characterized by the amount of translation and angulation at the fracture site. **A:** In a type I injury, the fracture line is either vertical or slightly off vertical *(arrows)*. **B:** In a type II injury, the fracture line is relatively vertical with wide separation of the fragments *(arrows)*. These are characterized by more than 3 mm of translation and significant angulation as well. They frequently demonstrate a compression of the anterosuperior corner of the body of C-3 as a result of the flexion force that caused the anterior translation *(star)*. In this case, avulsion of the anterosuperior corner of the body has occurred. **C:** Type IIA traumatic spondylolisthesis is different in its mechanism from type I and II injuries. Frequently, the fracture lines are more oblique *(arrows)* and are not located as close to the junction of the body and the pedicle as in the type I and II injuries. **D:** Type III traumatic spondylolisthesis of the axis combines fractures of the neural arch with facet injuries at C2–C3. The first type is a bilateral facet dislocation at C2–C3 *(star)* with a type I Hangman's fracture at the base of the body–pedicle junction *(arrowhead)*. (From Levine AM, Eismont FJ, Garfin SR, Zigler JE. *Spine Trauma*. Philadelphia: W. B. Saunders Co., 1998, with permission.)

differentiate it from a reduced type II. In order to undergo flexion-extension radiographs, patients must be awake, alert, and neurologically intact, and able to perform the flexion extensor maneuver themselves. Atypical hangman's fractures may require axial images from a CT scan to fully appreciate the direction and extent of the fracture lines. Finally, in type III injuries, a CT scan with reconstructions may be necessary to characterize the facet component of the injury.

Treat type I injuries nonoperatively with a rigid collar for 8 to 12 weeks. Late-onset degenerative arthritic changes can occur in up to 30% of patients because the initial injury causes severe impaction forces across the facet joint, which can be destructive to the articular cartilage. Patients with type I injuries do not go on to spontaneous ankyolsis across the C2–C3 disc, as is seen in type

II injuries. Treat type II injuries with significant amounts of displacement or angulation initially by reduction using skeletal traction in a slight amount of extension followed by a halo vest for 12 weeks. It is not uncommon for some reduction to be lost in the halo vest, but this loss of reduction usually does not lead to any long-term consequences. If the displacement is in the range of 6 to 7 mm, alignment is maintained with a period of 4 to 6 weeks in halo traction, followed by another 6 weeks in the halo vest. Alternatively, after reduction in traction a direct osteosynthesis of the fracture can be accomplished with a lag screw. Treat type IIA injuries with a halo vest placed in compression and extension. This is achieved by placing the halo vest on the patient in a routine fashion and then using the bolts on the uprights to compress the ring down toward the vest.

Type III fracture pattern injuries, in contrast, require immediate surgery. When this fracture pattern is identified, closed reduction should not even be attempted because it is rarely achieved and is potentially dangerous. Even if it is achieved, the remaining instability present is enough to warrant arthrodesis. A preoperative MRI is performed to evaluate the C2–C3 disc. The goal of surgical treatment is to stabilize the C2–C3 facet joint. This can be accomplished with a C2–C3 posterior plate with a C-2 pedicle screw and a lateral mass screw at C-3.

Reduction and Stabilization of a Type III Hangman's Fracture

- Carry out a fiberoptic, awake intubation and turn the patient prone on a Stryker frame. Check the patient's neurologic status and induce general anesthesia. Check lateral position on fluoroscopy or plain radiographs. High-quality biplanar flouroscopy is required to monitor the trajectory of the screws.

- Make a standard approach to the posterior cervical spine from the occiput down to C3–C4 level and expose the C2–C3 and C3–C4 facet joints. Use an elevator to dissect the medial aspect of the C-2 pedicle.

- The facet joint at C1–C2 does not need to be disrupted, but dissection from posterior to anterior toward the facet will usually demonstrate the fracture of the pedicle.

- Then carry out the reduction of the unilateral or bilateral facet dislocation at C2–C3. Place towel clips on the spinous processes of C-2 and C-3. Spread the spinous processes apart with a slight amount of flexion. This should unlock the jumped facets. Apply a posterior translation force to the C-2 spinous process as the towel clamps are brought together to achieve the final reduction.

- A bilateral subluxation is generally easier to reduce than a unilateral subluxation because of the increased ligamentous damage. Traction is not effective in this situation because the break in the pars of C-2 prevents any force from being transmitted to the C2–C3 joint level. Rarely, the C2–C3 facets need to be unlocked manually.

- Place a Freer or small Cobb elevator into the facet joint and gently elevate the C-2 facet until it becomes level with the C-3 facet. Then apply a posterior translation force to the towel clip on C-2 as the elevator is slowly removed to achieve reduction. After reduction is obtained, the C2–C3 joint must be stabilized. A standard interspinous process wiring or C2–C3 lateral mass plating can be used; however, the pedicle fracture would then be treated as a type II Hangman's fracture with 12 weeks in a halo vest.

- An alternative method of fixation is to insert a C-2 pedi-

cle screw to secure the pedicle fracture (Fig. 139.15*A* to *D*) (72). If this technique is used, a partially threaded lag screw must be placed so that the threads are beyond the fracture site to prevent any distraction.

- Before beginning screw insertion, take care that the fracture is as reduced as possible and that a #4 Penfield elevator can be placed along the medial border of the pedicle for guidance.

- Verify the trajectory of the pedicle and the location of the vertebral arteries on a preoperative CT scan. Palpate the medial wall and gently retract the epidural soft tissue medially. The fracture site and posterior body should be seen. Then pass a drill, starting at the center of the facet and directed along the pedicle into the body beyond the fracture site.

- Select a plate of the appropriate length and contour to fit the lateral masses of C-2 and C-3.

- Place a partially threaded screw through the plate across the pedicle fracture. The threads should be beyond the fracture site, and no distraction of the pedicle fracture should be observed.

- Place a standard C-3 lateral mass screw through the plate.

- A rigid collar for 12 weeks is needed for postoperative immobilization.

Surgery is warranted for the other types of fracture patterns only if there is an associated cervical fracture that requires fixation, if conservative treatment fails, or if the use of a halo is contraindicated. A C-2 pedicle screw (Fig. 139.15*A* to *D*) can be used and offers immediate stability to the fracture. The starting point for the screw is just medial to the C2–C3 facet joint on the inferior edge of the lamina. Check the starting point on a lateral fluoroscopic view. A preoperative CT scan is necessary to identify the angle of the pedicle and the location of the vertebral artery. Use a rigid collar for 8 weeks for postoperative immobilization. Anterior arthrodesis for this injury has also been used with mixed results (40,41,87).

The results of treatment are related to the injury type. For type I fractures, union rates approach 98%. Recognition of other associated injuries is important because these fractures can occur with posterior arch fractures or odontoid fractures. The result of these combined injuries follows that of the associated fracture. The most common long-term problem of type I fractures is arthritic degeneration of the C2–C3 facet joint, which occurs in approximately 10% of injuries. For type IA fractures, the results are related to the fracture pattern but generally are similar to type I fractures. For type II fractures, displacement of 5 mm or more between the anterior and posterior fragments yields a high incidence of nonunion, although more than 70% go on to develop anterior fusions of the disc space. Injuries with symptomatic nonunion and large gaps are generally not amenable to C-2 pedicle screw fixation and

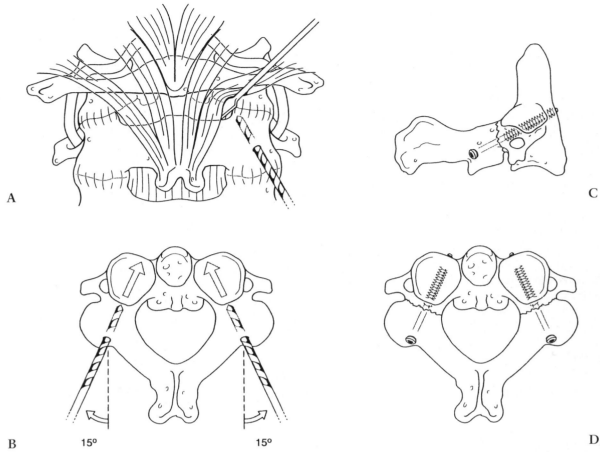

Figure 139.15.   **A:** The surgical technique for osteosynthesis of a traumatic spondylolisthesis of the axis. See the text for a description of the technique. **B:** Orientation of the drills along the pedicle in an axial plane. Slight convergence of the screws is desirable. **C:** Orientation across the fracture line from the posterior fracture to the anterior fragment. A partially threaded screw, with usually about 15 mm of thread and 20 mm of shank, is desirable. The proximal fragment can be overdrilled and lagged to the anterior fragment. **D:** The final axial view.

require an anterior C2–C3 fusion. The results of type III fractures depend on the severity of the commonly associated head injuries and neurologic deficits. The overall success rate of fusion after reduction is achieved is quite high.

Extension Teardrop Fractures   Although a number of different types of "teardrop fractures" have been described since the term was first used by Schneider and Kahn in 1956 (76) the two most common types are the flexion variant, which occurs in the lower cervical spine, and the extension type, which occurs predominantly in the upper cervical spine. The extension type of injury results from a hyperextension and axial loading mechanism and may be observed in combination with posterior arch fractures of the atlas and traumatic spondylolisthesis of the axis. The injury can be easily diagnosed on a lateral

roentgenogram of the cervical spine. The triangular fragment usually comprises approximately 50% of the height and 50% of the width of the body. The vertebral body of C-2 remains in normal alignment with the body of C-3, but the avulsed fragment is rotated anteriorly (Fig. 139.16). This is in contradistinction to flexion teardrop injuries, in which the fragment remains in relatively normal orientation to the bodies above and below and the affected body is rotated posteriorly.

These injuries are uniformly stable, although they may occur in combination with unstable contiguous injuries in the upper cervical spine. If they occur alone or in combination with a stable injury collar, immobilization is sufficient to achieve a satisfactory result. If they occur in combination with an unstable injury, the treatment of the second injury determines the overall treatment.

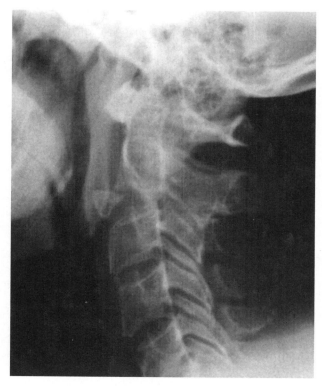

Figure 139.16. Extension teardrop fracture.

PITFALLS AND COMPLICATIONS

The most important aspect of the management of upper cervical spine fractures is diligent and thorough follow-up of the patients after treatment. Progressive deformities and neurologic deficits are more easily dealt with when recognized early. Union must always be verified with maximum flexion-extension radiographs after treatment.

Because the treatment of many of these fractures requires the use of a halo vest, take care in its proper placement and in follow-up. Complications include pin loosening, bone erosion, skull perforation, pin track infections, and cerebrospinal fluid leaks. If a circumferential collar is used, injury to the greater occipital nerve must be recognized because loss of sensation in this area can lead to occipital decubitus ulcers.

Although posterior wiring techniques are successful, the nonunion rates may be as high as 10%. Take care also with the passage of sublaminar wires because neurologic injuries have been reported. Mechanical testing has shown the transarticular screw to be more stable than wiring techniques. The procedure is difficult, but the early concerns of neurologic injury and the sequelae of perforation of one vertebral artery are not as formidable as they were previously thought to be. Clearly, if a vertebral artery injury does occur on one side, do not attempt screw placement on the other side for any reason. Screw malpositions have occurred in approximately 16% of cases, but complications attributable to this problem are rare (less than 2%) and include hypoglossal nerve irritation from excessive screw length, instability from the screws not crossing the joint, and screw breakage.

Anterior odontoid screws are extremely difficult to use and can cause spinal cord injury, cranial nerve injury, and loss of fixation. Other technical problems include incomplete fracture reduction with residual posterior angulation, incorrect screw entry site, and posterior screw angulation. Because of these problems, only experienced spine surgeons should use transarticular or anterior odontoid screws.

The occipitocervical fusion with plate and screws has added significant benefits to traditional wiring techniques. Complications are associated with the placement of the Magerl screw, as described previously. Leakage of CSF is not uncommon with the placement of bicortical occipital screws, but no persistent leaks or significant problems have been reported.

AUTHORS' PERSPECTIVE

Injuries of the upper cervical spine encompass a wide spectrum of not only fractures but also patterns of instability that result from ligamentous disruption. The most critical features of the treatment of these injuries are to appreciate the true nature of the instability and the pertinent regional anatomy. Injuries of the upper cervical spine have often been treated more aggressively than necessary (e.g., halo vest for a posterior arch fracture or a Type I hangman's fracture). Surgery is often not necessary if appropriate use of nonoperative modalities are employed.

More recently, however, innovative surgical techniques have appeared that have been applicable to the upper cervical spine injuries. The Magerl C1–C2 transarticular screw fixation has simplified fixation for several different types of injuries. However, the rationale for surgery has sometimes been the desire not to use a halo as the immobilization device. Clearly, the risks and benefits have to be discussed with the patient in an objective fashion before the final treatment decision is made. For example, elderly patients have been reported to have difficult times tolerating a halo as an immobilization device, and physicians have resorted to operative procedures that also have high rates of morbidity. For example, the use of an anterior dens screw in the elderly patient with a Type II fracture without neurologic deficit may have more morbidity than halo immobilization. More recent studies suggest that less rigid immobilization may yield acceptable patient outcomes without either the risks of surgery or a halo. Accurate assessment of the true significance of the injury and its effect on spine stability will ultimately yield the best patient outcomes.

REFERENCES

Each reference is categorized according to the following scheme: *, classic article; #, review article; !, basic research article; and +, clinical results/outcome study.

+ 1. Aebi M, Etter C, Cosica M. Fractures of the Dens: Treatment with Anterior Screw Fixation. *Spine* 1989;14:1065.

+ 2. Alker GH, Oh YS, Leslie FV, et al. Postmortem Radiology of Head and Neck Injuries in Fatal Traffic Accidents. *Radiology* 1975;114:611.

+ 3. Anderson LD, D'Alonzo RT. Fractures of the Odontoid Process of the Axis. *J Bone Joint Surg [Am]* 1974;56:1663.

+ 4. Anderson PA, Montesano PX. Morphology and Treatment of Occipital Condyle Fractures. *Spine* 1988;13:731.

+ 5. Apple JS, Kirks DR, Merten DF, et al. Cervical Spine Fractures and Dislocations in Children. *Pediatr Radiol* 1987;17:45.

+ 6. Apuzzo MLJ, Heiden JS, Weiss MH, et al. Acute Fractures of the Odontoid Process: An Analysis of 45 Cases. *J Neurosurg* 1978;48:85.

+ 7. Berkheiser EJ, Seidler F. Nontraumatic Dislocations of the Atlantoaxial Joint. *JAMA* 1931;96:517.

+ 8. Böhler J: Anterior stabilization for acute fractures and non-unions of the dens. J. Bone Joint Surg Am 64:18, 1982.

+ 9. Botte MJ, Byrne TP, Garfin SR. Application of the Halo Fixation Device Using an Increased Torque Pressure. *J Bone Joint Surg [Am]* 1987;69:750.

+ 10. Botte MJ, Byrne, TP, Garfin SR. Use of Skin Incisions in the Application of Halo Skeletal Fixator Pins. *Clin Orthop* 1989;246:100.

+ 11. Bracken MB, Shepard MJ, Holford PR, et al. Administration of Methylprednisolone for 24 or 48 Hours or Tirilizad Mesylate for 48 Hours in the Treatment of Acute Spinal Cord Injuries: Results of the Third National Acute Spinal Cord Injury Randomized Controlled Study—National Acute Spinal Cord Injury Study. *JAMA* 1997;277:1597.

+ 12. Brooks A, Jenkins E. Atlantoaxial Arthrodesis by the Wedge-compression Method. *J Bone Joint Surg [Am]* 1978;60:279.

+ 13. Bucholz RW, Burkhead WZ. The Pathological Anatomy of Fatal Atlanto-occipital Dislocations. *J Bone Joint Surg [Am]* 1979;61:248.

+ 14. Clark CR, White AA. Fractures of the Dens. *J Bone Joint Surg [Am]* 1985;67:1340.

+ 15. Clyburn TA, Lionberger DR, Tullos HS. Bilateral Fracture of the Transverse Process of the Atlas. *J Bone Joint Surg [Am]* 1982;64:948.

+ 16. Crisco JJ III, Oda T, Panjabi MM, et al. Transections of the C1-C2 Joint Capsular Ligaments in the Cadaveric Spine. *Spine* 1991;16(Suppl):S474.

+ 17. Davis D, Bohlman H, Walker AE, et al. The Pathological Findings in Fatal Craniospinal Injuries. *J Neurosurg* 1971;34:603.

+ 18. Dickman CA, Mamourian A, Sonntag VKH, et al. Magnetic Resonance Imaging of the Transverse Atlantal Ligament for the Evaluation of Atlantoaxial Instability. *J Neurosurg* 1991;75:221.

+ 19. Dunn ME, Seljeskog EL. Experience in the Management of Odontoid Process Injuries: An Analysis of 128 Cases. *Neurosurgery* 1986;18:306.

+ 20. Dvorak J, Hayek J, Zehnder R. CT-functional Diagnostics of the Rotatory Instability of the Upper Cervical Spine: II. An Evaluation on Healthy Adults and Patients with Suspected Instability. *Spine* 1987;12:726.

! 21. Dvorak J, Panjabi M, Gerber M, et al. CT-functional Diagnostics of the Rotatory Instability of the Upper Cervical Spine: I. An Experimental Study on Cadavers. *Spine* 1987;12:197.

! 22. Dvorak J, Panjabi M. Functional Anatomy of the Alar Ligaments. *Spine* 1987;12:183.

! 23. Dvorak J, Schneider E, Saldinger P, et al. Biomechanics of the Craniocervical Region: The Alar and Transverse Ligaments. *J Orthop Res* 1988;6:452.

! 24. Ebraheim NA, Lu J, Bijani A, et al. An Anatomic Study of the Thickness of the Occipital Bone: Implications for Occipitocervical Instrumentation. *Spine* 1996;21:1725.

+ 25. Effendi B, Roy D, Cornish B, et al. Fractures of the Ring of the Axis: A Classification Based on the Analysis of 131 Cases. *J Bone Joint Surg [Br]* 1981;63:319.

+ 26. Eismont FJ, Bohlman HH. Posterior Atlanto-occipital Dislocation with Fractures of the Atlas and Odontoid Process. *J Bone Joint Surg [Am]* 1978;60:397.

+ 27. Ersmark H, Kalen R. Injuries of the Atlas and Axis: A Follow-up Study of 85 Axis and 10 Atlas Fractures. *Clin Orthop* 1987;217:257.

+ 28. Etter C, Coscia M, Jaberg H, et al. Direct Anterior Fixation of Dens Fractures with a Cannulated Screw System. *Spine* 1991;16(Suppl 3):S25.

* 29. Fielding JW, Cochran GVB, Lawsing JF, et al. Tears of the Transverse Ligament of the Atlas. *J Bone Joint Surg [Am]* 1974;56:1683.

* 30. Fielding JW, Hawkins RJ, Ratzan SA. Spine Fusion for Atlantoaxial Instability. *J Bone Joint Surg [Am]* 1976;58:400.

* 31. Fielding JW, Hawkins RJ. Atlantoaxial Rotatory Fixation. *J Bone Joint Surg [Am]* 1977;59:37.

32. Fielding JW, Hawkins RJ. Roentgenographic Diagnosis of the Injured Neck. *Instruct Course Lect* 1976;25:149.

+ 33. Fielding JW, Stillwell WT, Chynn KY, et al. Use of Computed Tomography for the Diagnosis of Atlantoaxial Rotatory Fixation. *J Bone Joint Surg [Am]* 1978;60:1102.

+ 34. Francis WR, Fielding, JW, Hawkins RJ, et al. Traumatic Spondylolisthesis of the Axis. *J Bone Joint Surg [Br]* 1981;63:313.

* 35. Gallie W. Fractures and Dislocations of the Cervical Spine. *Am J Surg* 1939;46:495.

! 36. Garfin SR, Botte MJ, Centeno RS, et al. Osteology of the Skull as it Affects Halo Pin Placement. *Spine* 1985; 10:696.

! 37. Goel VK, Winterbottom JM, Schulte KR, et al. Ligamentous Laxity Across C0-C1-C2 Complex: Axial-torque Rotation Characteristics Until Failure. *Spine* 1990;15:990.

+ 38. Grob D, Dvorak J, Panjabi MM, et al. Posterior Occipitocervical Fusion: A Preliminary Report of a New Technique. *Spine* 1991;16:17.

+ 39. Grob D, Dvorak J, Panjabi MM, et al. The Role of Plate and Screw Fixation in Occipitocervical Fusion in Rheumatoid Arthritis. *Spine* 1994;19:2545.

+ 40. Hadley MN, Browner C, Sonntag VKH: Axis Fractures: A Comprehensive Review of Management and Treatment in 107 Cases. *Neurosurgery* 1985;17:281.

+ 41. Hadley MN, Dickman CA, Browner CM, et al. Acute Axis Fractures: A Review of 229 Cases. *J Neurosurg* 1989;71:642.

+ 42. Han SY, Witten DM, Mussleman JP. Jefferson Fracture of the Atlas. *J Neurosurg* 1976;44:368.

+ 43. Hays MB, Alker GJ. Fractures of the Atlas Vertebra: The Two-part Burst Fracture of Jefferson. *Spine* 1988;13:601.

! 44. Heller JG, Alson MD, Schafler MB, et al. Quantitative Internal Dens Morphology. *Spine* 1992;17:861.

45. Jarrett PJ, Whitesides TE Jr. Injuries of the Cervicocranium. In Browner BD, Jupiter JB, Levine AM, et al, eds. *Skeletal Trauma: Fractures, Dislocations, Ligamentous Injuries,* Vol 1. Philadelphia: WB Saunders Co., 1992:668.

+ 46. Jeanneret B, Magerl F. Primary Posterior Fusion of Cl-2 in Odontoid Fractures: Indications Technique, and Results of Transarticular Screw Fixation. *J Spinal Disord* 1992;5:464.

+ 47. Jeanneret B, Vernet O, Frei S, Magerl F: Atlantoaxial Mobility after Screw Fixation of the Odontoid: A Computed Tomographic Study. *J Spinal Disord* 1991;4:203.

* 48. Jefferson G. Fracture of the Atlas Vertebra. *Br J Surg* 1920;7:407.

* 49. Jefferson G. Fractures of the First Cervical Vertebra. *Br Med J* 1927;July 30:153.

+ 50. Kowalski HM, Cohen WA, Cooper P, et al. Pitfalls in the CT Diagnosis of Atlantoaxial Rotary Subluxation. *AJR* 1987;149:595.

+ 51. Lee C, Woodring JH, Goldstein SJ, et al. Evaluation of Traumatic Atlanto-occipital Dislocations. *Am J Neuroradiol* 1987;8:19.

+ 52. Lee S, Joyce S, Seeger J. Asymmetry of the Odontoid-lateral Mass Interspaces: A Radiographic Finding of Questionable Clinical Significance. *Ann Emerg Med* 1986;15:1173.

+ 53. Lesoin F, Blondel M, Dhellemmes P, et al. Post-traumatic Atlanto-occipital Dislocation Revealed by Sudden Cardiorespiratory Arrest. *Lancet* 1982;2:447.

+ 54. Leventhal MR, Maguire JK Jr, Christian CA. Atlantoaxial Rotary Subluxation in Ankylosing Spondylitis: A Case Report. *Spine* 1990;15:1374.

+ 55. Levine AM, Edwards CC. Fractures of the Atlas. *J Bone Joint Surg [Am]* 1991;73:680.

+ 56. Levine AM, Edwards CC. The Management of Traumatic Spondylolisthesis of the Axis. *J Bone Joint Surg [Am]* 1985;67:217.

57. Levine AM, Edwards CC. Treatment of Injuries in the Cl-C2 Complex. *Orthop Clin North Am* 1986;17:31.

+ 58. Lipson SJ. Fractures of the Atlas Associated with Fracture of the Odontoid Process and Transverse Ligament Ruptures. *J Bone Joint Surg [Am]* 1977;59:940.

* 59. Magerl F, Seemann PS. Stable Posterior Fusion of the Atlas and Axis by Transarticular Screw Fixation. In: Kehr P, Weidner A, eds. *Cervical Spine.* Berlin: Springer-Verlag, 1986:322.

+ 60. Maiman DJ, Larson SJ. Management of Odontoid Fractures. *Neurosurgery* 1982;11:471.

+ 61. Martel W. The Occipito-atlantoaxial Joints in Rheumatoid Arthritis and Ankylosing Spondylitis. *AJR* 1961;86:223.

62. McGuire RA, Harkey HL. Unstable Jefferson's Fracture Treated with Transarticular Screws. *Orthopedics* 1995;18:207.

+ 63. Ono K, Yonenobu K, Fuji T, et al. Atlantoaxial Rotatory Fixation: Radiographic Study of its Mechanism. *Spine* 1985;10:602.

! 64. Panjabi M, Dvorak J, Duranceau J, et al. Three Dimensional Movements of the Upper Cervical Spine. *Spine* 1988;13:726.

+ 65. Paramore CG, Dickman CA, Sonntag V. The Anatomic Suitability of the C1-C2 Complex for Transarticular Screw Fixation. *J Neurosurg* 1996;85:221.

+ 66. Parke WW. The Vascular Relations of the Upper Cervical Vertebrae. *Orthop Clin North Am* 1978;9:879.

! 67. Paul LW, Moir WW. Non-pathologic Variations in Relationship of the Upper Cervical Vertebrae. *AJR* 1949;62:519.

+ 68. Penning L. Paravertebral Hematoma in Cervical Spine Injury: Incidence and Etiologic Significance. *AJR* 1981;136:553.

! 69. Penning L, Wilmink JT. Rotation of the Cervical Spine. A CT Study in Normal Subjects. *Spine* 1987;12:732.

+ 70. Phillips WA, Hensinger RN. The Management of Rotatory Atlantoaxial Subluxation in Children. *J Bone Joint Surg [Am]* 1989;71:664.

+ 71. Powers B, Miller MD, Kramer RS, et al. Traumatic Anterior Atlanto-occipital Dislocation. *Neurosurgery* 1979;41:12.

+ 72. Roy-Camille R, Saillant G, Bouchet T. Technique du Vissage des Pedicules de C2. In: Roy-Camille R, ed. *Cinquiemes Journees d'Orthopedie de la Pitie, Rachis Cervical Superieur.* Paris: Masson, 1986:41.

+ 73. Sakou T, Kawaida H, Morizino Y, et al. Occipitoatlantoaxial Fusion Utilizing a Rectangular Rod. *Clin Orthop* 1989;239:136.

! 74. Schaffler MB, Alson MB, Heller JG, et al. Morphology of the Dens: A Quantitative Study. *Spine* 1992;17:738.

+ 75. Schlicke LH. A Rational Approach to Burst Fractures of the Atlas. *Clin Orthop* 1981;154:18.

+ 76. Schneider RC, Kahn EA. Chronic Neurological Sequelae of Acute Trauma to the Spine and Spinal Cord, Part I: The Significance of the Acute Flexion or "Teardrop"

Fracture Dislocation of the Cervical Spine. *J Bone Joint Surg [Am]* 1956;28A:985.

+ 77. Segal LS, Grimm JO, Stauffer ES. Non-union of Fractures of the Atlas. *J Bone Joint Surg [Am]* 1987;69:1423.

+ 78. Shkrum MJ, Green RN, Nowak ES. Upper Cervical Trauma in Motor Vehicle Collisions. *J Forensic Sci* 1989; 34:381.

+ 79. Sonntag VK, Dickman CA. Craniocervical Stabilization. *Clin Neurosurg* 1993;40:243.

+ 80. Spence KF, Decker S, Sell KW. Bursting Atlantal Fracture Associated with Rupture of the Transverse Ligament. *J Bone Joint Surg [Am]* 1970;52:543.

+ 81. Starr JK, Eismont FJ. Atypical Hangman's Fractures. *Spine* 1993;18:1954.

! 82. Steel HH. Anatomical and Mechanical Considerations of the Atlantoaxial Articulations. *J Bone Joint Surg [Am]* 1968;50:1481.

+ 83. Stewart GC Jr, Gehweiler JA Jr, Laib RH, et al. Horizontal Fracture of the Anterior Arch of the Atlas. *Radiology* 1977;122:349.

* 84. Sudeck P. Torsion Dislocation of Atlas. *Dtsch Z Chir* 1924;183:289.

+ 85. Templeton PA, Young JWR, Mirvis S, et al. The Value of Retropharyngeal Soft Tissue Measurements in Trauma of the Adult Cervical Spine. *Skeletal Radiol* 1987;30:1.

+ 86. Traynelis VC, Marano GD, Dunker RO, et al. Traumatic Atlanto-occipital Dislocation. *J Neurosurg* 1986;65: 863.

+ 87. Tuite GF, Papadopoulos MD, Sonntag VK. Caspar Plate Fixation for the Treatment of Complex Hangman's Fractures. *Neurosurgery* 1992;30:761.

+ 88. Wang G-J, Mabie KN, Whitehill R, et al. Nonsurgical Management of Odontoid Fractures in Adults. *Spine* 1984;9:229.

+ 89. Werne S. Studies in Spontaneous Atlas Dislocation. *Acta Orthop Scand* 1957;23(Suppl):1.

+ 90. Wertheim SB, Bohlman HH. Occipito-cervical Fusion. Indications, Techniques, and Results in 13 patient. *J Bone Joint Surg [Am]* 1987;69:833.

+ 91. Wetzel FT, La Rocca H. Grisel's Syndrome: A Review. *Clin Orthop* 1989;240:141.

92. White AA III, Panjabi MM. *Clinical Biomechanics of the Spine*. Philadelphia: JB Lippincott, 1991.

+ 93. White GM, Healy WI. Tumor-associated Atlantoaxial Rotatory Fixation: A Case Report. *Spine* 1987;12:406.

+ 94. Zimmerman E, Grant J, Vise WM, et al. Treatment of Jefferson Fracture with a Halo Apparatus. *J Neurosurg* 1976;44:372.

CHAPTER 140

FRACTURES AND DISLOCATIONS OF THE CERVICAL SPINE FROM C-3 TO C-7

Michael J. Goebel, Charles Carroll, IV, and Paul C. McAfee

Traumatic injuries to the cervical spine, a common cause of death and disability, range in severity from simple soft-tissue injuries to severe fractures or dislocations with paralysis or death. Cervical spine injuries are often first detected in the emergency room and must be carefully evaluated and managed to minimize adverse sequelae. Early diagnosis, immobilization, preservation or restoration of spinal cord function, and stabilization are the keys to successful management of these injuries.

As many as one third of all cervical spine injuries result from motor vehicle accidents, one third from falls, and the remainder from athletic injuries, falling objects, or fired projectiles (9). Most injuries occur to young and active persons in adolescence or early adulthood. The second-largest group comprises adults in their sixth or seventh decades. In this age group, preexisting spondylosis or stenosis may predispose these patients to severe injuries despite a relatively small amount of force being imparted to the cervical spine.

M. J. Goebel: Blue Ridge Bone and Joint, Asheville, North Carolina, 28801.
C. Carroll, IV: Department of Clinical Orthopaedic Surgery, Northwestern University Medical School, Chicago, Illinois, 60611.
P. C. McAfee: Division of Spinal Surgery, St. Joseph's Hospital, Baltimore, Maryland, 21204.

The formation of spinal cord injury centers has allowed progress in emergency care, medical and surgical intervention, and rehabilitation of the patient who has sustained a spine and/or spinal cord injury. A team approach is important to obtain optimal results. The therapeutic goals are to preserve life, maintain or restore neurologic function, provide stabilization of the cervical spine, and allow optimal rehabilitation. These goals are attainable if appropriate care is provided.

PRINCIPLES OF TREATMENT

INITIAL CARE

Care for a patient with a suspected cervical spine injury begins at the scene of the accident. Carefully move the patient to safety and then immobilize her on a long backboard and apply a rigid cervical collar. Stabilize the head by placing sandbags along each side or use tape to secure the forehead to the board. Paramedics or other emergency management team members often perform the initial assessment and resuscitation.

On arrival to the emergency department, continue resuscitation. Follow advanced trauma life support (ATLS) guidelines. If an airway needs to be secured, take care to prevent further cervical injury by utilizing fiberoptic nasotracheal intubation whenever possible. This technique minimizes movement of the injured cervical spine. Intravenous access is mandatory for fluid resuscitation in cases of neurogenic shock.

Obtain a history from the patient, the paramedics, or witnesses to determine the mechanism of injury and the circumstances surrounding the accident. A history of loss of consciousness is important, as the patient may not be able to accurately recall the events as they occurred. In addition, there is a high correlation between head trauma and cervical spine injuries. Make note of the initial neurologic assessment, with attention to any paralysis.

While the history is being obtained, perform a physical exam. The observation of craniofacial trauma can be important in the assessment of the mechanism of injury. If the patient is conscious, gently palpate the anterior and posterior cervical spine to determine the site of pain or swelling. Palpate the posterior elements in the midline posteriorly, noting any increase in the interspinous distance. Palpate the anterior vertebral bodies in the interval between the sternocleidomastoid and the trachea.

Perform a detailed neurologic examination. Note the general state of consciousness as well as respiratory status. The C-3 to C-5 levels innervate the diaphragm. Cord injury above the C-5 level may lead to respiratory failure. If the patient is conscious, perform motor, sensory, and reflex examination of the upper and lower extremities. The American Spine Injury Association (ASIA) spinal cord injury assessment form (Fig. 140.1) provides an excellent checklist to ensure completeness. Use rectal tone and perianal sensation to assess for the presence of sacral sparing. Document the absence or presence of the bulbocavernosis reflex for the determination of spinal shock.

In Bohlman's evaluation of 300 cervical spine injuries, 100 were initially missed at the time of presentation (7). Delay in diagnosis ranged from 1 day to 1 year. The common causes for lack of recognition were concomitant closed head injuries, multiple traumatic injuries, alcohol intoxication, and initial misdiagnosis such as cerebrovascular accidents. An alteration in consciousness contributed to the lack of proper evaluation and failure to take appropriate radiographs. Patients with these injuries often do not complain of pain, and facial and neck lacerations may detract from the evaluation of the cervical spine. Nevertheless, the physician always must suspect a cervical spine injury any time there is associated head trauma (7, 18).

RADIOGRAPHIC EVALUATION

As part of the initial trauma assessment, obtain the lateral view of the cervical spine, anteroposterior (AP) view of the chest, and AP view of the pelvis. Approximately 80% of cervical spine fractures can be diagnosed on the initial lateral view if it is adequately done (49,53). Once the patient is stabilized, complete the remaining views of the cervical spine trauma series. This includes the AP, openmouth odontoid, and bilateral obliques or pillar views. The lateral view must extend to the C7–T1 level to be considered complete (7,36). A swimmer's view may be required to visualize the C7–T1 level in patients with short necks. If visualization still remains questionable, perform a computed tomography (CT) scan (59).

Scrutinize all radiographs carefully for abnormal alignment or fractures. The presence of retropharyngeal softtissue swelling is important and may indicate adjacent fractures or ligamentous injuries (20). Loss of facet parallelism, facet overlap, or widening of the distance between adjacent vertebrae may also indicate ligamentous injury. If abnormalities are noted, a CT scan is helpful in defining the compromised structures and the presence of bone or disc fragments within the spinal canal. Ligamentous injuries are best visualized by magnetic resonance imaging (MRI) performed within the first 72 hours (23,45).

ANATOMY

The vertebrae from C-3 to C-7 are anatomically similar. Little inherent stability is achieved from the interrelationships of the osseous structures, and therefore the integrity of the supporting ligaments is very important (34,40). The anterior and posterior longitudinal ligaments span the length of this region and are firmly adherent to the annulus

STANDARD NEUROLOGICAL CLASSIFICATION OF SPINAL CORD INJURY

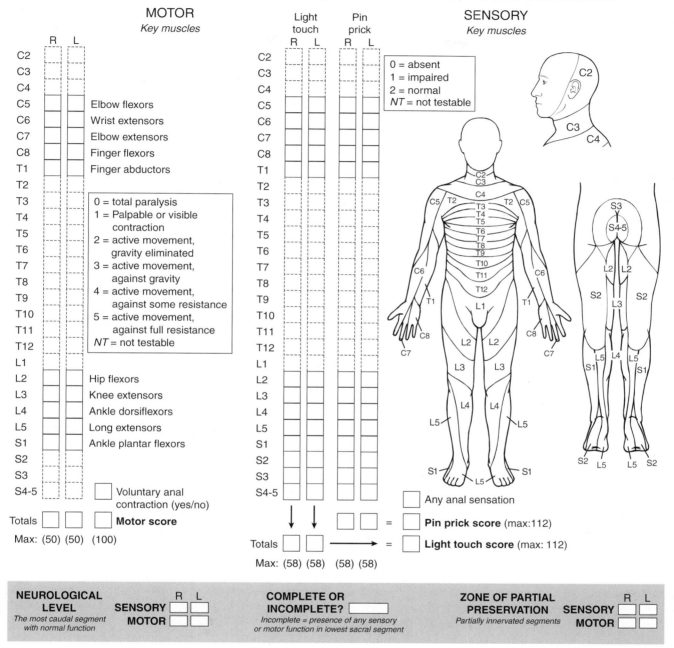

Figure 140.1. American Spine Injury Association (ASIA) spinal cord injury assessment form. (Redrawn with permission from the American Spine Injury Association. *Standard Neurological Classification of Spinal Cord Injury*, revised. Chicago: American Spine Injury Association, 1992.)

fibrosis at each level. These ligaments, along with the annulus, are the primary stabilizers of the anterior column. Posteriorly, the interspinous, supraspinous, and facet joint capsules comprise the primary ligamentous stabilizers. The ligamentum flavum becomes important at the extremes of motion (56).

The anterior structures, including the anterior longitudinal ligament and the annulus fibrosis, act as a tension band during extension. Similarly, the posterior longitudinal ligament, supraspinous and interspinous ligaments, and facet capsules act as a tension band in flexion (57). Flexion compresses the anterior column and tensions the posterior column, whereas extension tensions the anterior column and compresses the posterior column. Thus, the anterior and posterior columns are reciprocally affected by sagittal plane motion (27).

Approximately 50% of the flexion and extension arc of the cervical spine is achieved through the occipital cervical articulation. The remainder occurs through the lower cervical vertebrae, ranging from 8° to 17° at each motion segment. Rotation is equally shared between the atlantoaxial joint and the lower cervical vertebrae. Lateral bending in the subaxial region ranges from 4° to 11° at each segment (58).

CLASSIFICATION

The most widely used classification system of lower cervical spine injuries was published by Allen et al. in 1982 (3). In a retrospective review of 165 cases of lower cervical spine injury, they developed a mechanistic system of classifying closed indirect fractures and dislocations.

Injuries are divided into six groups, each named according to the dominant force vector leading to failure and the position of the cervical spine at the time of injury (Fig. 140.2). The groups include compressive flexion, vertical compression, distractive flexion, compressive extension, distractive extension, and lateral flexion. The three most common groups are compressive flexion, distractive flexion, and compressive extension. The least common are distractive extension and lateral flexion, with vertical compression falling between. *Compressive* indicates that compression accounts for the initial structural failure in a motion segment, whereas *distractive* indicates that tension is the dominant force. The use of *flexion* or *extension* denotes the position of the cervical spine at the time of injury (3).

Each group is then classified into various stages, with the higher stages reflecting a greater degree of instability (3). Although the degree of neurologic injury cannot be correlated with the staging, the risk of injury is certainly greater in the advanced stages.

Compressive Flexion
Five stages are recognized in the compressive flexion (CF) group. The force vector is directed anteriorly and inferi-

orly. In CFS1 injuries, mild blunting of the anterior-superior vertebral body is noted, caused by impression of the more superior vertebrae. In CFS2, the anterior vertebral body loses additional height and becomes wedged, but still without disruption of the posterior ligamentous structures. In CFS3, a fracture line passes obliquely from the anterior vertebral surface to the inferior endplate without displacement. CSF4 injuries have subluxation and displacement of the posterior vertebral wall into the spinal canal, but not exceeding 3 mm. CFS5 injuries involve severe displacement of the body fragment into the canal, as well as increased interspinous distance, facet subluxation, and posterior longitudinal ligament disruption (3).

CFS1 and CFS2 injuries are usually stable and can be treated nonoperatively (47). CFS3–5 injuries may be unstable, and operative intervention may be required to limit late instability (12,13).

Distractive Flexion
Four stages are recognized within the distractive flexion (DF) group. The force vector is directed anteriorly, away from the trunk, with the neck flexed. In DFS1 injuries, posterior ligamentous disruption with facet subluxation and increased interspinous distance is noted. DFS2 represents a unilateral facet dislocation and DFS3 a bilateral facet dislocation. In DFS4, the superior vertebral body is displaced anteriorly, the full width of the body, creating a "floating" vertebra (3).

All distractive flexion injuries should be considered potentially unstable, although DFS1 injuries can commonly be treated nonoperatively. DFS2–4 commonly require operative intervention to prevent late instability (5,7,22,44).

Compressive Extension
Five stages are recognized in the compressive extension (CE) group, although the distinction between the latter stages remains unclear. Unilateral vertebral arch fracture with or without displacement is found in CES1 injuries. Bilateral involvement distinguishes CES2. In CES3–5, comminution of the lamina and lateral masses occurs with vertebral or disc space separation. In CES5, complete anterior displacement of the superior vertebral body is noted (3).

CES1 and some CES2 injuries may be treated nonoperatively. However, the higher stages, especially CES5, usually require operative stabilization.

Vertical Compression
Three stages are recognized in the vertical compression (VC) group, in which the force vector is axial. In VCS1 injuries, a fracture occurs through either the superior or the inferior endplate. VCS2 involves a fracture through both endplates, but with minimal displacement. In VCS3, further compression causes the fracture fragments to displace peripherally, possibly through a tear of the posterior longitudinal ligament (3).

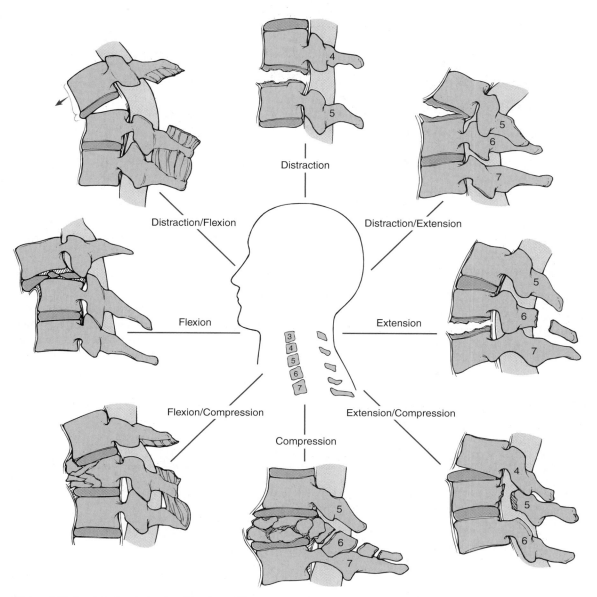

Figure 140.2. Mechanistic classification of lower cervical spine injury. (Modified from Allen BL, Ferguson RL, Lehmann TR, O'Brien RP. A Mechanistic Classification of Closed, Indirect Fractures and Dislocations of the Lower Cervical Spine. *Spine* 1982;7:1, with permission.)

The majority of these injuries have a high rate of healing when treated nonoperatively. However, VC3 injuries with canal compromise require operative decompression and stabilization (1,2).

Distractive Extension

Two stages are identified in the distractive extension (DE) group, in which the force vector is directed posteriorly, away from the trunk, with the head in extension. DES1 injuries involve either a transverse fracture through the vertebral body or disruption of the anterior ligamentous complex. DES2 consists of failure of the posterior ligamentous structures with displacement of the superior vertebral body into the canal (3).

DES1 injuries involving fracture of the vertebrae often heal nonoperatively without deformity. DES2 injuries, however, often require operative intervention.

Lateral Flexion

Two stages are identified in the lateral flexion (LF) group, in which the force vector is directed laterally. In LFS1 injuries, an ipsilateral vertebral body fracture and neural arch fracture are noted, without displacement. LFS2 progresses to displacement (3). Treatment depends on the extent of the injury, but most LFS1 injuries may be treated nonoperatively.

CRITERIA FOR INSTABILITY

White and Panjabi (55) have defined clinical instability as the "loss of the ability of the spine under physiologic loads to maintain relationships between vertebrae in such a way that there is neither initial nor subsequent damage to the spinal cord or nerve roots, and in addition, there is neither development of incapacitating deformity nor severe pain." In this definition, physiologic loads are those incurred during normal daily activity. Incapacitating deformity is defined as gross deformity that the patient finds intolerable. Severe pain is that which cannot be controlled by nonnarcotic medications.

In an effort to systemize this evaluation of clinical instability, White et al. (58) devised a checklist, incorporating both clinical and radiographic parameters. Radiographic parameters for ligamentous instability were established through biomechanical studies. Using fresh cadaveric specimens, serial sectioning of the posterior and anterior ligamentous structures was performed. Abnormal motion of the adjacent vertebrae was then measured. In an otherwise intact spine, instability was defined as translatory displacement of two adjacent vertebrae greater than 3.5 mm, or angulation greater than 11° compared with adjacent motion segments. Based on these and other results, a comprehensive checklist was developed for assessing traumatic instability.

According to this checklist, both clinical and radiographic findings are assigned point values. Assign two points each for anterior elements destroyed or unable to function, posterior elements destroyed or unable to function, relative sagittal plane translation greater than 3.5 mm, relative sagittal plane rotation greater than 11°, positive stretch test, or spinal cord damage. Assign one point each for nerve root damage, abnormal disc space narrowing, or dangerous loading anticipated. If the total point value is equal to or greater than five, assume instability of the motion segment (54).

Although checklists may be useful in the systematic determination of spinal instability, each case should be assessed individually; the importance of certain criteria may vary depending on the specific situation. Of prime importance is spinal cord integrity. When spinal cord injury is caused by extruded bone fragments, or deformity resulting from ligamentous disruption, assume instability. Evidence of isolated nerve root compromise is a weaker indicator of instability.

The stretch test can be particularly useful for evaluating the integrity of the ligamentous structures of the middle and lower cervical spine. This test is performed as follows:

- Apply traction through the use of secure skeletal fixation or a head halter device.
- To reduce frictional forces, place a roller under the patient's head.
- Place the radiographic plate 14 inches from the patient's spine and the tube 72 inches from the plate.
- Take an initial radiograph to ensure no occiput to C-1 to C-2 subluxation.
- Add a 10-pound weight and obtain a lateral radiograph.
- Repeat this process, increasing the traction by 10-pound increments until reaching one third of the body weight, or 65 pounds, whichever is less.
- After each additional weight application, check the patient for any change in neurologic status. If there is a change in status, stop the test. The test is then considered to be positive.

Radiographs are evaluated for any abnormal separation of the anterior or posterior elements. An abnormal test is indicated by differences either greater than 1.7 mm of interspace separation or 7.5° of change in the angle between vertebrae (35). An interval of at least 5 minutes should be allowed between incremental weight applications to allow for creep of the viscoelastic structures. The test is contraindicated in a spine with obvious clinical or radiographic instability.

INDICATIONS FOR TREATMENT

Management of lower cervical spine injuries must proceed in an orderly fashion to minimize morbidity and mortality. At the time of initial evaluation and resuscitation, immobilize the injured spine as medical stabilization is implemented. Assess spinal alignment and correct it if necessary. Perform operative decompression if indicated and consider the long-term stability of the injured spine. If the injured segment or multiple segments are unstable, operative stabilization is necessary.

If significant malalignment is noted on initial radiographs, realignment is indicated to relieve any pressure on the neural elements, limiting ischemia and edema formation. Exactly what constitutes significant malalignment is debatable; however, sagittal translation greater than 3.5 mm or angulation greater than 11° would seem reasonable. In addition, realignment or traction would also be indicated in injuries in which extruded bone or disc fragments were contributing to spinal cord or nerve root compromise, even though no significant angulation or translation were present. Reduction can usually be established by skeletal traction with tongs in the skull (16).

- After the tongs are applied in a sterile fashion, apply an initial weight of 10 pounds of traction with appropriate analgesia.

- Perform a detailed neurologic examination and obtain a lateral radiograph.
- Perform careful evaluation of the occiput to C-1 to C-2 levels to ensure no concomitant injury to this region.
- If reduction is not achieved, add weight in 5-pound increments and repeat the process each time.
- Once reduction is obtained, reduce the weight to 15–20 pounds and obtain a repeat radiograph to confirm maintenance of reduction.
- Continue traction until a definitive treatment plan is chosen.

If closed treatment with traction of up to two thirds of body weight or 65 pounds (whichever is less) is unable to achieve adequate reduction, operative intervention is usually required. In cases of facet dislocation, closed manipulative reduction may be an option when traction alone fails to reduce the dislocation. This should be performed only by surgeons experienced in these techniques to minimize the risk of, or exaggeration of, neurologic injury.

Cervical vertebral body dislocations are associated with substantial disruption of the anterior and posterior ligamentous structures and clinical instability. Patients who are undergoing realignment in traction must be constantly monitored and examined to prevent iatrogenic injury to the neural elements resulting from excessive stretching across injured segments. Traction weights should begin at 5 pounds and progress cautiously in order to ensure that overdistraction does not occur.

INDICATIONS FOR NONOPERATIVE TREATMENT

In patients with no compression of the neural elements and in whom the stability of the spine has not been jeopardized, a course of bracing in a rigid orthosis for 6–12 weeks may be appropriate. Injuries included in this category are mild compression fractures of the anterior elements and isolated fractures of the posterior elements or lateral masses. Mild vertical compression fractures may require halo immobilization. Follow-up radiographs must be obtained at regular intervals to assess healing. If instability is noted on follow-up radiographs, operative intervention is required.

INDICATIONS FOR URGENT OPERATIVE INTERVENTION

In general, early operative intervention for lower cervical spine injuries is indicated in all cases for which decompression is necessary to restore or preserve spinal cord func-

tion, and if stabilization is required to prevent further cord or root injury (8,42). Schneider et al. (43) formulated their criteria for urgent operative intervention in patients who had sustained cervical spinal cord injuries. The criteria they deemed important included documented progression of neurologic signs and complete block of the subarachnoid space on myelography. Cooper and Ransohoff (15) included any myelographic evidence of spinal cord compression by hematoma or by bone or disc elements after alignment had been optimized.

Urgent operative intervention is not indicated in a patient with a complete neurologic deficit with loss of motor function distal to the injured segment. Such a patient is unlikely to achieve functional recovery, and operative intervention to stabilize the spinal column may be delayed until he is medically stable. However, urgent decompression of compromised nerve roots may be required in some such patients to preserve an additional neurologic level. Urgent stabilization of the spinal column may also be necessary to facilitate the treatment of other system injuries.

 ## SURGICAL TECHNIQUES

When operative intervention is required, the choice of the procedure depends on the nature of the injury and the goals of the surgeon. In general, approach the fracture from the site of major instability (47,51,55). If the injury involves the anterior longitudinal ligament, vertebral body, or disc, an anterior approach is most appropriate. If there is posterior ligamentous involvement or posterior element fractures, a posterior approach is preferred. Sometimes, combined anterior and posterior approaches are required (17). Perform a stabilization procedure at the site of decompression.

POSTERIOR INSTRUMENTATION OPTIONS

The two most common posterior stabilization methods use posterior cervical wires or cables and lateral mass plates. In recent years, multistrand stainless steel or titanium cables have replaced traditional stainless steel wires. Multiple studies have shown that cables are stronger, more flexible, and more fatigue resistant than wires (19, 28,46). However, the cables are also more expensive. In addition, the added bulk of the crimping device may detract from its use in certain situations. Most posterior wiring techniques require intact posterior arches and spinous processes across the levels to be fused. To provide suffi-

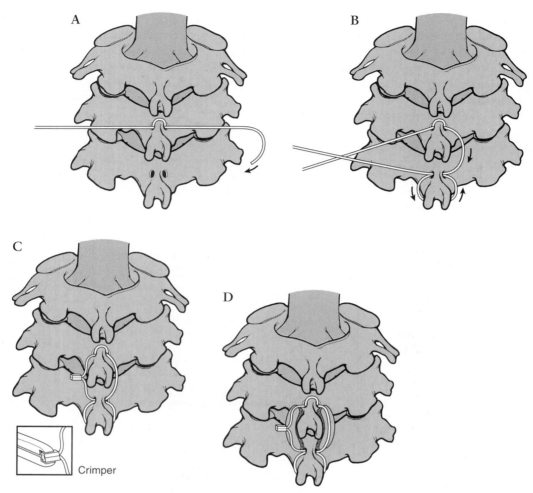

Figure 140.3.   Interspinous technique using flexible multiple cables. **A:** Pass cable 1, near to far, through the C-4 drill hole. Loop it around cephalad edge of the C-4 spinous process, and then pass through the hole again, near to far. **B:** Then pass cable 1, far to near, through the C-5 hole, loop it around the caudal edge of the C-5 spinous process, and then pass it through the hole again, far to near. **C:** Apply crimp to achieve single interspinous wiring. **D:** The bone is then in place under the parallel interspinous portions of the cable.

cient spinal stability, the anterior column should be capable of weight bearing, and excessive rotational forces must be avoided (14,24). When these conditions are not present, lateral mass plates are preferred (31). However, it should be kept in mind that a real risk to the spinal cord, nerve roots, and vertebral arteries exists with lateral mass plating. Posterior cervical wiring techniques have fewer risks and years of proven success (11,52).

Most posterior wiring techniques used today have evolved from the interspinous technique reported by Rogers in 1942 (39). In his description, a wire was passed through and around the base of adjacent spinous processes. Corticocancellous bone grafts were placed under the wires, across the interlaminar space to facilitate fusion. Figure 140.3 diagrams the use of a flexible multistrand cable in a procedure similar to that presented by Rogers (see Rogers's technique in the next section).

Bohlman's triple-wire technique is a modification of Rogers's, in which an additional two wires are used to secure the bone graft to the lamina and spinous processes (30). Bohlman's modification results in increased flexural and torsional stiffness that is superior to Rogers's wiring technique and to sublaminar wiring techniques (Figs. 140.4–140.6).

When the lamina and spinous processes are compromised by injury or decompression, Rogers's and Bohlman's techniques cannot be used. An alternative to lateral mass plating is facet wiring, reported by Robinson and Southwick in 1960 (38), and modified by Callahan in 1977 (Fig. 140.7) (11). In this technique, the articular processes are denuded and wires are passed through the inferior articular processes, which are then secured to overlying bone graft. In the case of rotational instability, or when there is a one-level lamina fracture, oblique facet wiring is an option (Fig. 140.8) (10,21). Wires are placed through the inferior facet as described later in the facet wiring technique, but then secured to the next inferior spinous process instead of overlying bone graft. Bilateral wiring from the facets to the inferior spinous process is recommended.

Lateral mass plating is considerably more demanding than posterior wiring techniques. Plates are fixed to the lateral masses by screws placed at each level. Two methods of screw placement are commonly used, the original technique described by Roy-Camille et al. (41) and the Magerl technique (29). Of the two techniques, Magerl's is more commonly used because it provides a stronger and stiffer construct (Fig. 140.9) (32).

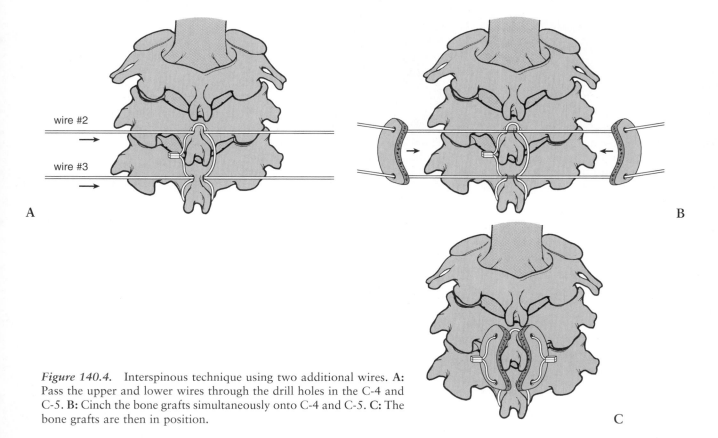

Figure 140.4. Interspinous technique using two additional wires. **A:** Pass the upper and lower wires through the drill holes in the C-4 and C-5. **B:** Cinch the bone grafts simultaneously onto C-4 and C-5. **C:** The bone grafts are then in position.

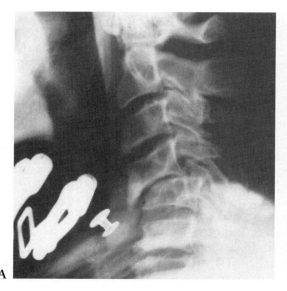

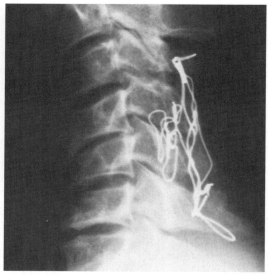

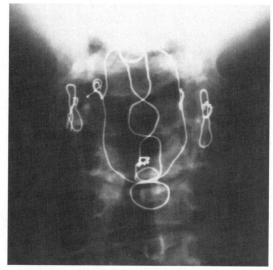

Figure 140.5.   **A:** Lateral radiograph of a 40-year-old lumberjack struck on the back of his neck by a falling tree. There is anterior subluxation of C-4 on C-5. The anterior subluxation was not adequately held despite the application of a halo vest. **B:** Lateral radiograph after posterior reduction and triple-wire stabilization from C-3 to C-6. Notice that there are two wires linking the facet joints at C4–C5 and a midline tethering wire bridging the base of the spinous processes from C-3 to C-6. There are no sublaminar wires. **C:** AP radiograph showing the lateral interfacet wires and the midline tethering wires. The patient at 1-year follow up was neurologically completely intact and his spine was completely fused. He returned to work as a lumberjack doing heavy manual labor.

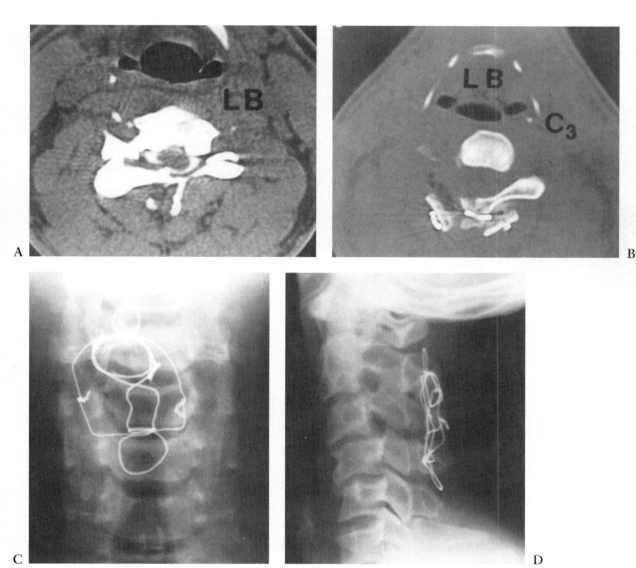

Figure 140.6. **A:** Axial CT image of a 25-year-old man who sustained a diving injury. The patient has a fracture dislocation of the left C-3 facet joint. The inner aspect of the lamina is seen compressing the posterior aspect of the spinal cord. He had numbness on the left side of his neck in the C-3 nerve distribution. In addition, he was hyperreflexic throughout, secondary to a myelopathic lesion. **B:** The patient underwent a posterior decompression and triple-wire stabilization from C-2 to C-4. This axial postoperative CT image shows the posterior wiring and bone graft that stabilized the spine. Notice the adequacy of the decompression of the spinal canal. **C:** AP radiograph of the triple-wire stabilization technique from C-2 to C-4. The lateral wires hold two corticocancellous bone grafts in compression against the posterior aspects of the lamina at C-2 and C-4. **D:** Postoperative lateral radiograph shows a solid fusion from C-2 to C-4 with good spinal alignment aside from the patient's original 15% subluxation at C3–C4. The patient was neurologically completely intact, and his spine was stable at long-term follow-up.

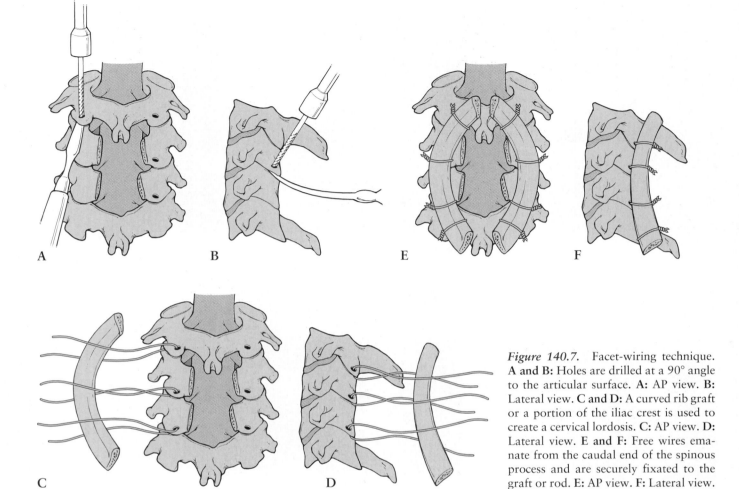

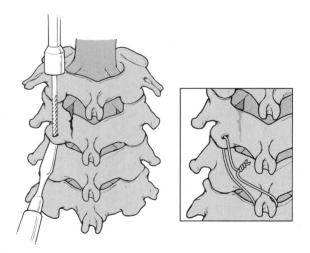

Figure 140.7. Facet-wiring technique. **A and B:** Holes are drilled at a 90° angle to the articular surface. **A:** AP view. **B:** Lateral view. **C and D:** A curved rib graft or a portion of the iliac crest is used to create a cervical lordosis. **C:** AP view. **D:** Lateral view. **E and F:** Free wires emanate from the caudal end of the spinous process and are securely fixated to the graft or rod. **E:** AP view. **F:** Lateral view.

Figure 140.8. Oblique facet wiring. A small drill is used to create a hole in the inferior articular process at a 90° angle to the articular surface. (*Inset*) Wires in place in the drill holes after being tightened and securely fixated.

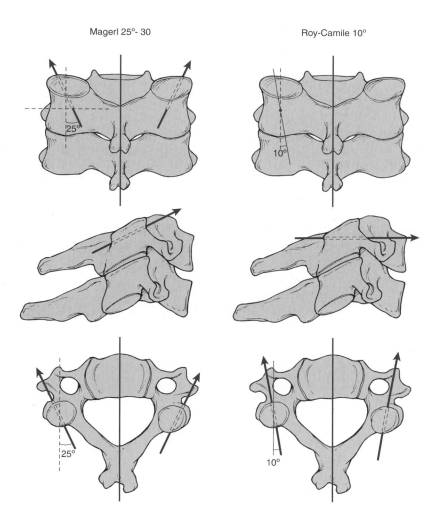

Magerl 25°- 30   Roy-Camile 10°

Figure 140.9. Screw direction for the Magerl and Roy-Camille techniques.

POSTERIOR FUSION

If the patient was previously placed in tongs, maintain traction throughout the case. Fiberoptic intubation is preferred to minimize any movement of the unstable spine.

- Following intubation, turn the patient prone on a spine-turning frame. If possible, keep her awake until after she is prone to monitor for any neurologic changes. Intraoperative neurologic monitoring [e.g., for somatosensory evoked potential (SSEP)], is helpful in identifying changes.
- Hold her face in a Mayfield head holder or other similar device.
- Tuck her arms at her sides. With 3-inch tape, secure her shoulders down to the foot of the bed with a gentle longitudinal pull. This permits radiographic visualization of the lower cervical spine.
- Obtain a preoperative radiograph in the prone position to verify spinal alignment.
- Shave and prepare the neck from the occiput to the midscapular region as well as the posterior iliac crest for bone graft harvesting.
- Make a midline incision overlying the injured area and use the cautery knife to expose the tips of the spinous processes.
- Dissect the subperiosteal soft tissues off the posterior elements to the lateral border of the articular masses.
- Take care to avoid undue pressure over the compromised levels.
- If the injured levels are difficult to identify intraoperatively, use radiographic localization.
- Decompress the areas dictated by the preoperative studies, and perform one of the following fusion techniques.
- After the stabilization procedure, obtain a radiograph to assess the reduction and to confirm the levels of fusion.
- Close the wound in layers over a drain.
- Continue prophylactic antibiotics for 24–48 hours.
- Continue postoperative traction for 24–48 hours, and then immobilize the neck with a hard collar or two

poster orthosis, depending on the adequacy of the stabilization construct.

Rogers's Technique

- Using a burr, make a hole in the midportion of the base of each spinous process to be included in the fusion. Avoid penetration of the laminae.
- Place a pointed towel clip through each hole to confirm adequate room for passage of the cable.
- Pass the cable through the hole in the most superior spinous process, and then wrap the cable around the spinous process and reenter the hole from the same direction (Fig. 140.3). This creates a tethering loop around the spinous process, decreasing the chance of the cable cutting out of the bone.
- From the opposite direction, pass the wire through the next spinous process to be included in the fusion, and follow a similar technique.
- Both ends of the cable should end on the same side of the patient. Tighten the construct and secure with the crimping device.
- Cut the cables flush with the crimp.
- Measure the length of the graft needed with a malleable probe.
- Harvest the corticocancellous graft from the posterior iliac crest. An oscillating saw minimizes the risk of microfractures in the graft. A piece that is the proper length and width can be split into two pieces for each side of the fusion.
- Using a saw, split the graft longitudinally.
- Before the graft is placed, remove all the soft tissue covering the lamina and roughen the bone surfaces with a burr to allow fusion to occur.
- Place the bone grafts underneath the cables, spanning the interlaminar space.

Bohlman's Triple-Wire Technique

- Place the first cable as described for Rogers's technique.
- Place the remaining two cables through and around the most superior and inferior spinous processes to be included in the fusion (Figs. 140.4–140.6).
- Burr holes toward each end of the previously harvested corticocancellous grafts.
- In addition to roughening the surface of the lamina, include the portion of the spinous process that will be in contact with the graft as well.
- Place the cables through each end of the graft and tighten them simultaneously, orienting the graft into its most stable configuration.
- Crimp and cut the cables as in Rogers's technique.
- Pack extra bone along the sides of the grafts if needed.

Facet Wiring Technique

- Identify each articular facet to be included in the fusion.
- Using a small, thin elevator, pry open the joint and rotate the elevator to maintain exposure of the joint surfaces (Fig. 140.7).
- Denude the surfaces with a burr to facilitate fusion.
- Drill a 3 mm hole at 45° off the horizontal through the inferior facet.
- Pass a cable through this hole from a posterior to anterior direction and grasp it from within the joint to deliver it into the field.
- Repeat this process bilaterally at each level to be included in the fusion.
- Use a burr to gently roughen the posterior surfaces of the lateral masses to be fused.
- Secure the corticocancellous grafts to the lateral masses by tightening and crimping the cables.
- Holes may be drilled though the grafts for more secure fixation.

Oblique Facet Wiring

- Drill a hole through the inferior articular facet as described for facet wiring.
- Burr an additional hole through the base of the next inferior spinous process (Fig. 140.8).
- After passing the cable through the facet, pass it through and around the spinous process.
- Tighten and secure as previously noted for other techniques.
- Apply bone graft wherever possible.

Lateral Mass Plating

- Using the Magerl technique, identify the four borders of each lateral mass to be included in the fusion. The medial border is the valley at the junction of the lamina and the facet. The lateral border is the far edge of the articular mass. The superior and inferior borders are the respective facet joints. The starting point is 1–3 mm medial to the center of the four borders of the lateral mass (Fig. 140.9).
- Direct the drill bit 30° to 40° superiorly, parallel to the facet joints, and 25° to 30° laterally. Use bicortical purchase and breach the far cortex by the "loss of resistance" technique with an oscillating drill. A depth gauge accurately assesses the length of screw needed, which is generally 16–22 mm. The vertebral artery is located directly anterior to the valley at the junction of the lamina and articular mass. Avoid this artery by aiming the screws laterally. Avoid the nerve roots by keeping the screws within the articular masses, aiming parallel to the articular surfaces.
- Place the most superior screw in the construct, as described for the Magerl oblique facet wiring technique.
- Drill the pilot hole with a 2 mm drill bit, aiming parallel to the articular surfaces and approximately 25° laterally.
- Place the appropriate-length plate over the lateral masses to be included in the fusion.

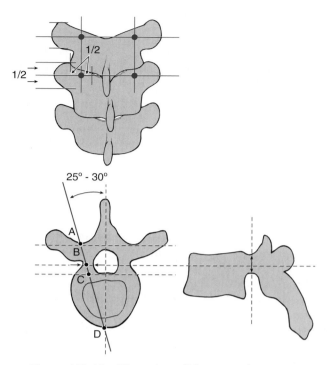

Figure 140.10. Thoracic pedicle screw placement.

- Use the depth gauge to measure the length of the hole.
- Insert the appropriate-length screw and tighten moderately.
- Screw placement for the remaining articular masses will be somewhat dictated by the plate hole configuration. Place the remaining screws in a fashion similar to the first one.
- Tighten all screws securely at the end of the procedure.
- Denude the joints with a burr and apply local bone graft prior to plate placement.

In cases of spinal instability across the cervicothoracic junction, extension of the posterior plating construct to the upper thoracic vertebrae can be achieved. Fixation to the thoracic spine may be through the use of pedicle screws or hooks, depending on which plate or plate–rod construct is utilized. If pedicle screws are desired, the placement technique must be changed from that used for lateral mass screws (Fig. 140.10). Aim the upper thoracic pedicle screws 25° to 30° medially, with the starting point at the intersection of the midportion of the facet joint and the midportion of the transverse process. Thoracic pedicle screw placement is demanding and should be performed only by surgeons experienced in these techniques.

ANTERIOR INSTRUMENTATION

In the early 1950s, Robinson began his work on anterior approaches to the cervical spine in animals and cadavers (37). Currently, the Robinson anterolateral approach between the carotid sheath and the esophagus is optimally suited for access to levels C-3 to C-7. With exacting technique, it is possible to reach as superior as the second cervical vertebra and as inferior as the second thoracic vertebra. In fracture management, this approach is suited for decompression of herniated disc material and of retropulsed fragments from compressed vertebral bodies.

Anterior plates are commonly used for stabilization after decompression for traumatic injuries. Without instrumentation, loss of reduction and graft displacement occur in up to 64% of anterior decompression and strut graft reconstructions (2,6,26,48). The first-generation anterior cervical plates required bicortical purchase of the screws because there was no mechanism for locking the plate–screw interface. This problem was solved with the second-generation plates, which do not require bicortical purchase of the screws and have a rigid plate–screw interface. Morscher et al. (33) established the concept of the cervical locking plate—that is, a rigid plate–screw interface. A variety of second-generation systems are available today.

ANTERIOR FUSION

- If the patient has previously been placed in traction, maintain traction for the remainder of the case.
- Use fiberoptic equipment to insert a nasotracheal or endotracheal tube, avoiding manipulation of the unstable cervical spine during intubation.
- Position the patient carefully on the operative table. Tuck his arms at his sides and tape his shoulders down to the foot of the bed to permit radiographic visualization of the lower cervical levels.
- Obtain a preoperative lateral radiograph to check alignment.
- Prepare the skin aseptically from the chin to the nipple line bilaterally, as well as the anterior iliac crest for graft harvesting.
- Identify the carotid tubercle of the C-6 vertebra (Chassaignac's tubercle) for orientation purposes. If this is not palpable, the hyoid bone overlies C-3, thyroid cartilage is at C-4 to C-5, and cricoid cartilage localizes C-6. Use these landmarks to adjust the position of the skin incision in relation to the injured level.
- Make a transverse incision on the left or right side of the neck, whichever is preferred, extending from the midline to just past the anterior border of the sternocleidomastoid. Alternatively, use an oblique incision along the anterior border of the sternocleidomastoid to approach several levels (Figs. 140.11, 140.12). The rationale for approaching on the left side of midline is that the recurrent laryngeal nerve ascends in the neck on the left side between the trachea and the esophagus, having branched off from its parent nerve, the vagus, at the

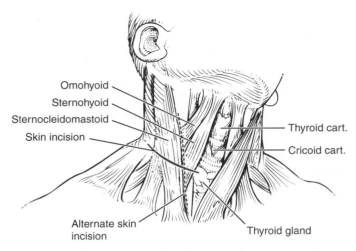

Figure 140.11. Longitudinal and transverse incisions allow the necessary exposure to the anterior cervical spine.

level of the arch of the aorta. On the other hand, the right recurrent laryngeal nerve travels alongside the trachea in the neck after passing beneath the right subclavian artery. In the lower part of the neck, the right recurrent laryngeal nerve is vulnerable to injury as it passes from the subclavian artery to the tracheoesophageal groove. Its course in the groove is also more variable on the right than on the left. Therefore, there is theoretically less risk to the recurrent laryngeal nerve by using the left-sided approach. However, the approach on the left has the possibility of injuring the thoracic duct, which enters the jugular vein–subclavian vein junction at the base of the neck on the left.

- Identify and elevate the platysma, incising it in line with the incision using Metzenbaum scissors.
- Next, incise the superficial layer of the deep cervical

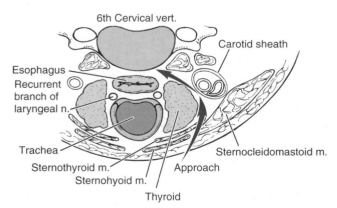

Figure 140.12. The anterior spine can be visualized with dissection in the plane between the thyroid and the carotid sheath, which should be gently retracted laterally.

fascia along the anterior border of the sternocleidomastoid. Proper exposure is necessary to facilitate mobilization of the underlying structures. The omohyoid muscle traverses the field and can be retracted or divided as necessary.

- Palpate the arterial pulse to identify the carotid artery within its investing sheath.
- The middle layer of the deep cervical fascia is the next important layer to be divided. Divide it longitudinally, medial to the carotid sheath. Identify the carotid artery (by using your fingers), and protect it as this layer of fascia is divided. Retract the artery laterally, along with the internal jugular vein, vagus nerve, and phrenic nerve.
- Carry blunt dissection through the loose areolar tissue to the anterior cervical spine.
- Identify the esophagus medially, and retract it with a blunt Richardson retractor. Use a thyroid retractor to retract the carotid sheath and sternocleidomastoid laterally.
- Identify and protect the recurrent laryngeal nerve, which descends along the carotid sheath and ascends between the trachea and esophagus. This structure can be injured with sharp retractors or prolonged pressure.
- The midline of the anterior cervical spine can be palpated, as well as the anterior carotid tubercle at C-6. This landmark can be helpful in localizing the injured vertebrae. Transect the alar and prevertebral fascia vertically in the midline, revealing the underlying anterior longitudinal ligament. The longus colli is visible along the lateral aspects of the anterior cervical vertebrae.
- Perform subperiosteal dissection to the lateral edge of the vertebrae of the injured levels.
- Confirm the appropriate level with an intraoperative radiograph.
- After radiographic verification of the appropriate level, perform a decompressive procedure at the injured levels. Incise the disc with a #11 blade and remove it with curets and rongeurs. Complete excision of the disc is essential to gauge the proper depth to the posterior longitudinal ligament. If a corpectomy is required, excise each adjacent disc first and then remove the intervening bone. The posterior longitudinal ligament is usually disrupted in unstable injuries. Remove all bony fragments within the canal under direct visualization. Take care to avoid bone or disc excision lateral to the uncovertebral joints, to avoid injury to the vertebral arteries.
- After completing the decompression, use a burr to roughen the endplates to be included in the fusion to expose bleeding cancellous bone. Make a small trough in each endplate to accommodate pegs fashioned on either end of the tricortical iliac crest bone graft. Insert the graft with the pegs in the vertebral bodies with the cortical surfaces placed posteriorly to give maximal stability and to prevent collapse.

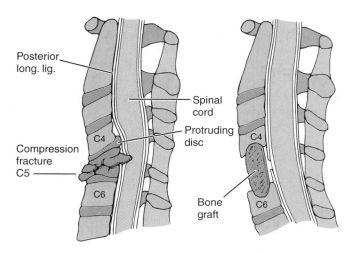

Figure 140.13. **A:** Decompression of the cervical cord should include excision of the discs above and below the burst fracture and the appropriate vertebral body. **B:** The endplates should be undermined to allow the tricortical iliac crest graft to be countersunk.

- After placement, obtain a radiograph to confirm reduction and placement (Fig. 140.13).
- An anterior cervical plate may be added based on the amount of instability. Choose the length of the plate by using the provided template. Place the plate in the appropriate position, spanning the grafted area. Be sure that the longitudinal center of the plate is midline, not displaced to one side or another.
- Position the drill guide in its correct orientation, as dictated by the manufacturer's instructions. Usually, the drill guide is aimed medially 20°, with the sagittal angle determined by the position of the plate. Drill to a preselected depth, taking care to remain in bone at all times.
- After tapping, place the screw and tighten moderately. Place two screws in each vertebral body at the ends of the construct. Additional screws may be added in the graft. Tighten all screws and engage the locking mechanism. Radiographic confirmation of correct screw placement is advised.
- Place a large Penrose drain into the depths of the wound. Close the platysma with interrupted sutures and the skin with subcuticular sutures. Keep a tracheostomy set at bedside for 48 hours in case of hematoma formation, which may obstruct the airway. Remove drains at 48 hours.
- Keep the patient in traction overnight, and then place the neck into a hard cervical collar or halo, depending on the amount of instability and the stabilization achieved. Continue immobilization for 3 months or until union is achieved.

PITFALLS AND COMPLICATIONS

Complications associated with the care of patients with lower cervical spine injuries can be numerous and involve many systems. Comprehensive care must be given to prevent or minimize these complications, especially those that may be iatrogenic in origin.

NEUROLOGIC

It is essential to identify cervical spine injuries in trauma victims at the time of initial evaluation to prevent neurologic injury. Keep the patient immobilized at all times to prevent further injury to the spinal cord or nerve roots. Placement of an orthosis or halo apparatus must be done in an organized and efficient fashion to avoid further damage.

Ascending paralysis in the spinal cord–injured patient is rare. However, overdistraction in a circumferential injury pattern may be one cause. This is more common in patients with associated cervical spondylosis and ankylosing spondylitis. It can be seen at any time after injury and is usually secondary to ascending central necrosis of the gray matter, with an enlarging central syrinx. The diagnostic modality of choice is MRI.

SPINAL DEFORMITY

Reduce any fractures and dislocations as expeditiously as possible by traction or operative means. If the deformity is not reduced, additional spinal cord or nerve root injury can occur by compression or edema. In addition, compression of the radicular arteries to the cord can precipitate ischemia and further worsen the neurologic injury.

Monitor the neurologic status of the patient at the time of the reduction because disc material and bone fragments may be pushed into the canal, causing further neural injury. If the reduction is performed nonoperatively, serial neurologic examinations provide adequate information regarding neurologic function. If operative reduction is required, neurologic monitoring (e.g., SSEPs or an electromyogram) is useful. Should a neurologic deficit occur following a closed or intraoperative reduction, operative decompression of the affected area is indicated.

If no neurologic deficit is noted initially with a unilateral or bilateral facet dislocation, a prereduction MRI is beneficial to identify extrusion of the disc material into the canal (22). If this is found, the authors recommend an anterior discectomy prior to reduction to minimize iatrogenic injury to the cord. A delay of reduction to perform imaging is of little benefit to the patient with a spinal cord injury (25). In cases with concomitant spinal cord injury, perform MRI after reduction. Carefully evaluate chronic dislocations with an intact neurologic status prior to any treatment. Operative fusion in the dislocated position may be required to prevent neurologic injury caused by reduction.

Carefully follow all fractures and dislocations treated nonoperatively or operatively to monitor for late instability and deformity. Should this occur, operative intervention is required.

PULMONARY

In patients with high cervical lesions, hypoventilation may result from paralysis of the intercostal muscles and diaphragm. Hypoxia can ensue, requiring ventilatory support. Atelectasis and pneumonia are common causes of morbidity and mortality and must be treated aggressively.

Because patients with spinal cord injuries lose vasomotor tone and use of their upper and lower extremities, venous thrombosis and pulmonary embolism may be a problem. Emphasis should be placed on the prevention of venous thrombosis with compression pump stockings and other modalities. The use of prophylactic anticoagulants is controversial.

GASTROINTESTINAL

In his review of 300 patients with cervical spine injuries, Bohlman (7) found gastrointestinal hemorrhage to be a common problem. This occurred most commonly 10–14 days after injury and was highly associated with the use of steroids. Recovery in the groups treated with steroids did not differ from that in the group treated without steroids.

Other factors play a role in gastrointestinal complications, including excessive gastric secretions, gastric stasis, and immobilization of the patients. Prophylactic care, including H_2 blockers, can be useful in the prevention of upper gastrointestinal hemorrhage.

OPERATIVE

Bacterial contamination in anterior or posterior operations can cause sepsis or wound infections, which may result in cervical osteomyelitis, meningitis, and death.

In anterior procedures, the esophagus can be injured by retraction or with instrumentation such as drill bits or screws. This may result in dysphagia, fistula formation, and infection.

An injury to the carotid artery can produce massive hemorrhage.

Do not use methylmethacrylate in fractures other than those of pathologic bone. Bone cement does not fuse with bone, and fixation loosens with time, resulting in instability. Increased infection rates have been associated with the use of cement.

Decompressive laminectomy for relief of anterior compression is usually not helpful and may cause increased neurologic deficit. Laminectomy can decrease stability and does not permit retrieval of anterior fragments from the canal. Because sublaminar wires take up space within the canal and can injure the spinal cord, they are contraindicated in cervical spinal trauma.

If reduction of a dislocation is performed when the patient is asleep, spinal cord monitoring may help detect the rare complication of retropulsion of a ruptured disc causing spinal cord compression. If monitoring is not used, an intraoperative wake-up test may be performed. If there is a change in the neurologic status during or after a posterior procedure, perform anterior decompression without delay.

Nonunion with the posterior triple-wiring technique within the C-3 to C-7 levels is rare. In a review of 100 consecutive patients, no nonunions or increased neural deficits were noted (52). Similar rates of fusion have been reported with anterior instrumented fusions (4,33,50).

BRACING

Patients who have neurologic deficits secondary to spinal cord injury must be followed for skin breakdown if they are placed in a two-poster orthosis or a halo jacket. Their insensate skin can break down easily. The two-poster orthosis and Philadelphia collar can cause breakdown over the chin region and therefore must be carefully applied and followed.

Potential complications of halo jackets are numerous. Pressure sores must be prevented. Pin placement and care are important when the ring is applied. Retorque the halo pins the day after application and check them for looseness periodically thereafter. Pay constant attention to the screws and rods to prevent loss of reduction.

Obtain radiographs periodically to assess the position of bone grafts and to look for loss of reduction. Before removing a halo jacket, obtain flexion and extension radiographs, after the connecting bars are loosened, to assess fusion and stability.

REFERENCES

Each reference is categorized according to the following scheme: *, classic article; #, review article; !, basic research article; and +, clinical results/outcome study.

+ 1. Aebi M, Mohler J, Zach G, Morscher E. Indication, Surgical Technique and Results of 100 Surgically Treated Fractures and Fracture Dislocations of the Cervical Spine. *Clin Orthop* 1986;203:244.

+ 2. Aebi M, Zuber K, Marchesi D. The Treatment of Cervical Spine Injuries by Anterior Plating. *Spine* 1991;16:38.

* 3. Allen BL, Ferguson RL, Lehmann TR, O'Brien RP. A Mechanistic Classification of Closed, Indirect Fractures and Dislocations of the Lower Cervical Spine. *Spine* 1982;7:1.

4. Bassett T, Zdeblick TA. Complications of Cervical Spine Instrumentation. *Tech Orthop* 1994;9:8.

+ 5. Beyer CA, Cabanela ME, Bergquist TH. Unilateral Facet Dislocations and Fracture-Dislocations of the Cervical Spine. *Orthopedics* 1992;15:311.

+ 6. Boehler J, Gaudernak T. Anterior Plate Stabilization for Fracture-Dislocations of the Lower Cervical Spine. *J Trauma* 1980;20:203.

* 7. Bohlman HH. Acute Fractures and Dislocations of the Cervical Spine: An Analysis of 300 Hospitalized Patients and Review of the Literature. *J Bone Joint Surg Am* 1979;61:1119.

+ 8. Bohlman HH, Anderson PA. Anterior Decompression and Arthrodesis of the Cervical Spine. *J Bone Joint Surg Am* 1992;74:671.

9. Bohlman HH, Boada E. Fractures and Dislocations of the Lower Cervical Spine. In: The Cervical Spine Research Society, eds. *The Cervical Spine.* Philadelphia: JB Lippincott, 1983:232.

+ 10. Cahill DW, Bellegarrigue R, Ducker TB. Bilateral Facet to Spinous Process Fusion: A New Technique for Posterior Spinal Fusion after Trauma. *Neurosurgery* 1983;13: 1.

+ 11. Callahan RA, Johnson RM, Margolis RN, et al. Cervical Facet Fusion for Control of Instability Following Laminectomy. *J Bone Joint Surg Am* 1977;59:991.

12. Capen DA, Nelson RW, Zigler J, et al. Surgical Stabilization of the Cervical Spine: A Comparative Analysis of Anterior and Posterior Spine Fusions. *Paraplegia* 1987; 25:111.

+ 13. Capen DA, Zigler J, Garland DE. Surgical Stabilization in Cervical Spine Trauma. *Contemp Orthop* 1987;14: 25.

! 14. Coe JD, Warden KE, Sutterlin CE, McAfee PC. Biomechanical Evaluation of Cervical Spinal Stabilization Methods in a Human Cadaveric Model. *Spine* 1989;14: 1122.

15. Cooper PR, Ransohoff J. Surgical Treatment. In: The Cervical Spine Research Society, eds. *The Cervical Spine.* Philadelphia: JB Lippincott, 1983:305.

+ 16. Cotler JM, Herbison GJ, Nasuti JF, et al. Closed Reduction of Traumatic Cervical Spine Dislocation Using Traction Weights up to 140 Pounds. *Spine* 1993;18:386.

17. Cybulski GR, Douglas RA, Meyer PR, Rovin RA. Complications in Three Column Cervical Spine Injuries Requiring Anterior-Posterior Stabilization. *Spine* 1992;17: 253.

+ 18. Davis D, Bohlman HH, Walker AE, et al. The Pathologic Findings in Fatal Craniospinal Injuries. *J Neurosurg* 1971;34:603.

! 19. Dickman CA, Sonntag VK. Wire Fixation of the Cervical Spine: Biomechanical Principles and Surgical Techniques. *BNI Quarterly* 1993;9:2.

20. Dunn EJ, Blazar S. Soft Tissue Injuries of the Lower Cervical Spine. *Instr Course Lect* 1987;36:499.

! 21. Edwards CC, Matz SO, Levine AM. The Oblique Wiring

Technique for Rotational Injuries of the Cervical Spine. *Orthop Trans* 1986;10:455.

+ 22. Eismont FJ, Aruna MJ, Green BA. Extrusion of an Intervertebral Disc Associated with Traumatic Subluxation or Dislocation of Cervical Facets. *J Bone Joint Surg Am* 1991;73:1555.

+ 23. Forster BB, Koopmans RA. Magnetic Resonance Imaging of Acute Trauma of the Cervical Spine: Spectrum of Findings. *Can Assoc Radiol J* 1995;46:168.

+ 24. Gill K, Paschal S, Corin J, et al. Posterior Plating of the Cervical Spine. *Spine* 1988;13:813.

+ 25. Hadley MN, Fitzpatrick BC, Sonntag VK, Browner CM. Facet Fracture Dislocation Injuries of the Cervical Spine. *Neurosurgery* 1992;30:661.

+ 26. Hamilton A, Webb JK. The Role of Anterior Surgery for Vertebral Fractures With or Without Cord Compression. *Clin Orthop* 1994;300:79.

+ 27. Harris JH. Radiographic Evaluation of Spinal Trauma. *Orthop Clin North Am* 1986;17:75.

! 28. Huhn SL, Wolf AL, Ecklund J. Posterior Spinal Osteosynthesis for Cervical Freacture/Dislocation Using a Flexible Multistrand Cable System: Technical Note. *Neurosurgery* 1991;29:943.

+ 29. Jeanneret B, Magerl F, Haterward E. Posterior Stabilization of the Cervical Spine with Hook Plates. *Spine* 1991; 16:56.

! 30. McAfee PC, Bohlman HH, Wilson WL. The Triple-wire Fixation Technique for Stabilization of Acute Fracture-Dislocations: A Biomechanical Analysis. *Orthop Trans* 1985;9:142.

! 31. McGuire R. Biomechanics of Cervical Spine Fixation. *Tech Orthop* 1994;9:30.

! 32. Montesano PX, Juach EC, Anderson PA, et al. Biomechanics of Cervical Spine Internal Fixation. *Spine* 1991;16: 10.

+ 33. Morscher E, Sutter F, Jenny H, Olerud S. Die Vordere Verplattung der Halswirbelsaule mit dem Hohlschrauben-Plattensystem aus Titanium. *Chirurg* 1986;57:702.

34. Norton WL. Fractures and Dislocations of the Cervical Spine. *J Bone Joint Surg Am* 1962;44:115.

! 35. Panjabi MM, White AA, Keller D, et al. Stability of the Cervical Spine Under Tension. *J Biomech* 1978;11:189.

+ 36. Reid DC, Henderson R, Saboe L, Miller JD. Etiology and Clinical Course of Missed Spine Fractures. *J Trauma* 1987;27:980.

* 37. Robinson RA, Smith A. Anterolateral Cervical Disc Removal and Interbody Fusion for Cervical Disc Syndrome. *Bull Johns Hopkins Hosp* 1955;96:223.

+ 38. Robinson RA, Southwick WO. Indications and Techniques for Early Stabilization of the Neck in Some Fracture Dislocations of the Cervical Spine. *South Med J* 1960;53:565.

+ 39. Rogers WA. Treatment of Fracture-Dislocation of the Cervical Spine. *J Bone Joint Surg Am* 1942;24:245.

40. Rogers WA. Fractures and Dislocations of the Cervical Spine. *J Bone Joint Surg Am* 1957;39:341.

* 41. Roy-Camille R, Saillant G, Mazel C. Internal Fixation of the Unstable Cervical Spine by a Posterior Osteosynth-

esis with Plates and Screws. In: The Cervical Spine Research Society, eds. *The Cervical Spine*. Philadelphia: JB Lippincott, 1989:390.

+ 42. Schlegel J, Bayley J, Yuan H, Fredricksen B. Timing of Surgical Decompression and Fixation of Acute Spinal Fractures. *J Orthop Trauma* 1996;10:323.

+ 43. Schneider RC, Crosby EC, Russo RH, Gosch HH. Traumatic Spinal Cord Syndromes and Their Management. *Clin Neurosurg* 1972;20:424.

+ 44. Shapiro SA. Management of Unilateral Locked Facet of the Cervical Spine. *Neurosurgery* 1993;33:832.

+ 45. Silberstein M, Tress BM, Hennessy O. Prevertebral Swelling in Cervical Spine Injury: Identification of Ligament Injury with Magnetic Resonance Imaging. *Clin Radiol* 1992;46:318.

+ 46. Songer MN, Spencer DL, Meyer PR, Jayaraman G. The Use of Sublaminar Cables to Replace Luque Wires. *Spine* 1991;16:S418.

47. Stauffer ES. Management of Spine Fractures C3-C7. *Orthop Clin North Am* 1986;17:45.

+ 48. Stauffer ES, Kelley EG. Fracture-Dislocation of the Cervical Spine: Instability and Recurrent Deformity Following Treatment by Anterior Interbody Fusion. *J Bone Joint Surg Am* 1977;59:45.

+ 49. Streitwieser DR, Knopp R, Wales LR, et al. Accuracy of Standard Radiographic Views in Detecting Cervical Spine Fractures. *Ann Emerg Med* 1983;12:538.

+ 50. Suh PB, Kostuik JP, Esses SI. Anterior Cervical Plate Fixation with the Titanium Hollow Screw Plate System. *Spine* 1990;15:1079.

! 51. Ulrich C, Woersdoerfer O, Kalff R, et al. Biomechanics of Fixation Systems to the Cervical Spine. *Spine* 1991; 16:S4.

+ 52. Weiland DJ, McAfee PC. Posterior Cervical Fusion with Triple-Wire Strut Graft Technique: One Hundred Consecutive Patients. *J Spinal Disord* 1991;4:15.

+ 53. West OC, Anbari MM, Pilgram TK, Wilson AJ. Acute Cervical Spine Trauma: Diagnostic Performance of Single-View Verses Three-View Radiographic Screening. *Radiology* 1997;204:819.

! 54. White AA, Panjabi MM. *Clinical Biomechanics of the Spine*. Philadelphia: JB Lippincott, 1978:223.

! 55. White AA, Panjabi MM. *Clinical Biomechanics of the Spine*. Philadelphia: JB Lippincott, 1990.

56. White AA, Panjabi MM, Posner I, et al. Spinal Stability: Evaluation and Treatment. *Instr Course Lect* 1983;32.

! 57. White AA, Panjabi MM, Saha S, Southwick WO. Biomechanics of the Axially Loaded Cervical Spine: Development of a Clinical Test for Ruptured Ligaments. *J Bone Joint Surg Am* 1975;57:582.

58. White A, Southwick W, Panjabi M. Clinical Instability in the Lower Cervical Spine: A Review of Past and Current Concepts. *Spine* 1976;1:15.

+ 59. Woodring JH, Lee C. The Role and Limitations of Computed Tomographic Scanning in the Evaluation of Cervical Trauma. *J Trauma* 1992;33:698.

## CHAPTER 141

THORACOLUMBAR FRACTURES: EVALUATION, CLASSIFICATION, AND INITIAL MANAGEMENT

Robert F. McLain and Daniel R. Benson

To treat spinal column injuries properly, the physician must recognize life-threatening injuries and treat them appropriately, provide initial supportive care at the same time diagnostic studies are initiated, and protect the neural elements until definitive treatment can be provided. Whether acting in concert with a team of trauma specialists or alone in the emergency department, an orderly, stepwise approach to assessment and management will improve overall outcome and ensure that serious injuries are not missed.

In providing initial care to a spine-injured patient, the physician must perform the following procedures:

- Assess vital functions—airway, bleeding, circulation.
- Protect the spine while managing initial shock or life-threatening injuries.

- Initiate a diagnostic workup for suspected spinal injury.
- Stabilize the spinal column to protect the neural elements during further evaluation and any emergency procedures.

Once the patient is hemodynamically stable and the fracture is identified and classified, the surgeon can prepare a treatment plan based on the fracture pattern, the severity of injury, and the patient's overall condition.

INITIAL ASSESSMENT AND THE FUNDAMENTALS

In trauma management, the first priority is to preserve the patient's life. In some cases, the threat to life is evident (e.g., from hemorrhage, visceral trauma), but in others it is not.

Unstable thoracolumbar fractures are usually high-energy injuries. Anywhere from 40% to 80% result from

R. F. McLain: Department of Orthopaedics, The Cleveland Clinic Foundation, Cleveland, Ohio, 44195.

D. R. Benson: Department of Orthopaedics, University of California, Davis Medical School, Sacramento, California, 95817.

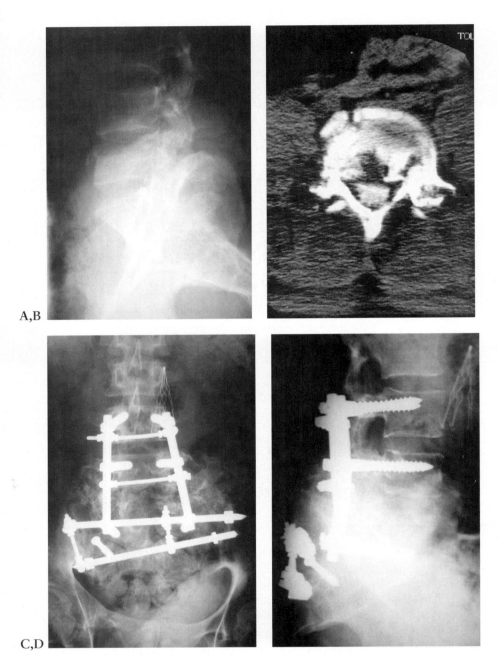

A,B

C,D

Figure 141.1. Spinal trauma—a high-energy injury. **A:** Lateral radiograph of an 18-year-old man crushed under a wall, forced into extreme hyperflexion. He had massive thoracic injuries, a splenic laceration, and a progressive cauda equina injury. Radiograph demonstrates L-5 burst fracture. Pelvic radiographs also demonstrated bilateral sacroiliac fracture–dislocations. **B:** CT scan shows comminuted lumbar fracture, with retropulsed vertebral body fragment abutting the volar surface of the laminae. **C,D:** AP and lateral radiographs after emergent stabilization and resuscitation. The patient underwent multiple procedures under the initial anesthetic, including splenectomy, chest tube placement, L-5 vertebrectomy, cauda equina decompression, posterior spinal stabilization L-4 to sacrum, placement of vena caval filter, and posterior stabilization of the pelvic disruption. This aggressive approach provided enough spinal column stability to allow early mobilization and aggressive pulmonary toilet. Four years after this massive injury, the patient was ambulatory with an ankle–foot orthosis, had mild back pain, and had returned to college.

motor vehicle accidents, involving drivers and passengers of automobiles, riders of motorcycles, and pedestrians (1, 7,17,18,20,23,25,29). Other causes of spine fractures include falls from height, penetrating trauma, and crush injuries, such as those sustained by a worker caught beneath a collapsing structure. In these kinds of injuries, polytrauma is common (Fig. 141.1). In our experience, patients with unstable thoracolumbar fractures suffer an average of two other major injuries in addition to their spinal fracture; some patients may present with as many as six associated injuries (20).

THE CHEST

Common injuries associated with thoracolumbar and thoracic fracture reflect the forces of blunt trauma and rapid deceleration. Intrathoracic injuries include the following:

- Pneumo- and hemothorax associated with rib fractures or bronchial disruption
- Myocardial or pulmonary contusion
- Great vessel injury from blunt trauma or rapid deceleration

- Hemopericardium and cardiac tampanade
- Diaphragmatic rupture and acute hiatal hernia

A plain chest radiograph will confirm the presence of a hemo- or pneumothorax or a diaphragmatic rupture, and it may show widening of the mediastinum associated with a great-vessel injury. If multiple rib fractures are seen, particularly first rib and clavicle fractures, consider getting an angiogram to study the aortic arch.

Tension pneumothorax can be rapidly fatal, as can cardiac tampanade. Rapid placement of a chest tube will resolve the pneumo- or hemothorax, with immediate improvement of oxygenation and cardiac output. Pericardiocentesis will decompress the cardiac tampanade with rapid improvement in circulatory function. These injuries are often associated with thoracic fractures and fracture–dislocations. A quick assessment of bilateral breath sounds and heart sounds should identify either problem. In a tension pneumothorax, breath sounds are absent or diminished on the injured side, and the esophagus and trachea are displaced toward the normal lung. In cardiac tampanade, there are indistinct heart sounds, and the neck veins are distended. Cardiac output is impaired in either case, and the patient manifests signs of shock and cyanosis.

THE ABDOMEN

Pay particular attention to patients with seat-belt injuries. The association of lap-belt abrasions with the classic flexion–distraction fracture should alert the physician to a high likelihood of intra-abdominal injury (12). Because this fracture occurs as the body is flexed forward over the lap-belt, visceral injuries are found in 40% to 60% of patients (10,27). Solid viscera may be injured directly when they are compressed between the body wall and the lap-belt, or they may be torn from their attachments when the body is suddenly and rapidly decelerated. Hollow viscera may be ruptured, perforated, or torn from their mesenteries. Obtain a general surgical assessment whenever a flexion–distraction injury is suspected. A rigid abdomen, falling hematocrit, and abdominal pain or tenderness are clear indications for emergent peritoneal lavage and laparotomy. In the stable patient with no symptoms of shock, an abdominal computed tomography (CT) scan may be used to rule out an abdominal injury. Intra-abdominal injuries are also common in thoracolumbar injuries.

THE EXTREMITIES

Because most unstable thoracic and thoracolumbar fractures are high-energy injuries, it is not surprising that they are commonly associated with additional skeletal injuries:

- Fractures of the femurs, tibias, and feet are common.

- Fractures of humeri and forearm bones are less common.
- Major pelvic fractures are not common and are usually seen only after massive trauma.
- Hemorrhage from multiple long-bone fractures can be severe, resulting in shock (3).

THE HEAD AND NECK

Injuries to the head and neck should be carefully assessed in the emergency room, and the cervical spine should be protected throughout the initial evaluation and emergency procedures (19). Unconscious, obtunded, or intoxicated patients cannot provide a dependable history or reliably report pain or numbness. These patients should be protected as though a cervical injury existed (2,24). Plain radiographs will demonstrate the majority of bony injuries but may not reveal soft-tissue disruptions; retropharyngeal hematoma indicates significant soft-tissue injury and mandates a formal cervical workup (30). Head injuries may be evaluated by a magnetic resonance imaging (MRI) or CT scan prior to anesthesia if surgery is needed, or they may be held under observation if otherwise stable.

SHOCK

Shock may be seen for a variety of reasons. Hemorrhagic, hypovolemic shock is the most serious, and it must be recognized and corrected quickly. Young patients manifest tachycardia and peripheral vasoconstriction as primary symptoms; hypotension may not be seen until shock is severe and vascular collapse occurs. Older patients generally do not compensate well, and tachycardia and hypotension may both appear early on.

- Place a Foley catheter to monitor urine output.
- Rapidly assess common sites of blood loss—open wounds, intra-abdominal and intrathoracic hemorrhage, and long-bone and pelvic fractures.
- Institute fluid resuscitation immediately.

Neurogenic shock results from loss of normal vasomotor tone. Patients present with hypotension and tachycardia although they have warm, well-perfused skin and peripheral tissues. They may not respond to fluid bolus, and vasopressors may be needed.

Shock may result from any condition that reduces cardiac output, including cardiac tampanade, tension pneumothorax, myocardial injury, or myocardial infarction. In every case, rapid vascular access and fluid resuscitation are the vital initial treatments for spinal trauma patients.

PROTECTING THE PATIENT

Once the potentially life-threatening injuries have been addressed or ruled out, the next priority is to stabilize and protect the patient's spine so that a more formal evaluation and workup can be carried out without injuring the spinal cord. This is particularly important in the polytrauma patient who may be unconscious, may require anesthesia and surgical care, and must be moved repeatedly to manage other life-threatening injuries. Plain radiographs of the cervical spine are mandatory before intubating the patient, and if injury is seen or suspected, a fiberoptic nasotrachial intubation is the safest.

Transfer of the patient is safest on a spine board or slide board, and it should always be done with sufficient personnel to make the transfer smoothly and without struggling. When log-rolling the patient, the team must coordinate efforts to see that the shoulders and pelvis move together as a unit. If the patient is hemodynamically stable and does not require emergency procedures, he may be transferred to a firm mattress and maintained under strict spinal precautions until the workup is completed. Precautions include strict supine positioning, log-rolling side to side every 2 hours for skin care, and periodic reexamination of neurologic status. Head-injured and combative patients may need to be sedated and intubated to avoid self-inflicted spinal cord injury.

INITIAL SPINAL EVALUATION

With the patient hemodynamically and mechanically stabilized, return to the spinal injury assessment. Obtain a complete history, paying close attention to reports of transient paresthesias, acute back or neck pain, or temporary weakness or paralysis at the time of injury. Record the location and radiation of pain symptoms, as well as any radicular symptoms. Any history of previous injury, fracture, or pain symptoms should be noted. A global examination of motor and sensory function should rapidly focus on any areas of deficit. If the patient cannot cooperate with the exam, carefully observe and note spontaneous movements and withdrawal responses. Carry out a rectal exam to assess rectal tone, voluntary rectal control, and the bulbocavanosus reflex. If the patient is neurologically normal, log-roll him to one side so that the spine can be palpated for step-offs, tenderness, or kyphosis. Note the condition of the skin over the symptomatic area. If a neurologic deficit exists, obtain radiographs of the symptomatic level before moving the patient.

If a spinal cord injury is identified, start the patient on high-dose steroids to attempt to facilitate recovery (4). Steroids have been shown to improve spinal cord recovery relative to placebo and naloxone therapy, and they are thought to combat abnormal biochemical processes brought on by thromboxanes and prostaglandins released at the site of injury. Steroids must be given within 8 hours of injury to have any beneficial effect. Patients treated with high-dose steroids may be exposed to an increased infection rate and risk of gastrointestinal hemorrhage.

DIAGNOSTIC WORKUP

A formal physical examination and history may not be possible until the patient has been stabilized hemodynamically and has recovered from initial resuscitation. When the patient is alert and cooperative, a formal motor, sensory, and reflex examination should be repeated, and a detailed history of the accident obtained.

The history should focus on three issues: mechanism of injury; presence or absence of neurologic symptoms, and past history of spinal trauma, surgery, or symptoms. In high-energy injuries, it is often difficult to determine exactly what forces acted on the spine to produce fracture, but knowledge of the injury mechanism can help identify associated injuries and provide clues to the level of instability to be expected. A lap-belted patient in a motor vehicle accident may present with a straightforward flexion–distraction injury, for instance, whereas a patient ejected from the vehicle or from a motorcycle frequently will present with a more complex fracture pattern consistent with the combination of torsional and axial loading forces experienced when striking the ground. If the forces involved in the fracture were rather low, an underlying pathologic process must be considered. If the forces involved were very high, and multiple injuries were sustained, the risk of prolonged recumbency to the patient's life must be considered in timing a surgical procedure.

If the patient can recall the event, it is important to elicit any history of transient paresthesias or paralysis from the time of injury. Even if the patient's symptoms resolved quickly, they suggest that some level of root or cord injury occurred at the time of the injury; therefore, assume that the spinal fracture is unstable. If the patient cannot give the details of the event, careful scrutiny of field notes can provide important clues to whether the patient had abnormal findings at the accident site. These notes are often gross evaluations only, however, and a patient with a severe cauda equina injury can still "move all four extremities."

A history of previous trauma, surgery, or symptoms is important to understanding the current injury. Lower extremity weakness due to old injury or spinal disease can confuse the diagnostic picture after an acute injury, and a preexisting deformity—compression fracture, spondylolisthesis, or kyphosis—can be difficult to differentiate from a new injury. Furthermore, the surgical approach to the multiply operated back will be more demanding and may require different instrumentation than for an ordinary fracture.

The physical examination for the spinal-injured patient centers around a careful, complete neurologic assessment.

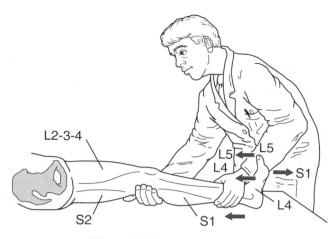

Figure 141.2. Motor testing.

Having examined the musculoskeletal system in the emergency department, carefully reexamine the extremities for tenderness and pain, and examine the back again to determine the level of discomfort and the presence of step-offs or gaps between the spinous processes, and to assess the skin over the area of injury.

Document a complete motor and sensory examination. Test each motor group for the lumbar and sacral plexuses independently and compare to the contralateral group (Fig. 141.2). Motor strength is recorded on six-point scale:

5 full strength adequate to powerfully resist the examiner
4 power to resist but not overcome the examiner
3 power to overcome gravity
2 power to move the joint but not to overcome gravity
1 capacity to contract the muscle without functional power
0 no motor function at all

When extremity injuries are present, make an educated assessment as to whether the patient is clinically weak or limited in effort by pain. Also determine whether the pattern of weakness is consistent with a cord lesion, a root lesion, or a peripheral nerve injury.

The sensory examination begins at the chest wall and seeks a level of anesthesia, root by root, down to the sacrum. Patients with thoracic cord injuries will have an anesthetic level at or just below their fracture. If the anesthetic level and the recognized fracture do not coincide, obtain an MRI to determine the actual cause of the cord impairment. Sensation in the lower extremities follows a dermatomal pattern; test each dermatome for light-touch and pin-prick sensation (Fig. 141.3).

Check reflexes at both the knees and the ankles. The bulbocavernosus reflex, an involuntary contraction of the rectal sphincter, can be triggered either by gently squeezing the glans penis or glans clitoris or by gently tugging on the Foley catheter. If this reflex is absent, the patient either is in spinal shock or has suffered an injury to the caudal segments of the conus medullaris. Hyperactive reflexes suggest disinhibition due to a cord-level injury. Absent reflexes in an isolated distribution suggest an incomplete injury or root lesion. Complete absence of reflexes may be due to either spinal cord shock or a complete cauda equina injury. Spinal cord shock occurs at the time of injury and may persist for 72 hours. While the patient is in spinal cord shock, the neurologic examination remains unreliable—an incomplete injury may appear complete due to the overriding effects of cord shock. Once shock resolves and caudal reflexes return, the examination provides clear prognostic information: Incomplete injuries have potential for improvement, complete injuries have almost none. The bulbocavernosus reflex is the most reliable level for testing reflex return because it tests the most caudal segment of the spinal cord.

The rectal examination deserves special comment. The most caudal motor and sensory unit in the body is the rectum, the function of which is crucial to independent social activity. Carry out an independent examination of rectal tone, sensation, and reflex activity. Do not rely on emergency department records if there is any concern of neurologic injury. Explain the purpose of the examination to the patient, who may be anxious over repeated exams. Document resting tone, voluntary contraction, perianal sensation, and bulbocavernosus reflex.

Plain radiographs should include anteroposterior (AP) and lateral views of the thoracic spine and/or the lumbosacral spine, depending on the symptomatic level (16). On occasion, standard thoracic films will cut off T12–L1, and lumbosacral films will start at L-1, giving an inadequate view of the most frequently injured level. If fracture of the thoracolumbar junction is suspected, repeat AP and lateral radiographs, centered at the T-12 level. In stable fractures (compression fractures, mild burst fractures, and mild flexion–distraction injuries), plain radiographs are sufficient to allow definitive treatment, and no further diagnostic studies are needed. In unstable spine fractures, however, additional imaging studies are often indicated.

Unstable fractures (severe burst fractures, fracture-dislocations, significant flexion–distraction injuries, and any fracture with a neurologic deficit) require further study to assess the extent of bony disruption, spinal cord impingement, canal compromise, and/or cord injury. A CT scan provides the most definitive information on bony characteristics, such as fracture pattern and comminution (8,11,15). The axial cuts of the CT scan can completely miss flexion–distraction injuries, however. An MRI is superior for soft-tissue details such as cord injury, cord compression, disc herniation, and ligamentous disruption (28). The MRI has the added benefit of scanning the entire thoracolumbar spine, and it can pick up noncontiguous

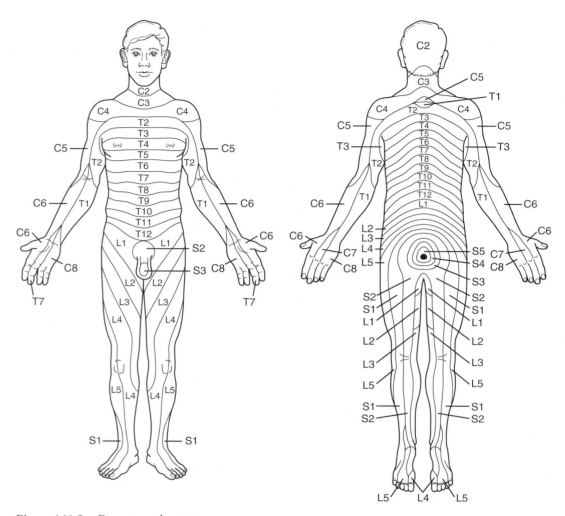

Figure 141.3. Dermatomal patterns.

fractures, cord injury, and epidural hematoma at levels other than that of the primary fracture. Longitudinal MRI cuts show the soft-tissue disruption and bony separation of flexion–distraction injuries well.

Myelography, the gold standard for assessing neural compromise just a decade ago, is now replaced by the MRI in all but a few cases. When an MRI is contraindicated (e.g., intraocular fragments, cardiac valves), CT myelography is an appropriate but more invasive alternative.

There are two absolute indications for ordering MRI or myelography in the acutely injured patient:

- Any patient with a progressive neurologic deficit needs emergent imaging.
- Any patient whose neurologic level does not coincide with the recognized injury needs further evaluation for an unrecognized fracture or disc disruption.

Plain tomography is sometimes useful for evaluating the cervicothoracic junction when a CT scan cannot be obtained immediately. Flexion–extension studies or nuclear medicine scans have little role in acute trauma. There is no role for electrodiagnostic testing in the acute management of spine trauma patients.

FRACTURE CLASSIFICATIONS

Once the diagnostic evaluation is complete, the fracture can usually be classified according to one of a number of schemes. Holdsworth first characterized spinal fractures according to a two-column—anterior and posterior—model of the spinal column (13,14). This model has since given way to the three-column model of Denis, which considers the vertebral body, anulus, and posterior longitudinal ligament to be the middle column, a discrete unit separate from the anterior and posterior stabilizers (5,6,22) (Fig. 141.4).

The first consideration is whether to classify a specific

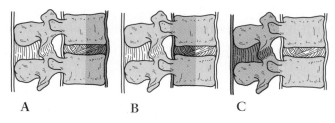

Figure 141.4. Three-column model of Denis. **A:** Anterior column. **B:** Middle column. **C:** Posterior column.

injury as stable or unstable. Unstable injuries include all those with any of the following:

- Three-column disruption
- Greater than 50% collapse of anterior cortex
- Greater than 25° of focal kyphosis
- Any extent of neurologic deficit

Although all stable injuries may be treated nonoperatively, not all unstable injuries need to be treated operatively. A simple algorithm for treatment is indicated in Fig. 141.5.

After assessing the level of instability, classify the fracture according to fracture type and severity. The Denis fracture classification (Table 141.1) depends on information about the fracture pattern, the mechanism of injury, and the deforming forces that caused the fracture. The differences between severe burst fractures and rotational fracture–dislocations, and severe seat-belt injuries and flexion–distraction fracture–dislocations are subtle, and of limited importance: These severe injuries are all clearly unstable, and all require operative treatment.

COMPRESSION FRACTURES

Compression fractures are common injuries, occurring with moderate trauma in young patients and minimal to no trauma in elderly, osteoporotic patients. The anterior column collapses under an axial or flexion load, with fracture of one or both endplates, but the middle and posterior columns are undamaged. These stable injuries are appropriately treated with a removable brace and symptomatic care. Observe patients with advanced osteoporosis for progressive collapse; severe compression fractures may warrant a CT examination to rule out a burst component.

BURST FRACTURES

Burst fractures occur when the vertebral body is exposed to higher axial or flexural loads at a high loading rate. These fractures are commonly the result of motor vehicle accidents, falls from height, or crush injuries. The anterior cortex fails in compression, and either one or both endplates are fractured. The middle column is also fractured, and a portion of the posterior vertebral body is retropulsed backward into the canal. Depending on the severity of the fracture, the posterior elements may be fractured as well. Determine the need for surgical treatment by the extent of vertebral comminution, the extent of canal compromise, and the status of the posterior column structures (21). Burst fractures may be subdivided by fracture pattern:

- Type A fractures occur with axial loading, with fractures of both upper and lower endplates.
- Type B fractures are the most common (50%), with fracture of only the upper endplate.

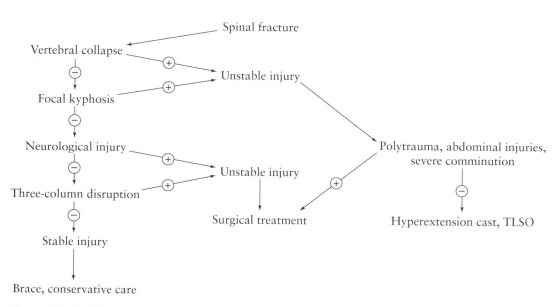

Figure 141.5. Treatment algorithm for thoracolumbar fractures.

Table 141.1.   *Denis Fracture Classification*

Fracture type	Subtype	Deforming forces	Columns injured	Stability
Compression		Axial loading	1: Anterior	Stable
Burst fracture	Type A	Axial loading	2: Anterior and middle	Unstable
	Type B	Flexion, axial loading	2: Anterior and middle	Possibly unstable
	Type C	Flexion, axial loading	2: Anterior and middle	Possibly unstable
	Type D	Axial loading, rotation	3: Anterior, middle, posterior	Unstable
	Type E	Lateral compression	2–3: Anterior, middle, posterior	Possibly unstable
Seat-belt		Flexion–distraction	2: Posterior and middle	Unstable
Fracture–dislocation	Flexion–rotation	Hyperflexion–rotation	3: Anterior, middle, posterior	Unstable
	Shear	Extension, translation	3: Anterior, middle, posterior	Unstable
	Flexion–distraction	Hyperflexion–distraction	3: Anterior, middle, posterior	Unstable

- Type C fractures, with disruption of the lower endplate, are uncommon.
- Type D fractures have a rotational displacement of one body relative to the other on AP radiographs.
- Type E fractures are lateral compression injuries, with traumatic scoliosis (Fig. 141.6).

Canal compromise is most accurately assessed on a CT scan, by comparing the AP diameter of the normal spinal canal at an adjacent level to the reduced diameter at the level of the retropulsed fragment (26). The ratio of the injured to the intact diameters provides the percent compromise (Fig. 141.7). The greatest compromise occurs at the level of the pedicles and upper vertebral body. In type A and B burst fractures, the central portion of the posterior cortex and body is driven back into the canal between the two pedicles, which then prevent the fragment from reducing. Because of the differing volumes of neural tissue in the canal at different levels, compromise of greater than 50% may produce symptoms at the thoracolumbar junction, whereas compromise of 85% or more may be well tolerated at the lumbosacral junction (9). A CT scan will also demonstrate the presence and extent of posterior element disruptions (Fig. 141.8). Three-column injuries are

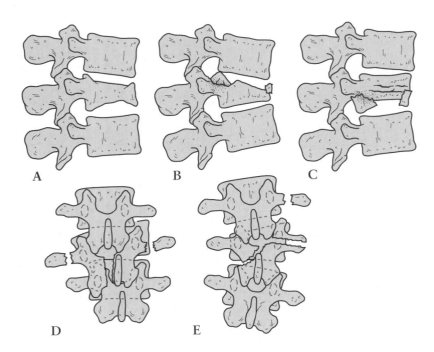

Figure 141.6.   Burst fracture patterns.

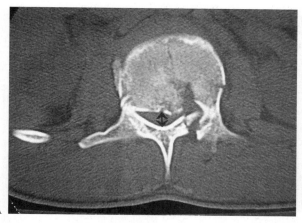
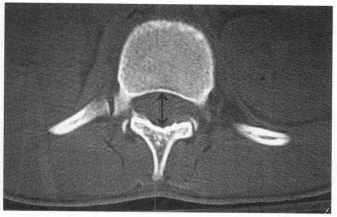

Figure 141.7. Canal dimension at injured level (**A**) is compared to adjacent normal level (**B**) to determine percent canal compromise.

inherently more unstable than two-column injuries, and the inability to load the posterior facet joints in a hyperextension cast may exclude nonoperative care for some patients.

FLEXION-DISTRACTION FRACTURES

Flexion-distraction, or seat-belt fractures may be either one- or two-level injuries (5,10,12,27). The classic one-level injury is the Chance fracture. The mechanism of injury involves the patient being thrown forward across an intact lap-belt, resulting in a hyperflexion force acting around a center of rotation *anterior* to the spinal col-

umn—at the belt itself. This results in distraction forces at all three columns of the spine: (a) The posterior elements are torn apart through either the facet joints or the bone itself, (b) the middle column is torn apart through either the posterior disc or the posterior vertebral body, and (c) the anterior column is either disrupted (in severe injuries) or left as a hinge that cannot resist either flexion or rotational displacement. Plain radiographs demonstrate the gap between the spinous processes and the disruption of the pedicle in most cases (Fig. 141.9) but may show minimal displacement when the patient is supine because the fracture tends to reduce in this position. An MRI shows the injury clearly.

The violent compression of viscera between the spinal

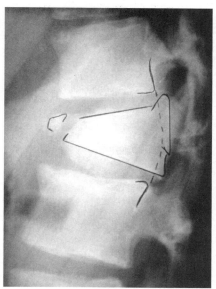
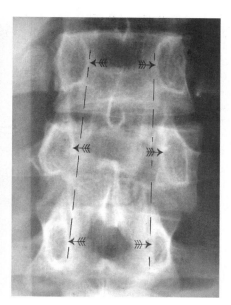

A,B

Figure 141.8. Radiographic characteristics of burst fractures. **A:** Lateral view demonstrates fracture of anterior cortex and superior endplate, with resulting focal kyphosis. The posterosuperior portion of the vertebral body can be seen retropulsed into the spinal canal, with loss of normal concave contour of the posterior vertebral body. **B:** AP radiograph demonstrates the increased intrapedicular distance associated with a burst fracture; the distance between the L-1 pedicles is significantly greater than for the levels either above or below, indicating a complete disruption of anterior, middle, and posterior columns.

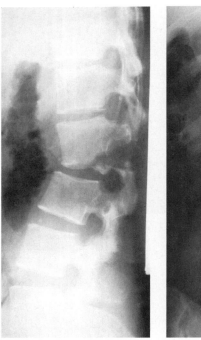
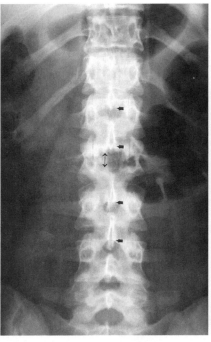
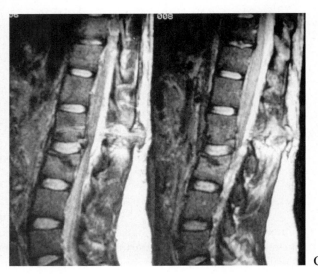

A,B   **C**

Figure 141.9.   Radiographic characteristics of seat-belt fractures. **A:** Lateral radiograph of severe flexion–distraction injury, taken in sitting position. The patient was admitted following a head-on motor vehicle accident and treated for abdominal contusions, splenic rupture, and rupture of the colon. Injury was not apparent on supine radiographs. **B:** AP radiograph shows wide spacing between spinous processes at the level of injury. **C:** MRI confirms extensive soft-tissue disruption including rupture of the lumbodorsal fascia.

column and lap belt can rupture hollow viscera, lacerate solid viscera (liver and spleen), and avulse major vascular pedicles. Unrecognized, any of these injuries can prove rapidly fatal; it is therefore necessary that any patient with a seat-belt injury be carefully assessed by a general surgeon for acute or occult intra-abdominal injury.

Single-level injuries pass through the posterior ligamentous structures and the underlying disc at the same level, or through the posterior lamina, pedicle, and vertebral body in the same transverse plane (Fig. 141.10). These injuries disrupt only a single motion segment. Two-level injuries begin posteriorly at one level of lamina or facet joint, then proceed anteriorly in an oblique fashion so that the injury passes out of the vertebral body into an adjacent disc or through the disc into an adjacent body. In these injuries, two adjacent motion segments are disrupted, and stabilization requires addressing both levels of injury.

FRACTURE–DISLOCATIONS

Fracture–dislocations are, by definition, three-column injuries. They are highly unstable, usually associated with neurologic injury, and often associated with other musculoskeletal and visceral injuries. The neurologically intact

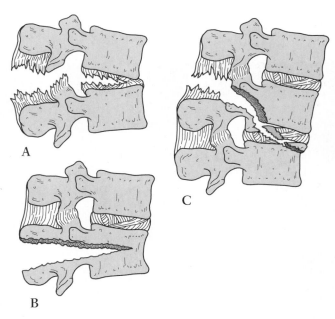

Figure 141.10.   Seat belt-fractures. **A:** Injury to soft-tissues only. **B:** Bony chance fracture. **C:** Mixed injury.

patient must be carefully protected during any necessary testing or emergent operative procedures, and the spine must be stabilized at the first reasonable opportunity to allow mobilization and prevent paralysis. In the patient with neurologic deficit, postural reduction may improve alignment and reduce neural compression, and longitudinal traction may allow manual reduction of a displaced fracture–dislocation. Neither will reduce neural compression by retropulsed vertebral fragments, however, and direct decompression is indicated for those patients with an incomplete injury and hopes of improvement.

Flexion–rotation fracture–dislocations (Fig. 141.11) are caused by hyperflexion and rotation forces such as

seen when a patient is ejected from a vehicle at high speed. When the vertebral body is fractured, this injury may be indistinguishable from a severe type D burst fracture. Shear fractures are more uncommon injuries and occur in the absence of axial loading or flexion–extension forces. Translational forces occurring when the subject is struck squarely from the side, front, or back act to shift one vertebral body relative to the next by shearing through bony articulations and ligamentous structures. Flexion–distraction fracture–dislocations occur when all three columns fail in hyperflexion. These injuries are often not distinguishable from severe seat-belt injuries.

A key consideration in fracture–dislocations is that all three columns are unstable in both axial loading *and in longitudinal traction.* Instrumentation systems that depend on distraction forces to secure hook purchase cannot be safely applied in these injuries, and any system incorrectly applied may overdistract the fracture and stretch the neurologic elements, precipitating or worsening the neurologic injury.

 AUTHORS' PERSPECTIVE

Successful fracture treatment begins with a careful and comprehensive initial evaluation. The key to success is, as always, to look at the whole patient—never allowing a single, dramatic injury to distract attention from more subtle, and potentially more dangerous, injuries. Once the patient is hemodynamically stable, and the fracture is recognized and classified, prepare a treatment plan based on the fracture pattern, the severity of injury, and the patient's overall condition. The options for nonoperative and operative treatment are extensive, and the correct choice for any patient must be determined by weighing all the above considerations, as well as the surgeon's experience, against the potential risks of treatment.

REFERENCES

Each reference is categorized according to the following scheme: *, classic article; #, review article; !, basic research article; and +, clinical results/outcome study.

+ 1. Benson DR, Burkus JK, Montesano PX, et al. Unstable Thoracolumbar and Lumbar Burst Fractures Treated with the AO Fixateur Interne. *J Spinal Disord* 1992;5: 335.

* 2. Bohlman HH. Treatment of Fractures and Dislocations of the Thoracic and Lumbar Spine. *J Bone Joint Surg Am* 1985;67:165.

3. Bone LB. Management of Polytrauma. In: Chapman MW, ed. *Operative Orthopaedics*, 2nd ed. Philadelphia: JB Lippincott, 1993.

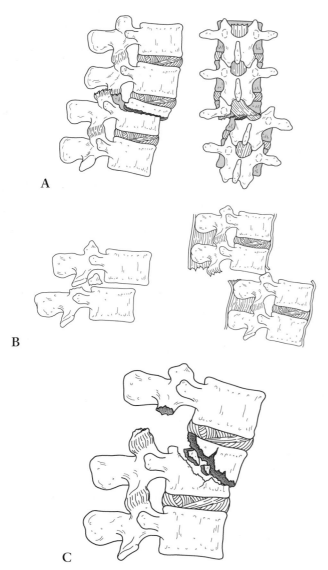

Figure 141.11. Fracture dislocations. **A:** Flexion-rotation. **B:** Shear. **C:** Flexion-distraction.

+ 4. Bracken MB, Shepard MJ, Collins WF, et al. A Randomized, Controlled Trial of Methylprednisolone or Naloxone in the Treatment of Acute Spinal Cord Injury. Results of the Second National Acute Spinal Cord Injury Study. *N Engl J Med* 1990;322:1405.

* 5. Denis F. The Three Column Spine and Its Significance in the Classification of Acute ThoracoLumbar Spinal Injuries. *Spine* 1983;8:817.

* 6. Denis F. Spinal Instability as Defined by the Three Column Spine Concept in Acute Trauma. *Clin Orthop* 1984; 189:65.

+ 7. Dickson JH, Harrington PR, Erwin WD. Results of Reduction and Stabilization of the Severely Fractured Thoracic and Lumbar Spine. *J Bone Joint Surg Am* 1978; 60:799.

+ 8. El-Khoury GY, Kathol MH, Daniel WW. Imaging of Acute Injuries of the Cervical Spine: Value of Plain Radiography, CT, and MR Imaging. *AJR Am J Roentgenol* 1995;164:43.

+ 9. Finn CA, Stauffer ES. Burst Fractures of the Fifth Lumbar Vertebra. *J Bone Joint Surg Am* 1992;74:398.

* 10. Gertzbein SD, Court-Brown CM. Rationale for the Management of Flexion Distraction Injuries of the Thoracolumbar Spine Based on a New Classification. *J Spinal Disord* 1989;2:176.

+ 11. Golimbu C, Firooznia H, Rafii M, et al. Computed Tomography of Thoracic and Lumbar Spine Fractures That Have Been Treated with Harrington Instrumentation. *Radiology* 1984;151:731.

* 12. Gumley G, Taylor TK, Ryan MD. Distraction Fractures of the Lumbar Spine. *J Bone Joint Surgery Br* 1982;64: 520.

* 13. Holdsworth FW. Fractures, Dislocations, and Fracture-Dislocations of the Spine. *J Bone Joint Surg Br* 1963;45: 6.

* 14. Holdsworth FW, Chir M. Fractures, Dislocations, and Fracture-Dislocations of the Spine. *J Bone Joint Surg Am* 1970;52:1534.

* 15. Keene JS. Radiographic Evaluation of Thoracolumbar Fractures. *Clin Orthop* 1984;189:58.

+ 16. Keene JS, Goletz TH, Lilleas F, et al. Diagnosis of Vertebral Fractures: A Comparison of Conventional Radiography, Conventional Tomography, and Computed Axial Tomography. *J Bone Joint Surg Am* 1982;64:586.

+ 17. McBride GG. Cotrel-Dubousset Rods in Spinal Fractures. *Paraplegia* 1989;27:440.

+ 18. McBride GG. Cotrel-Dubousset Rods in Surgical Stabilization of Spinal Fractures. *Spine* 1993;18:466.

+ 19. McLain RF, Benson DR. Missed Cervical Dissociation —Recognizing and Avoiding Potential Disaster. J Emergency Medicine, In Press, 1998.

+ 20. McLain RF, Benson DR. Thoracolumbar Fractures Treated with Segmental Fixation. Unpublished data.

* 21. McLain RF, Sparling E, Benson DR. Early Failure of Short Segment Pedicle Instrumentation for Thoracolumbar Fractures. *J Bone Joint Surg Am* 1993;75:162.

! 22. Panjabi MM, Oxland TR, Kifune M, et al. Validity of the Three-column Theory of Thoracolumbar Fractures. A Biomechanic Investigation. *Spine* 1995;20:1122.

+ 23. Place HM, Donaldson DH, Brown CW, Stringer EA. Stabilization of Thoracic Spine Fractures Resulting in Complete Paraplegia. A Long-term Retrospective Analysis. *Spine* 1994;19:1726.

24. Reid DC, Henderson R, Saboe L, Miller JDR. Etiology and Clinical Course of Missed Spine Fractures. *J Trauma* 1987;27:980.

25. Saboe LA, Reid DC, Davis LA, et al. Spine Trauma and Associated Injuries. *J Trauma* 1991;31:43.

+ 26. Shuman WP, Rogas JV, Sickler ME, et al. Thoracolumbar Burst Fractures: CT Dimensions of the Spinal Canal Relative to Postsurgical Improvement. *AJR Am J Roentgenol* 1985;145:337.

* 27. Smith WS, Kaufa H. Patterns and Mechanisms of Lumbar Injuries Associated with Lap Seat Belts. *J Bone Joint Surg Am* 1969;51:239.

+ 28. Tarr RW, Drolshagen LF, Kerna TC. MRI of Recent Spinal Trauma. *J Comput Assist Tomogr* 1987;11:412.

+ 29. Tasdemiroglu E, Tibbs PA. Long-term Follow-up Results of Thoracolumbar Fractures after Posterior Instrumentation. *Spine* 1995;20:1704.

+ 30. Vandermark RM. Radiology of the Cervical Spine in Trauma Patients: Practice, Pitfalls, and Recommendations for Improving Efficiency and Communication. *AJR Am J Roentgenol* 1990;155:465.

## CHAPTER 142

OPERATIVE TREATMENT OF THORACIC AND THORACOLUMBAR FRACTURES

Robert F. McLain and Daniel R. Benson

INTRODUCTION

Since the early 1980s, operative treatment has moved to the forefront of fracture management in the spine. Techniques and implants have evolved to provide better results with decreased morbidity and mortality (1,9,11,13,17),

R. F. McLain: Director, Spine Research, Department of Orthopaedics, The Cleveland Clinic Foundation, Cleveland, Ohio, 44195.
D. R. Benson: Department of Orthopaedics, University of California, Davis, Sacramento, California, 95817.

and current operative management more rapidly returns the patient to work and satisfactory function (9,10,20, 86). Changes in health care management and patient expectations have made prolonged bed rest or immobilization unacceptable (12). Improved imaging, a better understanding of fracture and implant biomechanics, and the introduction of a variety of new anterior and posterior fixation devices allow surgeons to plan definitive stabilizing procedures for any fracture pattern, allowing rapid mobilization and return to function. Hence, patients who cannot be mobilized in a cast or brace within a few days of their injury are often more reasonably treated with surgery.

The goals of treatment, operative or otherwise, remain to

1. Protect neural elements, restore/maintain neurological function;
2. Prevent or correct segmental collapse and deformity;
3. Prevent spinal instability and pain;
4. Permit early ambulation and return to function; and
5. Restore normal spinal mechanics.

NONOPERATIVE TREATMENT

Only 20% to 30% of spine fractures require surgery. The rest can be treated nonoperatively in a brace, molded orthosis, or hyperextension cast. Single-column injuries (e.g., compression fracture, laminar fracture, spinous process fracture) are treated in an off-the-shelf brace that encourages normal spinal alignment and limits extreme motion (Fig. 142.1). More significant compression fractures may be treated in a molded orthosis. Two-column injuries, including severe compression fractures, mild to moderate burst fractures, and bony Chance fractures, are too unstable to be braced but may well be reduced and maintained at bed rest or in a hyperextension cast. Previous studies (84) have shown that even severe burst fractures can be treated with a regimen of bed rest, postural reduction, and casting. Bony remodeling reduces residual canal compromise by more than 50% over the course of a year (71) (Fig. 142.1), making surgical treatment unnecessary in many patients, including those with retropulsed fragments in the spinal canal. Recumbent treatment, although effective, is very expensive and rarely reimbursed or permitted in managed care systems. Hyperextension casting, on the other hand, allows immediate mobilization and early return to independent function.

The hyperextension cast can be used in many patients with severe compression fractures or burst fractures. Figure 142.2 shows an example of closed reduction and casting for thoracolumbar fractures.

- Place the patient on a modified fracture table (Fig. 142.2A). Suspend the patient on a narrow, midline, taut canvas support in cervical halter traction, with arms out to the side, knees flexed, and feet resting on the support to give the patient a sense of balance.
- Apply a vertically directed force that will achieve hyperextension at the fracture site (Fig. 142.2B). Once maximum hyperextension is achieved through this means, relax the horizontal canvas support and place additional traction on the iliac crests.
- After satisfactorily positioning the patient on the table, wrap the torso with Webril (Fig. 142.2C). Pad the bony prominences additionally with foam and apply the cast.

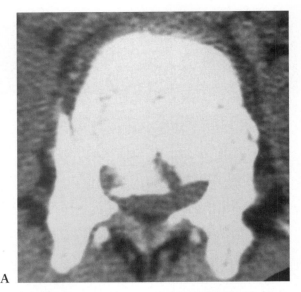

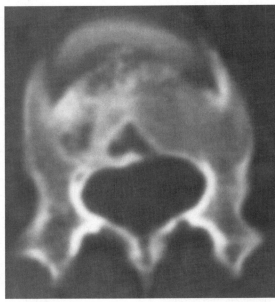

Figure 142.1.   Fracture remodeling. **A:** Thoracic level burst fracture. With nonoperative treatment, normal remodeling mechanisms tend to restore canal diameter compromised by retropulsed bony fragments. **B:** Resorption of the retropulsed vertebral body results in a "heart-shaped" canal with near-normal anteroposterior (AP) diameter 1 year later. (Courtesy Joseph Mumford, MD, Topeka, KS.)

- Note the extreme hyperextension placed into the cast, as well as the large anterior abdominal hole that has been created (Fig. 142.2D, E). Send the patient to the x-ray department for postreduction and casting x-ray studies. If satisfactory alignment has been achieved, allow the patient to ambulate immediately.

If the posterior elements are intact, axial loads are

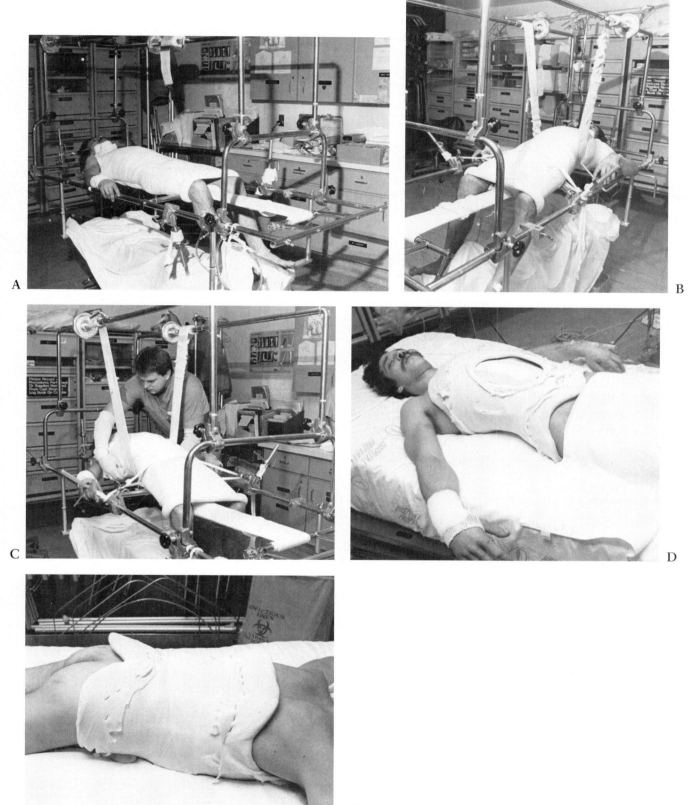

Figure 142.2. Closed reduction and hyperextension casting of thoracolumbar fractures.

transferred posteriorly through the facet joints, allowing immediate weight bearing and good restoration of sagittal alignment and vertebral body height. In Chance fractures, hyperextension closes the posterior defect and approximates the fracture margins. The cast cannot be placed until the abdomen is cleared and any ileus or distention has subsided, however, limiting its use in polytrauma patients. Patients with abdominal trauma, prolonged ileus, chest trauma, or multiple extremity fractures may not be suitable for casting for some time after admission. Once the abdomen is cleared and a well-molded cast is applied, the patient may begin transfers and ambulation. Braces and removable orthoses cannot generate the hyperextension forces necessary to maintain sagittal alignment and should not be considered substitutes for a well-molded hyperextension cast. Also see Chapter 10.

Operative treatment offers significant advantages over casting or recumbency (18,32,43,44,52,53). First, immediate spinal stability is provided for patients who can tolerate neither a cast or prolonged recumbency. Prolonged recumbency in multiply injured patients predisposes them to severe and life-threatening complications. Prompt surgical stabilization allows the patient to sit upright, transfer, and start rehabilitation earlier, with fewer complications (14,31,42). Second, surgical treatment more reliably restores sagittal alignment, translational deformities, and canal dimensions than does cast treatment. And, finally, surgical decompression more reliably restores neurologic function and decreases rehabilitation time (16,23,52,72).

INDICATIONS

COMPRESSION FRACTURES

Compression fractures are usually single-column injuries, are typically stable, and rarely cause neurologic injury. A hyperextension orthosis or chair-backed brace is sufficient to allow ambulation and return to limited activity. Fractures with more than 50% collapse of the anterior vertebral body or with more than 20° of sagittal angulation are considered potentially unstable. A computed tomography (CT) scan may be necessary to distinguish these injuries from a burst fracture. Severe compression fractures can be treated with a hyperextension cast, although some may require posterior instrumentation and fusion.

BURST FRACTURES

Stable burst fractures (two-column injuries) may be treated in a hyperextension cast if the patient has no abdominal or thoracic injuries. Unstable injuries typically require operative reduction and stabilization.

Burst fractures that are considered unstable include

- Greater than 50% axial compression.
- Greater than 20° angular deformity.
- Multiple contiguous fractures.
- Neurologic injury—complete, incomplete, or root.
- Three-column injuries and dislocations.
- Patients with extensive associated injuries.
- Greater than 50% canal compromise at L-1 and 80% compromise at L-5.

Neurologically Intact

In patients with no neurologic injury, treatment decisions are based on issues of mechanical stability and sagittal alignment primarily, and canal compromise secondarily. In the thoracic region, sagittal deformities are corrected by longitudinal distraction, which may also indirectly reduce some retropulsed vertebral fragments from the spinal canal. In the lumbar region, forceful distraction tends to reduce lumbar lordosis, introducing sagittal imbalance and a flat back. Forceful distraction in a patient with a three-column injury may inadvertently lengthen the spinal column and stretch the spinal cord, causing neurologic injury. Segmental spinal systems now allow segmental distraction within the construct while neutralizing construct length and sagittal alignment (Fig. 142.3). The segmental

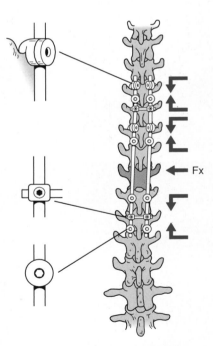

Figure 142.3. Segmental fixation allows the surgeon to neutralize the overall length of the spinal segment, preventing overdistraction, and segmentally distract or compress segments within the construct to either decompress the fracture site or compress an anterior graft.

fixation system allows multiple points of fixation, to distribute reduction forces more evenly. Posterior systems cannot resist sagittal deforming forces if the anterior spinal column is deficient, however (70). Thoracolumbar and lumbar fractures with severe collapse and vertebral comminution tend to lose correction over time unless anterior instability is corrected. Patients with sagittal collapse tend to have more pain and may develop new neurologic symptoms if kyphosis progresses (27,70).

Canal compromise should be assessed in every burst fracture, but it becomes the primary concern only when a high degree of compromise is recognized. Residual compromise greater than 50% is worrisome at the T12–L1 level, where the conus medullaris and cauda equina fill the spinal canal (Fig. 142.4). Small increments of axial or sagittal collapse can compromise neurologic elements, and anterior decompression and stabilization should be considered for both mechanical and neurologic reasons. On the other hand, 80% to 85% canal compromise may be well tolerated in the lower lumbar spine, where only a few roots remain in the otherwise capacious canal (40). Retropulsed bony fragments reabsorb and remodel over time, and do not need to be addressed in their own right (70). Sagittal collapse and kyphosis of a moderate degree is usually well tolerated in the thoracic region, and does not require aggressive reconstruction. Lower lumbar burst

fractures are also well tolerated, and most have a satisfactory outcome without reconstruction. Canal compromise, sagittal imbalance, and segmental kyphosis are all poorly tolerated at the thoracolumbar junction, which is, unfortunately, the most common site of fracture.

Neurologically Compromised

In patients with a neurologic injury, operative treatment is carried out to protect residual function, restore neurologic deficits, and allow early mobilization and rehabilitation without a cast. If the cord or cauda equina injury is incomplete, neurologic decompression can significantly improve the eventual outcome (16,33,61), assuming that there is significant residual compression at the time of surgery (Fig. 142.5). If no residual compression exists, posterior stabilization is carried out alone. If the neurologic injury is complete, anterior surgery will not improve the chance of neurological improvement but may be indicated to treat sagittal deformity or instability. Posterior instrumentation is usually adequate to allow immediate transfers and early rehabilitation.

FLEXION-DISTRACTION INJURIES

Flexion-distraction injuries may occur through bone or soft tissue, and may involve one or multiple motion

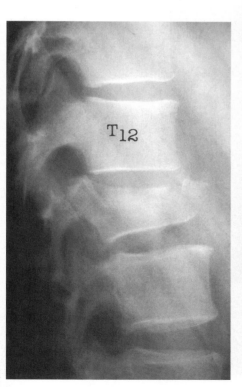 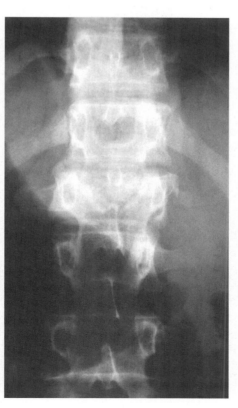

A,B

Figure 142.4. Burst fracture: 32-year-old man fell 35 feet, sustaining severe L-1 burst fracture (Denis type B) and an open tibial shaft fracture. **A, B:** Lateral and AP radiographs demonstrate loss of vertebral height and widening of the pedicles, with little kyphosis. Cortical retropulsion is difficult to appreciate on plain radiograph. *(continued)*

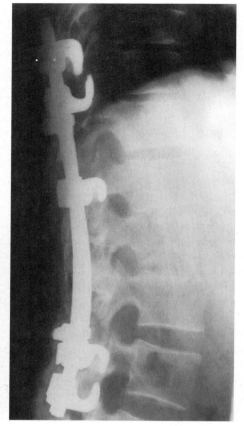

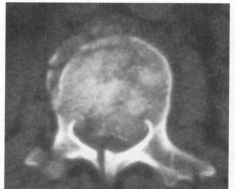

C,D

Figure 142.4. (continued) C: Computed tomography demonstrates severe comminution and canal compromise. A fracture of the lamina is also seen. Even though the patient was neurologically intact, the 75% compromise at the L-1 level seen here was considered too severe, and the spine, unstable. D: Anterior vertebrectomy was followed by strut graft reconstruction, restoring anterior column support and thoracolumbar alignment. Posterior segmental instrumentation stabilizes the spine; the intermediate, down-going hook compresses and entraps the anterior strut. The patient had a full recovery and returned to work and sports without restrictions.

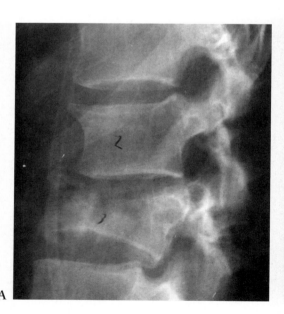

A

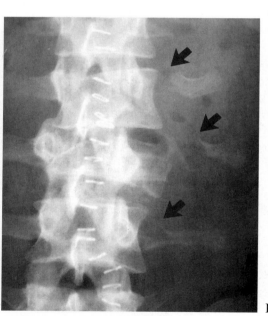

B

Figure 142.5. Burst fracture-contiguous levels: 18-year-old man, status post motor vehicle accident, sustained L-2 and L-3 burst fractures with incomplete cauda equina injury. A, B: Lateral and AP radiographs. Multiple transverse process fractures suggest extent of soft-tissue trauma. (continued)

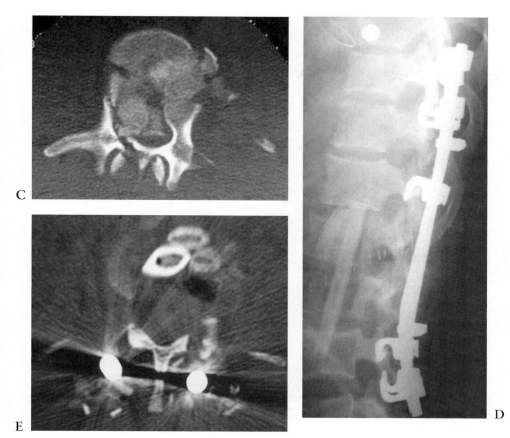

Figure 142.5. *(continued)* C: CT of L-3 demonstrates greater than 80% canal compromise, laminar fractures, and extensive comminution. L-2 was less disrupted but unable to support an anterior strut. D: Lateral radiograph following L-2 partial and L-3 total vertebrectomy, followed by fibular autograft reconstruction. Construct was stopped at L-4 to spare the subjacent discs. At 4-year follow-up, the patient had normal neurologic function and minimal, intermittent back pain. E: Postoperative CT of patient following anterior decompression and reconstruction with autograft fibula and rib. The entire vertebral body has been removed from pedicle to pedicle, and all fragments have been removed from the canal. The patient had full neurologic recovery.

segments (24–26,44,79). Two-column injuries occurring through bone heal reliably and may well be treated in a hyperextension cast. Ligamentous injuries do not heal reliably and more often result in residual instability and pain. These injuries are best treated with a short compression construct and posterior fusion, as are patients with abdominal injuries in patients who cannot tolerate a cast (Fig. 142.6).

Three-column flexion-distraction injuries are highly unstable. The incidence of spinal cord injury is high, as is the incidence of intra-abdominal injury, necessitating a more aggressive surgical approach. Pedicle instrumentation or extended segmental constructs are often needed to stabilize these fractures.

FRACTURE-DISLOCATIONS

Fracture-dislocations are the result of high-energy trauma (motor vehicle accidents and falls from height) and are typically associated with severe neurologic damage and multiple associated injuries (67,74,75). Complete spinal cord lesions do not improve with surgery, but mortality and morbidity are both improved by early mobilization and rehabilitation. Cauda equina lesions are less predictable than thoracic lesions (some improvement may be seen), and restoration of spinal alignment is indicated to stabilize the spine and to decompress entrapped and compressed roots.

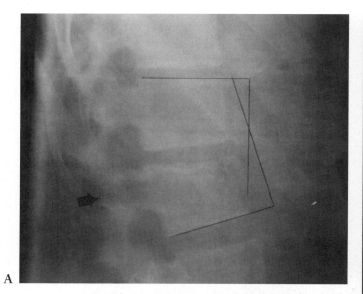

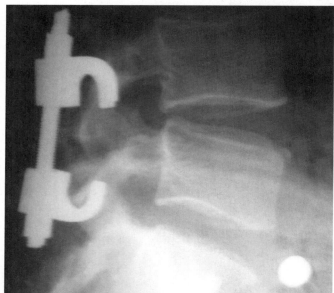

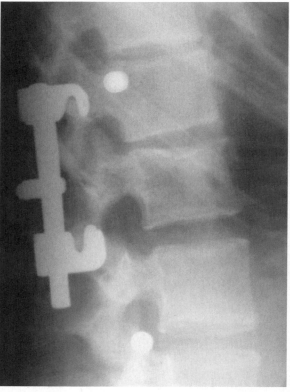

Figure 142.6. Flexion-distraction injury—Chance fracture: 23-year-old with seat belt injury. The patient was neurologically intact but sustained severe internal injuries requiring colostomy. **A:** Lateral radiograph demonstrates focal kyphosis, expanded vertebral height, and transpedicular fracture line associated with Chance fracture. **B:** Because of abdominal injuries, casting was not possible. Operative reduction and fusion were carried out using a segmental fixation system. Reduction was obtained by positioning the patient in lordosis, manipulating the spinous processes to reduce displacement, and sequentially compressing the rod/hook construct until the fracture was closed and facets tightly compressed. **C:** A similar fracture treated with threaded Harrington compression rods.

SURGICAL TIMING

The patient's overall condition must be considered in making a surgical decision. Delaying treatment affords no benefit to the patient but may allow the surgeon to assemble a more skilled team of personnel. If the patient is stable, neurologically intact, and not suffering from multiple injuries, it is safe and reasonable to schedule surgery for the next elective opportunity. On the other hand, morbidity or mortality are not increased by taking the patient to the operating room on an emergent basis, and in some instances, an emergent stabilization may prove instrumental in the patient's overall management.

Patients with thoracic fracture-dislocation associated with severe chest trauma and pulmonary contusion may deteriorate rapidly after hospitalization. Recumbency frequently leads to hypoventilation, pneumonia, and sepsis, irrespective of antibiotic prophylaxis, making delayed stabilization impossible. Pneumonia and respiratory insufficiency will not clear until the patient can be set upright, so a vicious circle is initiated that may take weeks to resolve or may even take the patient's life. Early stabilization

Table 142.1. Polytraumatized Patients Undergoing Surgical Decompression or Stabilization on an Emergent or Routine Basis

	Emergent surgery (<24 hours after surgery)	Routine surgery (24–72 hours after surgery)
N	14	13
Mean age, years	27.5 (16–46)	30.0 (18–58)
Mean ISS	42 (27–75)	36 (27–50)
Mean time to OR	9.7 hours	35.0 hours
Mean EBL, posterior	1432 ml	1600 ml
Perioperative mortality	1/14 (7%)	1/13 (7.7%)
ARDS, sepsis, DVT, PE	0/14	1/13

ARDS, adult respiratory distress syndrome; DVT, deep venous thrombosis; EBL, estimated blood loss; ISS, Injury Severity Score; PE, pulmonary embolism.

(12 to 24 hours) allows aggressive pulmonary toilet, upright positioning, and limits time on the ventilator and in the intensive care unite (ICU), reducing the likelihood of nosocomial infection. Indications for urgent or emergent stabilization include

- Severe chest trauma, pulmonary contusion.
- Polytrauma, with multiple injured systems or long-bone fractures.
- Progressive neurologic deficit.
- Fracture dislocation in a patient already undergoing emergency surgery.
- Fracture dislocation or deformity threatening skin breakdown.

In a recent review of polytraumatized spine fracture patients, perioperative and postoperative morbidity were not increased by emergent stabilization, but neurologic improvement was increased and life-threatening complications were reduced (70a) (Table 142.1). Note that overall mortality is this study was significantly less than predicted by the high Injury Severity Score (ISS), where an ISS of greater than 40 typically results in a 50% mortality rate in this age group.

INSTRUMENTATION OPTIONS

Because the decision to operate is usually predicated on the presence of spinal instability, instrumentation is almost always incorporated into the surgical plan. The type of instrumentation used depends on the injured level, the fracture pattern, the need for anterior stabilization or decompression, and the surgeon's level of experience and training.

Options for instrumentation include

- Nonsegmental rod/hook systems (Harrington rod).
- Hybrid systems (Luque; Harrington rod with sublaminar wires).
- Segmental systems.
  - rod/hook constructs
  - extended pedicle screw constructs
  - short-segment pedicle instrumentation (SSPI)
  - compression instrumentation
- anterior screw/plate or screw/rod instrumentation

HARRINGTON RODS

Harrington rods have been largely replaced by segmental spinal systems but can still play a role in fracture stabilization, primarily in the thoracic spine. Applied properly, Harrington distraction rods can reduce angular deformity, restore vertebral body height, and provide adequate stiffness to allow early mobilization (5,41,52,54). Fixation is dependent on strong distraction forces between the superior and inferior hooks, however, and constructs must span a number of vertebrae to provide optimal corrective forces. Constructs that span three levels above and two below the injury are biomechanically superior to shorter constructs. Three-column spinal injuries cannot resist the distraction forces of the Harrington rod, however, and rods placed in these injuries will either overdistract the spinal column or will not be firmly fixed.

Harrington rods also break in 7% to 10% of cases, usually at the junction of the ratchet and the main rod body (60). Because there are only two points of fixation on each rod, forces tend to concentrate at those points, and lamina fracture or hook dislodgement are frequent, leading to complete loss of fixation (32,36,82).

HYBRID CONSTRUCTS

Adding sublaminar or spinous process wires significantly improves fixation of the Harrington rod and limits the risk of hook displacement (55). Spinous process wires are less likely to pull sublaminar hooks into the canal, but well-fitted hooks are unlikely to displace with either technique (Fig. 142.7). These constructs are best suited to fractures of the midthoracic spine, where extended fusions are relatively well tolerated. Although the addition of sublaminar segmental wires has improved the sagittal and torsional stiffness of Harrington constructs (3,19,63,81,85), it has not eliminated rod breakage. Luque instrumentation may prove useful in some thoracic fractures but does not provide sufficient axial stability to treat burst fractures.

SEGMENTAL SPINAL INSTRUMENTATION

Segmental spinal instrumentation has improved treatment results for a variety of spinal disorders. Originally intended for scoliosis patients, segmental hook and rod systems have now been used to successfully treat trauma, infections, tumors, and degenerative disorders (51,59,76). Clinical series have documented the efficacy and technical demands of segmental systems in scoliosis, kyphosis, and congenital deformities, and have provided the clinician with enough information to develop rational and reliable treatment plans. Such principles have not been as well established for fracture treatment, however.

Segmental instrumentation is being used with increasing frequency for thoracic and thoracolumbar spine fractures, but only a handful of clinical studies have been published to support this application (47,64,80). McBride reported good results in thoracic and thoracolumbar fractures treated with longer hook and rod constructs (64, 65), and SSPI constructs have been endorsed for treatment of lumbar fractures (7,20). Enthusiasm for SSPI has been tempered somewhat by recent studies identifying a high rate of screw failure in unstable fractures (4,8,69,70), however.

Segmental rod/hook constructs take advantage of three-point bending mechanics to reduce and maintain thoracic kyphosis and prevent translation of disrupted vertebral segments. The success of this strategy has been documented in nonsegmental systems (Harrington rods), and a number of construct patterns have been presented for segmental systems (64,65,80). Although they use the same basic reduction strategy as the Harrington rod, seg-

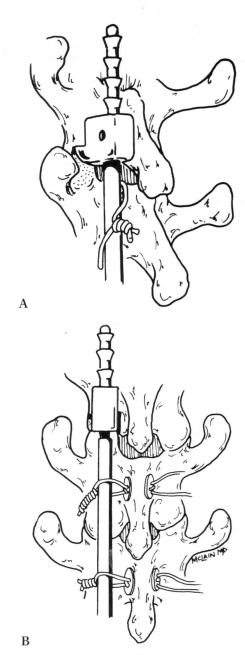

A

B

Figure 142.7. Harrington rod fixation for thoracic fractures. Harrington rods, supplemented with sublaminar wires (**A**) or interspinous wires (**B**), provide sufficient rigidity and stability to treat many thoracic level fractures and fracture dislocations.

mental rod/hook systems offer several unique advantages over first-generation instrumentation systems (6,39,49):

• Proximal and distal hook pairs (claws) provide more stable fixation than the Harrington hooks they replaced.
• Segmental systems are not dependent on strong distraction forces for purchase.

- Contact between the rod and the lamina still provides correcting forces in the sagittal plane.
- Segmental systems allow placement of intermediate hooks, thus distributing corrective forces over more laminae and reducing the likelihood of hook pull-out or fixation failure.
- Segmental constructs are stiffer than Harrington rods in both axial and torsional loading.

PEDICLE SCREW FIXATION

Pedicle screws allow the surgeon to instrument vertebrae with absent or fractured laminae directly. They provide three-column fixation in unstable injuries and limit the length of fusion in the lumbar spine (50). Pedicle screws may be used exclusively or in combination with hook constructs to address a wide variety of fracture patterns. Combined (or "extended") constructs are particularly useful at the thoracolumbar junction. Here, the thoracic spine is relatively immobile and tolerant of fusion. Extending the construct into these segments incurs little mechanical cost and provides more extensive fixation. This improved proximal fixation allows the surgeon to apply enough corrective force to restore sagittal alignment, an imperative at the thoracolumbar junction. Pedicle screws are then applied in the upper lumbar segment to limit the length of the construct, minimizing interference with lumbar motion segments. Extending fusion into the lower lumbar spine does alter mechanics and predisposes patients to junctional pain and subsequent degeneration.

The extended construct often incorporates an intermediate hook applied just above the fracture and just below the upper claw, and directed either cranially or caudally, depending on the situation. In most constructs, a narrow-width hook is placed up-going under the lamina of the vertebra two levels above the fracture. With the upper and lower fixation points locked in place to neutralize the construct length, this hook allows segmental distraction of the fracture to improve vertebral height and decompress the spinal canal indirectly without overdistracting the spine. In anterior and posterior reconstructions, this additional hook may be directed downward to compress and capture the anterior strut graft.

SSPI allows rigid fixation of short segments of the lumbar spine and provides sagittal, axial, and torsional stability superior to rod/hook constructs or sublaminar wiring (49,50). Fixation is not dependent on intact lamina, so there is no need to extend the fusion in cases of laminar fracture or laminectomy. Because distraction is not needed to correct the axial deformity, the risk of either overdistracting the disrupted segment or producing a flat-back syndrome is lessened. Both the surgical and mechanical disturbance to the adjacent lumbar segments is minimized. Nevertheless, SSPI is limited in its ability to maintain sagittal correction in severe burst fractures (7,69,70). If the anterior and middle spinal columns cannot share axial loads,

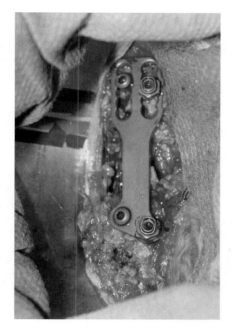

Figure 142.8. Anterior instrumentation for burst fracture treatment.

the bending moments generated at the pedicle screw hub result in a high rate of bending failure or fracture. Once initial bending has occurred, progressive collapse is more likely, with progressive loss of lordosis in some patients.

ANTERIOR PLATES AND SCREWS

A number of anterior fixation systems have been developed over the past 10 years, all based on the principle of anterolateral screw fixation coupled with longitudinal plates or rods (Fig. 142.8). These devices can span multiple segments and can be applied from the midthoracic region down to the L-5 vertebral body. They are intended to augment anterior column reconstruction, providing torsional and translational stability while sharing axial loads with a strut graft or cage (see Chapter 137). When posterior soft tissues and structures are intact, an anterior reconstruction and instrumentation may be adequate to stabilize the spine. If the posterior elements are disrupted, however, the anterior construct is likely to fail unless posterior instrumentation is carried out as well.

 SURGICAL TECHNIQUES

Instrumentation provides little benefit unless the spinal alignment is corrected at the time of fixation. Failure to correct sagittal alignment will result in a fixed kyphotic deformity, predisposing the patient to dysfunction, pain, and instrumentation failure, and necessitating late revision and reconstruction. Failure to correct translational deformity will result in a residual stenosis at the level of offset, and may predispose the patient to nonunion and treatment failure.

POSTURAL REDUCTION OF FRACTURE

The residual deformity in compression, burst, and many dislocation injuries is kyphosis. If this deformity is allowed to persist, it will become fixed and irreducible, but immediately after fracture, fragments are typically mobile and amenable to indirect reduction.

■ If nonoperative treatment is planned, place the patient supine over a bolster until provisional healing has occurred (84) or until the patient is ready for casting. For operative care, accomplish reduction by properly positioning the patient on the surgical frame.
■ Return fractures of the thoracic spine to normal kyphosis by placing the patient on a Wilson frame, adjusted to fit the patient's chest wall. Avoid hyperextension.
■ Reduce fractures of the lower lumbar spine on either a Wilson or a fracture frame.
■ Carry out instrumentation of the shortest possible segment with the hips extended and the torso positioned comfortably on the frame of choice.

Fractures at the thoracolumbar junction are most problematic for the following reasons: (1) The injured segments are junctional between the rigid thoracic spine and the well-supported lumbosacral vertebrae. (2) The neural elements at risk include the conus medullaris and entire cauda equina. (3) Residual deformity is poorly tolerated, and mechanical imbalance predisposes the patient to pain and construct failure.

■ Position the patient gently and carefully in the prone position, with support under the iliac crests distally and the anterior chest wall proximally. Allow the abdomen and midtrunk to hang free.
■ Options for positioning include transverse bolsters, the Relton-Hall type frame, and the Jackson turning frame. The Jackson turning frame allows the surgeon to position bolsters, arm boards, and headrest with the patient supine and awake, then turn the frame and patient as a unit without further repositioning (Fig. 142.9). A Wilson frame attachment is also available.
■ As the abdomen and lower torso hang free, normal lumbar lordosis is accentuated, reducing the kyphotic deformity.
■ Because postural reduction does not completely reduce the kyphosis of a severe burst fracture, it is incumbent on the physician to recognize residual deformity intra-

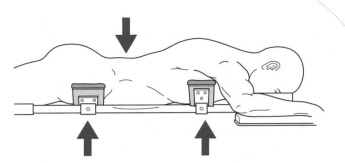

Figure 142.9. Postural reduction of burst and flexion-distraction injuries. Normal thoracolumbar lordosis can be restored by placing patient on a spinal frame supporting the torso and pelvis and allowing the abdomen to hang free. Further elevating the thighs will increase the lordosis in segments adjacent to the fracture, which helps in restoring normal alignment.

operatively and manually restore thoracolumbar alignment at least to neutral position.

OPEN REDUCTION OF FRACTURE

To complete reduction of a burst fracture, it may be necessary to manipulate the spine operatively. Two options are available. First, *in situ* contouring of the implants can restore lordosis to segments that are not completely reduced passively.

■ Contour standard rod and screw or plate and screw constructs *in situ* to restore sagittal balance, or contour the rod before placement and then insert and rotate it into sagittal orientation to increase lordosis. Take care not to overpower and damage the implants, however.
■ Supplement pedicle screws by offset laminar hooks before attempting vigorous contouring.
■ Implants designed specifically for fracture reduction are available; they are designed to neutralize construct length at the same time that manipulation of the pins corrects sagittal collapse (7,30,37,38).

Short-Segment Pedicle Instrumentation

Correction of residual kyphosis is important in the thoracolumbar region. Transpedicular instrumentation systems limit the extent of the spinal fusion to a few levels, and allow direct reduction of deformity. Figure 142.10 illustrates the use of SSPI:

■ After obtaining the best postural reduction, place screws according to anatomic landmarks and fluoroscopic control (step A).
■ Apply the fixation rod and carry out gentle axial distraction to restore the normal height and alignment of the posterior elements (step B).
■ Restore lordosis by levering the dorsal extensions of

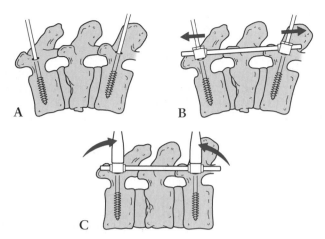

Figure 142.10. Short-segment pedicle instrumentation. See text.

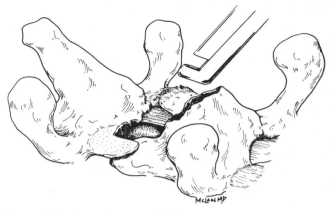

Figure 142.12. Reduction of fracture-dislocation. When simple distraction cannot easily reduce a dislocated facet in a neurologically intact patient, resection of the overlapping articulation with a Kerrison rongeur or burr will allow gentle reduction.

the screws together to distract the anterior and middle columns back to their normal height (step C). The sagittal rotation force applied at the screw-rod connection will further lengthen the posterior column as well, so avoid overdistraction during step B.

■ Then tighten the locking nuts to fix both the axial and the sagittal correction.

Transpedicular Bone Graft

The second option is to reduce the vertebral collapse directly through a posterolateral approach. Using this method, the surgeon elevates the depressed endplate through a transpedicular approach and reinforces the fracture site with a transpedicular bone graft (Fig. 142.11).

■ To restore the anterior weight-bearing column without strut–graft reconstruction, carry out a transpedicular reduction and grafting.
■ Using a specially designed instrumentation set (Synthes NA, Paoli, PA), directly elevate the fractured endplate using a transpedicular approach.
■ Impact fracture fragments into the fracture defect or remove them through a transpedicular decompression.
■ Impact additional graft, harvested from the pelvis using an acetabular reamer, into the anterior half of the vertebral body using a transpedicular funnel and stylet.

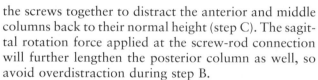

Figure 142.11. Transpedicular bone graft. See text.

Irreducible facet dislocations may require an operative reduction to restore alignment. Fracture-dislocations are usually reduced easily because the soft tissues are completely disrupted. If part of the facet capsule or posterior longitudinal ligament is intact, manual reduction is more difficult. In such a case, in a neurologically intact patient, use a burr to take down the locked facet and allow a gentle reduction without overdistracting the spine (Fig. 142.12).

FUSION TECHNIQUE

Because segmental instrumentation allows the surgeon to instrument only those segments intended for fusion, the routine practice is to fuse all instrumented segments. Long rod/short fusion constructs have been only marginally successful at protecting lumbar segments in fracture patients (3), and newer systems allow surgeons to avoid instrumenting the lower lumbar spine altogether. This technique eliminates the need for a second surgery to remove the hardware and avoids concerns over degenerative changes seen in immobilized, unfused facet joints (21,56).

■ Observe meticulous fusion technique to avoid pseudarthrosis.
■ After stabilizing the fractured segment, decorticate laminae, and transverse processes, take down the facet joints, and liberally dress the lateral and dorsal surfaces with autologous iliac crest graft.
■ Concentrate corticocancellous strips of autograft bone across the fractured segment and around the construct ends, which are typical areas of fusion failure.
■ Take care to preserve the adjacent facet joints and avoid extending the fusion beyond the instrumented segments.

STABILIZATION TECHNIQUES

Thoracic Spine

- Stable thoracic compression and burst fractures may be treated in a Jewett brace or thoracolumbar sacral orthosis (TLSO) with good results.
- Multilevel compression or burst fractures will collapse into further kyphosis; instrument either with a Harrington rod and Drummond wires or with a segmental rod/hook construct. If the Harrington system is used, follow the old rule of "three above, two below," with spinous process wires placed at each intact laminar level.
- Contour the rods to fit the thoracic kyphosis better but leave them somewhat straighter than the desired alignment to provide a third reduction force where the rod contacts the spinal laminae.

Segmental instrumentation can be placed in a variety of ways, depending on the fracture level and pattern.

- For compression fractures, place a simple transversopedicular claw (Fig. 142.13) above and below the fracture level.
- In more severe fractures, use additional claws and intermediate hooks to provide secure fixation and allow intersegmental distraction.
- The rod/hook construct should take advantage of three-point bending mechanics to reduce and maintain thoracic kyphosis and prevent translation of disrupted vertebral segments.

The proximal and distal "claws" provide more stable fixation than the Harrington hooks they replace and are not dependent on strong distraction forces for fixation. The additional hooks applied in segmental constructs distribute corrective forces over more laminae, reducing the likelihood of hook pull-out and fixation failure.

- Arrange hooks to accommodate the regional anatomy and the fracture pattern, as long as at least two hooks are applied on either side of the fracture (Fig. 142.14A–D).
- In upper thoracic fractures, place supplemental hooks caudal to the injury to avoid a bulky construct under the thinner soft tissues of the upper back.
- In lower thoracic injuries, place the supplemental hooks cranial to the fracture site.
- Never place supplemental hooks at the laminae just above the fractured vertebra, because this places the hook directly opposite any bone fragment retropulsed into the spinal canal.
- In osteoporotic bone or in face of transverse process fractures, substitute laminolaminar claws for transversopedicular claws.

Thoracolumbar Junction

- SSPI allows direct reduction of sagittal deformity and translation while instrumenting the shortest possible segment of the lumbar spine.
- Treat thoracolumbar and lumbar fractures with pedicle screws placed immediately above and below the fractured segment.
- In cases of severe axial instability, place offset laminar hooks at the level above the cranial hooks and at the level of the caudal hooks.

If the anterior and middle columns cannot withstand axial loads, a large bending moment is generated at the

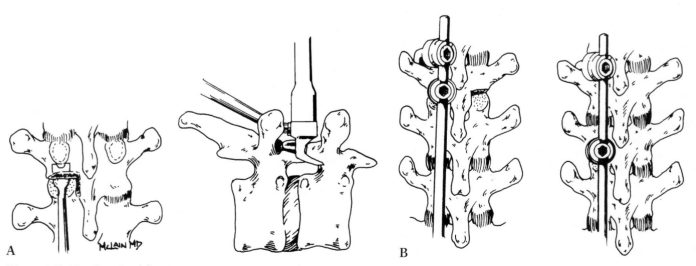

Figure 142.13.   Proximal fixation patterns. **A:** Proximal transversopedicular claw constructs mirror those applied in adult deformities. **B:** In osteoporotic bone, or when the transverse process has been broken, a laminolaminar claw can be substituted.

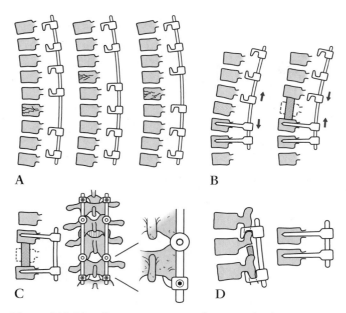

Figure 142.14. Construct patterns for posterior instrumentation: Four basic construct patterns have been applied in thoracic, thoracolumbar, and lumbar fractures, with or without anterior reconstruction. **A:** Upper and lower hook patterns used primarily in the thoracic segments but sometimes in the thoracolumbar segments. These consist of claw configurations above and below the fractured level, with supplemental hooks applied as an additional claw above the fracture in lower thoracic fractures (1), below the fracture in upper thoracic fractures (2), and across the fracture in the midthoracic region (3). **B:** Extended pedicle screw patterns used at the thoracolumbar junction. Pedicle screws placed below the fractured level are supported by offset laminar hooks or additional screw fixation at the level below. Proximal fixation is provided by a claw construct carried to the lower thoracic segment. A supplemental hook is placed above the fracture, providing distraction against the lumbar screws when an indirect reduction is desired (1), and compressing the anterior graft when a direct decompression has been performed (2). **C:** Short-segment pedicle instrumentation (SSPI) patterns used in thoracolumbar and lumbar fractures to limit fusion. Specifically designed constructs are available, or SSPI constructs can be designed from standard instrumentation sets. If the anterior column is unstable, protect posterior screws with an anterior strut (1), or with offset hooks applied above and below the screws (2). **D:** Compression construct patterns. Flexion distraction injuries are generally treatable with a simple posterior compression construct (1). If a fracture dislocation has occurred, pedicle screw instrumentation may be required to combat translational and rotational displacements (2).

pedicle screw hub, resulting in a high rate of bending failure. Acute bending failure occurs before a solid arthrodesis has occurred and before anterior column structures have regained enough strength to share compressive loads. Failure during this period results in progressive collapse of the spinal segment, progressive kyphosis, and clinical

symptoms. Ebelke et al. (34) found that transpedicular bone grafting eliminated pedicle screw failure in their series (see the section entitled Transpedicular Bone Graft), and similarly, patients with an intact or restored anterior column do not experience screw-bending failure (70).

If care is taken to protect pedicle screws in patients with anterior column instability, SSPI is still an ideal approach for selected patients (Fig. 142.15A, B). Do not attempt *in situ* contouring of the rod unless offset laminar hooks are applied to supplement screw fixation. These hooks provide improved clinical results (4,39) and have been shown to improve construct stiffness and to reduce screw bending moments significantly both in sagittal loading and *in situ* contouring (22,83).

Extended pedicle screw constructs are intended to address thoracolumbar fractures with as little alteration of lumbar spinal mechanics as possible (Fig. 142.16).

■ Extend the fixation construct into the lower thoracic region to apply sufficient corrective force to reverse sagittal deformity and restore neutral or lordotic alignment.

■ Use pedicle screws just below the level of fracture to limit the extent of lumbar dissection and fusion (47, 70). Pedicle screws may be supplemented with offset hooks.

The weak link in the extended construct, as in the short-segment construct, is the pedicle screw itself. Unless they are supplemented with an offset laminar hook, additional levels of fixation, or an anterior reconstruction, the pedicle screws are exposed to large cantilever bending loads (73, 78). These forces are concentrated at the screw hub, a natural stress riser, and the contact point between the screw and the lamina (22,45,68,70). Screw breakage that occurs after healing is complete is often asymptomatic (62). Bending failure that occurs before the fracture has consolidated results in progressive material failure and sagittal collapse, and can occur even in braced patients (20,29,58). Patients treated with supplemental offset hooks or with an anterior reconstruction do not develop segmental collapse.

An incomplete neurologic deficit is a relative indication for anterior decompression. It should be recognized, however, that canal compromise can be improved through indirect reduction (77,86), and that bony remodeling improves canal diameter over time irrespective of treatment (71). Still, persistent neural compression can inhibit neurologic recovery (46), and anterior decompression can provide dramatic neurologic improvement in many patients (57,61). Because functional outcome is more clearly related to the residual neurologic deficit than to any other parameter, we continue to emphasize the need to maximize early neurologic recovery. This entails early recognition, rapid resuscitation, corticosteroid therapy, and sur-

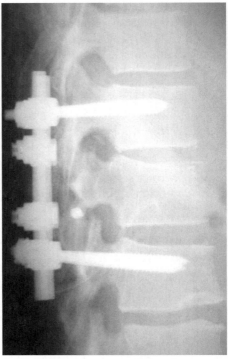
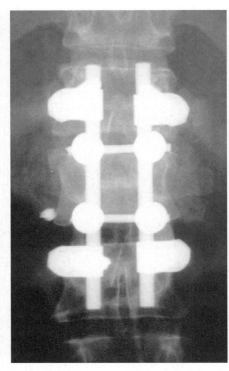
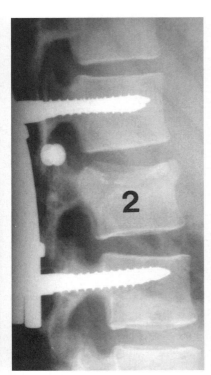

A,B   C

Figure 142.15.   Short-segment pedicle instrumentation. **A, B:** Lateral and AP views of 38-year-old patient with an L-1 burst fracture and marked sagittal collapse. Synthes Universal System fracture module was applied to correct kyphosis and anterior vertebral collapse. **C:** Similar fracture pattern treated with Cotrel-Dubousset segmental instrumentation. Because anterior column disruption was not severe, offset hooks were not applied.

gical decompression when the patient is hemodynamically stable (12,15,23).

- Carry out anterior decompression at the thoracolumbar level through a combined thoracoabdominal approach, providing access to the entire thoracolumbar segment.
- A T-11 retroperitoneal approach may expose all of L-1 and most of T-12 but access to the fractured vertebra and, particularly, to the canal will be hampered by the intact diaphragm (see Chapter 138).
- After completing the surgical approach, identify the fractured vertebral body by inspection and confirm the level radiographically.
- After double-ligating the segmental vessels at the level of the fracture and both vertebral bodies to be instrumented, peel the psoas back from the vertebral body with a Cobb elevator.

    After elevating the psoas muscle back to the level of the neural foramen, completely debride the disc spaces above and below the fracture of disc material, removing the outer annulus circumferentially to the far side.

- Debride the posterior annulus back to the rim of the vertebral body and release it with a small curved curet. The discectomies should be relatively bloodless. Release as much of the fractured vertebra as is possible.
- Once the discs are gone, remove the fractured body piecemeal, taking the near and anterior cortices with double action rongeurs.
- Remove bone back to the posterior cortex with rongeurs and a high-speed burr, until the bell of the near pedicle is exposed and the posterior vertebral cortex has been identified.
- Usually, there will be one large fragment of bone locked between the pedicles, attached to the posterosuperior annulus. Insinuate a fine, curved curet between the bell of the pedicle and the back rim of this fragment to draw it out of the canal.
- Once this edge is freed from the overhanging pedicle, deliver the whole fragment anteriorly with the curet and pituitaries.
- Significant bleeding may be encountered as the posterior cortex is pulled away from the posterior longitudinal ligament (PLL) and the nutrient vessels (Fig. 142.17). Use bipolar cautery and thrombin-soaked gel foam to control this hemorrhage.

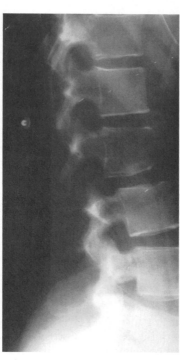
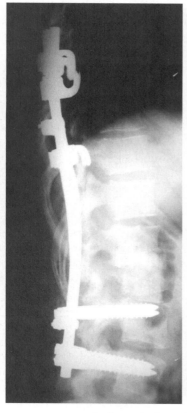
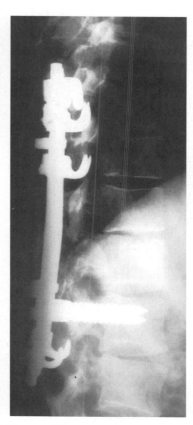

A,B　　　　　　　　　　　　　　　　　　　　　　　　　　　　　　　　　　**C**

Figure 142.16. Extended pedicle screw constructs. **A:** Lateral view of 18-year-old patient with L1–L2 fracture-dislocation and incomplete cauda equina syndrome. **B:** Extended construct using pedicle screws at L-2 and L-3 to stabilize the spinal column, with a down-going supplemental hook to compress the anterior strut graft. **C:** Extended pattern using supplemental offset hooks to protect pedicle screws. Intermediate hooks are directed cranially to decompress the fracture site indirectly.

- On completion of the vertebrectomy, the dura should be visible from endplate to endplate and from pedicle to pedicle.
- Then prepare the endplates for reconstruction.

Lumbar Spine

Whether for simple stabilization or for instrumentation after decompression, SSPI performs well in fractures of the lumbar spine below L-2. Of the few burst fractures of the lower lumbar spine that require surgical treatment, half will undergo anterior decompression for cauda equina compression, followed by strut graft reconstruction (70). Patients with no neurologic injury typically require posterior SSPI alone. If there is severe vertebral comminution, however, anterior reconstruction may be needed to prevent progressive sagittal collapse (66).

Flexion-distraction injuries through soft tissues or multilevel injuries may benefit from internal fixation by one

of two techniques: compression hook constructs or pedicle screw fixation.

- Reduce transverse disruptions by positioning the patient prone on transverse bolsters or the Jackson frame.
- Use a limited exposure of the fracture site, extending to the cranial rim of the first intact lamina above the injury and to the caudal rim of the intact lamina below the injury.
- Debride the disruption of bone fragments, hematoma, and disrupted ligamentum flavum, joint capsule, and muscle. This will prevent the soft tissues from infolding into the canal when the injury is reduced.
- After determining that the facet joints are reduced and the laminar edges aligned, apply a compression construct, with a hook above and one below the intact laminae.
- A Harrington compression rod may be used with two

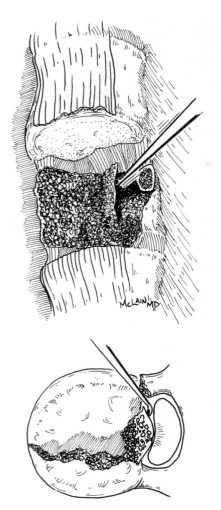

Figure 142.17.   Reduction of retropulsed fragments.

opposing laminar hooks, or a rod/hook combination from any segmental system (44,48,79).

■ For more unstable injuries or frank dislocations, pedicle screw instrumentation provides three-column fixation to control axial, translational, and rotational displacements.

Anterior reconstruction of lumbar fractures may follow a decompressive procedure or may be carried out primarily to address axial instability. Anterior plate fixation may be adequate to immobilize the spine in some cases in which the posterior elements have not been injured. In cases in which laminar fractures or soft-tissue disruption have rendered the posterior column incompetent, reinforce anterior reconstruction with concomitant posterior instrumentation. Likewise, anterior reconstruction at the lumbosacral junction will require a posterior instrumentation, because no suitable fixation of the sacrum yet exists.

Lumbosacral Junction

Surgical treatment of L-5 burst fractures is rarely necessary (40); the spinal canal is large compared with the volume of its contents, and sagittal imbalance is more easily compensated for than at the thoracolumbar junction.

Traumatic spondylolisthesis is an uncommon injury, occasionally associated with sacral fractures or sacral facet fractures. Progressive deformity or onset of neurologic symptoms requires surgical stabilization, typically with lumbosacral pedicle screw instrumentation. Noninstrumented fusion is an option, but progression of the slip may occur even when fusion is successful.

Severe burst fractures are occasionally associated with pelvic and sacral injuries. These injuries are the result of high-energy trauma, and the patients are severely traumatized. Urgent spinal stabilization is indicated to allow safe treatment of multiple injuries, with early mobilization and aggressive pulmonary therapy. If decompression is needed anteriorly, blood loss may be severe.

■ Repair dural tears primarily or with a fascial graft, and reconstruct the vertebrectomy with a tricortical strut or cage.
■ Standard anterior instrumentation is not possible because screw fixation to the sacrum is both difficult and tenuous. Immediate posterior instrumentation to prevent graft displacement is indicated, when possible.
■ Coordinate reconstruction of pelvic fractures or sacral disruptions with spinal care.

Sacral Fractures

Sacral fractures occur most often in patients with pelvic ring fractures, either in association with sacroiliac (SI) joint injuries or as discreet sacral fractures. The treatment of sacral fractures in the context of pelvic trauma is discussed in Chapter 17. There are six basic fracture patterns, as shown in Table 142.2.

Injuries of types 4, 5, and 6 have a high incidence of root and cauda equina injury. Residual compression may result in persistent neurologic deficit requiring surgical treatment. Patients with persistent radiculopathy following fracture should undergo a fine-cut CT scan of the sacrum. Neural foraminae with greater than 50% canal compromise may be indicated for surgical decompression (24, 28,35).

■ Position the patient prone with the abdomen free and a bolster under the pelvis.
■ Expose the sacral lamina through a midline incision and perform an L5–S1 laminotomy.
■ Then unroof the dural sac by laminectomy down to the S-3 level.
■ Identify the involved root (typically S-1) and follow it laterally into the foramen.
■ Take the interval between S-1 and S-2 down to the dorsal aspect of the ventral cortex.
■ Debride the fracture fragments, fibrous tissue, and hematoma away from the undersurface of the nerve root

Table 142.2. Sacral Fracture Patterns

Fracture type	Description	Stability	Nerve injury (%)	Treatment
1	SI joint avulsion	Often highly unstable	21	Unstable—ORIF SI joint
2	Alar fracture	Stable if impacted	10	Protected weight bearing
3	Transforaminal	Unstable if displaced	17	Closed reduction, percutaneous SI screws
4	Transforaminal, extending into canal	Unstable if displaced	60	Closed reduction, percutaneous SI screws
5	Transverse	Highly unstable	50	Bed rest; decompression for neurologic deficit
6	Bilateral transforaminal	Highly unstable	60	Bed rest; decompression for neurologic deficit

ORIF, open reduction and internal fixation.

using down-biting curets, pituitary rongeurs, and small osteotomes.

■ Carry out debridement to the anterior aperture of the neuroforamen, or until the compression is relieved and the nerve root is free and mobile.
■ Fixation of the fracture is usually not possible. Limit the patient's weight bearing until the fracture has united; patient should avoid sitting for up to 2 months.

Transverse Sacral Fractures When a transverse sacral fracture is encountered, laminectomy alone may not be enough to decompress the nerve roots, which are often tented over the kyphotic deformity. This bony prominence must be removed.

■ To avoid injuring these roots, carry out a lateral approach to the anterior from between the exposed nerve roots at the level of fracture, usually between S-1 and S-2.
■ Use narrow osteotomes and down-biting curets to fragment the retropulsed bone, and decompress the cauda equina.
■ Once the kyphotic ridge has been removed, the nerve roots should be freely mobile.

PITFALLS AND COMPLICATIONS

Unless basic biomechanical rules are understood and followed, serious complications can occur following spinal stabilization. Reduction of fractures and fracture-dislocations through distraction is a routine manuever, but overdistraction can widely displace bony elements and stretch the spinal cord, causing serious neurological injury. Also, posterior reconstruction of severe burst fractures without restoring the anterior weight-bearing column exposes instrumentation systems to excessive cantilever-bending forces, resulting in acute pedicle screw-bending failure, or late collapse and fatigue failure. If the normal thoracolumbar lordosis is not restored at the time of surgery, the forces of weight bearing will fall anterior to the lumbar spine and pelvis, imparting an exaggerated flexion moment on the fracture and fixation construct, again predisposing to instrumentation failure. Finally, failure to expose the thecal sack completely—from pedicle to pedicle and endplate to endplate—during an anterior decompression may result in persistent neurologic impairment.

SUMMARY

With newer, segmental instrumentation systems, our ability to address the individual "personality" of each spine fracture has improved. Segmental constructs and pedicle fixation have improved fixation strength and construct stiffness, allowing us to get patients out of bed, into rehabilitation, and home more rapidly and with better long-term results. Newer implant systems must still be applied with full attention to fracture type and biomechanical principles, or implant failure is sure to occur. Technique and implant design cannot alter the damage done to the spinal cord at injury either, and functional outcomes are most profoundly dependent on neurologic integrity. Further research in spinal cord recovery and regeneration holds the greatest promise for future victims of major spinal trauma.

REFERENCES

Each reference is categorized according to the following scheme: *, classic article; #, review article; !, basic research article; and +, clinical results/outcome study.

1. Aebi M, Etter C, Kehl T, Thalgott J. The Internal Skeletal Fixation System: A New Treatment of Thoracolumbar Fractures and Other Spinal Disorders. *Clin Orthop* 1988;227:30.

+ 2. Akbarnia BA, Crandall DG, Burkus K, Matthews T. Use of Long Rods and a Short Arthrodesis for Burst Fractures of the Thoracolumbar Spine. A long-term follow-up study. *J Bone Joint Surg [Am]* 1994;76:1629.

+ 3. Akbarnia BA, Fogarty JP, Tayob AA. Contoured Harrington Instrumentation in the Treatment of Unstable Spinal Fractures. The Effect of Supplementary Sublaminar Wires. *Clin Orthop* 1984;189:186.

+ 4. Argenson C, Lovet J, de Peretti F, et al. The Treatment of Spinal Fractures with Cotrel-Dubousset Instrumentation. Results of the First 85 Cases. Scoliosis Research Society/European Spine Meeting. *Orthop Trans* 1990;14:776.

! 5. Ashman RB, Birch JG, Bone LB, et al. Mechanical Testing of Spinal Instrumentation. *Clin Orthop* 1988;227:113.

6. Benli IT, Tandogan NR, Kis M, et al. Cotrel-Dubousset Instrumentation in the Treatment of Unstable Thoracic and Lumbar Spine Fractures. *Arch Orthop Trauma Surg* 1994;113:86.

+ 7. Benson DR, Burkus JK, Montesano PX, et al. Unstable Thoracolumbar and Lumbar Burst Fractures Treated with the AO Fixateur Interne. *J Spinal Disord* 1992;5:335.

+ 8. Benzel EC. Short-segment Compression Instrumentation for Selected Thoracic and Lumbar Spine Fractures: The Short-rod/Two-claw Technique. *J Neurosurg* 1993;79:335.

+ 9. Bernard TN, Whitecloud TS III, Rodriguez RP, Hadad RJ Jr. Segmental Spinal Instrumentation in the Management of Fractures of the Thoracic and Lumbar Spine. *South Med J* 1983;76:1232.

* 10. Bohlman HH. Treatment of Fractures and Dislocations of the Thoracic and Lumbar Spine. *J Bone Joint Surg* 1985;67A:165.

11. Bohlman HH, Freehafer A, Dejak J. The Results of Treatment of Acute Injuries of the Upper Thoracic Spine with Paralysis. *J Bone Joint Surg Am* 1985;67:360.

* 12. Bone, LB. Management of Polytrauma. In: Chapman MW, ed. *Operative Orthopaedics*, 2nd ed. Philadelphia: J.B. Lippincott Co., 1993:299.

+ 13. Bosch A, Stauffer ES, Nickel VL. Incomplete Traumatic Quadriplegia: A Ten-year Review. *JAMA* 1971;216:473.

* 14. Bostman OM, Myllynen PJ, Riska EB. Unstable Fractures of the Thoracic and Lumbar Spine: The Audit of an 8-year Series with Early Reduction using Harrington Instrumentation. *Injury* 1987;18:190.

* 15. Bracken MB, Shepard MJ, Collins WF, et al. A Randomized, Controlled Trial of Methylprednisolone or Naloxone in the Treatment of Acute Spinal Cord Injury. Results of the Second National Acute Spinal Cord Injury Study. *N Engl J Med* 1990;322:1405.

+ 16. Bradford DS, McBride GG. Surgical Management of Thoracolumbar Spine Fractures with Incomplete Neurologic Deficits. *Clin Orthop* 1987;218:201.

17. Bradford DS, Thompson RC. Fractures and Dislocations of the Spine. *Minn Med* 1976;59:711.

18. Broom MJ, Jacobs RR. Current Status of Internal Fixation of Thoracolumbar Fractures. *J Orthop Trauma* 1989;3:148.

+ 19. Bryant CE, Sullivan JA. Management of Thoracic and Lumbar Spine Fractures with Harrington Distraction Rods Supplemented with Segmental Wiring. *Spine* 1983;8:532.

+ 20. Carl AL, Tromanhauser SG, Roger DJ. Pedicle Screw Instrumentation for Thoracolumbar Burst Fractures and Fracture-dislocations. *Spine* 1992;17(Suppl):S317.

* 21. Casey MP, Jacobs RR, Asher MA. *The Rod-Long-Fuse-Short Technique in Treatment of Thoracolumbar and Lumbar Spine Fractures.* Transactions of the 19th annual meeting of the Scoliosis Research Society, Orlando, 1984.

! 22. Chiba M, McLain RF, Yerby SA, et al. Short-segment Pedicle Instrumentation. Biomechanical Analysis of Supplemental Hook Fixation. *Spine* 1996;21:288.

+ 23. Clohisy JC, Akbarnia BA, Bucholz RD, et al. Neurologic Recovery Associated with Anterior Decompression of Spine Fractures at the Thoracolumbar Junction (T12–L1). *Spine* 1992;17(Suppl):S325.

* 24. Davis AG. Fractures of the Spine. *J Bone Joint Surg* 1929;11:133.

* 25. Denis F. The Three Column Spine and Its Significance in the Classification of Acute ThoracoLumbar Spinal Injuries. *Spine* 1983;8:817.

* 26. Denis F. Spinal Instability as Defined by the Three Column Spine Concept in Acute Trauma. *Clin Orthop* 1984;189:65.

+ 27. Denis F, Armstrong GWD, Searls K, Matta L. Acute Thoracolumbar Burst Fractures in the Absense of Neurological Deficit: A Comparison Between Operative and Non-operative Treatment. *Clin Orthop* 1984;189:142.

+ 28. Denis F, Davis S, Comfort T. Sacral Fractures: An Important Problem: Retrospective Analysis of 236 Cases. *Clin Orthop* 1988;227:67.

+ 29. Devito DP, Tsahakis PJ. *Cotrel-Dubousset Instrumentation in Traumatic Spine Injuries. The 6th Proceeding of the International Congress on Cotrel-Dubousset Instru-*

mentation. Montpellier, France: Sauramps Medical, 1989:41.

+ 30. Dick, W. The Fixateur Interne as a Versatile Implant for Spine Surgery. *Spine* 1987;12:882.

31. Dickman CA, Yahiro MA, Lu HT, Melkerson MN. Surgical Treatment Alternatives for Fixation of Unstable Fractures of the Thoracic and Lumbar Spine. A Meta-analysis. *Spine* 1994;19(Suppl):2266.

* 32. Dickson JH, Harrington PR, Erwin WD. Results of Reduction and Stabilization of the Severely Fractured Thoracic and Lumbar Spine. *J Bone Joint Surg [Am]* 1978; 60:799.

+ 33. Dimar Jr 2nd, Wilde PH, Glassman SD, et al. Thoracolumbar Burst Fractures Treated with Combined Anterior and Posterior Surgery. *Am J Orthop* 1996;25:159.

* 34. Ebelke DK, Asher MA, Neff JR, Kraker DP. Survivorship Analysis of VSP Spine Instrumentation in the Treatment of Thoracolumbar and Lumbar Burst Fractures. *Spine* 1991;16(Suppl):428.

+ 35. Epstein NE, Epstein JA, Carras R. Unilateral S-1 Root Compression Syndrome Caused by Fracture of the Sacrum. *Neurosurgery* 1986;19:1025.

* 36. Erwin WD, Dickson JH, Harrington PR. Clinical Review of Patients with Broken Harrington Rods. *J Bone Joint Surg* 1980;62A:1302.

+ 37. Esses SI, Botsford DJ, Kostuik JP. Evaluation of Surgical Treatment for Burst Fractures. *Spine* 1990;15:667.

+ 38. Esses SI, Botsford DJ, Wright T, et al. Operative Treatment of Spinal Fractures with the AO Internal Fixator. *Spine* 1991;16(Suppl):S146.

! 39. Farcy J-P, Weidenbaum M, Michelsen CB, et al. A Comparative Biomechanical Study of Spinal Fixation Using Cotrel-Dubousset Instrumentation. *Spine* 1987;12:877.

* 40. Finn CA, Stauffer ES. Burst Fractures of the Fifth Lumbar Vertebra. *J Bone Joint Surg* 1992;74A:398.

+ 41. Flesch JR, Leider LL, Erickson DL, et al. Harrington Instrumentation and Spine Fusion for Unstable Fractures and Fracture-dislocations of the Thoracic and Lumbar Spine. *J Bone Joint Surg [Am]* 1977;59:143.

+ 42. Fletcher DJ, Taddonio RF, Byrne DW, et al. Incidence of Acute Care Complications in Vertebral Column Fracture Patients with and without Spinal Cord Injury. *Spine* 1995;20:1136.

+ 43. Gaines RW, Humphreys WG. A Plea for Judgement in Management of Thoracolumbar Fractures and Fracture-dislocations. *Clin Orthop* 1984;189:36.

44. Gertzbein SD, Court-Brown CM. Rationale for the Management of Flexion-distraction Injuries of the Thoracolumbar Spine Based on a New Classification. *J Spinal Disord* 1989;2:176.

+ 45. Gillet P, Meyer R, Fatemi F, Lemaire R. *Short Segment Internal Fixation Using CD Instrumentation with Pedicular Screws: Biomechanical Testing. The 6th Proceeding of the International Congress on Cotrel-Dubousset Instrumentation.* Montpellier, France: Sauramps Medical, 1989:19.

+ 46. Golimbu C, Firooznia H, Rafii M, et al. Computed Tomography of Thoracic and Lumbar Spine Fractures that Have Been Treated with Harrington Instrumentation. *Radiology* 1984;151:731.

+ 47. Graziano GP. Cotrel-Dubousset Hook and Screw Combination for Spine Fractures. *J Spinal Disord* 1993;6: 380.

* 48. Gumley G, Taylor TK, Ryan MD. Distraction Fractures of the Lumbar Spine. *J Bone Joint Surg [Br]* 1982;64: 520.

! 49. Gurr KR, McAfee PC, Shih C. Biomechanical Analysis of Posterior Instrumentation Systems after Decompressive Laminectomy. An Unstable Calf-spine Model. *J Bone Joint Surg* 1988;70A:680.

! 50. Gurr KR, McAfee PC, Shih C. Biomechanical Analysis of Anterior and Posterior Instrumentation Systems after Corpectomy. A Calf-spine Model. *J Bone Joint Surg* 1988;70A:1182.

+ 51. Gurr KR, McAfee PC. Cotrel-Dubousset Instrumentation in Adults. A Preliminary Report. *Spine* 1988;13: 510.

+ 52. Jacobs RR, Asher MA, Snider RK. Thoracolumbar Spinal Injuries: A Comparative Study of Recumbent and Operative Treatment in 100 Patients. *Spine* 1980;5:463.

+ 53. Jacobs RR, Casey MP. Surgical Management of Thoracolumbar Spinal Injuries. *Clin Orthop* 1984;189:22.

+ 54. Jacobs RR, Nordwall A, Nachemson, A. Reduction, Stability, and Strength Provided by Internal Fixation Systems for Thoracolumbar Spinal Injuries. *Clin Orthop* 1982;171:300.

+ 55. Johnston CE, Ashman RB, Sherman MC, et al. Mechanical Consequences of Rod Contouring and Residual Scoliosis in Sublaminar Segmental Instrumentation. *J Orthop Res* 1987;5:206.

! 56. Kahanovitz N, Bullough P, Jacobs RR. The Effect of Internal Fixation without Arthrodesis on Human Facet Joint Cartilage. *Clin Orthop* 1984;189:204.

+ 57. Kostuik JP. Anterior Fixation for Burst Fractures of the Thoracic and Lumbar Spine with or without Neurological Involvement. *Spine* 1988;13:286.

+ 58. Kramer DL, Rodgers WB, Mansfield FL. Transpedicular Instrumentation and Short-segment Fusion of Thoracolumbar Fractures: A Prospective Study Using a Single Instrumentation System. *J Orthop Trauma* 1995;9: 499.

+ 59. Markel DC, Graziano GP. A Comparison Study of Treatment of Thoracolumbar Fractures Using the ACE Posterior Segmental Fixator and Cotrel-Dubousset Instrumentation. *Orthopaedics* 1995;18:679.

+ 60. McAfee PC, Bohlman HH. Complications Following Harrington Instrumentation for Fractures of the Thoracolumbar Spine. *J Bone Joint Surg [Am]* 1985;67:672.

* 61. McAfee PC, Bohlman HH, Yuan HA. Anterior Decompression of Traumatic Thoracolumbar Tractures with Incomplete Neurological Deficits Using a Retroperitoneal Approach. *J Bone Joint Surg* 1985;67A:89.

! 62. McAfee PC, Weiland DJ, Carlow JJ. Survivorship Analysis of Pedicle Spinal Instrumentation. *Spine* 1991; 16(Suppl):S422.

! 63. McAfee PC, Werner FW, Glisson RR. A Biomechanical Analysis of Spinal Instrumentation Systems in Thoracolumbar Fractures. Comparison of Traditional Harrington Distraction Instrumentation with Segmental Spinal Instrumentation. *Spine* 1985;10:204.

+ 64. McBride GG. Cotrel-Dubousset Rods in Spinal Fractures. *Paraplegia* 1989;27:440.

+ 65. McBride GG. Cotrel-Dubousset Rods in Surgical Stabilization of Spinal Fractures. *Spine* 1993;18:466.

! 66. McCormack T, Karaikovic E, Gaines RW. The Load Sharing Classification of Spine Fractures. *Spine* 1994; 19:1741.

+ 67. McEvoy RD, Bradford DS. The Management of Burst Fractures of the Thoracic and Lumbar Spine. Experience in 53 Patients. *Spine* 1985;10:631.

! 68. McKinley TO, McLain RF, Yerby SA, et al. The Effect of Pedicle Morphometry on Pedicle Screw Loading in Unstable Burst Fractures: A Synthetic Model. *Spine* 1997;22:246.

+ 69. McKinley LM, Obenchain TG, Roth KR. *Loss of Correction: Late Kyphosis in Short Segment Pedicle Fixation in Cases of Posterior Transpeduncular Decompression. The 6th Proceeding of the International Congress on Cotrel-Dubousset Instrumentation.* Montpellier, France: Sauramps Medical, 1989:37.

* 70. McLain RF, Sparling E, Benson DR. Early Failure of Short Segment Pedicle Instrumentation for Thoracolumbar Fractures. *J Bone Joint Surg* 1993;75A:162.

+ 70a. McLain RF, Benson DR. Urgent Surgical Stabilization of Spinal Fractures in Polytraumatized Patients. *Spine* 1999;24:1646.

* 71. Mumford J, Weinstein JN, Spratt KF, Goel VK. Thoracolumbar Burst Fractures. The Clinical Efficacy and Outcome of Nonoperative Management. *Spine* 1993;18: 955.

+ 72. Osebold WR, Weinstein SL, Sprague BL. Thoracolumbar Spine Fractures. Results of Treatment. *Spine* 1981; 6:13.

! 73. Panjabi MM, Oxland TR, Kifune M, et al. Validity of the Three-column Theory of Thoracolumbar Fractures. A Biomechanic Investigation. *Spine* 1995;20:1122.

+ 74. Place HM, Donaldson DH, Brown CW, Stringer EA. Stabilization of Thoracic Spine Fractures Resulting in Complete Paraplegia. A Long-term Retrospective Analysis. *Spine* 1994;19:1726.

+ 75. Saboe LA, Reid DC, Davis LA, et al. Spine Trauma and Associated Injuries. *J Trauma* 1991;31:43.

+ 76. Sasso RC, Cotler HB. Posterior Instrumentation and Fusion for Unstable Fractures and Fracture-dislocations of the Thoracic and Lumbar Spine. A Comparative Study of Three Fixation Devices in 70 Patients. *Spine* 1993;18: 450.

! 77. Shuman WP, Rogers JV, Sickler ME, et al. Thoracolumbar Burst Fractures: CT Dimensions of the Spinal Canal Relative to Postsurgical Improvement. *AJR Am J Roentgenol* 1985;145:337.

! 78. Slosar PJ Jr, Patwardhan AG, Lorenz M, et al. Instability of the Lumbar Burst Fracture and Limitations of Transpedicular Instrumentation. *Spine* 1995;20:1452.

+ 79. Smith WS, Kaufer H. Patterns and Mechanisms of Lumbar Injuries Associated with Lap Seat Belts. *J Bone Joint Surg* 1969;51A:239.

+ 80. Stambough JL. Cotrel-Dubousset Instrumentation and Thoracolumbar Spine Trauma: A Review of 55 Cases. *J Spine Disord* 1994;7:461.

+ 81. Sullivan JA. Sublaminar Wiring of Harrington Distraction Rods for Unstable Thoracolumbar Spine Fractures. *Clin Orthop* 1984;189:178.

+ 82. Tasdemiroglu E, Tibbs PA. Long-term Follow-up Results of Thoracolumbar Fractures after Posterior Instrumentation. *Spine* 1995;20:1704.

! 83. Yerby S, Ehteshami J, McLain RF. Offset Laminar Hooks Decrease Bending Moments on Pedicle Screws During In-Situ Contouring. *Spine* 1997;22:376.

* 84. Weinstein JN, Collalto P, Lehmann TR. Thoracolumbar "Burst" Fractures Treated Conservatively: A Long-term Follow-up. *Spine* 1988;13:33.

! 85. Wenger DR, Carollo JJ. The Mechanics of Thoracolumbar Fractures Stabilized by Segmental Fixation. *Clin Orthop* 1984;189:89.

+ 86. Willen J, Lindahl S, Nordwall A. Unstable Thoracolumbar Fractures. A Comparative Clinical Study of Conservative Treatment and Harrington Instrumentation. *Spine* 1985;10:111.

CHAPTER 143
CERVICAL DISC DISEASE

Louis G. Jenis and Howard S. An

The pathoanatomy of disc degeneration or spondylosis of the cervical spine can be considered part of the normal aging process. The progressive deterioration that develops is commonly found in asymptomatic individuals but also may lead to neurocompression, radiculopathy, and myelopathy. The presentation of these syndromes depends on the specific structures compromised by the degenerative process. Treatments of axial neck pain, radicular arm pain, and myelopathy are based on a clear understanding of the natural history of the disorders and available therapeutic options. This chapter reviews the pathophysiology of cervical spondylosis and relates it to the development of clinical manifestations, including the evaluation as well as the nonoperative and operative management of such problems.

CERVICAL ANATOMY/PATHOANATOMY

An understanding of normal and pathologic cervical anatomy is essential to appreciate the role of management of the symptomatic patient. The cervical spine comprises seven vertebrae, each possessing five articulations (Fig. 143.1). The cranial two vertebrae, the atlas and axis, are anatomically unique, whereas the third through the seventh (subaxial) vertebrae are more typical. The first two are rarely involved in the degenerative process and are

L. G. Jenis: New England Baptist Spine Center, New England Baptist Hospital; and Department of Orthopaedic Surgery, Tufts University School of Medicine, Boston, Massachusetts, 02120.
H. S. An: Department of Orthopaedic Surgery, Rush–Presbyterian–St. Luke's Medical Center, Chicago, Illinois, 60612.

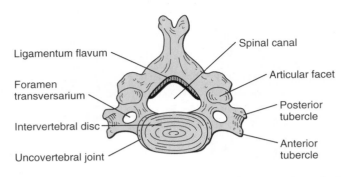

Figure 143.1. Cross-sectional diagram of a normal cervical vertebra. Note the articulations of zygapophyseal facet joints and uncovertebral joints of Luschka.

more commonly affected by inflammatory processes such as rheumatoid arthritis (see Chapter 154).

The subaxial vertebral bodies increase in size from cephalad to caudad and are greater in the transverse than in the anteroposterior (AP) dimension (46). The superior endplate surface is concave, whereas the inferior surface is convex. Uncovertebral joints of Luschka or uncinate processes project from the superoposterior corner of each vertebral body and form a synovium-lined articulation with the corresponding vertebra (32). Short, small pedicles arise from the posterior vertebral body and extend posterolaterally to the lateral masses. The lateral masses are unique to the cervical spine and form superior and inferior articulations via synovium-lined facet joints. The laminae extend posteromedially from the lateral masses and form into the spinous process, which in the cervical spine are ordinarily bifid.

SOFT DISC HERNIATION

The lordosis typically seen in the cervical spine is achieved through the shape and configuration of the intervertebral discs. These discs make up nearly 22% of the overall length of the cervical spine (46). They are thicker in height in the anterior aspect of the intervertebral space supporting the lordotic curvature. The intervertebral discs increase range of motion between the vertebral bodies and distribute forces over the length of the spine (46).

The intervertebral disc consists of the central gelatinous nucleus pulposus, the outer annular fibrosis, and the superior and inferior endplate cartilage. The annulus is composed of alternating layers of collagen fibers running in oblique directions. A normal functioning disc will disperse forces by initial expansion of the nucleus pulposus and stretching of the annular fibers. This process essentially converts an axial load into horizontal forces absorbed by the annulus (46).

The neuroforamina are clinically important parts of the cervical spine. The neuroforamina are confined zones for the exiting nerve roots, bordered anteriorly by the lateral aspect of the intervertebral disc and the uncovertebral joint, superiorly and inferiorly by the pedicles, and posteriorly by the articular masses, notably the superior articular facet. Pathologic conditions involving these structures can lead to critical stenosis of the foramen and nerve root compression.

SPONDYLOSIS

The change from normal anatomy to an aging spondylotic cervical spine is subtle and is part of the degenerative cascade. The initial alterations are suspected to occur within the intervertebral disc leading to secondary changes in the surrounding facet joints and soft-tissue structures. Diminished water content along with changes in the ratio of proteoglycan to collagen, and keratin sulfate to chondroitin sulfate are early manifestations of degeneration (60). Because of this, the nucleus pulposus no longer can generate the hydrostatic intradiscal force required to expand the annular fibers. This subjects the annular fibers to compression and shear forces, causing weakening and tearing in the outer layers. Disc protrusion or frank herniation may ensue, with or without neurocompression.

Disc dehydration also results in loss of height. This is more prominent in the anterior disc space because the uncovertebral joints impact on the posterior vertebral bodies as collapse occurs, preventing further posterior disc height loss. The combined effect leads to the characteristic loss of cervical lordosis on lateral plain radiographs (48).

Approximation of the vertebral bodies alters the biomechanical forces placed on the uncovertebral joints and articular facet joints. Osteophytic spurring, often referred to as hard disc, may develop, leading to encroachment on the neuroforamina. Similarly, reactive bone forms along the posterior vertebral bodies as the margins come into greater contact when higher forces are applied. A spondylotic transverse bar may subsequently form, in combination with bulging of the posterior disc and stretching of the posterior longitudinal ligament. Further collapse of the anterior column height leads to buckling of the ligamentum flavum into the spinal canal, most notably during neck extension. This combination of events may lead to spondylosis-induced compromise of the AP diameter of the canal.

As the cervical discs degenerate, there are several potential sources of pain. Distortion of the intervertebral disc may lead to stretching or compression of the sinuvertebral nerve and finer nerve endings, with subsequent symptoms (54). Additionally, distortion or injury of innervated areas such as the apophyseal facet joints, ligamentous structures, and posterior musculature may produce pain.

There are several sites within the spinal canal where neurocompression may occur. Radiculopathy may occur

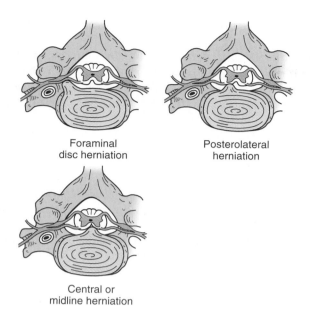

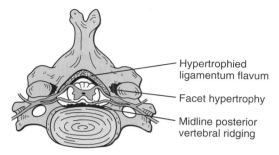

Figure 143.4.   Spondylosis leading to spinal cord compression secondary to hypertrophied ligamentum flavum and spondylotic ridging.

Figure 143.2.   Depiction of types of "soft disc" herniation causing impingement on the exiting nerve root or spinal cord.

from posterolateral soft disc herniation either contained by the posterior longitudinal ligament (PLL) or as free material extruded into and sequestered within the canal (Fig. 143.2). In addition, foraminal stenosis from the changes previously described may also lead to impingement on the exiting nerve root (Fig. 143.3).

The pathophysiology of myelopathy involves many factors (7,8). The stenotic spinal canal may lead to neurologic dysfunction via compression of the anterior spinal artery with cord ischemia or mechanical deformation of the spinal cord from direct pressure, and/or dynamic compression (Fig. 143.4). Hyperextension may cause the lax and hypertrophied ligamentum flavum to buckle, compressing

the spinal cord against the anterior spondylitic bar. Another mechanism of dynamic compression occurs in flexion, where the spinal cord is stretched over the anterior bony prominences. Occasionally, a midline soft disc herniation may cause cord compression and myelopathy combined with a degree of nerve root compression, leading to a myeloradiculopathy.

OSSIFICATION OF THE POSTERIOR LONGITUDINAL LIGAMENT

Finally, myelopathy may stem from cord compression secondary to ossification of the PLL (OPLL). The ossified mass arising from the PLL has been classified as *continuous*, extending over several vertebral bodies; *segmental*, ossification at the level of the posterior vertebral bodies only; *mixed* continuous and segmental; and *localized*, with ossification at the level of the disc only (13).

NATURAL HISTORY OF CERVICAL DISC DISEASE

NECK PAIN

Because of the numerous etiologies that can produce symptoms, establishing a prognosis for a patient with axial neck pain can be difficult. The natural history of neck pain has been evaluated by Gore et al. (30), who performed a retrospective review of patients with neck pain followed clinically and radiographically over a 10-year period. Of these patients, 79% had diminished pain and 43% had nearly complete relief of symptoms. However, nearly one third of the study group reported persistent moderate to severe pain. Outcome could not be correlated with radiographic or clinical findings, making outcome projections difficult for patients with neck pain.

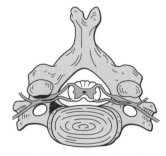

Diagram depicting facet hypertrophy and uncovertebral spurring causing foraminal stenosis

Figure 143.3.   Nerve root impingement secondary to a "hard disc" from spondylosis and foraminal stenosis.

RADICULOPATHY

The natural history of cervical radiculopathy has been well described. Lees and Turner reported on the long-term follow-up of patients with spondylosis and confirmed that 30% experienced intermittent radicular symptoms and 25% had persistent pain (45). Progression from radiculopathy to myelopathy is unusual, and most likely these are distinct entities (25). In general, there is agreement that nonoperative treatment may alleviate symptoms of cervical spondylitic radiculopathy (CSR) in the short term, but over a long period of time symptoms frequently recur. Gore et al. retrospectively reviewed patients with cervical radiculopathy treated conservatively and noted that 50% had persistent symptoms at 15-year follow-up (30).

MYELOPATHY

Cervical spondylotic myelopathy (CSM) is associated with an insidious onset of symptoms and, in general, neurologic function undergoes episodes of worsening with intervening stable periods (42). However, there are no pathognomonic findings to predict the progression of symptoms (49). Clarke and Robinson evaluated the natural history of CSM prior to treatment and concluded that 75% in their cohort experienced episodic worsening of symptoms; 20% showed slow, steady progression without intervening stabilizing periods; and 5% experienced rapid onset of the disease process and progression (18). Progression to total disability is unusual, although slight incremental neurologic deterioration may occur with time, resulting in upper and lower extremity functional deficits. As the neurologic deficit worsens, improvement of disability becomes more unlikely and complete recovery even less likely.

CLINICAL EVALUATION

The clinical evaluation of a patient with cervical degenerative disorders requires interpretation of the patient's complaints, meticulous examination, and appropriate selection of diagnostic tests. To perform a complete evaluation of a patient's complaints, first determine if the problem involves neck pain, arm pain, or a combination of both, or whether there is a myelopathic component. A detailed history is the initial step in evaluating a patient with cervical degenerative disc disease. Obtain a complete description of the symptomatology, including the onset, quality, and location of pain; inciting and alleviating factors; temporal nature; degree of impairment; and any associated symptoms.

Axial neck pain may be discogenic or musculogenic in origin, or it may be related to shoulder, occipitocervical, myofascial, or visceral pathology. To differentiate the potential multiple sources of neck pain, establish whether the symptoms are mechanical (increased with activity and diminished with rest or positioning) or nonmechanical (no relief with positional changes or rest). Nonmechanical neck pain may be related to tumor or infection, and such processes should be carefully sought out. A history of deep-seated aching pain that occurs only at night and is absent or markedly diminished during the day is suggestive of neoplasm or infection. Mechanical neck pain is commonly discogenic in origin and exacerbated with neck extension and rotation toward the side that is more symptomatic. Patients may describe pain referred to the shoulder, upper arm region, or interscapular area. Patients with upper cervical degeneration may also experience occipital or temporal pain, or retro-ocular headaches. Musculogenic pain, as from an acute or chronic muscle strain, is more often exacerbated with neck flexion and rotation, leading to increased symptoms on the opposite side of head rotation.

Radicular symptoms may be caused by a soft lateral disc herniation, chronic disc degeneration with osteophytic spurring, or segmental instability. The majority of patients present with a monoradiculopathy, although several roots can be involved. Symptoms consist of sharp, lancinating, radiating arm pain associated with various degrees of dysesthesia, paresthesia, and numbness along a dermatomal pattern consistent with distribution of the involved nerve root.

The symptoms may be exacerbated or relieved by several provocative tests. Typically, patients will describe an increase in pain with Valsalva activities and with neck extension or turning the head toward the symptomatic side. A Spurling's sign is indicative of radiculopathy. This is elicited by neck hyperextension and rotation toward the symptomatic side, resulting in reproduction of the pain. This maneuver serves to diminish the available area in an already compromised neuroforamen, leading to further nerve root compression. A less reliable provocative sign is the axial compression test, in which compression on the vertex of the skull may diminish the height of the foramen and also symptoms. The shoulder abduction sign is a test that relieves symptoms of compression by lessening nerve root stretch with placement of the ipsilateral hand on top of the head. Patients may present with this as the only upper extremity position that provides relief or comfort.

The history and examination identify the level of radiculopathy. Typically, the patterns of pain distribution that patients describe are imprecise because of anatomic variations, involvement of multiple levels, or the presence of chronic conditions. Upper cervical nerve root compression is less common than lower levels; however, it must be considered in the differential diagnosis of recalcitrant neck pain.

Radiculopathy of the C-3 or C-4 roots will manifest as neck pain radiating to the trapezial, shoulder, and anterolateral area of the chest. The symptoms are described as pain with variable degrees of paresthesia but without a specific motor deficit. A more classic presentation occurs with compression of the lower cervical nerve roots. A C-5 radiculopathy produces radiating pain down the lateral aspect of the shoulder and proximal arm with associated sensory changes and/or increased fatigue or weakness of shoulder abduction. The C-5 root solely innervates the deltoid, whereas the biceps has dual innervation from C-5 and C-6.

A C-6 radiculopathy produces neck pain radiating down the biceps and anterior arm to the radial aspect of the forearm and index finger and thumb. The biceps and wrist extensors may demonstrate weakness. The extensor carpi radialis longus and brevis are innervated by C-6, and the extensor carpi ulnaris is primarily C-7. Therefore, wrist extensor weakness may reflect compression of either C-6 or C-7. The brachioradialis reflex is most directly affected with C-6 compression with subtle changes noted in the biceps reflex due to its dual innervation.

Compressive pathology of the C-7 nerve root presents with pain along the posterior shoulder and arm, radiating to the posterolateral aspect of the forearm to the long finger. Inconsistent symptoms involving the index and ring digits as well as the first web space may also be detected. The triceps muscle is affected, resulting in a diminished reflex and elbow extensor weakness. Triceps weakness is an infrequent complaint, unless the patient is physically active.

A C-8 radiculopathy is characterized by pain referred to the ulnar aspect of the forearm, small finger, and ulnar half of the ring finger. The findings are primarily below the elbow, with most dysfunction noted as numbness along the ulnar digits and weakness in finger adduction, abduction, and flexion. In chronic C-8 root compression, intrinsic muscle atrophy may be seen.

The symptoms of cervical myelopathy are variable and complaints may be vague, so myelopathy is not easily picked up on the initial examination (17,23). Symptoms and findings can include gait difficulties, spasticity, decreased manual dexterity, paresthesias in the extremities, urinary urgency or frequency, and specific extremity or generalized weakness (52). In contrast to cervical radiculopathy, pain is not a common presenting finding. Depending on the site of anatomic spinal cord compression, the symptoms may be quite variable.

The gait disturbance may be an early presenting complaint. Patients describe insidious and slowly progressive stumbling or generalized gait disturbances. Patients may initially become aware of these changes from family members who note a shuffling gait or frequent falls. The characteristic stooped, wide-based gait of the elderly is the common end result. Involvement of the upper extremities may occur concomitantly or follow the gait changes, with complaints of clumsy or numb hands. Weakness of the

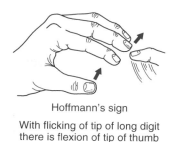

Hoffmann's sign

With flicking of tip of long digit there is flexion of tip of thumb

Figure 143.5. Hoffmann's reflex is indicative of cervical cord impingement. The reflex is positive if the fingers and thumb react in flexion when the long finger distal interphalangeal joint is flicked into extension.

hand manifests as decreased grip strength. Manual dexterity will often suffer and progress until the patient lacks the ability to complete routine activities such as buttoning a shirt, counting change, or writing. Several researchers have noted characteristic hand dysfunction in cervical myelopathy. For example, Ono et al. reported on the myelopathic hand syndrome, describing the finger escape sign and grip and release test (53). The finger escape sign is positive when the patient is asked to hold all the digits of her hand in an adducted and extended position and the two ulnar digits fall into abduction and flexion with time. In the grip and release test, the patient is asked to rapidly form a fist and then release all digits into extension repeatedly. A patient without myelopathy should be able to perform this test 20 times in a 10-second period.

Physical examination of a myelopathic patient consists of thorough neurologic and other special testing. The presence of lower extremity clonus and Babinski extensor plantar responses should be noted. The Hoffmann's reflex (finger and thumb interphalangeal flexion with sudden long finger distal interphalangeal joint extension) when present, and especially when asymmetrical, is strongly suggestive of cervical myelopathy (Fig. 143.5). Other tests that may be noted include an inverted radial reflex, a scapulohumeral reflex, and Lhermitte's sign (43).

DIAGNOSTIC TESTING

Improved neuroradiologic imaging has led to a better understanding of the pathologic process of cervical radiculopathy and myelopathy. Several techniques are available for the evaluation of the symptomatic patient. Each modality has its own inherent strengths and weaknesses, and often combinations of examinations are required.

For initial radiographic evaluation, take AP, lateral, and oblique views and when instability is suspected, perform dynamic lateral images in flexion–extension. Evaluate findings such as disc space narrowing, developmental canal stenosis, subluxations and malalignments, and vertebral osteophtye formation in light of symptoms. Abnormal findings on plain radiographs may not be the cause of the clinical picture; therefore, further correlative studies may be necessary prior to recommending specific treatment. Changes on plain radiographs may also confirm the clinical suspicion of typical degenerative disease and reassure the clinician and the patient that appropriate therapy is being followed.

Water-soluble myelography has been used to evaluate cervical radiculopathy and myelopathy. The AP view demonstrates the exiting nerve roots to the level of the pedicle. A filling defect is a typical finding of nerve root compression. The lateral view may detect spinal cord compression by the disc or posterior vertebral osteophytes and/or hypertrophied ligamentum flavum. Current practice includes myelography followed by computed tomography (CT), which permits visualization of osseous compressive structures, especially in the neuroforamina (4). However, CT-myelography infers neural compression by deformity of the dural sac or nerve roots and cannot directly determine the etiology of contrast blockade.

Magnetic resonance imaging (MRI) does provide direct information about nerve root or spinal cord compression. The advantage of MRI in detecting direct compression is the intrinsic "contrast" available from the cerebrospinal fluid (CSF), as seen on T2-weighted images. This is the most sensitive modality for assessing the morphology of the spinal cord and its relation to the spinal canal. MRI also shows intramedullary cord changes, which may relate to disease prognosis (64). However, MRI is less sensitive in detecting foraminal stenosis and does not demonstrate cortical margins as well as CT-myelography.

Electromyography/nerve conduction studies (EMG/NCS) may be utilized to confirm suspected radiculopathy or may be used as an additional modality to further elucidate the cause of symptoms in a patient with atypical findings. These tests may be most useful when attempting to differentiate root compression and a peripheral neuropathy. Nuclear medicine bone scanning, local diagnostic injections, discography, and CSF analysis have a limited role in the diagnostic process.

NONOPERATIVE TREATMENT

Most patients with symptoms of neck pain with or without radiculopathy can be managed nonoperatively. The initial treatment of moderate to severe symptoms should consist of a soft collar, nonsteroidal anti-inflammatory agents (NSAIDs), and physical therapy modalities, including traction, particularly when radicular signs are present. The limited use of a soft collar may help to decrease the dynamic compression of an irritated nerve root and permit the pain from fatigue or spasm in the paraspinal muscles

to resolve. Prolonged use of a collar is not recommended because of the risk of paraspinal muscle atrophy. Restrict activities to avoid neck extension and heavy lifting during the acute period. Aspirin, ibuprofen, or NSAIDs may provide pain relief. Use narcotic pain medications sparingly, especially in elderly patients. Occasionally, a brief tapered course of oral cortisone may alleviate symptoms of radiculopathy. Physical therapy modalities such as heat and ultrasound may improve acute symptoms, but it is unclear whether they have any effect on natural history. Manual or home traction may provide relief of nerve root compression through distraction of the intervertebral foramen.

As in the lumbar spine, epidural steroid injections (ESI) may be recommended for treatment of the inflammatory component of cervical radiculopathy. The role of ESI is controversial, and the literature lacks well-designed studies documenting their efficacy. Before recommending ESI, weigh the short-term relief of symptoms against possible risks and complications of needle placement (15,65).

Patients with symptoms of myelopathy may be immobilized in a soft collar to prevent dynamic spinal cord compression. However, this is a temporizing measure only and is not definitive treatment.

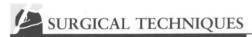

SURGICAL TECHNIQUES

NECK PAIN

The indications for surgery in patients with neck pain secondary to spondylosis, canal stenosis, or discogenic neck pain are limited. Whitecloud and Seago reported 70% good-to-excellent results from anterior interbody fusion for patients with concordant neck pain on discography (68). However, others have found that fusion for discogenic neck pain based on provocative testing yields results that are not much improved from the natural history of the disorder (22). Conservative management for these individuals remains the treatment of choice.

Recalcitrant neck pain from degenerative spondylolisthesis or retrolisthesis is rare in the cervical spine. Instability suggested on dynamic flexion–extension radiographs may be managed by either anterior or posterior segmental fusion.

CERVICAL RADICULOPATHY

The indications for operative intervention in cervical radiculopathy include (a) failure of a 3-month trial of nonoperative treatment to relieve persistent or recurrent radicular arm pain with or without neurologic deficit, and (b) a progressive neurologic deficit (9,27). Neuroradiographic findings must be consistent with the clinical signs and

Table 143.1. Indications for the Operative Treatment of Cervical Radiculopathy

Anterior cervical discectomy and fusion
    Radiculopathy with significant degenerative neck pain
    Bilateral radiculopathy
    Presence of localized kyphosis
    Anterior plating recommended for three levels, or two
        levels with high risk for nonunion

Anterior corpectomy with strut graft fusion
    As an alternative to two-level discectomy and fusion
        procedure, partial anterior corpectomy and strut
        graft fusion can be done to improve fusion rates with
        only two surfaces of fusion between the graft and the
        endplate
    Posterolateral soft disc herniation at two levels
    Spondylotic radiculopathy at two levels
    Migrated disc fragment behind vertebral body; requires
        corpectomy to the dura

Posterior laminotomy/foraminotomy
    Unilateral radiculopathy without significant neck pain
    Absence of localized kyphosis
    C7–T1 level that would be difficult to approach in cer-
        tain patients with short necks

Laminectomy
    Multiple-level radiculopathy
    Bilateral radiculopathy at multiple levels
    Maintenance of cervical lordosis
    Absence of significant neck pain
    Ankylosed or stiff spine

Laminoplasty
    Unilateral, multilevel radiculopathy
    Congenital cervical stenosis
    Maintenance of cervical lordosis
    Absence of significant neck pain

symptoms, and the duration and magnitude of symptoms must be sufficient to justify surgery.

The operative approaches utilized for radiculopathy include anterior decompression with discectomy [anterior cervical discectomy without fusion (ACD)] with or without interbody fusion (ACDF/ACD), anterior corpectomy with fusion (ACF), posterior laminotomy with foraminotomy, or laminectomy or laminoplasty with or without fusion (Table 143.1).

Anterior Cervical Discectomy and Fusion

Surgical exposure of the anterior aspect of the cervical spine is a relatively safe procedure that takes advantage of normal anatomic fascial planes during the approach (55–57).

■ Place the patient in the supine position with a small roll placed under the shoulder blades to drop the shoulders from the field and to present the anterior neck favorably. Strap the shoulders at the side with minimal traction to allow visualization of the lower cervical spine on lateral radiographs.

■ Apply skull traction via a chin halter device or with Gardner-Wells tongs. Keep head rotation to a minimum because deep dissection will depend on identifying the vertebral midline to prevent inadvertent injury to adjacent structures. The reverse Trendelenburg position facilitates venous drainage and results in less bleeding during surgery.

■ The superficial anatomic landmarks for incision include the hyoid bone overlying C-3, thyroid cartilage overlying the C4–5 interspace, and cricoid cartilage overlying the C-6 level. Use transverse incision for exposure in most cases when one or two discs are to be exposed. When three or more levels are approached, use a longitudinal incision along the anterior border of the sternocleidomastoid muscle. The transverse incision is preferred for its cosmetic appeal and access to the anterior spine, whereas the longitudinal incision serves to improve visualization of the region over multiple levels and avoids excessive retraction that may otherwise be necessary.

■ Place the transverse incision along the anterior neck from the midline to the anterior border of the sternocleidomastoid in Langer's lines.

■ Divide the superficial fascia and platysma muscle exposing the middle layer of the cervical fascia.

■ Bluntly dissect the pretracheal fascia and palpate the carotid pulse.

Dissection through the pretracheal fascia places several structures at risk. The superior and inferior thyroid arteries extend through the pretracheal fascia from the carotid artery to the midline. The superior and inferior thyroid arteries travel at the C3–C4 and C6–C7 levels, respectively. The intervening area provides a relatively avascular plane for dissection. The recurrent laryngeal nerves are also at risk during the anterior approach. The right recurrent laryngeal nerve ascends in the neck after passing around the subclavian vessels and courses medially and cranially at the C6–C7 level, often along with the inferior thyroid artery. The left recurrent laryngeal nerve ascends after curving around the aortic arch along the tracheoesophageal groove in a more midline and protected position. A left-sided procedure may be safer, especially when lower cervical segments are approached. However, the thoracic duct is often visible on the left at the C7–T1 level and must be protected.

■ Retract the sternocleidomastoid muscle and the carotid sheath along with its contents (common carotid artery, internal jugular vein, and vagus nerve) laterally, and retract the midline structures, including the trachea, esophagus, and thyroid gland medially.

■ Complete blunt dissection through the deeper levels to the prevertebral fascia and vertebral bodies.

■ Once the midline is identified, incise the prevertebral fascia and elevate the medial edges of the longus colli muscles.

■ Place blunt self-retaining retractors under the leading edges of the muscle. Take care to avoid dissecting along the longus colli muscle because injury to the cervical sympathetic plexus is likely.

■ Identify the vertebral bodies by their concave appearance and the discs by their more convex contour.

■ Localize the disc space with a radiopaque marker and lateral radiograph.

■ Incise the disc with an annulotomy blade and perform the decompression.

■ Remove the disc contents and endplate cartilage to the PLL (Fig. 143.6*A–C*). The proper technique of discectomy involves removal of disc material in a posterior to anterior direction and lateral to medial away from the vertebral arteries. Use thorough evaluative preoperative imaging to determine the presence of a sequestered disc behind the PLL. Palpate the PLL for the presence of a rent that may also indicate a sequestered fragment. In the event that a rent is noted, or if an expected disc fragment is not identified, remove the PLL with Kerrison rongeurs or curets. Beware of routine removal of the PLL, because reports of postoperative epidural hematoma have been associated with this technique (70).

■ Removal of endplate and uncovertebral osteophytes is controversial. The proposed benefits of fusion without spur resection are that disc space distraction reduces

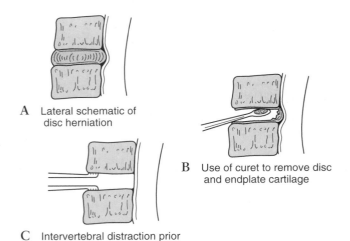

A Lateral schematic of disc herniation

B Use of curet to remove disc and endplate cartilage

C Intervertebral distraction prior to graft insertion

Figure 143.6. Anterior cervical discectomy with distraction of the interspace and removal of disc to the posterior longitudinal ligament. See text for details.

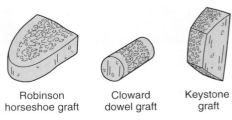

Robinson horseshoe graft   Cloward dowel graft   Keystone graft

Figure 143.7. Types of anterior cervical grafts used in interbody arthrodesis.

ligamentum flavum buckling and increases neuroforaminal area. It is believed that fusion will arrest spur progression, and stability may allow for resorption over time. However, this is not a consistent phenomenon, and the location and size of the offending spur must be carefully considered when performing decompression for spondylitic radiculopathy. Exposure of the uncinate processes is critical to safely remove osteophytes.

■ Utilize a high-speed burr to excise the spur from medial to lateral. Judge the adequacy of foraminotomy by the ability to place the tip of a curet anterior to the exiting nerve root without significant resistance.

Several techniques of anterior interbody fusion in the cervical spine have been described; they differ by graft configuration (Fig. 143.7).

Robinson Technique The Robinson interbody fusion technique involves the placement of a tricortical iliac crest wedge graft into the disc space for bony healing.

■ The graft height should be 2 mm greater than the preexisting disc height, or at least 5 mm, to obtain adequate compressive strength and to enlarge the neural foramina (1). Overdistraction of the disc space by greater than 4 mm of the preexisting height may result in graft collapse and pseudarthrosis (14). Achieve distraction of the disc space with skull traction, laminar spreader, vertebral screws, or combinations of these.

■ Burr the endplates to create a flat surface on both sides of the intervertebral space. Additionally, small holes may be created in the endplates to promote vascularization of the graft.

■ After measuring the depth and width of the disc space, harvest the tricortical graft from the anterior iliac region. Obtain the graft with an oscillating bone saw, because graft weakening has been associated with the use of osteotomes (37).

■ Contour the graft to fit into the disc space and insert it with the leading cortical edge anteriorly and inset 2 mm beyond the vertebral bodies. The graft may also be inserted in the reverse position, with the leading cortex directed posteriorly, to maximize posterior disc space and foraminal distraction. This has been shown to be an acceptable alternative to the more traditional graft position. The graft should be stable with compression after removal of all traction devices.

Cloward Technique   The Cloward technique utilizes a bicortical dowel-shaped graft (19). The technique requires the use of specialized instruments including drills, guards, and a dowel cutter.

Simmons Technique   The Simmons technique for interbody fusion utilizes a keystone-shaped graft (59).

■ After completion of the discectomy, remove bone from the inferior aspect of the superior vertebral body and the superior aspect of the inferior vertebral body with specialized osteotomes.

■ The end of the vertebra is beveled to an angle of between 14° and 18°, as recommended by Simmons and Bhalla (59). Maximally distract the neck and measure the graft site.

■ Harvest a rectangular iliac crest graft and contour to match the beveled surfaces of the vertebral bodies.

■ After the graft is impacted in the host bed, release the traction, thus locking the graft in place.

Bailey and Badgley Technique   The Bailey and Badgley technique involves developing an anterior trough in the vertebral bodies to accomplish fusion (3).

■ Make a trough ½ inch wide and ³⁄₁₆ inch in depth along the full length of the vertebrae to be fused.

■ Remove the intervening disc and endplate cartilage to a depth of ³⁄₁₆ inch and impact a unicortical iliac crest graft into place. Insert the graft with the neck in extension and, after placement, flex the neck to achieve stability.

The Cloward and the Bailey and Badgley techniques have the disadvantage of having no direct nerve root decompression, and thus are seldom used today.

Because iliac crest bone harvesting has an associated morbidity, the use of allograft bone has become a popular method of interbody fusion. In one study, although nonunion rates and graft collapse were more common in ACDF with freeze-dried tricortical iliac crest allograft, the clinical results were similar to ACDF with autogenous bone graft (77). Fibular allograft has also been shown to provide results similar to autograft, with acceptable single-level fusion rates and the absence of donor site pain (74). Other studies have found a higher radiographic nonunion rate with allograft and greater clinical improvement when autograft is used (44). Therefore, the results of using allograft bone are difficult to evaluate. One-level fusion with allograft may be acceptable, but graft collapse and radiolucencies may persist.

The presence of fusion following discectomy has not been uniformly correlated with a favorable clinical outcome, nor has nonunion consistently resulted in a clinical failure (16). The fact that a pseudarthrosis may be associated with a good clinical result led to the concept of ACD. A major advantage of ACD is the lack of donor site complications. However, the disadvantage is postoperative neck pain, which may become severe and is more common than when ACDF is performed (71). Postdiscectomy collapse and angular kyphosis may also occur, leading to recurrent nerve root compression if posterior osteophytes are not widely resected at the index procedure. Bilateral foraminotomies must be performed to prevent contralateral radiculopathy due to resultant disc space collapse. If ACD is to be performed, it most likely should be limited to soft disc herniations and avoided in patients with evidence of spondylosis who require disc space distraction.

Anterior Cervical Corpectomy

A partial or complete anterior corpectomy and strut graft fusion (ACF) may be necessary in situations in which disc herniation is associated with a sequestered fragment that has migrated behind the vertebral body. Subtotal anterior corpectomy and fusion may also be performed when two-level disc disease is present. The theoretical advantage of ACF over two-level ACDF resides in the number of sites that must fuse.

■ Accomplish anterior cervical corpectomy by discectomy above and below the vertebra in question. Then excise the vertebral body with rongeurs or a high-speed burr to the posterior cortex.

■ Next, remove the posterior shell with angled curets directed away from the dura.

■ Traction or distraction may then be applied to restore sagittal plane alignment at the decompressed level.

■ Harvest an iliac crest strut graft and insert it into the prepared endplates, and countersink it slightly into the vertebral bodies. Assess stability of the graft with traction released and, if necessary, consider application of a rigid external orthosis, halo, or internal fixation such as an anterior cervical plate.

Posterior Decompression

Posterior decompression for cervical radiculopathy can be performed with laminotomy and foraminotomy, laminectomy, or laminoplasty (Figs. 143.8, 143.9). Careful patient positioning is required to minimize the risk of neurologic injury and to maximize exposure of the required level.

Laminoforaminotomy

■ Stabilize the head in the prone position with Mayfield skull tongs, leaving the face free without sources of pressure. The reverse Trendelenburg position promotes

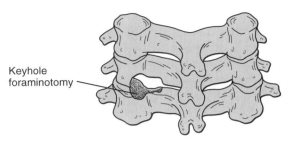

Keyhole
foraminotomy

Posterior cervical exposure

Figure 143.8. Posterior laminotomy and foraminotomy depicting thinning of the lamina and facet joint with nerve root decompression.

epidural venous drainage. The posterior approach to the cervical spine utilizes an internervous plane in the midline which separates the muscles from the segmental innervation supplied by the right and left posterior rami of the cervical nerves.

■ Incise the ligamentum nuchae in the midline and carry the subperiosteal dissection down the spinous processes and corresponding laminae. In the cervical spine, the laminae do not override each other as much as in the thoracic spine; therefore, the interlaminar space may be inadvertently penetrated if caution is not taken during the exposure.

■ Carry dissection out to the lateral edge of the lateral masses and preserve the facet joint capsule if no fusion is required or anticipated.

■ Remove portions of the inferior and superior laminae at the level of the specific nerve root compression and perform partial facetectomy with a high-speed burr.

■ To prevent iatrogenic instability, remove no more than 50% of the facet (78). The lamina and thinned bone should be gently lifted off the nerve and spinal cord with small angled curets.

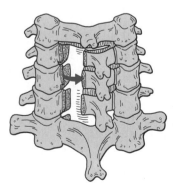

Opening door laminoplasty

Figure 143.9. Open-door laminoplasty depicting hinged lamina and spinal canal decompression.

■ Assess foraminotomy by placing a blunt probe or Woodson dental instrument into the neuroforamen to judge its patency.

■ If disc removal is deemed necessary, expose the nerve root and cauterize the surrounding venous plexus. Gently retract the nerve root cephalad and remove the disc tissue.

Laminectomy   Laminectomy is an option for treating multilevel spondylotic radiculopathy with anterior bony ankylosis when cervical lordosis has been preserved.

■ Perform laminectomy by thinning the cortices at the junction of the laminae and lateral masses bilaterally with a power burr.

■ Use a small Kerrison rongeur to complete the cut and a small angled curet to elevate the laminae.

■ Cauterize the adherent underlying venous plexus to minimize epidural hematoma formation.

■ Loss of the posterior structural support of the bony elements may increase the risk of subsequent vertebral subluxation and kyphotic deformity, especially in younger patients, in whom fusion should be considered at the time of decompression.

Laminoplasty   Laminoplasty may be used in the treatment of multilevel spondylotic radiculopathy with predominantly unilateral symptoms. There are several methods of laminoplasty, which vary by location of the hinge and means of maintaining the open position (36).

■ As in laminectomy, perform laminoplasty by thinning the cortex at the lamina and lateral mass junction with a high-speed burr bilaterally to the inner cortex.

■ Thin the hinged side without completing the cut while completing the osteotomy on the opening side.

■ Gently open the lamina either with towel clips placed through the respective spinous processes or with a vertebral spreader placed into the defect. Fracture the thinned inner cortex of the hinged side and hold the posterior elements open.

CERVICAL MYELOPATHY

The surgical indications for the treatment of cervical myelopathy are not as well defined as they are for the treatment of cervical radiculopathy. A patient with mild, nonprogressive myelopathy that is long-standing and does not cause significant disability can be observed closely. Operative intervention is recommended for (a) progressive myelopathy, (b) moderate or severe myelopathy that is stable and of short duration (less than 1 year), and (c) mild myelopathy that affects routine activities of daily living. The age of the patient or severity of the disease should not serve as a contraindication for surgery; it must be conveyed to the patient that the goal of surgery is to prevent neurologic worsening.

Table 143.2. *Indications for the Operative Treatment of Cervical Myelopathy*

Anterior cervical discectomy and fusion
    Myelopathy with one- (or more) level disease due to disc herniation
    Anterior plating recommended for multilevel cases

Anterior corpectomy with strut graft fusion
    Myelopathy due to disc or osteophyte posterior to the vertebral body at multiple levels
    Loss of cervical lordosis
    Presence of significant neck pain

Laminectomy
    Cord compression at three or more levels
    Maintenance of cervical lordosis
    Ankylosed, stiff spine
    Absence of significant neck pain
    Concomitant fusion recommended if there is vertebral subluxation or instability, or significant neck pain

Laminoplasty
    Continuous OPLL at multiple levels
    Congenital cervical stenosis
    Maintenance of cervical lordosis
    Absence of significant neck pain

OPLL, ossification of the posterior longitudinal ligament.

Based on the clinical and radiographic evaluation, decide whether to approach the area of compression with an anterior technique, a posterior technique, or a combination (Table 143.2). The factors that are critical in this decision process are the site of compression, presence or absence of spinal stability, sagittal alignment of the cervical spine, and extent of the disease process (41).

The presence of primarily anterior compression of the spinal cord limited to the intervertebral disc space without intervening stenosis of the canal at the vertebral body level indicates an anterior decompression. Anterior decompression can be performed with ACDF using the techniques described. Remove the spondylotic ridge, as well as any other areas of spur formation deemed clinically significant that may require hemicorpectomy. If multilevel disease is present, consider anterior corpectomy and strut graft fusion. When compressive pathology is present at the disc level as well as posterior to the vertebral body, as with OPLL, then an ACDF will increase the AP diameter at the disc level only and not the remainder of the spinal canal. Anterior corpectomy allows more complete decompression.

If myelopathy is present along with a kyphotic alignment, an anterior decompression is also indicated. This is best performed with ACF to realign and decompress the spine. When accompanied by significant subluxations, kyphosis may need to be approached from a combined ante-

rior and posterior direction. In the presence of spondylotic spurring and a congenitally tight spinal canal over several segments, consider the posterior approach. A compression ratio of less than 0.5 (sagittal diameter divided by the transverse diameter of the spinal cord) may also indicate a posterior decompression (43). This can be performed with laminectomy or laminoplasty, as previously described.

Anterior corpectomy is performed through a transverse or longitudinal incision, based on the number of levels involved. Decompression of the spinal cord is accomplished by removal of the middle third of the vertebral body. Recommendations for safe decompression to within 5 mm of the transverse foramen allow removal of disc or bone 7.5 mm lateral to the midline at C-3 and 9.5 mm at C-6, which can be estimated intraoperatively (63). Because patient anatomy varies, evaluate this on an individual basis based on the preoperative imaging studies. In anterior decompression for OPLL, a "floating procedure" may be performed (72). The anterior ossified mass is not actually removed but rather is released from its surrounding attachments. The localized OPLL segment mass migrates anteriorly and allows decompression of the spinal cord. Because it is possible to encounter absence of the dura or coalescence of dura and PLL in the anterior approach to OPLL, this form of decompression is often recommended (61).

Strut graft fusion is performed with iliac crest when up to two vertebral bodies are removed, but because of its curvature this graft is less useful when longer struts are needed. In corpectomies of three or more levels, a fibular graft is indicated. The iliac crest graft has more exposed cancellous sites for incorporation, but the fibula is mechanically stronger.

SPINAL INSTRUMENTATION

The role of instrumentation in the surgical management of cervical radiculopathy and myelopathy is less clear than in traumatic conditions (Fig. 143.10). In degenerative disc disease, various studies suggest that nonunion rates and graft dislodgement increase with the number of levels operated on (9,76). The goals of applying instrumentation are to provide immediate stability, increase fusion rate, prevent loss of fixation of the bone graft, improve postoperative rehabilitation, and possibly avoid the requirements for an external orthosis (34).

Animal studies have not shown evidence of improved fusion rates of three-level ACDF with plating (76). Avascularity beneath the plate has also been detected, although its significance is unclear. It is doubtful that anterior plating for single-level ACDF increases fusion rate (21). The potential benefits of instrumentation may not outweigh the risks in these situations. Whether multiple-level ACDF fusion is improved by instrumentation remains to be deter-

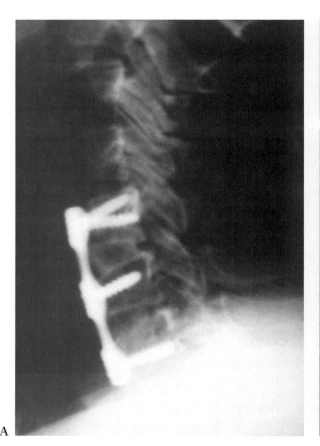

A

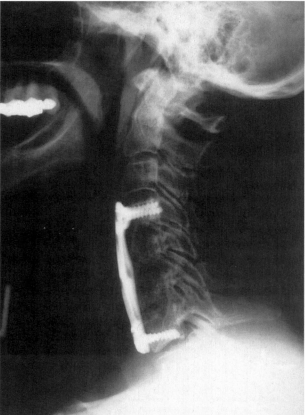

B

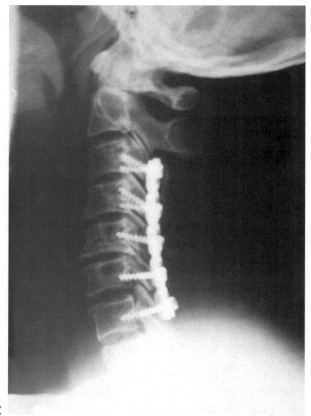

C

Figure 143.10.   **A:** Lateral radiograph shows interbody fusion at C5-6 and C6-7 with segmental plating from C-5 to C-7 (the Peak Polyaxial Anterior Cervical Plate, Depuy-Acromed, Cleveland, OH). This patient, who had a history of cigarette smoking, underwent anterior fusion with plating for cervical radiculopathy with neck pain. The plate was used to improve fusion. **B:** Lateral radiograph shows strut grafting and anterior plating from C-4 to C-7 (the Orion Plate, Sofamor-Danek, Inc., Memphis, TN). This patient underwent anterior corpectomy and fusion for cervical spondylotic myelopathy. **C:** Lateral radiograph shows laminectomy and lateral mass plating from C-3 to C-7 (Axis Plate, Sofamor-Danek, Inc., Memphis, TN). This patient underwent the procedure for myelopathy due to multilevel cervical spondylosis.

mined, and presently no guidelines are available for their use. Two-level ACDF has a higher pseudarthrosis rate than single levels, and instrumentation is often used in certain situations such as patients who are actively smoking. Although rare, three-level ACDF may be accompanied by anterior plating; however, no scientific data support its use. The main use of anterior plating in ACF is to prevent graft dislodgement. When long graft constructs are used, a plate may be inserted at the inferior vertebra as a buttress where graft displacement most commonly occurs (75).

The role of posterior instrumentation in degenerative conditions is also controversial. Posterior decompressive laminectomy may require concomitant fusion in patients with preexisting instability based on imaging studies. Whether the addition of instrumentation such as lateral mass plating or facet joint wiring increases fusion rate while improving the postoperative course is unknown.

POSTOPERATIVE MANAGEMENT—RESULTS

Patients who undergo anterior cervical spine surgery are allowed to gradually increase their postoperative activities and are encouraged out of bed with directed therapy as needed. Liquids are started with a gradual advance to solids as tolerated. Brace management is controversial and dealt with on an individualized basis. Patients recovering from one- or two-level ACDF may be treated in a rigid or soft orthosis based on their surgeon's preference. We recommend rigid external orthoses in ACDF, especially when multilevel decompression and fusion are performed in the absence of anterior plating. Such devices include Philadelphia collars or, in severely osteoporotic individuals, halo-vest immobilization. External wear may continue for 6–12 weeks based on radiographic progression of the fusion and the patient's comfort level. A gradual weaning process may follow from a rigid to a soft collar to no immobilization. A soft collar is all that is needed for posterior laminotomy, laminectomy, or laminoplasty when performed in the absence of fusion.

Postoperative results of surgical treatment of cervical radiculopathy and myelopathy vary, depending on the type of approach utilized and the severity of the disease. Literature review is depicted in Tables 143.3 and 143.4. Limitations in drawing firm conclusions from previous reports stem from the lack of uniform patient population, inclusion of different disease processes in the same analysis (soft versus hard disc), and inconsistency of establishing successful results. Overall, the surgical treatment of radiculopathy yields satisfactory results in greater than 90% of patients. Although controversial, it appears that patients who attain a solid fusion do have better outcomes than those with a pseudarthrosis. The results of treatment of myelopathy also are variable, as depicted by the numer-

Table 143.3. *Results of Surgical Treatment of Cervical Radiculopathy*

Author (ref.)	Patients (N)	Technique	Results	Notes
Robinson et al. 1962 (57)	55 (none radicular)	ACDF	G-E 94% 1-level, 73% 2-level, 50% 3-level	13% nonunion; no correlation between nonunion and outcome
Connolly et al. 1965 (20)	63	ACDF	70% satisfactory	21% nonunion
Williams et al. 1968 (69)	60 (45 radicular)	ACDF	G-E 73%	10% nonunion
DePalma et al. 1972 (24)	229	ACDF	G-E 63%	12.9% nonunion; no correlation with outcome
Aronson 1973 (2)	88	ACDF	100% improvement	0% nonunion
White et al. 1973 (66)	65	ACDF	G-E 68%	25% nonunion, correlated with outcome

(continued)

Table 143.3. (continued)

Author (ref.)	Patients (N)	Technique	Results	Notes
Gore and Sepic 1984 (29)	146	ACDF	76% relief of symptoms	—
Herkowitz et al. 1990 (35)	33	ACDF PLF	G-E 94% G-E 75%	—
Krupp et al. 1990 (40)	230	PLF	G-E 98%	—
Bosacco et al. 1992 (11)	232	ACDF	G-E 87%	6.5% nonunion
Bohlman et al. 1993 (9)	122 (with fusion)	ACDF	G-E 93%	Improved results
Brigham and Tsahakis 1995 (12)	43	ACDF with anterior foraminotomy	G-E 93%	7% nonunion

ACDF, anterior cervical discectomy and fusion; *PLF*, posterior laminoforaminotomy; *G-E*, good to excellent.

Table 143.4. *Results of Surgical Treatment of Cervical Myelopathy*

Authors (ref.)	Patients (N)	Technique	Results	Notes
Bohlman 1977 (6)	17	ACDF	82% improved	—
Lunsford et al. 1980 (47)	32	Ant. decompression	50% improved	—
Zhang et al. 1983 (79)	121	ACDF, 3 or more levels	90% improvement	—
Boni et al. 1984 (10)	29	Ant. decompression, osteophyte removal	G-E 53%	—
Hanai et al. 1986 (31)	30	Ant. decompression, osteophyte removal	5-point improvement on motor/sensory/ bladder scale	—
Yang et al. 1987 (73)	214	ACDF, 3 or more levels	90% improvement	—
Bernard and Whitecloud 1987 (5)	21	Ant. decompression, fibular strut graft	76% improved 1 grade	—
Saunders et al. 1991 (58)	40	Ant. decompression	57.5% improved	15% failure rate; 47.5% complication rate
Ebersold et al. 1995 (26)	84	51, laminectomy 33, ant. decompression	68% improved 73% improved	Increased duration of symptoms Likely late deterioration
Kimura et al. 1995 (39)	29	Laminoplasty	G-E 58%	—
Nagata et al. 1996 (50)	173	96, laminectomy 77, ant. decompression	Improvement in younger patients, fewer levels, milder disease	

ACDF, anterior cervical discectomy and fusion; *ant.*, anterior; *G-E*, good to excellent.

ous techniques utilized to decompress the spinal cord. Overall, patients with greater neurologic deficits tend to experience less improvement in symptoms following surgery than those with more acute and less severe neurologic findings.

PITFALLS AND COMPLICATIONS

The anterior surgical approach to cervical disc disease involves dissection and retraction of numerous vital vascular, respiratory, neural, and intestinal structures. An overall 0.2% incidence of neck site complications based on an extensive review of published series has been reported in one series (67). It is with an understanding of the potential complications that may occur that improvements in techniques and results may follow.

The incidence of *vocal cord paralysis* from recurrent laryngeal nerve injury ranges from 1% to 11% of all neurologic injuries (33). The possible causes are traumatic division, stretch injury, compression from postoperative swelling, and injury from thermal necrosis. Injury is much more likely during a right-sided approach because the right subclavian is occasionally anomalous. In these cases, the right recurrent laryngeal nerve, having no vessel to follow, may cross the surgical field directly and may be easily injured during exposure to the mid-cervical spine. The injury is manifested as a hoarse, weak voice with a risk of aspiration due to the inability to completely close the larynx. When symptoms persist for longer than 6 weeks, referral to an otolaryngologist is recommended for evaluation and possible vocal cord injection.

Sympathetic chain injury is also uncommon and manifests as ipsilateral miosis, ptosis, and anhidrosis. Treatment options are limited.

Midline soft tissue injury to the trachea, esophagus, and pharynx are likewise unusual. *Dysphagia* following anterior cervical surgery is common and is estimated to occur transiently in 8% of patients. When persistent symptoms develop, evaluation should include a lateral radiograph to check bone graft position. *Esophageal lacerations* occur in 0.25% to 0.7% of patients (38). When identified, immediate primary repair should be performed, the wound appropriately drained, and the patient started on broad-spectrum antibiotics.

Vascular injuries during the surgical approach or decompression are rare but can have devastating sequelae. The structures that may potentially be injured include the carotid sheath contents, superior and inferior thyroid arteries, and vertebral artery. Avoid overzealous retraction and use blunt-edged retractors to reduce the risk of injury to these vessels. Knowledge of the anatomy of the vertebral artery and its relationship to the lateral disc space and

vertebral body, as well as maintaining midline orientation during decompression, all serve to minimize the risk of injury estimated to occur in 0.3% to 0.5% of patients (62). The thoracic duct is at some risk during left-sided approaches to the cervicothoracic junction. If a chylous effusion is encountered, injury to the duct must be suspected.

Spinal cord injury is perhaps the most devastating complication that can occur in anterior cervical surgery. An incidence of 0.1% to 0.64% has been reported in the literature (28). The literature indicates that the drill and dowel technique and the presence of myelopathy are the major risk factors for neurologic injury. In addition, neck manipulation during intubation, cervical malalignment following decompression and grafting, and postoperative epidural hematoma must all be considered in the evaluation of the patient with postoperative neurologic deterioration. Management should include maintenance of normotensive blood pressure, administration of steroids, and imaging studies to assess for possible graft dislodgement (28). If compressive pathology is identified, rapid reexploration and decompression are indicated.

Pseudarthrosis rates following anterior grafting procedures range from 0% to 26% (19,20,24,55,57,66,69). Estimates for fusion for single-level, two-level, and three-level ACDF are 88% to 90%, 73% to 80%, and 70%, respectively (9,76). Even though bony union may not occur, a stable fibrous union can develop and account for the lack of symptoms in some patients with pseudarthrosis. However, several reports have found better clinical results when solid fusion is attained (9,55,66).

Bone graft site complications are not infrequent, with a near 20% incidence reported (67). Injury to superficial nerves may result in numbness or pain with neuroma formation. Superior gluteal artery injury has also been reported in iliac crest bone harvest as well as iliac crest fracture.

Complications associated with the posterior approach to cervical degenerative disc disease may also occur. The risk of *hematoma* can be diminished with strict attention to dissection within the ligamentum nuchae and subperiosteally along the laminae. Reattachment of the paraspinal muscles, especially to the C-2 spinous process, may prevent loss of cervical lordosis following posterior decompression (51).

Neurologic injuries are rare during the posterior approach, although they are more common than with anterior surgery (28). Avoidance of placement of instruments into the spinal canal and thinning of the cortex with a high-speed burr followed by the use of curets during decompression may diminish the risk of neurologic injury.

AUTHORS' TECHNIQUES

The clinical syndromes of neck pain, radiculopathy, and myelopathy require extensive preoperative evaluation, and when indicated, surgery must be directed at the specific pathology leading to symptoms (Tables 143.1, 143.2). We manage cervical radiculopathy based on the number of levels involved and the degree of neck pain present. Significant neck pain and up to two levels of radicular symptoms are managed with anterior cervical discectomy and fusion. Radiculopathy without significant neck pain is managed with posterior laminoforaminotomy. In the uncommon situation in which a migrated disc fragment is located behind the vertebral body, a subtotal corpectomy followed by strut graft fusion is the preferred treatment. Radiculopathy involving three levels or greater is managed by laminoforaminotomy or laminoplasty for unilateral and laminectomy for bilateral symptoms. Laminectomy is frequently accompanied by lateral mass plating if there is associated instability. Another option is multilevel anterior discectomy and fusion with plating. For these multilevel cases, the anterior approach is preferred if there is loss of cervical lordosis, and the posterior approach is preferred if there is maintenance of lordosis.

Our approach to the treatment of myelopathy considers the site of spinal cord compression and the sagittal alignment of the cervical spine. Single- or two-level disease is treated with anterior decompression and fusion either with ACDF, if impingement is at the disc level, or with subtotal corpectomy if compression is behind the vertebral body. Multiple-level compression at greater than two levels is managed with anterior decompression and fusion or posterior decompression, depending on the pathology identified. Myelopathy with cervical kyphosis is approached with anterior decompression and strut graft fusion. Laminoplasty or laminectomy plus lateral mass plating and fusion is recommended for three- (or more) level disease with maintenance of cervical lordosis. If there is significant neck pain in addition to myelopathy, fusion is preferred over laminoplasty. Combined anterior and posterior decompression and fusion may be performed when severe circumferential cord compression is present.

CONCLUSIONS

When evaluating patients with cervical degenerative conditions, the physician must be attentive to symptoms and signs of radiculopathy and myelopathy. Appropriate selection of imaging and other diagnostic tests is important for making the correct diagnosis and for cost-effectiveness. The treatment of patients with cervical disc disease is largely nonoperative. Only those patients who failed conservative treatment should undergo surgery for symptomatic relief of radicular arm pain or improvement of neurologic deficits. Patients with cervical spondylotic myelopathy should be treated more aggressively to prevent permanent loss of neurologic function. The choice of anterior versus posterior approach depends on the pa-

tient's symptoms, the location of neural compression, the sagittal alignment, the number of levels involved, and the surgeon's preference.

REFERENCES

Each reference is categorized according to the following scheme: *, classic article; #, review article; !, basic research article; and +, clinical results/outcome study.

! 1. An H, Evanich C, Nowicki B, Haughton V. Ideal Thickness of Smith-Robinson Anterior Cervical Fusion. *Spine* 1993;18:2043.

+ 2. Aronson N. The Management of Soft Cervical Disc Protrusions Using the Smith-Robinson Approach. *Clin Neurosurg* 1973;20:253.

* 3. Bailey R, Badgley C. Stabilization of the Cervical Spine by Anterior Fusion. *J Bone Joint Surg Am* 1960;42:565.

4. Bell G, Ross J. The Accuracy of Imaging Studies of the Degenerative Cervical Spine: Myelography, Myelo-Computed Tomography, and Magnetic Resonance Imaging. In: Weisel S, ed. *Seminars in Spine Surgery—Cervical Disc Disease.* Philadelphia: WB Saunders, 1995:9.

+ 5. Bernard T, Whitecloud T. Cervical Spondylotic Myelopathy and Myeloradiculopathy—Anterior Decompression and Stabilization with Autogenous Fibula Strut Graft. *Clin Orthop* 1987;221:149.

* 6. Bohlman H. Cervical Spondylosis with Moderate to Severe Myelopathy: A Report of 17 Cases Treated by Robinson Anterior Cervical Discectomy and Fusion. *Spine* 1977;2:151.

7. Bohlman H. Cervical Spondylosis and Myelopathy. *Instr Course Lect* 1995;44:81.

8. Bohlman H, Emery S. The Pathophysiology of Cervical Spondylosis and Myelopathy. *Spine* 1988;13:843.

+ 9. Bohlman H, Emery S, Goodfellow D, Jones P. Robinson Anterior Cervical Discectomy and Arthrodesis for Cervical Radiculopathy. *J Bone Joint Surg Am* 1993;75:1298.

+ 10. Boni M, Cherubino P, Benazzo F. Multiple Subtotal Somatatectomy: Technique and Evaluation of a Series of Thirty-nine Cases. *Spine* 1984;9:358.

+ 11. Bosacco D, Berman A, Levenberg R, Dosacco S. Surgical Results in Anterior Cervical Discectomy and Fusion Using a Countersunk Interlocking Autogenous Iliac Crest Bone Graft. *Orthopedics* 1992;15:923.

+ 12. Brigham C, Tsahakis P. Anterior Cervical Foraminotomy and Fusion: Surgical Technique and Results. *Spine* 1995;20:766.

13. Brower R. Ossification of the Posterior Longitudinal Ligament: Clinical Manifestations and Surgical Treatment. In: Weisel S, ed. *Seminars in Spine Surgery—Cervical Disc Disease.* Philadelphia: WB Saunders, 1995:33.

! 14. Brower R, Herkowitz H, Kurz L. Effect of Distraction on the Union Rate of Smith-Robinson Type Anterior Cervical Discectomy and Fusion. Presented at the Cervical Spine Research Society Annual Meeting, Palm Desert, CA, 1992.

+ 15. Castagnera L, Maurette P, Pointillart V, et al. Long Term Results of Cervical Epidural Steroid Injection With and Without Morphine in Chronic Cervical Radicular Pain. *Pain* 1994;58:239.

16. Chestnut R, Abitol J, Garfin S. Surgical Management of Cervical Radiculopathy. Indications, Techniques, and Results. *Orthop Clin North Am* 1992;23:461.

17. Clark C. Cervical Spondylotic Myelopathy: History and Physical Findings. *Spine* 1988;13:847.

* 18. Clarke E, Robinson P. Cervical Myelopathy: A Complication of Cervical Spondylosis. *Brain* 1956;79:483.

* 19. Cloward R. The Anterior Approach for Removal of Ruptured Cervical Discs. *J Neurosurg* 1958;15:602.

+ 20. Connolly E, Seymore R, Adams J. Clinical Evaluation of Anterior Cervical Fusion for Degenerative Cervical Disc. *J Neurosurg* 1965;23:431.

+ 21. Connolly P, Esses S, Kostuik J. Anterior Cervical Fusion Outcome. Analysis of Patients Fused With and Without Anterior Cervical Plates. *J Spinal Disord* 1996;9:202.

+ 22. Connor P, Darden B. Cervical Discography Complications and Efficacy. *Spine* 1993;18:2035.

* 23. Crandall P, Batzdorf U. Cervical Spondylotic Myelopathy. *J Neurosurg* 1966;25:57.

* 24. DePalma A, Rothman R, Lewinneck R. Anterior Interbody Fusion for Severe Cervical Disc Degeneration. *Surg Gynecol Obstet* 1972;134:755.

25. Dillin W, Booth R, Cuckler J, et al. Cervical Radiculopathy—A Review. *Spine* 1988;11:988.

+ 26. Ebersold M, Pare M, Quast L. Surgical Treatment of Cervical Spondylotic Myelopathy. *J Neurosurg* 1995;82:745.

27. Fischgrund J, Herkowitz H. Anterior Surgical Procedures for Cervical Spondylotic Radiculopathy and Myelopathy. In: An H, ed. *Surgery of the Cervical Spine*. Baltimore: Williams and Wilkins, 1994:195.

28. Flynn T. Neurologic Complications of Anterior Cervical Interbody Fusion. *Spine* 1982;7:536.

+ 29. Gore D, Sepic S. Anterior Cervical Fusion for Degenerated or Protruded Discs. *Spine* 1984;9:667.

* 30. Gore D, Sepic S, Gardner G, Murray M. Neck Pain: A Long Term Follow-up of 205 Patients. *Spine* 1987;12:1.

+ 31. Hanai K, Fujiyoshi F, Kamei K. Subtotal Vertebrectomy and Spinal Fusion for Cervical Spondylotic Myelopathy. *Spine* 1986;11:310.

32. Hayashi K, Yabuki T. Origin of the Uncus and of Luschka's Joint in the Cervical Spine. *J Bone Joint Surg Am* 1985;67:788.

+ 33. Heeneman H. Vocal Cord Paralysis Following Approaches to the Anterior Cervical Spine. *Laryngoscope* 1973;83:17.

34. Herkowitz H. Internal Fixation for Degenerative Cervical Spine Disorders. In: Weisel S, ed. *Seminars in Spine Surgery—Cervical Disc Disease*. Philadelphia: WB Saunders, 1995:57.

+ 35. Herkowitz H, Kurz L, Overholt D. Surgical Management of Cervical Soft Disc Herniation: A Comparison between the Anterior and Posterior Approach. *Spine* 1990;15:1026.

+ 36. Hirabayashi K, Watanabe K, Wakano K, et al. Expansive Open-Door Laminoplasty for Cervical Spinal Stenotic Myelopathy. *Spine* 1983;8:693.

! 37. Jones A, Dougherty P, Sharkey N, Benson D. Iliac Crest Bone Graft: Osteotome Versus Saw. *Spine* 1993;18:2048.

+ 38. Kelley M, Rizzo K, Spigel J, Zwillenberg D. Delayed Esophageal Perforation: A Complication of Anterior Spine Surgery. *Ann Otol Rhinol Laryngol* 1991;100:201.

+ 39. Kimura I, Shingu H, Nasu Y. Long Term Follow-up of Cervical Spondylotic Myelopathy Treated By Canal Expansive Laminoplasty. *J Bone Joint Surg Br* 1995;77:956.

+ 40. Krupp W, Schatke H, Muke R. Clinical Results of the Foraminotomy as Described by Frykholm for the Treatment of Lateral Cervical Disc Herniation. *Acta Neurochir* 1990;107:22.

41. Kurz L, Herkowitz H. Surgical Management of Myelopathy. *Orthop Clin North Am* 1992;23:495.

42. LaRocca H. Cervical Spondylotic Myelopathy: Natural History. *Spine* 1988;13:854.

43. Law M, Bernhardt M, White A. Evaluation and Management of Cervical Spondylotic Myelopathy. *Instr Course Lect* 1995;44:99.

+ 44. Lee S, Connolly K, Incorvania B, et al. Anterior Cervical Fusion Using Allograft Versus Autograft Bone. Presented at the Cervical Spine Research Society Annual Meeting, Baltimore, MD, 1994.

* 45. Lees F, Turner J. Natural History and Prognosis of Cervical Spondylosis. *Br Med J* 1963;2:1607.

46. Lestini W, Weisel S. The Pathogenesis of Cervical Spondylosis. *Clin Orthop* 1989;239:69.

+ 47. Lunsford L, Bissoneete D, Zorub D. Anterior Surgery for Cervical Disc Disease. Part 2: Treatment of Cervical Spondylotic Myelopathy in 32 Cases. *J Neurosurg* 1980;53:12.

48. McNab I. Symptoms in Cervical Disc Degeneration. In: Sherk H, ed. *The Cervical Spine*, 2nd ed. Philadelphia: Lippincott, 1989:599.

49. Montgomery D, Brower R. Cervical Spondylotic Myelopathy—Clinical Syndrome and Natural History. *Orthop Clin North Am* 1992;23:487.

+ 50. Nagata K, Ohashi T, Abe J, et al. Cervical Myelopathy in Elderly Patients: Clinical Results and MRI Findings Before and After Decompression Surgery. *Spinal Cord* 1996;34:220.

! 51. Nolan J, Sherk H. Biomechanical Evaluation of the Extensor Musculature of the Cervical Spine. *Spine* 1988;13:9.

* 52. Nurick S. The Pathogenesis of the Spinal Cord Disorder Associated With Cervical Spondylosis. *Brain* 1972;95:87.

+ 53. Ono K, Ebara S, Fiji T, et al. Myelopathy Hand—New Signs of Cervical Cord Damage. *J Bone Joint Surg Br* 1987;69:215.

54. Parke W. Correlative Anatomy of Cervical Spondylotic Myelopathy. *Spine* 1988;13:831.

* 55. Riley L, Robinson R, Johnson K. The Results of Anterior Interbody Fusion of the Cervical Spine. *J Neurosurg* 1969;30:127.

\# 56. Robinson R, Riley L. Techniques of Exposure and Fusion of the Cervical Spine. *Clin Orthop* 1975;109:78.

* 57. Robinson R, Walke A, Ferlic E, Wiecking D. The Results of Anterior Interbody Fusion of the Cervical Spine. *J Bone Joint Surg Am* 1962;44A:1569.

\+ 58. Saunders R, Bernini P, Shireffs T, Reeves A. Central Corpectomy for Cervical Spondylotic Myelopathy: A Consecutive Series with Long Term Follow-up Evaluation. *J Neurosurg* 1991;74:163.

* 59. Simmons E, Bhalla S. Anterior Cervical Discectomy and Fusion. *J Bone Joint Surg Br* 1969;51:255.

! 60. Simpson J, An H. Degenerative Disc Disease of the Cervical Spine. In: An H, ed. *Surgery of the Cervical Spine.* Baltimore: Williams and Wilkins, 1994:181.

\+ 61. Smith M, Bolesta M, Levanthal M, Bohlman H. Postoperative Cerebrospinal Fluid Fistula Associated with Erosion of the Dura. *J Bone Joint Surg Am* 1992;74:270.

\+ 62. Smith M, Emery S, Dudley A, et al. Vertebral Artery Injury during Anterior Decompression of the Cervical Spine—A Retrospective Review of Ten Patients. *J Bone Joint Surg Br* 1993;75:410.

! 63. Vaccarro A, Ring D, Scuderi G, Garfin S. Vertebral Artery Location in Relation to Vertebral Body as Determined by Two-Dimensional Computed Analysis Evaluation. *Spine* 1994;19:2637.

\+ 64. Wada E, Ohmura M, Yonenobu K. Intramedullary Changes of the Spinal Cord in Cervical Myelopathy. *Spine* 1995;20:2226.

\+ 65. Waldman S. Complications of Cervical Epidural Nerve Blocks with Steroids: A Prospective Study of 790 Consecutive Blocks. *Reg Anesth* 1989;14:149.

* 66. White W, Southwick W, Deponte R. Relief of Pain by Anterior Cervical Spine Fusion for Spondylosis. *J Bone Joint Surg Am* 1973;55:525.

\# 67. Whitecloud T. Complications of Anterior Cervical Fusion. *Instr Course Lect* 1978;30:223.

\+ 68. Whitecloud T, Seago R. Cervical Discogenic Syndrome: Results of Operative Intervention in Patients with Positive Discography. *Spine* 1987;12:313.

\+ 69. Williams J, Allen M, Harkess J. Late Results of Cervical Discectomy and Interbody Fusion: Some Factors Influencing Results. *J Bone Joint Surg Am* 1986;50:277.

\+ 70. Wilson CUH. Postoperative Epidural Hematoma as a Complication of Anterior Cervical Discectomy. *J Neurosurg* 1978;49:288.

\+ 71. Yamamoto I, Ikeda A, Shibuya R, et al. Clinical Long Term Results of Anterior Cervical Discectomy without Interbody Fusion for Cervical Disc Disease. *Spine* 1991; 16:272.

\+ 72. Yanagi T, Yamamura K, Ando K, Sobve I. Ossification of the Posterior Longitudinal Ligament of the Cervical Spine. *Clin Neurol* 1967;7:727.

\+ 73. Yang K, Lu X, Cai Q, et al. Cervical Spondylotic Myelopathy Treated by Anterior Multilevel Decompression and Fusion. *Clin Orthop* 1987;221:161.

\+ 74. Young W, Rosenwasser R. An Early Comparative Analysis of the Use of Fibular Allograft versus Autograft Iliac Crest Graft for Interbody Fusion after Anterior Cervical Discectomy. *Spine* 1993;18:1123.

\+ 75. Zdeblick T, Bohlman H. Cervical Kyphosis and Myelopathy. Treatment by Anterior Corpectomy and Bone Grafting. *J Bone Joint Surg Am* 1989;71:170.

! 76. Zdeblick T, Cooke M, Wilson D, et al. Anterior Cervical Discectomy, Fusion, and Plating—A Comparative Animal Study. *Spine* 1993;18:1974.

\+ 77. Zdeblick T, Ducker T. The Use of Freeze-dried Allograft Bone for Anterior Cervical Fusions. *Spine* 1991;16:726.

! 78. Zdeblick T, Zou D, Warden K, et al. Cervical Stability after Foraminotomy: A Biomechanical In Vitro Analysis. *J Bone Joint Surg Am* 1992;74:22.

\+ 79. Zhang Z, Yin H, Yang K, et al. Anterior Intervertebral Disc Excision and Bone Grafting in Cervical Spondylotic Myelopathy. *Spine* 1983;8:16.

## CHAPTER 144

LUMBAR DISC HERNIATION

Dan M. Spengler

This chapter focuses on the evaluation and management of the patient with low back pain or sciatica, or both, that results from a herniation of a lumbar disc. The gold standard technique using open lumbar discectomy with loupe magnification is presented. In addition, the technical options for removing a lateral extraforaminal disc herniation are also discussed, as are pitfalls and complications. The most important concern regarding the management of lumbar disc herniation is selection of the appropriate patient for surgery than it is the technique for removal, assuming that a competent surgeon performs an adequate decompression.

ETIOLOGY OF LUMBAR HERNIATION

This is a multifactoral problem and we still do not understand the precise cause for lumbar disc herniation in any given patient. Why is it that one person develops a lumbar disc herniation and another person does not? Patients with lumbar disc herniations are commonly seen in clinical practice. Fortunately, the majority of these patients re-

spond to nonoperative management and do not require surgical removal of the disc. The reason for this improvement remains elusive, although recent work by Haro et al. (6) suggests that a local inflammatory process in the epidural space may stimulate host macrophages to resorb the displaced disc tissue.

From a biomedical perspective, Farfan (4) has shown that lumbar disc herniation may be reflective of high stresses at the posterolateral region of the disc secondary to torsion. These high loads cause fatigue failure of the annulus fibrosis that enables the inner nucleus pulposus to penetrate the laminations of the annulus gradually until a herniation occurs (4). Because the region of the disc with the highest torsional stresses is adjacent to the nerve root, these posterolateral herniations nearly always affect the exiting root or the central thecal sac. Less commonly, the disc may protrude into the extraforaminal area and produce compromise of the more proximal exiting root (e.g., L-4 for a lateral L4–L5 herniation).

Many authors have examined various factors that may represent predictors or risk factors for a lumbar disc herniation (2,3,9,15–17). The factors that seem to emerge as possibly being predictive include tall men, heavy women, individuals with a small spinal canal, and those who work in an environment with considerable vibration, such as that of airplane pilots and heavy equipment operators (2).

D. M. **Spengler:** Vanderbilt University Medical Center, Department of Orthopaedics, Nashville, Tennessee, 37232.

NATURAL HISTORY

In a controlled, prospective long-term study, Weber (20) randomized 126 patients between surgical and nonsurgical treatments. At 1 year, those in the surgical group had fewer pain complaints. At 4 years, there was no statistically significant difference between the two groups. Weber was not a surgeon, and he had no bias toward the efficacy of surgery. One can conclude that surgical intervention should be limited to patients with a significant neurologic deficit or to those patients who are unable to engage in the lifestyle they desire because of sciatica. Weber (20) also demonstrated that less than 2% of the patients in both groups remained symptomatic at the end of 10 years.

ASSESSMENT AND DIAGNOSIS

In patients with the acute onset of sciatica, perform a general history and physical examination. If no findings are identified that suggest another disease process, and the history and physical exam are consistent with a lumbar disc herniation without major neurologic compromise, initiate nonoperative treatment without imaging studies. Many patients improve rapidly and do not require further diagnostic testing. Those patients who do not improve within 30 days and who wish a prompt resolution to their problem warrant a thorough assessment. Plain radiographs with an anteroposterior (AP) and lateral flexion-extension views are useful to document hypermobility patterns or any spinal deformity. Obtain an magnetic resonance imaging (MRI) scan to characterize any disc pathology, localize any herniation, and exclude other conditions such as a spinal cord tumor or tethered cord. If the MRI reveals herniations at numerous disc levels, or if the patient has a contraindication to MRI (e.g., claustrophobia, intracranial vascular clips), obtain a computed tomography (CT) scan or myelogram.

I also request my patients to complete a pain drawing

Table 144.1. *Objective Patient Evaluation System*

Category	Maximum points allowed for category	Points assigned to parameters
I. Neurologic signs	25	
Consistent weakness associated with positive results on EMG		25
Normal EMG		10
• Atrophy more than 2 cm		10
• Absent or asymmetric reflex		
Patients younger than 50 years of age (add 5 points if EMG results are positive)		20
Patients older than 50 years of age (add 15 points if EMG results are positive)		10
• No clinical signs: positive findings on EMG		15
II. Sciatic tension signs	25	
• Positive crossed straight-leg-raising sign		20
• Pelvic tilt (pelvic list)		15
• Dysrhythmia of the lumbar paraspinal muscles with motion		15
• Positive ipsilateral straight-leg raising		5
III. Personality factors (MMPI Scores)	25	
• Normal (includes depression)		25
• Abnormal (impulsive/schizophrenic)		10
• Elevated hysteria (more than 1 SD and less than 2 SD)		10
• Conversion reaction or hysteria (more than 2 SD)		0
IV. Lumbar myelography/CT scan/MRI	25	
• Positive results that correlate with clinical findings		25
• Equivocal nerve root asymmetry		10
• Positive results, but no correlation with clinical findings (excludes spinal stenosis)		0
• Normal		0
Total	100	

Adapted from Spengler DM, Freeman D. Patient Selection for Lumbar Discectomy. *Spine* 1979;4:129, with permission.
EMG, Electromyogram; MMPI, Minnesota multiplastic personality inventory; SD, standard deviation; CT, computed tomography.

to evaluate the psychological characteristics of the patient. The pain drawing has been shown to correlate well with more formalized psychological testing (13). Psychological factors have been shown to be important predictors of outcome and, therefore, are of value to the surgeon (19).

I continue to formulate my surgical recommendation for patients by using the objective patient evaluation system (OPES) (19) (Table 144.1). If a patient has less than 50 points on this system, I recommend nonoperative management. More recently, we have found that even patients who have lumbar disc herniation with more than 50 points on the OPES will not necessarily achieve a "good outcome," as we previously reported (11). If the patient has engaged an attorney to assist with a compensation claim or if the patient has an attorney who is involved in a civil claim, such as for a car accident, the likelihood for a good clinical outcome drops approximately 30% (11).

Patients who present with profound neurologic deficits, such as complete foot drop or cauda equina syndrome, require prompt imaging studies and early surgical decompression. These patients will not be discussed in this chapter because the focus here is on elective lumbar discectomy.

NONOPERATIVE MANAGEMENT

In approaching patients with lumbar disc herniations, it is imperative to formulate a good nonoperative treatment plan. The initial goal is to control symptoms. Once symptoms are controlled, start an activation program. Such a program should include both an aerobic conditioning component and trunk muscle strengthening. In the majority of patients, symptoms can be controlled with nonsteroidal anti-inflammatory drugs (NSAIDs), acetaminophen (Tylenol), or salicylates. Narcotic medications are occasionally necessary in the first few days of the acute phase, but do not use narcotics for long-term pain control. Steroid dose packs have not been shown to be effective in a controlled study (5). Bed rest may be useful for 1 to 2 days but no longer. As the patient improves, implement a self-guided or supervised physical therapy program to enhance aerobic activity and to improve trunk strength. I prefer resistive exercise equipment such as Cybex, Nautilus, and therabands to strengthen both trunk flexors and extensors. Limit range of motion to 30° of flexion and 30° of extension if resistive equipment is used. If the patient demonstrates good progress, he or she can resume full activities at approximately 3 months after onset, assuming that there is full compliance with an activation program.

Although I do use epidural injections in selected patients with back or radicular pain, I avoid these injections in a patient with lumbar disc herniation, especially if a neural deficit is present. No prospective study has demonstrated success with the use of epidural injections in patients with a lumbar disc herniation.

AUTHOR'S PERSPECTIVE

My indications for lumbar discectomy are based on the OPES (Table 144.1) (19). I recommend an elective discectomy only if the patient has failed to respond to a minimum of 30 days of nonoperative management. The patient must demonstrate that his or her quality of life is sufficiently impaired to warrant an elective spinal procedure. Finally, the patient must have a minimum of 50 points on the OPES (19). The technique that I select for surgery has nothing to do with the indications. Once I am comfortable that the patient understands the diagnosis and alternate treatment options, I select the optimal procedure for the patient based on the preoperative imaging studies as well as my knowledge and experience.

I believe that the gold standard surgical procedure for patient management remains open laminotomy with discectomy using loupe magnification (7,16). I perform the approach unilaterally if the symptoms are unilateral. If the patient has a central herniation with bilateral symptoms, I use a bilateral approach with bilateral removal of the disc nucleus. If a massive extruded disc is apparent on imaging studies, a hemilaminectomy may be necessary to provide sufficient longitudinal decompression to be able to safely mobilize the affected nerve root or thecal sac.

In the patient who demonstrates a far lateral or extraforaminal disc herniation, there are two options. An intervening hemilaminectomy may be performed so that the lateral herniation can be clearly visualized between the exiting nerve root above and the exiting nerve root below (18). Thus, for a far lateral disc herniation at L4–L5, expose both the L-4 and the L-5 nerve roots. Some surgeons prefer an extraforaminal approach (21,22). In this approach, make an incision lateral to the midline in the region of the transverse processes and facet joints. Carry the dissection through the intertransverse muscles and ligament to expose the lateral disc and exiting nerve root. Gain adequate exposure to understand the pathologic process clearly because the nerve root may be displaced from the normal course (3).

Microdiscectomy has been touted by several authors, most notably McCulloch and Young (12), who have written an entire text dealing with the nuances of this technique. Although lumbar microdiscectomy remains an appropriate technique to remove a lumbar disc herniation, I continue to prefer the open laminectomy approach with loupe magnification. Potential benefits of lumbar microdiscectomy would include a smaller incision, more focused lighting, and not wearing loupes and a fiberoptic headlight. Disadvantages include a higher incidence of dural tears and a more limited exposure, which might contribute to overlooking foraminal stenosis. Length of stay, blood loss, and time to full recovery are not different between the two procedures. I have no objection to these techniques but prefer the open-loupe technique. Our patients do not require blood transfusions. Our average hospital stay has been reduced to a 23-hour admission for the majority of patients with primary lumbar disc herniations.

Percutaneous techniques for lumbar disc removal are of interest and deserve our continued study to determine their usefulness once more clinical outcome studies are reported by noninventors. Kambin and Zhou (8) have demonstrated the clinical feasibility of a percutaneous approach by being able to remove the herniated portion of the disc and visually freeing the nerve root. This was a clear advance over the original automated percutaneous approach, which removed the central disc without addressing the posterolateral herniation. Revel et al. (14) demonstrated automated percutaneous lumbar discectomy to be ineffective in a randomized clinical trial. Treatment was considered successful in 61% of the 72 patients in the chymopapain group, with 44% of the 69 patients in the percutaneous discectomy group. At 1 year, overall success rates were 66% in the chemonucleolysis group and 37% in the automated percutaneous group. Within 6 months of treatment, 7% of the patients in the chemonucleolysis group and 33% in the discectomy group underwent subsequent open surgery. Although complication rates were low, 42% of the chemonucleolysis group continued to complain of significant low back pain.

More recently, Foley and Smith (4a) have described the MicroEndoscopic Discectomy (MED) system, which seems appropriately designed for patients with a soft herniation in close relationship to the nerve root. The visualization and lighting are superb. Before widespread endorsement, however, further clinical study is required to ascertain the indications, contraindications, and complications.

Chemonucleolysis with chymopapain continues to be used sparingly in various centers around the world, but few centers employ this technique in the United States. Although the concept makes some sense, the enzyme uses the central nucleus as the primary substrate without necessarily affecting the protruded portion of the disc. In addition, an enzymatic reaction is difficult to standardize with a set dosage because the composition of the substrate varies widely among patients. For example, the ratio of collagen to nucleus pulposus varies considerably among different age groups. Finally, as noted in the Rand (14) study, only 66% of the patients improved using chymopapain as compared with 85% to 90% in open discectomy (19).

 SURGICAL TECHNIQUES

I perform all lumbar disc procedures under general inhalation anesthesia. Once anesthesia has been administered, place the patient prone on a Jackson table with slight hip flexion. This table enhances intraoperative positioning by accommodating a wide range of patient sizes. The abdominal viscera hang free without pressure on the venous plexus. The knees are well supported, and the lumbar spine can be flexed adequately. Transient paresthesias in the lateral femoral cutaneous nerve distribution are common postoperatively. In addition, some patients complain of mild postoperative discomfort over the greater trochanter. To prevent irritation of the brachial plexus, the arms must not be elevated excessively in relation to the trunk.

HINTS AND TRICKS

The extent of the exposure depends on a number of factors: patient size, size and location of the lumbar herniation, and patient age. For a patient who is in excellent health and good physical condition, I recommend a unilateral approach. Place a small vertical incision over the appropriate vertebral interspace and perform only unilateral paraspinous stripping. Another option is to strip the paraspinal muscles bilaterally but to perform only a unilateral laminotomy. An older patient with significant degenerative changes may require bilateral stripping of the paraspinal muscles in addition to partial resection of the adjacent spinous processes. A patient with a large herniation and a neurologic deficit may require bilateral paraspinous stripping plus a partial or complete laminectomy to gain sufficient visualization to safely remove the herniation without incurring additional neurologic injury. No study has shown any adverse outcomes with a more generous exposure, so I believe that it is always better to err on the side of too generous rather than too small an approach. Greater retraction may be required when attempting to remove a large disc herniation through a small exposure. The technique that is illustrated describes a more generous exposure to illustrate better the anatomic details for an axillary lumbar disc herniation. A range of options exists regarding the extent of the exposure, depending on the above-mentioned parameters.

As an example, I describe the approach to the right L4–L5 disc level for the treatment of L-5 radiculopathy.

- Once the patient is properly positioned and carefully checked for pressure areas, especially the eyes, prepare and drape the lower back in sterile fashion.
- Palpate the iliac crests to locate the suspected L4–L5 level.
- Compare the clinically observed level of the iliac crests with preoperative radiographs, and label the level with a marking pencil.
- Make a vertical midline incision over the appropriate spinous processes.
- After the skin incision is made, complete the remaining portion of the dissection to the bony lamina using electrocautery.
- Extend the dissection to the lumbodorsal fascia. Identify the spinous processes of L-4 and L-5, and use the cautery unit to incise the fascia directly over the spinous processes. Use pickups to apply tension or a Cobb elevator as a gentle retractor.
- Dissect the fascia away from the spinous processes of L4–L5 and the inferior portion of L-3. By using Cobb elevators, carefully strip the paraspinous muscles from the spinous process to the lamina.
- Take care to maintain a subperiosteal approach. Blood loss is markedly reduced by avoiding the muscle envelope.
- Once the periosteum is stripped, insert a self-retaining retractor. Irrigate the wound and clearly identify the interlaminar space of L4–L5.

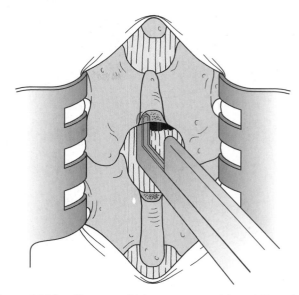

Figure 144.2. Use an upbiting rongeur with a 45° angle to resect additional bone in the midline from the inferior portion of the L-4 lamina. Resect a section of bone that is approximately 2 to 3 mm in length superior to the midline raphe of the ligamentum flavum.

- Place a towel clip through a spinous process, and obtain a lateral radiograph to confirm the level.

- Once you are satisfied that you are operating at the proper level, continue dissection by partially resecting the inferior portion of the L-4 spinous process and the superior portion of the L-5 spinous process:
- Examine the interlaminar space. With a Penfield 1 elevator, strip the ligamentum flavum from the inferior and anterior surface of the lamina of L-4 (Fig. 144.1).
- Use a Harper 45 rongeur to excise part of the middle portion of the L-4 lamina (Fig. 144.2).
- Carry the dissection cephalad until the midline raphe of the ligamentum flavum can be identified.
- Insert a Penfield 3 elevator in the midline from proximal to distal immediately anterior to the ligamentum flavum (Fig. 144.3). Using a #15 blade knife, divide the ligamentum flavum in the midline.
- Carry the dissection laterally toward the lateral recess, again using the Penfield 1 or Penfield 3 elevator to protect the underlying dura (Fig. 144.4). Dissection can be accomplished using either a scalpel, curets, or a rongeur with a 45° angle.
- Once the bulk of the ligamentum flavum has been removed, examine the epidural fat and dura to determine the degree of lateral wall dissection necessary to identify and retract the displaced nerve root safely.
- In this chapter, I have chosen to depict a less common form of disc herniation to emphasize the pitfalls of root

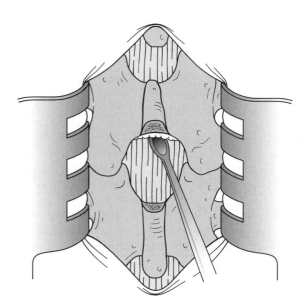

Figure 144.1. Use a Penfield 1 elevator or curved curet to remove the ligamentum flavum from the anteroinferior surface of the lamina of L4.

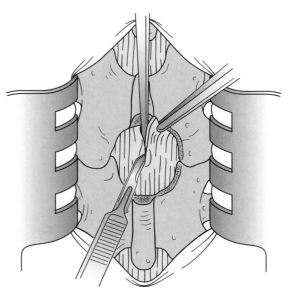

Figure 144.3. Pass a Penfield 3 elevator from proximal to distal, and divide the ligamentum flavum on top of the elevator to minimize the possibility of injury to the dura.

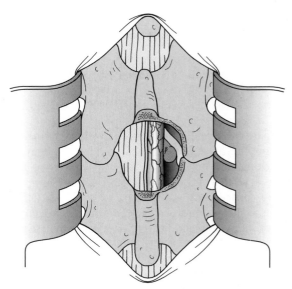

Figure 144.5. Expose the contents of the vertebral canal after resection of the ligamentum flavum from the right side and after lateral wall resection using an upbiting rongeur with a 45° angle. A disc herniation medial to the nerve root was illustrated intentionally to emphasize the point that the surgeon can mistake the lateral border of the dura for the lateral border of the nerve root. The nerve root must be clearly visualized.

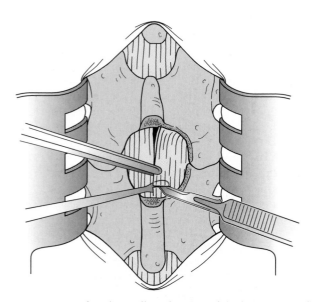

Figure 144.4. After the midline division of the ligamentum flavum, use a Penfield 1 or 3 elevator to protect the contents of the spinal canal while the flavum is resected further using a #15 blade scalpel. Other options are to use a small curet or to elevate the flavum and remove it with an upbiting rongeur with a 45° angle.

injury (Fig. 144.5). When the disc herniation is medial to the root, the lateral portion of the dura may be misinterpreted as being the lateral border of the nerve root. Such a misinterpretation can result in division of the nerve root or at least injury to the nerve root. Take extreme care to identify the nerve root.

- Resection of the lateral wall of the spinal canal using a rongeur with a 45° angle is necessary in most cases.
- Once the nerve root is identified and the disc herniation is visualized, remove a portion of the herniation. Then medially displace the root and excise the remaining portion of the displaced disc (Fig. 144.6).
- A disc herniation is categorized as being extruded when the annulus is disrupted, and the herniated portion of the disc is categorized as being protruded when the annulus is intact but eccentrically displaced. The term sequestered is applied to a free fragment of intervertebral disc lying in the spinal canal with no defect evident in the annulus fibrosus. Seventy-five percent of lumbar disc herniations are of the extruded variety, whereas sequestered disc fragments are far less common (less than 5%).
- Dissect from the medial portion of the dura laterally, using a Penfield 4 elevator in the dominant hand and a Freer elevator in the other hand. Take extreme care to identify the displaced nerve root. Use of surgical loupes with 2.5 magnification and a fiberoptic headlight is essential for optimal visualization in this operation. Once

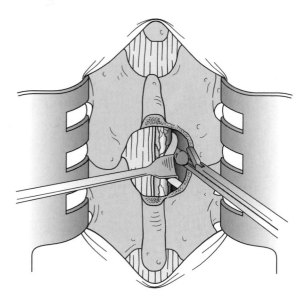

Figure 144.6. Gently elevate the nerve root with a Freer elevator and a Penfield 4 elevator, and retract it medially over the displaced disc tissue. A Love root retractor can be used as illustrated to displace the root dura medially. Then remove the extruded disc with a small pituitary rongeur.

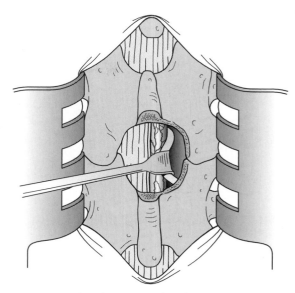

Figure 144.7. After disc removal, it should be easy to displace the involved nerve root 1 cm medially. Should the root remain fixed, additional exploration of the foramina and the vertebral canal is necessary.

the nerve can be displaced medially, insert a Love root retractor to displace the nerve root and dura gently medially, so that the extruded disc herniation can be excised (Fig. 144.6). A sharp incision into the annulus is seldom necessary because the pseudomembrane overlying an extruded disc can nearly always be dissected using a Penfield 4 elevator. In protruded disc herniation, however, the annulus must be incised.

- Once the disc has been removed, free the nerve root of tension and carefully inspect the neural foramina. The nerve root should be able to be displaced at least 1 cm medially (Fig. 144.7).
- Take care to ensure that no disc material is present between the annulus and the posterior longitudinal ligament.
- Once the disc has been excised, irrigate the wound and place an interposition membrane of Gelfoam or fat over the laminotomy. At present, I prefer to use Gelfoam (Fig. 144.8).
- Then close the wound in layers. Use figure-8 sutures to achieve watertight closure of the fascia; I prefer subcuticular stitches for the skin.
- Apply a dry, sterile bandage.
- Gently straighten and rotate the patient onto the stretcher for extubation. Following extubation, take the patient to the recovery room. Blood transfusion is seldom necessary for a primary lumbar discectomy because blood loss usually averages less than 100 ml.

I have used this technique successfully for the past 15 years with no incidence of recurrent disc herniation over that reported by others (2%).

FAR LATERAL AND INTRAFORAMINAL DISCS

Far lateral and intraforaminal disc lesions cannot be easily removed through a midline approach (Fig. 144.9). Al-

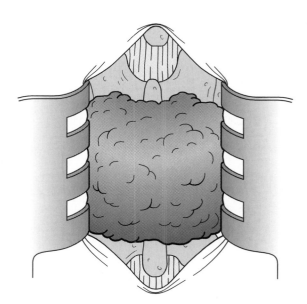

Figure 144.8. An interposition membrane of Gelfoam; many surgeons prefer fat grafts.

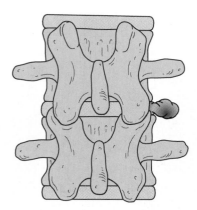

Figure 144.9. Far lateral disc lesion. Note the relationship of the disc to the transverse processes.

though taking down the entire facet is one alternative advocated by some (1), the extraforaminal approach has been advocated by Wiltse (21,22). The proponents of going from the midline through the facets suggest that instability is not a subsequent problem and believe the nerve root can be more easily identified. Furthermore, they believe the surgeon can have greater confidence of complete decompression. However, many do not share this view.

The paramedian approach popularized by Wiltse (21, 22) is a muscle-splitting approach.

■ Make the incision 5 cm from the midline, followed by blunt dissection of the paraspinal muscles (Fig. 144.10).

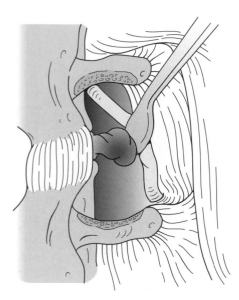

Figure 144.10. The annulus is incised, the nerve root is retracted laterally, and the disc is removed with a pituitary rongeur.

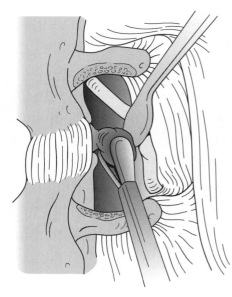

Figure 144.11. Nerve identified and retracted at a 45° angle.

■ At this point, take radiographs to verify the level and clear the transverse processes of soft tissues.
■ Enter the intertransverse ligaments and fascia with a knife or curet, then remove those structures between the transverse processes.
■ Identify the nerve, which is usually 2 to 4 mm anterior to the fascia and directed at a 45° angle (Fig. 144.11).
■ Follow the nerve medially and identify the disc.
■ If a free fragment is present, remove it. If only a bulge is present, incise the annulus and remove easily identifiable fragments. When the nerve root is easily mobile, sufficient disc has been removed.
■ If the lesion is intraforaminal, take down a portion of the facet laterally to expose the nerve root canal. McCulloch and Young (12) point out, however, that this procedure is rarely necessary because of the the usual anatomic location of these lesions.
■ Closure in both instances is routine, using a free fat graft or Gelfoam to cover the nerve.

POSTOPERATIVE CARE AND REHABILITATION

In most patients, the preoperative radicular symptoms are improved when they awaken in the recovery room. On the evening of surgery, the patient is permitted to stand. By the first postoperative day, the patient is allowed to ambulate. If a dural leak occurs, ambulation is delayed by 24 to 48 hours. An abdominal binder is used for 4 weeks as partial protection for the patient. Rehabilitation is initiated 4 weeks after surgery and continued indefinitely. Patients are advised to maintain ideal weight and to develop good abdominal and trunk extensor muscle tone. Aerobic activity is encouraged and is initiated 4 weeks following surgery. Patients are discharged from follow-up approximately 12 months after surgery.

◤ PITFALLS AND COMPLICATIONS

The primary consideration is the selection of appropriate patients for surgical repair of lumbar disc herniations. The use of an objective method to accomplish this, as described in this chapter, will lessen the incidence of negative explorations (19), which is less than 2% in my experience. Although technical errors infrequently account for persistent pain after surgery, such errors invariably compromise the outcome. In a patient with established disc herniation, exploration at the wrong intervertebral level will not benefit the patient (10). Avoid this mistake by taking an intraoperative radiograph to confirm the appropriate level. If a disc herniation is not found, consider exploring additional levels after an intraoperative radiograph to confirm the proper level. Explorations at the wrong level are more common in patients who have transitional lumbar vertebrae.

Poor technique can prolong postoperative pain. Because excessive traction of neural tissue can cause irreversible nerve damage, use loupe magnification and fiberoptic lighting. These technologies have done much to minimize injury to neural tissue. Likewise, the use of an interpositional membrane (either free fat grafts or Gelfoam) at the completion of surgical exploration may minimize long-term perineural scar formation. Presently, newer antiadhesion barriers are being investigated in the United States. Experience in Europe has suggested that such barriers may lessen scarring within the spinal canal and perhaps even enhance clinical outcome. Additional evaluations are necessary to support these early but exciting assertions scientifically.

Technical errors can also result when the surgeon fails to detect a fragment of disc tissue that has migrated from the level of herniation, either cephalad in the canal or laterally into the extraforaminal area, trapping nerve roots (10). Because the only patients who should undergo surgery are those with objective findings, explore the canal thoroughly if no specific pathologic changes are encountered at the suspected level. Because the nerve root should be able to be displaced easily for a distance of approximately 1 cm medially, a nerve root that is tight in the canal and cannot be displaced suggests either a sequestered fragment along the nerve root or a stenotic lateral recess (10). Gently palpate the cauda equina to ensure that an intradural disc herniation is not present. Although a neoplasm involving the neural elements of the lumbar spine is always

a possibility, it is distinctly uncommon. The most likely neoplastic lesion encountered in the lumbar vertebral canal is a metastatic extradural lesion.

Hemostasis is essential in lumbar disc surgery. With proper technique, blood loss should be minimal, rarely exceeding 150 ml. Generally, epidural bleeding is easily controlled with bipolar coagulation, packing, or both.

Always be prepared to expand the surgical exposure. A straightfoward unilateral lumbar disc herniation rarely requires a complete laminectomy; however, when the surgical findings do not explain the preoperative symptoms, more open exposure is necessary.

Inadequate exposure can also present problems. Identify the dura and the nerve root, and expose the lateral wall adequately before examining the nerve root. Attempting to extract a large, extruded fragment through a small incision may traumatize the involved nerve root unnecessarily.

This point is especially important when dealing with a patient who presents with a cauda equina syndrome or a large central herniation without neurologic involvement. In these situations, remove the ligamentum flavum on both sides of the spine. Because the dura mater will be displaced posteriorly, a careful dissection is essential to avoid injury. A laminectomy may be the most appropriate exposure to ensure adequate visualization of the thecal sac and the exiting nerve roots on both sides. Often, the most appropriate beginning may be to perform an annulotomy and discectomy on the side with least herniation to debulk the herniation and to provide easier access to the root under maximal tension.

In patients older than 40 years of age, exploration of the neural canal must include a careful assessment of the lateral recess to interpret pathologic changes accurately. Performing a discectomy in a patient who also has lateral entrapment of the nerve root will not reduce the patient's symptoms. Careful probing of the neural foramina at the completion of the lumbar discectomy will locate the narrowing of the neural foramina. If stenosis of the lateral recess is the only manifestation, lumbar discectomy may not be necessary.

As with any surgical procedure, a list of potential complications that might occur would be exhaustive. Dural tears may occur during a lumbar discectomy. Such tears are more common in patients who undergo surgery for spinal stenosis or revision procedures. I recommend primary repair of dural tears with 5-0 Dermalon. Injuries to the iliac arteries and veins and viscera, including any structure from the appendix to the ureter, have been reported in association with a lumbar discectomy (15). Errors in diagnosis may occur. The patient may have symptoms suggestive of a lumbar disc herniation, which may, in fact, be related to intra-abdominal pathologic processes such as an aneurysm or a malignancy. Minimize these unusual complications by performing a thorough diagnostic assessment and decision analysis before a decision to operate on the spine. With proper patient selection and careful operative technique, lumbar disc surgery is highly successful and yields gratifying results for both the patient and the surgeon.

REFERENCES

Each reference is categorized according to the following scheme: *, classic article; #, review article; !, basic research article; and +, clinical results/outcome study.

+ 1. Abdullah, AF, Wolber PG, Warfield JR, Gunadi IK. Surgical Management of Extreme Lateral Lumbar Disc Herniations: Review of 138 Cases. *Neurosurgery* 1988;22:648.

+ 2. Battie MC. *The Reliability of Physical Factors as Predictors of the Occurrence of Back Pain Reports.* Goteborg, 1989.

+ 3. Epstein JA. Discussion on Extreme Lateral Lumbar Disc Herniation. *J Spinal Disord* 1989;2:138.

4. Farfan H. *Mechanical Disorders of the Low Back.* Philadelphia: Lea and Febiger, 1973.

4a. Foley KT, Smith MM. Image-guided spine surgery. *Neurosurg Clin NAM* 1996;7:171.

+ 5. Haimonvic, IC, Beresford, HR. Dexamethasone Is Not Superior to Placebo for Treating Lumbosacral Radicular Pain. *Neurology* 1986;36:1593.

+ 6. Haro H, Shinomiya K, Komori H, et al. Unregulated Expression of Chemokines in Herniated Nucleus. *Spine* 1996;21:1647.

7. Holmes HE, Rothman RH. Technique of Lumbar Laminectomy. *Instr Course Lect* 1979;28:200.

+ 8. Kambin P, Zhou L Arthroscopic Discectomy of the Lumbar Spine. *Clin Orthop* 1997;337:49.

+ 9. Kane W. *Incidence of Lumbar Discectomy.* Presented at the 6th Annual Meeting of the International Society for the Study of the Lumbar Spine, New Orleans Louisiana, 1980.

+ 10. MacNab, I. Negative Disc Exploration. An Analysis of the Causes of Nerve Root Involvement in Sixty-eight Patients. *J Bone Joint Surg* 1971;53-A:891.

+ 11. Klekamp J, McCarty E, Spengler D. Results in Elective Lumbar Discectomy for Patients Involved in the Workers' Compensation System. *J Spinal Disord* 1998;II:277.

12. McCulloch J, Young P. *Essentials of Spinal Microsurgery.* Philadelphia: Lippincott-Raven, 1998.

+ 13. Ransford AO, Cairns D, Mooney V. The Pain Drawing as an Aid to the Psychological Evaluation of Patients with Low-back Pain. *Spine* 1976;1:127.

+ 14. Revel M, Payan C, Vallee C, et al. Automatic Percutaneous Discectomy versus Chemonucleolysis in the Treatment of Sciatica. *Spine* 1993;18:1.

+ 15. Spangfort EV The Lumbar Disc Herniation: A Computer-aided Analysis of 2,504 Operations. *Acta Orthop Scand* 1972;142(Suppl):1.

16. Spengler DM. Lumbar Discectomy. In: Chapman MW, ed. *Operative Orthopaedics,* Vol 3. Philadelphia: Lippincott, 1988:2055.

+ 17. Spengler DM, Freeman C, Westbrook R, Miller JW. Low Back Pain Following Multiple Lumbar Spine Procedures. *Spine* 1980;5:356.

18. Spengler DM, Frymoyer J., eds. Indications and Techniques. In: *The Adult Spine.* New York: Raven Press, 1991.

+ 19. Spengler, DM, Ouellette E, Battie M, Zeh J. Elective Discectomy for Herniation of a Lumbar Disc. *J Bone Joint Surg Am* 1990;72:230.

+ 20. Weber H. Lumbar Disc Herniation: A Controlled, Prospective Study with Ten Years of Observation. *Spine* 1983;8:131.

+ 21. Wiltse LL. Discussion on Extreme Lateral Lumbar Disc Herniation. *J Spinal Disord* 1989;2:134.

22. Wiltse LL, Watkins RG, Collis JC, eds. *Lumbar Discectomy and Laminectomy.* Rockville, MD: Aspen, 1987.

CHAPTER 145
DEGENERATIVE DISC DISEASE

Eeric Truumees and Harry N. Herkowitz

The term *degenerative disc disease* (DDD) has been used to describe a wide variety of morphologic and radiographic changes in the adult lumbosacral spine. The North American Spine Society Consensus Committee on Nomenclature (16) defined disc degeneration as follows:

> Changes in a disc characterized by desiccation, fibrosis, or cleft formation in the nucleus; fissuring or mucinous degeneration of the annulus; defects and sclerosis of the endplates; and/or osteophytes at the vertebral apophysis.

The committee noted, "The term *degeneration* does not imply an etiology. Depending on age, degree, and type of change . . . the changes of disc degeneration may be clinically insignificant." Degenerative disc *disease*, on the other hand, is broadly defined as "a clinical syndrome characterized by manifestations of disc degeneration and symptoms thought to be related to those changes." The authors point out that "causal connections between degenerative changes and clinical symptoms are often difficult clinical distinctions."

In this chapter, *degenerative disc disease* refers to a continuum of nonradicular, mechanical pain disorders of presumably degenerative origin. Specifically excluded are those disc pathologies with neurologic impingement, such as disc displacement, spinal stenosis, and deforming degenerative conditions, such as degenerative scoliosis and spondylolisthesis.

E. Truumees and H. N. Herkowitz: Section of Spinal Surgery, William Beaumont Hospital, Royal Oak, Michigan, 48073.

Degenerative disc disease as a clinical entity remains controversial for five principal reasons:

1. A confusing and contradictory nomenclature
2. The similarity of "pathologic" changes to those of normal aging
3. The difficulty in accurately identifying the source of pain
4. Our limited understanding of the etiology and natural history of this process
5. Historically low success rates from surgical intervention for patients with DDD

PATHOPHYSIOLOGY AND PATHOMECHANICS

BACK PAIN

The social impact and suffering that results from back pain cannot be overestimated. With a lifetime incidence of 60% to 80%, low back pain (LBP) generates at least 15 million office visits per year (23). In fact, low back complaints are the leading compensable cause of injury in the workplace. In the United States, $24 billion a year is spent on the evaluation and direct management of patients with back pain. Indirect costs include work and productivity losses, and they account for an additional $27 billion annually (28).

Typically, back pain has a benign course. Within 3 months of the onset of symptoms, 95% of patients return to their previous employment. The 5% of patients with residual symptoms after 3 months, however, incur 85% of the costs. Moreover, the probability of returning to work falls with increasing duration of disability. After 2 years off work, less than 2% will return. Therefore, the early detection of those patients in whom LBP is more likely to become chronic would be of tremendous clinical and social benefit.

Adult LBP can arbitrarily be divided into five categories:

1. Referred back pain
2. LBP with radiculopathy or myelopathy
3. LBP with deformity, such as scoliosis, kyphosis, or spondylolisthesis
4. LBP in the context of fractures, tumors, or infections
5. Mechanical LBP without the features already noted

Before focusing on the spine and its related structures, consider other potential sources of referred pain. Included in the first LBP group are intra-abdominal and retroperitoneal pathologies such as abdominal aortic aneurysm and endometriosis. In groups 2 through 4, symptoms more readily correlate with evident spinal pathology; as a result, treatment of these patients is satisfying and, overall, associated with good results.

The fifth group, patients with mechanical LBP only, includes several benign conditions, most likely representing ligamentous and muscular strain, mechanical stress from poor posture, or facet joint irritation. More chronic and disabling degenerative disc conditions, however, are included as well. In these patients, uncertain identification of the pain generator is associated with vague diagnostic groupings and failed surgical management. Included among these is DDD.

The multiple and synonymous terminology reflects an incomplete understanding of the pathophysiology and natural history of DDD. Moreover, because the "pathoanatomic" changes noted in DDD do not qualitatively differ from those of normal aging, the appropriateness of the appellation *disease* is intensely debated.

NOCICEPTION IN THE DISC

It is theorized that in DDD, pain arises in the disc. Historically, while the lumbar facets, posterior longitudinal ligament, dura, dorsal root ganglion, and myofascial structures of the lumbar spine have been recognized as pain-generating structures, the disc was felt to be aneural. More recently, however, nociceptive fibers have been identified in the outer annulus (22,30,47).

In one study, pain was generated by applying pressure to the disc during operations under local anesthesia (15). In another study, back pain resolved with procaine injection into the disc (75). Kuslich et al. (47) used a progressive local anesthesic technique to gauge pain response in different tissues in 193 consecutive laminectomies. Stimulation via blunt probe or unipolar electrocautery on the facet cartilage and synovium never caused pain. Also, no pain followed stimulation of the lamina, spinous process, ligamentum flavum, lumbar fascia, and uncompressed roots. Stimulation of the facet capsule, however, was associated with sharp, localized pain in 30%. This pain did not match the patient's preoperative symptoms. Stimulation of a compressed root resulted in sciatic pain in 79%. Finally, LBP similar to preoperative symptoms was noted in 70% of patients after stimulation of the posterior annulus or posterior longitudinal ligament (PLL). Local anesthetic injection obliterated the pain.

Nociceptive free nerve endings of the recurrent sinuvertebral nerve most likely carry these impulses. The sinuvertebral nerve, first described by Von Luschka, consists of a postganglionic derivative of rami communicantes that branches into segments. These segments ascend and descend into one or more adjacent levels (30,78) (Fig. 145.1). The branches accompany the venous plexus into the vertebral endplates and terminate in nociceptive free nerve endings in both the PLL and outer lamina of the annulus (51). In histometric studies, the outer third of the annulus has been found to contain nerve endings with nociceptive neurotransmitters [substance P, calcitonin, vasoactive intestinal peptide (VIP)] (54). Further, nociceptive fibers may *grow into* diseased discs (22). Theoretically, a small tear of the outer annulus may cause pain, even with a normal nucleus pulposus.

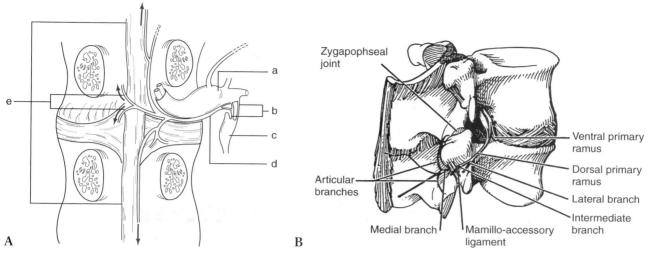

Figure 145.1. The course of the sinuvertebral nerve (24,37). **A:** The sinuvertebral nerve shown on a cutaway drawing. **B:** The branches of the invertebral nerve shown on a lateral view of an intact spine. **a:** Dorsal root ganglion. **b:** Rami communicantes. **c:** Autonomic ganglion. **d:** Sinuvertebral nerve. **e:** Terminal branches of the nerve (may ascend or descend one or two vertebral levels).

Disc degeneration may indirectly stimulate pain receptors elsewhere. Disc height collapse may produce nociceptive signals from the facet mechanoreceptors by abnormal loading. Such mechanical derangement has been associated with abnormal intervertebral motion and has been termed *lumbar segmental instability.*

A degenerated disc may also indirectly cause pain by extrusion of nuclear material, a source of neural irritation and inflammation (54). The potential sources of pain in the lumbar spine are illustrated in Figure 145.2.

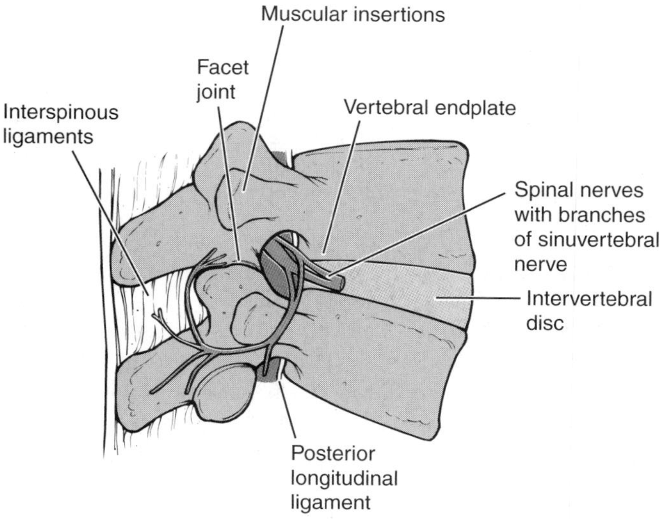

NORMAL AGE-RELATED CHANGES IN THE DISC

During an individual's lifetime, intervertebral disc composition changes greatly. Given that certain degenerative phenomena may lead to pain, it is necessary to have a clear understanding of what changes constitute normal degeneration.

At birth, the disc surface area is 50% nucleus pulposus (NP) and 50% annulus. The notochordal cells of the NP are gradually replaced by chondrocytes throughout the early teenage years. This replacement is associated with annular thickening (Fig. 145.3). The demarcation between

Figure 145.2. Various potential pain generators in the lumbar spine.

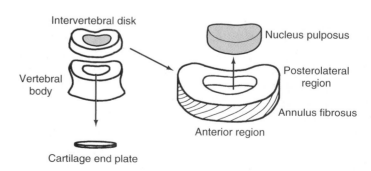

Figure 145.3. Schematic of basic intervertebral disc anatomy.

the annulus and the nucleus becomes less distinct. The older NP has a higher collagen content with more structured fibers. In these fibers, the ratio of type II to type I collagen increases (51).

Proteoglycan metabolism changes with age as well. Chondroitin-4-sulfate and chondroitin-6-sulfate concentrations decrease, and the ratio of keratin sulfate to chondroitin sulfate increases. Keratin sulfate has a smaller hydrophilic potential and a reduced tendency to form stable aggregates with hyaluronic acid. Dehydration, in turn, decreases the disc's resistance to axial loading (20).

As desiccation continues, clefts can be identified that originate in the central portion of the dehydrated NP. One hypothesis holds that these clefts eventually migrate toward the peripheral annulus and endplate and cause tears. Annular tears are classified by Vernon-Roberts (20) as peripheral, circumferential, and radiating. Circumferential and radiating tears are associated with degenerative changes in the endplate and NP.

With maturity, the vascular supply to the disc is obliterated. In adults, the disc is the largest avascular structure in the body. Thereafter, disc nutrition requires diffusion through the vertebral endplates (80%) and outer annulus (20%) (25).

Some authors have differentiated age related changes from pathological degeneration. One study found that altered collagen staining patterns and increases in lipofuscin and amyloid can be used to differentiate aged from degenerated discs (20). Further, this cycle of degeneration may be self-promoting, that is, small annular tears lead to further nuclear degeneration in animal models (47,54). Vascular ingrowth may also mark degenerated and herniated discal tissues (41).

At present, there is no clear boundary between these aging changes and disc degeneration. While some authors claim a quantitative if not qualitative difference between aged and degenerated discs, all discs degenerate with age. Miller et al. (55) reported evidence of disc degeneration by the age of 50 in 90% of 600 autopsy specimens. Holt (39) found evidence of disc degeneration on the plain radiographs of 80% of adults studied, although 53% had no history of LBP.

ETIOLOGY

While it appears that all intervertebral discs degenerate with age, the degree and rate of this degeneration vary significantly from individual to individual. The underlying reasons for this variability are only partly known.

The Hirsh theory of disc degeneration holds that insufficient nutrition, impaired waste transport, and traumatic mechanical factors combine with a genetic and hormonal proclivity to cause desiccation and annular tearing. Severe degeneration is associated with increased lactate metabo-

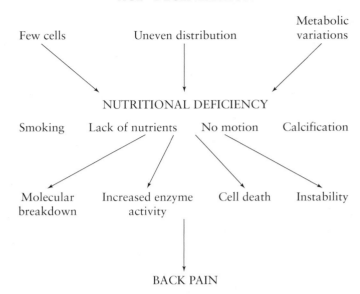

Figure 145.4. The role of nutritional deficiency in the etiology of discogenic back pain. With advancing age, disc cells diminish in number and distribution and undergo metabolic variations. As a consequence, disc nutrition diminishes. These changes are accelerated by systemic factors such as overall nutritional status, smoking, motion, and endplate or disc calcification. Ultimately, cell death, increased enzyme activity, molecular breakdown, and instability ensue.

lism, decreased pH, accumulation of proteolytic enzymes, and chondrocyte necrosis (Fig. 145.4) (37).

Various clinical factors have been implicated in precocious degeneration. Smoking and a familial tendency toward degeneration have long been established as contributing factors (68). Twins demonstrate similar degeneration patterns (3). In one study of 15-year-olds, LBP, decreased activity, and decreased spinal range of motion predicted later DDD (66). Anatomically, no association between DDD and facet tropism can be demonstrated (6). The endplate irregularities of thoracolumbar Scheuermann's disease, however, may be related to DDD (35).

PATHOPHYSIOLOGY OF DDD

If disc degeneration is a programmed, physiologic phenomenon influenced by heredity and environment, it is incumbent upon the clinician to ascertain when these changes constitute a disease. Benign age-related phenomena have been differentiated from pathologic phenomena on the basis of three factors: impaired function, structural changes, and an association with pain.

Yong-Hing and Kirkaldy-Willis (86) described a three-joint complex in the spinal column, with the disc anteri-

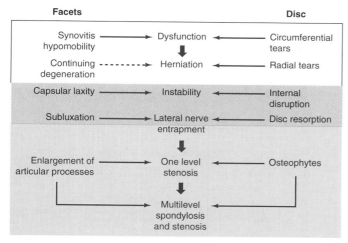

Figure 145.5. The Kirkaldy-Willis (86) states of lumbar degeneration, including (left side) the events that occur in the facets and (right side) intervertebral discs and associated syndromes.

orly and the two facet joints posteriorly. They theorized that benign microscopic alterations progress to pathologic degeneration in stages. In this way, circumferential annular tears progress to radial tears. Radial tears, in turn, engender further disc degeneration or frank disc herniation. The ensuing loss of disc height alters facet joint mechanics, and facet cartilage disruption or destruction may take place. Coincidentally, the decrease in the intervertebral height causes buckling of the ligamentum flavum and facet overriding or enlargement. These changes may, singly or in combination, cause narrowing of the neuroforaminal and central canals. So, while disc degeneration manifests as mechanical LBP in some patients, others will experience neurologic claudication or radiculopathy from frank disc herniation (Figs. 145.5, 145.6).

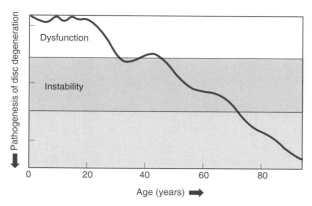

Figure 145.6. The natural history of lumbar degeneration (Yong-Hing K, and Kirkaldy-Willis WH: The Pathophysiology of Disc degeneration of the Lumbar Spine. *Ortho Clin North Am* 1983;14:59).

Yong-Hing and Kirkaldy-Willis (86) then proposed three stages of degeneration of the intervertebral disc.

I. Microscopic alterations of disc consistent with aging
II. Increased spinal mobility
III. Stabilization of the functional spinal unit (discs anterior and facets posteriorly)

Vernon-Roberts (20) showed that many of these changes are present in nearly all middle-aged people and are not necessarily associated with back pain. Thus, the issue of when degenerative changes represent a disease remains unresolved. While data are lacking, it has been suggested that younger patients with relatively precocious disc degeneration do not tolerate these changes as well as older adults. Whether this perceived difference stems from higher functional demands or from a subtle difference in disc mechanics is not known. It is reasonable, however, to identify DDD as a chronic, mechanical LBP *syndrome* associated with changes in the structural and functional integrity of one or more intervertebral discs.

TYPES OF DDD

At present, DDD can be characterized by one of several associated terms, listed in Table 145.1. While some authors use these terms to refer to the same global discogenic pain syndrome, others view them as a means to differentiate among subgroups of patients. The divisiveness and misapplication of nomenclature further confuses any evidence-based appraisal of DDD, and its incidence, pathophysiology, and natural history.

Three subtypes may be identified as points in a continuum. First, *internal disc disruption* (IDD) refers to a painful annular tear in the absence of bony changes or disc height loss. As such, IDD must not be confused with disc protrusions, which are normal hydrodynamic findings (5).

Next, *lumbar spondylosis* (LS) refers to mechanical back pain in association with disc height loss, sclerosis,

Table 145.1. Named Discogenic Disorders
Lumbar segmental instability
Degenerative disc disease
Black or dark disc disease
Discogenic back pain
Anterior column disease
Internal disc disruption
Isolated disc resorption
Lumbar spondylosis

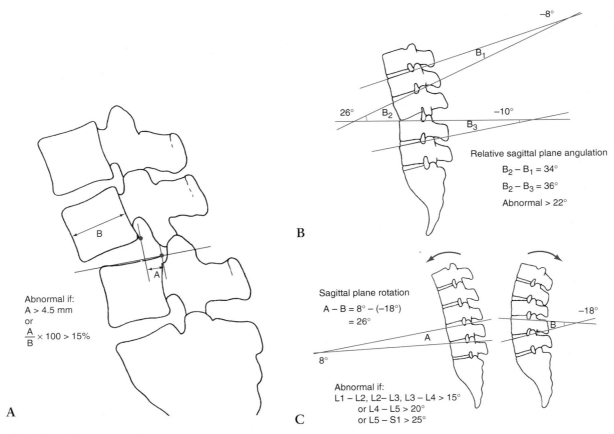

Figure 145.7.   **A:** The White and Panjabi (83) method for measuring sagittal plane translation. Greater than 4.5 mm (or 15% of vertebral body) of motion is considered abnormal. **B:** Method of measuring static sagittal plane angulation. Greater than 22° of relative angulation (i.e., angulation greater than that seen in the levels above and below) is considered abnormal. **C:** Method of measuring sagittal plane rotation on flexion–extension radiographs. Cobb measurements taken in extension are subtracted from those in extension. Abnormal values are greater than 15° at L1-2, L2-3, and L3-4, and greater than 20° at L4-5 and 25° at L5–S1.

and osteophyte formation. LS is the most frequently described form of DDD, and it is the entity most authors are describing when they use the more global term *DDD*.

Finally, *lumbar segment instability* (LSI), which represents a progressive relaxation of facet capsules and ligamentous restraints, occurs in the context of chronically compromised disc biomechanics. White and Panjabi (83) define lumbar instability as more than 4.5 mm of translation, 15° to 25° of angular motion between adjacent segments on flexion–extension radiographs, or both (Fig. 145.7). It is not clear, however, that the chronic increase in intervertebral motion seen in degenerative lumbar diseases may be mechanically equated with traumatic spinal instability. Therefore, some authors classify this abnormality with degenerative spondylolisthesis and degenerative scoliosis, which have a similar pathogenesis. Others feel that all the subtypes of DDD represent a painful "microinstability" of the motion segment (48).

NATURAL HISTORY OF DDD

The critical question of why most degenerated discs are asymptomatic remains to be answered. Even in those patients with degenerative changes, severe back pain, and positive discography, pain may spontaneously improve. In one series, 25 patients who had not had surgery were positive on a single-level discogram. When they were evaluated after an average of 4.9 years, 68% had improvement without surgery (70). Of the 32% who were unimproved, 66.7% had an underlying psychiatric diagnosis. In the absence of a more complete understanding of the natural history of this disorder, appropriate evaluation of surgical outcomes is extremely difficult.

In summary, while knowledge of the benign degeneration of the aging spine continues to grow, surprisingly little is known about disc degeneration as a disease process (Table 145.2) (78).

Table 145.2. What We Do Not Know about Disc Degeneration as a Disease

Why are some people symptomatic and others are not?

What is the incidence and prevalence of disc degeneration as a disease?

Which disc level is the source of the problem in a given patient?

What is the natural history of disc disease in any given patient?

In which patients can the natural history of DDD can be reliably improved with surgical intervention?

EVALUATION AND IMAGING

HISTORY

When evaluating a patient with chronic LBP, DDD remains a diagnosis of exclusion. A thorough history and physical examination are mandatory.

In patients with "red flags" such as very young or old age, nonmechanical pain, constitutional symptoms, and trauma, perform a thorough radiologic and serologic evaluation for infection, tumor, and fractures (Table 145.3). Other important considerations include intra-abdominal and intrapelvic pathology. Posterior penetrating ulcers, pancreatitis, renal disease, abdominal aortic aneurysm, and endometriosis are all known causes of severe, referred pain to the back.

Pay careful attention to historical clues as well as to significant social and psychological issues. Ask specific questions regarding drug and alcohol intake, mood, sleep disturbance, pending litigation, and job satisfaction.

In patients with pain of degenerative etiology, first exclude those with radicular or myelopathic signs and symptoms. Similarly, the evaluation of patients with significant thoracolumbar deformities such as scoliosis, hyperlordosis, and kyphosis is considered elsewhere (see Chapters 153, 155, 156, 159, 160, and 161). For example, spondylolisthesis, another disorder of genetic and environmental stress, is the most common structural abnormality in the adult spine (see Chapter 162). Spondylolisthesis is related to LBP in 5% of the population (21).

The evaluation of the remaining group of patients with isolated, mechanical LBP is challenging. The difficulty in identifying a specific pain generator accounts for the fact that only 15% of patients are given a definitive diagnosis. Physically and radiographically abnormal structures may not cause symptoms. On the other hand, grossly and radiographically normal structures may be associated with severe pain in certain individuals.

Muscular etiologies account for the vast majority of

patients reporting acute LBP. Patients with myofascial pain are especially difficult to distinguish from those with "discogenic pain" when radiographic signs of disc degeneration are present. However, myofascial pain tends to have an acute onset and a relatively brief duration. The pain is localized to a specific paraspinal area, and muscle spasm is evident. In most cases, while some DDD patients identify a specific, traumatic event (such as bending, lifting, or twisting) with symptom onset, their pain is midline and does not resolve but rather worsens over time.

The pain described by patients with DDD is mechanical in that it is aggravated by activity, particularly flexion. Relative rest temporarily ameliorates symptoms. Patients with lumbar segmental instability may complain of a catch with flexion and extension (Fig. 145.8). DDD patients may also report having difficulty when getting up from a chair. In an attempt to splint the back, some will use upper extremity leverage, pressing their arms against their thighs, when arising.

Pain related to DDD may predate or postdate an episode of sciatica. Often, DDD patients report having had prior discectomy or chymopapain injections (20). Further, the disc collapse associated with LS may result in forami-

Table 145.3. Historical Elements Requiring Thorough Evaluation ("Red Flags")

Age <20 or >50 years

Progressive neurologic deficit

Gait disturbance, history of falls

Bowel or bladder difficulties

Cancer

Infection

Major trauma

Prior spine surgery

Immunocompromised status

History of intravenous drug abuse

Metabolic bone disease

Peripheral vascular disease

Genitourinary or gynecologic complaints

Nonmechanical pain pattern (worse when supine or at night)

Psychosocial overlay (e.g., depression, active legal proceedings)

Constitutional symptoms (malaise, fever, chills, weight loss)

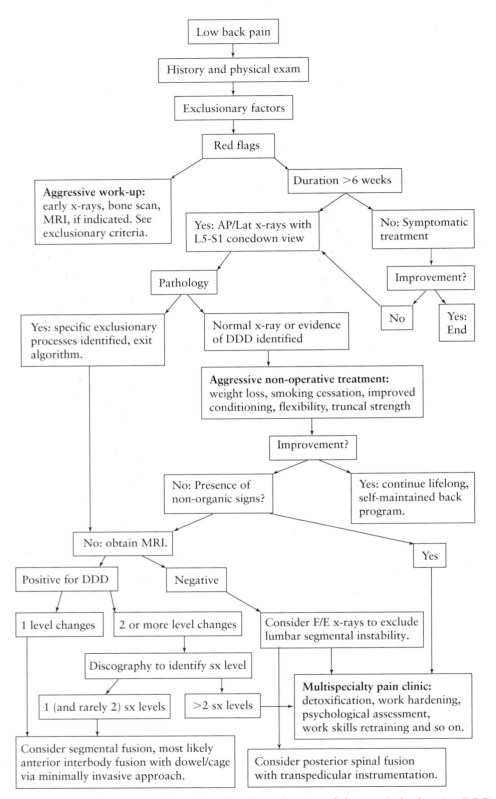

Figure 145.8. A suggested algorithm for the evaluation of discogenic back pain. *DDD*, degenerative disc disease; *F/E*, Flexion/Extension; *SX*, symptomatic.

nal stenosis and mild radiculopathies (48). Other patients followed for axial spinal pain will later present with acute radicular complaints and imaging studies consistent with disc herniation. Diagnosis and treatment for these patients is discussed in Chapter 144.

Degenerative discs may be associated with referred, sclerotomal pain to the buttocks and posterior thigh. However, it is very difficult or impossible to localize the symptomatic disc level on the basis of history or physical exam alone.

PHYSICAL EXAMINATION

The examination of DDD patients is generally nonspecific. These patients exhibit no point tenderness or paraspinal spasms. They often report pain or difficulty with flexion and rotation maneuvers of the spine, however. Normal neurologic findings including sensory, motor, and reflex exams are expected. Particular attention must be paid to Waddell's signs (Table 145.4) (79), which suggest psychological overlay.

Moreover, unexpected findings on physical examination such as anal sphincter laxity or major muscle weakness should be construed as red flags and investigated accordingly.

PLAIN RADIOGRAPHY

The ubiquity of painless LS limits the specificity of plain radiography in DDD. In the absence of red flags, radiographs are indicated only after a trial of symptomatic

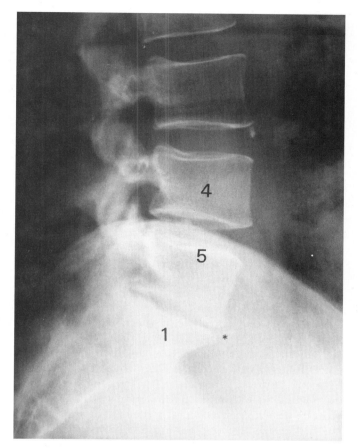

Figure 145.9. Plain radiographic findings of DDD: disc space loss, endplate sclerosis, and osteophyte formation.

Table 145.4. *Waddell's Nonorganic Physical Signs*

Tenderness: pain at the tip of the tailbone; pain, numbness, or giving way of the whole leg; pain to light touch

Simulation: pain with light axial loading of head or shoulders; pain with pelvic rotation through the hips; reproduction of pain with rolling of lumbar skin

Distraction: no pain with a sitting straight-leg raise (SLR), pain with a supine SLR

Regional: nonanatomic distributions of weakness or sensory changes (especially in a stocking distribution)

Overreaction: moaning, trembling, collapsing, sweating, emergency admissions

From Waddell G, McCullough JA, Kummel E, et al. Nonorganic Physical Signs in Low Back Pain. *Spine* 1980;5:117.

---

treatment. In patients failing to improve with these modalities, begin radiologic assessment with plain anteroposterior (AP) and lateral views of the lumbosacral spine. Oblique views and a lateral L5–S1 cone-down view are often helpful. The principal purpose of these studies in the early management of mechanical back pain is to exclude spondylolisthesis and the less benign entities mentioned previously.

Patients with internal disc derangement will have no plain radiographic changes. The cardinal findings of LS are endplate sclerosis and loss of disc space. Radiographs may also show a loss of lordosis, subluxations, vacuum phenomenon, and osteophytes (Fig. 145.9). Radiography, however, can be misleading: Frymoyer et al. (24) showed that signs suggestive of disc degeneration were present in 90% of adults studied, whereas 53% had no history of LBP (Table 145.5).

It should be noted that the presence of nitrogen gas bubbles (the vacuum phenomenon) in degenerative discs probably excludes the diagnosis of discitis, as infection by gas-forming organisms are exceedingly rare.

Table 145.5. Plain Radiographic Findings of DDD

IDD	Lumbar spondylosis	Lumbar segmental instability
None	Endplate sclerosis Loss of disc space Loss of lordosis Vacuum phenomenon Osteophytes	None, any, or all of those in lumbar spondylosis Subluxations

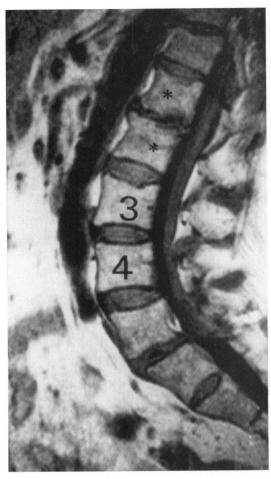

Figure 145.10. Sagittal T1-weighted MRI depicting disc degeneration at L1–L2 with endplate sclerosis (*asterisk*).

In patients with normal findings on static radiography, obtain flexion–extension radiographs to exclude subtle instability patterns. Relatively subtly increased intervertebral motion can be associated with pain. In these patients, discography may be useful to establish a pain generator. Some authors assign no clinical importance to lumbar segmental motion (24,32).

Radionucleotide bone scans have only a minor role in the evaluation of disc degeneration by excluding other suspected pathologic processes, such as tumor, infection, or spondylolysis. Computed tomography (CT) may demonstrate degenerative changes in the lumbar spine, but is not particularly useful in the evaluation of patients with DDD.

MAGNETIC RESONANCE IMAGING

In the evaluation of DDD, magnetic resonance imaging (MRI) is the most commonly employed imaging modality. In that MRI can directly measure water content of the disc, it is the only imaging technique that can detect biochemical changes in the nucleus (56,61). The normal, hydrated NP has an increased proton signal on T2 images. With increasing desiccation, this signal blends with that of the surrounding annulus. With further degeneration, a dark, isointense signal may be seen on T2 (Figs. 145.10, 145.11). An increased T2 signal may be noted in some areas, where it is thought to represent free fluid in annular tears and fissures (87). Aprill and Bogduk (1) described a high-intensity zone (HIZ) representing a tear of the outer annulus. In their study, these HIZ lesions were associated with painful, concordant discography. Subsequent reports as to the significance of these lesions have been mixed (64).

Aside from the discs themselves, changes in endplate morphology adjacent to degenerating discs may have clinical significance (56). These changes were first described by Modic et al. (57) and can be divided into three types. Type I reflects an acute disruption and fissuring of endplates, which leads to ingrowth of vascularized fibrous tissue into the adjacent vertebral body marrow. This tissue exhibits a diminished signal on T1 images and increased signal on T2 images.

In chronic degeneration, the hematopoietic (red) peridiscal marrow undergoes fatty degeneration. Here, a type II pattern is exhibited with an increased T1 and an isointense or slightly hyperintense T2 signal. While type II changes tend to remain stable, type I changes have been shown to develop into type II. Type III changes probably reflect extrinsic bone sclerosis as seen on plain radiographs. Dense bone in the vertebral endplates yields a hypointense signal on both T1 and T2 images (Table 145.6).

Just as the pathologic changes of disc degeneration are likely to be a normal part of aging, the MRI findings associated with the changes described by Modic and Ross (56) frequently do not correlate with LBP. In 1990, Boden et al. (5) found that MRI evidence of degenerative discs was present in 34% of patients 20–29 years old, and in 93% of patients 60–80 years old.

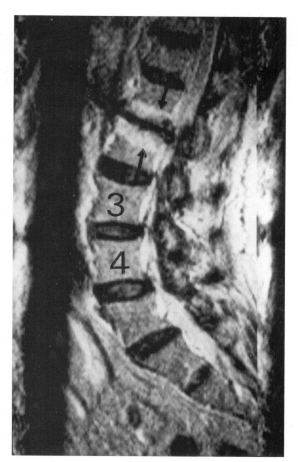

Figure 145.11. Sagittal T2-weighted MRI depicting black disc at L1–L2 with typical endplate changes (*arrow*).

Table 145.7. **Information Available from Discography**
Patient's pain response at the involved level
Pain response at control levels
Disc morphology
Disc pressure and injectant volume

DISCOGRAPHY

Although discography is controversial, it represents the only provocative method available to assess patients with a possible discogenic pain generator. In theory, fluid injected into the disc increases endplate pressures. These transferred pressures may cause pain (34). Abnormal pressure transmission may account for the small subset of patients with normal MRI findings and positive discography. Properly performed, discograms *may* be able to directly identify a cause-and-effect relationship between radiographic signs of degenerated discs and clinical symptoms of lumbar pain.

Morphologic information is available from the discogram or a postdiscography CT (Table 145.7, Fig. 145.12). Abnormal radiographic findings with leakage of dye were seen in 37% of an asymptomatic population, so the study is positive only if the radiographic changes correlate with a concordant pain response. A concordant response requires replication of the patient's usual pain with injection at the degenerated level, and no pain at adjacent, control levels (Table 145.8).

In one large series, Holt (38), having found that a high percentage of previously asymptomatic volunteers had

Table 145.6.	**Modic Changes**			
	MRI image			
Stage	T_1	T_2	*Tissue*	*Clinical correlation*
I	D	I	Vascular fibrous tissue	Acute annular tearing, endplate fissure
II	I	D	Fatty replacement	Chronic marrow of disuse
III	D	D	Endplate sclerosis	Chronic spondylosis

D, decreased; I, increased; MRI, magnetic resonance imaging.
From Modic MT, Ross JS. Magnetic Resonance Imaging in the Evaluation of Low Back Pain. *Orthop Clin North Am* 1991;22:283.

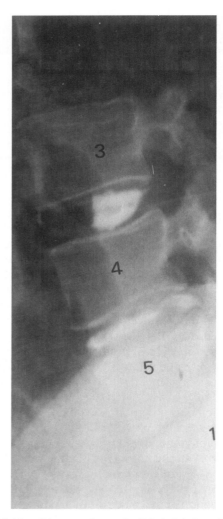

Figure 145.12. Discography at the L3-4, L4-5, and L5–S1 interspaces. Note the normal appearance of the control L3-4 level and the abnormal morphology below.

Table 145.8.   Key Elements of Discographic Technique

Nonirritating, radiopaque contrast

Nonsedated patients

Independent observer of pain response

Injection into both degenerated and one or two nondegenerated "control" levels

Paraspinal, not transdural, approach

positive discography, considered the test unreliable. This study was later criticized by Simmons et al. (69), who noted that injections without fluoroscopic guidance often pressurize the sensitive annulus rather than the nucleus. Further, the contrast material used, diatrizoate meglumine, has been found to be irritating and painful. Later, the Holt study was repeated using modern techniques by Walsh et al. (80), who injected a nonionic, water-soluble contrast agent under fluoroscopic guidance. The study was considered positive only if the disc was radiographically abnormal and a concordant pain response reported. A false-positive rate of 0% with a specificity of 100% was noted in 10 asymptomatic volunteers.

Calhoun et al. (8) found that 89% of 137 patients with positive provocative discography had significant and sustained benefit from fusion at the indicated level. Of 20 patients fused without a positive discogram, only 52% enjoyed postoperative pain relief.

Given the overall controversy surrounding discography, it can be expected that recommendations regarding its role in patient assessment also vary. Some report that a negative MRI may miss clinically significant DDD (7). Others report that positive discography in the context of a negative MRI is associated with inferior results after fusion (27).

Schneiderman et al. (67) found a high correlation between MRI and discographic findings. They reported on 101 disc levels in 36 patients with LBP of longer than 2 months' duration. In each patient, both MRI and discography were performed and blindly reviewed by a neuroradiologist. MRI was accurate in predicting discographic disc morphology 99% of the time. Only one disc level with a normal MRI signal had an abnormal discogram. Of 49 levels with decreased signal on MRI, only two were normal on discogram. The authors found that concordant pain with discography was helpful in the assessment of abnormal discs identified by MRI, but they felt that discography was not indicated in the presence of a normal MRI. Simmons et al. (69), on the other hand, found only a 55% correlation between the tests. They wrote that discography is the only dynamic test available for disc evaluation and thus the only study that can determine which abnormal discs are truly symptomatic.

Horton and Daftari (40) found that, in many cases, MRI could not reliably predict or replace discography. They divided the MRI signal of lumbar discs into dark, white, and speckled patterns, and they characterized the posterior annulus as flat, bulged, or torn. Most dark or torn discs demonstrated positive discography, whereas white or flat discs were very likely to be negative on discography. The intermediate MRI patterns had uncertain correlation with discographic findings, however.

At present, we feel that discography should be performed only as a preoperative test in psychologically normal patients with positive MRI findings, and after aggressive, nonsurgical measures have failed. Discography is probably not warranted in patients with single-level changes. In patients with multilevel or equivocal MRI findings, we use a discogram to detect the symptomatic level.

IMMOBILIZATION TECHNIQUES

Various braces and supports have been recommended to provide pain relief in DDD (14,60,65). The underlying hypothesis is that bracing will simulate effects of fusion by restricting segmental motion. In general, such bracing is not justified, in that the braces most commonly recommended are unreliable in restricting lumbar spinal motion (17,65). Adequate immobilization of the lower lumbosacral spine requires a pantaloon brace.

PSYCHOLOGICAL ASSESSMENT

Ultimately, the treatment of DDD is directed only at pain, the perception of which is quite variable. Depression and anxiety are quite common in DDD patients and are associated with heightened pain perception (77). Historically, it has been difficult to establish whether the pain preceded the psychological disturbance. However, in a series of 200 patients with chronic back pain, 77% met the American Psychiatric Association's Diagnostic and Statistical Manual of mental disorders (DSM III-R) lifetime criteria for psychiatric illness, and 59% met criteria for current, active psychiatric illness (63). In this study, the authors concluded that psychiatric illness (particularly anxiety and substance abuse disorders) often preceded the onset of back pain.

Indications of somatic fixation on the Minnesota Multiphasic Personality Inventory (MMPI) include abnormal elevations of the hypochondriasis and hysteria scales, above that of the depression scale. On this inventory, somatic fixation tends to be predictive of poor surgical outcomes (84). Patients with low hypochondriasis and hysteria scores had 90% good to excellent results 1 year after surgery, while patients with higher scores had only a 10% rate of good to excellent results (84). Southwick and White (71) reported that patients in the latter category were more likely to have positive discograms at nondegenerated levels.

SUMMARY OF THE ASSESSMENT STRATEGY

While certain radiologic findings are consistent with disc degeneration, there are no findings pathognomonic for DDD. As in any degenerative condition of the spine, begin the evaluation with a complete history and physical exam. Pursue atypical pain and other red flags vigorously. Then, assuming limited findings on physical exam, commence

further management with a rigorous nonoperative management regimen.

Only patients failing this management after a 2-month trial require plain radiographic evaluation. While the changes on plain radiographs associated with disc degeneration do not necessarily confer a diagnosis, use plain radiography to exclude other potentially serious causes of pain. If these radiographs are negative, obtain flexion–extension lateral radiographs to rule out subtle instability.

In all cases, pay careful attention to psychosocial factors. A long period of evaluation and nonoperative management affords the surgeon an opportunity to get to know the patient well. Obtain an MMPI if there are any doubts as to the psychological profile. A motivated, professionally satisfied patient is the ideal candidate for further evaluation and possible surgical treatment.

The MRI is the study of choice in the evaluating the intervertebral disc. In the context of unresponsive mechanical pain in a psychologically normal individual, single-level degenerative changes may warrant consideration of operative treatment. Perform multilevel discography if several levels are involved or MRI findings are equivocal. Consider surgery only for those patients demonstrating one (possibly two) levels of concordant pain with no pain at control levels. Discography is at present not indicated in patients with a normal MRI.

NONOPERATIVE TREATMENT

Treat the vast majority of patients with mechanical LBP nonoperatively (4). Begin treatment at the initial patient encounter and, should the pain fail to improve, continue it through the protracted evaluation period. During this period, optimize the patient's physiologic status through cessation of smoking, increasing spinal flexibility, and increasing aerobic exercise tolerance. Consider only patients actively participating in a surgeon-directed rehabilitation program for invasive presurgical testing, such as discography.

Specifically, institute a focused program of physical therapy including strengthening and stretching. Some have found that flexion exercises exacerbate discogenic pain. Specific abdominal strengthening and trunk-stabilizing exercises, such as abdominal crunches with flexed hips and knees, however, can be performed with limited lumbar flexion. Extension exercises and low-impact aerobic exercises, such as swimming and cycling, are often recommended and well tolerated.

For patients whose pain prevents them from being able to begin conditioning and strengthening exercises, start a course of acetaminophen or nonsteroidal anti-inflammatory drugs (NSAIDs). Muscle relaxants may be useful in the setting of acute LBP but are not recommended for patients with chronic difficulties (5).

Chiropractic care may also have a role in the management of acute LBP episodes, although no convincing evidence of efficacy in the context of chronic LBP is available. Further, as in acute back pain, extended periods of bed rest have no role in the management of DDD patients. Several clinical trials have studied the role of bracing. The Quebec Task Force on Spinal Disorders found insufficient scientific evidence to support the efficacy of a lumbar corset or support (5,14,89).

Other nonoperative modalities such as traction, massage, and acupuncture for chronic, mechanical LBP are not supported by the scientific literature (89).

Consider a multidisciplinary pain clinic for patients who fail to adequately participate in a nonoperative regimen. In such a setting, detoxification, psychological assessment, work hardening, work skills retraining, tricyclic antidepressant medication, and other modalities may be effectively applied to improve the patient's pain and functional status.

OPERATIVE TREATMENT

In general, offer surgery only to those patients for whom operative results would represent an improvement over the natural history of DDD. Since the natural history of DDD remains to be elucidated, balance any recommendations for surgery carefully against surgical risks and the significant possibility of failure to obtain clinical improvement.

Presently, 50% to 80% clinical success rates are reported for the various operative modalities in DDD. There are no data to suggest that the various subtypes of DDD require different approaches to surgical management.

Different outcomes measures have been used in the past to quantify acceptable surgical results. Often, failures result from unrealistic expectations on the part of both physician and patient. One factor is "fusion disease," described by Zdeblick (89). The stripping and retraction required for posterior spinal fusion procedures may cause permanent fibrosis and ischemic injury of the extensor musculature. Long periods of intense manual labor may be impossible even in the presence of a solid bony union.

While fusions for multiple-level DDD typically fail, single-level (and occasionally double-level) fusions for DDD may be considered if the following prerequisites have been met (36):

- Pain and disability are present for at least 1 year.
- There is failure of aggressive physical conditioning and conservative treatment of more than 4 months duration.
- There is single-level disc degeneration on MRI with concordant pain response on discography.
- There is absence of psychiatric or secondary gain issues.

The aim of surgery for DDD is to decrease pain by limiting mechanical stimuli across the painful motion segment. The least controversial procedures achieve this goal by solid arthrodesis. Several methods currently advocated to promote such a fusion will be described next.

POSTEROLATERAL SPINAL FUSION

Posterolateral spinal fusion was previously the gold standard for the surgical treatment of discogenic back pain (36,62). The advantage of the posterior approach is that fusion can be performed in the absence of the posterior element; the risk of injury to the neural elements is low; and because the graft is placed away from midline, there is less risk of iatrogenic spinal stenosis.

Reported results of uninstrumented fusion have been contradictory. Stauffer and Coventry (73) reported 89% good results, and they achieved an 80% fusion rate by radiographic criteria; there was a high correlation between successful fusion and the clinical result. Dawson et al. (11) reported a 92% rate of solid fusion, with a 70% to 90% clinical success rate. Those undergoing a fusion above the lumbosacral motion segment were found to have a 45% pseudarthrosis rate, however.

Others have noted poor results with fusion. Finlayson et al. (18) performed a posterolateral fusion for DDD in 20 patients with concordant discography. While 11 felt the operation was worthwhile, only six had a good outcome as measured by impairment, disability, and work status. Parker et al. (62) reported a prospective, consecutive series of patients with discogenic LBP undergoing posterolateral fusion. They observed only 39% good to excellent results, with 13% fair and 48% poor results. Poor results were associated with workers' compensation status, pseudarthrosis, and being out of work longer than 3 months Greenough et al. (29) concluded that posterolateral fusion was an acceptable treatment for discogenic back pain only in very carefully selected patients.

Pedicle screw instrumentation has been added to posterolateral fusion procedures in an attempt to decrease pseudarthrosis rates (Figs. 145.13, 145.14). Data from fusion procedures for degenerative spondylolisthesis suggest increased fusion rates but no effect on clinical outcome (19). Instrumentation is associated with higher costs and complication rates. One recent series noted 10% of patients had instrumentation-related problems. Yet, biomechanical studies suggest that pedicle screw constructs are superior in stabilizing the nonosteoporotic spine (31). These constructs may confer immediate stability to motion segments and allow an expedited postoperative recovery. This added stiffness and faster recovery interval may be more important in the younger population with DDD than in the older patient with degenerative spondylolisthesis.

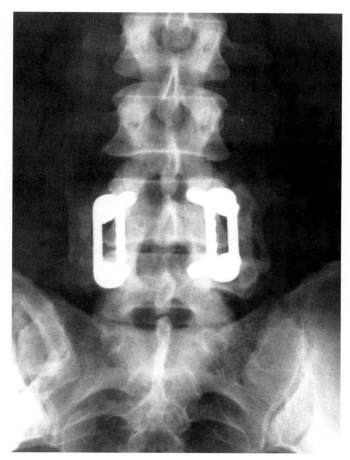

Figure 145.13. Postoperative AP radiograph after single-level L4-5 posterior fusion with instrumentation.

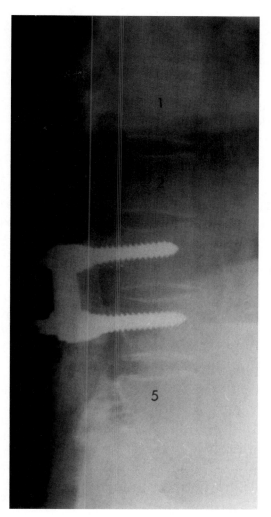

Figure 145.14. Postoperative lateral radiograph depicting fusion with instrumentation at L3-4.

Pseudarthrosis rates in noninstrumented fusions range from 35% to 68%. Instrumented fusions have pseudarthrosis rates reported from 0% to 33%. Increased rates of 75% to 95% significant clinical improvement are also reported in patients undergoing instrumented fusions, versus 59% to 70% in those fused without instrumentation (3,88). In patients undergoing fusion for discogenic pain, solid fusion is associated with increased return-to-work rates as well (11). Posterolateral fusions undertaken to treat DDD should probably be undertaken with rigid, transpedicular instrumentation, particularly in the revision situation (85).

ANTERIOR LUMBAR INTERBODY FUSION

There are two common approaches to anterior lumbar interbody fusion (ALIF). The first, the open retroperitoneal approach, employs a 5–10 cm incision to directly access the anterior spine. A complete discectomy may then be undertaken and a variety of implants, including allo-graft rings and threaded cages, placed into the disc space. Various endoscopic methods of threaded cage placement have been described as well. These approaches use relatively straightforward techniques for access, but they do not include a complete discectomy. Moreover, the threaded cage techniques require violation of the vertebral endplate. While these newer approaches may be less invasive, long-term data regarding fusion rates and implant stability are not available.

Historically, ALIF has been reserved as a salvage procedure for patients failing multiple posterior procedures (27). More recently, increased ease of access and concerns over extensor muscle retraction in a relatively young patient population have renewed interest in this approach. Moreover, some authors, citing the disc as the primary source of pain, recommend its complete extirpation (27, 29,43,58,59,72,82,89,90).

The advantages of ALIF include the following:

- Complete excision of disc material
- Placement of the graft under compression
- Availability of a large surface area for graft incorporation
- Availability of a virgin operative site if there has been a prior posterior spinal fusion
- Avoidance of extensor muscle injury ("fusion disease")

Advocates of ALIF report that even after solid posterior arthrodesis, flexion may occur through the fusion mass. This slight movement may cause continuing pain in the intervening degenerated discs. Weatherly et al. (81) reported complete relief of pain after ALIF in four patients with solid posterolateral fusion and concordant discograms at the previously fused level. Because ALIF places the fusion mass at the center of motion of the spine, it more rigidly immobilizes the spine once it is solid (33,90).

Results of ALIF have included highly variable fusion rates from 18% to 96% (26). However, the pseudarthrosis rate is generally felt to be lower than that for one-level posterolateral fusions or posterior lumbar interbody fusions (76,85). Similar variability in rates of pain relief and return to work have been reported. Ostensibly, this variability is caused by differences in surgical indications and techniques.

Several distinct operative techniques have been described for ALIF (see Chapter 146). Traditionally, corticocancellous bone from the iliac crest was placed in the disc space and maintained in position with a screw and washer. This approach was sometimes associated with graft collapse and pseudarthrosis. Allograft rings were then recommended and, subsequently, threaded cage techniques.

The cited advantages of threaded cages include structural support for the anterior column, indirect decompression of the foramina and nerve roots by distraction of the disc space, the potential for bony ingrowth through the cage, and the possibility of minimally invasive implantation (90). While clinical results are preliminary, early series demonstrate good mechanical stability with these constructs (52). Figure 145.15 shows sample cases.

When considering the more recently described endoscopic methods of ALIF, it is important to remember that they represent only a new technique, not a new operation. Therefore, operative indications remain the same. There are proposed benefits of an endoscopic approach, however. Preliminary studies suggest shorter hospital stays, decreased morbidity, and earlier return to work with minimally invasive techniques (52,53).

At present, several endoscopic techniques are evolving. The transperitoneal approach with gas insufflation serves as a direct extension of conventional laparoscopic surgery (90). This technique allows direct access to L5–S1, L4–L5, and occasionally L3–L4. Proposed advantages include ease of organ retraction, more rapid exposure of the spine, increased working space, and decreased bleeding. Disadvantages include the requirement for expensive trocars with diaphragms and other special instruments, as well as the potential for air leakage and a carbon dioxide venous embolism.

A gasless approach has been devised wherein the working space is maintained by lifting the anterior abdominal wall with a fan-like retractor. This approach allows the use of conventional instruments and avoids carbon dioxide effects and expensive valves. The procedure is associated with increased time for exposure, limited lateral vision, and an overall more technically difficult approach. Therefore, an intermediate, combined insufflated and gasless technique was devised, in which insufflation is used for the initial spine exposure. Retractors and Steinmann pins are placed, and then conversion to gasless technique is undertaken.

For a retroperitoneal approach utilizing the potential space between the spine and the abdominal cavity, make a 2.5 cm flank incision by splitting the anterior lateral abdominal muscles. After an initial finger dissection, enlarge the space with a retroperitoneal balloon. Again, the laparoscopic retractor with a hydraulic arm is employed to create a tent-like effect. Further peritoneal reflection can then be carried out under direct vision. This procedure provides access from T-12 to S-1. Further, conventional instruments may be used and the procedure can be converted from a pure percutaneous endoscopic to an endoscopic-assisted anterior approach should the degree of difficulty be increased. Some authors report difficulty obtaining a direct frontal approach to the disc space with this technique, however.

GLOBAL FUSIONS

Global (360°) fusions were previously recommended for multilevel involvement and postlaminectomy patients. Kozack and O'Brien (44) reported a series of 69 patients with global fusions for DDD. Fusion levels were determined by provocative discograms. With one- and two-level procedures, 90% fusion rates were achieved. Three-level and greater procedures were associated with 77% fusion rates. Overall, 80% had acceptable clinical results. O'Brien et al. (59) described a global fusion procedure for 150 patients with severe disability due to back pain or with previous failed operations. With posterior instrumentation, they noted an 86% success rate.

Lower pseudarthrosis rates, usually 5% to 10%, were the principal justification for the added surgical morbidity of these combined procedures (44,76). More recently, concerns regarding the effectiveness of threaded cages as stand-alone devices has intensified the debate over the need for posterior stabilization.

A variation on this theme involves an endoscopic anterior fusion with a percutaneous posterior stabilization

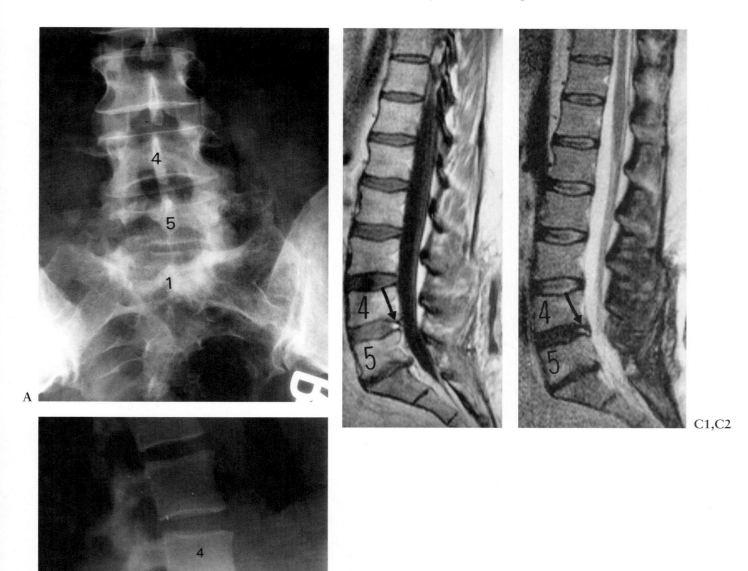

Figure 145.15. Case example. **A:** Preoperative AP radiograph of the lumbar spine depicting loss of disc space height and L5–S1. **B:** Lateral radiograph showing disc degeneration at L5–S1. **C1:** Sagittal T1-weighted MRI demonstrating disc degeneration at L4-5 and L5–S1 with an annular tear evident at L4-5 (*arrow*). **C2:** Sagittal T2-weighted MRI in the same patient. *(continued)*

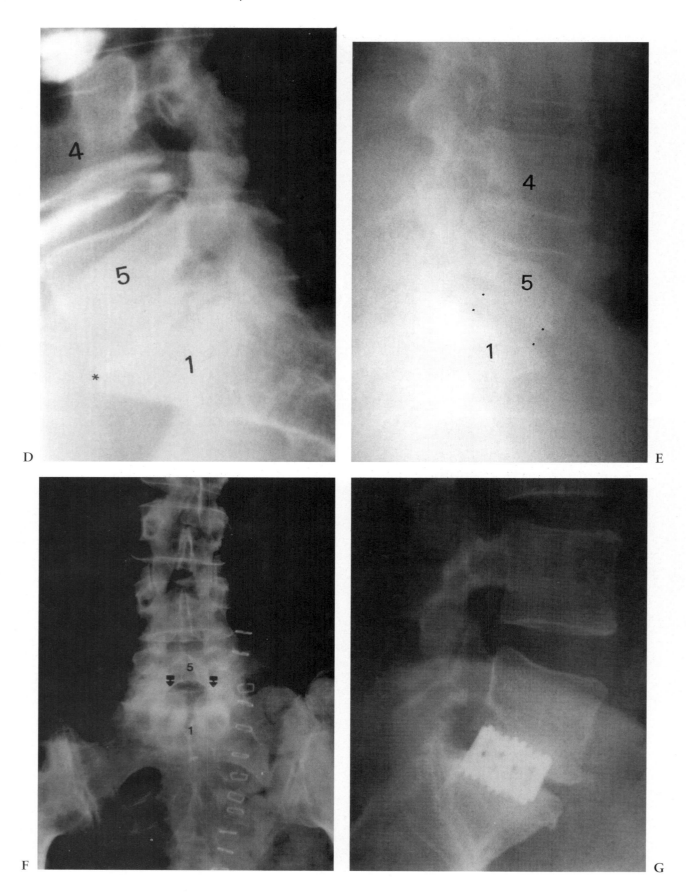

procedure with pedicle screws or translaminar facet screws, but there are no reports of long-term results.

POSTERIOR LUMBAR INTERBODY FUSION

A method of achieving an anterior arthrodesis with posterior stabilization in a single surgical approach is the posterior lumbar interbody fusion (PLIF). A wide posterior decompression is performed, allowing retraction of the dural sleeve and nerve roots for complete disc excision and anterior column fusion.

The PLIF was introduced by Cloward in 1945 to treat lumbar disc ruptures (9). He stated that PLIF was indicated for "the treatment of low back pain with or without sciatica due to lumbar disc disease." This procedure has also been recommended for spondylolisthesis, lumbar scoliosis, osteomyelitis, lumbar kyphosis, and to increase posterior fusion rates in high-risk patients (e.g., smokers and diabetics).

In each case, the addition of an anterior load-sharing graft may enhance the fusion rate, stabilize the construct, and protect the posterior spinal implant by load sharing. In patients with deformity, the PLIF may aid in correction by partial anterior release. Most commonly, however, PLIF procedures are performed for discogenic back pain.

Cloward (9) summarized the PLIF as able to address "all sources of pathologic change of the motion segment in one operation, through one incision." Yet, after initial enthusiasm, use of the PLIF declined due to high rates of pseudarthrosis and graft dislodgement. More recently, the advent of transpedicular instrumentation led to a resurgence of interest in PLIF. Steffee and Sitkowski (74) reported 104 fusions performed without graft dislocation, pseudarthrosis, or infection.

Reported advantages of PLIF include near total disc excision, restoration of disc height and normal sagittal contour, root decompression, solid mechanical arthrodesis, immediate load-sharing with structural support, large surface area for fusion between the vertebral endplates, fusion under compression, and avoidance of an additional anterior approach.

Disadvantages include graft displacement, pseudarthrosis, anterior and posterior destabilization, increased bleeding, dural tears, risk to nerve roots, and risk of epidural fibrosis from root retraction (36).

Ma (50) reported 100 consecutive PLIFs for back or leg pain, spondylolisthesis, or failed back syndrome. There was an 11% reoperation rate: six for pseudarthrosis, three for bone graft extrusion, one bone graft fracture, and one hematoma. Others have reported good to excellent results in 89%, with a fusion rates of 73% to 95% and an 82% return-to-work rate (49,76).

Of particular concern is the trauma to the nerve roots from wide retraction. Epidural fibrosis may develop into a chronic radiculopathy for which there is presently no satisfactory solution. Harms et al. (33) recently popularized a variant of the PLIF procedure that avoids significant retraction on the thecal sac. This posterolateral approach to the disc space relies on facet excision and has been termed the transforaminal lumbar interbody fusion (TLIF). While transpedicular instrumentation is recommended for the midline laminotomy version of the PLIF, it is mandatory here.

Transforaminal lumbar interbody fusion preserves the anterior and posterior ligamentous complex, thereby maintaining a tension band for compression of the graft and prevention of retropulsion. While long-term outcome reports are not yet available, some authors noted the proximity of the dorsal root ganglion and the potential for chronic, neurogenic pain after even minor trauma to this structure.

Posterior lumbar interbody fusion is contraindicated in patients with preexisting, significant epidural fibrosis and those with significant osteopenia. Aside from the more typical complications such as bleeding, infection, and pseudarthrosis (mentioned later), the unique complications possible with PLIF deserve special mention here. With standard PLIF procedures, damage to nerve roots remains a principal concern. The surgeon must be careful about overdistraction, particularly in patients with nerve root anomalies. New or increased deficits occur in 0.5% to 4% of patients after PLIF (48). The upper (exiting) root traverses the interspace just out of direct view in the lateral recess and can be damaged when grafts are inserted in the disc space.

Steffee and Sitkowski (74) report that a failed PLIF has

Figure 145.15. (continued) **D:** Discography was performed at the L3-4, L4-5, and L5–S1 levels. Concordant pain was noted at the L5–S1 level (*asterisk*). While the L4-5 annular tear is again appreciated on discography, this level was not painful to dye injection. **E:** Lateral radiograph demonstrating corticocancellous autograft ALIF at L5–S1 (*dots* outline the anterior and posterior extent of the graft). **F:** An immediately postoperative AP radiograph of another patient with allograft dowel placement via a mini-open ALIF approach. **G:** Lateral radiograph of another patient with BAK cage placement.

"a worse outcome than failure of any other fusion procedure." They report that exploration of patients with a post-PLIF chronic radiculopathy reveals epidural fibrosis for which there is no satisfactory salvage. Careful attention to the tension placed on the cauda and nerve roots may diminish the incidence of these problems.

Neural structures may also be injured with posterior bone graft migration. The subtotal discectomy required for a PLIF procedure risks penetration of the anterior annulus with attendant anterior vessel damage, a potentially catastrophic complication.

Revision options in failed PLIF are limited. A noninstrumented PLIF may be converted to an instrumented PLIF. A failed instrumented PLIF is most often revised with an attempted anterior fusion (82).

With the rising popularity of anterior approaches in the treatment of lumbar disc disease, the role of PLIF or TLIF is not entirely clear. For example, the importance of "fusion disease" in these relatively young patients remains to be established (42). Certain criteria, however, may reasonably aid in the selection between ALIF and PLIF (Table 145.9).

Because PLIF is a relatively difficult surgery to revise, present recommendations for PLIF include lumbar disc disease with sciatica (10) and certain revision situations in which an anterior/posterior fusion through a single incision is desirable.

Table 145.9. Soft Selection Criteria to Decide Between ALIF and PLIF

Situation	Relative preference
Posterior decompression needed	PLIF
Previous retroperitoneal approach	PLIF
Pedicle screw instrumentation needed	PLIF
Male patient, to avoid retrograde ejaculation	PLIF
Previous laminectomy or discectomy	ALIF
Nerve root anomaly present (retraction more difficult)	ALIF
Loss of lumbar lordosis	ALIF
Technical ease at L5–S1	ALIF
Foraminal stenosis without central or lateral stenosis	ALIF
Large cage needed for stabilization	ALIF

ALIF, anterior lumbar interbody fusion; PLIF, posterior lumbar interbody fusion.

SUMMARY OF TREATMENT OPTIONS

We feel that a posterior fusion with instrumentation is the gold standard for the rare patient with true lumbar segmental instability. Those patients with painful lumbar spondylosis LS are best served with a disc ablative procedure such as ALIF and PLIF. Circumferential fusions should be reserved for patients with significant canal pathologies, where revision is required, and other situations in which additional stabilization is required.

We favor ALIF because of the destabilizing effects of PLIF and its potential for nerve root injury, epidural fibrosis, and "fusion disease." The advent of transforaminal interbody fusion procedures may decrease the risk of the PLIF technique, but firm evidence is not available. As more information regarding the long-term results of interbody cage placement becomes available, treatment recommendations will no doubt be revised.

SURGICAL TECHNIQUES

Two surgical procedures commonly employed to treat DDD in its various forms are discussed here: posterior lumbar fusion (with and without instrumentation) and PLIF. ALIFs, either through traditional open or laparoscopic techniques, are increasingly favored for patients with these disorders and are covered in Chapter 146.

POSTEROLATERAL SPINAL FUSION

Before undertaking a posterior spinal fusion for DDD, carefully review your patient selection criteria. Be sure the patient is well informed as to the risks and the potential for an unsatisfactory clinical outcome. Pay careful attention to patient physiology by the following measures:

- Discontinue aspirin and NSAIDs.
- Ensure a good nutritional status.
- Have the patient stop smoking and other tobacco use.
- Recommend preoperative blood donation and institute prophylactic antibiotics.

A posterolateral fusion begins with proper patient positioning. Choose a frame or bolsters that allow the abdominal contents to be free of compression and maintain proper lumbar lordosis (Fig. 145.16).

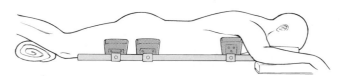

Figure 145.16. Proper positioning on a frame that decompresses the abdomen and avoids pressure points is critical to the success of any lumbar fusion procedure.

- Freedom of abdominal contents will decrease epidural venous engorgement and blood loss.
- A Foley catheter similarly decreases intra-abdominal pressure by preventing bladder distention.
- Carefully pad all bony prominences and avoid pressure over the eyes.
- Use a radiolucent turning frame in procedures in which multiplanar image intensification is anticipated.
- Maintain the patient's core body temperature with ventral and lower-extremity air-circulating devices.

As in all spine surgery, a headlight and loupes increase the effectiveness of the exposure. Intraoperative neural monitoring may be used to stimulate pedicle screws during placement to detect pedicular penetration.

Spine fusion procedures may be associated with significant blood loss. Intraoperative blood salvage is occasionally useful. More important, anticipate and control bleeder sites as you encounter them. Three fairly constant bleeding points include the pars interarticularis artery, the artery of Macnab (transverse process artery), and the sacral arteries.

- The pars artery is encountered during the initial exposure. Emerging from a recess inferior to the facet, it wraps around the pars.
- A curved bayonet may help control the artery of Macnab, which lies on the upper aspect of the junction of the transverse process.
- The sacral arteries protrude from the posterior sacral foramina and are difficult to control without inserting bipolar cautery or forceps into the bony recess. Often, temporary packing with Gelfoam will provide adequate hemostasis.
- Begin the exposure by centering a 6–10 cm midline skin incision just cranial to the involved level (Fig. 145.17).
- Inject a dilute epinephrine solution into the skin and subcutaneous tissue to decrease bleeding.
- Use electrocautery to proceed through the subcutaneous tissue to the fascia.
- Expose a 0.5 cm portion of the fascia on either side of the midline to aid subsequent closure. Avoid extensive fascial stripping, which increases dead space.
- Enter the deep space over the spinous processes in a subperiosteal fashion. Use the Cobb elevator for countertraction.
- Carry the subperiosteal dissection over the laminae to the facets with the electrocautery. Do not violate the facet capsules at this point.
- Insert a Penfield #4 elevator (Fig. 145.18) under a lamina and obtain a radiograph. Confirm operative levels and mark the superior level by resecting a portion of the spinous process with a rongeur.
- Expose the laminae one level above and one level below the anticipated level of fusion. Leave the facets intact at these levels. This additional dissection will reduce

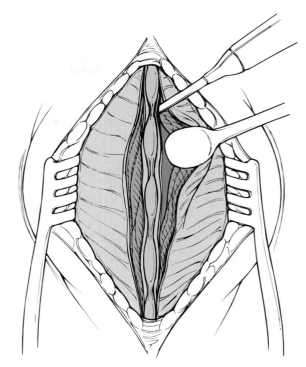

Figure 145.17.　Initiation of a midline subperiosteal approach.

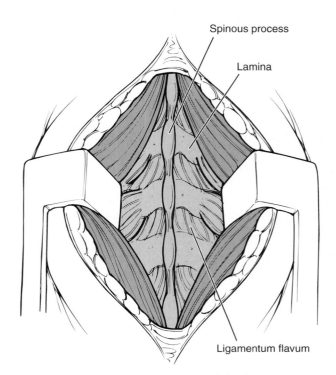

Figure 145.18.　Exposure of the facets.

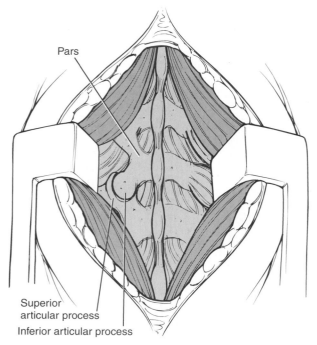

Figure 145.19. Exposure of the transverse processes and pars interarticularis.

gently. Then add corticocancellous strips and compress gently into position.

■ For each level to be included in the fusion, remove the entire facet joint capsule and denude the cartilage from the facet.

■ Close the wound in layers to create a watertight fascial closure. Place a drain in the deep space.

HINTS AND TRICKS

To diminish operative morbidity in posterior approaches, do the following:

• Periodically release the retractor to reestablish muscle vascularity.

• Handle muscle carefully to minimize devascularization and necrosis.

• Make the exposure generous to minimize the required retractor tension.

• Use Gelfoam or bipolar cautery over the pars, transverse processes, neural foramen, and dorsal sacral foramen.

• Prevent overcauterization to minimize injury to nearby neural structures.

---

tension over the transverse process exposure at the operative level.

■ Bluntly dissect over the facets with a Cobb elevator and a sponge at the operative level.

■ Then expose the lateral pars interarticularis and transverse processes with electrocautery. The transverse processes lie immediately adjacent to the facets. Be careful not to penetrate the intertransverse membrane (Fig. 145.19).

If no midline decompression is required, consider a bilateral Wiltse (paramedian) approach. A larger midline skin incision and subcutaneous dissection is required. Make the fascial incisions two finger breadths lateral to the midline bilaterally. Then bluntly dissect down to the lateral facets between the multifidus and longissimus muscles. This approach is covered more extensively in Chapter 138.

■ Remove all soft tissue from the posterior aspect of the transverse processes, outer facets, and pars. If the fusion includes S-1, clear the sacral ala. Complete soft-tissue removal will double the area available for bone graft. Preparation of the graft bed is the most important part of any fusion procedure.

■ Decorticate the lateral pars, the transverse process, and the lateral wall of the facets.

■ Lay autologous cancellous bone into place and impact

INSTRUMENTED POSTERIOR SPINAL FUSION

Employ the same initial steps as in a noninstrumented fusion. Do not insert pedicle screws prior to complete exposure of the posterior elements. Decortication of the transverse processes and bone graft insertion are more easily and completely accomplished prior to hardware insertion. Many surgeons, however, prefer to decorticate after instrumentation to diminish blood loss.

Several useful techniques for entry-point localization and pedicle-screw placement have been described. Thorough knowledge of pedicular anatomy is critical. Various radiographic techniques of localization are now available, but none replaces a firm grasp of the relationships of the posterior elements to one another.

The pedicle lies along the midline axis of the transverse process. The outer border of the facets describes a line roughly conforming to the lateral border of the pedicle. The lateral border of the pars defines the medial pedicular border. The accessory process is often identified at the junction of the facet and the transverse process. This process serves as a useful entry point (Fig. 145.20A).

While multilevel fusions are generally not recommended for DDD, instrumentation in these cases is placed at each level in an effort to reduce micromotion. How much segmental stiffness is required to achieve fusion and eliminate pain is not established (45); however, given that

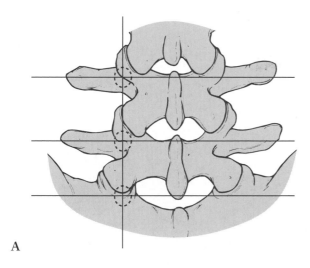

A

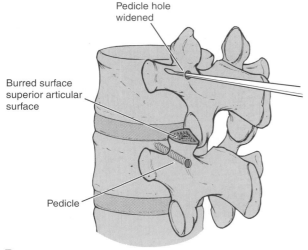

Pedicle hole
widened

Burred surface
superior articular
surface

Pedicle

B

Figure 145.20. **A:** Anatomy of pedicle location. See text for details. **B:** Sounding the pedicle with a probe or curret.

micromotion has been hypothesized as a cause of pain in four screw micromotion-segment constructs (81), maximizing points of fixation is recommended. Screw placement is abandoned if preoperative imaging demonstrates thin pedicles. Similarly, if difficulties with cortical breech are noted intraoperatively, abandonment of that point of fixation is recommended.

- Carefully review the preoperative MRI or CT scan to confirm the extent of convergence of the pedicle at each level, as well as the length and size of screw necessary.
- In general, screws should converge by 5° at the thoracolumbar junction. This convergence increases to 10° at L-2 and 15° at L-5.
- Use the localization lateral radiograph to define the proper attitude of the pedicle in the cranial and caudad planes.

- Most often, an L-3 pedicle screw is inserted perpendicular to the floor. Angle superior screws progressively more cranially. Angle inferior screws progressively more caudally.
- Decorticate the pedicle entry site with a burr.
- Enter the pedicle with a curet or pedicle probe. Gently work this device anteriorly into the vertebral body (Fig. 145.20*B*).
- Check for cortical penetration with a ball-tip probe. If a midline decompression has been performed, the pedicle may also be palpated from within the canal. If necessary, place markers and confirm radiographically.
- Tap the hole and insert the screw (Fig. 145.20*B*). The optimal depth of screw placement has not been determined, but pullout strength increases linearly with depth of penetration (46). We estimate 75% penetration using lateral fluoroscopy to increase purchase while minimizing risk to anterior vascular structures.
- Once the screws and bone graft have been placed, affix a plate or rod according to the manufacturer's instructions.
- Be careful to maintain proper lumbar lordosis.
- Undertake closure over a drain with watertight fascial closure, and follow with a layered closure of the subcutaneous tissues and skin.

SACRAL FIXATION

Sacral fixation remains the weak link in posterior fixation systems (13). Large constructs extending to the sacrum require additional fixation. The combination of large forces transmitted to the sacrum and the size and bone content of the sacral pedicle may render S-1 screws inadequate as the sole point of inferior fixation. In the degenerative conditions described in this chapter, however, smaller, single-level constructs are recommended. In these cases, simple transpedicular instrumentation is usually successful. The sacral pedicle requires larger screws.

- Locate the S-1 pedicle at the intersection of a horizontal line connecting the inferior aspect of the lumbosacral facets, and a vertical line tangential to the lateral border of the superior facet.
- Insert the screws above and in line with the first sacral foramen. Converge the screws and incline them superiorly, parallel with the lumbosacral disc space.

Medial angulation allows longer screws with superior fixation strength, although iliac crest overhang may limit optimal screw trajectory. In the case of tenuous fixation, additional cortical purchase is recommended to prevent "windshield-wipering." Options include careful perforation of the anterior cortex or of the L5–S1 disc space (Fig. 145.21).

When considering penetration of the anterior sacral cortex, recognize the possibility of significant individual

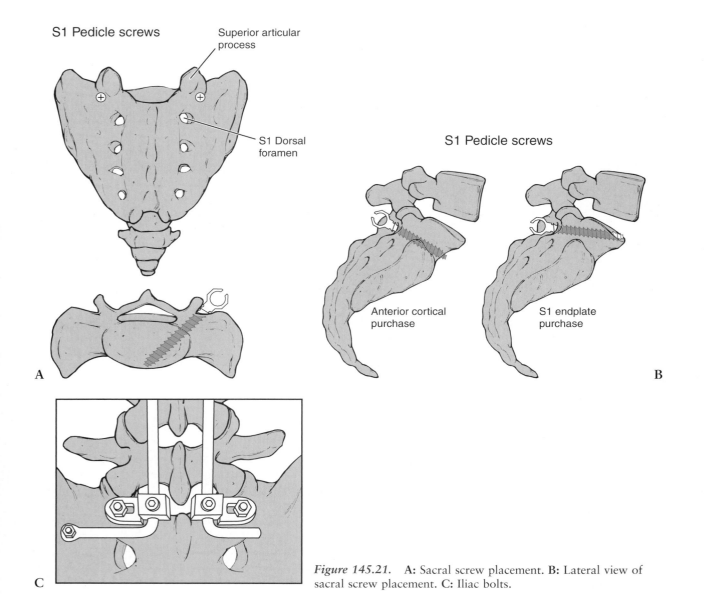

Figure 145.21. **A:** Sacral screw placement. **B:** Lateral view of sacral screw placement. **C:** Iliac bolts.

anatomic variability (13). Differences in sacral bony anatomy are associated with differences in vascular tree branching patterns and in the location of the neural foramina. Assess the morphology and choose an optimal trajectory from preoperative CT or MRI scans.

The medial sacral promontory is the safest place to penetrate the anterior cortex. More lateral sacral screws may hit the lumbosacral plexus, which is affixed to the bone here. Lateral trajectories also risk injury to the iliac veins, particularly on the left.

Other options for fixation below the lumbosacral interspace include S-2 pedicle screws, sacroiliac bolts, and sacral rods. S-2 screws are easily inserted along the intermediate sacral crest midway between the first and second dorsal foramina, but they are considered biomechanically

weak. Cortical penetration at this level risks injury to the sigmoid colon.

Postoperative bracing is not usually recommended, and genuinely effective bracing requires a pantaloon extension. Sacral fixation techniques are further discussed in Chapters 156, 159, and 160.

POSTERIOR LUMBAR INTERBODY FUSION

Carry out the initial stages of PLIF (10,48,74) in the same manner as posterolateral fusion. Careful positioning is critical. Lumbar lordosis and abdominal decompression are important. Some authors feel the knee–chest position adequately maintains lordosis while maximizing hip and knee flexion. Hip and knee flexion ensure decreased tension on the nerve roots, which may allow greater thecal sac retraction for PLIF surgery.

Although PLIF was originally described without instrumentation, this is not recommended. The wide posterior exposure necessary for a safe PLIF produces increased instability with increased rates of pseudarthrosis and graft dislodgement.

Classically, a PLIF is performed in three steps: laminotomy, removal of the intervertebral disc, and spinal fusion.

- Perform a standard 10 cm midline exposure of the posterior elements (as described previously) with a wide laminotomy at the level of interest.
- Preserve the superior portion of the superior lamina and the inferior portion of the inferior lamina with portions of the spinous processes. Muscular attachment sites and interspinous ligaments to levels above and below operative level are thereby preserved.
- Remove the inferior third of the inferior facet, and the medial two thirds of the superior facet to the level of the pedicle. Visualize the lateral half of the intervertebral disc as well as the cranial and caudal nerve roots.
- The medial facet resection can be more aggressive if a combined posterior fusion and instrumentation is planned (Fig. 145.22).

- Next, insert pedicle screws as described previously to allow placement of a working plate or rod.
- Distract the disc space with a lamina spreader and hold the distraction with the working plate. Minimize the force placed through the screws themselves.
- Retract and protect the dural sac and nerve roots. Take great care to prevent overdistraction of the neural structures. Ensure adequate mobilization of the thecal sac to the midline from either side.
- Meticulously cauterize the epidural venous plexus over the posterior annulus with bipolar cautery.
- Make box annulotomies with a knife, and aggressively clean the disc space on both sides of the thecal sac.
- Curet the endplates to remove the annulus and endplate cartilage.

A number of techniques are described for preparing the disc space. Specialized instruments are particularly useful. If they are not available, curets, pituitary rongeurs, and osteotomes may be used. The goal is to clear 80% to 90% of the disc space. Better preparation of the graft site yields a larger area of bony contact with the graft and increases the chance of successful fusion.

- Insert an 8 mm intradiscal shaper parallel to the end-

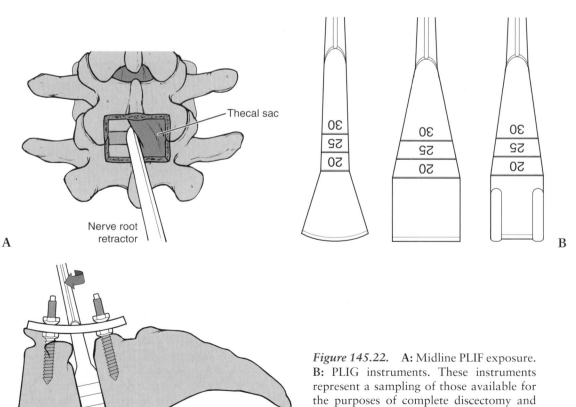

Figure 145.22. **A:** Midline PLIF exposure. **B:** PLIG instruments. These instruments represent a sampling of those available for the purposes of complete discectomy and disc space distraction. **C:** Obtaining distraction through the disc space.

plates. The shaper has a blunt end to protect the annulus anterolaterally.

- Rotate the shaper to allow its side cutting flutes to remove disc material and cartilaginous endplate. Repeat this step on the opposite side.
- Increase the shaper size by increments of 1 mm. Although these instruments are graduated, the disc space depth varies from 25 to 35 mm and it is necessary to pay careful attention to the depth of insertion at all times.
- Avoid the anterior portion of the disc space beneath the anterior longitudinal ligament to minimize the chances of a catastrophic vascular injury.

Numerous techniques are also described for the posterior grafting of the anterior column (Fig. 145.23). With disc space distraction maintained, various graft materials may be inserted. These include dowels, corticocancellous ramps, titanium plugs, and metal or carbon fiber cages of the vertical (e.g., the Harms cage, DePuy-Acromed, Raynham, MA) or the horizontal variety (e.g., the BAK, Sulzer-Spinetech Minneapolis, MN) (12).

Cages are designed to prevent postoperative collapse by providing a structural support to the interspace while the cancellous graft material becomes incorporated. The use of morcelized cancellous bone rather than corticocancellous pieces may minimize donor site morbidity. Specialized instrumentation has been developed for the posterior insertion of threaded interbody cages. While the specific instruments vary by the system used, the concepts are the same. The larger size of these implants requires a larger laminotomy or complete laminectomy and facetectomy. Base implant sizing on preoperative templating. Furthermore, the larger size of the instrumentation warrants a heightened awareness of the position of and tension on the dura and nerve roots.

- In some systems (e.g., the BAK), a drill tube is available to dock onto the disc space posteriorly. This allows insertion of the remainder of the instrumentation in a relatively safe fashion. The instrumentation includes distraction plugs or other devices to open the disc space, reamers to remove disc and endplate tissue, taps to prepare the threaded cage path, and cage inserters.

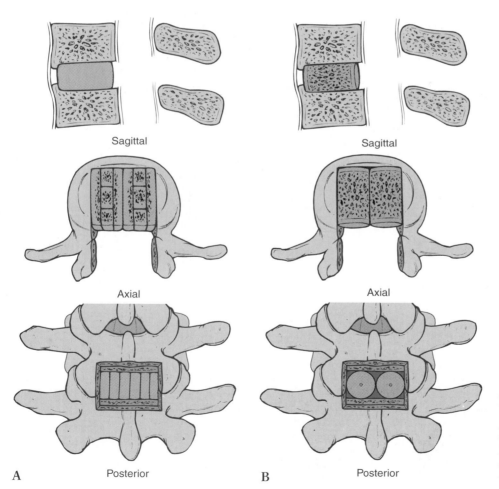

Sagittal

Axial

A   Posterior

Sagittal

Axial

B   Posterior

Figure 145.23. Bone grafting options in PLIF. **A:** Sagittal, axial, and posterior views (from top to bottom) of Cloward's (9) tricortical rectangular graft technique. **B:** Similar views of threaded bone dowels used to obtain a PLIF.

- When using this instrumentation, avoid long periods of traction on the dural sleeve with the tube in place.
- Remember to tightly pack the cage with autograft.
- Insert remaining autograft around the cage in the disc space. If individual bone pieces are used, pack the anterior disc space first, then pack medially under the thecal sac, then laterally.
- In all cases, countersink the graft material 3–5 mm to prevent canal encroachment.
- Some authors recommend placing a fat graft anteriorly between the dura and the grafts.
- Once maximal fill of the disc space has been achieved, remove the distractive forces to allow compression of the graft. With transpedicular instrumentation, further compression is achieved across the screws before final tightening. In all cases, make sure that appropriate lordosis is maintained.

TRANSFORAMINAL LUMBAR INTERBODY FUSION

The TLIF variant (33) of the standard PLIF procedure requires a wide, unilateral approach to the disc space at its posterolateral aspect.

- First remove the inferior facet of the superior vertebra with an osteotome. Then remove the superior facet of the inferior vertebra (Fig. 145.24).
- Identify and protect the exiting and traversing nerve roots.
- After the pedicles have been identified, insert pedicle screws. Distract the disc space with an intervertebral

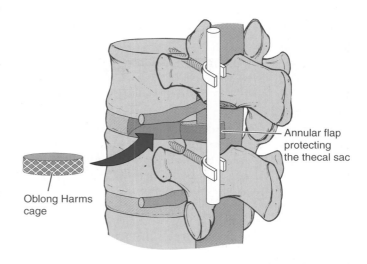

Figure 145.25. Once a subtotal discectomy has been performed through a posterolateral annulotomy, bone graft is packed into the disc space anteriorly. Next, oblong, autogenous bone-graft-filled Harms cages are tamped across the disc space.

spreader and maintain the distraction with working plates or rods affixed to the screws.
- Perform an annulotomy by creating a medially based annular flap. This flap may aid in thecal sac protection.
- Perform a complete discectomy, as described previously, and increase disc space distraction after the annulotomy.
- Tamp loose, morcelized, autogenous graft into the anterior disc space.
- Insert additional graft into an oblong 10–12 mm Harms cage (Fig. 145.25). Tamp the cage across the disc space to the contralateral side with either a straight or an angled impactor.
- Insert a second cage ipsilaterally.
- When packing extra bone graft around the insertion site, be sure that the nerve root is protected.
- Once grafting is completed, compress the posterior instrumentation.

REHABILITATION AND POSTOPERATIVE PRINCIPLES

Regardless of the approach, early mobility is a prime postoperative goal.

- Mobilize patients to a chair the evening after surgery. No braces are employed.
- Request physical therapy assistance for ambulation and transfer techniques in the early postoperative period. Most patients can comfortably ambulate by the third day after surgery. Typically, young DDD patients rarely require assistive devices.

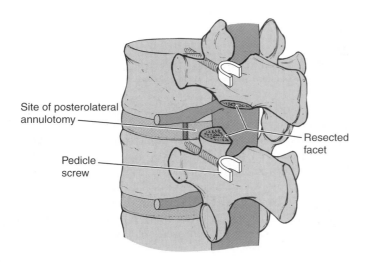

Figure 145.24. Facet resection and interspace distraction through pedicle screws allows access to the disc without significant retraction of the thecal sac.

- Early postoperative restrictions include limitations on bending, lifting, and twisting, but other gentle activities are encouraged.
- After posterior fusion, remove drains and Foley catheters on the first postoperative day.
- At present, we use 24–48 hours of postoperative antibiotics.

Most patients are ready for discharge by the third postoperative day. See them for a wound check and staple removal at 7–14 days after surgery. Subsequent visits include 6- and 12-week checks. Obtained radiographs at these intervals to assess the status of the fusion.

The schedule for return to work and sporting activities is individualized on the basis of clinical status, radiographic union, and the nature of the activities involved. Early return with limited duty is preferred to lengthy sick leave.

After solid fusion is achieved, aerobic activities, spinal flexibility, and truncal strength and stability are important, life-long aspects of the patient's personal fitness regime. Further specific physical therapy is not usually needed, however.

Some patients may not be able to return to physically demanding occupations. Early intervention with skills retraining and a realistic outlook are crucial to optimal functional recovery.

PITFALLS AND COMPLICATIONS

It is important to appreciate the scope and magnitude of potential pitfalls before selecting one of these procedures. Perisurgical problems include general surgical complications and specific procedure-related complications. The latter are detailed in their respective sections. Also, see Chapter 147.

General complications can be divided temporally into preoperative, intraoperative, and postoperative problems. Preoperative problems include the following:

- Wrong patient. Patient selection cannot be overemphasized.
- Wrong level. Correct identification of a pain generator amenable to surgical treatment is fraught with difficulty and remains the biggest hurdle in the treatment of patients with disc degeneration.
- Wrong surgery. Fusion procedures, particularly disc ablative procedures, are the only acceptable surgical modalities for DDD patients.
- Wrong doctor. Anterior and posterior spinal fusion procedures are technically demanding and should be practiced only by surgeons with special training.

Intraoperative complications are often site specific. An-

terior and posterior approaches have a unique complement of attendant problems.

Adjacent segment degeneration is a significant problem in young, active patients with stiff spinal segments. While risks and pathomechanics are not entirely understood, some patients will require extension of fusion in the future for painful degeneration above or below the index fusion.

The risks of pseudarthrosis relative to each procedure have been discussed. In general, grafts under compression have lower pseudarthrosis rates. But anterior column applications require structural graft or cage support. Autogenous structural grafts have higher harvest morbidity. Allografts may have higher collapse potential. Further, autogenous bone harvest is recommended in each of these procedures. The morbidity of bone graft harvest, covered in Chapter 9, should not be underestimated.

Failure to improve despite solid fusion is most often related to poor patient selection or misidentification of the pain generator. In some cases, a solid posterior fusion may allow painful micromotion of the painful disc anteriorly (as described in the section on ALIF).

Benign postoperative urinary retention is common, but cauda equina syndrome and other postsurgical causes must be excluded. Further, indwelling catheters or repeated instrumentation of the genitourinary tract may lead to urinary tract infection and subsequent sepsis.

Ileus may be seen after posterior spine surgery, but it is more common after transperitoneal approaches or those retroperitoneal approaches that violate the peritoneum.

Deep vein thrombosis and pulmonary embolism, while less common than after hip and knee procedures, have rates similar to those in most general surgery procedures. Use of intermittent pneumatic compression stockings after surgery is recommended as a mechanical prophylaxis against this potentially fatal complication.

 ## AUTHORS' PERSPECTIVE

Recent studies demonstrate that the disc may be a source of back pain via nocireceptors and mechanoreceptors in the annulus and chemical irritants from the NP. The changes ascribed to DDD, however, are similar to the changes of normal aging. Moreover, a clear understanding of the pathophysiology and natural history of this pain complex is lacking. Given the ubiquity of back pain in society at large, isolating those symptom patterns and imaging findings consistent with a surgically treatable pain syndrome has been fraught with failure. A range of painful degenerative lumbar conditions exists. These entities have been grouped as degenerative disc disease or subclassified with names such as internal disc disruption, lumbar segmental instability, and lumbar spondylosis. These distinctions are largely conjectural and almost nothing is known about their natural histories.

Evaluation of DDD requires exclusion of other causes of pain. Begin investigation with a thorough history and physical examination. In the absence of red flags, a long trial of nonoperative treatment is indicated. Should symptoms continue, a progressive preoperative evaluation including MRI and psychosocial assessment is mandatory. Based on these studies, discography may be indicated to identify concordant pain at abnormal levels seen on MRI.

Then, only after rigorous selection criteria are fulfilled, may a patient be considered for surgery. Lumbar fusion remains the treatment of choice. In any operative procedure, the known benefits must outweigh the risks. As the benefits of fusion for DDD have not been clearly established, a great deal of further study is required before routine operative intervention can be recommended for these patients.

In some circumstances, dual-level surgery may be justified. However, results of multilevel fusion for painful disc degeneration are abysmal, and it is best avoided. Multidisciplinary pain clinics remain a viable alternative.

Questions surrounding surgical approach are rapidly evolving. Presently, minimally invasive anterior approaches with threaded cages appear promising, but significant long-term data are lacking. PLIF techniques are also frequently employed. A transforaminal posterior interbody fusion may be a sensible approach in certain patients. As with any major posterior lumbar procedure, however, the long-term effects of "fusion disease" in an otherwise active patient population must be considered. With reasonable results reported for each of the various anterior and posterior procedures, the surgeon should ultimately choose that technique with which she is most comfortable. The most important factor in clinical success with this group of patients remains patient selection.

REFERENCES

Each reference is categorized according to the following scheme: * classic article; #, review article; !, basic research article; and +, clinical results/outcome study.

+ 1. Aprill C, Bogduk N. High Intensity Zone. A Diagnostic Sign of Painful Lumbar Disc on Magnetic Resonance Imaging. *Br J Radiol* 1992;65:361.

! 2. Battie MC, Haynor DR, Fisher LD, et al. Similarities in Degenerative Findings on Magnetic Resonance Images of the Lumbar Spines of Identical Twins. *J Bone Joint Surg Am* 1995;77:1662.

+ 3. Bernhard M, Swatz D, Clothiaux P, et al. Posterolateral Lumbar and Lumbosacral Fusion With and Without Pedicle Screw Internal Fixation. *Clin Orthop* 1992;284:109.

4. Bigos SJ. A Literature-based Review as a Guide for Generating Recommendations to Patients Acutely Limited by Low Back Symptoms. In: American Association of Orthopaedic Surgeons, eds. *Orthopaedic Knowledge Update: Spine*. Rosemont, IL: AAOS, 1997:A15.

* 5. Boden SD, Davis DO, Dina TS, et al. Abnormal Magnetic Resonance Scans of the Lumbar Spine in Asymptomatic Subjects. A Prospective Investigation. *J Bone Joint Surg Am* 1990;72:403.

! 6. Boden SD, Riew KD, Yamaguchi K, et al. Orientation of the Lumbar Facet Joints. Association with Degenerative Disc Disease. *J Bone Joint Surg Am* 1996;78:403.

+ 7. Brightbill TC, Pile N, Eichelberger RP, Whitman M Jr. Normal Magnetic Resonance Imaging and Abnormal Discography in Lumbar Disc Disruption. *Spine* 1994;19:1075.

+ 8. Calhoun E, McCall I, Williams I, et al. Provocative Discography as a Guide to Planning Operations on the Spine. *J Bone Joint Surg Br* 1988;70:267.

* 9. Cloward R. The Treatment of Ruptured Lumbar Intervertebral Discs by Vertebral Body Fusion. *J Neurosurg* 1953;10:154.

* 10. Cloward R. Posterior Lumbar Interbody Fusion Updated. *Clin Orthop* 1982;193:16.

11. Dawson EG, Lotysch M, Urist MR. Intertransverse Process Lumbar Arthrodesis and Autogenous Bone Graft. *Clin Orthop* 1981;154:90.

+ 12. Enker P, Steffee A, McMillin C, et al. Artificial Disc Replacement. Preliminary Report with a Minimum 3 Year Follow-up. *Spine* 1993;18:1061.

! 13. Esses SI, Botsford DJ, Huler RJ, Raushning W. Surgical Anatomy of the Sacrum. A Guide for Rational Screw Fixation. *Spine* 1991;16:S283.

+ 14. Esses S, Botsford D, Kostuik J. The Role of External Spinal Skeletal Fixation in the Assessment of Low Back Disorders. *Spine* 1989;14:594.

! 15. Falconer M, McGeorge M, Begg A. Observations of the Cause and Mechanism of Symptom Production in Sciatica and Low Back Pain. *J Neurol Neurosurg Psychiatry* 1948;11:13.

16. Fardon DF, Herzog RJ, Mink JH, et al. Nomenclature of Lumbar Disc Disorders. In: In: American Association of Orthopaedic Surgeons, eds. *Orthopaedic Knowledge Update: Spine*. Rosemont, IL: AAOS, 1997:A3.

! 17. Fidler MW, Plasmans C. The Effect of Four Types of Support on the Segmental Mobility of the Lumbosacral Spine. *J Bone Joint Surg Am* 1983;65:943.

+ 18. Finlayson D, Birche M, Morris E, et al. Is There a Place for Fusion in Simple Backache? *J Bone Joint Surg Br* 1985;67:151.

+ 19. Fischgrund JS, MacKay M, Herkowitz HN, et al. Degenerative Lumbar Spondylolisthesis with Spinal Stenosis. A Prospective, Randomized Study Comparing Decompressive Laminectomy and Arthrodesis With and Without Instrumentation. *Spine* 1997;22:2807.

20. Fraser RD, Bleasel JF, Moskowitz RW. Spinal Degeneration: Pathogenesis and Medical Management. In: Frymoyer JW, Ducker TB, Hadler NM, et al., eds. *The Adult Spine: Principles and Practice*, 2nd ed. New York: Lippincott-Raven, 1997.

* 21. Frederickson BE, Baker D, McHolicle WJ, et al. Natural History of Spondylolysis and Spondylolisthesis. *J Bone Joint Surg Am* 1984;66:699.

! 22. Freemont AJ. Nerve Ingrowth into Diseased Intervertebral Disc in Chronic Back Pain. *Lancet* 1997;350:178.

! 23. Frymoyer J, Cats-Baril W. An Overview of the Incidence and Costs of Low Back Pain. *Orthop Clin North Am* 1991;22:263.

! 24. Frymoyer JW, Newberg JA, Pope MH, et al. Spine Radiographs in Patients with Low Back Pain. An Epidemiologic Study in Men. *J Bone Joint Surg Am* 1984;66:1048.

+ 25. Frymoyer JW, Selby DK. Segmental Instability. Rationale for Treatment. *Spine* 1985;10:280.

+ 26. Fujimaki A, Crock H, Bedbrook G. The Results of 150 Anterior Lumbar Interbody Fusion Operations Performed by Two Surgeons in Australia. *Clin Orthop* 1982;165:164.

+ 27. Goldner J, Urbaniak J, McCollum D. Anterior Disc Excision and Interbody Spinal Fusion for Chronic Low Back Pain. *Orthop Clin North Am* 1971;2:54.

\# 28. Grazer K, Holbrock T, Kelsey J, Stauffer R, eds. *The Frequency of Occurrence, Impact, and Cost of Musculoskeletal Conditions in the United States.* Chicago, IL: American Association of Orthopaedic Surgeons, 1984.

+ 29. Greenough CG, Taylor LJ, Fraser RD. Anterior Lumbar Fusion. A Comparison of Noncompensation and Compensation Patients. *Clin Orthop* 1994;300:30.

! 30. Groen G, Baljet B, Drukker J. The Nerves and Nerve Plexuses of the Human Vertebral Column. *Am J Anat* 1990;188:282.

! 31. Guss K, McAfee P, Shih C. Biomechanical Analysis of Posterior Instrumentation Systems after Decompressive Laminectomy. *J Bone Joint Surg Am* 1988;70:680.

\# 32. Hanley EN. The Indications for Lumbar Spinal Fusion With and Without Instrumentation. *Spine* 1995;20:143S.

\# 33. Harms J, Jeszensky D, Stoltze D, Bohm H. True Spondylolisthesis Reduction and Monosegmental Fusion in Spondylolisthesis. In: Bridwell KH, DeWald RL, eds. *Textbook of Spinal Surgery*, 2nd ed. Philadelphia: Lippincott-Raven, 1997:1337.

! 34. Heggeness MH, Doherty BJ. Discography Causes End Plate Deflection. *Spine* 1993;18:1050.

! 35. Heithoff KB, Gundry CR, Burton CV, Winter RB. Juvenile Discogenic Disease. *Spine* 1994;19:335.

\# 36. Herkowitz HN, Sidhu KS. Lumbar Spine Fusion in the Treatment of Degenerative Conditions. Current Indications and Recommendations. *J Am Assoc Orthop Surg* 1995;3:123.

! 37. Hirsh C, Ingelmark BE, Miller M. The Anatomical Basis for Lowback Pain. *Acta Orthop Scand* 1948;18:132.

* 38. Holt E. The Question of Lumbar Discography. *J Bone Joint Surg Am* 1968;50:720.

* 39. Holt L. Cervical, Dorsal and Lumbar Spinal Syndrome. *Acta Orthop Scand* 1954;17:65.

* 40. Horton W, Daftari T. Which Disc as Visualized by MRI is Actually a Source of Pain? *Spine* 1992;17:51.

! 41. Kauppila LI. Ingrowth of Blood Vessels in Degenerative Discs. Angiographic and Histochemical Studies of Cadaver Spines. *J Bone Joint Surg Am* 1995;77:26.

! 42. Kawaguchi Y, Matsui H, Tsuji H. Changes in Serum Creatine Phosphokinase MM Isoenzyme after Lumbar Spine Surgery. *Spine* 1997;22:1018.

+ 43. Knox BD, Chapman TM. Anterior Lumbar Interbody Fusion for Discogram Concordant Pain: *J Spinal Disord* 1993;6:242.

+ 44. Kozack J, O'Brien J. Simultaneous Combined Anterior and Posterior Fusion. An Independent Analysis of a Treatment for the Disabled Low Back Pain Patient. *Spine* 1990;15:322.

! 45. Krag MH. Biomechanics of Thoracolumbar Spinal Fixation. *Spine* 1991;16:584.

! 46. Krag MH, Beynnon BD, Decoster TA, Pope MH. Depth of Insertion of Transpedicular Vertebral Screws into Human Vertebrae: Effect upon Screw–Vertebra Interface Strength. *J Spinal Disord* 1988;1(4):287.

! 47. Kuslich S, Stephan D, Ulstrom C. The Tissue Origin of Low Back Pain and Sciatica. *Orthop Clin North Am* 1991;22:181.

\# 48. Lanzino G, Shaffrey CI, Ray CD. Posterior Lumbar Interbody Fusion. In: Benzel E, ed *Spine Surgery: Techniques, Complication Avoidance, and Management.* Philadelphia: Churchill-Livingstone, 1999.

+ 49. Lin PM, Cautini RA, Joyce MF. Posterior Lumbar Interbody Fusion. *Clin Orthop* 1983;180:154.

+ 50. Ma G. Posterior Lumbar Interbody Fusion with Specialized Instruments. *Clin Orthop* 1985;193:57.

! 51. Malinsky J. The Ontogenetic Development of Nerve Terminations in the Intervertebral Discs of Man. *Acta Anat* 1959;38:96.

+ 52. Matthews HH, Evans MT, Molligan HJ, Long BH. Laparoscopic Discectomy with Anterior Lumbar Interbody Fusion. A Preliminary Review. *Spine* 1995;20:1797.

+ 53. McAfee PC, Regan JR, Zdeblick T, et al. The Incidence of Complications in Endoscopic Anterior Thoracolumbar Spinal Reconstructive Surgery. A Prospective Multicenter Study Comprising the First 100 Cases. *Spine* 1995;20:1624.

! 54. McCarron RF, Wimpee MW, Hudkins P, et al. The Inflammatory Effect of Nucleus Pulposus. A Possible Element in the Pathogenesis of Low Back Pain. *Spine* 1987;12:760.

! 55. Miller J, Schmatz C, Schultz A. Lumbar Disc Degeneration Correlation with Age, Sex, and Spine Level in 600 Autopsy Specimens. *Spine* 1988;13:173.

\# 56. Modic MT, Ross JS. Magnetic Resonance Imaging in the Evaluation of Low Back Pain. *Orthop Clin North Am* 1991;22:283.

\# 57. Modic MT, Steinberg PM, Ross JS, et al. Degenerative Disc Disease. Assessment of Changes in Vertebral Body Marrow with MR Imaging. *Radiology* 1988;166:193.

+ 58. Newman MH, Grinstead GL. Anterior Lumbar Interbody Fusion for Internal Disc Disruption. *Spine* 1992;17:831.

+ 59. O'Brien J, Dawson M, Heard C, et al. Simultaneous Combined Anterior and Posterior Fusion. *Clin Orthop* 1986;203:191.

+ 60. Orderburg G, Nskog J, Sjostrom L. Diagnostic External Fixation of the Lumbar Spine. *Acta Orthop Scand* 1993;64:94.

+ 61. Paajanen H, Erkintalo M, Kuusela T, et al. MR Study of Disc Degeneration in Young Low Back Pain Patients. *Spine* 1989;14:982.

+ 62. Parker LM, Murrell SE, Boden SC, Horton WC. The Outcome of Posterolateral Fusion in Highly Selected Patients with Discogenic Low Back Pain. *Spine* 1996;21:1909.

+ 63. Polatin PB, Kinney RK, Gatchel RJ, et al. Psychiatric Illness and Chronic Low Back Pain. The Mind and the Spine. Which Goes First? *Spine* 1993;18:66.

! 64. Raininko R, Manninen H, Battie MC, et al. Observer Variability in the Assessment of Disc Degeneration on Magnetic Resonance Images of the Lumbar and Thoracic Spine. *Spine* 1995;20:1029.

+ 65. Rask B, Dall BE. Use of the Pantaloon Cast for the Selection of Fusion Candidates in the Treatment of Chronic Low Back Pain. *Clin Orthop* 1993;288:148.

+ 66. Salminen JJ, Erkintalo M, Laine M, Pentti J. Low Back Pain in the Young. A Prospective Three-year Follow-up Study of Subjects With and Without Low Back Pain. *Spine* 1995;20:2101.

+ 67. Schneiderman G, Flannigan B, Kingston S, et al. Magnetic resonance Imaging in the Diagnosis of Disc Degeneration. Correlation with Discography. *Spine* 1987;12:276.

+ 68. Simmons ED Jr, Guntupalli M, Kowalski JM, et al. Familial Predisposition for Degenerative Disc Disease. A Case Control Study. *Spine* 1996;21:1527.

* 69. Simmons J, Aprill C, Dwyer A, Brodsky A. A Reassessment of Holt's Data on "The Question of Lumbar Discography." *Clin Orthop* 1988;237:120.

+ 70. Smith SE, Darden BV, Rhyne AL, Wood KE. Outcome of Unoperated Discogram Positive Low Back Pain. *Spine* 1996;20:1997.

71. Southwick SM, White AA. The use of Psychological Tests in the Evaluation of Low Back Pain. *J Bone Joint Surg Am* 1983;65:560.

+ 72. Stauffer R, Coventry M. Anterior Interbody Lumbar Spine Fusion: Analysis of Mayo Clinic Series. *J Bone Joint Surg Am* 1972;54:756.

+ 73. Stauffer R, Coventry M. Posterolateral Lumbar Spine Fusion—Analysis of Mayo Clinic Series. *J Bone Joint Surg Am* 1972;54:1195.

+ 74. Steffee A, Sitkowski D. Posterior Lumbar Interbody Fusion and Plates. *Clin Orthop* 1988;227:99.

75. Steindler A, Luck J. Differential Diagnosis of Pain Low in the Back. *JAMA* 1938;110:106.

76. Steinmann JC, Herkowitz HN. Pseudarthrosis of the Spine. *Clin Orthop* 1992;284:80.

77. Sternbach R, Wolf SR, Murphy R, Akeson W. Aspects of Chronic Back Pain. *Psychosomatics* 1973;14:52.

78. Videman T, Battie MC. Epidemiology of Disc Disease. In: Weisel S, ed. *The Lumbar Spine*, 2nd ed. Philadelphia: Saunders, 1996:16.

* 79. Waddell G, McCullough JA, Kummel E, et al. Nonorganic Physical Signs in Low Back Pain. *Spine* 1980;5:117.

! 80. Walsh T, Weinstein J, Spratt K, Lehmann T. Lumbar Discography in Normal Subjects. *J Bone Joint Surg Am* 1990;72:1081.

* 81. Weatherly C, Prickett C, O'Brien J. Discogenic Pain Persisting Despite Solid Posterior Fusion. *J Bone Joint Surg Br* 1986;68:142.

+ 82. Wetzel FT, Larocca H. The Failed Posterior Lumbar Interbody Fusion. *Spine* 1991;167:83.

! 83. White AA, Panjabi MM, eds. *Clinical Biomechanics of the Spine*, 2nd ed. Philadelphia: Lippincott, 1990:345.

+ 84. Wiltse L, Rocchio P. Preoperative Psychological Tests as Predictors of Success of Chemonucleolysis in the Treatment of Low Back Pain Syndrome. *J Bone Joint Surg Am* 1975;57:478.

+ 85. Wood GW, Boyd RJ, Carothers TA, et al. The Effect of Pedicle Screw/Plate Fixation on Lumbar/Lumbosacral Autogenous Bone Graft Fusions in Patients with Degenerative Disc Disease. *Spine* 1995;20:819.

* 86. Yong-Hing K, Kirkaldy-Willis WH. The Pathophysiology of Disc Degeneration of the Lumbar Spine. *Orthop Clin North Am* 1983;14:59.

! 87. Yu S, Haugton VM, Sether LA, et al. Criteria for Classifying Normal and Degenerated Lumbar Intervertebral Discs. *Radiology* 1989;170:523.

+ 88. Zdeblick TA. A Prospective, Randomized Study of Lumbar Fusion—Preliminary Results. *Spine* 1993;18:983.

89. Zdeblick TA. The Treatment of Degenerative Lumbar Disorders. A Critical Review of the Literature. *Spine* 1995;20:126S.

+ 90. Zucherman JF, Zdeblick TA, Bailey SA, et al. Instrumented Laparoscopic Spinal Fusion. Preliminary Results. *Spine* 1995;20:2029.

## CHAPTER 146

ANTERIOR LUMBAR INTERBODY FUSION

Thomas A. Zdeblick

Perhaps no topic has generated as much interest in orthopaedic spine surgery over the past 10 years as anterior lumbar interbody fusion (ALIF). Although anterior fusions have been performed on the spine for more than 50 years, it is only recently that interest in the procedure has exploded. Traditionally, anterior or anterolateral approaches to the lumbar spine were performed for tumor, trauma, or infections. In these cases, debridement, strut grafting, and occasionally anterior fixation were used to decompress the spinal canal or stabilize the anterior spinal column. The advantages of these procedures included direct spinal canal decompression and reconstruction of the weight-bearing capability of the anterior column. Another advantage is that they avoid injury to posterior muscles.

The avoidance of posterior muscle dissection is important. Often, when posterolateral fusions were performed for degenerative disc problems, patients would have continued complaints of fatigue and weakness in the lumbar spine. Some of these symptoms may have been due to injury to the paraspinal muscles leading to "fusion disease" (19). In addition, over the past several decades, much research has pointed to the disc as a predominant source of chronic low back pain (see Chapter 144). Fusion procedures that eliminate discs entirely may offer advantages that more traditional posterior fusions do not. For both of these reasons, the indications for ALIF have greatly expanded over the last decade.

INDICATIONS

Lumbar interbody fusion is indicated in selected patients with degenerative disc disease, internal disc derangement, spondylolisthesis, pseudarthrosis, and, occasionally, scoliosis, trauma, or infection. Each case must be evaluated on an individual basis to determine the appropriateness of surgical intervention.

DEGENERATIVE DISC DISEASE

Degenerative disc disease shows radiographic changes of disc-space narrowing, endplate sclerosis, osteophyte for-

T. A. Zdeblick: Professor and Chair, Orthopedic Surgery, University of Wisconsin, Madison, Wisconsin 53792.

mation, and occasionally vacuum phenomena within the disc space. Magnetic resonance imaging (MRI) corroborates this diagnosis, revealing "Modic" changes in the endplates surrounding the degenerative disc (14). Many of these changes can be traced to a previous episode of disc herniation that had been treated either with or without surgery. Often, in these cases, the sciatica has resolved but has been replaced by persistent chronic midline low-back pain.

Many patients with degenerative disc disease complain of pain over the sacroiliac joints, particularly if the L5–S1 disc space is involved. Most patients with degenerative disc disease can be successfully treated with an aggressive physical therapy program that includes trunk stabilization exercises and nonimpact aerobics. In the majority, symptoms improve, and patients decide to live with a low-level midline low-back ache. Other modalities that may be helpful include short-term periods of bracing, administration of nonsteroidal antiinflammatory medication, and occasionally manipulation. Epidural steroid injection, prolonged bed rest, transcutaneous electrical nerve stimulation units, and passive modalities such as heat, massage, or ice have not been proven to be of benefit.

Before offering surgery, evaluate a patient's psychological profile. Office findings of pain behaviors, Waddell's signs, chronic narcotic use, or excessive secondary gain are contraindications for surgical treatment (see Chapter 144). In addition, evaluate the adjacent discs. Ideally, only a one- or two-level fusion should be performed for degenerative disc disease. Fusion of more than two levels leads to less satisfactory clinical results. MRI of the adjacent disc is an excellent screening test. With normal MRI findings, it is safe to assume that the adjacent disc can be left unfused. If MRI is abnormal, then discography may be indicated to evaluate adjacent levels for fusion.

INTERNAL DISC DERANGEMENT

Patients with a normal radiographic examination but abnormal MRI may have internal disc derangement (IDD). The MRI abnormalities of IDD include decreased signal intensity within the disc nucleus on T2-weighted images, annular tears (with or without enhancement), and high-intensity-zone lesions. In these cases, initiate a similar nonoperative treatment program before considering surgical therapy. Should patients satisfy diagnostic criteria and fail to improve with adequate conservative measures over 3–4 months, then discography is indicated for confirmation of the diagnosis. A positive discogram should include reproduction of the patient's symptoms upon injection, abnormal morphology with dye leakage through annular disruptions, and normal adjacent-level injections without pain reproduction (3). A patient who meets all of these criteria may be a candidate for ALIF surgery (1,6).

Other treatment modalities may include steroid injec-

tion within the disc, thermal repair of the disc annulus, or annular debridement. ALIF surgery, however, has the longest history of successful results in the treatment of this condition. It must always be kept in mind, however, that success is not universal in the treatment of patients with IDD. Many clinical reports document success rates in the 50% to 70% range (1,6–9). Patient selection is critical. Offer ALIF only to highly motivated patients with single-level disease who have no psychological overlay, secondary-gain issues, or chronic narcotic use. Only strict selection criteria will lead to an acceptable success rate from surgery.

SPONDYLOLISTHESIS

Often, degenerative spondylolisthesis with spinal stenosis does not require ALIF. Most patients with this condition can be successfully treated with posterior decompression and posterolateral fusion techniques (19). In adult isthmic spondylolisthesis, however, ALIF plays an important role (see Chapter 162).

My approach to adult isthmic spondylolisthesis has evolved over the years. In patients in whom reduction of a spondylolisthesis is planned, anterior interbody support is necessary to prevent late hardware failure or pseudarthrosis. In patients with spondylolisthesis with a well preserved disc space and translational motion on flexion–extension films, anterior interbody support in addition to posterior fixation is necessary to achieve a high incidence of solid fusion. In patients with a collapsed disc space with degenerative changes, as well as isthmic spondylolisthesis, fusion with either anterior procedures alone or posterior procedures alone may be successful. Interbody fusion cages alone have successfully been used in this subset of spondylolisthesis patients. Exercise caution, however, when using cages alone for a spondylolisthesis patient who has a preserved disc space and hypermobility. In these cases, it is often difficult to obtain stability through the use of anterior cages alone.

DEFORMITY

In selected cases of scoliosis and kyphosis in which correction will be performed, anterior release and interbody fusion are indicated. In addition, for patients with traumatic endplate disruption or disc space infection, debridement and interbody fusion are helpful. Finally, in cases of previous pseudarthrosis of a posterolateral fusion, interbody fusion is often the only means of obtaining a solid arthrodesis. In addition, it avoids dissection through a previously scarred posterior paraspinal muscle approach.

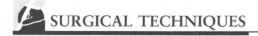 **SURGICAL TECHNIQUES**

Anterior lumbar interbody fusion surgery can be performed through a variety of surgical approaches. Open

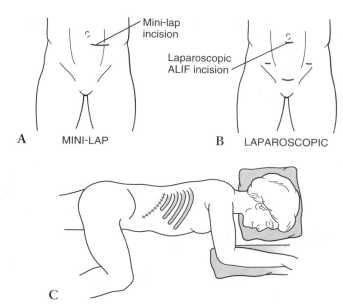

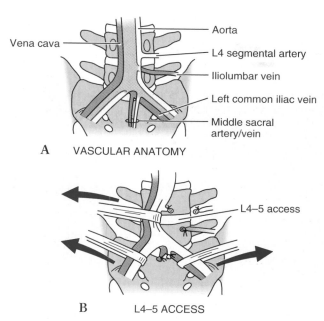

Figure 146.1. Skin incisions utilized in anterior lumbar surgery. **A:** A skin incision utilized in the minilap retroperitoneal approach. A vertical paramedian incision may also be used. In this approach, the anterior rectus sheath is divided in line with the skin incision, the rectus abdominis muscle protected, and the preperitoneal space developed lateral to the peritoneal contents. **B:** The laparoscopic transperitoneal technique utilizes small skin incisions for the placement of the viewing camera (periumbilical portal), 5 mm incisions for lateral retractors, and a 15–20 mm incision for the placement of the fusion cages. This incision is typically placed in the suprapubic location for the L5–S1 disc space. **C:** Approach the lumbar interbody spaces laterally through a flank approach. Position the patient laterally with the ipsilateral hip flexed to relax the psoas muscles. Make a flank incision paralleling the twelfth rib. The position will vary, depending on the level for the fusion. For L-1 burst fractures, a typical incision will overly the eleventh rib. For L-2 or L-3 access, a twelfth rib incision is useful, and an incision midway between the iliac crest and the twelfth rib is useful for the L3–4 space.

approaches include the transperitoneal, anterior retroperitoneal, and retroperitoneal flank approaches. For endoscopic techniques, the anterior transperitoneal laparoscopic approach has become popular, as has the retroperitoneal endoscopic approach using balloon insufflation or gasless techniques. All of these approaches require an excellent knowledge of the anatomy surrounding the middle and low lumbar spine (Fig. 146.1).

Surgeons must be familiar with the vascular anatomy, including the bifurcation of the aorta and vena cava and the surrounding veins such as the iliolumbar vein or segmental vessels, as well as the path of the ureters and the left-sided placement of the sigmoid colon. In addition, the locations of the nerve roots as they exit the foramina and of the presacral parasympathetic plexus should be well

known. Surgeons unfamiliar with this vascular anatomy or unwilling to handle complications from injuries to these and other important structures should enlist the help of a vascular or general surgeon in exposing the anterior lumbar spine (see Chapter 138).

OPEN TECHNIQUES

Open Transperitoneal Approach

The open transperitoneal approach is the oldest and most traditional approach to the anterior lumbar spine.

- Make a midline vertical skin incision, and split the fascia between the rectus abdominis muscles (Fig. 146.2).
- Enter the peritoneal cavity, and retract the small bowel superiorly and the sigmoid colon to the left laterally.
- Typically, the aorta and vena cava bifurcate at the level of the L-5 vertebra. There is considerable variation, however, so check the preoperative MRI to confirm the level.

Figure 146.2. **A:** Normal vascular anatomy of the anterior lumbar spine. Typically, the vena cava bifurcates at a higher point than the aorta. Usually, it bifurcates at the L4–5 disc space, and the aorta bifurcates over the L-5 body. The iliolumbar vein is a branch of the left common iliac vein and runs in an inferior direction at approximately 40°. **B:** Access to the L5–S1 disc space is typically between the bifurcation of the vessels. Ligation and control of the middle sacral artery and vein is necessary for complete disc exposure. At L4–5, the most common access pathway is to the left of both of the great vessels, with retraction in a left-to-right direction. This requires control and ligation of the iliolumbar vein for complete vessel mobility. Use blunt dissection only at both levels to prevent damage to the presacral nerve plexus.

■ To expose the L5–S1 disc space, incise the posterior peritoneum vertically overlying the disc space. This incision can be safely made between the bifurcation of the aorta and vena cava.

■ The presacral plexus of nerves runs directly over the L5–S1 annulus at this level. To minimize damage to this plexus, infiltrate the retroperitoneal space with saline, using a fine needle, before dividing the posterior peritoneum.

■ Cut the peritoneum without cautery, and dissect over the disc space bluntly to minimize the risk of damage to the nerve plexus. In men, retrograde ejaculation may result if this plexus of nerves is damaged.

■ Ligate the middle sacral artery and vein, which are adherent to the annulus, before exposing the disc.

■ At L4–5, access to the disc space is more difficult. Study the vascular anatomy preoperatively on the patient's MRI scan (Fig. 146.2). Occasionally, the L4–5 disc space can be approached between the bifurcation of the vessels. Most commonly, however, a left-to-right path to the L4–5 disc space is recommended. In this manner, the aorta and vena cava are both retracted from the left to the right across the L4–5 disc space. This retraction is only possible after the iliolumbar vein is ligated. This vein descends at a 45° angle from the vena cava, angling toward the psoas muscle on the left side.

■ Once it is ligated, adequate mobility of the great vessels is usually obtained. If possible, avoid dissection between the aorta and vena cava.

■ The presacral plexus nerves are particularly vulnerable during dissection between the great vessels.

■ At L3–4 disc space, the aorta and vena cava are more mobile, although segmental vessels need to be ligated to obtain exposure.

■ After exposure is obtained, it is mandatory that the vascular structures be protected throughout the fusion procedure. I prefer to drive four Steinmann pins covered with a red rubber catheter into the endplates above and below the disc space to be worked on. These four pins serve as self-retaining retractors, providing a safe zone in which to perform the fusion. Other retraction systems are available, as well as self-retaining blades that may be staked through the vertebral endplates.

■ Take particular care to avoid injury to the vena cava and common iliac veins. Once exsanguinated by the retraction, they are difficult to visualize and are prone to injury.

■ Transperitoneal exposures of the lumbar spine above

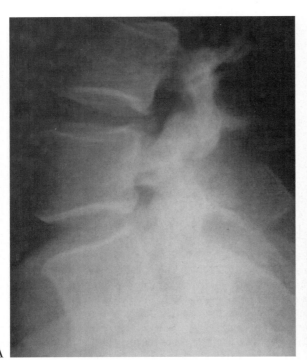 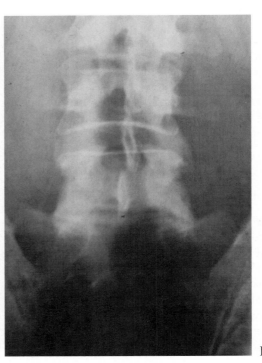

A   B

Figure 146.3. Anteroposterior (**A**) and lateral (**B**) radiographs of a 39-year-old man with persistent low-back pain. He had a history of remote sciatica, which resolved but has now developed into persistent low-back pain despite maximal physical therapy. These radiographs show classic changes of degenerative disc disease: a narrowed disc space, sclerotic endplates, and marginal osteophyte formation. The L4–5 disc was normal on MRI, and thus no discography was indicated.

L-3 are difficult because of the renal and mesenteric vessels. At these levels, the flank retroperitoneal approach offers a lateral exposure of the lumbar vertebral bodies. This approach is most useful when debridement for infection, trauma, or tumor is required. When corpectomy is necessary, a lateral plate device is useful for stability and can best be placed from a lateral approach. If debridement and grafting alone are being performed, the anterolateral or anterior approach is adequate.

Flank Approach

The flank approach involves an oblique incision centered over the area of pathology of the lumbar spine. It parallels the twelfth rib and is anywhere from 4 to 8 in (10–20 cm) long, depending on the size of the patient.

- Use fluoroscopy to center this incision directly over the level of pathology.
- Should exposure of the low lumbar spine be required as well, curve the incision across the lateral aspect of the abdomen.
- After incising the skin, divide the external oblique, internal oblique, and transversalis muscle layers in line with the incision.
- Take care when dividing the transversalis to ensure that the reflection of the peritoneum is free.
- Once the transversalis fascia is divided, enter the retroperitoneal space, which is behind the fascia surrounding the kidney and thus is truly behind Girota's fascia.
- After entering the retroperitoneal space, identify the psoas muscle, and take care to preserve the ilioinguinal nerve lying on its surface.
- The origin of the psoas muscle is usually at the L-1 body, and each of the lumbar nerve roots as they exit the foramina run in the substance of the psoas muscle. For this reason, the psoas must be retracted in an anterior-to-posterior direction to expose the appropriate disc space.
- Perform this exposure, using elevators and cautery, controlling segmental vessel as needed.

This approach gives excellent visualization of the lateral aspect of the disc and vertebral body; it is limited posteriorly by the level of the nerve at the foramen and anteriorly by the great vessels. If necessary, dissect the anterior longitudinal ligament free from the vertebral bodies, and carry out subperiosteal dissection around to the opposite side of the vertebral body. This maneuver permits complete release of all soft-tissue structures in cases of deformity.

Anterior Rectus–sparing Retroperitoneal Approach

My preferred approach for ALIF is the anterior rectus-sparing retroperitoneal approach. In this approach, none of the muscles of the abdominal wall is divided, and therefore quick recovery is possible. I prefer a transverse incision.

- Begin in the midline, and extend the incision to the left for approximately 3–4 in (7.5–10 cm).
- Divide the anterior rectus sheath, and retract the rectus muscle from the midline to the left.
- Identify the posterior rectus sheath and the arcuate line.
- Use blunt dissection beneath the arcuate line to enter the preperitoneal space, and continue the dissection laterally to the left until you are lateral to the peritoneal contents and the psoas muscle can be identified.
- Place a retractor to pull the peritoneal contents toward the midline to expose the retroperitoneal space overlying the spine.
- Identify the left ureter, and protect it throughout the procedure. In general, in cases involving the L3-4 or L4-5 disc space, the ureter will be retracted toward the midline with the visceral peritoneum. At the L5-S1 space, the ureter will usually be on the left side of the incision and will be retracted laterally.
- Identify the sympathetic chain running on the psoas muscle and protect it.
- The dissection at this point proceeds in much the same fashion as previously described (see "Open Transperitoneal Approach" above).
- Bluntly dissect the tissues lateral to the aorta and vena cava at the L4–5 space or between the great vessels at L5–S1.
- At L4–5, ligate the iliolumbar vein to allow exposure.
- At L5–S1, ligate the middle sacral artery and vein to allow blunt dissection to proceed along the annulus.
- Several self-retaining retraction systems are available for use through this "minilaparatomy (minilap)" approach.

ENDOSCOPIC TECHNIQUE

In 1993, I began performing laparoscopic transperitoneal fusion of the lumbar spine and developed this approach along with Dr. David Mahvi, my general surgery colleague (13,20). The L5–S1 level lends itself to an endoscopic approach because of its easy accessibility between the bifurcation of the great vessels (Fig. 146.4).

- Give a light bowel preparation the night before surgery.
- Facilitate exposure by placing the patient in the Trendelenburg position and allowing abdominal insufflation, which causes the small bowel to drift toward the diaphragm. It precludes the need for retraction of the abdominal contents; thus postoperative ileus is eliminated.
- Usually, the laparoscopic camera is placed in a periumbilical incision.
- Place two 5 mm portals laterally, midway between the

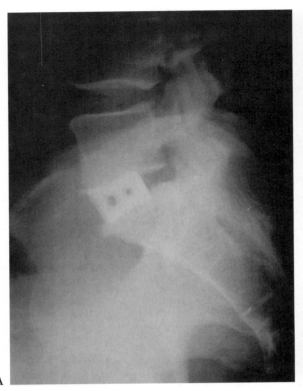
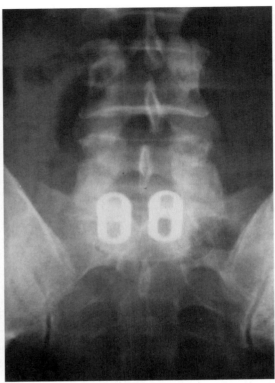

A   B

Figure 146.4.   Laparoscopic transperitoneal fusion access route. Surgery consisted of anterior discectomy at L5–S1, distraction, and insertion of two tapered (LT) cages (Lumer Tspered, Sofamon Danek, Memphis, TN) at the L5–S1 disc space. Note the restoration of foraminal height and sagittal contour.

umbilicus and the pubis, to allow retraction or suction as needed.

- Finally, place a suprapubic portal in line with the disc space. At the L5–S1 level, this is often two to three fingerbreadths above the pubic symphysis. At L4–5, it is usually midway between the umbilicus and pubic symphysis.
- Drain the bladder with a Foley catheter before placing this portal.
- The sigmoid colon may need to be retracted toward the left and will usually stay in this position throughout the procedure. The remainder of the dissection proceeds in much the same fashion as previously described (see "Open Transperitoneal Approach" above).
- Incise the posterior peritoneum vertically overlying the disc space. For the L5–S1 space, it is done just to the right of the midline or, for L4–5, just to the left of the aorta.
- Bluntly dissect the tissues in the retroperitoneal space. Often, the presacral plexus of nerves can be visually identified. Bluntly retract the nerves.
- At L5–S1, the middle sacral artery and vein lie in a plane adherent to the anterior annulus. Coagulate them with bipolar cautery.

- At L4–5, identify the iliolumbar vein coming off the vena cava at a 45° angle and heading inferiorly and laterally toward the psoas muscle. Ligate this vein, and retract the great vessels in a left-to-right direction to expose the annulus of the disc. Specially made vein retractors placed laparoscopically through the portals facilitate retraction of the great vessels.

The advantages of endoscopy are better visualization with magnification of the vascular structures and rapid patient recovery. Contraindications to the transperitoneal endoscopic technique include multiple abdominal adhesions, previous anterior spine surgery, and severe sacral tilt such that the L5–S1 disc space is not accessible. It is strongly recommended that this surgery be done with a general surgeon who has laparoscopic experience.

Endoscopic techniques utilizing retroperitoneal dissection have also been performed. Transfeldt et al. (18) and Thalgott et al. (17) described techniques whereby a small lateral incision is made through the oblique muscles and a balloon is placed in the retroperitoneal space. This balloon is then inflated, dissecting free the retroperitoneal cavity. Once the peritoneal reflection is dissected toward the midline, an anterolateral skin incision is made to expose the disc space.

This approach can also be carried out without balloon dissection, using a gasless system in which the anterior abdominal wall is lifted with a retractor system. My experience with this technique is that it can cause abdominal wall discomfort and slower patient recovery. In all of these endoscopic systems, the cost of disposable equipment and the time required for surgeons to learn the procedure must be balanced against the more traditional open or mini-open approaches. My current approach is as follows:

- At L5–S1 disc space, the laparoscopic transperitoneal approach is safe and quick and allows excellent visualization of the space.
- For multilevel fusions or fusion at L4–5, I now prefer a minilap-type open retroperitoneal exposure. It gives more reliable control of the bifurcation of the great vessels at the L4–5 space.

FUSION OPTIONS

Interbody fusion of the lumbar spine can be performed with a variety of methods. Most surgeons prefer to remove the entire disc before fusion. This requires a rectangular block-style incision of the annulus, removal of the annulus, and removal of all disc material including endplate cartilage through the use of a combination of curets, rongeurs, and elevators. In general, the annulus is left intact laterally and posteriorly. In some endoscopic techniques, trephine-style discectomies are preferred because it is risky to use curets and elevators in endoscopy. These techniques

also preserve more of the anterior annulus, which helps ensure cage stability.

Surgical options for fusion include iliac crest or other autogenous bone graft, allograft bone consisting of femoral rings or fibula, and processed allografts consisting of threaded cortical dowels combined with autograft cancellous bone. Metallic options include the placement of a lateral plate overlying the disc space and bone graft, as well as devices placed within the disc space itself. These devices include anteriorly placed threaded cylindrical cages, anteriorly placed threaded tapered cages, laterally placed cages, lateral cages plus lateral plates, and upright cages placed within the disc space (Fig. 146.5). Other materials that have been used include carbon fiber cages and ceramic spacers.

The principles of cage interbody fusion include the following:

- Disc space distraction to cause tension in surrounding ligamentous structures, which increases stability
- Preparation of the endplates to expose cancellous bone, as well as providing an endplate substrate for weight bearing
- Provision of enough bony surface area to heal from one endplate through the bone graft to the other endplate
- Realignment of the spine to its optimal lordotic sagittal balance
- Production of a solid, long-term arthrodesis.

With current short-term follow-up, it appears that cage interbody fusion is successful in meeting these goals (13).

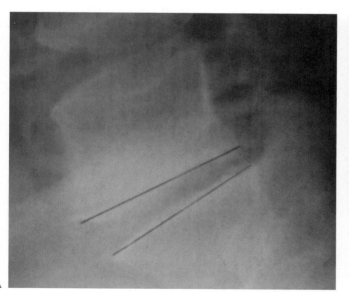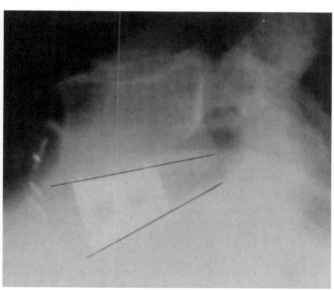

A   B

Figure 146.5. The use of tapered interbody fusion cages at L5–S1 permits the restoration of both height and lordosis. Preoperative (**A**) and postoperative (**B**) lateral radiographs demonstrate the lordosis obtained in a 48-year-old man with degenerative disc disease.

Several principles must be kept in mind, however, when interbody fusion cages are used. Disc spaces that have not undergone any degree of collapse are difficult to further distract. Therefore, the tall mobile disc space may not be an ideal candidate for cage-only fusion procedures. In addition, forceful distraction is required, and if the endplate bone is not strong enough to resist the distractive force, subsidence and instability will result. For this reason, do not use cages in patients with osteoporosis. Finally, most cage systems are designed for two cages to be implanted side by side. Although some biomechanical studies suggest that a single cage may lead to short-term stability, it is my feeling that there is inadequate surface area to ensure long-term arthrodesis.

The RAY cage (Surgical Dynamics, Minneapolis, MN) and the BAK device (Spinetech, Minneapolis, MN) were the initial threaded interbody fusion cages (10). They have been used with both posterior and anterior interbody fusion techniques. When used anteriorly, these systems restore lordosis through patient positioning and the placement of a tapered distraction plug.

- After the disc space is distracted, prepare the endplate on each side of the disc by passing a reamer to remove endplate cartilage, bone, and disc material. Then tap each side and place two threaded devices.
- Take great care, when placing cages, to identify the midline of the spine so that cages are not placed eccentrically.
- Determine the appropriate size cages from the radiographs and preoperative templates.
- A tapered threaded device has been designed that more accurately matches the anatomy of the L5–S1 disc space. It appears that a greater amount of lordosis can be obtained through the use of tapered cages with a minimal amount of endplate resection (16).

In general, threaded cages placed anteriorly can restore the stability of the lumbar spine without the need for supplementary posterior fixation. They have successfully been used in patients with degenerative disc disease or spondylolisthesis with a degenerated disc space. I do not recommend the use of cages alone in cases of spondylolisthesis with a tall mobile disc space.

Lateral cages have been placed both openly and endoscopically in the lumbar spine. Often, a single threaded cylindrical lateral cage is utilized. Although some authors have had success with this technique, others have shown that additional bone grafting is necessary to provide an adequate surface area for healing. In addition, LeHuec (11) designed a combined lateral cage and plate system to increase the rate of fusion.

Harms first introduced upright titanium mesh cages. Typically, two upright cylinders of titanium mesh are cut to fit the disc space and then driven into the space to provide support for the endplate and for healing potential. Harms recommended that posterior instrumentation be used to supplement ALIF with upright cages. Brantigan and Steffee (2) designed upright carbon fiber cages. While these were also met with worldwide acceptance and a high degree of success, most authors would agree that the upright carbon fiber cage is not stable enough to be used as a stand-alone device. Fraser (5) recommends that posterior fusion, as well as facet screw instrumentation, be utilized to augment the interbody carbon fiber cage.

The use of spinal cages is evolving rapidly. Surgeons must evaluate each patient on an individual basis to determine which particular device is most appropriate.

PITFALLS AND COMPLICATIONS

Anterior lumbar surgery is never easy and requires adequate surgical planning and preoperative preparation. An accurate understanding of the vascular and neurologic anatomy is a requirement for the performance of these procedures. The assistance of a general or vascular surgeon may be necessary to obtain adequate and safe exposure. Preoperative preparation consisting of a light bowel regime (e.g., GOLYTELY and Fleet enema) will make retraction of intestinal structures easier. Preoperative examination of the patient's abdomen and flank for prior incisions and potential adhesions is necessary. Preoperative evaluation of MRI or computed tomography to assess variations in the vascular anatomy is important, as it directs which approach will used for the portion of the spine to be fixed.

Vascular complications are certainly the most serious and life-threatening. The incidence of injury to the aorta, vena cava, or iliac vessels is estimated at 1% to 3% for anterior approaches (7,9). These injuries may be life-threatening and need to be dealt with calmly and with assistance. Obtain immediate control with tamponade. If the procedure is being done endoscopically, immediate laparotomy is recommended.

The assistance of a vascular surgeon is highly recommended for repair of the great vessels. The most common areas of vascular injury are the left common iliac vein at the L5–S1 level and the left side of the vena cava at the L4–5 level. At L4–5, there are several small perforating veins that may come from the posterior surface of the vena cava. They may need to be coagulated and divided before the vena cava is retracted, to prevent their avulsion. As mentioned earlier, control and ligation of the iliolumbar vein will greatly assist in vena cava mobilization.

Arterial occlusion due to embolization of plaques has also been reported (18). Anterior approaches to the lumbar spine in elderly patients are hazardous and must be done only when absolutely necessary and with caution. In many of these patients, the arterial system is much less mobile, and retraction may dislodge plaques. Always do a postoperative vascular examination, and if pulses are absent or the limb is cool, obtain an immediate consultation with a vascular surgeon. Routine anticoagulation has not been found to be necessary in ALIF surgery. However, if a major vessel must be repaired, postoperative anticoagulation may be necessary.

Neurologic complications include damage to the presacral plexus, nerve root injury, and violation of the spinal canal. As mentioned, the parasympathetic nerves that run within the presacral plexus are vulnerable to injury. They run along the aorta and vena cava and then between the bifurcation as they pass distally. For work along the L4-5 or L5–S1 disc spaces, it is mandatory that only blunt dissection be used and that no monopolar electrocautery be used. The incidence of retrograde ejaculation following ALIF has been estimated to be from 1% to 4%.

It appears that the incidence of neurologic injury is slightly higher in endoscopic procedures than in the open retroperitoneal approach. Early in any surgeon's experience, there is certainly a higher incidence of retrograde ejaculation. Fortunately, most cases of retrograde ejaculation are temporary and resolve within 4–6 months. It is assumed that they are due to stretch injury that occurs during exposure of the disc space. Should the patient not recover from retrograde ejaculation, urologic consultation is recommended.

The nerve roots are vulnerable after they exit the neuroforamina and proceed toward the psoas muscle. If the midline is not adequately evaluated and fusions are performed far lateral to the disc space, the nerve root is vulnerable to injury. Bone grafts or cages that are placed too laterally or too deeply may impinge on the neuroforamen of the level above. It is imperative to use fluoroscopy at some point to locate the midline of the disc space and maintain orientation as to the right and left margins of the disc space.

Cages or grafts that are placed too deeply may impinge on the spinal canal, causing cauda equina injury. Once again, fluoroscopic control of the implantation of interbody fusion devices should help eliminate this complication.

Abdominal-wall complications related to the approach may occur. The epigastric vessels must be either retracted or controlled, or a postoperative abdominal-wall hematoma may occur. Overzealous retraction of the rectus abdominis may lead to a stretch injury and cause weakness of the abdominal wall. During a flank approach, repair each layer independently to prevent weakening of the abdominal wall.

Pseudarthrosis of an ALIF may occur. Although the incidence of a pseudarthrosis after a 360° fusion is performed is exceedingly low, ALIF alone does carry a risk of pseudarthrosis. With the use of only iliac crest autograft, the pseudarthrosis rate was estimated at 30% to

35% (4,7). Femoral allograft rings have shown to have a pseudarthrosis rate approaching 20% (12). Threaded cortical bone dowels appear to have a much lower pseudarthrosis rate, but follow-up is too short to be conclusive.

Threaded interbody fusion cages have been reported to have a 90% fusion rate in the early BAK and RAY cage studies (10). Recent reports show a higher pseudarthrosis rate, however, which may be secondary to poor surgical indications or poor surgical technique (15). Should pseudarthrosis occur and the cages or bone dowels remain in an acceptable position, I recommend proceeding with a posterior instrumented fusion at that level. It will often resolve the patient's symptoms and may lead to healing of the interbody fusion. If a cage or bone dowel should migrate and cause neurologic symptoms, it should be removed at the time of revision surgery. Revision anterior interbody surgery is dangerous and should be approached with caution. Vascular structures often become adherent to the previously operated disc space, and the presence of a vascular surgeon is necessary for these challenging cases.

Finally, the incidence of persistent pain after ALIF has been estimated to be 10% to 20%. The exact cause is unknown and may be related to patient selection. This fact alone indicates that the treatment of low-back pain with interbody fusion is evolving. Keep in mind that the exact cause of each patient's low-back pain may be unknown.

 AUTHOR'S PERSPECTIVE

The use of ALIF techniques provides numerous advantages. Restoration of the weight-bearing column, provision of a greater surface for fusion to occur, and the ability to recreate the normal sagittal position of the spine are among its greatest advantages. If complications should occur, however, many of these advantages are lost. To obtain a high clinical and radiographic success rate, strict adherence to the details of the surgical approach and the fusion technique are required.

REFERENCES

Each reference is categorized according to the following scheme: *, classic article; #, review article; !, basic research article; and +, clinical results/outcome study.

+ 1. Blumenthal SL, Baker J, Dossett A, Selby DK. The Role of Anterior Lumbar Fusion for Internal Disc Disruption. *Spine* 1988;13:566.
+ 2. Brantigan JW, Steffee AD. A Carbon Fiber Implant to

Aid Interbody Lumbar Fusion: Two-year Clinical Results in the First 26 Patients. *Spine* 1993;18:2106.

+ 3. Crock HV. Internal Disc Disruption: A Challenge to Disc Prolapse Fifty Years on. *Spine* 1986;11:650.

+ 4. Dennis S, Watkins R, Landaker S, et al. Comparison of Disc Space Heights after Anterior Lumbar Interbody Fusion. *Spine* 1989;18:876.

+ 5. Fraser R. Personal communication.

+ 6. Gill K, Blumenthal SL. Functional Results after Anterior Lumbar Fusion at L5-S1 in Patients with Normal and Abnormal MRI Scans. *Spine* 1992;17:940.

+ 7. Goldner J, Urbaniak J, McCollum D. Anterior Disc Excision and Interbody Spinal Fusion for Chronic Low Back Pain. *Orthop Clin North Am* 1971;2:544.

+ 8. Knox BD, Chapman TM. The Anterior Lumbar Interbody Fusion for Discogram Concordant Pain. *J Spinal Disord* 1993;6:242.

+ 9. Kozak JA, Heilman AE, O'Brien JP. Anterior Lumbar Fusion Options: Technique and Graft Materials. *Clin Orthop* 1994;300:45.

+ 10. Kuslich SD, Dowdle JA. Two-year Follow-up Results of an Interbody Fusion Device. Presented at the Ninth Annual Meeting of the North American Spine Society, Minneapolis, MN, October 19–21, 1994.

+ 11. LeHuec JC. Lateral Cage Endoscopic Fusion. Presented at the Thirteenth Annual Meeting of the North American Spine Society, San Francisco, CA, October 27, 1998.

+ 12. Loguidice VA, Johnson RG, Guyer RD, et al. Anterior Lumbar Interbody Fusion. *Spine* 1988;13:366.

+ 13. Mahvi DM, Zdeblick TA. A Prospective Study of Laparoscopic Spinal Fusion. *Ann Surg* 1996;224:85.

+ 14. Modic MT, Steinberg PM, Ross JS, et al. Degenerative Disc Disease: Assessment of Changes in Vertebral Marrow. *Radiology* 1988;166:193.

+ 15. O'Dowd JK, Lam K, Mulholland RC, BAK Cage: Nottingham Results. Presented at the Thirteenth Annual Meeting of the North American Spine Society, San Francisco, CA, October 28, 1998.

+ 16. Orr RD, Andres B, Checovich M, Zdeblick TA. Results of Anterior Spinal Fusion with the Tapered Interbody Fusion (TIF) Device. Presented at the Thirteenth Annual Meeting of the North American Spine Society, San Francisco, CA, October 28, 1998.

+ 17. Thalgott JS, Chin AK, Ameriks JA. Minimally Invasive 360° Fusion. Presented at the Thirteenth Annual Meeting of the North American Spine Society, San Francisco, CA, October 28, 1998.

+ 18. Transfeldt E, Escobar G, Garvey T. Complications of View-assisted Spine Surgery. Presented at the Thirteenth Annual Meeting of the North American Spine Society, San Francisco, CA, October 28, 1998.

+ 19. Zdeblick TA. A Prospective Randomized Study of the Surgical Treatment of L5-S1 Degenerative Disc Disease. Presented at the Tenth Annual Meeting of the North American Spine Society, Washington, DC, October 20, 1995.

+ 20. Zuckerman JF, Zdeblick TA, Bailey SA, et al. Instrumented Laparoscopic Spinal Fusion: Preliminary Results. *Spine* 1995;20:2029.

CHAPTER 147
SPINAL STENOSIS

Gordon R. Bell

Spinal stenosis describes a clinical syndrome of back, buttock, or leg pain with characteristic provocative and palliative features. The term "stenosis" denotes a narrowing or constriction of a tubular structure. Sachs and Fraenkel (103a) were among the first to relate symptoms of sciatica to neural compression within the spinal canal. Subsequent descriptions of this condition described acquired (degenerative) bony compression and congenital narrowing of the spinal canal. Van Gelderen (114a) proposed hypertrophied ligamentum as a potential cause of spinal stenosis and reported on two patients with this condition. The clinical features of the syndrome of spinal stenosis and its relationship to congenital narrowing were described in detail by the Dutch surgeon Verbiest, who also demonstrated mechanical compression of neural structures by myelography (116). Kirkaldy-Willis et al. further defined the pathoanatomy of spinal stenosis and helped correlate pathologic changes with symptoms (62).

ASSESSMENT

CLASSIFICATION

The etiology of spinal stenosis is most commonly either congenital (developmental), acquired (degenerative), or a combination of both (Table 147.1) (2). The majority of cases of spinal stenosis are acquired, being caused by degenerative changes occurring in the three-joint complex consisting of the intervertebral disc and the two facet joints. In some cases, such degenerative changes may be

G. R. Bell: Vice-Chairman, Department of Orthopaedic Surgery, Head, Section of Spinal Surgery, Cleveland Clinic Foundation, Cleveland, Ohio, 44195.

Table 147.1.   *Classification of Spinal Stenosis*

I. Congenital/developmental stenosis
  A. Idiopathic (hereditary)
  B. Achondroplastic

II. Acquired stenosis
  A. Degenerative
    1. Central
    2. Peripheral (lateral recess, neural foramen)
    3. Degenerative spondylolisthesis
  B. Combined congenital and degenerative stenosis
  C. Spondylolytic/spondylolisthetic
  D. Iatrogenic
    1. Postlaminectomy
    2. Postfusion
    3. Postchemonucleolysis
  E. Posttraumatic
  F. Metabolic
    1. Paget's disease
    2. Flourosis

From Arnoldi C, Brodsky A, Cauchoix J, et al. Lumbar Spinal Stenosis and Nerve Root Entrapment Syndromes. *Clin Orthop* 1976;115:4, with permission.

superimposed on a pre-existing congenital stenosis. Variations in the shape, as well as the size, of the spinal canal may predispose the patient to spinal stenosis, with a trefoil canal being associated with lateral recess stenosis more commonly than a round or oval canal.

CLINICAL EVALUATION

History

Spinal stenosis is an anatomic description that should not be confused with *neurogenic claudication*, although the two terms are often used interchangeably. Spinal stenosis refers to morphology, not symptoms. Neurogenic claudication, also known as *pseudoclaudication*, is a clinical syndrome with symptoms of leg pain that are associated with walking (116). Neurogenic claudication should also be distinguished from vascular claudication, which has a different etiology and slightly different clinical features (Table 147.2).

Spinal stenosis is a condition of middle age and older, and is typically due to age-related degenerative changes of the lumbar spine (Table 147.3). The onset of symptoms is usually insidious and without associated trauma. A history of antecedent low back pain (LBP) is common, partly because of age-related spondylosis.

Neurogenic claudication is defined as lower extremity pain, paresthesias, or weakness associated with walking or standing (57). Pain is the predominant symptom, being present in up to 94% of patients, with numbness (63%) and weakness (43%) being less common. Bilateral involvement is common. Patients with neurogenic claudication may present with either unilateral radicular pain or with diffuse, nondermatomal symptoms beginning in the buttocks and extending a variable distance into the legs. Radicular pain is typically dermatomal in distribution and is often unilateral. It is the presenting type of symptom in 6% to 13% of symptomatic patients. It is often seen with lateral recess stenosis, foraminal stenosis, or with concom-

Table 147.2.   *Vascular Versus Neurogenic Claudication*

Evaluation	Vascular	Neurogenic
Walking distance	Fixed	Variable
Palliative factors	Standing at rest	Sitting/bending
Provocative factors	Walking/exercise	Walking/standing
Walking uphill	Painful	Painless
Bicycle test	Positive (painful)	Negative (painless)
Pulses	Absent	Present
Skin	Loss of hair/shiny	Normal
Weakness	Rarely	Occasionally
Back pain	Occasionally	Commonly
Back motion	Normal	Limited
Pain character	Cramping/distal-to-proximal	Numbness/aching/proximal-to-distal
Atrophy	Uncommon	Occasionally

Table 147.3. *Comparative Features of Lumbar Disc Herniation versus Spinal Stenosis*

	Lumbar disc herniation	Lumbar spinal stenosis
Age (years)	<50	>50
Sex	Male	Female
Onset	Acute	Insidious
Pain	Radicular/dermatomal	Referred/diffuse
Provocative factors	Sitting	Standing/walking
Palliative factors	Standing	Sitting
Weakness	Common	Uncommon
Sensory changes	Common	Uncommon
Tension sign	Present	Absent
Neurological findings	Present	Absent

itant disc herniation. The presence of a symptomatic disc herniation in a patient with a narrowed spinal canal and spinal stenosis is not uncommon. Patients with either developmental or degenerative stenosis are more likely to develop symptomatic radiculopathy in the presence of a small disc herniation or even disc bulging (42,94).

Symptoms are typically produced by standing or walking and are relieved by sitting or bending forward (Table 147.2). Patients may preferentially assume a stooped-over posture when walking, or even standing, in order to ameliorate symptoms (5). Other leg symptoms such as weakness or numbness may also occur in association with prolonged standing or walking. Night pain is uncommon, although it has been described in patients with lateral recess stenosis (54). Unusual symptoms, such as priapism associated with intermittent claudication during walking, have also been reported.

The relationship of symptoms to posture can be explained by the variation of canal size with posture (5,47, 122). Cadaveric studies have demonstrated that the spinal canal cross-sectional area, midsagittal diameter, and subarticular sagittal diameter are significantly reduced in extension (standing) and are increased with flexion (sitting) (47). Associated neural compression was also found to be greater in extension than in flexion (47).

In vivo studies relating posture to epidural pressure measurements have shown that epidural pressures at the level of stenosis were higher in the standing posture compared with those in the lying and sitting postures. Furthermore, local epidural pressures were increased with extension and decreased with flexion (47).

Neurogenic claudication should be distinguished from vascular claudication (Table 147.2). Although both condi-

tions may present with leg pain associated with walking, it is only patients with neurogenic claudication who have leg pain resulting from standing. Leg pain associated with neurogenic claudication is highly position dependent. Vascular claudication, on the other hand, is unaffected by positions of lumbar flexion or extension. Leg pain from vascular claudication may be produced by cycling in a sitting position (27). Patients with vascular claudication typically have leg pain while walking uphill, whereas patients with a neurogenic etiology do not have this pain owing to the slightly flexed posture of the lumbar spine associated with this activity. Patients with neurogenic claudication may actually have increased leg pain when walking down an incline owing to increased associated lumbar lordosis.

A summary of the pertinent historical features of spinal strenosis are listed below:

- Demographics
  - Typically middle aged or older, unless congenital
  - Female > male (3:1 to 5:1)
- Leg pain > LBP
- May have long history of antecedent LBP
- Leg pain
  - Referred or radicular
  - Pseudoclaudication (neurogenic claudication)
    - Provoked by standing or walking
    - Relieved by sitting or leaning ("grocery cart sign")
- Differential diagnosis
  - Peripheral neuropathy (not activity related; burning dysesthesia)
  - Vascular claudication versus neurogenic claudication (Table 147.2)
  - Hip arthropathy ("Hip-spine syndrome")

Physical Examination

Begin the examination of the patient with spinal stenosis by observing the patient, both at rest and during walking. Because symptoms are typically induced by the normal lordotic posture associated with walking or standing, the patient often preferentially assumes a slightly flexed posture in order to relieve neural compression causing leg pain. Flattening of the lower lumbar spine, owing to reduction in lumbar lordosis, may also be observed. With progressive ambulation, the patient may become increasingly more kyphotic in posture. This represents a conscious, or subconscious, attempt to decrease root compression by increasing canal or foraminal size. Back range of motion will likely be reduced as a result of age-related arthrosis.

Lumbar spinal stenosis is usually unaccompanied by hard neurologic signs (Table 147.3) (5,57,102). Tension signs, such as straight leg raising sign or femoral nerve stretch test, are uncommon with spinal stenosis unless it is associated with a disc herniation. Deep tendon reflexes, particularly at the ankle, may be normal, symmetrically reduced, or absent in the older patient. Therefore, the presence of diminished reflexes is usually not clinically significant unless it is asymmetric. Sensory findings, such as diminution of pinprick sensation, are uncommon with spinal stenosis. The presence of paresthesias should raise the suspicion of an underlying peripheral neuropathy.

The pathology of spinal stenosis comprises both a *fixed*, anatomic lesion as well as a *dynamic* component. Because of the dynamic nature of spinal stenosis, symptoms or objective neurologic findings are not usually elicited until these dynamic factors are invoked. Therefore, resting neurologic examination is usually normal. The most common neurologic finding is weakness of the extensor hallucis longus (EHL). Patient symptoms may sometimes be provoked by either walking or lumbar hyperextension. Indeed, reproduction of leg pain by hyperextension of the back may be the only objective finding (5). Signs and symptoms may also occasionally be elicited by examining the patient immediately after walking to the point of producing leg pain. Under such circumstances, mild muscle weakness or diminution of a tendon reflex may be detected. Profound muscle weakness is uncommon unless stenosis is accompanied by concomitant disc herniation. Long tract findings of spasticity, hyperreflexia, and clonus suggest superimposed cervical or thoracic myelopathy.

When examining the patient, rule out other potential causes for leg pain such as hip arthropathy or peripheral vascular disease. Include an examination of peripheral pulses and an examination of the hip. In addition to reproduction of the patient's pain by hip range of motion, the presence or absence of a hip flexion contracture should also be determined because its presence may not only help explain a patient's symptoms but also has therapeutic implications.

Radiographic Evaluation

Correlate the objective clinical findings with the radiographic findings in order to determine the significance, if any, of the radiographic finding and the patient's symptoms. Precise correlation between objective clinical findings and diagnostic imaging has been shown to have a high positive predictive value for good clinical outcome in patients undergoing surgery for symptomatic lumbar disc herniation. This poses somewhat of a problem in the diagnosis of lumbar spinal stenosis, in which objective neurologic findings are usually absent and the clinical diagnosis is made by patient symptoms rather than clinical findings (53).

Overemphasis on the radiographic component of patient evaluation can lead to a poor outcome following surgery, because radiographic abnormalities, including neural compression, are found in a significant proportion of asymptomatic individuals (13,45a,50,120). Unless there is concern for the presence of tumor or infection, avoid diagnostic imaging when the history or objective clinical findings do not support a compressive or mechanical cause for the patient's pain. Extensive diagnostic imaging can be delayed until the patient is a clear candidate for surgery.

Conventional Radiography   Plain radiography is insensitive in predicting symptoms of either LBP or radicular leg pain (37,71). It has been estimated that only one in 2,500 lumbar radiographs yields clinically unsuspected findings in patients 20 to 50 years of age. Numerous studies have reported age-related degenerative x-ray changes to be present equally in both asymptomatic and symptomatic populations (37). Only the study by Frymoyer et al. (37) reported a statistically significant correlation between symptoms and any degenerative finding, that being an association between LBP and disc space narrowing or traction spurs at the L4–L5 interspace only.

Plain radiography is still an important preoperative tool. Obtain radiographs in all patients undergoing surgery for spinal stenosis. Look for unsuspected bony pathology, such as spina bifida occulta, on plain radiographs of patients undergoing lumbar surgery. In addition, the presence of transitional vertebrae should be identified when present, thereby alerting the surgeon to the possibility of errors in intraoperative localization.

Obtain *standing* lumbar x-ray studies for all patients undergoing surgical decompression for spinal stenosis to identify unrecognized degenerative spondylolisthesis or degenerative scoliosis, which could be undetectable on supine films. Preoperative identification of such pathology may influence the type of the planned surgery, such as the need for concomitant fusion with decompression. Furthermore, failure to identify a pre-existing degenerative spondylolisthesis preoperatively might lead to the erroneous conclusion that a slip seen on a postoperative x-ray study is iatrogenic.

Dynamic Radiography (Flexion-extension X-ray Studies)
Many authors believe that dynamic radiographs are more useful than static x-ray studies in making a radiographic diagnosis of instability (14,41,81). Even with these radiographs, however, there is no uniformly accepted method of measurement of such instability (105). Shaffer et al. reported that the Morgan and King method of measuring from the anterior aspect of the vertebral body was the most reproducible method to measure translation (105). Other authors have described angulation, in addition to translation, as being indicative of radiographic instability (14,41).

As with routine radiographs, there exists a spectrum of normal translation and angulation that can exist in the absence of symptoms (14,41). Over 90% of asymptomatic volunteers exhibit between 1 and 3 mm of translation on flexion extension radiographs, and the mean dynamic sagittal rotation from flexion to extension ranges from 7.7° to 9.4° at each lumbar level (14). For translation, a dynamic change of greater than 4 mm is considered abnormal. Because plain radiographs do not visualize neural structures, they generally fail to provide an explanation for radicular pain.

Myelography As opposed to computed tomography (CT) or magnetic resonance imaging (MRI), both of which *directly* visualize neural compression, myelography provides *indirect* evidence of nerve root compression by demonstrating changes in the contour of normal contrast-filled structures. As such, the exact nature of compression may be unclear and could, therefore, result in diagnostic confusion. For example, lateral indentation of the dye column due to facet arthropathy could easily be confused with that due to a lateral disc herniation or to a ganglion cyst from a facet joint.

Current myelographic techniques employ *water-soluble* agents that permit better visualization of subtle pathology than did older *oil-based* agents. Myelography is superior to routine CT in its ability to image the entire thoracolumbar spine, thereby revealing unsuspected lesions at the thoracolumbar junction. This is particularly important with conditions such as spinal stenosis, in which compressive findings are often present diffusely throughout the lumbar spine, including the upper lumbar region, which is not routinely imaged by conventional CT.

Another advantage of myelography over CT or MRI is its superior ability to visualize neural compression associated with scoliosis afforded by its coronal imaging capabilities. The presence of a three-dimensional deformity such as scoliosis makes visualization of neural compression by CT or MRI more difficult than with myelography.

Because the dura ends at the level of the dorsal root ganglion (DRG) (21), which is located at the level of the pedicle, myelographic dye cannot extend beyond that point and myelography is unable to detect foraminal disc herniations, lateral stenosis, or the so-called far out syndrome, which is diagnosed more accurately by CT or MRI (121). The far-out syndrome typically occurs in the elderly patient with degenerative scoliosis or in the younger patient with a grade II or higher isthmic spondylolisthesis. The L-5 nerve root is compressed far laterally by either the L-5 transverse process or kinking beneath the L-5 pedicle.

Another disadvantage of myelography over CT is its inability to detect pathology below the level of a complete block to dye flow (43). This may occur in cases of severe spinal stenosis, such as with a high-grade L4–L5 degenerative spondylolisthesis. Under such circumstances, dye must be introduced both below and above the level of the block, or as is more commonly done, an adjunctive study such as MRI or CT must be used (43).

Postoperative imaging of the instrumented spine by CT or MRI is difficult owing to significant metal artifact associated with the use of stainless steel spinal instrumentation. This problem is partially obviated by the use of myelography, which is not associated with image distortion.

Hitselberger and Witten reported that 24% of asymptomatic patients undergoing oil-based contrast studies for suspected acoustic neurilemmoma had abnormal lumbar myelography (45a). This finding underscores the importance of correlating radiographic abnormalities with clinical findings.

The reported accuracy of water-soluble nonionic lumbar myelography in the diagnosis of lumbar nerve root compression ranges from 67% to 100%, depending on the criteria employed for diagnosing nerve root compression, whether or not surgical confirmation of compression was used as the standard, and whether or not the tests were interpreted without knowledge of clinical symptoms or objective neurologic findings (10,41,48,49,112). Most studies report the diagnostic accuracy of myelography for spinal stenosis to be between 70% and 90%.

Computed Tomography and Postmyelography Computed Tomography Unlike myelography, CT visualizes the neural structures *directly*, and therefore provides more accurate knowledge of the nature of the compressing lesion. Advantages of CT over myelography include its noninvasive nature, less ionizing radiation, and a better ability to visualize lateral pathology such as lateral or foraminal disc herniation or foraminal stenosis. Because CT is usually performed without sagittal reformation, it provides imaging in only one plane and routinely images only a limited segment of the spine. Therefore, CT misses proximal lumbar pathology, such as a high lumbar disc herniation, proximal stenosis, or other significant pathology (e.g., a thoracolumbar tumor) unless it is specifically oriented to those levels. Because spinal stenosis is a global condition, commonly involving upper lumbar segmental levels as well as lower lumbar levels, routine use of only CT as the primary imaging tool would result in some missed diagnoses.

As with routine radiography and myelography, lumbar CT abnormalities are common in asymptomatic subjects. Wiesel et al. (120) reported that 35.4% of asymptomatic individuals in their study group had an abnormal CT scan. Reported accuracy of CT in the diagnosis of nerve root compression from disc herniation or stenosis ranges from 72% to 100% (10,48,49,112).

The accuracy of CT can be enhanced by the simultaneous use of water-soluble contrast agents (intrathecal contrast-enhanced CT or myelo-CT). The incremental benefit provided by combining both procedures is so great that they are usually performed sequentially as part of a single study for spinal stenosis. Postcontrast CT allows distinction between the disc margin, thecal sac, and ligamentum flavum, three structures that can blend together in a tight spinal canal in which normal tissue-separating fat is absent. It is invaluable in visualizing a stenotic spine associated with a complete myelographic block, as in severe lumbar stenosis associated with degenerative spondylolisthesis (43). Correlation between contrast-enhanced CT and myelography ranges between 75% and 96%, with myelo-CT invariably being the more accurate study (43, 48,49,112).

Magnetic Resonance Imaging   MRI images the spine by a matrix of numbers that have been assigned a shade of gray based on the intensity of a radio wave signal emanating from the tissue (7,8). In the lumbar spine, T1-weighted sagittal and axial sequences of approximately 4 mm slice thickness and sagittal gradient echo (GE) sequences are performed most commonly. Typically, osseous structures appear as areas of relative signal void, with cortical bone having a low intensity on MRI, and cancellous bone having a higher signal intensity owing to its fat content. The distinction between a small cortical bone osteophyte and a small disc herniation on T1-weighted sagittal image may be difficult, and precise differentiation between the two features may require CT. The nucleus pulposus is best visualized by T2-weighted spin echo (SE) sequences, which reflect the degree of hydration of the disc. With aging and disease, there is decreased signal intensity due to changes in total hydration within the disc (13). The T2 image tends to overemphasize the size of a disc herniation and, therefore, can overestimate its potential significance.

MRI, like myelography, can image the entire spine and can detect unsuspected pathology such as high-lumbar disc herniation, proximal stenosis, or thoracolumbar spinal tumor. MRI is noninvasive and eliminates the potential risk and associated discomfort associated with my-

elography. Like CT, MRI visualizes the spine *directly*, providing detail as to the etiology of neural compression and can accurately image lateral pathology. Unlike routine CT, however, MRI provides sagittal visualization of the spine and, therefore, provides imaging in orthogonal planes. Furthermore, MRI uses parasagittal views, which provide sequential visualization of neural foramina and can detect foraminal entrapment better than routine CT. This feature is particularly valuable for imaging spinal stenosis, in which neural entrapment within or beyond the neural foramen can be well visualized. MRI distinguishes between the disc and neural tissue better than nonenhanced CT but generally does not distinguish between bony and soft-tissue compression as well as CT. When this distinction is deemed important, as it sometimes is in cases of spinal stenosis, CT or contrast-enhanced CT is sometimes needed.

As with plain radiography and CT, abnormal MRI findings are common in asymptomatic individuals. In one study of asymptomatic subjects, the lumbar MRI images of 22% of those younger than age 60 and 57% of those older than age 60 were abnormal, showing disc herniation or spinal stenosis (13). Approximately 90% of those older than 80 years of age showed some element of lumbar disc degeneration, as demonstrated by decreased signal on T2-weighted images. The reported accuracy of MRI, when compared with documented intraoperative lumbar nerve root compression, is comparable to that of contrast-enhanced CT (myelo-CT) (9,49).

NATURAL HISTORY

The true natural history of spinal stenosis is unclear, because good studies documenting the course of nontreatment are lacking. This is partly because most patients with this condition receive some form of conservative or surgical treatment, and those with severe stenosis are ultimately operated on (12). Several reported studies have described the clinical features of spinal stenosis, or its surgical treatment, and have included some patients who received no treatment (51). Approximately 20% of those receiving no treatment experienced progression of their symptoms.

The largest and best study of the natural course of lumbar spinal stenosis was published by Johnsson et al. (52), who reported on 32 patients with spinal stenosis followed for an average of 49 months. These patients were described as having "conservative treatment (i.e., no treatment)" because either the patient refused to undergo surgery or the anesthesiologist refused to administer anesthesia. Therefore, these patients had indications for surgery but were not operated on. At final follow-up, based on the clinical examination, 41% of patients were improved and 18% were worse. Based on subjective symptoms, only 15% were improved and 15% were

Table 147.4. *Final Outcome for Untreated Spinal Stenosis by VAS[a], Clinical Exam, and Walking Capacity*

	Worse (%)	Unchanged (%)	Improved (%)
VAS	15	70	15
Clinical exam	18	41	41
Walking capacity	30	33	37

[a] VAS, Visual analog scale.
From Johnsson K, Rosen I, Uden A. The Natural Course of Lumbar Spinal Stenosis. *Clin Orthop* 1992;279;82, with permission.

worse. Changes in the patients' walking capacities were equally distributed among improved, worse, and unchanged (Table 147.4). When the final outcome was compared with the anteroposterior (AP) diameter of the dural sac, as measured on water-soluble contrast myelography, patients with narrow AP diameters had a tendency not to improve. This study concluded that the majority of patients with spinal stenosis who did not undergo surgery remained unchanged at 4 years of follow-up and severe progression was unlikely.

Johnsson et al. (51) compared the outcome of a group of 44 patients treated with surgical decompression with that of 19 patients treated without surgery (Table 147.5). The authors referred to the nonsurgical group as both *untreated* and *conservatively treated*, leaving unanswered what, if any, treatment this group did receive. Nevertheless, the authors found that only 32% of the nonsurgical patients had improved at an average follow-up of 31 months. In the *surgical* group, 59% of the patients reported improvement. Although 59% of the group who had received surgery improved, a greater percentage of the surgical group were worse at follow-up compared with patients who had not undergone surgery (25% versus 10%). This study concluded that nonsurgical treatment produced reasonably good results in approximately one third of patients, with only a 10% chance of deterioration during the 2- to 3-year follow-up period. This study, however, was not prospective nor randomized, making comparison between the two groups difficult. In the absence of randomization, it is not known whether the conservatively treated patients were comparable to the surgical group.

A recent attempt at meta-analysis of the literature on surgery for spinal stenosis failed to identify a single randomized trial comparing surgery with conservative treatment (113). A recent report evaluating the outcome of patients treated with aggressive nonsurgical measures (therapeutic exercises and epidural steroids, if necessary) suggested that such treatment could be very effective (103). Fifty-two patients were followed for 2 to 8 years. Thirty-three patients (63%) reported a tolerable pain level without major restriction in daily activities or use of narcotic analgesics; 36 patients (69%) reported "no or minimal restriction in walking tolerance," although 25 patients (48%) reported "difficulty in standing for long periods." None of the patients experienced any neurologic loss. Four of the 52 patients (8%) required surgery for presumed failure of nonsurgical measures. The exclusion criteria for this study included patients with pre-existing disease (comorbid conditions) or with a "compliance issue that prevented participation in a therapeutic exercise program." In addition, it did not compare conservative treatment methods with surgery and could not, therefore, offer any comparative data regarding optimal treatment of this condition.

Standard modalities commonly employed to treat spinal stenosis include nonsteroidal anti-inflammatory medications, analgesics, oral and epidural steroids, physical therapy, bracing, and calcitonin (109).

Table 147.5. *Comparison of Surgical Versus Nonsurgical Treatment of Lumbar Spinal Stenosis*

	Worse (%)	Unchanged (%)	Improved (%)
No surgery	10	58	32
Surgery	25	16	59

From Johnsson K, Uden A, Rosen I. The Effect of Decompression on the Natural Course of Spinal Stenosis. A Comparison of Surgically Treated and Untreated Patients. *Spine* 1991;16(6):615, with permission.

SURGICAL TECHNIQUES

Surgery for lumbar spinal stenosis may be broadly divided into decompressive procedures without concomitant fusion and decompression with fusion. Surgical decompression may vary from limited procedures, such as single-level unilateral laminotomy for focal neural compression, to global procedures, such as multilevel bilateral laminectomy with bilateral facetectomies. Types of fusion procedures include anterior lumbar interbody fusion (ALIF), posterior lumbar interbody fusion (PLIF), posterior fusion, posterolateral (also known as intertransverse or bilateral lateral) fusion, or combinations of these procedures (see Chapters 145 and 146). Indirect neural decompression may occur following ALIF or PLIF if disc-space distraction occurs, thereby enlarging the central or foraminal canal. Fusion may be augmented by the use of spinal instrumentation, either anterior fixation devices or posterior devices such as those using pedicle screw fixation.

COMORBIDITY AND SURGICAL OUTCOME

Comorbidity refers to the presence and severity of conditions other than the disorder under study or treatment (56). The relationship between comorbidity and outcome is more commonly applied to surgical than medical outcomes. Comorbidity typically increases with age and is associated with a poor outcome for many medical and surgical conditions (20,25,107). Sick people have a higher mortality rate, a higher complication rate, and a lower level of function than do healthy patients. It is imperative to take this factor into account when assessing and comparing outcomes between treatment groups. If such factors are not taken into account, differences in outcome between treatment groups could reflect differences in patient comorbidities rather than differences as a result of treatment.

Rates of hospital morbidity and mortality following lumbar spinal surgery are greater with increasing age of the patient (25). Complications are more frequent with advancing patient age, increasing the complexity of both diagnosis and surgical treatment. The study by Deyo et al. (25) reported an overall mortality of 0.07% for 18,122 hospitalizations between 1986 through 1988. The mortality increased with age, increasing to 0.6% (ninefold increase) in patients older than 75 years of age. The overall complication rate of 9.1% increased to 17.7% in patients 75 years of age or older.

As would be expected, an increase in comorbidity is often associated with more in-hospital complications and perioperative mortality. This finding is independent of age alone. Oldridge et al. (86) found an age-related increase in mortality only for patients older than 80 years of age. There was, however, a significant increase in in-hospital and 1-year cumulative mortality associated with increasing number of comorbidities.

In a retrospective review of 88 patients undergoing laminectomy for spinal stenosis, Katz (56) concluded that the long-term outcome was generally less favorable than had been previously reported (Table 147.6). By 1 year after surgery, 6% of patients had a second operation and, by the time of the last follow-up, 17% had a repeat surgery. Only 40% of patients with the highest comorbidity score had a good outcome at the time of final follow-up compared with 75% of patients who had the lowest comorbidity score (P = 0.004). The most common comorbidities

Table 147.6.   Long-Term Outcome Following Surgery for Spinal Stenosis

	One-year follow-up (%)	Final follow-up (%)
Poor outcome	11	43
Severe pain	7	30
Reoperation	6	17
Limited function	8	35
Inability to walk 50 feet	8	21

From Katz, Lipson S, Larson M, et al. The Outcome of Decompressive Laminectomy for Degenerative Lumbar Stenosis. *J Bone Joint Surg* 1991;73A:809, with permission.

were osteoarthritis (32%), cardiac disease (22%), rheumatoid arthritis (10%), and chronic pulmonary disease (7%). Their data suggested that the effect of comorbidities was additive, because no single comorbidity was significantly associated with worse outcome. In a subsequent study by the same authors, comorbidity was found to be the second most important determinant of disability in lumbar canal stenosis, with complaints of predominantly LBP (as opposed to leg pain) preoperatively being the most important contributor to disability (55,58).

LAMINECTOMY

The gold standard surgical procedure for spinal stenosis is decompressive laminectomy. This procedure may involve either *bilateral laminectomy* or *hemilaminectomy*. For bilateral laminectomy, the lamina and ligamentum flavum are removed on both sides of the stenotic level or levels to the lateral recess. Decompression begins at the most distal extent of neural compression and proceeds in a caudal-to-cranial direction. Although the L5–S1 level is rarely compressed centrally, owing to the capacity of the spinal canal at that level, decompression is most safely initiated at that level rather than at L4–L5, the most commonly involved level, which is often severely stenotic. Perform decompression sequentially, from medial to lateral.

▪ Position the patient in a kneeling position to allow the abdomen to hang freely in order to reduce abdominal compression and thereby reduce epidural bleeding. Prepare and drape the lumbosacral spine and expose the posterior elements from facet joint to facet joint laterally along the entire length of the intended decompression.

- Begin with a midline decompression. This is generally performed from the left side of the operating table (i.e., on the patient's left side) for a right-handed surgeon and on the right side by a left-handed surgeon.
- Use either 45° or 90° Kerrison rongeurs. In areas where stenosis is not severe, use a relatively large rongeur, such as a 4 mm Kerrison rongeur, to remove the thickened lamina.
- In areas of severe stenosis, however, use of such large instruments risks injury to underlying neural structures. Under these circumstances, it is safer to first thin the lamina with either a Lexsell rongeur or a high-speed power burr. Then use smaller instruments, such as 2 mm or 3 mm Kerrison ronguers, to complete the midline decompression.
- Maintain proper orientation during the procedure by identifying the level of the pedicle, because this defines the level of the nerve root. If in doubt as to the proper level, confirm with an intraoperative radiograph with a bent probe beneath the pedicle, within the neural foramen.
- Decompress the lateral recess next. Extend the decompression laterally until the lateral edge of the root is visualized and determined to be free of pressure. Take care to preserve the pars interarticularis to minimize the risk of producing instability by inadvertent sacrifice of the superior articular facet. Preserve the facet joint by using oblique-angled (45°) Kerrison rongeurs or by the use of osteotomes to undercut the facet joint (39,104).
- Finally, perform lateral decompression of the foraminae. Once the shoulder of the nerve root is identified and decompressed, follow it from its origin through the neural foramen.
- It is generally safer to proceed in a cranial-to-caudal manner in order to minimize risk of inadvertently cutting across the root, which can occur when performing the lateral decompression from a distal-to-proximal direction. Occasionally, the use of a right- or left-angled Kerrison rongeur can be helpful for foraminal decompression.
- Assess the adequacy of decompression within the neural foramen both visually and by palpation. Use a bent probe, such as a bent #4 Penfield elevator or a properly contoured ball probe, to determine the presence or absence of nerve root compression within the neural foramen. Decompression is generally complete when a bent probe can be passed out the foramen both dorsal and ventral to the nerve root, and the root can be gently retracted approximately 1 cm medially.

Following midline and lateral decompression, check for the presence or absence of a concomitant disc herniation, which might contribute to neural compression. Such herniations may be located either posterolaterally, foraminally, or extraforaminally. Unless the disc is contributing to definite neural compression, it is generally best to avoid discectomy in the presence of laminectomy because subsequent instability is more likely to occur when both anterior and posterior supporting structures are violated. When laminectomy is accompanied by discectomy, consider performing an arthrodesis at the time of surgery.

Because spinal stenosis is a global degenerative process, encompassing multiple levels and involving nerve roots bilaterally, multilevel bilateral laminectomy is commonly required. There is, however, some debate as to whether it is more appropriate to decompress only the symptomatic level and side, or whether all stenotic levels should be decompressed. The argument against decompression of asymptomatic root levels or sides is the risk of producing symptoms at a previously asymptomatic level or side. On the other hand, failure to decompress a stenotic but asymptomatic level or side risks progression of the degenerative process with the development of more severe and potentially symptomatic stenosis. In addition, the natural tendency for degenerative changes to progress over time makes it possible that, in time, asymptomatic stenotic levels will eventually become stenotic. Indeed, several studies have reported long-term deterioration following initially successful surgical decompression (18,19,56,60,90–92).

HEMILAMINECTOMY

Hemilaminectomy involves unilateral, rather than bilateral, removal of bone and ligamentum flavum. Because the spinous processes, interspinous ligaments, and supraspinous ligaments are preserved medially, normal stabilizing structures are retained with less risk of development of postoperative instability. Take care to preserve the pars interarticularis laterally in order to minimize risk of postoperative instability (16,106). Hemilaminectomy is appropriate for patients with unilateral symptoms from stenosis. A disadvantage of this procedure is the relative difficulty of performing contralateral decompression and also in obtaining enough medial exposure to perform an adequate ipsilateral decompression in patients with foraminal stenosis. The presence of an intact spinous process and interspinous or supraspinous ligament complex makes it difficult to angle the Kerrison rongeur laterally enough to insert the jaw of the rongeur into the depths of the neural foramen. Under such circumstances, removal of the midline spinous process and interspinous or supraspinous ligament complex may be necessary in order to allow the proper angulation of the rongeur to perform the foraminal decompression. In addition to preserving midline stabilizing structures, hemilaminectomy also avoids exposure of, and potential injury to, the contralateral facet joint. Because the integrity of the unexposed contralateral facet is maintained, more aggressive decompression of a nerve root by partial, or even total, ipsi-

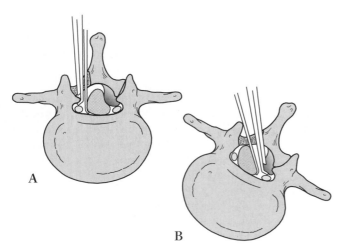

Figure 147.1. **A:** Axial representation of hemilaminotomy showing ipsilateral decompression of the nerve root. The operating table can be tilted toward the surgeon to facilitate visualization of the contralateral spinal canal. A Kerrison rongeur is shown decompressing the nerve root within the lateral recess, while a Penfield retractor is protecting the common dural sac medially. **B:** Axial representation of hemilaminotomy showing contralateral decompression of nerve root. The operating table is tilted away from the surgeon. The Kerrison rongeur is shown decompressing the opposite nerve root, while the Penfield retractor is gently moving the common dural sac medially to facilitate visualization of the contralateral nerve root.

lateral facetectomy need not necessarily be accompanied by a fusion.

Contralateral nerve root decompression may be accomplished through a unilateral hemilaminectomy approach by tilting the table away from the operating surgeon (Fig. 147.1). Particularly when used in conjunction with an operating microscope, which provides excellent illumination and which can be angled to visualize the opposite side, contralateral decompression can be accomplished without the need for removal of stabilizing midline structures (spinous processes and interspinous or supraspinous ligaments). The contralateral neural foramen can be visualized and decompressed, and its more distal portion can be palpated with a long bent probe such as a #4 Penfield elevator or a contoured probe. Although offering the advantage of preserving normal, noncompressing midline structures and minimizing scar tissue on the opposite side, this technique is more demanding than bilateral laminectomy because decompression is performed through a more limited exposure and the determination of adequate foraminal patency is more dependent on feel (palpation) than by direct visualization. In addition, there is a greater potential for dural laceration from the Kerrison rongeur when working through a small opening. Should such a dural tear occur, its repair often necessitates complete (bilateral) laminectomy with adequate exposure of the dural rent.

RESULTS OF DECOMPRESSIVE LAMINECTOMY

A recent review of the literature for spinal stenosis surgery failed to identify even a single randomized trial comparing surgery and conservative treatment (Table 147.7) (113). Turner et al. (113) attempted a meta-analysis of the literature on surgical outcomes for spinal stenosis, but the poor scientific quality of the literature precluded the authors from conducting the intended meta-analysis. Even using the authors' own ratings, the average proportion of good-to-excellent outcomes was only 72%. This study found no statistically significant relationship between outcome and patient age, gender, presence of prior back surgery or number of levels operated on. In those studies reporting on only patients with degenerative spondylolisthesis, the outcome was better. There was no statistically significant difference in outcome between decompression with or without associated fusion. This observation is particularly significant in light of the reported increased morbidity associated with lumbar fusion (114).

In contrast, the prospective cohort study of Atlas et al. (3) reported the 1-year outcome of patients with spinal stenosis treated surgically or nonsurgically in the state of Maine and found that at 1 year, 55% of the surgical patients reported definite improvement in their predominant symptom, compared with only 28% of the nonsurgical group. Surgery was found to increase the relative odds of "definite improvement" 2.6 fold compared with nonsurgical treatment.

In a large retrospective series Katz et al. (60) followed 88 patients for a period of 2.8 to 6.8 years (Table 147.6). Outcome assessment included a questionnaire in which the patients rated their outcomes in terms of pain and function. The authors reported a surprisingly high failure rate, with 11% of patients reporting a poor outcome at 1 year and 43% reporting poor outcome at final follow-up. Six percent of patients had repeat lumbar surgery

Table 147.7.   Results of Decompression of Spinal Stenosis without Fusion: Meta-Analysis of Literature 1970–1993 (11 Articles)

Total no. of patients	Satisfactory	Unsatisfactory	Progressive slip
216	140 (69%)[b]	75 (31%)[b]	67 (31%)[a]

[a] Reported in only 9 of 11 Articles.
[b] Weighted pooled proportion.
From Mardjetko SM, Connolly PJ, Shott S. Degenerative lumbar Spondylolisthesis. A Meta-Analysis of Literature 1970–1993. *Spine* 1994;19(20S):2556S, with permission.

within the first year and 17% had additional surgery by the time of last follow-up. The authors concluded that the long-term outlook for patients undergoing decompressive laminectomy for spinal stenosis is guarded owing to progressive deterioration of the results over time. They suggested that more extensive bone removal may be indicated at the time of initial surgery.

The authors also reported a high initial success rate following surgery, but by 5 years, the failure rate had reached 27%, with a predicted failure rate of 50% within the anticipated life expectancy of most patients. More than half (62%) of these failures were due to subsequent neurologic symptoms, with an equal incidence of recurrent stenosis at the same level and stenosis at a new level. Because of the high rate of failure from recurrent stenosis, the authors recommended that all levels of impending stenosis be decompressed along with the symptomatic levels.

ALTERNATIVES TO LAMINECTOMY

Despite the fact that some studies report deterioration of standard bilateral decompressive laminectomy over time, more limited alternatives to decompressive laminectomy and hemilaminectomy have been espoused in order to avoid removal of normal, noncompressing structures and thereby minimize risk of postoperative instability (18,54, 60,91). Such procedures include *hemilaminotomy, wide fenestration,* and *laminoplasty.* Hemilaminotomy involves a more limited decompression than hemilaminectomy (Fig. 147.2). Rather than removing an entire hemilamina, hemilaminotomy removes only the ligamentum flavum and adjacent portions of two hemilaminae responsible for neural compression. This procedure is more commonly performed in younger patients with unilateral focal stenosis in whom extensive laminectomy carries the risk of instability. It may also be considered in older patients who do not have extensive global stenosis.

- In the absence of significant underlying congenital stenosis, neural compression is generally due to buckling of the ligamentum flavum, which is usually secondary to collapse of the intervertebral disc, and to hypertrophy of the facet joint, which occurs as a result of subsequent instability. Decompression of only these structures should, therefore, relieve symptoms of neural compression.
- Because the superior attachment of the ligamentum flavum is approximately at the midpoint of the deep surface of the superior hemilamina, resect the distal half of the superior hemilamina in order to remove the proximal extent of the ligamentum (Fig. 147.2A).
- Remove the inferior portion of the superior hemilamina and the superior portion of the inferior hemilamina, together with the intervening ligamentum flavum (Fig. 147.2B).

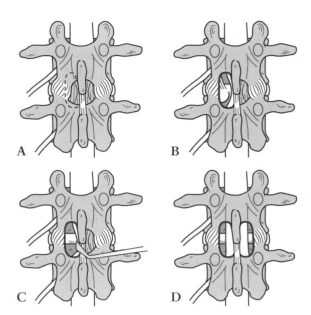

Figure 147.2. Posterior view of a hemilaminotomy to decompress nerve root. **A:** Dotted line on left represents the inferior portion of the superior lamina, which is resected in order to decompress the dural sac. This allows identification of the origin of the ligamentum flavum, which attaches approximately half way up the deep surface of the lamina. **B:** Diagram showing the resected distal portion of the superior lamina and ligamentum flavum to reveal the underlying dura. The common dural sac is deviated medially by an underlying disc herniation. **C:** The common dural sac is gently retracted medially to facilitate lateral decompression of the facet joint or disc. **D:** Diagram showing bilateral hemilaminotomies with preservation of midline laminae and ligamentous complex.

- Perform lateral decompression by partial facetectomy as with bilateral laminectomy or hemilaminectomy (Fig. 147.2C).
- Like hemilaminectomy, contralateral decompression with preservation of spinous processes and midline supraspinous or interspinous ligaments can be performed by tilting the operating table away from the surgeon and by undercutting the medial and contralateral ligamentum flavum with a 45° Kerrison ronguer.

Wide fenestration is a procedure described for central stenosis in which only the medial portion of the inferior facets and adjacent ligamentum flavum is removed (69, 83,123). Care is taken to remove only pathologic anatomy and to preserve the interspinous or supraspinous ligament complex and spinous processes, which make up the midline stabilizing structures. This may be performed by using bilateral laminotomies at one or more segmental levels, removing the ligamentum flavum (Fig. 147.2D). In a 5-year follow-up study of this procedure, 82% of patients had good or excellent early surgical outcomes, but results deteriorated to 71% satisfactory by 4 years postoperatively (83).

Laminoplasty is an alternative to laminectomy that was originally advocated for active manual workers (76,77). This procedure is similar to cervical laminoplasty and involves hinging open the lamina on one side and inserting the excised spinous processes into the open hinge in order to keep it patent. There is not sufficient experience with this technique to provide outcomes assessment.

LAMINECTOMY AND FUSION FOR SPINAL STENOSIS

The role of fusion in the treatment of spinal stenosis is somewhat controversial. For stenosis not associated with degenerative spondylolisthesis or other deformity, most studies report that simple decompression is the preferred method of surgical treatment. For patients with associated degenerative spondylolisthesis, concomitant fusion is generally recommended (30,44). The issue of using supplementary spinal instrumentation is yet unresolved (32, 125).

In a recent prospective, randomized study of 45 patients undergoing either decompression alone or decompression with fusion for spinal stenosis without associated instability, there was no significant difference in outcome between fused and unfused groups (Table 147.8) (40). Overall, 78% of patient-reported and 80% of examiner-rated results were rated very good or good. When broken down by type of procedure performed, there were no significant differences in outcome between the three groups with regard to pain relief. The authors concluded that surgical decompression changed the natural history of spinal stenosis, resulting in generally favorable outcome and improved quality of life in the majority of patients. They further concluded that arthrodesis was not justified in the absence of radiographically proven segmental instability because there was no statistical difference in outcome between the three treatment groups.

SPINAL STENOSIS WITH DEGENERATIVE SPONDYLOLISTHESIS

Degenerative spondylolisthesis was first described in 1930 by Junghanns who coined the term *pseudospondylolisthesis* to describe the presence of forward slippage of a vertebral body in the presence of an intact neural arch (54a). The clinical and pathologic features of this entity were further defined by Macnab, who described the condition as "spondylolisthesis with an intact neural arch" (70). The term *degenerative spondylolisthesis* was originally used by Newman and Stone and is the terminology most commonly used to describe the anterior slippage of one vertebral body on another in the presence of an intact neural arch (84a).

Degenerative spondylolisthesis may be a source of both LBP and leg pain and may contribute to radicular or referred leg pain in a characteristic pattern of neurogenic claudication (36). The diagnosis is typically made on lateral radiographs, but it may have a dynamic component to it such that the slip may reduce in the supine position and, therefore, may be readily apparent only on stress radiographs. Such radiographs may include standing lateral views, sitting or standing flexion-extension views, or distraction compression radiography (14,41).

As with spinal stenosis generally, little is known of the natural history of degenerative spondylolisthesis. Mardjetko et al. (74) attempted a meta-analysis of the literature from 1970 to 1993. Only three papers, reporting on 278 patients, described the natural history of degenerative spondylolisthesis (33,78,96). Overall, 90 of these 278 patients (32%) achieved satisfactory results untreated (Table

Table 147.8. *Comparison of Decompression, Decompression and Fusion, and Limited Decompression and Fusion in Spinal Stenosis: Percentage of Good to Excellent Results*

Evaluator	Decompression without fusion (%)	Decompression and fusion (most stenotic segment only) (%)	Decompression and fusion (all decompressed levels) (%)
Patient	13/15 (87)	12/15 (80)	10/15 (67)
Examiner	13/15 (87)	12/15 (80)	11/15 (73)

From Grob D. Humke T, Dvorak J. Degenerative Lumbar Spinal Stenosis: Decompression with and without Arthrodesis. *J Bone Joint Surg* 1995;77A:1036, with permission.

Table 147.9. Non-Operative/Natural History of Degenerative Spondylolisthesis (Three Studies Reviewed)			
No. of patients	Satisfactory	Unsatisfactory	Progressive
278	90 (32%)	188 (68%)	12[a]

[a] Reported in only one of three studies.
From Mardjetko S, Connolly P, Shott S. Degenerative Lumbar Spondylolisthesis. A Meta-Analysis of Literature 1970–1993. *Spine* 1994;19:2256S, with permission.

Table 147.10. Results of Decompression without Fusion: Meta-Analysis of Literature 1970–1993 (11 Articles)			
Total no. of patients	Satisfactory	Unsatisfactory	Progressive slip
216	140 (69%)[b]	75 (31%)[b]	67 (31%)[a]

[a] Reported in only 9 of 11 articles.
[b] Weighted pooled proportion.
From Mardjetko SM, Connolly PJ, Shott S. Degenerative Lumbar Spondylolisthesis. A Meta-Analysis of Literature 1970–1993. *Spine* 1994;19:2556S, with permission.

147.9). Matsunaga et al. (78) presented a study of 40 patients who received no treatment and who were followed for at least 5 years (range: 5 to 14 years.; mean: 8.25 year). Progressive slip was noted in 12 patients (30%), although no correlation was noted between slip progression and worsening of symptoms. Only 4 of 40 patients (10%) showed clinical deterioration over the course of the study, all of whom were in the group of 28 patients showing no slip progression over the follow-up period. Interestingly, none of the 12 patients with slip progression deteriorated clinically. Therefore, the majority of the patients in this study showed a slight improvement in their clinical symptoms over time, although only 1/3 were felt to have satisfactory function at final follow-up.

RESULTS OF DECOMPRESSION WITHOUT FUSION

Although current thinking generally favors concomitant fusion for spinal stenosis associated with degenerative spondylolisthesis, decompression without fusion is also a viable therapeutic option (Table 147.10) (74). Overall, 69% of patients from Mardjetko's meta-analysis reported satisfactory outcome with decompression without fusion, with 31% having an unsatisfactory result and 31% having progression of their slip. There was generally no correlation between clinical outcome and amount of slip progression except in the study by Bridwell et al., which showed a positive correlation between the two (15).

A recent report by Epstein and Epstein (29) reviewed 290 patients undergoing decompression without fusion for degenerative spondylolisthesis. Only patients with a "stable" slip, as defined by a slip having less than 4 mm translation and less than 10° to 12° angulation on dynamic lateral radiographs, were included. Two hundred and fifty patients had one-level listhesis and 40 had a two-level slip. Decompressive procedures included laminectomy in 249 patients and fenestration procedures in 41 patients.

Fenestration procedures typically involved bilateral laminotomy with partial medial facetectomy and foraminotomy. At an average 10-year follow-up (range: 1 to 27 years), 69% of patients exhibited excellent, 13% good, 12% fair, and 6% poor outcome. The authors concluded that 82% excellent or good outcome was very acceptable in their elderly population (average age: 67 years old), in whom fusion is associated with higher morbidity and mortality (26).

Poor surgical outcome following laminectomy without fusion was reported in the prospective randomized study by Herkowitz and Kurz (44) comparing decompression alone with combined decompression and noninstrumented fusion (Table 147.11). In the decompression group, only 11 of 25 patients (44%) had a satisfactory result. This group of patients was found to have significantly more LBP and leg pain than their fused counterparts. Furthermore, the mean slip increased from an average of 5.3 mm preoperatively to 7.9 mm postoperatively. Other authors have reported a similar experience (15,30).

RESULTS OF DECOMPRESSION WITH NONINSTRUMENTED FUSION

The role of fusion in the surgical treatment of spinal stenosis associated with degenerative spondylolisthesis is less controversial than the role of fusion in the treatment of other degenerative back conditions (80,115). Caputy and Luessenhop (18) reported a retrospective review of 96 patients undergoing decompressive surgery for spinal stenosis who were followed for at least 5 years. The treatment failed in 16 patients because of recurrent neural involvement, and it failed in 10 patients because of LBP (total failures = 26). The authors concluded that because of the higher incidence of recurrent symptoms in patients with pre-existing degenerative spondylolisthesis, all patients with an associated slip should undergo fusion of the listhetic level.

Table 147.11. *Prospective, Randomized Comparison of Decompression versus Decompression and Noninstrumented Spinal Fusion for Degenerative Spondylolisthesis*

Result	Arthrodesis (no. = 25)	No arthrodesis (no. = 25)
Excellent	11 (44%)	2 (8%)
Good	13 (52%)	9 (36%)
Fair	1 (4%)	12 (48%)
Poor	0 (0%)	2 (8%)
Mean Increase in Slip (preop to postop)	0.5 mm	2.6 mm (P = 0.002)

From Herkowitz HN, Kurz LT. Degenerative Lumbar Spondylolisthesis with Spinal Stenosis. A Prospective Study Comparing Decompression with Decompression and Intertransverse Process Arthrodesis. *J Bone Joint Surg* 1991;73A:802, with permission.

In their prospective and randomized study comparing decompression alone with decompression and noninstrumented spinal fusion in the treatment of degenerative spondylolisthesis with spinal stenosis, Herkowitz and Kurz (44) reported superior results when concomitant fusion was performed with the decompression (Table 147.11). The reported outcome for the arthrodesis group was excellent in 44% and good in 52% (96% excellent or good total results), whereas in the nonarthrodesis group, only 8% reported an excellent outcome and 36% reported a good outcome (44% excellent or good total results) (P = 0.0001). There was a significant increase in the preoperative slip in patients not receiving an arthrodesis compared with those undergoing fusion (P = 0.002). Interestingly, 36% of those undergoing attempted arthrodesis were noted to have a pseudarthrosis, all of whom had either an excellent or a good result. This study concluded that the results of surgical decompression with *in situ* arthrodesis are superior to those of decompression alone. The authors further concluded that the decision for concomitant arthrodesis should be based purely on the presence or absence of a preoperative slip rather than on other preoperative factors, such as the age or sex of the patient or the disc height, or on intraoperative factors such as the amount of bone resected during the decompression.

The prospective randomized study by Bridwell et al. (15) included a subgroup of 11 patients undergoing decompression and noninstrumented fusion. Of the 10 patients available for follow-up, only 3 (30%) reported improved functional outcome and seven had an increase in their preoperative spondylolisthesis.

Postacchini and Cinotti (90) reported on bone regrowth occurring an average of 8.6 years after surgical decompression for spinal stenosis (92). Although all 16 patients with degenerative spondylolisthesis showed some bone regrowth, the degree of regrowth was more severe in the six patients who did not undergo arthrodesis. Furthermore, the proportion of satisfactory results was significantly higher in patients who had spinal fusion (Table 147.12). Although this study was nonrandomized and retrospective, it suggested that arthrodesis stabilizes the spine, resulting in less bone regrowth and superior long-term results.

RESULTS OF DECOMPRESSION WITH INSTRUMENTED FUSION

Zdeblick (125) reported a prospective and randomized study of 124 patients undergoing either instrumented or

Table 147.12. *Relationship Between Outcome and Fusion in Patients with Degenerative Spondylolisthesis*

	No. of patients	Excellent	Good	Fair	Poor
Fusion	10	3	5	2	0
No Fusion	6	0	2	1	3

From Postacchini F, Cinotti G. Bone Regrowth After Surgical Decompression for Lumbar Spinal Stenosis. *J Bone Joint Surg* 1992;74B:862.

noninstrumented fusion for a variety of diagnoses. The overall fusion rate for the noninstrumented group was 65%; for the semirigid fixation group, the fusion rate was 77%; and for the rigid fixation group, it was 95%. A trend for better clinical outcome with increasing rigidity of fixation was also observed. Seventy-one percent of the noninstrumented patients, 89% of the semirigid group, and 95% of the rigid group reported excellent or good results. For the subgroup of patients with degenerative spondylolisthesis, 65% of the noninstrumented patients fused compared with 50% of the semirigid fixation group, and 86% of the rigid fixation group had a good or excellent result. Subsequent studies have also reported superior results with concomitant arthrodesis and decompression for spinal stenosis with degenerative spondylolisthesis (18, 44,60,90).

The historical cohort study of spinal fusion using pedicle screw fixation reported by Yuan et al. (124) involved a retrospective, multicenter study of 2,684 patients with degenerative spondylolisthesis. Solid radiographic fusion was noted in 89% of patients undergoing pedicle screw fixation compared with 70% of those without instrumentation. Clinical outcome was also better in the group of patients undergoing instrumented fusion.

Nork et al. (85) reported a retrospective study of 30 patients undergoing decompression and instrumented fusion for degenerative spondylolisthesis. Outcome was determined by fusion rate, a functional questionnaire, and the SF-36 survey. Both the rate of fusion and patient satisfaction was 93%. Thirteen patients (43%) had complications, including dural tears (three patients), excessive blood loss (two patients), pseudarthrosis (two patients), pulmonary embolus (PE) (one patient), deep infection (one patient), urinary tract infections (3 patients), and unstable angina (one patient).

A recent randomized prospective study of posterolateral lumbar fusion, with and without pedicle screw instrumentation, for a variety of conditions concluded that the addition of instrumentation did not produce an incremental clinical benefit to that obtained from noninstrumented fusion, although there was a slight nonsignificant trend toward a higher fusion rate in the instrumented fusion group (34). This study, involving a mean clinical follow-up of 40 months, prospectively examined 71 patients undergoing posterolateral fusion for either failed back surgery syndrome (FBSS), degenerative disc disease, isthmic spondylolisthesis, or degenerative spondylolisthesis. For the 10 patients who had degenerative spondylolisthesis, five underwent instrumented fusion and five underwent fusion *in situ*. Eighty percent of the patients with degenerative spondylolisthesis undergoing instrumented fusion achieved an excellent or good outcome, compared with 40% of those without instrumentation. For the small subgroup of 10 patients with degenerative spondylolisthesis, the clinical outcome appeared to be better than that of the overall population studied, although this subgroup was too small to establish statistical significance.

There does not appear to be a clear consensus as to the optimal way to treat the patient with degenerative spondylolisthesis. Most studies suggest that patients undergoing concomitant fusion do better when decompression is accompanied by fusion (44). It is less clear, however, whether or not the fusion should be augmented with instrumentation (32). It would seem reasonable that if there is clear evidence of instability on flexion-extension radiographs, the immediate stability provided by instrumentation would warrant the additional time, expense, and potential morbidity associated with its use. On the other hand, the indication for its use in the patient with a collapsed disc space and no motion at the spondylolisthetic level is less clear.

AUTHOR'S PREFERRED TREATMENT

As noted earlier, the optimal surgical treatment of spinal stenosis, particularly when it is associated with degenerative spondylolisthesis, is still somewhat controversial. One area of controversy is the recommended extent of surgical decompression. Because spinal stenosis is a *global* degenerative condition, there are frequently many segmental levels showing radiographic central stenosis, with bilateral foraminal stenosis also being common. Clearly, decompression of every level showing any degree of radiographic stenosis is not always required. Obviously, all symptomatic levels should be decompressed. The extent of surgical decompression of asymptomatic levels, however, depends on many factors. As described earlier, many long-term studies suggest that restenosis at previously decompressed levels, or the development of symptomatic stenosis at previously nonoperated stenotic levels, is a common reason for failure of surgery for spinal stenosis. Therefore, when in doubt, it is generally more prudent to decompress a suspicious segmental level than not to decompress. I generally decompress all moderately and severely stenotic levels. When diffuse degenerative changes produce moderate or severe multilevel stenosis, I prefer to decompress the involved levels by unilateral or bilateral laminotomies, rather than by complete laminectomies. This approach reduces the need for concomitant fusion, and it preserves the uninvolved laminae and ligamentous structures, thereby and minimizing the risk of developing late instability.

During the course of surgery, it is sometimes unclear to the surgeon whether or not to decompress an adjacent level above or below the operated level. When this occurs, the degree of central stenosis of the adjacent segment can be gauged by passing a small catheter proximally or distally beneath the lamina. Difficult passage of the catheter mandates decompression of the involved level.

The decision of whether or not to perform fusion on a patient with stenosis associated with degenerative spondylolisthesis can be difficult in the elderly patient with multiple comorbidities. As noted previously, many studies suggest that patients have better clinical outcomes when decompression is accompanied by arthrodesis. The issue of whether or not to augment the fusion with segmental (pedicle) instrumentation is not yet resolved (32,34,125). The decision to fuse must be balanced against the increased morbidity associated with arthrodesis in the elderly patient (26). In the younger, healthy patient with spinal stenosis associated with degenerative spondyloli-

sthesis, I will generally fuse the listhetic level, usually with segmental fixation. In elderly, debilitated, or low-demand patients, arthrodesis may not be required. This is particularly true when the listhetic level is associated with decreased disc height, spur formation, subchondral sclerosis, or ligament ossification. These degenerative changes may help stabilize the listhetic level and minimize the risk of slip progression. Under such conditions, I consider unilateral or bilateral laminotomies in order to preserve uninvolved stabilizing structures.

There are several techniques for orienting the pedicle screws for segmental fixation (Fig. 147.3). Roy-Camille et al. (99,100) described a *straight-ahead* method, in which the entry point of the pedicle screw is at the junction

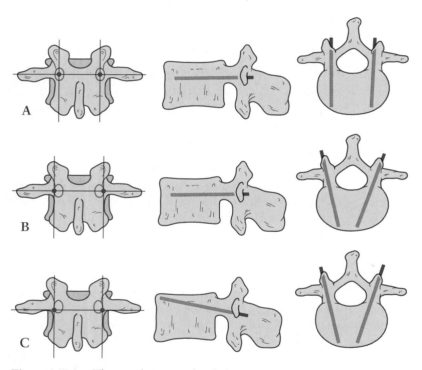

Figure 147.3.   Three techniques of pedicle screw insertion. **A:** The straight-ahead method of Roy-Camille. With this technique, the screw is inserted at the junction of a line bisecting the transverse axis of the transverse process and a line bisecting the facet joint. The pedicle screw is oriented parallel to both the sagittal plane and the superior and inferior vertebral endplates. **B:** The inward method of Magerl. The pedicle screw entry point is slightly more laterally located than that described by Roy-Camille. The screw entry point is at the junction of a line intersecting the transverse axis of the transverse process and a line along the lateral aspect of the facet joint. The screw orientation is parallel to the superior and inferior vertebral end plates but is oriented medially so that it is oblique to the sagittal plane. **C:** The author's preferred up-and-in method, as described by Krag. The entry point for the pedicle screw is at the junction of a line running slightly inferior to the transverse axis of the transverse process and a line along the lateral aspect of the facet joint. The screw is oriented slightly cephalad and is angled medially to the sagittal plane. By making the pedicle screw entry point slightly more caudal than with the other methods, this technique minimizes damage to the superior facet joint by the head of the screw and reduces the risk of subsequent adjacent level degeneration. The screw must be angled superiorly in order to maintain its path within the pedicle.

of a line bisecting the transverse axis of the transverse process and a line bisecting the facet joint (Fig. 147.3*A*). The pedicle screw is oriented parallel to both the sagittal plane and the superior and inferior vertebral end plates. Another technique is the *inward* method described by Magerl (72,73), in which the pedicle screw entry point is slightly more lateral than that described by Roy-Camille. The entrance point is at the junction of a line intersecting the transverse axis of the transverse process and a line along the lateral aspect of the facet joint (Fig. 147.3*B*). The screw orientation is parallel to the superior and inferior vertebral end plates but is oriented medially so that it is oblique to the sagittal plane.

The method I prefer is the *up-and-in* method described by Krag and others (Fig. 147.3*C*) (64,65,68). The entry point for the pedicle screw is at the junction of a line running slightly inferior to the transverse axis of the transverse process and a line along the lateral aspect of the facet joint. The screw is oriented slightly cephalad and is angled medially to the sagittal plane. The up-and-in method is particularly useful in minimizing damage to the superior facet joint. By making the pedicle screw entry point slightly more caudal than the other methods, damage to the facet joint by the head of the screw is minimized and the risk of subsequent adjacent level degeneration is theoretically less. The screw must be angled superiorly in order to maintain its path within the pedicle.

In summary, I favor decompression and fusion with pedicle fixation in active, healthy, physiologically young patients with spinal stenosis associated with degenerative spondylolisthesis who have relatively few degenerative changes promoting stability at the level of the slip. I usually manage the elderly, low-demand patient with multiple comorbidities who has significant associated degenerative changes at the listhetic level by limited decompression without fusion.

◤ PITFALLS AND COMPLICATIONS

Complications related to surgical decompression for spinal stenosis may be either *general* in nature, sharing features in common with all types of spinal surgery, or they may be *specific* and related only to spinal stenosis decompression. Those that are specific to only spinal stenosis decompression include complications related to posterior approaches for spinal stenosis decompression and those complications associated with spinal fusion.

GENERAL COMPLICATIONS

All lumbar spine surgery, and indeed all surgeries generally, share certain broad groups of potential complica-

tions, which can be thought of as occurring either *preoperatively, intraoperatively, or postoperatively.*

Preoperative Complications

Preoperative factors that are important determinants of surgical outcomes involve primarily surgical decision making, and therefore, complications of this process can be thought of as being judgment errors of patient selection. In general, surgery is more reliable in producing relief of leg pain than LBP. The difficulty with surgery for LBP lies not with the technical aspects of the surgical procedures but with the difficulty in determining the genesis of the back pain. Discography has been advocated as a diagnostic test for determining the source of pain (22). The role of discography is controversial and may not accurately predict the painful level, even when the pain might be coming from the disc (46). See Chapters 144 and 145 for more details.

Intraoperative Complications

Anesthetic complications related to spinal surgery are comparable to the complications associated with other nonspinal surgery. These complications include airway complications; fluid management problems, including shock, fluid overload, and transfusion reactions; pulmonary complications; cardiac risks related to perioperative myocardial infarction, cardiogenic shock, or congestive heart failure; and vascular complications related to blood loss, hypertension, hypotension, and thrombotic or embolic phenomena.

Posterior decompression for spinal stenosis poses particular problems related to positioning of the patient in the prone position, which is the least physiologic position for the patient under general anesthesia (118). These problems include potential difficulties with ventilation and airway management. In addition, there is the risk of pressure to sensitive structures such as the eyes, which can result in blindness. Pressure can result in compression of various neural structures, which can result in temporary or permanent nerve palsies. These structures include the sciatic nerve or its branches from prolonged pressure of the buttocks against a buttress while in the kneeling position, the ulnar nerve at the elbow, the anterior interosseous nerve in the cubital tunnel, the axillary nerve (84), brachial plexus from excessive shoulder abduction (23), and cervical area from prolonged positioning of the neck in a rotated position.

The optimum patient position for surgery is one in which the abdomen is hanging free in order to reduce inferior vena cava (IVC) pressure and thereby minimize intraoperative bleeding. This may be accomplished by placing the patient in a kneeling or a knee-chest position, or by placing the patient prone with the abdomen hanging freely. *In vivo* IVC pressure measurements have shown that pressure in the IVC is 1.5 times greater when the patient is in the prone position than when the patient is on a frame that allows the abdomen to hang freely. Problems associated with the kneeling position include sciatic nerve palsy, deep venous thrombosis (DVT), and compartment syndrome. Ophthalmic complications associated with spinal surgery have only recently been recognized and reported (66,82). Such complications include posterior optic nerve ischemia (66,82), occipital lobe infarcts, central retinal vein thrombosis (82), and cerebral ischemia (82). Although the etiology of the diminished visual acuity or blindness associated with these conditions is not always clear, identifiable causes include prolonged operative time, hypotension, blood loss, and direct pressure on the eye.

Anesthetic problems related to spinal anesthesia include persistent spinal fluid leak from spinal needle puncture and hypotension from venous pooling of blood in the lower extremities. The advantage of spinal anesthesia in posterior spinal surgery is that some of the positioning complications previously described can be obviated by having the patient remain awake and in control of the head and upper extremities. This approach minimizes the risk of pressure on the eyes, compression to the ulnar nerve at the elbow, and brachial plexus palsies.

The syndrome of inappropriate antidiuretic hormone (SIADH) secretion is a condition characterized by the release of antidiuretic hormone (ADH) from the posterior pituitary gland in the absence of the usual osmometric or volumetric stimulus of dehydration or hypovolemia. This results in failure to excrete free water, resulting in dilutional hyponatremia. SIADH is known to occur in many conditions, including surgery, and has also been reported during and following spinal surgery (7). It is thought that ADH secretion reaches its maximum during surgery, and that the syndrome gradually resolves by approximately the third postoperative day. It is imperative to distinguish between SIADH and hypovolemia as a cause of low urine output because SIADH demands treatment by fluid restriction whereas low urine output from hypovolemia requires fluid administration. SIADH should always be considered as a cause of low urine output and dilutional hyponaetremia during and immediately after surgery.

Postoperative Complications

Some postoperative complications are common to many surgical procedures, including spinal surgery. These include *metabolic* problems such as postoperative confusional states and SIADH, *pulmonary* conditions such as atelectasis and pneumonia, *genitourinary* complications such as urinary retention, and *gastrointestinal* problems such as ileus and stress ulcer.

Although they are uncommon, some spinal conditions such as cauda equina syndrome may predispose the patient to urinary retention owing to impairment in function of the nervous supply to the bladder. When urinary reten-

tion is due to acute cauda equina compression, prompt surgery is imperative. Chronic urinary retention may require either intermittent straight catheterization or an indwelling catheter. The presence of a urinary catheter, particularly a long-standing indwelling catheter, may predispose the patient to a urinary tract infection requiring treatment with antibiotics.

Postoperative ileus is a condition that can occur following any surgery, and is common following large posterior spinal procedures such as multilevel decompressions for spinal stenosis and instrumented lumbar fusions. When the intertransverse membrane is violated during posterolateral fusion, bleeding into the retroperitoneal space may occur, and ileus is more likely.

DEEP VENOUS THROMBOSIS AND PULMONARY EMBOLUS

PE is the third most common cause of death in the United States, accounting for up to 200,000 deaths annually. In hospitalized patients, PE is the most common preventable cause of hospital death with pulmonary emboli detectable in more than one quarter of all routine autopsies. The etiology of pulmonary embolism includes the immobilization associated with hospitalization as well as factors related to surgery itself, which produce a hypercoagulable state. DVT is the precursor to PE in 90% of cases and is common in hospitalized patients. The risk of DVT following general surgery ranges between 5% and 63% and is particularly high with certain orthopaedic conditions, such as fracture of the hip, and following some orthopedic procedures, particularly total hip and total knee arthroplasty, in which the incidence of DVT following unprotected joint replacement is as high as 60% to 80%.

Although it is uncommon, DVT has been reported to occur following scoliosis surgery. DVT following routine spinal decompressions, however, was thought to be a rare occurrence. More recently, DVT has been recognized following spinal surgery (108,119). Using postoperative duplex scanning, the incidence of DVT in unprotected patients undergoing posterior lumbar surgery has been reported to be 14% (119). The use of elastic compression stockings or intermittent pneumatic compression stockings (PCS) has been shown to reduce the incidence of DVT diagnosed by duplex scanning to 0.9% to 6% (108). Bell et al. reported the incidence of venographically proven DVT following unprotected surgery for lumbar disc herniation or spinal stenosis performed under spinal anesthesia to be 25.8% (6A). This rate is significantly higher than that reported using duplex scanning as the method of diagnosis, thereby reflecting the greater accuracy of venography in diagnosing DVT (30a,30b,119). Prophylaxis with PCS reduced the incidence to 4.5% in patients receiving spinal anesthesia. PCS seemed to provide no significant protection from DVT in patients receiving general anesthesia, in whom the incidence of DVT was 13.6% in unprotected spinal surgery and 8.1% with PCS protection. This study suggested that the best combination of type of anesthesia and DVT prophylaxis in terms of prevention of DVT was spinal anesthesia with PCS. The worst combination was spinal anesthesia without PCS. See Chapter 5 for more details as well as recommendations for treatment

SPECIFIC COMPLICATIONS RELATED TO POSTERIOR DECOMPRESSION FOR SPINAL STENOSIS

Both laminectomy and laminotomy share common bony, soft-tissue, and neural anatomy, and therefore, share a common list of potential complications. These complications include inadequate neural decompression, recurrent stenosis, incidental durotomy, neural injury, epidural hematoma, neural compression from either fat grafts or other barriers to scar formation, vascular injury, and late instability.

INADEQUATE NEURAL DECOMPRESSION

Although it is not a complication in the usual sense of the term, failure to obtain symptomatic relief of radicular leg pain that is not due to an error in surgical decision making should be considered at least an adverse effect of surgery. Its avoidance requires precise correlation of the preoperative imaging study with the clinical picture and surgical anatomy, and demands that surgery be continued until the offending neural compression is found. It also requires a thorough knowledge of surgical anatomy and of the potential sources and sites of neural compression, as described by MacNab (70). In addition, it is imperative that the surgeon have a precise understanding of the potential anatomic variations in the location of disc herniations so that he will know precisely where to look for neural compression, particularly when the predicted pathology is not found (110).

It is important for the surgeon to recognize and look for additional sites of neural compression that may account for inadequate relief following decompression of only one site. This condition is sometimes referred to as a "double crush phenomenon" and is thought to be at least partially due to venous congestion of the neural segment located between the two sites of compression resulting in a compartment syndrome–like condition of the intervening segment. Multiple sites of compression are common with spinal stenosis, which is a global condition frequently involving multilevel, bilateral neural compression. Sites of compression include central compression of the cauda equina and lateral compression, either within the lateral recess, within the neural foramen, or extrafo-

raminally. It is important to identify all clinically significant sites of neural compression and to decompress those levels adequately.

RECURRENT STENOSIS

Distinguishing recurrent symptoms due to neural compression from those due to scar formation is a complex decision-making process that requires a precise history and high-quality radiographic imaging. Failure to obtain even temporary pain relief following decompressive lumbar surgery suggests either inadequate neural decompression, irreversible neural damage already present at the time of surgery, or a nonspinal cause for the pain. A short pain-free interval of less than 6 months suggests development of scar formation as the cause of recurrent pain. Recurrence of pain following a long pain-free interval of more than 6 to 12 months suggests a new process such as a recurrent disc herniation or recurrent stenosis.

Because spinal stenosis may occur in association with disc herniation, recurrence of symptoms following decompression involving discectomy could be due to recurrent disc herniation. The overall reported incidence of recurrent disc herniation is approximately 3% (38). Its incidence following laminectomy or laminotomy associated with discectomy is unknown but could be even greater if decompression involved destabilization from facetectomy and resulted in instability (31).

Several studies have reported that the surgical results of spinal stenosis surgery deteriorate over time (18,56,60, 91). Although this may be due to many factors, such as associated comorbidity and advanced patient age, surgical and pathologic factors are also important. These factors include progression of degenerative changes at unoperated levels (60), regrowth of bone at the operated levels (90, 91), pre-existing instability (degenerative scoliosis or spondylolisthesis) (35), and development of postoperative instability [for example, due to resection of one or more facets at a single segmental level (1) or development of a facet fracture at the level of decompression during or following decompression (95)]. All of the above-mentioned factors can lead to recurrent LBP or radicular leg pain following decompressive surgery for spinal stenosis.

DUROTOMY

Incidental violation of the dura (durotomy) is a well-recognized complication of spinal surgery that has a reported incidence of 0.3% to 13%. It most commonly occurs when the edge of a biting instrument, such as a Kerrison rongeur, inadvertently grabs the dura and produces either a punctate hole in the dura or a frank laceration. Usually, the injury is noted immediately by the sudden appearance of cerebrospinal fluid (CSF) within the wound. Occasionally, however, the tear is not noted until sometime later by the clinical appearance of persistent spinal headache, the presence of CSF drainage from the wound, or by the onset of an obvious swelling in the patient's back suggesting a pseudomeningocele (75). The incidence of the latter complication has been estimated between 0.07 and 2 per cent.

Repair of Durotomy

When the durotomy is noted intraoperatively, repair the dura primarily (75,117).

- It is imperative that there be adequate exposure to visualize the full extent of the laceration and that adequate illumination and magnification be available with either an operating microscope or headlight and loupe magnification. This often requires wide decompression.
- To facilitate closure of the defect, place the patient in a slightly head-down (Trendelenberg) position in order to minimize the amount of CSF in the operative field. This approach not only provides a drier operative field but also minimizes the tendency for the individual roots of the cauda equina to float to the surface, which can result in their inadvertent injury during dural repair.
- For safe closures of large tears, place a small cottonoid patty over the exposed nerve roots for the initial portion of the repair and then remove it just before dural closure (28). For tears associated with loss of tissue, or for tears in difficult to repair locations, an autologous fat graft, a piece of autograft fascia (thoracolumbar fascia or fascia lata), or a freeze-dried fascia allograft may be required to close the defect (28). Perform a watertight closure with a running 5-0 or 6-0 nonabsorbable suture (e.g., silk or nylon).
- After meticulous closure, return the patient to a neutral or slightly head-up (reverse Trendelenberg) position and perform a Valsalva maneuver in order to assess the integrity of the closure. The use of a fibrin glue may also be considered for additional strength and integrity of the repair.
- The remainder of the surgical wound closure proceeds as usual, except that a drain is often not employed in order to minimize risk of development of a CSF fistula. Oversew the fascial closure with a running stitch to maintain a watertight closure of the fascia. Perform routine interrupted skin closure.
- If the dural closure is watertight, the patient may be ambulatory the day following surgery. If there is any doubt about the integrity of the closure, keep the patient on bed rest for 3 to 5 days (28).

If a postoperative dural leak is suspected due to persistent spinal headache or a pseudomeningocele, confirm the diagnosis by myelography or MRI, and return the patient to the operating room for dural repair and watertight closure (75). Alternatively, a subarachnoid drain can be inserted at the bedside and the patient placed on bed rest

until the leak subsides. This generally involves removal of approximately 300 ml of CSF in a sterile blood collection bag daily. The volume and rate of CSF removal is titrated by adjusting the height of the bag to produce the appropriate rate of CSF flow (63).

The long-term outcome of spinal surgery complicated by incidental durotomy is generally favorable (117). When identified intraoperatively and repaired primarily, perioperative surgical morbidity and long-term outcome is comparable to that of surgery not associated with incidental durotomy (117).

NERVE ROOT INJURY

Neural injury may occur due to direct trauma to the nerve root itself during surgery. This injury may be due to excessive neural retraction, contusion, laceration, or electrocauterization (111). The incidence of neurologic complications following lumbar spine surgery has been estimated to be 0.2%. Such injury may be suspected postoperatively by the presence of a new or increased objective neurologic deficit, or by the onset of new parasthesias. This condition, sometimes referred to as the "battered root," may occur either as an unavoidable consequence of severe neural compression or as a result of indelicate surgery (11). Meticulous surgical technique, therefore, is of paramount importance in order to minimize such complications. Adequate surgical exposure is imperative in order to minimize excessive neural retraction. In cases of a large midline disc herniation or a disc herniation associated with spinal stenosis, for example, a bilateral laminectomy rather than a keyhole laminotomy may be required in order to remove the disc fragment safely.

It is important to perform an anteroposterior x-ray study of the lumbar spine in order to identify bony anatomy that might be of surgical significance. Note the presence of spina bifida occulta or a pre-existing laminectomy defect, for example, on the preoperative radiograph because the presence of either of these features mandates cautious surgical exposure in order to minimize risk of damage to underlying dura and nerve roots. Carefully examine other pre-operative studies to identify other potentially significant anatomic variants, such as anomalous nerve roots, that could be injured during surgical decompression (111).

It is important always to visualize the lateral edge of the nerve root during surgical decompression to be sure that exposure is not inadvertently being performed in the axilla of a nerve root where accidental dural laceration and neural injury could occur and where repair of such injuries is particularly difficult. This is also important during revision lumbar surgery, in which dissection should usually be performed lateral to the root along the lateral edge of the bony canal to avoid a potentially dangerous midline scar. When performing lateral nerve root decompressions, work parallel, rather than perpendicular, to the long axis of the nerve root in order to minimize risk of cutting across a root.

SCAR TISSUE

Although scarring is a common event following all surgeries, it has been implicated as a potential cause for continued pain following spinal surgery. Postoperative scar tissue may be located either intradurally *(arachnoiditis)* or extradurally *(epidural fibrosis)*. Arachnoiditis is an inflammation of the pia-arachnoid membrane that surrounds the cauda equina or spinal cord (17). It can result in surgical failure and continued pain following decompressive surgery. Its etiology is often unclear, but it has been associated with many conditions, including oil-based myelographic contrast agents and prior surgery (93). The exact mechanism by which arachnoiditis occurs following surgery is not completely understood, but it is thought to be more likely to occur following dural laceration in which blood gains entry into the dural sac and mixes with neural elements. It is also associated with intraoperative trauma to neural structures. Arachnoiditis exists as a spectrum of severity, from mild pia-arachnoid thickening to severe scarring with complete blockage of the flow of contrast agents or spinal fluid. Diagnosis can be made by water-soluble myelography, MRI, or post-contrast CT in which the individual nerve roots of the cauda equina appear clumped together rather than as well-defined structures. Surgical treatment of arachnoiditis is not indicated because surgery rarely produces any significant pain relief and may be complicated by further damage to neural structures and more scarring (17).

Epidural fibrosis is extradural, rather than intradural, scar tissue in which adhesive constrictions can form around neural tissue. It commonly arises from contact with the paraspinal musculature and is probably a relatively frequent event following spinal surgery. Although such scar tissue can result in postoperative pain, symptoms are relatively infrequent. When postoperative pain exists, the primary differential diagnosis is between scar and recurrent disc herniation. Radiographic distinction between these two conditions is best made with gadolinium-enhanced MRI or post-contrast CT (97).

Efforts to prevent postoperative scar formation include delicate surgical technique with adequate illumination and magnification, meticulous hemostasis and drainage, and the use of some form of an interposition membrane as a barrier to scar formation. These barriers include a thin layer of fat or synthetic agents such as an absorbable gelatin sponge. The use of a free fat graft has been considered the gold standard interposition membrane, although use of large grafts has been associated with postoperative cauda equina syndrome (79).

SUPERFICIAL WOUND INFECTION

Postoperative spine infections may be divided into either *superficial* or *deep* infections. Although the treatment for both types of infections is often similar (i.e., debridement and antibiotic therapy), it is useful to make this distinction because duration of treatment (e.g., short-term antibiotics for superficial infections versus long-term intravenous antibiotics for deep infections), morbidity, and long-term outcome are often very different for the two types.

Superficial wound infections are located beneath the dermis and subcutaneous tissue but superficial to the deep thoracolumbar fascia and are characterized by tenderness and localized erythema. They usually have associated drainage and fluctuance, although in milder cases consisting only of cellulitis these may be absent. Patients may be febrile but usually show no other systemic signs of illness (67). Laboratory data usually show elevation of the erythrocyte sedimentation rate (ESR) and C-reactive protein (CRP), although the white blood cell count (WBC) is usually within normal limits.

Treatment of superficial wound infections consists of local wound care, ranging from simple packing of a small area of localized infection, followed by a short course of oral antibiotics, to more aggressive surgical debridement of necrotic tissue with short-term parenteral antibiotics. In cases requiring surgery, the wound can usually be closed primarily, although delayed closure is an option if there is any question about the adequacy of the debridement. The use of short-term suction-irrigation tubes is at the discretion of the surgeon, although they are usually not required.

DEEP WOUND INFECTIONS

As opposed to superficial infections, in which the diagnosis is usually readily apparent, deep infections may be difficult to diagnose and a high index of suspicion is often required (67). Because delay in diagnosis is common, the amount of tissue necrosis is often extensive. Symptoms include disproportionate back pain or leg pain. This may follow a relatively painless and uneventful immediate postoperative period. The patient may feel and look ill and may exhibit generalized malaise. Fever is often present but may be deceptively low grade. If an epidural abscess is present, radicular leg pain and neurologic deficit may occur. Although the patient may exhibit a leukocytosis, elevation of the WBC count is frequently absent. The ESR and CRP are usually elevated.

Radiographic imaging studies are usually required to confirm the diagnosis. MRI provides the best and most useful information by revealing both the presence and extent of a deep abscess. Typically, an abscess is demonstrated by the presence of a well-demarcated area of increased signal intensity on the T2-weighted image. When

MRI is not available, diagnosis may be confirmed radiographically by the presence of a circumscribed area of fluid density visualized by CT. If a deep abscess is strongly suspected, diagnosis may be confirmed by aspiration, with subsequent culture and sensitivity of any fluid obtained (61).

Treat deep wound infection aggressively with surgical debridement of all necrotic tissues, followed by appropriate parenteral antibiotics. Begin surgical exposure of the affected area with careful sequential debridement, and irrigate each layer before proceeding to the next deeper layer to avoid inadvertent contamination of potentially unaffected deeper tissues. If the infection extends deeply into the laminectomy site, take care to remove any fat graft or absorbable gelatin sponge material. Following removal of infected or suspicious tissues, thoroughly irrigate the wound with pulsatile lavage. Do not remove rigid fixation and bone graft from an instrumented spinal fusion because this may increase the risk of subsequent pseudarthrosis. Loose hardware, on the other hand, no longer performs its function of providing stability to the spine and, therefore, should be removed and thoroughly debrided. Place a drain and close the wound meticulously. Tightly close the deep fascia with interrupted absorbable suture oversewn with a continuous running stitch. Close the wound primarily, particularly in the presence of spinal fixation hardware, unless there is infection from a particularly virulent organism. This may require extensive undermining of wound margins in order to avoid tension on friable wound edges. It is usually advisable to close the wound using large throws of a sturdy, nonabsorbable suture rather than staples. Use of suction-irrigation tubes for a few days may be considered, although this is usually not necessary.

EPIDURAL ABSCESS

Epidural abscess, because of its risk of paresis or frank paralysis, is one of the most feared complications of spinal surgery. Fortunately, it is a rare occurrence following spinal surgery, with only 16% of epidural abscesses resulting from postoperative infection (4). Signs and symptoms are obvious and constitute a typical presentation (4). Patients nearly always have significant back pain, and often present with obvious neurologic findings such as nuchal rigidity and weakness or paralysis of the lower extremities. The patient appears to be much sicker than with either postoperative discitis or vertebral osteomyelitis and typically has a fever. Both the WBC and acute phase reactants are elevated. MRI is the diagnostic imaging modality of choice and clearly visualizes the abscess as a discreet, well-circumscribed entity within the subarachnoid space. It clearly delineates the upper and lower extent of the abscess and, therefore, is invaluable in the preoperative planning of the extent of decompression.

Treatment of an epidural abscess must be prompt and decisive: surgical evacuation of the abscess and any adjacent necrotic tissue, followed by parenteral antibiotics. The preferred surgical approach is generally posterior, although an anterior approach may be indicated in the presence of a significant kyphotic deformity in which bony collapse has compromised the neural structures and simultaneous anterior reconstruction and bone grafting are required to restore stability.

EPIDURAL HEMATOMA

Epidural hematoma causing symptomatic neurologic compression is another devastating complication of spinal surgery. Fortunately, the risk of this complication can be minimized by meticulous attention to preoperative, intraoperative, and postoperative detail. *Preoperatively,* advise the patient to stop all nonsteroidal anti-inflammatory drugs (NSAIDS) for approximately 1 week before surgery. In addition, it is important that the patient is not hypercoagulable. When indicated, check the prothrombin time (PT), partial thromboplastin time (PTT), bleeding time, platelet count, and platelet function. *Intraoperatively,* position the patient with the abdomen hanging freely in order to minimize epidural venous congestion. Keep the blood pressure below 100 mm Hg systolic, if possible, in order to minimize bleeding. Use electrocautery, and seal raw bone surfaces with bone wax to minimize bleeding during the surgical exposure. Control epidural bleeding with bipolar electrocoagulation. At the end of the surgery, when the deep paraspinal muscle retractors are removed, check the muscle walls for persistent bleeding, because prolonged muscle retraction may temporarily occlude potentially significant muscle bleeders that could begin bleeding after muscle layer closure. In general, I prefer to use a drain postoperatively in order to minimize the formation of postoperative hematoma. *Postoperatively,* leave the drain in place for 24 to 48 hours or until the amount of collected blood is less than approximately 30 ml per 8-hour shift. I do not prescribe NSAIDS during the immediate postoperative period (during the first 48 hours) in order to minimize bleeding from the fresh wound.

A characteristic clinical feature of epidural hematoma is the presence of severe pain that appears out of proportion to what is normally expected. This is usually associated with a progressive neurologic deficit. Depending on the extent and location of the surgical exposure and the magnitude of the hematoma, the neurologic deficit may be focal and unilateral, or it may be widespread and may involve multiple muscle groups in both legs.

The key to diagnosis of this condition is having a high index of suspicion. Confirm the diagnosis with MRI, myelography, or CT. Once the diagnosis is suspected, immediately return the patient to the operating room for decompression and drainage of the hematoma.

COMPRESSION BY FAT GRAFTS OR SYNTHETIC SCAR BARRIERS

Postoperative neurologic compression may be due to structures other than epidural hematoma. The use of free fat grafts as a barrier to scar formation has been associated with symptomatic neurologic compression mimicking epidural hematoma (79). Although this risk can be minimized with the use of a smaller (3 to 5 mm thick) piece of fat, the fear of epidural compression by fat graft has led some surgeons to abandon fat grafts in favor of other synthetic scar barrier substances. Even these substitutes, however, may cause neural compression if proper care is not exercised. For multilevel laminectomy requiring the use of a lengthy piece of scar barrier material, I prefer an absorbable gelatin sponge material rather than fat because the fat could theoretically become balled up and exert focal compression on the underlying dura, and result cauda equina syndrome.

VASCULAR COMPLICATIONS

Vascular injuries associated with posterior lumbar spinal procedures are nearly always associated with surgical discectomy, rather than laminectomy. Vascular injury occurs most commonly at L4–L5, followed by L5–S1 (24). Although to some extent this reflects the most common levels of spinal surgery, regional differences in vascular anatomy of the lower lumbar spine also play a role. Injury of a major abdominal vessel typically occurs from aggressive use of the pituitary rongeur, with penetration through the anterior annulus.

Such injuries may be recognized early or late. Brisk bleeding from acute laceration of a major abdominal vessel presents early as hypotension and abdominal distention and is associated with a high mortality rate. The mortality rate from arterial injuries has been reported to be 78%, whereas that for venous injuries is 89% (24). Vascular injuries may be recognized late by the development of high-output cardiac failure or abdominal bruits from formation of an arteriovenous fistula. Arteriovenous fistula formation is the most common result of a vascular injury. It occurs most commonly between the right common iliac artery and vein (29.1%), between the left common iliac artery and vein (25.5%), the right common iliac artery and the IVC (21.8%), and the right common iliac artery and left common iliac vein (12.7%). Late arteriovenous fistula formation is more compatible with long-term survival, with mortality reported between 9% and 11% (24).

POSTOPERATIVE INSTABILITY

Instability following surgical decompression is usually an iatrogenic complication of spinal surgery. Such instability

can occur in either the anteroposterior plane (spondylolisthesis), in the mediolateral plane (lateral listhesis and scoliosis), or in both planes simultaneously. In general, the risk of postoperative anteroposterior instability can be minimized by maintaining the integrity of at least one facet joint at the level decompressed (1). In other words, if a unilateral complete facetectomy is performed on one side, then the integrity of the opposite facet must be maintained. Similarly, if half of one facet is removed during a surgical decompression, then at least half of the contralateral facet joint should be spared. If a total of more than one facet is removed during a decompression, consider prophylactic fusion of that level.

When decompressing a stenotic level associated with a degenerative spondylolisthesis, concomitant fusion should generally be performed because surgical outcome has been shown to be better with fusion than with decompression alone (44). This seems to occur even in the absence of solid bony arthrodesis, suggesting that even the presence of a stable pseudarthrosis results in better clinical outcome than when no fusion is attempted. This is thought to be due to a reduced risk of a subsequent increase in the slip, although a direct relationship between increase in magnitude of a subsequent slip and poorer surgical outcome has not been demonstrated. Although the use of segmental spinal fixation with pedicle screws has been shown to increase the rate of fusion compared with posterolateral fusion without instrumentation, there is no convincing evidence that such instrumentation leads to better clinical outcome (32).

Isthmic spondylolisthesis with frank fracture of the pars interarticularis may also occur in the absence of prior slip as a result of surgical decompression. In such cases, the patient presents with evidence of a *de novo* spondylolisthesis occurring either at one of the levels decompressed or at a level above the level of decompression. The presumed mechanism is either a mechanical stress fracture or perhaps an impairment of the blood supply to the affected level (16,106). Instability may also occur as a result of fracture of the facet joint following decompressive surgery.

▲ AUTHOR'S PERSPECTIVE

Spinal stenosis is a common pathologic clinical entity that is largely degenerative in nature, although it may have a predisposing congenital component to it. It may be accompanied by other structural changes (degenerative spondylolisthesis) producing instability. The natural history of spinal stenosis is unclear, but it appears that approximately 20% of patients worsen over time, 40% improve slightly, and 40% remain unchanged.

The surgical treatment of spinal stenosis involves decompression of the symptomatic level or levels. At the time of decompression of symptomatic levels, the role of surgical decompression of clinically asymptomatic levels that show compression on imaging studies is controversial. However, because long-term failures are frequently characterized by restenosis at previously decompressed levels, or by the development of symptoms at levels that were previously stenotic but asymptomatic, it is better to decompress any questionable levels. Such decompression may be performed through laminectomy or may be more limited in extent by multilevel laminotomies.

The role of fusion depends on whether or not there is associated spondylolisthesis. In general, fusion is indicated for spinal stenosis associated with degenerative spondylolisthesis. The indications for the use of concomitant segmental (pedicle) fixation are unclear, but we use fixation more commonly in relatively young, active, healthy patients who lack significant degenerative changes at the level of the slip. Patients with more severe degenerative changes, particularly if they are elderly and of low demand, may do well with focal decompression (laminotomies) without fusion.

REFERENCES

Each reference is categorized according to the following scheme: *, classic article; #, review article; !, basic research article; and +, clinical results/outcome study.

! 1. Abumi K, Panjabi M, Dramer K, et al. Biomechanical Evaluation of Lumbar Spinal Stability after Graded Facetectomies. *Spine* 1990;15:1142.

* 2. Arnoldi C, Brodsky A, Cauchoix J, et al. Lumbar Spinal Stenosis and Nerve Root Entrapment Syndromes. Definition and Classification. *Clin Orthop* 1976;115:4.

+ 3. Atlas S, Deyo R, Keller R, et al. The Maine Lumbar Spine Study, Part III. *Spine* 1996;21:1787.

+ 4. Baker AS, Ojemann RG, Swartz MN, et al. Spinal Epidural Abscess. *N Engl J Med* 1975;293:463.

5. Bell GR. Diagnosis of Lumbar Disc Disease. *Seminars in Spine Surgery* 1994;6:186.

6. Bell GR. Degenerative Lumbar Spinal Stenosis: Natural History and Results of Simple Decompression and Decompression and Fusion for Degenerative Spondylolisthesis. In *Low Back Pain: A Scientific and Clinical Overview.* 1996,663.

+ 6a. Bell GR, Boumphrey F, Piedmont M, et al. The Incidence and Prophylaxis of Deep Venous Thrombosis (DVT) Following Spinal Surgery. Presented at 20th Annual Meeting of the International Society for the Study of the Lumbar Spine. Marseilles, France 1993.

! 7. Bell GR, Gurd AR, Orlowski JP, et al. The Syndrome of Inappropriate Antidiuretic Hormone Secretion Following Spinal Fusion. *J Bone Joint Surg* 1986;68A:720.

8. Bell GR, Modic MT. Radiology of the Lumbar Spine.

In: Rothman RH, Simeone FA, eds. *The Spine*, 3rd ed. Philadelphia: W.B. Saunders Company, 1992:125.

9. Bell GR, Ross JS. Imaging Studies of the Spine. In: *Orthopaedic Knowledge Update: Spine. American Academy of Orthopaedic Surgeons (AAOS).* Rosemont, IL: 1997:41.

+ 10. Bell GR, Rothman RH, Booth RE, et al. A Study of Computer-assisted Tomography. *Spine* 1984;9:552.

* 11. Bertrans G. The Battered Root Problem. *Orthop Clin North Am* 1975;6:305.

+ 12. Blau J, Logue V. Intermittent Claudication of the Cauda Equina. An Unusual Syndrome Resulting from Central Protrusion of a Lumbar Intervertebral Disc. *Lancet* 1961;1:1082.

! 13. Boden SD, Davis DO, Dina TS, et al. Abnormal Magnetic-resonance Scans of the Lumbar Spine in Asymptomatic Subjects. A Prospective Investigation. *J Bone Joint Surg* 1990;72A:403.

! 14. Boden SD, Wiesel SW. Lumbosacral Segmental Motion in Normal Individuals: Have We Been Measuring Instability Properly? *Spine* 1990;5:571.

+ 15. Bridwell K, Bridwell KH, Sedgewick TA, O'Brien MF, et al. Role of Fusion and Instrumentation in the Treatment of Degenerative Spondylolisthesis. *J Spinal Disord* 1993;6:461.

+ 16. Brunet J, Wiley J. Acquired Spondylolysis after Spinal Fusion. *J Bone Joint Surg Br* 1984;66:720.

+ 17. Burton C. Lumbosacral Arachnoiditis. *Spine* 1978;3:24.

* 18. Caputy A, Luessenhop A. Long-term Evaluation of Decompressive Surgery for Degenerative Lumbar Stenosis. *J Neurosurg* 1992;77:669.

+ 19. Chen Q, Baba H, Kamitani K, et al. Postoperative Bone Re-growth in Lumbar Spinal Stenosis. A Multivariate Analysis of 48 Patients. *Spine* 1994;19:2144.

+ 20. Cinotti G, Postacchini F, Weinstein J. Lumbar Spinal Stenosis and Diabetes. Outcome of Surgical Decompression. *J Bone Joint Surg Br* 1994;76:215.

! 21. Cohen MS, Wall EJ, Brown RA, et al. Cauda Equina Anatomy. II: Extrathecal Nerve Roots and Dorsal Root Ganglia. *Spine* 1990;15:1248.

+ 22. Collis JS, Gardner WJ. Lumbar Discography—an Analysis of One Thousand Cases. *J Neurosurg* 1962;19:452.

+ 23. Cooper DE, Jenkins RS, Bready L, et al. The Prevention of Injuries of the Brachial Plexus Secondary to Malposition of the Patient During Surgery. *Clin Orthop* 1988;228:31.

+ 24. DeSaussure RL. Vascular Injury Coincidence to Disc Surgery. *J Neurosurg* 1959;16:222.

+ 25. Deyo R, Cherkin D, Loeser J, et al. Morbidity and Mortality in Association with Operations on the Lumbar Spine. *J Bone Joint Surg* 1992;74A:536.

+ 26. Deyo R, Ciol M, Cherkin D, et al. Lumbar Spinal Fusion. A Cohort Study of Complications, Reoperations, and Resource Use in the Medicare Population. *Spine* 1993;18:1463.

+ 27. Dyck P, Doyle JB. "Bicycle test" of Van Gelderen in Diagnosis of Intermittent Cauda Equina Compression. *J Neurosurg* 1977;46:667.

+ 28. Eismont FJ, Wiesel SW, Rothman RH. Treatment of Dural Tears Associated with Spinal Surgery. *J Bone Joint Surg* 1981;63A:1132.

+ 29. Epstein N, Epstein J. Decompression in the Surgical Management of Degenerative Spondylolisthesis: Advantages of a Conservative Approach in 290 Patients. *J Spinal Disord* 1998;11:116.

+ 30. Feffer H, Weisel S, et al. Degenerative spondylolisthesis: To fuse or not to fuse. *Spine* 1985;10:286.

+ 30a.Ferree B, Stern P, Jolson R, et al. Deep Venous Thrombosis after Spinal Surgery. *Spine* 1993;18:315.

+ 30b.Ferree BA, and Wright AM. Deep Venous Thrombosis Following Posterior Lumbar Spinal Surgery. *Spine* 1993;18:1079.

+ 31. Finnegan WJ, Tenlin JM, Mavel JP, et al. Results of Surgical Intervention in the Multiply Operated Back Patient. *J Bone Joint Surg* 1979;61A:1077.

+ 32. Fischgrund J, Mackay M, Herkowitz H, et al. Degenerative Lumbar Spondylolisthesis with Spinal Stenosis: A Prospective, Randomized Study Comparing Decompressive Laminectomy and Arthrodesis with and without Spinal Instrumentation. *Spine* 1997;22:2807.

+ 33. Fitzgerald J, Newman P. Degenerative Spondylolisthesis. *J Bone Joint Surg* 1976;58B:184.

+ 34. France JC, Yaszemski MJ, Lauerman WC, et al. A Randomized Prospective Study of Posterolateral Lumbar Fusion. Outcomes with and without pedicle screw instrumentation. *Spine* 1999;24:553.

+ 35. Frazier D, Lipson S, Fossel A, et al. Associations between Spinal Deformity and Outcomes after Decompression for Spinal Stenosis. *Spine* 1997;22:2025.

\# 36. Frymoyer J. Degenerative Spondylolisthesis: Diagnosis and Treatment. *J Am Acad Orthop Surg* 1994;2:9.

! 37. Frymoyer JW, Newberg A, Pope MH, et al. Spine Radiographs in Patients with Low-back Pain. *J Bone Joint Surg Am* 1984;66A:1048.

+ 38. Garfin SR, Glover M, Booth RE, et al. Laminectomy: A Review of the Pennsylvania Hospital Experience. *J Spinal Disord* 1988;1:116.

+ 39. Getty C, Johnson J, Kirwan E, et al. Parial Undercutting Facetectomy for Bony Entrapment of the Lumbar Nerve Root. *J Bone Joint Surg* 1981;63B:330.

+ 40. Grob D, Humke T, Dvorak J. Degenerative Lumbar Spinal Stenosis Decompression with and without Arthrodesis. *J Bone Joint Surg* 1995;77A:1036.

! 41. Hayes MA, Howard TC, Gruel CR, et al. Roentgenographic Evaluation of Lumbar Spine Flexion-extension in Asymptomatic Individuals. *Spine* 1989;14:327.

! 42. Heliovaara M, Vanharanta H, Korpi J, et al. Herniated Lumbar Disc Syndrome and Vertebral Canals. *Spine* 1986;11:433.

+ 43. Herkowitz H, Garfin S, Bell G, et al. The Use of Computerized Tomography in Evaluating Non-visualized Vertebral Levels Caudal to a Complete Block on a Lumbar Myelogram. *J Bone Joint Surg* 1987;69A:218.

+ 44. Herkowitz H, Kurz L. Degenerative Lumbar Spondylolisthesis with Spinal Stenosis: A Prospective Study Comparing Decompression with Decompression and Intertransverse Process Arthrodesis. *J Bone Joint Surg* 1991;73A:802.

* 45. Hirsch C, Nachemson A. The Reliability of Lumbar Disc Surgery. *Clin Orthop* 1963;29:189.

+ 45a.Hitselberger WE, Witten RM. Abnormal Myelograms in Asymptomatic Patients. *J Neurosurg* 1968;28:204.

* 46. Holt EP. The Question of Lumbar Discography. *J Bone Joint Surg* 1968;50A:720.

! 47. Inufusa A, An H, Lim T, et al. Anatomic Changes of the Spinal Canal and Intervertebral Foramen Associated with Flexion-extension Movement. *Spine* 1996;21:2412.

+ 48. Jackson RP, Becker GJ, Jacobs RR, et al. The Neuroradiographic Diagnosis of Lumbar Herniated Nucleus Pulposus: I. A Comparison of Computed Tomography (CT), Myelography, CT-myelography, Discography, and CT-discography. *Spine* 1989;14:1356.

+ 49. Jackson RP, Cain JE Jr, Jacobs RR, et al. The Neuroradiographic Diagnosis of Lumbar Herniated Nucleus Pulposus: II. A Comparison of Computed Tomography (CT), Myelography, CT-myelography, and Magnetic Resonance Imaging. *Spine* 1989;14:1362.

! 50. Jensen MC, Brant-Zawadzki MN, Obuchowski N, et al. Magnetic Resonance Imaging of the Lumbar Spine in People without Back Pain. *N Engl J Med* 1994;331:69.

+ 51. Johnsson K, Uden A, Rosen I. The Effect of Decompression on the Natural Course of Spinal Stenosis. A Comparison of Surgically Treated and Untreated Patients. *Spine* 1991;16:615.

* 52. Johnsson KE, Rosen I, Uden A. The Natural Course of Spinal Stenosis. *Clin Orthop* 1992;279:82.

+ 53. Jonsson B, Annertz M, Sjoberg C, et al. A Prospective and Consecutive Study of Surgically Treated Lumbar Spinal Stenosis. Part I: Clinical Features Related to Radiographic Findings. *Spine* 1997;22:2932.

+ 54. Jonsson B, Stromqvist B. Symptoms and Signs in Degeneration of the Lumbar Spine. A Prospective, Consecutive Study of 300 Operated Patients. *J Bone Joint Surg* 1993;75:381.

+ 54a.Junghanns H. Spondylolisthesen Ohne Spalt in Zwischengelenksteuck. *Archiv fuer Orthopadische Unfallchirurgie* 1930;29:118.

! 55. Katz J. Lumbar Spinal Fusion. Surgical Rates, Costs and Complications. *Spine* 1995;20(Suppl):78S.

+ 56. Katz J. Comorbidity and Outcome in Degenerative Lumbar Spinal Stenosis. Low Back Pain: A Scientific and Clinical Overview. 1996;41:689.

+ 57. Katz J, Dalgas M, Stucki G, et al. Degenerative Lumbar Spinal Stenosis. Diagnostic Value of the History and Physical Examination. *Arthritis Rheum* 1995;38:1236.

+ 58. Katz J, Lipson S, Brick G, et al. Clinical Correlates of Patient Satisfaction after Laminectomy for Degenerative Lumbar Spinal Stenosis. *Spine* 1995;20:1155.

+ 59. Katz J, Lipson S, Chang L, et al. Seven- to 10-year Outcome of Decompressive Surgery for Degenerative Lumbar Spinal Stenosis. *Spine* 1996;21:92.

+ 60. Katz J, Lipson S, Larson M, et al. The Outcome of Decompressive Laminectomy for Degenerative Lumbar Stenosis. *J Bone Joint Surg [Am]* 1991;73:809.

+ 61. Keller RB, Pappas AM. Infections after Spinal Fusion

3842   *Section VIII* ■ *The Spine*

Using Internal Fixation Instrumentation. *Orthop Clin North Am* 1972;3:99.

* 62. Kirkaldy-Willis W, Paine K, Cauchoix J, et al. Lumbar Spinal Stenosis. *Clin Orthop* 1974;99:30.

+ 63. Kitchel SH, Eismont FJ, Green BA. Closed Subarachnoid Drainage for Management of Cerebrospinal Fluid Leakage after an Operation on the Spine. *J Bone Joint Surg* 1989;71A:984.

64. Krag MH. Lumbosacral Fixation with the Vermont Spinal Fixator. In: Lin PM, Gill K, eds. *Lumbar Interbody Fusion: Principles and Techniques of Spine Surgery.* Rockville, MD: Aspen, 1988.

! 65. Krag MH. Spinal Instrumentation. Biomechanics of Transpedicle Spine Fixation. In: *The Lumbar Spine,* 2nd ed. Philadelphia: W.B. Saunders Company, 1996: 1177.

+ 66. Lee A. Ischemic Optic Neuropathy Following Lumbar Spine Surgery. Case Report. *J Neurosurg* 1995;83:348.

67. Lestini WF, Bell GR. Spinal Infections: Patient Evaluation. *Seminars in Spine Surgery* 2:244-256; 1990.

68. Levine AM, Edwards CC. Low Lumbar Burst Fractures. *Orthopaedics* 1988;11:1427.

+ 69. Lin PM. Internal Decompression for Multiple Levels of Lumbar Spinal Steonosis: A Technical Note. *Neurosurgery* 1982;11:546.

* 70. MacNab I. Spondylolisthesis with an Intact Neural Arch—the So-called Pseudo-spondylolisthesis. *J Bone Joint Surg* 1950;32B:325.

71. MacNab I. The Traction Spur: An Indication of Segmental Instability. *J Bone Joint Surg Am* 1971;53A: 663.

72. Magerl F: External Spinal Skeletal Fixation. In: Weber BG, Magerl F, eds. *The External Fixator.* New York: Springer-Verlag, 1985.

73. Magerl FP. Stabilization of the Lower Thoracic and Lumbar Spine with External Skeletal Fixation. *Clin Orthop* 1984;189:125.

+ 74. Mardjetko S, Connolly P, Shott S. Degenerative Lumbar Spondylolisthesis: A Meta-analysis of Literature, 1970–1993. *Spine* 1994;19(Suppl):2256S.

75. Marshall LF. Cerebrospinal Fluid Leaks: Etiology and Repair. In: Rothman RH, Simeone FA, eds. *The Spine,* 3rd ed. Philadelphia: W.B. Saunders, 1992.

+ 76. Matsui H, Kanamori M, Ishihara H, et al. Expansive Lumbar Laminoplasty for Degenerative Spinal Stenosis in Patients below 70 Years of Age. *Eur Spine J* 1997; 6:191.

+ 77. Matsui H, Tsuji H, Seido H, et al. Results of Expansive Laminoplasty for Lumbar Spinal Stenosis in Active Manual Workers. *Spine* 1992;17(Suppl):S37.

+ 78. Matsunaga S, Sakou T, et al. Natural History of Degenerative Spondylolisthesis: Pathogenesis and Natural Course of the Slippage. *Spine* 1990;15:1204.

+ 79. Mayer P, Jacobsen F. Cauda Equina Syndrome after Surgical Treatment of Lumbar Spinal Stenosis with Application of Free Autogenous Fat Graft. A Report of Two Cases. *J Bone Joint Surg* 1989;71:1090.

+ 80. McCulloch J. Microdecompression and Uninstrumented Single-level Fusion for Spinal Canal Stenosis

with Degenerative Spondylolisthesis. *Spine* 1998;23: 2243.

! 81. Morgan FP, King T. Primary Instability of Lumbar Vertebrae as a common Cause of Low Back Pain. *J Bone Joint Surg Am* 1957;39B:6.

+ 82. Myers M, Hamilton S, Bogosian A, et al. Visual Loss as a Complication of Spine Surgery. A Review of 37 Cases. *Spine* 1997;22:1325.

+ 83. Nakai O, Ookawa A, Yamaura I. Long-term Roentgenographic and Functional Changes in Patients Who Were Treated with Wide Fenestration for Central Lumbar Stenosis. *J Bone Joint Surg* 1991;73A:1184.

+ 84. Nambisan RN, Karkousis CP. Axillary Compression Syndrome with Neurapraxia due to Operative Positioning. *Surgery* 1989;105:449.

* 84a. Newman P, Stone K. The Etiology of Spondylolisthesis. *J Bone Joint Surg* 1963;45B:39.

+ 85. Nork SE, Serena SH, Workman KL, et al. Patient Outcomes after Decompression and Instrumented Posterior Spinal Fusion for Degenerative Spondylolisthesis. *Spine* 1999;24:561.

+ 86. Oldridge N, Yuan Z, Stoll J, Rimm A. Lumbar Spine Surgery and Mortality among Medicare Beneficiaries, 1986. *Am J Public Health* 1994;84:1292.

! 87. Olmarker K, Rydevik B, Holm S. Edema Formation in Spinal Nerve Roots Induced by Experimental, Graded Compression. An Experimental Study on the Pig Cauda Equina with Special Reference to Differences in Effects between Rapid and Slow Onset of Compression. *Spine* 1989;14:569.

! 88. Parke WW, Watanabe R. The Intrinsic Vasculature of the Lumbosacral Spinal Nerve Roots. *Spine* 1985;10: 508.

! 89. Parke WW. The Significance of Venous Return Impairment in Ischemic Radiculopathy and Myelopathy. *Orthop Clin North Am* 1991;22:213.

+ 90. Postacchini F, Cinotti G. Bone Regrowth after Surgical Decompression for Lumbar Spinal Stenosis. *J Bone Joint Surg* 1992;74B:862.

+ 91. Postacchini F, Cinotti G, Gumina S, et al. Long-term Results of Surgery in Lumbar Stenosis. 8-year Review of 64 Patients. *Acta Orthop Scand* 1993;251(Suppl): 78.

+ 92. Postacchini F, Cinotti G, Perugia D, et al. The Surgical Treatment of Central Lumbar Stenosis. Multiple Laminotomy Compared with Total Laminectomy. *J Bone Joint Surg* 1993;75B:386.

+ 93. Quiles M, Marchisello PS, Tsairis P. Lumbar Adhesive Arachnoiditis: Etiologic and Pathologic Aspects. *Spine* 1978;3:45.

! 94. Ramani P. Variations in Size of the Bony Lumbar Canal in Patients with Prolapse of Lumbar Intervertebral Discs. *Clin Radiol* 1976;27:301.

+ 95. Rosen C, Rothman S, Zigler J, et al. Lumbar Facet Fracture as a Possible Source of Pain after Lumbar Laminectomy. *Spine* 1991;16(Suppl):S234.

+ 96. Rosenberg N. Degenerative Spondylolisthesis: Surgical Treatment. *Clin Orthop* 1976;117:112.

+ 97. Ross JS, Masaryk TJ, Modic MT. MR Imaging of Lumbar Arachnoiditis. *Am J Neuroradiol* 1987;8:885.

+ 98. Rothman S, Glenn W Jr, Kerber C. Postoperative Fractures of Lumbar Articular Facets: Occult Cause of Radiculopathy. *AJR Am J Roentgenol* 1985;145:779.

99. Roy-Camille R. *Experience with Roy-Camille Fixation for the Thorocolumbar and Lumbar Spine. Acute Spinal Injuries: Current Management Techniques. University of Massachusetts Continuing Medical Education Course.* Sturbridge, MA: University of Massachusetts, 1987.

100. Roy-Camille R, Saillant G, Mazel C. Internal Fixation of the Lumbar Spine with Pedicle Screw Plating. *Clin Orthop* 1986;203:7.

! 101. Rydevik BL, Brown MD, Lundborg G. Pathoanatomy and Pathophysiology of Nerve Root Compression. *Spine* 1984;9:7.

! 102. Rydevik BL, Pedowitz RA, Hargens AR, et al. Effects of Acute, Graded Compression on Spinal Nerve Root Function and Structure. An Experimental Study of the Pig Cauda Equina. *Spine* 1991;16:487.

103. Saal JA, Saal JA, Parthasarathy R. *The Natural History of Lumbar Spinal Stenosis. The Results of Non-operative treatment.* Presented at Tenth Annual Meeting of the North American Spine Society (NASS). Washington, D.C., 1995.

* 103a. Sachs B, Fraenkel J. Progressive ankylotic rigidity of the spine (spondylose rhizomelique). *J Nerve Ment Dis* 1900;27:1.

+ 104. Sanderson P, Getty C. Long-term Results of Partial Undercutting Facetectomy for Lumbar Lateral Recess Stenosis. *Spine* 1996;21:1352.

! 105. Shaffer WO, Spratt KF, Weinstein J, et al. The Consistency and Accuracy of Roentgenograms for Measuring Sagittal Translation in the Lumbar Vertebral Motion Segment: An Experimental Model. *Spine* 1990;15:741.

+ 106. Sienkiewicz P, Flatley T. Postoperative Spondylolisthesis. *Clin Orthop* 1987;221:172.

+ 107. Simpson J, Silveri C, Balderston R, et al. The Results of Operations on the Lumbar Spine in Patients Who Have Diabetes Mellitus. *J Bone Joint Surg* 1993;75:1823.

+ 108. Smith M, Bressler E, Lonstein J, et al. Deep Venous Thrombosis and Pulmonary Embolism after Major Reconstructive Operations on the Spine. A Prospective Analysis of Three Hundred and Seventeen Patients. *J Bone Joint Surg* 1994;76:980.

109. Spivak J. Current Concepts Review. Degenerative Lumbar Spinal Stenosis. *J Bone Joint Surg* 1998;80A:1053.

110. Stambough JL. Surgical Technique for Lumbar Discectomy. *Seminars is Spine Surgery* 1989;1:47.

111. Stambough JL, Simeone FA. Neurogenic Complications in Spine Surgery. In: Rothman RH, Simeone FA, eds. *The Spine*, 3rd ed. Philadelphia: W.B. Saunders, 1992.

+ 112. Tchang SP, Howie JL, Kirkaldy-Willis WH, et al. Computed Tomography Versus Myelography in Diagnosis of Lumbar Disc Herniation. *J Can Assoc Radiol* 1982;33:15.

113. Turner J, Ersek M, Herron L, et al. Surgery for Lumbar Spinal Stenosis: Attempted Meta-analysis of the Literature. *Spine* 1992;17:1.

114. Turner JA, Ersek M, Herron L, et al. Patient Outcomes after Lumbar Spinal Fusions. *JAMA* 1992;268:XX.

+ 114a. Van Gelderen C. Ein orthotisches (Lordotisches) Kaudasyndrom. *Acta Psychiatr Neurol* 1948;23:57.

+ 115. Vaccaro A, Garfin S. Degenerative Lumbar Spondylolisthesis with Spinal Stenosis, a Prospective Study Comparing Decompression with Decompression and Intertransverse Process Arthrodesis: A Critical Analysis. *Spine* 1997;22:368.

* 116. Verbiest H. A Radicular Syndrome from Developmental Narrowing of the Lumbar Vertebral Canal. *J Bone Joint Surg* 1954;36B:230.

+ 117. Wang JC, Bohlman HH, Riew KD. Dural Tears Secondary to Operations on the Lumbar Spine. Management and Results After a Two-Year-Minimum Follow-up of Eighty-eight Patients. *J Bone Joint Surg* 1998;80A:1728.

+ 118. Ward CF. Complications of Positioning for Spine Surgery. In: Garfin SR, ed. *Complications of Spine Surgery.* Baltimore: Williams & Wilkins, 1989.

+ 119. West J, Anderson L. Incidence of Deep Vein Thrombosis in Major Adult Spinal Surgery. *Spine* 1992;17(Suppl):S254.

! 120. Wiesel SW, Tsourmas N, Feffer HL, et al. A Study of Computer-assisted Tomography: I. The Incidence of Positive CAT Scans in an Asymptomatic Group of Patients. *Spine* 1984;9:549.

+ 121. Wiltse LL, Guyer RD, Spencer CW, et al. Alar Transverse Process Impingement of the L5 Spinal Nerve: The Far-out Syndrome. *Spine* 1984;9:31.

! 122. Yoshida M, Shima K, Taniguchi Y, et al. Hypertrophied Ligamentum Flavum in Lumbar Spinal Canal Stenosis. Pathogenesis and Morphologic and Immunohistochemical Observation. *Spine* 1992;17:1353.

+ 123. Young S, Veerapen R, O'Laoire S. Relief of Lumbar Canal Stenosis Using Multilevel Subarticular Fenestrations as an Alternative to Wide Laminectomy: Preliminary Report. *Neurosurgery* 1988;23:628.

+ 124. Yuan HA, Garfin SR, Dickman CA, Mardjetko SM. A Historical Cohort Study of Pedicle Screw Fixation in Thoracic, Lumbar, and Sacral Spinal Fusions. *Spine* 1994;19(Suppl):2279S.

+ 125. Zdeblick T. A Prospective, Randomized Study of Lumbar Fusion: Preliminary Results. *Spine* 1993;18:983.

CHAPTER 148

FAILED AND REVISION CERVICAL SPINE SURGERY

Eeric Truumees and Robert F. McLain

Cervical spine surgery is usually successful. The population of chronic, failed cervical spine surgery patients is smaller than for the lumbar spine. However, cervical spine surgery is becoming more common. Fusion procedures increased 70% between the periods of 1979–1981 and 1988–1990 (11). With this increase, more complications will be encountered and the need for revisions will rise. This chapter will focus on pseudarthrosis, residual compression, postlaminectomy kyphosis, hardware failure, and progressive or adjacent segment degeneration.

E. Truumees: Department of Spinal Surgery, William Beaumont Hospital, Royal Oak, Michigan, 48073.
R. F. McLain: Department of Orthopaedics, The Cleveland Clinic Foundation, Cleveland, Ohio, 44195.

CAUSES OF FAILURE

PATIENT-RELATED FACTORS

Patients with active medicolegal issues or complex, unresolved psychosocial problems are less likely to achieve a satisfactory outcome from primary cervical spine surgery. Unrealistic expectations and poor compliance with postoperative care also reduce the chances for successful postsurgical outcome. Nutrition, smoking, diabetes, and steroid use all have implications in wound healing, bony fusion, and recovery.

Poor patient selection will predispose to failure of primary cervical surgery and will make revision surgery even more difficult. When failure is the result of, or compounded by, any of these factors, the issues must be addressed before surgical revision is likely to succeed.

3845

SURGEON-RELATED FACTORS

Preoperative factors leading to poor outcome include errors in diagnosis, surgical timing, and intended procedure. Common errors of surgical judgment include choosing the wrong approach, selecting improper fusion levels, or recommending improper postoperative care. These errors will be considered in terms of their outcome: deformity, pseudarthrosis, or inadequate decompression. Perioperative events, including infection, dural leak and pseudomeningocele, and hematoma are not uncommon causes of clinical failure and must be evaluated before planning a revision procedure.

Pseudarthrosis

Pseudarthrosis complicates both anterior and posterior fusion procedures, but it is not always the cause of postoperative neck pain. Anterior cervical discectomy (ACD), without fusion, relieves radicular and axial neck pain in many patients. The success of ACD highlights the fact that nonunion is not always painful (26). Nonetheless, the most common cause of axial pain or radicular symptoms after anterior cervical discectomy and fusion (ACDF) is still pseudarthrosis (36,41). Published reviews of ACDF outcomes report pseudarthrosis in up to 26% of patients (13,22,32,36). Patients at increased risk for pseudarthrosis after ACDF include those undergoing multilevel, individual fusions and those fused with allograft (20,48).

In their analysis of anterior cervical fusion, Lowery et al. (22) defined pseudarthrosis as having the following components:

- Continued or worsening axial pain 6 months after the index procedure
- Complete radiolucency at the host–graft interface
- Vertebral body motion of >2 mm on flexion–extension films

Symptomatic pseudarthroses were seen mainly at the interface between the graft and the vertebral body below. Only 9% of patients with pseudarthrosis felt better after their initial surgery; 27% felt the same, and 64% felt worse.

The literature regarding pseudarthrosis after posterior cervical fusion is relatively sparse. Posterior fusions do not enjoy the biological advantage of grafting under compression, but overall, fusion rates are felt to be high. Reported pseudarthrosis rates following traditional wiring techniques range from 0% to 50% (16), but it can be expected in 10% of patients. Outcomes after rigid posterior plating are reported with rates of 0% to 1.4% pseudarthrosis (16).

Residual Compression

Residual compression of the neural elements is a common cause of failure in both anterior and posterior cervical spine procedures (29). The diffuse nature of degenerative changes in the cervical spine sometimes requires more global or comprehensive procedures than the surgeon is initially willing to entertain. Residual compression after an index spine procedure may result from any of the following:

- Failure to perform a complete decompression at the injured/involved level
- Failure to decompress adjacent involved levels
- Migration of graft or fixation materials into the canal or foramen
- Wrong-level surgery

After ACDF, posterior osteophytes in the region of the posterior longitudinal ligament (PLL) may be a significant source of residual compression (44). Some surgeons feel that posterior osteophytes will resorb after successful fusion. Therefore, they avoid PLL resection and the dangers of operating near the spinal cord. However, the extent of osteophyte resorption is controversial. Recent studies have noted little remodeling or resorption after solid ACDF (32,38). Some authors have advocated more complete decompression in this area through PLL resection and direct visualization with an operating microscope or loupes (19).

Similarly, persistent neural compression following fracture may impair neurologic recovery. While stabilization alone affords some protection of neurologic tissues, adequate decompression of bony and soft-tissue elements increases neurologic recovery (31).

Postlaminectomy Kyphosis

Postlaminectomy kyphosis is a focal and often dramatic angulation of the cervical spine occurring after posterior decompression (21). Wide decompression necessarily sacrifices all or part of the facet and eliminates the attachments for the posterior spinal musculature. Bilateral facetectomy of more than 25% of the facet increases cervical motion in all planes and should prompt posterior fusion to prevent deformity (27,28). After extensive laminectomy, glacial progression toward scoliosis or kyphosis occurs in 30% to 50% of younger patients, and fusion is indicated (39).

Risk factors for postoperative kyphosis include (21) the following:

- Young age (into third decade)
- Preoperative deformity [particularly S-shaped or kyphotic deformities (25)]
- Removal of more than four laminae
- Destruction of facets
- Tumors
- Removal of C-2 posterior elements (major semispinalis insertion)
- Paralysis with paraspinal muscle weakness
- Anterior instability following fracture

Hardware Failure

If due consideration is given to the biomechanical status of the cervical spine and its relationship to the construct employed, the likelihood of failure of most modern instrumentation is small. Fixation failure reflects the types of failure already described:

- Persistent pseudarthrosis results in fatigue failure or failure at the host–hardware interface.
- Underestimated or unrecognized biomechanical loads cause acute failure.
- Aggressive postoperative mobilization, particularly in osteopenic bone, causes acute or progressive hardware loosening.
- Noncompliant patients can accelerate all these processes, particularly when smoking retards the healing process.
- Progressive destruction by tumor or infection further destabilizes the spine.

Progressive or Adjacent-Segment Degeneration

Cervical spine fusion may accelerate degeneration of neighboring, unfused levels (3). These changes may reflect local biomechanical alterations that result from an existing fusion (adjacent segment degeneration) or may simply reflect the natural history of that patient's cervical spondylosis. As such, this degeneration may take the form of recurrent stenosis, recurrent disc herniation, or degenerative disc disease. Up to 89% of ACDF patients report symptomatic degeneration at long-term follow-up (17, 43). Anecdotal evidence suggests that fusions ending at C-5 or C-6 are particularly associated with recurrent axial neck pain, perhaps because of the increased segmental motion at these levels (40).

In patients with continued pain despite a solid arthrodesis, rule out inadequate decompression first. Then evaluate radicular or myelopathic symptoms for evidence of foraminal or canal stenosis or recurrent disc herniation. In patients with predominantly axial pain, assessment of the cervical discs above and below the fusion mass remains controversial. Some authors recommend cervical discography with anterior fusion for concordant pain (33).

PREOPERATIVE ASSESSMENT AND PLANNING

PRESENTATION

Failed Cervical Spine Surgery

Patients with failed cervical spine surgery present with the following:

- Residual axial pain
- Recurrent or residual myelopathy
- Recurrent or residual radiculopathy
- Development or progression of deformity

Evaluation algorithms are presented in Figures 148.1–148.3.

Pseudarthrosis

Patients with pseudarthrosis typically present with the following:

- Axial neck pain
- Recurrent radiculopathy or myelopathy from regrowth of posterior osteophytes
- Deformity from failure of intended fusion after wide posterior decompression

Inadequate Decompression or Adjacent-level Degenerative Disc Disease

Patients with inadequate decompression or progressive or adjacent-level degenerative disc disease present with the following:

- Neural compression after cervical spine surgery, most commonly related to inadequate decompression, recurrent disc herniation, or recurrent stenosis
- Radicular pain (radiculitis), one of the earliest symptoms of neural compression; often relieved by distraction and increased with axial loading
- Weakness and sensory changes, presenting in a radicular pattern (radiculopathy) with increasing compression
- In advanced cases, lower motor neuron findings, including weakness and diminished reflexes, at the level of compression; below the compression, upper motor neuron signs, including hyperreflexia and spasticity
- Ataxia, clumsiness, diffuse lower extremity weakness, and bowel and bladder problems (i.e., myelopathy) after cervical spine surgery, often related to the following:
  Large central disc (less common)
  Severe, unaddressed osteophytosis (with normal or stenotic canal)
  Hardware displacement
  Postoperative deformity

Postlaminectomy Kyphosis

Patients with postlaminectomy kyphosis present with a history of prior posterior cervical spine surgery and an often subtle, progressive pattern of pain and neurologic change (18):

- Neck pain (75%)
- Severe neck deformity (30%)
- Progressive myelopathy (90%)
- Radiculopathy (50%)

Hardware Failure

Hardware failure may result in any of the symptoms described in this section. In dramatic cases, patients com-

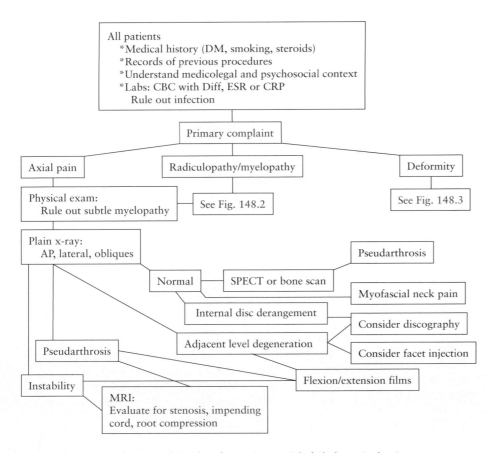

Figure 148.1.   Evaluation algorithm for patients with failed cervical spine surgery.

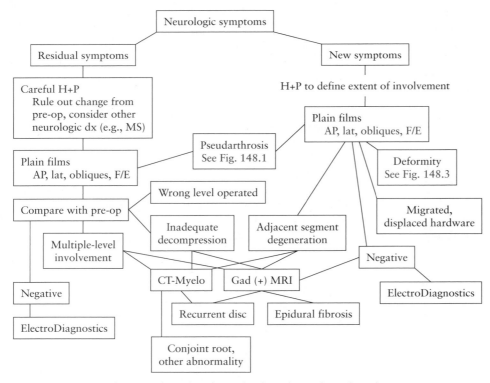

Figure 148.2.   Evaluation algorithm for radiculopathy and myelopathy.

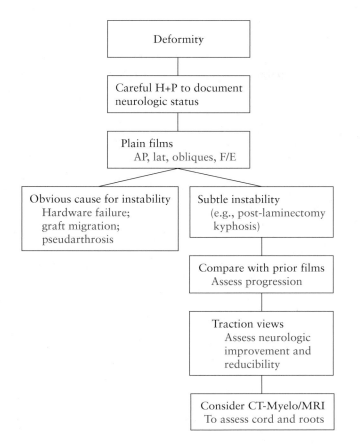

Figure 148.3. Evaluation algorithm for postsurgical deformity.

plain of tracheal or esophageal impingement. Sudden changes in alignment, neurologic status, or pain often indicate failure of hardware. Patients may be aware of a "pop" or acute onset of instability. However, slow pull-out of lateral mass plates, for example, can present with slowly increasing deformity, such as is seen in postlaminectomy kyphosis.

HISTORY AND PHYSICAL EXAMINATION

Understand the patient's spine thoroughly before making treatment decisions. First, obtain complete records of previous procedures and determine the following:

- What types of postoperative immobilization were employed?
- What was the condition of the bone?
- Was allograft or autograft employed?
- Was the PLL resected?

A complete motor and sensory examination is critical. Patients with prior cervical spine surgery are likely to dem-

onstrate complex abnormalities. Perform a detailed and stepwise assessment of sensory, motor, and reflex abnormalities, as well as a careful search for evidence of myelopathy to define new or residual neurologic deficits. Note bowel or bladder changes, gait disturbance, and the unilaterality or bilaterality of symptoms. The following may be a useful checklist:

- Recognize possible aberrant innervation patterns (23).
- Map complex sensory deficits on the skin with a skin marker.
- Chart complex motor and reflex changes.
- Distinguish cervical problems from those of shoulder, cardiac, cranial, or peripheral origin.
- Assess the location and healing of the prior incision(s).
- Assess cervical range of motion (ROM) and neck and body posture.
- Note areas of tenderness and spasticity of paravertebral and anterior strap muscles.

IMAGING STUDIES

Compare plain anteroposterior (AP), lateral, and oblique views with prior studies to assess progression of spondylosis, fusion, deformity, or hardware migration. New degeneration most often presents with narrowing of adjacent disc heights and increase in osteophyte formation. Space available for the cord, from the posterior vertebral body to its lamina, is normally over 17 mm; an AP diameter of less than 13 mm suggests spinal cord compression (12). Oblique views assess the fusion mass, intervertebral foramina, pedicles, and facets, and they show persistent compression due to uncovertebral joint spurring.

If postoperative instability or pseudarthrosis is suspected, flexion–extension lateral films are useful. Dynamic x-rays are also helpful in evaluating new instability secondary to adjacent-level degenerative disc disease. In a patient with postoperative deformity, 5 pounds of axial traction may be used to determine reducibility (15).

Correlate radiographic findings with presenting complaints and physical exam. For example, pseudarthrosis is often difficult to identify. As in the lumbar spine, shingling of the bone mass may obscure the fusion defect (5). Therefore, clinical criteria (intractable neck pain with or without radicular symptoms) must be correlated with radiographic criteria (6). Radiographic signs of pseudarthrosis include the following (6):

- Gross motion at previous fusion site on dynamic radiographs
- Persistence of disc-space lucency
- Graft displacement or failure to incorporate
- No dissolution of endplates
- Hardware failure

Advanced imaging modalities may also prove useful.

Single photon emission computed tomography (SPECT) scanning employs a tomographic camera to remove three-dimensional superimposition from scintigraphic images, thereby improving image contrast and offering more complete spatial information than conventional bone scans. It is increasingly being used to demonstrate increased focal uptake at sites of pseudarthrosis (37).

Computed tomographic myelography demonstrates neural compression indirectly through contour of the dural sac. While myelography is invasive, it is helpful in the presence of spinal deformity. Further, it offers information on conjoint nerve roots and other pathologies not readily appreciated with magnetic resonance imaging (MRI) (23). When spinal instrumentation is in place, myelography may be the only way to visualize neural structures.

Magnetic resonance imaging elucidates disc degeneration and intrinsic changes in the cord. However, major abnormalities are commonly encountered in asymptomatic patients (1). In postoperative patients, gadolinium enhancement reveals recurrent discs as nonenhancing space-occupying lesions, which scar enhances.

Some authors advocate cervical discography for patients with undetermined axial pain, reporting 70% good to excellent results with anterior fusion after concordant discography (41). However, others cite higher failure rates, including one report of 54% fair to poor results (8). These authors cite a 13% complication rate with cervical discography, including one case of acute epidural abscess resulting in quadriplegia. Discography is likely to remain controversial for some time.

Finally, root injections are occasionally used to determine painful levels. Resolution or mitigation of pain indicates specific root-level pathology and the likelihood of surgical relief of symptoms following surgery.

TREATMENT

Principles and operative indications are the same as for patients requiring primary treatment. Early operative treatment should be considered in any patient demonstrating the following:

- Progressive motor or gait impairment
- Persistent disabling pain and weakness (3 months)
- Progressive deformity
- Instability
- Static neurologic deficits with significant axial or radicular pain

Surgery should not be contemplated in patients without consistent findings in both clinical examination and imaging studies. Pseudarthrosis alone, for example, is not an indication for revision surgery. Nonoperative treatment should be fully explored in the majority of "failed neck" patients.

NONOPERATIVE TREATMENT

A trial of nonoperative treatment (Fig. 148.4) is useful even in those patients for whom later surgery is felt to be unavoidable. During this period, develop rapport with the patient, document compliance with prescribed treatment, maximize medical status, and optimize nutritional and smoking status. In certain patients, urine nicotine levels may be obtained.

OPERATIVE PLANNING AND TREATMENT

The operated neck is different in many ways from the "untouched" spine:

- Prior decompression may have rendered the spine unstable.
- Prior fusions create significant lever arms that must be considered in any subsequent construct.
- Surgical soft-tissue injury from the prior surgery interferes with blood supply, healing potential, and local biomechanics.

While many authors report acceptable results with allograft use in both index and revision cervical spine procedures, the decreased vascularity and altered biomechanics of the revision situation are an indication for autograft bone (14).

Anterior Pseudarthrosis

Posterior Repair of Cervical Pseudarthrosis   Posterior fusion for symptomatic anterior pseudarthrosis was proposed by Riley and Robinson (30). The additional stabilization offered by posterior wiring encourages the anterior fusion mass to consolidate. This approach remains the gold standard today, with 94% to 100% union rates reported (4,13,20,34) (Fig. 148.5).

Several randomized, prospective series have been undertaken to compare anterior and posterior treatment of anterior pseudarthrosis (4,22,29). Interestingly, while over 80% of patients treated posteriorly felt better than before surgery, only 70% of those treated circumferentially reported symptomatic improvement. These results argue for a posterior approach unless specific hardware concerns require an anterior approach.

- Use a standard, midline approach to the involved level.
- Several wiring methods may be employed. If the spinous processes are intact, a triple wire technique provides good resistance to torsional and flexion forces (Fig. 148.6).
- If the posterior elements are absent or inadequate, lat-

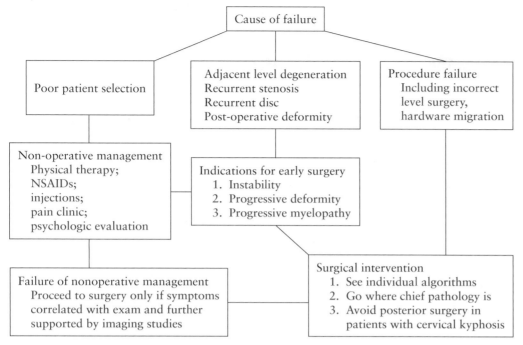

Figure 148.4. Algorithm for treatment of patients with failed anterior surgery.

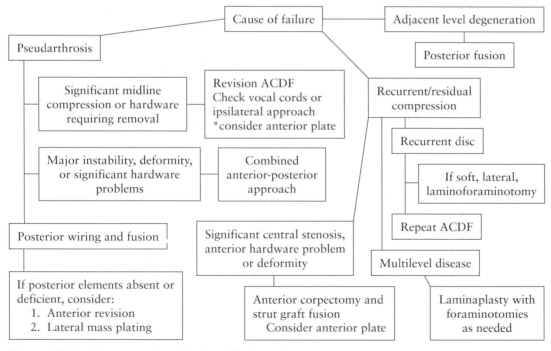

Figure 148.5. Treatment algorithm for failed anterior surgery.

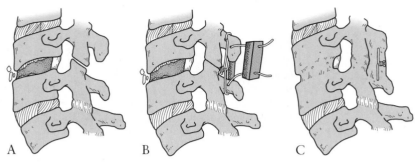

Figure 148.6.   Posterior stabilization for failed anterior cervical discectomy and fusion. **A:** Graft collapse and pseudarthrosis result in focal kyphosis, fragmentation, and instability. **B:** Posterior instrumentation and fusion are carried out without disturbing the anterior graft. The simplest approach is a triple wire technique using autograft bone. Approximate the spinous processes using an 18-gauge interspinous wire applied in a modified Rodger's technique. Apply the split autograft to either side of the intact spinous processes and compress the "sandwich" with a pair of 22-gauge wires. **C:** Posterior wiring will most often cause the anterior graft to consolidate at the same time the posterior fusion is healing.

eral mass plates provide greater resistance to torsional and extension forces.

■ Use lateral mass plates for multisegmental fusions as well.

■ Postoperative immobilization includes a Philadelphia collar for 6–12 weeks.

Anterior Repair of Cervical Pseudarthrosis   An anterior approach to failed anterior cervical fusion is often required in cases of residual radiculopathy, or failed or migrated hardware. Although repeat anterior surgery was felt to have lower success rates than posterior surgery, recent authors, citing modern anterior osteosynthesis techniques, report increased fusion rates with excellent and good results in 83% (9).

Proponents of the repeat anterior approach cite lower rates of wound problems, the biomechanical advantages of anterior column grafting, and the ability to explore the decompression site and to remove any remaining osteophytes. Anterior repair is being increasingly recommended for patients with collapse of a previous anterior graft in conjunction with pseudarthrosis.

Some authors recommend using a contralateral approach to avoid operating through the scarring on the previously approached side. Contralateral exposure should not be carried out until laryngoscopic evaluation of the vocal cords has confirmed that both cords are functioning normally. This approach limits the risk of sequential injury to both recurrent laryngeal nerves.

■ Use a transverse incision to approach the cervical spine in the standard fashion (see Chapter 138).

■ Locate the failed fusion intraoperatively by x-ray.

■ Next, place distraction pins into the superior and inferior vertebral bodies.

■ Once slight distraction is applied, excise residual graft, scar, and fibrous tissue with curets, rongeurs, and a high-speed burr.

■ Carefully contour the superior and inferior endplates with the burr.

For revision surgery, a tricortical block iliac crest autograft is preferred to dowel techniques.

■ Carefully measure the disc space for height, depth, and width.

■ Fashion the graft to fit the distracted disc space by cutting it 2–4 mm longer than the interspace is high.

■ The graft should be at least 5 mm thick to prevent resorption and restore disc space height.

■ To prevent microfracture, cut the iliac crest with a saw rather than osteotomes.

■ Carefully remeasure the graft depth. In smaller patients, a graft depth of 12–14 mm may cause cord impingement. Contour the graft so that it can be countersunk 2 mm below the anterior cortex without impinging on the back rim of the vertebral body.

Revision ACDF is a strong indication for anterior plate osteosynthesis. We use a unicortical fixation system with screws that lock to the plate.

■ Measure the sagittal depth of the vertebral body and preset the drill depth.

■ When drilling, be aware of the endplate angle to avoid penetrating the intervertebral disc space above or below the intended body.

■ Immediately mobilize the patient in a Philadelphia collar (usually worn for 6–12 weeks).

■ When plate fixation is impractical or bony purchase is tenuous, longer postoperative immobilization in a rigid collar or a four-poster brace is advocated. In some circumstances, adjuvant posterior fixation may be employed as well, as mentioned.

Inadequate Decompression

The principles of treatment of residual compression are fairly straightforward. If significant compression remains anteriorly, the approach must be anterior. If significant compression remains posteriorly, the approach must be posterior. Similarly, posterior hardware problems are addressed posteriorly, and so on.

Anterior decompression of residual or recurrent cervical spine disease is indicated in patients with less than three levels of disease. Occasionally, large central osteophytes will militate against posterior decompression in even multilevel spondylosis.

In patients with prior posterior procedures, an anterior procedure for recurrent or residual radiculopathy or myelopathy most often involves anterior corpectomy with strut graft fusion (Fig. 148.7). The likelihood of posterior

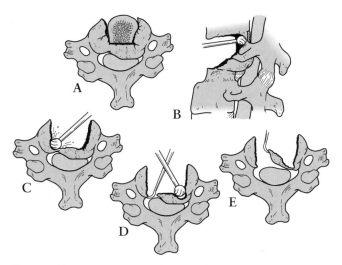

Figure 148.7. Treatment of residual cord compression after inadequate decompression. **A:** In patients who have undergone previous but inadequate surgical treatment, the original compressive lesion is densely consolidated, and access may be hindered by surgical scarring, old hardware, and, often, a well-integrated strut graft. **B:** Remove the strut graft with rongeurs and a high-speed burr, back to the posterior vertebral cortex. Study the preoperative CT scan to determine whether there is a distinct interval between the back of the graft and the residual vertebral body. **C:** Use a burr and microcurets to thin the posterior cortex in the lateral recess of the side with least compression. **D:** Enter the canal with a small curet or elevator directed toward the neural foramen and away from the cord. Thin the compressive mass with the burr, and use a diamond tip burr to thin the lateral recess to eggshell thickness. **E:** Use a small elevator or curet to reflect the residual bone fragments directly away from the canal and spinal cord. Dural adhesions may be divided with a fine Penfield elevator or microcuret.

instability represents a strong indication for anterior plate osteosynthesis in conjunction with well-fashioned struts. In patients with single-level and radicular findings, standard ACDF is recommended. Plate fixation may be helpful in these patients as well (7). Preoperative flexion–extension radiographs will better define the stability of the cervical spine.

Anterior Decompression Techniques for ACDF are discussed in Chapter 143. Anterior cervical corpectomy in the revision situation is discussed in the context of postlaminectomy kyphosis later. Key elements of the anterior decompression procedure include the following:

- Incise the annulus and remove adjacent discs with a pituitary rongeur and a small, angled curet.
- Remove the anterior portion of the vertebral body with rongeurs.
- Carefully thin the posterior cortices with a burr.
- Use a micro-Kerrison rongeur or curets to decompress the cord.
- Fashion a strut graft with iliac crest (two or fewer levels) or use allograft or autograft fibula.
- Contour and apply a plate.
- Use standard closure and postoperative immobilization (as described previously).

Postlaminectomy Kyphosis

Several approaches to postlaminectomy kyphosis have been described. They include anterior corpectomy and fusion, posterior fusion with lateral mass plates, and circumferential procedures (Fig. 148.8).

Correction of postlaminectomy kyphosis begins with preoperative traction. In most cases, moderate correction of the deformity is achieved and fusion is planned to the next normal level above and below the deformity (24,35).

A repeat posterior approach is often limited by inadequate bone stock, and corrective osteotomy through this approach is generally ineffective (2). Anterior cervical corpectomy with strut graft fusion and plating has become the favored approach in all cases without new posterior pathology (35,42,47).

A circumferential approach includes anterior corpectomy with posterior osteotomy and internal fixation (Fig. 148.9). This approach is particularly beneficial in patients with significant anterior instability as well. Generally, the circumferential approach allows for greater correction of the sagittal plane deformity. While reasoning of this surgical approach is sound, the added risks of a second operation make its use less compelling in the majority of postlaminectomy kyphosis patients (10,35).

Herman and Sonntag (18) found that anterior corpectomy and plate yielded a mean correction of only 16° of kyphosis, but that 95% of these patients reported improvement of their presenting complaints. The authors re-

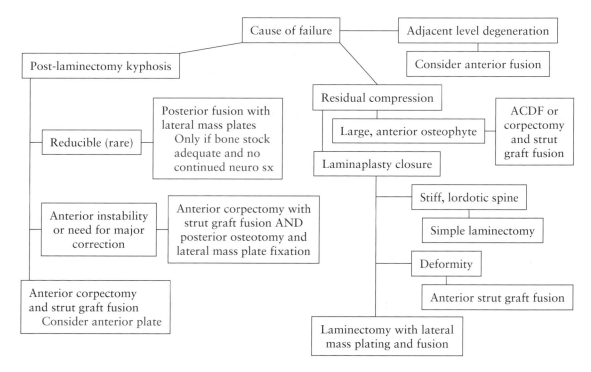

Figure 148.8. Algorithm for treatment of failed posterior cervical spine surgery.

port limited correction of the deformity due to fusions of the remaining levels at the facet and posterior element levels. Moreover, the goals of stabilization and prevention of further progression having been met, 10% reported complete relief of their symptoms and 55% noted substantial improvement.

Combined Approach for Postlaminectomy Kyphosis

- Begin the anterior approach with the patient supine. Tape the shoulders caudally and turn the head slightly away from the operative side. Place a bolster between the shoulders to provide mild hyperextension. A bolster may not be useful in patients with a fixed-flexion deformity due to the wedging of the vertebral bodies.
- A transverse incision may be used in most cases up to five levels. In longer procedures, an extensile incision along the anterior border of the sternocleidomastoid muscle can be used instead. A standard, left-sided approach is recommended.
- Use blunt, finger dissection to dissect the platysma from overlying and underlying tissues.
- Carefully develop the intervals between the tissue planes. This will increase the extensibility of the incision.
- The omohyoid may cross the surgical field, depending on the level of dissection. Division for increased exposure is rarely required.

A variable amount of scar may be seen anteriorly at the apex of the kyphosis (15). This scar may exert a tethering effect. Debridement of the scar will allow increased exposure of the anterior bodies. Overly aggressive lateral dissection threatens the sympathetic chain.

- To achieve correction of the deformity, completely excise the intercalary discs to the level of the PLL.
- Use a rongeur to remove large portions of the intervening bodies.
- Next, use a dental burr to remove bone laterally and posteriorly to the posterior cortex of the body.
- Use fine Kerrisons to remove the cortical wafer from the PLL.
- Once adequate decompression and visualization have been achieved, obtain radiographs to assess correction. Adjust the alignment and traction to achieve lordosis.
- Next, fashion an allograft or autograft fibular strut in the Whitecloud-LaRocca method with an H-shape. For less than two or three levels, iliac crest struts may be used. While crest graft offers a faster incorporation time, fibular graft is stronger in compression.
- Prior to insertion, undercut the endplates of the cranial and caudal vertebra with the burr. This allows the graft to be pushed into position cranially and, with a concurrent extension force on the neck, impacted into the caudal vertebra.

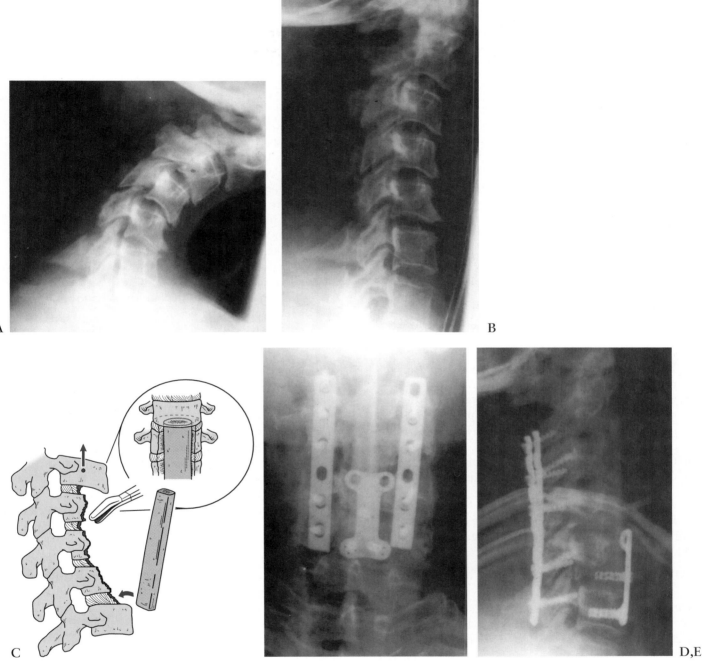

Figure 148.9. Postlaminectomy kyphosis. **A:** This patient presented with progressive pain and deformity 3 months after multilevel cervical laminectomy. The deformity was passively correctable, to a degree, and the patient was neurologically intact. **B:** After 48 hours in halo traction, significant correction was obtained and surgical treatment was initiated. **C:** A staged anteroposterior reconstruction was planned. A five-level anterior vertebrectomy was performed initially, reconstructed with an autograft fibular strut. **D,E:** Five days later, we performed a posterior instrumentation and fusion using lateral mass plates. The slight increase in cervical lordosis produced by the plates caused the anterior strut to loosen and shift. During the same surgical procedure, the graft was repositioned and a short anterior plate placed to buttress the distal pole of the graft. Fusion was successful and the excellent sagittal correction was fully maintained. Figures D & E show anteroposterior and lateral views 1 year after surgery.

- Release the extension moment provided by traction to lock the graft into place.
- Anterior plate osteosynthesis is recommended. In long constructs, a short anterior plate can be applied at the caudal vertebra to buttress the inferior pole of the graft.
- Screws are not placed into the graft because of the risk of graft fracture. A heavy suture may be passed around the graft and the plate to keep the graft from shifting posteriorly.

Once the anterior reconstruction is completed, the patient is turned and prepared for posterior instrumentation and fusion. While this procedure is not necessary in two- or three-level fusions, we routinely add posterior fusion to reconstructions of four or more levels, and to those with poor bone quality, translational instability, or risk factors for pseudarthrosis.

- Expose the posterior cervical spine in the usual fashion, taking care to document levels and protect levels not instrumented anteriorly.
- Use a burr to decorticate the laminae and facets, and remove articular cartilage from the facets with a small curet.
- Use a 2.0 mm drill to prepare pilot holes for lateral mass plating.
- Contour the lateral mass plate to *neutralize* the alignment obtained during the anterior procedure. Increasing lordosis at this point will tend to loosen the anterior construct.
- Graft the facet joints and apply the plates over the graft.
- Close in layers and apply a sterile dressing.

A hard cervical collar is used for 8–12 weeks. Halo immobilization for 12 weeks may be useful in patients with poor bone, previous failures, or multiple-level procedures. These patients may also benefit from a posterior stabilization procedure, often with lateral mass plates.

Hardware Failure

As in pseudarthrosis, not all failed hardware requires surgical intervention. In some cases, external immobilization can be used until fusion occurs. However, when failed hardware results in neurologic or soft-tissue compression, instability, or progressive deformity, surgical treatment is offered.

Anterior hardware impinging on anterior structures must be approached anteriorly. Failed posterior hardware may be approached posteriorly. However, in cases of poor bone quality, deformity, or three-column destabilization, circumferential stabilization procedures are recommended.

Take care when approaching displaced anterior hardware. The inflammation and tissue reaction around the old hardware will make the exposure difficult and will distort tissue planes. Inadvertent entry into the carotid sheath, esophagus, or thoracic duct can result in potentially lethal complications.

After hardware removal, spinal instability must be addressed. In some cases, postoperative halo immobilization suffices. Typically, however, revision internal fixation is employed in conjunction with postoperative immobilization (7).

Failed spinous process wires are easily removed and replaced with lateral mass plates. Sublaminar wires are more problematic, and they may be retained or removed. In cases where dense scar makes dissection difficult, the broken wire may be retightened around the intact lamina and left in place. If monofilament wire must be removed, contour the end to be pulled through the canal so that it can be pulled out smoothly. Place a Woodson or Penfield elevator between the wire and the thecal sack and extract the wire by winding the free end up with a needle-holder. Cut braided wires close to the lamina to remove as much of the frayed portion as possible before trying to remove them.

Adjacent-Level Degeneration and Recurrent Stenosis or Disc Herniation

Adjacent-level degeneration in the cervical spine is related to recurrent compression. Recurrence of stenosis or disc herniation often reflects the same global nature of cervical spondylosis seen in patients with recurrent axial symptoms. Whether or not surgical intervention accelerates degenerative changes at neighboring levels, principles regarding their treatment remain the same.

Treatment options for recurrent disc herniation include ACDF of the new level or posterior keyhole foraminotomy. There are proponents of each approach. In the patient with a previously operated neck, the same principles apply, with the caveat that repeat anterior surgery requires special attention to the status of the recurrent laryngeal nerves and vulnerable soft-tissue structures of the neck (as previously discussed).

When recurrent or residual root compression is the result of soft disc pathology at one or two levels, keyhole foraminotomy may be indicated. Most often, this is seen in patients with a prior ACDF and an incompletely excised disc, or with recurrent soft disc pathology at a neighboring level.

The advantages of keyhole foraminotomy include the avoidance of fusion-related problems and the need for only minimal laminar resection to expose the lateral edge of the dura. Disadvantages include its failure to decompress the cord and stabilize the spine. Laminoforaminotomy is contraindicated in patients with cervical kyphosis or major anterior cord compression (17).

As in primary cervical spine procedures, debate continues as to the best method to treat multilevel recurrent or residual stenosis. Laminaplasty is recommended for recurrent stenosis above and below a previously, anteriorly fused level, or in the case of disease affecting more than three levels (28). Others report success with vertebrectomy and strut graft fusion techniques (42).

Laminaplasty preserves the cervical facets and decreases the incidence of instability associated with multiple-level laminectomies. However, decompression may be incomplete if foraminal stenosis is not addressed. Contraindications include cervical deformity (especially kyphosis) and major anterior cord compression.

Anterior vertebrectomy and strut graft fusion is recommended for patients with recurrent or residual stenosis after laminectomy and in those patients who are not candidates for posterior decompressive laminaplasty.

In patients with no evidence of stenosis and predominantly axial pain, the possibility of adjacent-segment disc degeneration must be considered. Advocates of cervical discography recommend anterior fusion for concordant pain (41).

Keyhole Foraminotomy for Recurrent or Residual Disc Herniation

- With the patient prone, obtain precise radiographic localization prior to skin incision. Employ a standard midline approach with careful, unilateral exposure to the lateral aspect of the facet capsule.
- Thin the lateral portion of the lamina and the medial portion of the facet with a burr.
- Carefully develop the interval between the medial facet capsule and the ligamentum flavum with a fine curved curet or Penfield.
- Remove the medial 25% of the facet with Kerrison rongeurs. Remove the volar facet capsule to visualize the root and the lateral margin of the thecal sack.
- Expand the laminotomy over the junction of the root and dura taking care to preserve over 50% of the facet.
- If a contained herniation is found, incise the PLL to retrieve the fragment.
- Apply a collar for comfort for the first 2–3 weeks after surgery. If more than 50% of both facets, or more than 75% of one facet, is removed, consider fusion with lateral mass plates.

Laminaplasty for Multilevel Residual or Recurrent Stenosis

Open-book laminoplasty requires a wide exposure of the posterior elements and lateral masses of the involved cervical spine, as well as exposure of at least one normal level above and below the compression. The surgeon must elevate laminae at the margins of stenosis as well as those directly over the narrowed segment.

- Through a standard, midline approach, carefully elevate the paraspinal musculature to the lateral edges of the facets.
- Use a high-speed burr to cut longitudinal bone troughs through the lamina–facet junction.
- Use a fine Kerrison punch to complete the trough on the side of primary compression (i.e., at the greatest narrowing or most significant radiculopathy).
- Excise the ligamentum flavum and interspinous ligaments at the proximal and distal junctions of the laminaplasty segment with the normal spine.
- Apply gentle, sustained pressure on the spinous processes and upward on the open laminotomy to elevate the laminar flap on its intact cortical "hinge." Allow the intact lamina to deform plastically, being careful not to snap it off by applying too much force.
- Release dural adhesions to the lamina with a Penfield elevator.
- The lamina flap is then hinged wide open on the intact lamina in a staged fashion, moving cranially from the inferiormost hinged lamina. An elevation of 10–15 mm on the open side increases the sagittal diameter of the canal by 4–5 mm.

There are a number of techniques to keep the laminar flap open (Fig. 148.10). The laminae may be open with cadaver rib graft, as follows.

- Cut three grafts to length (12–14 mm).
- Cut a trough into each end of the graft.
- One graft is inserted between the lamina and lateral mass at C-3, C-5, and C-7.
- To avoid inadvertent fusion, care must be taken to avoid bone graft touching another level.

Often, the cervical spinous processes can be used for this purpose as well, as follows.

- To keep the graft from displacing, pass a heavy suture longitudinally through the cancellous bone of each spinous process or rib allograft. Pass the suture through a small drill hole in the laminar margin and through the medial edge of the facet, and tie it tightly to compress the graft strut between the lamina and the facet margin. The secured strut will keep the flap from closing.
- Supplemental foraminotomies may then be carried out to treat radiculopathy, as needed.
- Close the posterior wound over drains. Reattach the deep layer to the spinous processes at the margins of the laminaplasty. Immobilize in a Philadelphia collar for 6–12 weeks. Some authors recommend a CT scan at 8 weeks to check healing on the hinge side and ensure canal patency. Once healing is complete, physical therapy emphasizing cervical extension exercises is recommended.

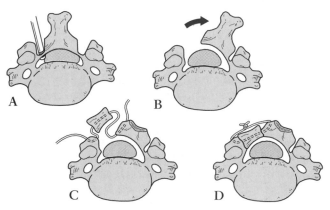

Figure 148.10. Trap-door laminoplasty for extensive stenosis or adjacent-level degeneration. **A:** Cut longitudinal troughs through the involved laminae using a high-speed burr. Troughs should be centered over the medial edge of the facet so that penetration exposes the lateral recess and not the cord. Complete the defect on the side of most compression using a small Kerrison. **B:** Thin the opposite lamina down to the volar cortex, then gradually elevate the opened side up and away from the facet, allowing time for the intact hinge to deform plastically. If the hinge is too stiff, thin it further. **C:** Use the spinous processes or an allograft bone strut to hold the laminoplasty open. Groove both ends of the graft to capture the cut edges of the lamina and the lateral mass. Use a small drill to make holes at the margins of both, and pass a heavy suture through the drill holes and lengthwise through the graft. **D:** Position the strut and allow the lamina to close down slightly to capture the strut. Tie the heavy suture over the outside of the graft to prevent it from migrating into the canal or dislodging and allowing the laminaplasty to close.

GENERAL REHABILITATION AND POSTOPERATIVE PRINCIPLES

Most patients have already been immobilized from their prior cervical spine procedure. Significant deficits in extensor muscle strength and flexibility are common. Therefore, a supervised isometric strengthening and ROM program is indicated prior to returning to unlimited activity. At 12 weeks, or when x-rays demonstrate adequate bony union, prescribe a twice-daily regimen of 10 minutes of neck muscle ROM and isometric strengthening. Weekly physical therapy supervision to monitor progress and add incremental exercises until functional strength and ROM are regained may be recommended.

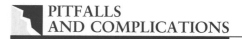

PITFALLS AND COMPLICATIONS

Prior surgery increases the likelihood of complications (Table 148.1). The hypovascular scar bed predisposes to

Table 148.1.   Complications of Revision Anterior Surgery

Vocal cord paralysis	15%
Pneumonia	10%
Deep venous thrombosis	5%
Reintubation	5%
Graft site problems	5%
Hardware failure	5%

From Coric D, Branch CL Jr, Jenkins JD. Revision of Anterior Cervical Pseudarthrosis with Anterior Allograft Fusion and Plating. *J Neurosurg* 1997;86(6):969, and Lowery GL, Swank ML, McDonough RF. Surgical Revision for Failed Anterior Cervical Fusions. Articular Pillar Plating or Anterior Revision? *Spine* 1995;20(22):2436.

infection or failure of healing. Some authors have reported complication rates for anterior surgery following failed posterior procedures similar to those reported in index anterior procedures (42,46,47). However, hardware problems are more likely in osteopenic bone and when normal anatomic landmarks are distorted.

Repeated dissection through anterior soft tissues increases the possibility of transient sore throat or swallowing difficulty. Further, dissection through scar requires meticulous attention to detail and great caution. Perforation of the esophagus is a life-threatening injury, and only one third are recognized at the time of surgery. Mortality for injuries recognized early is 15%. If recognized late, mortality rises to 30% (30,36).

The literature regarding incidence of vocal cord paralysis after revision anterior cervical spine surgery is varied (9,22). Although the ipsilateral operative approach requires dissection through scar, the contralateral approach should not be undertaken without confirming the function of both vocal cords through laryngoscopy.

Other problems related to anterior surgery could be increased in the revision situation as well. Horner's syndrome from injury to the sympathetic chain and overretraction of the longus colli is ostensibly more likely if the longus muscles are encased in scar, or the dissection difficult.

The most common complications of revision posterior cervical spine surgery are wound infection (1.2%) and failure of healing. Correction of identifiable nutritional deficiencies may decrease these problems. The incidence of dural tear also rises when dissecting through posterior scar (16).

REFERENCES

Each reference is categorized according to the following scheme: *, classic article; #, review article; !, basic research article; and +, clinical results/outcome study.

+ 1. Boden SD, McCoun PR, Davis DO, et al. Abnormal Magnetic Resonance Scans of the Cervical Spine in Asymptomatic Subjects. *J Bone Joint Surg Am* 1990;72:1178.

2. Bohlman HH, Dabb B. Anterior and Posterior Cervical Osteotomy. In: Bradford DS, ed. *Master Techniques in Orthopaedic Surgery: The Spine.* Philadelphia: Lippincott-Raven, 1997:75.

+ 3. Bohlman HH, Emery SE, Goodfellow DB, et al. Robinson Anterior Cervical Discectomy and Arthrodesis for Cervical Radiculopathy. Long-term Follow-up of One Hundred and Twenty-two Patients. *J Bone Joint Surg Am* 1993;75:1298.

+ 4. Brodsky AE, Khalil MA, Sassard WR, Newman BP. Repair of Symptomatic Pseudarthrosis of Anterior Cervical Fusion. Posterior versus Anterior Repair. *Spine* 1992;17:1137.

+ 5. Brodsky AE, Kovalsky ES, Khalil MA. Correlation of Radiologic Assessment of Lumbar Spine Fusions with Surgical Exploration. *Spine* 1991;16(suppl 6):S261.

+ 6. Brown MD, Malanin TI, Davis PB. A Roentgenographic Evaluation of Frozen Allografts vs Autografts in Anterior Cervical Spine Fusions. *Clin Orthop* 1976;199:231.

+ 7. Connolly PJ, Esses SJ, Kostuik JP. Anterior Cervical Fusion: Outcome Analysis of Patients Fused With and Without Anterior Cervical Plates. *J Spinal Disord* 1996;9:202.

+ 8. Connor PM, Darden BV II. Cervical Discography Complications and Clinical Efficacy. *Spine* 1993;18:2035.

+ 9. Coric D, Branch CL Jr, Jenkins JD. Revision of Anterior Cervical Pseudarthrosis with Anterior Allograft Fusion and Plating. *J Neurosurg* 1997;86:969.

+ 10. Cybulski GR, Douglas RA, Meyer PR Jr, et al. Complications in Three-column Cervical Spine Injuries Requiring Anterior-posterior Stabilization. *Spine* 1992;17:253.

+ 11. Davis H. Increasing Rates of Cervical and Lumbar Spine Surgery in the United States, 1979–1980. *Spine* 1994;19:1117.

+ 12. Epstein BS, Epstein JA, Jones MD. Cervical Spinal Stenosis. *Radiol Clin North Am* 1977;15:215.

+ 13. Farey ID, McAfee PC, Davis RF, Long DL. Pseudarthrosis of the Cervical Spine after Anterior Arthrodesis. *J Bone Joint Surg Am* 1990;72:1171.

+ 14. Fernyhough JC, White JI, LaRocca H. Fusion Rates in Multilevel Cervical Spondylosis Comparing Allograft Fibula with Autograft Fibula in 126 Patients. *Spine* 1991;16(suppl 10):S561.

+ 15. Fielding WJ, Tolli TC. Surgical Management of Postlaminectomy Kyphosis. *Semin Spine Surg* 1989;1:271.

+ 16. Heller JG, Silcox DH III, Sutterlin CE III. Complications of Posterior Cervical Plating. *Spine* 1995;20:2442.

+ 17. Herkowitz HN, Kurz LT, Overholt DP. Surgical Management of Cervical Soft Disc Herniation. A Comparison between Anterior and Posterior Approaches. *Spine* 1990;15:1026.

+ 18. Herman JH, Sonntag VK. Cervical Corpectomy and Plate Fixation for Postlaminectomy Kyphosis. *J Neurosurg* 1994;80:963.

+ 19. Kozak JA, Hanson GW, Rose JR, et al. Anterior Discectomy, Microscopic Decompression and Fusion. A Treatment for Cervical Spondylotic Radiculopathy. *J Spinal Disord* 1989;2:43.

+ 20. Lindsey RW, Newhouse KE, Leach J, Murphy MJ. Nonunion following Two-level Anterior Cervical Discectomy and Fusion. *Clin Orthop* 1987;223:155.

+ 21. Lonstein JE. Post-laminectomy Kyphosis. *Clin Orthop* 1977;128:93.

+ 22. Lowery GL, Swank ML, McDonough RF. Surgical Revision for Failed Anterior Cervical Fusions. Articular Pillar Plating or Anterior Revision? *Spine* 1995;20:2436.

! 23. Marzo JM, Simmons EH, Kallen F. Intradural Connections between Adjacent Cervical Spinal Roots. *Spine* 1987;12:964.

+ 24. Mikawa Y, Shikata J, Yamamuro T. Spinal Deformity and Instability after Multilevel Cervical Laminectomy. *Spine* 1987;12:6.

+ 25. Miyakazi K, Tada K, Matsuda T, et al. Posterior Extensive Simultaneous Multisegment Decompression with Posterior Lateral Fusion for Cervical Myelopathy with Cervical Instability and Kyphotic and/or S-shaped Deformities. *Spine* 1989;14:1160.

+ 26. Murphy MG, Gado M. Anterior Cervical Discectomy without Interbody Bone Graft. *J Neurosurg* 1972;37:71.

! 27. Nolan JP, Sherk HH. Biomechanical Evaluation of the Extensor Musculature of the Cervical Spine. *Spine* 1988;13:9.

+ 28. Nowinski GP, Visarius H, Nolte LP, Herkowitz HN. A Biomechanical Comparison of Cervical Laminaplasty and Cervical Laminectomy with Progressive Facetectomy. *Spine* 1993;18:1995.

+ 29. Raynor R. Anterior or Posterior Approach to the Cervical Spine. An Anatomical and Radiographic Evaluation and Comparison. *Neurosurgery* 1983;12:7.

+ 30. Riley LH, Robinson RA, Johnson KA, Walker E. The Results of Anterior Interbody Fusion of the Cervical Spine. *J Neurosurg* 1969;30:127.

+ 31. Robertson PA, Ryan MD. Neurologic Deterioration after Reduction of Cervical Subluxation. Mechanical Compression by Disc Tissue. *J Bone Joint Surg Br* 1992;74:224.

+ 32. Robinson RA, Walker AE, Ferlic DC, et al. The Results of an Anterior Interbody Fusion of the Cervical Spine. *J Bone Joint Surg Am* 1962;44:1569.

+ 33. Schellhaus KP, Smith MD, Gundry CR, Pollei SR. Cervical Discogenic Pain. Prospective Correlation of Magnetic Resonance Imaging and Discography in Asymptomatic Subjects and Pain Sufferers. *Spine* 1994;21:300.

+ 34. Shinomiya K, Okamoto A, Kamikozuru M, et al. An Analysis of Failures in Primary Cervical Anterior Spinal Cord Decompression and Fusion. *J Spinal Disord* 1993;6:277.

+ 35. Sim FH, Svien HJ, Bickel WH, et al. Swan-neck Deformity following Extensive Cervical Laminectomy. A Review of Twenty-one Cases. *J Bone Joint Surg Am* 1974; 56:564.

+ 36. Simmons EN, Bhalla SK. Anterior Cervical Discectomy and Fusion. *J Bone Joint Surg Br* 1969;51:225.

+ 37. Slizofski WJ, Collier BD, Flatley TJ, et al. Painful Pseud-arthrosis following Lumbar Spinal Fusion. Detection by Combined SPECT and Planar Bone Scintigraphy. *Skeletal Radiol* 1987;16:136.

+ 38. Stevens JM, Clifton AG, Whitiar P. Appearance of Posterior Osteophyte After Sound Anterior Interbody Fusion in the Cervical Spine. A High Definition CT Study. *Neuroradiology* 1993;35:227.

+ 39. Tachdjian MO, Matson DD. Orthopaedic Aspects of Intraspinal Tumors in Infants and Children. *J Bone Joint Surg Am* 1965;47:243.

40. White AA, Panjabi MM. *Clinical Biomechanics of the Spine*, 2nd ed. Philadelphia: JB Lippincott, 1990.

+ 41. Whitecloud TS, Seago RA. Cervical Discogenic Syndrome: Results of Operative Intervention in Patients with Positive Discography. *Spine* 1987;12:313.

+ 42. Whitecloud TS III. Anterior Surgery for Cervical Spondylotic Myelopathy. Smith-Robinson, Cloward and Vertebrectomy. *Spine* 1988;13:861.

+ 43. Winter CY, Brannstein EM, Bailey WR. Radiographic Changes following Anterior Cervical Fusion. *Spine* 1980;5:399.

+ 44. Wu W, Thuomas KA, Hedlund R, et al. Degenerative Changes following Anterior Cervical Discectomy and Fusion Evaluated by Fast Spin-echo MR Imaging. *Acta Radiol* 1996;37:614.

+ 45. Yonenobu K, Okada K, Fuji T, et al. Causes of Neurologic Deterioration following Surgical Treatment of Cervical Myelopathy. *Spine* 1986;11:818.

+ 46. Zdeblick TA, Bohlman HH. Cervical Kyphosis and Myelopathy. Treatment by Anterior Corpectomy and Strutgrafting. *J Bone Joint Surg Am* 1989;71:170.

+ 47. Zdeblick TA, Ducker TB. The Use of Freeze-dried Allograft Bone for Anterior Cervical Fusions. *Spine* 1991; 16:726.

CHAPTER 149

MANAGEMENT OF THE PATIENT WITH FAILED LOW-BACK SURGERY

William C. Lauerman and Sam W. Wiesel

Management of the patient with recurrent or residual back pain following previous surgery on the lumbar spine is a complex challenge. It is estimated that, in the United States alone, more than 300,000 lumbar laminectomies and 70,000 fusions are performed annually; at least 15% of these patients fail to achieve long-lasting pain relief (15, 36).

An individual in whom prior surgery has failed represents a unique challenge and opportunity; many patients

---

W. C. Lauerman: Associate Professor, Department of Orthopaedic Surgery, Chief, Division of Spine Surgery, Georgetown University Hospital, Washington, D.C., 20007.
S. W. Wiesel: Professor and Chairman, Department of Orthopaedic Surgery, Georgetown University Hospital, Washington, D.C., 20007.

can be made better with appropriate operative or nonoperative treatment, but there is a great chance of succumbing to the assumption that another operation, in the absence of objective indications, will be the solution to the patient's problem. The inherent complexity of these cases necessitates an approach to evaluation that is precise and unambiguous—one that, it is hoped, will lead to accurate identification of the source of the patient's pain and to appropriate treatment.

The best solution for failed low-back surgery is prevention. Although the technical aspects of performing surgery on the lumbar spine are very important, proper patient selection is probably the most important factor in avoiding postoperative failure (see Chapter 144). Long et al. (25) reviewed 78 patients with so-called failed back surgery syndrome (FBSS) in a chronic pain program. They noted that, when original records were reviewed from before the first operation, 68% of these patients failed to fulfill any objective criteria available in either the orthopaedic or neurosurgical literature for surgery. Fifty-six percent were found to have an underlying psychiatric abnormality.

They concluded that improper patient selection was the most common factor associated with failure. Thus, it is clear that the initial decision to operate is the most important one and should be arrived at only when clear identification of the source of the patient's pain is made and objective criteria for the proposed surgery are met. See the objective patient evaluation system in Chapter 144. Once low-back surgery has failed, the potential for a solution is limited.

In evaluating recurrent symptoms following surgery, distinguish between a mechanical source for the complaint from nonmechanical causes. The types of mechanical conditions that respond, in select cases, to revision surgery include recurrent disc herniation, discogenic pain, segmental instability of the spine, and spinal stenosis. Nonmechanical entities that can lead to recurrent symptoms include local scar tissue formation (either arachnoiditis or epidural fibrosis), abdominal or pelvic disorders, systemic medical diseases, or psychosocial instability. These nonmechanical problems will not be helped by additional spinal surgery.

The keystone of successful treatment is to obtain an accurate diagnosis. Although this factor is seemingly obvious, this essential step is often neglected and the rehabilitation of the patient is therefore inadequate.

EVALUATION AND IMAGING

A structured approach to the evaluation of the patient with recurrent symptoms following previous lumbar spine surgery is essential. Use a standardized form to detail the medical history and to list any and all previous back operations, including dates and the type of operation performed. Consider obtaining previous operative notes. The symptom complex before the original operation can help to determine the appropriateness of the procedure itself.

It is also useful to know the extent of postoperative pain relief and the length of the pain-free interval to determine the source of the patient's current pain. No relief of preoperative sciatica suggests failure to relieve root compression, which may be due to a retained disc fragment, surgery at the wrong level, or an improper original diagnosis. If the patient relates that the preoperative sciatica was relieved, note the percentage of relief and duration of that improvement. A pain-free interval of more than 6 months, and certainly more than 12 months, suggests that the patient's pain may be caused by recurrent

disc herniation. A pain-free interval lasting only 2 to 6 months, particularly with the gradual recurrence of symptoms, suggests that epidural fibrosis may be the cause of the pain (13).

Also, record the number of previous operations on the lumbar spine. It is well documented that each subsequent operation, almost regardless of the diagnosis or procedure, carries a poorer prognosis for an eventual good result. This fact alone does not mean that a patient's fifth or even sixth operation, in the presence of clear-cut objective indications of nerve root compression or instability, might not be beneficial. The surgeon and patient need to be aware, however, of the diminishing statistical likelihood of success with each successive surgery. It has been shown that second operations have only, on average, a 50% chance of success, and in patients undergoing a third or more operation, symptomatic worsening is as likely as symptomatic improvement (37).

Finally, evaluate the patient's pain pattern. If leg pain predominates, a herniated disc or spinal stenosis is most likely, although scar tissue is also a possibility. Predominance of back pain suggests segmental instability, discogenic back pain, or perineural scar tissue. Mechanical symptoms—with clear-cut worsening of the pain with sitting and standing, and relief at rest—point more toward instability or discogenic back pain, whereas pain at rest suggests scar tissue, or the remote possibility of tumor or infection. The presence of back and leg pain may be due to spinal stenosis or scar tissue.

On physical examination, note the neurologic findings and the existence of any tension signs, such as a positive straight-leg raise test or femoral nerve stretch test. Obtain the results of any dependable previous examination and compare the patient's preoperative and postoperative status. If the neurologic picture is unchanged from before the previous surgery, and tension signs are negative, mechanical pressure is unlikely. If, however, a new neurologic deficit has occurred since the last surgery, or if tension signs are present, nerve root compression is often found. The presences of a tension sign is not necessarily pathognomonic for mechanical nerve root compression because epidural or perineural fibrosis can result in a tension sign.

Finally, review previous imaging studies, including, when possible, those that led to the original decision for surgery. These studies may give valuable information as to the appropriateness of the original procedure, as well as the etiology of the current problem.

The most helpful initial study is plain radiography, which may reveal the extent of the laminectomy defect, the level of the previous operation, changes consistent with spinal stenosis, and evidence of instability on dynamic films. Perform plain films and dynamic films with the patient standing (weight bearing). Assess any evidence of abnormal motion, progressive deformity, or progressive anterolisthesis (Fig. 149.1). Plain radiographs, includ-

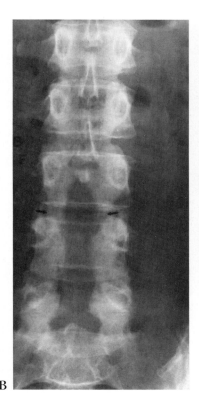
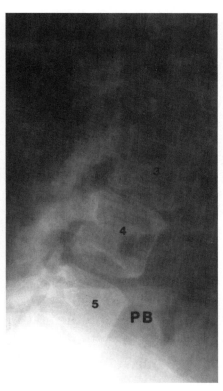

A,B

Figure 149.1. A 49-year-old woman approximately 1 year after a decompressive laminectomy, with worsening low-back pain and recurrent leg pain. **A:** The AP view demonstrates the extent of the laminectomy defect (*arrows*). **B:** On the lateral view, subluxation of L-3 on L-4, not present before surgery, is seen, demonstrating postlaminectomy instability.

ing dynamic views, also help assess the quality of any fusion mass that may be present. On a lateral view, a successful interbody fusion is indicated by the continuity of bone between the outer margins of the adjacent vertebral bodies. A posterior fusion mass can be difficult to evaluate, particularly at L5–S1; a Ferguson anteroposterior (AP) view (with the x-ray beam tilted cephalad 30° to run parallel to the L5–S1 disc space) highlights the fusion mass between the L-5 transverse processes and the sacral alae.

Indirect evidence of nonunion includes hardware failure such as screw loosening or breakage, rod breakage, progressive deformity across the fused levels, and evidence of motion on lateral flexion and extension views. Plain radiographs are relatively sensitive (90% to 95%) but fairly nonspecific (37% to 60%) in detecting pseudarthrosis following lumbar spine fusion (2,6).

In this setting, metrizamide myelography can still be of value. Although extradural compression is well seen on myelography, distinction between the presence of disc material and epidural scar formation is limited (8). Myelography is most helpful in confirming the diagnosis of arachnoiditis when it is otherwise uncertain.

Postmyelographic computed tomography (CT) has increased sensitivity for demonstrating changes of arachnoiditis. We still use it quite frequently in assessing spinal stenosis in a patient who has undergone previous surgery.

The size of the spinal canal, the presence of bony defects and the extent of posterior element resection, and hypertrophic bony changes causing stenosis are all well visualized (Fig. 149.2) (34).

CT scanning is quite useful in evaluating postoperative hardware placement. Although metallic scatter diminishes the quality of the images, careful scrutiny of the bony windows following plain CT scanning can usually establish whether or not a screw has broken out of the pedicle (usually medial) and is causing nerve root compression.

Magnetic resonance imaging (MRI) is, with rare exception, the most helpful diagnostic tool for imaging the lumbar spine that has previously undergone surgery. The most noteworthy use of MRI has been in the diagnosis of recurrent disc herniation, using images obtained before and after the injection of intravenous paramagnetic contrast material (Gadolinium-DTPA). MRI has 100% sensitivity, 71% specificity, and 89% accuracy (19). A nonenhancing soft-tissue mass causing nerve root compression is strongly suggestive of recurrent disc herniation, whereas Gd-DTPA enhancement suggests the presence of scar tissue (Fig. 149.3).

It should be noted that in the first 6 months following surgery, gadolinium-enhanced MRI frequently demonstrates pathologic changes and may suggest recurrent disc herniation, despite a good clinical result. Take care not to overinterpret gadolinium MRI in the early postoperative

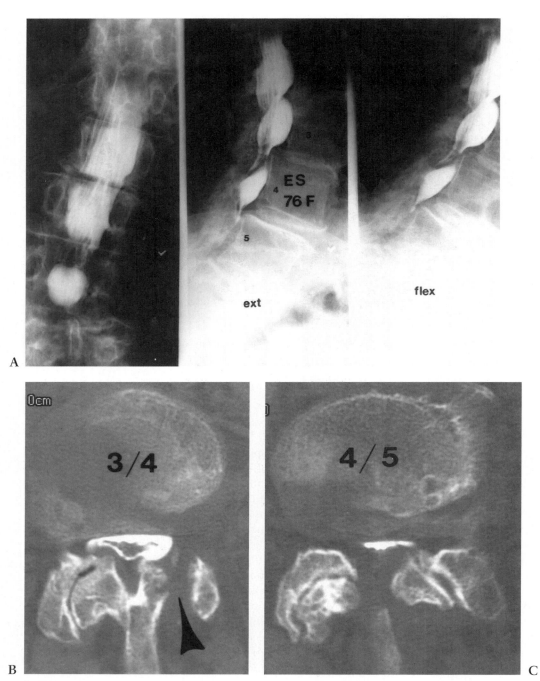

Figure 149.2. A 76-year-old woman, 9 months after a left L3–L4 hemilaminectomy, with persistent back and leg pain. This shows AP and lateral flexion and extension views with myelography (**A**) Multi-level stenosis, most severe at L3–L4 and L4–L5; (**B** and **C**) axial postmyelogram CT images, which clearly define the pathologic anatomy. The failure of the previous decompression to address the pathology is appreciated (*arrowhead*).

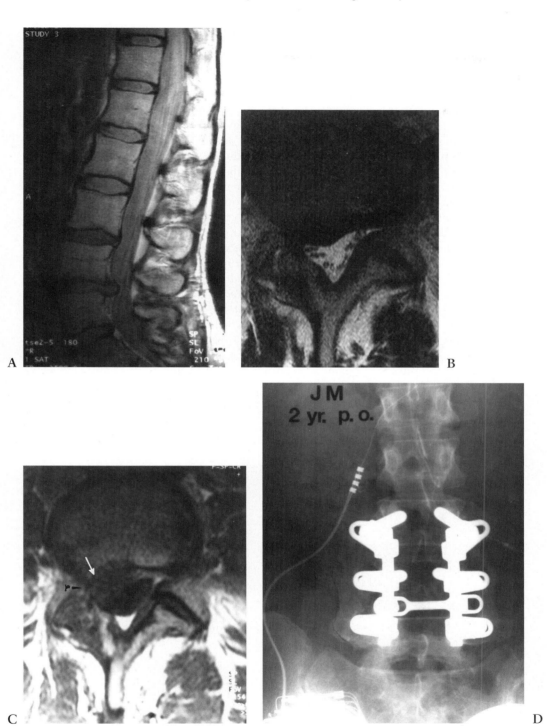

Figure 149.3. A 37-year-old woman with a history of three previous discectomies who had recurrent, severe right leg pain, numbness, and a positive straight-leg raising sign. (**A**) The sagittal MRI demonstrates an apparent disc herniation at L4–L5; (**B**) the axial T2 image, without contrast, through the L4–L5 disc space demonstrates a soft-tissue mass consistent with disc herniation; (**C**) the T1 image, following contrast administration. The absence of contrast-enhancement of the mass (*white arrow*) is diagnostic of recurrent disc herniation, rather than epidural fibrosis; (**D**) a solid fusion 2 years following repeat discectomy and fusion; the patient continued to have significant back pain.

period; overreliance on this study may lead to negative findings on repeat surgical exploration (4).

MRI is also extremely sensitive for identifying inflammatory processes such as discitis, and in fact, it is the test of choice when a postoperative disc space infection is suspected. Decreased signal intensity in the disc on the T1-weighted images and increased signal on the T2-weighted images, particularly with enhancement following Gd-DTPA injection, all suggest an inflammatory process (28).

A final use for MRI is for the definition of noninflammatory degenerative changes in the lumbar discs. Although the significance of disc degeneration in the lumbar spine remains controversial, MRI unquestionably gives the best picture of the discs involved with degenerative changes, the extent of disc desiccation, bulging, and reactive changes in the vertebral bodies. It may be beneficial in the evaluation of a patient with persistent mechanical back pain following a lumbar discectomy in whom discogenic back pain is considered a potential diagnosis (18).

Discography is occasionally used in the evaluation of the patient whose previous back surgery has failed. The indication for discography is to assess the reproduction of the patient's characteristic pain on disc injection and to compare it with the injection of control levels above and below. It should be stressed that, although discography gives a clear picture of abnormal disc morphology, this information rarely contributes meaningfully to surgical decision making and should not be used except in the context of reproduction of the patient's pain.

The role of discography in identifying the pain generator continues to be debated. Proponents believe that reproduction of pain during disc injection, in a manner and distribution concordant with the patient's characteristic pain complaints, identifies that disc as the source of the pain (Fig. 149.4). Conflicting reports regarding the specificity of discography have appeared, with Holt in 1968 reporting a false-positive rate of 37% (17), compared with Walsh et al., who recently noted no false-positive results in their study of normal subjects (38).

Suffice it to say that discography remains controversial, with its ability to predict the pain generator as well as to predict the results of surgical intervention still unproven. We agree with the North American Spine Society position statement on discography, which advocates discography only in the evaluation of a patient with unremitting spinal pain of more than 4 months' duration and only when the

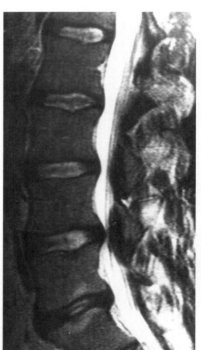
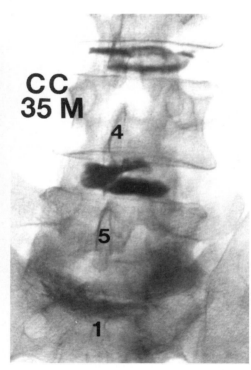
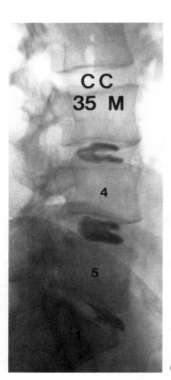

A,B   C

Figure 149.4.   A 35-year-old man, 3 years following right L5–S1 discectomy, with persistent incapacitating back and right buttock pain. (**A**) This is a T2-weighted MRI demonstrating degeneration of the disc, with reactive changes in the adjacent vertebrae; (**B** and **C**) AP and lateral discographic images. Injection of the L5–S1 disc reproduced the patients characteristic back and buttock symptoms, whereas injection at L4–L5 and L3–L4 discs was only minimally uncomfortable.

patient and physician have decided that surgical treatment is under consideration (29).

DIFFERENTIAL DIAGNOSIS

Burton et al. (7) have described the conditions that contribute to FBSS, including recurrent or persistent disc herniation (12% to 16%), lateral (58%) or central (7% to 14%) stenosis, arachnoiditis (1% to 16%), epidural fibrosis (6% to 8%), and instability (5%). Superimposed on many of these conditions is discogenic back pain, a relatively common cause of back or leg pain following surgery.

NONORTHOPAEDIC CONSIDERATIONS

First, rule out nonorthopaedic or systemic causes of pain such as pancreatitis, diabetes mellitus, or an abdominal aortic aneurysm. Other systemic disorders to be considered include fibromyalgia, ankylosing spondylitis, and osteoporosis or osteomalacia.

Also, assess the patient's psychosocial makeup. Identify specific factors such as alcoholism, drug dependence, depression, and the presence of compensation or litigation issues. Strongly weigh such factors when calculating the risk–benefit ratio of surgery. People with profound emotional disturbances and those involved in litigation rarely derive significant benefit from additional surgery (37). Even in the face of a specific orthopaedic diagnosis, make every attempt to address psychosocial problems such as drug dependence and depression before considering further surgery; in many cases, once a patient's underlying problem has been successfully treated, the somatic back complaints and disability improve.

HERNIATED INTERVERTEBRAL DISC

Three possibilities exist if the patient's pain is caused by a herniated disc. First, the disc that caused the original symptoms may not have been completely removed, as can occur if the surgery was performed at the wrong level, if inadequate decompression was performed, or if a fragment of disc material was simply left behind. The predominant complaint is leg pain, and the neurologic findings, tension signs, and radiographic pattern remain unchanged from presurgical findings. The distinguishing feature is that there is typically no pain-free interval; this patient will have awakened from surgery complaining of the same pain that he or she had preoperatively. Patients in this group are helped by a correctly performed discectomy.

A second possibility is a recurrent disc herniation at the previously decompressed level. In this case patients complain of recurrence of sciatica and have similar neurologic findings and tension signs. The distinguishing characteristic in this group is the presence of a well-defined pain-free interval that is usually of 6 months' duration or longer. The diagnosis is confirmed with gadolinium-enhanced MRI; a recurrent disc herniation is avascular, with only a thin enhancing rim at the periphery of the lesion (19). If nonoperative treatment fails, repeat discectomy is indicated in this group of patients.

Finally, a disc herniation may occur at a completely different level or on the opposite side. In this case, patients will also describe a pain-free interval of 6 months or longer following their original surgery. Otherwise the development of their symptoms, with leg pain predominating, is similar to that for a typical disc herniation. A tension sign is usually present, as are appropriate neurologic findings. A neurologic deficit should be different from that associated with the original operation, because the source of the pain is compression of a different nerve root. Repeat surgery in these patients has the same prognosis as a primary discectomy.

LUMBAR SPINAL STENOSIS

Lumbar spinal stenosis (LSS) in patients who have had previous back surgery can result in either back or leg pain but typically causes both. The etiology may be progression of the patient's underlying degenerative spine disorder, failure to decompress the patient's stenosis adequately at the time of the original operation, overgrowth of a previous posterior fusion mass, or transition syndrome.

Transition syndrome refers to the development of degenerative changes and frequently instability at a level adjacent to a previous lumbar fusion. The patient's report of a pain-free interval will vary when LSS is the cause of the symptoms; failure to recognize and relieve stenosis at the time of the original procedure may result in no pain-free interval whatsoever. Alternatively, a period of months or even many years may pass before stenosis develops in a patient who has undergone an otherwise successful operation.

In general, the history and physical examination of patients with postoperative LSS do not differ significantly from those of patients without prior surgery. Back and leg pain are typically seen. Worsening of the leg symptoms with walking or standing is a common finding, but not essential to the diagnosis, and many patients with LSS do not report neurogenic claudication. A normal neurologic examination is common, and neurologic findings, when present, are usually subtle. Tension signs are usually negative (14,33).

The plain radiographs can be suggestive of LSS, and they may display facet degeneration, decreased interpedicular distance, decreased sagittal canal diameter, and disc degeneration. Degenerative spondylolisthesis and degenerative scoliosis are commonly seen in patients with stenosis of the spinal canal and lateral recesses. Neuroradiographic imaging of the postoperative patient with suspected LSS may be accomplished using plain CT, postmyelographic CT, or MRI.

Advantages of MRI include the ability to image sagittal and parasagittal views of the thecal sac and foraminal narrowing, and to identify disc degeneration, which may be helpful in planning for a fusion. Its sensitivity in identifying other causes of back pain in this population, including metastatic disease and occult infection, is also an advantage. State-of-the-art technology in MRI has provided sufficient bony detail to diagnose adequately facet overgrowth, osteophyte formation, and other causes of LSS in most patients. This is our routine test of choice (Fig. 149.5). In some patients with previous surgery, however, it is helpful to use postmyelographic CT scanning, which still provides better bony detail and shows encroachment on the thecal sac and on the nerve roots in the lateral recesses and foramina. Postmyelographic CT is not as specific as MRI in identifying and differentiating postoperative scar tissue from normal soft tissue, when differentiation is a consideration (5).

The properly selected patient with symptomatic LSS, having failed nonoperative treatment, has at least a 70% chance of obtaining satisfactory results following surgery. If nonoperative treatment is unsuccessful, thorough decompression of any bony or soft-tissue compression is

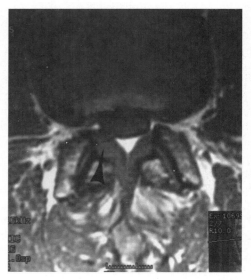

Figure 149.5. A 52-year-old man with recurrent back and right leg pain 8 years following a lumbar decompression and fusion from L4–S1. On T1-weighted axial MR images, right lateral recess stenosis at L2–L3 (*arrows*) is clearly demonstrated. Following repeat decompression and extension of his fusion to L-2 he had near-complete pain relief.

likely to relieve symptoms significantly. If, however, a significant component of the compression is due to epidural fibrotic scar, then the results of surgery are far less predictable. Patients undergoing repeat decompression who have either pre-existing instability or in whom instability may result from the decompression should also undergo a posterolateral fusion at the involved levels (20).

SEGMENTAL INSTABILITY

Lumbar instability is a poorly understood condition that can cause mechanical back pain following previous surgery. Instability results from the spinal motion segment's inability to bear physiologic loads; the result is abnormal motion between two vertebrae (42). Most commonly, it causes back pain, but leg pain or neurologic findings from dynamic stenosis may also be seen.

The diagnosis can be made on the basis of excessive motion on flexion and extension radiographs or by the development or worsening of spinal deformity (Fig. 149.6). Instability following lumbar spine surgery may be the result of a pre-existing condition, as in a patient with spondylolisthesis treated with decompression alone, or it may be the result of an excessively wide or aggressive decompression. It is not uncommon to see either frontal or sagittal plane instability occur in a patient who has had unilateral thinning of the inferior facet and pars, resulting in facet fracture (16). Unilateral facet resection is commonly believed to be benign, but this degree of resection in the presence of an incompetent disc, particularly after an extensive discectomy, may lead to instability. Another sign of instability would be painful motion occurring at the site of a pseudarthrosis.

Patients with instability complain predominantly of back pain, although 20% to 25% report radiating leg symptoms with weight bearing. The physical examination is frequently negative, although some patients have a characteristic reversal of normal spinal rhythm on return from forward bending (30). A key to diagnosis in these patients is the plain radiograph. Weight-bearing lateral flexion and extension views are diagnostic for instability when they demonstrate

- Sagittal plane translation greater than 12% of the AP diameter of the vertebral body,
- Relative sagittal plane rotation greater than 11°,
- Sagittal translation greater than 25% at L5–S1,
- Relative rotation greater than 19° (4).

Although these criteria represent absolute evidence of instability, indirect evidence may be seen in the patient who following surgery has developed

- Progressive deformity in either the sagittal or frontal planes;
- Short-segment angular collapse at the level of the decompression.

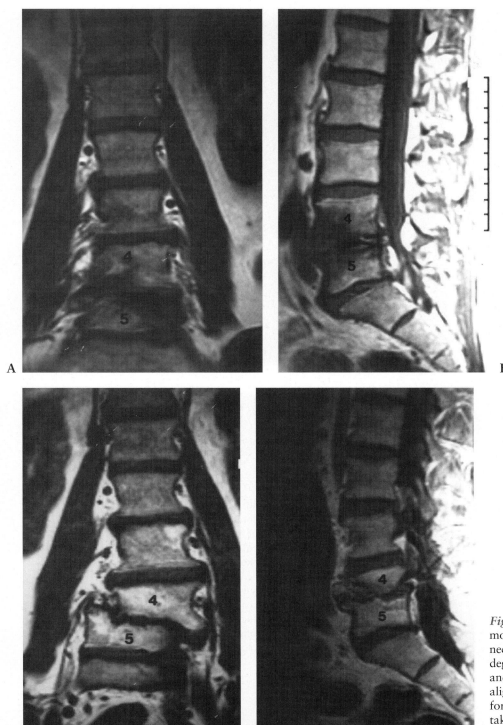

A

B

C,D

Figure 149.6. A 53-year-old man 18 months following a decompressive laminectomy at L4–L5, with discectomy, for degenerative stenosis. (**A** and **B**) Coronal and sagittal MRIs demonstrating the alignment of his lower lumbar spine before surgery; (**C** and **D**) similar images taken 16 months later, demonstrating progressive development of deformity, indicative of instability.

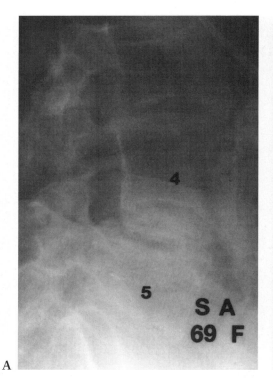

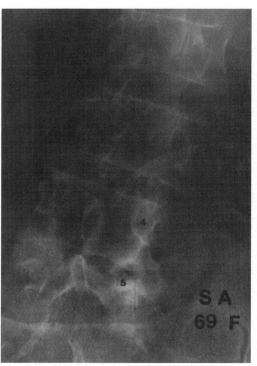

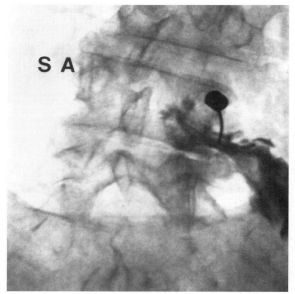

Figure 149.7. A 69-year-old woman who underwent two prior laminectomies at L4–L5 with no relief of her right buttock pain. (**A** and **B**) Lateral and PA views of the lumbar spine. The frontal view demonstrates asymmetric collapse on the right at L4–L5; (**C**) a captured image during selective nerve root infiltration of the L-4 root, which completely relieved her pain, strongly suggesting that L-4 root compression was the cause of the symptoms.

Frontal plane segmental collapse is seen commonly with postoperative instability and may result in dynamic stenosis, with leg pain resulting from root compression in the concavity of the collapse (Fig. 149.7). Scrutinize the plain AP radiograph for evidence of extensive or excessive resection of the posterior elements, such as the pars interarticularis and facet joints, which can lead to instability.

If there is radiographic evidence of instability in a symptomatic patient, spinal fusion, facet injections, or discography may help clarify the precise origin of the patient's symptoms. Rule out other possible causes of back pain before performing repeat surgery.

DISCOGENIC BACK PAIN

Degeneration of the disc may result in ongoing back pain in as many as 14% of patients who have had previous back surgery (15). Although the exact etiology of this pain may vary, a certain subset of patients is believed to suffer from primary disc-related or discogenic pain. The existence of this entity continues to be debated, as does a reliable method of diagnosis. The difficulty in arriving conclusively at the diagnosis of discogenic back pain is magnified in the patient who has had prior back surgery because of the potential contributions of instability, epidural fibrosis, and generalized deconditioning.

In our experience, the typical patient with discogenic back pain following previous surgery had a history of leg pain as well as significant back pain before the initial operation. A period of improvement in leg pain following the surgery is noted, but very often the back pain continues unabated or even worsens. Gradual worsening of the leg pain is frequently reported, although this symptom may be related to epidural fibrosis. The pain is typically relieved by rest. Generalized limitation of motion of the lumbar spine is seen on examination, but otherwise the physical examination is usually unremarkable.

Evaluate the patient radiographically with plain films including dynamic views to rule out instability. MRI, with or without gadolinium, may demonstrate disc degeneration at the previous surgical site, and possibly at other levels of the lumbar spine.

Modic et al. (27) have described three types of signal changes in the vertebral bodies adjacent to a degenerated disc degeneration. Type I changes show decreased T1 intensity and increased T2 intensity, which correlates histologically with disruption and fissuring of the endplate and vascularized fibrous tissue within the marrow of the vertebral body. These changes, which can be suggestive of vertebral osteomyelitis, can be differentiated from infection by the absence of increased signal intensity on T2-weighted images.

Type II changes have strong signal intensity on both T1- and T2-weighted images. Histologically, these changes represent yellow marrow replacement in the vertebral body. Finally, Type III changes show decreased signal intensity on both T1- and T2-weighted images, reflecting relative absence of marrow in the vertebral body; this finding correlates with bony sclerosis seen on plain radiographs. The significance of these discogenic changes in the vertebral bodies, as seen on MRI, has not been clearly defined; such changes, when present, would suggest that the intervening disc is the source of the pain.

Next, perform pain provocation discography. Because of the invasive nature of the procedure and the potential risks, in particular discitis, perform discography only in patient's in whom you are considering fusion and they have agreed to proceed. The morphologic picture seen with contrast injection typically correlates closely with the MRI of disc degeneration, but it is the patient's report of reproduction of his or her characteristic pain that is essential in attempting to determine that a given disc is the pain generator. Do not use extensive sedation during the test because it renders the patient's feedback meaningless. It is also important to inject three or even four levels to find at least one control level. If every level injected reproduces the patient's pain pattern, then the test result is unreliable, and surgery based on this discogram is less likely to result in adequate pain relief.

If one or two degenerated levels can be identified as clearly reproducing the patient's characteristic pain pattern, then the patient may be a candidate for surgery. It should be noted there is no conclusive evidence that a confirmatory discography can predict surgical success. The patient and surgeon should be aware that no spine-fusion technique for discogenic back pain has been conclusively shown to have a high success rate.

In the carefully selected patient, we favor interbody fusion (see Chapter 146) rather than relying solely on posterolateral fusion. These techniques are in evolution, but success depends on using abundant autologous iliac bone graft with adequate graft–endplate contact, adequate stabilization provided by the implant, and a minimum of destruction of normal anatomy. Available techniques include

- Transforaminal interbody fusion (TLIF) combined with transpedicular instrumentation,
- Anterior lumbar interbody fusion (ALIF), or
- Posterior lumbar interbody fusion (PLIF) with fusion cages packed with autologous bone, and
- ALIF with structural allograft replacement.

As of this writing, all of these procedures should be considered investigational. These are discussed in further detail in Chapter 146.

ARACHNOIDITIS AND EPIDURAL FIBROSIS

Arachnoiditis and epidural fibrosis are nonmechanical causes of back or leg pain in patients who have had previous back surgery. Scar tissue occurring beneath the dura is commonly referred to as arachnoiditis. Scar tissue can also form extradurally, compressing either the cauda equina or the nerve root, and is referred to as epidural fibrosis.

Arachnoiditis is strictly defined as an inflammation of the pia-arachnoid membrane surrounding the spinal cord or cauda equina (31). The condition may be present in varying degrees of severity, from mild thickening of the meninges to solid adhesions. The scarring may be severe enough to obliterate the subarachnoid space and block the flow of contrast agents. The etiology of this condition has been attributed to many factors; prior surgery and particularly a history of myelography with oil-based contrast are frequent precipitating factors. A dural tear with blood mixing with cerebrospinal fluid (CSF) or a postoperative infection may also play a role in its pathogenesis.

The exact mechanism by which arachnoiditis develops from these events is not clear. There is no uniform clinical presentation for arachnoiditis.

The patient's history usually reveals more than one previous operation and a pain-free interval lasting from 1 to 6 months. Often, the patient complains of back and leg pain. Physical examination is inconclusive; alteration in neurologic status may be on the basis of a previous operation. Myelography, CT, and MRI can all be helpful in confirming the diagnosis (43).

There is no effective treatment for arachnoiditis. Reconstructive or decompressive surgery has not proven effective in eliminating the scar tissue or significantly reducing the pain. Salvage procedures such as spinal cord stimulation or implantation of a morphine pump have been advocated, with some promising results reported (40).

Use nonoperative measures for most patients. Epidural steroids, transcutaneous nerve stimulation, operant conditioning, bracing, and patient education have all been tried. None leads to a cure, but all can provide symptomatic relief for varying periods of time. Patients should be detoxified from narcotics and encouraged to pursue physical activity as much as possible. Gabapentin (Neurontin) and amitriptyline (Elavil) are pharmacologic adjuncts that may be effective. Treating patients with arachnoiditis is a real challenge, and the physician must be willing to devote time and patience to achieve optimal results.

Formation of scar tissue outside the dura on the cauda equina or directly on the nerve roots is a common occurrence. This epidural scar tissue can act as a constrictive force around the neural elements and may cause postoperative pain. Although most patients have radiographic evidence of epidural scar tissue formation, only an unpredictable few become symptomatic.

Patients with epidural fibrosis may become symptomatic at almost any time, from several months to years after surgery. The onset is typically gradual, with complaints of back pain, leg pain, or both. Commonly the neurologic examination is normal, but the presence of a tension sign may occur due to nerve root constriction from fibrotic changes. The diagnosis is best differentiated from recurrent disc herniation or LSS by gadolinium-enhanced MRI.

As with arachnoiditis, there is no definitive treatment for epidural fibrosis. Prevention may be the best answer, and fat, Gelfoam, and other interpositional membranes have been suggested to minimize the formation of scar tissue following laminectomy (22). Once scar has formed, decompressive surgery with the goal of resecting scar tissue has not proven successful because of the almost inevitable recurrence of even worse fibrosis. It is our experience, however, that a fibrosed nerve root may be more susceptible to the deleterious effects of instability or stenosis than a nerve that has not been surgically treated.

DISCITIS

Discitis is an uncommon but debilitating complication of lumbar disc surgery. Its pathogenesis is postulated to be direct inoculation of the avascular disc space at the time of discectomy, but it is not completely understood (1,9). The onset of symptoms usually occurs 2 to 4 weeks following surgery.

Most patients complain of rapid onset of severe back pain. Pain is unremitting, even at rest, and sometimes extends to the buttocks. Pain does not usually follow a dermatomal pattern down the leg. The patient may have a low-grade fever. Physical examination usually reveals marked paraspinal spasm and rigidity, and pain is present with any type of motion. Straight-leg raising may be limited, but the presence of a true tension sign or new neurologic abnormality is unusual. Occasionally, a superficial wound infection is seen, but in most cases, wound healing has been uneventful.

If you suspect discitis, obtain blood cultures, a white blood cell count with a differential, erthrocyte sedimentation rate (ESR), and a C-reactive protein level. Plain radiographs are usually normal in the early stages; later, endplate erosion may be seen, but it may not be present for several weeks. Contrast-enhanced MRI is the test of choice in suspected disc space infection. Increased signal intensity in the disc space on T2-weighted images suggests discitis, which can be confirmed by enhancement of the disc space with use of gadolinium.

Treatment options include bed rest, bracing, antibiotics, or combinations thereof. Initially, place the patient on bed rest to immobilize the lumbar spine, with or without a brace or corset. Begin empiric antibiotic treatment and continue it for 6 to 12 weeks. Cefepime, a third-generation cephalosporin with improved staphylococcal coverage as well as pseudomonicidal properties, is administered, giving 1 to 2 g every 12 hours. If the patient fails to respond rapidly to antibiotics and immobilization or manifests constitutional signs and symptoms, perform a needle biopsy of the affected disc space. Open biopsy is reserved for patients who fail to respond to treatment, as evidenced by improvement in pain and decline of the ESR, or for patients with neurologic compromise (9). Once the patient is comfortable at bed rest and is afebrile, institute progressively increasing activity as symptoms allow. Most authors report good long-term results with resolution of infection and adequate pain control.

LUMBAR PSEUDARTHROSIS

Nonunion following fusion of the lumbar spine has been reported to occur in as many as 40% of cases. Risk factors include a history of cigarette smoking, multiple-level fusion, and instability that has not been adequately addressed with either internal or external immobilization at the time of fusion (32). Nonunion may occur with or without instrumentation, although the presentation may be somewhat delayed in cases in which rigid internal fixation is initially used. Patients with persistent symptoms due to pseudarthrosis complain primarily of back pain. Leg pain may be present, but direct causes of nerve root compression should be sought, and an assumption that the pseudarthrosis is the cause of the leg pain is frequently unwarranted.

A pain-free interval following surgery may be variable; patients may say that their symptoms never improved following surgery, or they may report many months or even years of relatively good pain relief. It should be noted that unlike a simple discectomy, in which it is not uncommon for the patient to describe truly complete relief of pain, patients who have undergone spine-fusion surgery, even when it is successful, rarely describe complete relief of their symptoms. Patients who have undergone internal fixation, however, are more likely to describe a clear-cut pain-free interval that begins to deteriorate when the implant either loosens (the most common mode of failure) or breaks.

Pseudarthrosis may result in instability and mechanical back pain. It has long been recognized, however, that the correlation between radiographic failure of fusion and symptoms is uncertain. It is very difficult to identify accurately the source of the patient's pain following lumbar fusion; solid fusion is no guarantee of pain relief, and many patients with an obvious nonunion do remarkably well.

It is essential to think twice before offering patients with a pseudarthrosis revision fusion. Undertaking repeat surgery for pseudarthrosis repair in the absence of motion at the affected level and without a thorough search for alternative causes for the patient's symptoms has limited chances for success. Most authors report compromised results after such surgery, particularly when leg pain is noted in the absence of a compressive etiology (24).

Begin evaluation of the patient with a possible pseudarthrosis with plain radiographs, including Ferguson AP and weight-bearing, dynamic lateral radiographs. Solid fusion, either posteriorly or anteriorly, should eliminate virtually all motion on flexion and extension views. Although the landmarks may be somewhat difficult to identify, careful scrutiny of dynamic views can usually identify whether or not motion is taking place (Fig. 149.8).

The AP views may be difficult to interpret, but many times, a serpiginous cleft in the fusion mass can be visualized. Although a number of other radiographic modalities, including CT scanning and single photon emission com-

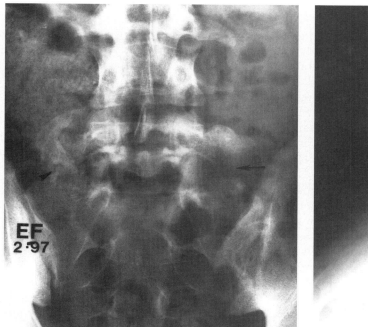
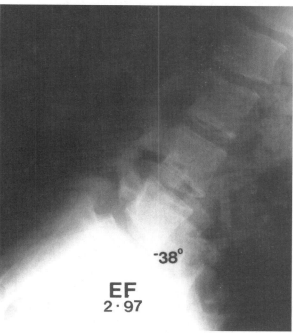

A   B

Figure 149.8. A 17-year-old man, 18 months following L5–S1 fusion for spondylolysis, who now reports worsening low-back pain. (**A**) A Ferguson AP view shows abundant fusion mass on the right, although a defect can be seen (*arrowhead*), whereas on the left, most of the graft has been resorbed (*arrow*). Lateral flexion and extension radiographs demonstrate 17° of angular motion; (**B**) clear-cut evidence of pseudarthrosis, which was confirmed at surgery; *(continued)*

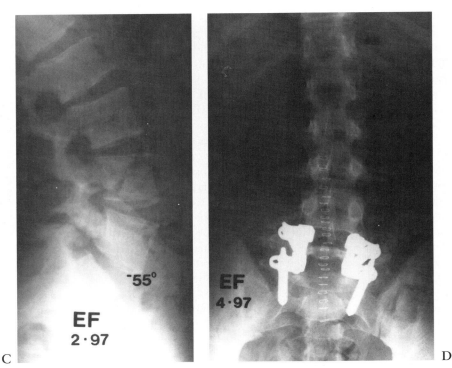

Figure 149.8. *(continued)* (**C**), clear-cut evidence of pseudarthrosis, which was confirmed at surgery; (**D**) revision fusion posteriorly, with transpedicular instrumentation, led to complete pain relief.

puted tomography (SPECT) scanning, have been suggested to diagnosis nonunion, we rely almost exclusively on plain radiographic findings of motion or progressive deformity to identify the patient who is likely to benefit from repeat surgery.

In many cases, it is difficult to identify a pseudarthrosis clearly; additionally, the correlation between pseudarthrosis and symptoms in a given patient is uncertain. For these reasons, an aggressive attempt at nonoperative treatment is indicated. When the nonsurgical approach is unsuccessful, revision surgery may be undertaken. A failure rate as high as 50%, both clinically and radiographically, has been reported, however. Lauerman et al. (24) reported improved results in patients who had undergone only one prior operation on the lumbar spine and in patients who had a clear-cut original indication for fusion, such as spondylolisthesis.

NONOPERATIVE TREATMENT

It is axiomatic that, for the patient with pain following previous surgery on the lumbar spine, there is always another operation that can be considered. Experience tells us, however, that the results following revision surgery on the lumbar spine are frequently unsatisfactory, and particularly when there is a history of two or more previous operations, the patient has a significant chance of being made worse rather than better with another surgery (37). In light of this, treat nonoperatively most patients who have failed prior surgery, even when it is possible to identify an etiology of their pain that is potentially amenable to surgery.

Nonoperative treatment involves generalized back care as well as some more specific interventions. Realistic goals for pain relief are essential. Close questioning of the patient often reveals that he or she is significantly better now than before the previous operation; any consideration of further surgery simply to "get rid of all of the pain" is likely to be unsuccessful and is unwarranted. Furthermore, it is apparent on questioning some patients that there has been almost no postoperative attempt at rehabilitation. These patients respond quite readily to a generalized back exercise and aerobic exercise program with judicious use of medication.

A generalized back treatment program consists of

- Weight reduction when appropriate;
- A defined program of aerobic exercise, particularly involving walking, riding an exercise bicycle, or swimming;

- A supervised program of active physical therapy consisting of specific back stretching and strengthening exercises; and
- Use of nonsteroidal anti-inflammatory medications.

Make every attempt to detoxify the patient from chronic narcotic usage. Elavil is useful for the patient with chronic pain and sleep disturbance, as are several other antidepressants. Neurontin, an antiepileptic, appears to be beneficial in some patients with chronic radicular pain.

Other psychopharmacologic agents are available for use in the patient with chronic pain and are becoming increasingly popular. It is up to the individual physician to decide to what extent his or her practice includes prescribing these medicines. The authors find it more effective, in most cases, to refer such patients to a pain management center for pharmacologic management. A final adjunct that is occasionally useful is external immobilization, which may be provided by something as simple as a lumbar corset or as elaborate as a custom-made polypropylene lumbosacral orthosis. It is widely believed that these devices decondition the lumbar musculature, although there is little objective evidence to document this belief. Corsets and orthotics do, however, provide significant pain relief for many patients, and they are particularly effective in elderly patients.

In patients with leg pain and evidence of epidural fibrosis or recurrent mechanical compression from stenosis or disc, a trial of lumbar epidural steroids is worthwhile. The long-term benefits are quite variable, but a certain percentage of patients will obtain lasting relief or will tolerate a more aggressive program of rehabilitation once the inflammatory radicular symptoms are controlled. Local trigger-point injections, facet joint blocks, and sacroiliac injection may also be tried, although none of these methods has consistently proven effective.

INDICATIONS FOR SURGERY

The principal indication for surgery in the patient with failed prior low-back surgery is persistent, unacceptable pain that has failed to respond to aggressive and persistent nonoperative treatment. In addition, it is explained by and correlates with either objective evidence of instability, mechanical nerve root compression, or both. The challenge in managing patients who have had prior back surgery, and the primary reason for the increased rate of failure with further surgeries, is the difficulty of clearly correlating the patient's pain with the radiographic findings. Adherence to guidelines that are as strict as or stricter than those used for primary surgery is essential. Our experience has been that attempts to extend these indications leads to consistently unsatisfactory results. Further, viewing fusion as a generically applicable salvage procedure for previously unsuccessful back surgery rarely results in significant and long-lasting pain relief.

Surprisingly good results can be obtained by operating on patients who fit into one of three categories. These include patients who have

1. Radicular leg pain and confirmatory evidence of nerve root compression on high-quality neuroradiographic imaging that demonstrates either recurrent disc herniation or LSS not caused by epidural fibrosis;
2. Back pain due to radiographically documented instability, as confirmed either by progressive deformity (scoliosis or spondylolisthesis), excessive motion on flexion and extension lateral radiographs, or a failed fusion with motion demonstrated on dynamic radiographs;
3. Back pain believed to be emanating from one or two painful degenerated discs, confirmed on pain-provocation discography.

Although the results are generally good when operating on this subset of patients, it should be stressed that only a relatively small percentage of patients with FBSS fit into one of these three categories.

Other indications for surgery in this patient population include the presence of a clearly documented progressive neurologic deficit. Although this condition is uncommon, it does occasionally occur, more often in elderly patients with severe stenosis. A progressive neurologic deficit is an indication for urgent surgery. Cauda equina syndrome, a distinctly rare occurrence in patients who have had unsuccessful back surgery, merits emergent imaging and surgical treatment. Finally, one occasionally encounters the patient with radiographic evidence of progressive spondylolisthesis or progressive collapsing scoliosis, which itself suggests the need for surgical stabilization. It rarely occurs in the absence of concurrent incapacitating pain but might be a situation in which a more aggressive approach is called for.

INSTRUMENTATION

Since the early 1980s, transpedicular instrumentation has gained increasing popularity in North America as an adjunct to lumbar fusion. This trend has, in several ways, complicated the approach to the treatment of patients whose back surgery has failed. First, an increasing number of patients are undergoing lumbar spine fusion, and unfortunately, in many cases, it has been carried out in the absence of traditional, objective indications. The usual result is failure. The presence of the implant itself raises several technical considerations relating to the possible need for repeat surgery, including the significance of screw breakage, implant loosening, infection, and malposition of one or more screws. Finally, adverse publicity related to these devices has led to a climate in which either medicolegal concerns or, at the least, undue patient anxiety further clouds a complicated clinical picture.

Pedicle screw instrumentation systems are composed of metal alloys that have a very low incidence of true allergy; therefore, allergy is rarely, if ever, the cause of pain. Failure can occur in one of several ways, but mechanical failure does not necessarily represent an indication for removal of the implant or revision surgery. Screw breakage is the most dramatic mode of failure, but with current technology, it is quite rare. A broken screw does not preclude the possibility of a successful fusion and, therefore, is not an absolute indication of clinical failure (26,39).

On the other hand, the patient who, having had good relief of back pain following an instrumented lumbar fusion, now has the sudden recurrence of pain and is noted to have new screw breakage may well have had a nonunion that was adequately stabilized when the implant was intact. Such a patient would benefit from revision fusion.

Another mechanism of failure is screw loosening in the pedicle and vertebral body. This is much more common than screw breakage. The loosening is seen as a small zone of radiolucency about the screw on routine radiographs. There is no clear-cut relationship between screw loosening and symptoms, and unless failure of fusion and motion on flexion and extension views are demonstrated, continued observation is indicated.

Finally, the risk of infection appears to be increased with the use of these bulky implants, and the rate of infection has been reported to be from 2% to 5% (35). Acute and subacute infection is readily diagnosed, but late infection may represent the source of recurrent back pain after a relatively long pain-free interval. Consider infection when evaluating the patient with the late onset of pain after an otherwise successful fusion. On CT scan, look for a fluid collection around the implant. Aspirate the wound to look for purulent fluid. Send any fluid aspirated for Gram's stain and culture.

In addition to disc herniation or stenosis adjacent to the fused levels, another possible source of nerve root compression in patients who have implants in place is a misplaced screw. Although most patients have symptoms early from a misplaced screw, it is not uncommon for radicular pain to develop weeks, months, or even years later (Fig. 149.9).

Thin-cut plain CT scanning of the lumbar spine, using bony windows, is a sensitive modality for identifying a screw placed outside the pedicle. Because screw misplacement is asymptomatic in as many as 20% of patients, close correlation between the patient's signs and symptoms and the root compromised by the screw in question is essential before deciding on repeat surgery (41). The most common location for screw impingement is medial to the pedicle, particularly at L-5, but it is important to check for the

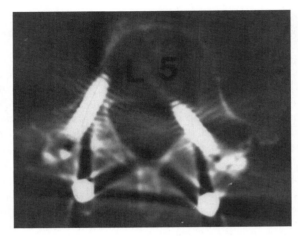

Figure 149.9. A 59-year-old woman who, 1 month following revision fusion with transpedicular instrumentation, reported worsening left leg pain and weakness. A plain CT scan demonstrates, on the bone windows, medial placement of the L-5 screw, correlating with her symptoms. Prompt screw removal led to complete resolution of her leg pain, although she had mild residual weakness.

possibility of an S-1 screw placed through the sacral ala, lateral to the sacral body, which brings it into proximity to the L-5 root, passing over the brim of the sacrum. Once the diagnosis of screw malposition, which is causing symptoms, has been made, screw removal is indicated.

Although transpedicular instrumentation may lessen the risk of pseudarthrosis, it certainly does not eliminate it (35). A rigidly fixed pedicle screw implant may temporarily provide stability to an unstable motion segment, but if solid bony fusion is not achieved, loosening commonly occurs. Therefore, mechanical back pain may recur after a pain-free interval. No radiographic modality has consistently proven accurate in diagnosing nonunion in the presence of a transpedicular implant (23). We rely on the presence or absence of motion on flexion and extension lateral views to decide whether further surgery in indicated.

One final indication for surgery in patients in whom pedicle screw instrumentation is present is routine implant removal. It is unusual for a patient to be so thin that the implants are palpable or cause pressure problems with sitting in a hard-backed chair. The role of routine implant removal is uncertain, and significant pain relief, if a solid fusion is present, occurs in only about one patient out of three (10). To the patient requesting implant removal, we explain the uncertainty regarding the chances for improvement of their pain as well as the fairly significant surgery required to remove these devices. If the patient wishes to proceed under these circumstances, we will remove the implants and explore the fusion. We inform our patients that if a pseudarthrosis is found, further bone grafting and revision instrumentation will be carried out.

SURGICAL TECHNIQUES

Operating on the lumbar spine after one or more previous surgeries can be a challenge. The technique of a repeat laminectomy or a repeat fusion is somewhat different from first-time surgery. The risk of complications is certainly greater, with the ever-present danger of a dural tear or neurologic injury.

REPEAT LAMINECTOMY

The goal of a laminectomy in repeat back surgery is the same as that for the initial procedure—to decompress the neural elements without injury or excessive hemorrhage. Unfortunately, once the spine has already undergone surgery, the anatomy is not as clear and a great deal of scar tissue can be present. Thus, several technical aspects of a repeat laminectomy are different from those of a primary procedure.

The first difference involves the operative approach: It is not possible to strip the paraspinal muscles away with impunity because of absence of the spinous processes, lamina, or ligamentum flavum at the sites of previous surgery.

- Begin the approach at a new level with normal anatomy and normal protection of the cauda equina. Find the normal depth of the posterior elements and cauda equina, and carefully extend the dissection into the area of the laminectomy defect.
- Working laterally, identify and expose the facet joints.
- Proceeding distally, define the pars interarticularis at the caudal base of the superior articular facet; follow the pars further distally and medially onto the remaining lamina and inferior articular facet of the next-lower facet joint.
- Carefully scrutinize the preoperative plain radiographs, CT scan, and MRI scan to determine the extent of previous resection. It is not uncommon to encounter a pars or facet fracture unexpectedly.
- Beginning at each facet joint, use sharp curets and a Penfield dissector to subperiosteally expose the remaining normal posterior elements while minimizing risk of injury to the dura and underlying cauda equina.

The surgeon may also be tempted, once the depth of the neural elements is determined, to remove the extradural scar tissue directly over the dura. This is a technically difficult procedure with the potential for a great deal of hemorrhage and a strong possibility of dural injury. Even if the scar tissue can be successfully removed, there is no reliable means available to prevent its regrowth. We recommend, for the most part, that extradural scar tissue be left intact; remove only the tissue covering the area of previously documented nerve root compression.

The object of the surgical procedure is to visualize the nerve roots laterally and remove any mechanical (nonscar) tissue pressure from them. Do so by extending the laminectomy from the new level down the lateral gutters, leaving the central scar tissue as is:

- Use sharp curets to follow the medial border of the laminectomy defect ventrally, developing a plane between the epidural scar tissue and the residual bone.
- Once this plane is developed, introduce a Kerrison rongeur at a 45° angle, and undercut the bony encroachment, usually arising from the medial overhang of the superior articular facet.
- Carry this decompression out proximally, distally, and laterally until all bony overgrowth has been removed back to the medial wall of the pedicle.
- You may also use an osteotome to remove the most medial portion of the facet, thereby gaining entry to the spinal canal and nerve roots.
- If the goal of the repeat procedure is decompression of recurrent stenosis, extend the laminectomy laterally to the pedicle on either side at whatever levels are radiographically involved.
- Leave the midline epidural fibrosis intact.
- If a central laminectomy is required either proximal or distal to the previous laminectomy, proceed in standard fashion, first developing the interval between the caudad half of the lamina and the underlying ligamentum flavum. Then resect the lamina piecemeal.
- Once normal dura is encountered proximally, reverse direction, working caudally to remove the intervening ligamentum flavum from the underlying dura.
- If, at the junction of the previous decompression and the ligamentum flavum, you find adherent scar tissue, leave a small amount of ligamentum flavum over the thecal sac if it cannot be safely dissected free.
- Address the nerve roots laterally, as previously described.

REPEAT DISCECTOMY

The use of Repeat surgery for a recurrent disc herniation is common. Many of the same caveats as described for repeat decompressive laminectomy apply. Usually, a recurrent disc herniation occurs in a patient who has had a previous relatively limited hemilaminotomy, with the majority of the posterior elements being preserved.

- Expose the affected side only by carefully dissecting along the involved laminae and following them laterally as they join to become the facet joint. Place a retractor lateral to the facet joint to visualize the previous laminotomy.
- As with a more extensive laminectomy, bear in mind at all times the risk of a dural tear when performing a repeat discectomy. This risk can be minimized, and safe entry into the canal achieved, by using sharp curets to

define clearly the remaining bony landmarks around the prior laminotomy.

- Scar tissue that is encountered can be thinned out, but as with a decompressive laminectomy, attempts to remove epidural fibrosis from the dura completely increase the risk of injury and are not indicated in most cases.
- Once the hemilaminotomy has been completely defined, use either a Kerrison rongeur or osteotome to remove a small portion of residual bone, first from the inferior facet of the cephalad level and then from the medial aspect of the superior facet of the caudad level.
- This new entry into the spinal canal and lateral recess is slightly more lateral to the original hemilaminotomy site. Extend the exposure until you are flush with the medial wall of the pedicle.
- The traversing nerve root is usually encased in a layer of scar tissue of variable thickness, but can be palpated with a Penfield dissector.
- Carefully dissect along the lateral border of the root to mobilize it and retract it medially. Expose the underlying disc.
- Although it can be fairly time consuming, careful mobilization of the nerve root is essential to avoid root injury.
- Once the root is safely retracted medially, expose the underlying disc and resect it in standard fashion.
- Whether or not to fuse in the face of a recurrent disc herniation is a highly controversial decision; we favor fusion when the patient has significant back pain or when there is any suggestion of instability. We are more inclined to fuse at the L4–L5 level than at L5–S1.
- A second recurrence (third disc herniation) merits strong consideration of fusion.

FUSION EXPLORATION AND REVISION

Do not undertake repeat surgery on the lumbar spine with the specific goal of repairing a nonunion unless other potential causes of pain have been excluded. We rarely undertake nonunion repair in cases in which evidence of motion on dynamic lateral x-ray studies or progressive deformity has not been documented. Once the decision has been made to proceed with revision fusion, several technical points facilitate the procedure.

- If there has been a prior laminectomy, expose carefully, starting at normal levels as described above.
- Carry the exposure lateral to the facet joints and out all the way to the tips of the transverse processes on each side.
- In cases in which there is a laminectomy defect from previous surgery and no further decompression is planned, use a paraspinal muscle-splitting approach, which affords excellent visualization of the facet joints,

pars interarticularis, and laterally placed fusion mass. It also facilitates pedicle screw placement.

- After exposure, carefully explore the fusion mass.
- In places where fixation devices are still in place, it is very difficult to determine whether the fusion is solid until the instrumentation is completely removed. Therefore, once exposure has been obtained, disassemble the implant and remove it piecemeal.
- Remove the fibrous scar tissue to visualize the fusion mass clearly.
- Use Cobb elevators and sharp curets to remove all soft tissue from the dorsal cortex of the fusion mass extending from cephalad to caudad and from the most medial extent to the lateral margins of the transverse processes and fusion mass.
- A well-consolidated fusion is easy to strip, although it is not uncommon to find islands of fibrous tissue surrounded by bridging trabecular bone. Soft tissues are attached strongly to nonunions and are difficult to strip.
- Once the fusion has been completely exposed, check not just for continuity but for adherence as well to the proximal and distal spinal elements; occasionally, well-formed bone is not adherent to the transverse process or, more commonly, the sacral ala.
- In order to verify the adequacy of fusion, take an osteotome and carefully remove the dorsal cortex of the fusion mass to verify that there is underlying cancellous bone in continuity with the transverse processes and alae.
- When a defect in the fusion mass is found, it is frequently narrow and wanders in a serpiginous fashion through the fusion. It can take fairly extensive exploration of a defect to document that it does indeed track through the entire fusion mass and allows motion.
- If the fusion is found to be solid, close the wound in standard fashion. If a defect in the fusion mass is found, use curets and a high-speed burr to remove all soft tissue from the dorsal aspect of the defect.
- Complete excision of all soft tissue is not necessary; remove the accessible dorsal soft tissue and decorticate the area around the defect. Then apply abundant autologous bone graft to the nonunion.
- Then stabilize the nonunions with a pedicle screw system and apply compression across the nonunion.
- Identification of the normal landmarks for pedicle screw placement can be difficult. Use interoperative fluoroscopy for identification of the appropriate starting point and path for the screws.

In addition to discovering a defect in an otherwise well formed fusion mass, nonunion is seen in many patients in whom there has been complete or near-complete resorption of the previously placed bone graft. It is more common in patients in whom an allograft is used and in smok-

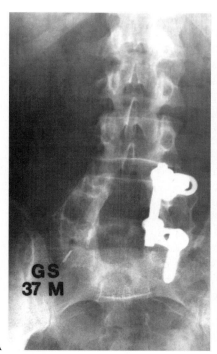
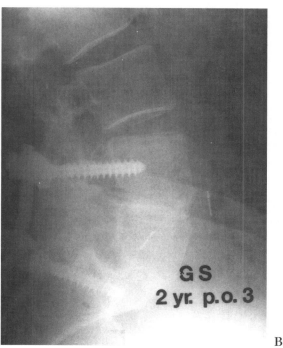

A   B

Figure 149.10.   A 37-year-old man 2 years following his third attempt at L4–L5 and L5–S1 fusion for isthmic spondylolisthesis. **A:** At the last posterior surgery, malpositioned left L-4 and L-5 screws were removed and it was elected only to instrument the right side. Because of the recurrent pseudarthrosis, and the ability to instrument only one side, it was elected to proceed with anterior interbody fusion, using a femoral ring allograft at both levels. **B:** At 2 years follow-up, solid fusion is seen, and the patient, who had not worked in 3 years, is minimally symptomatic and back to full-time employment.

ers. In these patients, it is usually readily apparent that the original fusion has failed.

- Thoroughly expose out to the tips of the transverse processes.
- Carefully decorticate the transverse processes and sacral ala.
- Apply a massive bone graft to provide the best chance for successful repair.
- In these cases, in which there is no stabilization from the original fusion, rigid internal fixation is essential.

Another alternative when considering repair of a previously failed fusion is interbody fusion. It can be performed through a transforaminal or posterior approach or, more commonly, through an anterior approach.

- Use allograft, if desired, as a block graft to provide stability, but supplement it with autologous bone from the iliac crest or from the adjacent vertebral body.
- We consider performing a combined posterior and anterior fusion in patients in whom a previously well-done fusion with rigid fixation has led to nonunion, in smokers, or in cases in which it is determined, at the time of posterior exploration, that there has been sufficient attenuation of the bone posteriorly to suggest that the chances of obtaining a solid fusion are minimal (Fig. 149.10).

POSTOPERATIVE MANAGEMENT

For the most part, postoperative management of patients undergoing revision low-back surgery is similar to that for primary surgery. Although the hospital stay is usually unchanged, the overall length of recovery can be prolonged compared with first-time surgery. The patient should be prepared for an extended time away from work or other pressing duties. Fixation after revision fusion may be less than ideal; therefore, we commonly supplement fixation with a brace. We use a physical therapist to mobilize the patient after surgery by facilitating transfers and ambulation; otherwise, we delay back rehabilitation for 3 to 4 months following surgery.

Try to detoxify patients from narcotics before surgery. The early postoperative period following a revision operation is not the time to withdraw narcotic medication.

Work with a pain management specialist to lessen narcotic usage gradually with a goal of discontinuing narcotic medication altogether by 6 to 12 months postoperatively. Although this is an extended period of time, it is impractical to assume that quicker withdrawal is possible.

◤ PITFALLS AND COMPLICATIONS

DURAL TEAR

The risk of encountering a dural tear is definitely greater in the patient who has undergone previous back surgery. Although each dural tear is different, certain basic principles always apply and certain steps should be followed.

A dural tear usually occurs as the surgeon is gaining visualization of, and entry into, the spinal canal. Although a large majority of dural tears do not result in any long-term morbidity, the repair of an intraoperative tear is time consuming and bears with it the potential for persistent CSF leakage, wound problems, and nerve root injury. The risk of dural tear is increased in repeat surgery because previous resection of the posterior elements obliterates the usual landmarks. Other risks include the difficulty of separating scar tissue from the dura to develop a plane between the thecal sac and nerve root, and the pathologic anatomy related to whatever is causing recurrent neural compression.

- Lessen the risk of dural injury by beginning the deep exposure of the posterior elements, proximally and distally, where there are retained normal spinous processes and laminae.
- Dissect proximally and distally along a normal lamina to the facet joints and then work caudally from the proximal end and distally from the cephalad end to expose the length of the entire laminectomy defect safely.
- Expose the preserved facet joints and pars interarticularis susperiosteally, and leave a layer of scar tissue over the dura.
- Use a curet to define the medial border of the retained posterior elements.
- Rather than try to directly peel off or resect scar tissue from the dura, resect a small amount of normal, retained lamina or medial facet to expose an area of spinal canal, thecal sac, or nerve root uninvolved with scar tissue. Entry to the canal in such a way usually permits decompression without dural injury.

If the goal of surgery is to remove epidural scar tissue that is contributing to the nerve root or thecal sac compression, then the technique described earlier is less likely to be adequate and the risk of a dural tear is increased.

Once a tear occurs, the wound usually fills quickly with CSF, obscuring the extent of the damage. The surgeon's first impulse is to try to see the tear by using suction in the approximate area of the problem. This is a mistake, because the individual nerve roots may be sucked out of the thecal sac, causing significant neurologic damage. Suction should be used only over a cottonoid so that no further damage to the nerve roots is done. After visualizing the tear, place a piece of Gelfoam over the injury site, cover it with a large cottonoid, and complete the original procedure. The patient's head may be tilted downward into the Trendelenburg position to decrease the flow of CSF into the wound.

Once the definitive procedure is completed, refocus on repair of the dural tear. The goal is to achieve a watertight closure; if not, a CSF fistula can form, raising the risk of meningitis or a subarachnoid cyst. A dry operative field with hemostasis maintained throughout the repair is essential. Similarly, achieve adequate exposure in both the cephalocaudad and mediolateral directions in order to define the extent of the tear adequately and to allow access for repair. Failure to maintain hemostasis and to obtain adequate exposure are the two most common causes of difficulty in repairing a dural tear. Magnification loupes and adequate lighting also facilitate the repair.

The actual technique of closure used depends on the size and location of the tear:

- For simple dural lacerations, we prefer 4-0 or 5-0 silk sutures on a tapered one-half circle needle. A running locking suture or simple sutures incorporating a free fat graft provide a watertight closure.
- If a tear is large or irreparable, harvest a fascial graft from the lumbodorsal fascia and suture it around the periphery of the defect with interrupted silk sutures.
- If the defect is in an inaccessible area, introduce a small tissue plug of muscle or fat through a second midline durotomy, pulling the tissue plug into the tear, thereby obliterating the tear from inside the dura (12).
- Use Fibrin glue to reinforce the dural repair if there is any question about the adequacy of the repair.
- Test the repair by placing the patient in the reverse Trendelenburg position and performing a Valsalva maneuver to increase intrathecal pressure. Close the fascia with a heavy, nonabsorbable suture, which must be watertight.

Most authors prefer not to use drains to avoid the possibility of the development of a draining fistula if there is persistent CSF leakage. Keep the patient on bed rest for at least 3 or 4 days to reduce pressure on the repair while it heals.

The diagnosis of a CSF leak in the postoperative period can be difficult to make. If relatively clear drainage occurs, consider the possibility of a dural leak. Similarly, a history of headaches when the patient sits or stands suggests CSF leakage. No completely reliable noninvasive diagnostic technique is available at present. The presence of glucose in the fluid draining from an incision is not a reliable determinant, because glucose is normally present in both non-inflammatory and inflammatory exudates. The best diagnostic test, a myelogram performed with water-soluble contrast medium, is recommended if a dural leak is suspected but the diagnosis is uncertain. Once a postoperative CSF leak is diagnosed, pursue aggressive treatment. In the early postoperative period, placement of a subarachnoid drain for 4 to 5 days has been reported with good results (21). If this procedure is unsuccessful or a leak is diagnosed late, timely return to the operating room for dural repair is in order.

 AUTHORS' PERSPECTIVE

We stress that an organized methodical approach to the evaluation of the patient who has had previous back surgery is essential. In many cases, the problem resulted from inadequate or incorrect indications for the original surgical procedure. In such patients, further exploratory surgery is not warranted and would lead only to further disability. Another surgery is indicated only when objective findings for a specific diagnosis are present.

In the few patients who do require an additional operation, it must be appreciated that the surgery is usually more extensive than the original operation with certain inherent risks. One must approach the spine at a new level to identify the normal anatomy of the neural elements and visualize the appropriate nerve root or roots laterally, leaving the midline epidural scar tissue intact.

If the dura is injured during the course of the procedure, repair it in a watertight fashion. If nonunion of a prior fusion is suspected, then carefully explore the fusion mass when a nonunion is found, perform a thorough decortication, removal of scar tissue, massive bone grafting, and rigid fixation.

Those involved with treatment of patients undergoing repeat back surgery must realize that the chance of returning these patients to a pain-free status is low. Depending on the type of previous surgery and the patient's symptoms, usually some form of permanent impairment persists. These patients need counseling and must be strongly encouraged to resume as functional a role as possible in society.

REFERENCES

Each reference is categorized according to the following scheme: *, classic article; #, review article; !, basic research article; and +, clinical results/outcome study.

+ 1. Bircher MD, Tasker T, Crashaw C, et al. Discitis Following Lumbar Surgery. *Spine* 1988;13:98.

+ 2. Blumell SC, Gill K. Can Lumbar Spine Radiographs Accurately Determine Fusion in Postoperative Patients? *Spine* 1993;18:1186.

+ 3. Boden SD, Davis DO, Dina TS, et al. Contrast-enhanced MR Imaging Performed After Successful Lumbar Disc Surgery: Prospective Study. *Radiology* 1992;182:59.

+ 4. Boden SD, Wiesel SW. Lumbosacral Motion in Normal Individuals: Have We Been Measuring Instability Properly? *Spine* 1990;12:571.

+ 5. Bolender NF, Schonstrom NSR, Spengler DM. Role of Computed Tomography and Myelography in the Diagnosis of Central Spinal Stenosis. *J Bone Joint Surg [Am]* 1985;67:240.

+ 6. Brodsky AE, Kovalsky ES, Khalil MA. Correlation of Radiographic Assessment of Lumbar Spine Fusions with Surgical Exploration. *Spine* 1991;16:261.

+ 7. Burton CV, Kirkaldy-Willis WH, Yong-Hing K, Heithoff KB. Causes of Failure of Surgery on the Lumbar Spine. *Clin Orthop* 1981;157:191.

+ 8. Byrd SE, Cohn ML, Biggers SL, et al. The Radiographic Evaluation of the Symptomatic Post-operative Lumbar Spine Patient. *Spine* 1985;10:652.

+ 9. Dall BE, Rowe DE, Odette WG, et al. Postoperative Discitis; Diagnosis and Management. *Clin Orthop* 1987; 224:138.

+ 10. Davne SH, Meyers DL. Results Following Removal or Revision of Lumbar Pedicle Screw Instrumentation. *Orthop Trans* 1994;18:257.

+ 11. Edwards CC, Weigel MC, Levine AM. Improved Results Treating Lumbosacral Nonunions with Compression Instrumentation. *Orthop Trans* 1988;12:131.

+ 12. Eismont FJ, Wiesel SW, Rothman RH. Treatment of Dural Tears Associated with Spinal Surgery. *J Bone Joint Surg* 1981;63-A:1132.

+ 13. Finnegan WJ, Fenlin JM, Marvel JP, et al. Results of Surgical Intervention in the Symptomatic Multiply-operated Back Patient. *J Bone Joint Surg* 1979;61-A:1077.

+ 14. Hall S, Bartleson JD, Onofrio BM, et al. Lumbar Spinal Stenosis: Clinical Features, Diagnostic Procedures, and Results of Treatment in 68 Patients. *Ann Int Med* 1985; 103:271.

+ 15. Hanley EN, Shapiro DE. The Development of Low Back Pain After Excision of a Lumbar Disc. *J Bone Joint Surg* 1989;71-A:719.

+ 16. Hazlett JW, Kinnard P. Lumbar Apophyseal Process Excision and Instability. *Spine* 1982;7:171.

+ 17. Holt E The Question of Lumbar Discography. *J Bone Joint Surg* 1968;50A:720.

+ 18. Horton W, Daftari T. Which Disc as Visualized by MRI Is Actually a Source of Pain? A Correlation Between MRI and Discography. *Spine* 1992;17:S164.

+ 19. Hueftle MG, Modie MT, Ross JS, et al. Lumbar Spine: Postoperative MRI with Gadolinium-DTPA. *Radiology* 1988;167:817.

+ 20. Johnsson KE, Wilner S, Johnsson K. Postoperative Instability After Decompression for Lumbar Spine Stenosis. *Spine* 1986;11:107.

+ 21. Kitchel SH, Eismont FJ, Green BA. Closed Subarachnoid

Drainage for Management of Cerebrospinal Fluid Leakage After an Operation on the Spine. *J Bone Joint Surg* 1989;71-A:984.

+ 22. Langenskydd A, Kiviluoto O. Prevention of Epidural Scar Formation After Operations on the Lumbar Spine by Means of Free Fat Transplants. *Clin Orthop* 1976; 115:92.

+ 23. Larsen JW, Rimoldi RL, Nelson RW, et al. Identification of Pseudarthrosis in the Presence of Pedicle Screw Instrumentation. *Orthop Trans* 1995;18:983.

+ 24. Lauerman WC, Bradford DS, Ogilvie JW, et al. Results of Lumbar Pseudarthrosis Repair. *J Spinal Discord* 1992;5:149.

+ 25. Long DM, Filtzer DL, BenDebba M, et al. Clinical Features of the Failed-back Syndrome. *J Neurosurg* 1988; 69:61.

+ 26. McAfee PC, Farey ID, Sutterlin CE, et al. Device-related Osteoporosis with Spinal Instrumentation. *Spine* 1989; 14:919.

27. Modic MT, Masaryk T, Paushter D. MRI of the Spine. *Radiol Clin North Am* 1986;24:A229.

+ 28. Modic MT, Pflanze W, Feiglin DH, et al. Magnetic Resonance Imaging of Musculoskeletal Infections. *Radiol Clin North Am* 1986;24:247.

+ 29. Mooney V. Position Statement on Discography. *Spine* 1988;13:1343.

+ 30. Paris SV. Physical Signs of Instability. *Spine* 1985;10: 277.

+ 31. Quiles M, Marchisello PJ, Tsairis P. Lumbar Adhesive Arachnoiditis: Etiologic and Pathologic Aspects. *Spine* 1978;3:45.

32. Reilly JP, O'Leary PF. Complications of Lumbar Spine Surgery. In: White AH, Rothman RH, Ray CD, eds. *The Lumbar Spine*. New York: Raven Press, 1987:357.

33. Spengler DM. Degenerative Stenosis of the Lumbar Spine. Current Concepts Review. *J Bone Joint Surg Am* 1987;69:305.

+ 34. Teplick JG, Haskin ME. CT of the Postoperative Lumbar Spine. *Radiol Clin North Am* 1983;21:395.

+ 35. Vaccaro AR, Garfin SR. Pedicle Screw Fixation in the Lumbar Spine. *J Am Acad Orthop Surg* 1995;3:263.

+ 36. Waddell G. Failures of Disc Surgery and Repeat Surgery. *Acta Orthop Belg* 1987;53:300.

+ 37. Waddell G, Kummel EG, Lotto WN, et al: Failed Lumbar Disc Surgery and Repeat Surgery Following Industrial Injuries. *J Bone Joint Surg* 1979;61:201.

+ 38. Walsh T, Weinstein J, Spratt K, et al. Lumbar Discography in Normal Subjects. A Controlled Prospective Study. *J Bone Joint Surg* 1990;72-A:1081.

+ 39. West JL, Bradford DS, Ogilvie JW. Results of Spinal Arthrodesis with Pedicle Screw-plate Fixation. *J Bone Joint Surg Am* 1991;73:1179.

40. Wetzel FT, LaRocca SH. Surgical Procedures for the Control of Chronic pain. In: Rothman RH, Simeone FA, eds. *The Spine,* 3rd ed. Philadelphia: W.B. Saunders, 1992:1982.

+ 41. Weinstein JN, Spratt KF, Spengler D, et al: Spinal Pedicle Fixation: Reliability and Validity or Roentgenogram-based Assessment and Surgical Factors on Successful Screw Placement. *Spine* 1988;13:1012.

42. White AA, Panjabi MM, Posner I. *Spinal Stability: Evaluation and Treatment. AAOS ICL XXX.* St. Louis: Mosby, 1981.

43. Wilkinson HA. Adhesive Arachnoiditis. In: Weinstein JN, Wiesel SW, eds. *The Lumbar Spine.* Philadelphia: W.B. Saunders, 1990;1872.

CHAPTER 150

PYOGENIC AND GRANULOMATOUS INFECTIONS OF THE SPINE

Munish C. Gupta and Daniel R. Benson

Tuberculosis played an important role in our learning about the treatment of infections of the spine. Tuberculosis patients with deformity and paralysis forced us to address this devastating process with aggressive surgical and medical treatment. Even with the decrease of tuberculosis in developed countries, the principles of treating infections, pyogenic or granulomatous, have been influenced by the experience of treating tuberculosis.

M. C. Gupta: Department of Orthopaedics, University of California, Davis, Sacramento, California 95817.
D. R. Benson: Department of Orthopaedics, University of California, Davis, Sacramento, California 95817.

Pyogenic infections have a spectrum of presentation from discitis in children, to osteomyelitis in adults, to postsurgical infections. The infection usually affects the vertebral body and disc and, less commonly, the posterior elements, except in cases of postsurgical infection (Fig. 150.1). The lumbar spine is the most common location of infection, followed by the thoracic spine; cervical spine infection is least common (132). The least common sites for spinal osteomyelitis are the occiput, atlas, and axis, with only a few isolated cases reported (178).

Hematogenous pyogenic osteomyelitis is characteristically a disease of men 50 years of age and older and is usually caused by *Staphylococcus aureus*. An increased

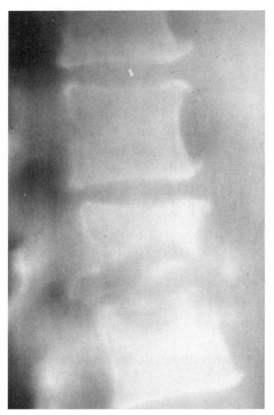

Figure 150.1. Hematogenous osteomyelitis most commonly invades first the anterior portion of the vertebral body, just adjacent to the endplate. Radiographic changes take time to appear and the usual picture is that of simultaneous involvement of two adjacent endplates with narrowing of the intervertebral disc space. This tomogram of the lumbar spine shows endplate destruction of the lower vertebral combine with loss of a good deal of the body of the upper vertebra.

incidence in younger male intravenous drug abusers has been noted. Pyogenic spinal osteomyelitis is usually monomicrobial, unless it is secondary to a systemic disease, in which case a polymicrobial infection is more common. There has been an increase in gram-negative infections compared with the more common gram-positive infections (19). The increased infection rates from gram-negative organisms may be due to wide use of broad-spectrum antibiotics.

Granulomatous infections of the spine, tuberculosis being the most common, readily infect the vertebral bodies and discs, with more than 50% of tuberculosis infections of bone occurring in the spine. The onset is insidious, with destruction of the vertebral bodies, discs, and ligaments if the disease progresses unchecked by medical and surgical treatment. As structural stability is destroyed, kyphosis combined with inflammatory debris and necrotic material can cause progressive paraplegia. Therefore, in the treatment of spinal infections, it is critical to make the diagnosis early so that antibiotic therapy or surgical debridement and fusion can be done before bony collapse and neurologic compromise occur.

ETIOLOGY: HEMATOGENOUS SPREAD

Hematogenous inoculation provides the most common source of organisms for both discitis and vertebral osteomyelitis. Other etiologies include surgery, direct spread from a pulmonary abscess, penetrating trauma, and soft-tissue deficits, such as a decubitus ulcer. Batson (10) demonstrated venous return from the pelvis into the venous plexus of the vertebral column. He theorized that the paravertebral venous reservoir could allow continued venous return and mixing in the setting of changing abdominal and intrathoracic pressures. In his view, these interconnecting venous systems provided an explanation for the presence of vertebral metastases in the absence of lung metastases.

Wiley and Trueta (168) doubted the importance of Batson's venous plexus, demonstrating by injection studies an arterial system of nutrient vessels that supplies the vertebral bodies under physiologic arterial pressures. They found that the richly vascular metaphyseal bone near the anterior longitudinal ligament correlates with the most common site of infections.

Ratcliffe (126) emphasized metaphyseal cancellous infarction caused by a septic embolus. The vascular anatomy of the spine, which changes as a child matures, provides the most likely explanation for the differences in spinal infections in children and adults, as well as for the characteristic locations of infections in the vertebral unit. The interosseous arteries in children are anastomotic; therefore, occlusion of a single nutrient artery leads to destruction of only a small portion of bone because of collateral flow. In adults, a larger portion of bone is destroyed because the interosseous arteries are end arteries, and septic thrombus spreads into peripheral interosseous arteries. The disc is avascular and is attacked by infection equally in all ages.

A process related to vertebral osteomyelitis is spinal epidural abscess (Fig. 150.2). Hlavin et al. (68) reported an incidence of this infection of 1.9 per 10,000 admissions per year. Spinal epidural abscess tends to occur in an older, more medically debilitated population and to be monomicrobial, despite its frequent occurrence in a more medically complex environment. The most common organism is *S. aureus*. Epidural abscess may be due to direct seeding from invasive procedures, such as spinal anesthesia or epidural steroid injection, may form adjacent to an area of osteomyelitis, or, less commonly, may occur from spontaneous hematogenous spread (2,27,107). The distribution

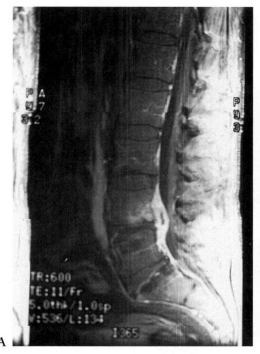
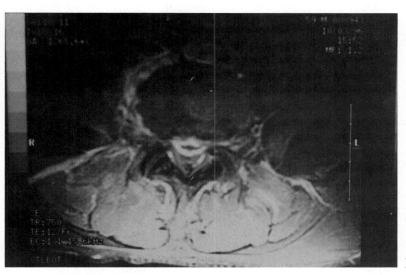

Figure 150.2. Epidural abscess formation occurs in about 15% of vertebral infections. MRI shows an epidural abscess compressing the thecal sac. **A:** Lateral view. **B:** Transverse section.

of this infection parallels the distribution of vertebral osteomyelitis: It is more common in the lumbar spine and less common in the thoracic and cervical segments (41).

While there are case reports of spinal infection following abdominal stab wounds and, rarely, gunshot wounds, the National Spinal Cord Injury Model System reported no cases of spinal infection in a series of 90 patients, despite a 20% incidence of alimentary perforation (64,65, 118,164).

RISK FACTORS

Risk factors for spinal osteomyelitis include diabetes mellitus; chronic steroid use; drug and alcohol abuse; rheumatoid arthritis; urinary, respiratory, or abdominal sepsis; previous surgery; dental infection or extraction; urinary tract manipulation; and any type of spinal needle procedure: acupuncture, spinal anesthesia, epidural catheters, or steroid injections (10,22,27,63,103,112,118,124,145, 148,165,166). Increasing age may be an independent risk factor, with the increasing incidence of gram-negative or anaerobic infections in elderly patients, often in the absence of any concomitant risk factors (23).

Malnutrition, urban overcrowding, and immunocompromising disease are prominent risk factors for granulomatous infection. Tuberculosis is found most commonly

in underdeveloped nations. Big cities in Western countries still have cases of tuberculosis in higher risk patients such as the homeless, immigrants, alcoholics, and other immunocompromised individuals such as those with human immunodeficiency virus infection (97). Other granulomatous infections have geographic risk factors, such as coccidioidomycosis in the San Joaquin Valley of California or histoplasmosis in the central United States.

PATHOPHYSIOLOGY: TUBERCULOSIS OF THE SPINE (POTT'S DISEASE)

Like any other osteoarticular tubercular lesion, spinal tuberculosis is the result of hematogenous dissemination from a primary infected visceral focus. The primary focus can be active or quiescent, apparent or obscure, and located in the lung, lymphatic system, kidney, or other viscus. In a typical lesion, the tuberculous bacilli find their way to the paradiscal area of two contiguous vertebrae, which supports the concept that the spread is via the arterial blood supply. Anterior extension of the lesion, with involvement of multiple vertebral bodies, is caused by extension of the abscess beneath the periosteum and anterior longitudinal ligament. The anterior and posterior longitudinal ligaments and periosteum are stripped from the ver-

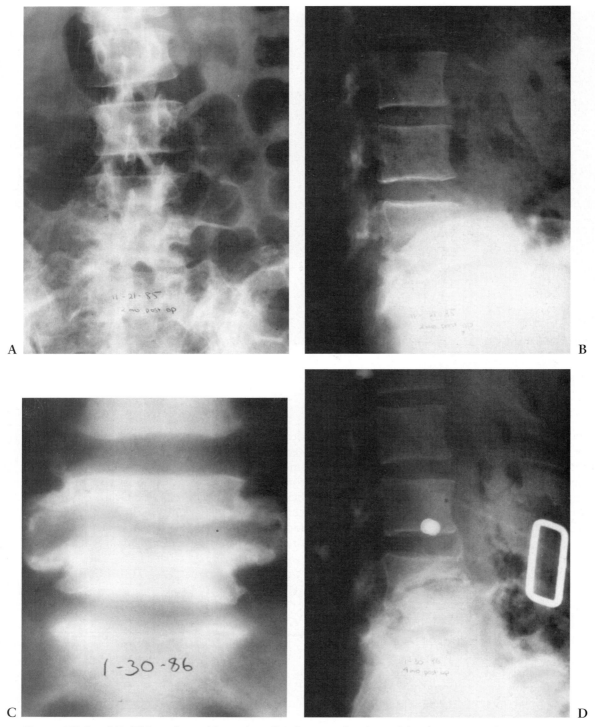

Figure 150.3. **A,B:** This patient with osteomyelitis has complete loss of the disc space with partial destruction of the contiguous vertebral bodies. The lateral x-ray (**B**) shows kyphotic angulation of L-4 in relation to L-5. This 70-year-old woman was having severe pain and muscle spasm. The physical examination revealed loss of L-5 nerve root function on the right. **C:** The patient elected nonoperative care. After a needle biopsy revealed the causative organism, she was treated with antibiotics and a body jacket. At 4 months, a tomogram of the involved level shows osteophyte formation that is starting to bridge the disc space. **D:** A lateral x-ray taken at 4 months reveals correction of the kyphotic angulation. After 2 months of bed rest, a body jacket was applied and molded in hyperextension. *(continued)*

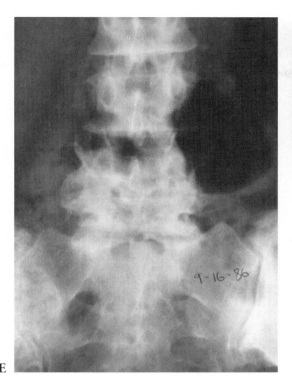
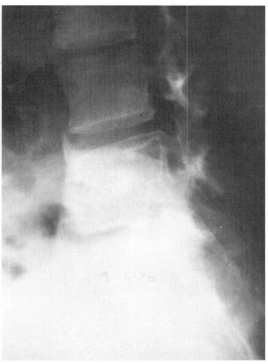

E   F

Figure 150.3. *(continued)* **E,F:** Radiographs taken after 1 year show fusion of L-4 to L-5. She returned to work as a farm wife, pain free and with resolution of the foot drop due to the L-5 root lesion. This patient shows that nonoperative treatment can be successful.

tebral bodies, which results in loss of periosteal blood supply and destruction of the anterolateral surfaces of several contiguous vertebrae.

Vertebral destruction takes place by bone lysis. Periosteal stripping combined with arterial occlusion due to endarteritis causes ischemic infarction leading in turn to necrosis of the involved bone. The body of the vertebra is thus softened and yields to compressive forces. The intervertebral disc is not involved primarily because it is avascular. However, involvement of the paradiscal regions of the vertebra compromises disc nutrition. A disc may then be invaded by the infectious process and destroyed. Radiographically, it is typical to see more than one vertebra involved (average, 3.4 vertebrae) (71). The most common finding is narrowing of the disc space and vertebral osteolysis. In more advanced disease, a paravertebral shadow is produced by extension of the tuberculous granulation tissue and formation of an abscess in the paravertebral region (Fig. 150.3); later, vertebral collapse and angulation of the spine occur.

DIAGNOSIS

The workup for suspected vertebral infection includes a history and physical examination, a complete blood cell count and erythrocyte sedimentation rate (ESR), venous blood cultures if temperature spikes are noted, nuclear medicine imaging (technetium Tc 99m or gallium Ga 65), plain radiographs, and magnetic resonance imaging (MRI) if symptoms are present for more than 1 month. Computed tomography (CT) may be useful for delineating bony destruction and can be used to guide needle biopsy. Lateral tomograms may also be indicated for preoperative evaluation, particularly to delineate bony destruction in the thoracic spine.

HISTORY AND PHYSICAL EXAMINATION

A significant delay of weeks to months is common in the diagnosis of vertebral osteomyelitis (46,163). This delay may be due to a lack of any distinctive early physical or radiographic findings or to a failure to look for spinal infection. Dramatic regional pain that is worsened by motion or compression is the most common symptom. The pain persists despite bed rest and is classically exacerbated with motion. Pain, particularly at night, may not be relieved with analgesics. Fever is not a consistent finding. Anorexia and weight loss have been noted, and although the presentation may be acute, the most typical presentation is subacute or chronic. Chills, night sweats, hemoptysis, or chronic bronchial cough are also suggestive of infection.

On physical examination, the most common finding is severe paraspinal muscle spasm associated with marked tenderness to palpation. A pseudoscoliosis due to spasm may be present. Loss of spinal motion is typical. Patients tend to splint and guard in an attempt to decrease pain; they may be unwilling to bear weight, particularly children. There may also be a mass and a concomitant deformity visible in the area of infection. Neurologic findings may vary from meningeal signs to mild weakness and, finally, paraplegia. One of the earliest findings of spinal cord involvement from tuberculosis is sustained clonus in the ankle.

LABORATORY DATA

The most consistent laboratory finding in the diagnosis of vertebral osteomyelitis is an elevated ESR, usually greater than 40 mm/h (Westergren method). However, Schofferman et al. (135) reported normal values for the ESR in seven of nine patients with occult infections by indolent organisms, such as diphtheroid or coagulase-negative staphylococci. Serial ESR readings are valuable for following a patient's response to intravenous antibiotic therapy (121). C-reactive protein (CRP) is an acute-phase protein synthesized by hepatocytes. An elevated CRP level is seen in various conditions, including infection, inflammation, and malignancy, as a response to tissue injury. Healthy individuals show only trace amounts of CRP. CRP levels rise after surgery but also drop quickly thereafter. An elevated CRP is more helpful for determining postoperative infection during the immediate postoperative period because the ESR can remain elevated at that time (96,151).

The peripheral white blood cell (WBC) count is unreliable. In a series of 38 patients with documented spinal infection, the average WBC count was only slightly increased over the usual high-normal value of 10,000 cells/mm^3 (162).

Blood cultures are an important part of the workup of vertebral osteomyelitis, particularly if the blood culture is obtained during a febrile episode (47,123). Negative culture results are common, however. The tuberculin purified protein derivative (PPD) test is usually positive in patients with tuberculosis. Before administering a PPD test, do an anergy battery to detect immune compromise.

ORGANISMS

By far the most common organism encountered in vertebral osteomyelitis is *S. aureus*. There has been a relative increase in other organisms over the last few years, particularly gram-negative organisms (163). *Pseudomonas aeruginosa* infections are often seen in the setting of intravenous drug abuse, trauma, or immune compromise (19).

Table 150.1. *Unusual Organisms Causing Pyogenic Vertebral Osteomyelitis*

Arconobacterium haemolyticum
Clostridium perfringens
Corynebacterium xerosis
Eikenella corrodens
Haemophilus aphrophilus
Haemophilus influenzae
Kingella kingae
Microorganism group Ve-1
Neisseria sicca
Pasteurella multocida
Peptostreptococcus spp.
Propionibacterium spp.
Pseudomonas cepacia
Salmonella spp.
Salmonella virchow
Serratia marcescens
Staphylococcus warneri
Streptococcus agalactiae
S. bovis
S. milleri
S. mutans
S. pneumoniae
S. sanguis
S. viridans
Torulopsis glabrata
Treponema pallidum
Yersinia enterocolitica

Staphylococcus epidermidis and *Enterococcus* species have also been noted with increasing frequency in postoperative infections (43). At least 27 other organisms have been found to cause vertebral osteomyelitis (Table 150.1). The most common granulomatous infection is tuberculosis.

Immunocompromised patients may present with uncommon or exotic pathogens, and often with multiple organisms. Oral flora is commonly cultivated from intravenous drug abusers and patients with dental abscesses or extensive oral surgery. Resistant strains of bacteria are of particular concern in chronically ill or hospitalized patients.

IMAGING STUDIES

The radiographic findings in pyogenic vertebral osteomyelitis tend to differentiate it from tuberculous involvement of the spine, which classically shows relative sparing of the disc space. With pyogenic vertebral osteomyelitis, the earliest x-ray finding is usually disc-space narrowing, which is noted at about 2–3 weeks after the onset of infection. Disc-space narrowing is followed by endplate erosion, then by progressive vertebral body destruction (Fig. 150.3) (121).

The next roentgenographic change seen is vertebral endplate sclerosis, with increased density noted in the subchondral bone secondary to deposition of new bone on the existing trabeculae and new subperiosteal bone formation (162). This subchondral sclerosis may be preceded by a period of relative radiolucency at about 6 weeks postinfection. The process of increasing postinfection sclerosis will then proceed and can ultimately lead to spinal fusion at about 6 to 24 months.

In tuberculous vertebral osteomyelitis, plain radiographs may not reveal disc-space narrowing until 24–36 months after the onset of the disease process. There may be loss of vertebral density, but reactive new bone is rarely seen and fusion is rarely noted. With tuberculous vertebral infection, a common finding is a large paravertebral soft-tissue mass with calcifications, which is often noted on plain radiographs and CT. This is relatively pathognomonic for tuberculosis. Vertebral pyogenic osteomyelitis, as well as vertebral discitis, tends to be more common in the lumbar spine, less common in the thoracic spine, and least common in the cervical spine. In contrast, tubercular spondylitis is most common in the thoracic spine and at the thoracolumbar junction.

Lateral tomograms may be useful to highlight subtle plain radiographic findings. They can be particularly helpful in imaging the thoracic spine and cervicothoracic junction (Fig. 150.4).

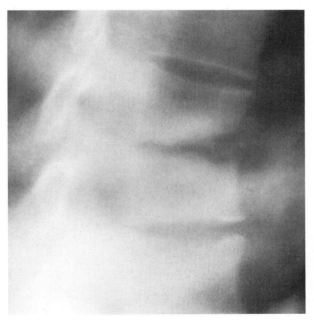

Figure 150.4. Lateral tomogram illustrates endplate destruction in this thoracic infection. Without special studies such as tomography, these lesions can be difficult to visualize.

Computed tomography also has an important role in diagnosis (1,95,161) and is particularly useful when used with myelography (Fig. 150.5) (18). However, in infected patients, myelography carries the risk of possible intrathecal spread of the infection. Bone density can be followed with CT and may give some clue as to whether the infection is progressing or resolving. Increasing bone density has been noted after successful treatment of vertebral body osteomyelitis with antibiotics (83).

CT-guide needle biopsy allows accurate placement within the vertebral body and disc in both pediatric and adult patients (58,72,111). The yield of needle biopsy in producing infectious organisms, however, has been reported to be as low as 50% (6).

Technetium bone scintigraphy is positive in most patients with active vertebral osteomyelitis, but false-positive results have been reported, particularly in the elderly population (3,134). Gallium scan has also been used to image pyogenic vertebral osteomyelitis. Haase et al. (62) described a butterfly appearance of pyogenic vertebral osteomyelitis on gallium scan; the butterfly shape, reflecting soft-tissue uptake, appears on either side of the spine on an anteroposterior view. Bruschwein (21a), reporting on a review of 100 consecutive patients with spinal infections studied with gallium scanning, found a sensitivity of 89%, a specificity of 85%, and an accuracy of 86% (9). Indium-labeled leukocyte imaging of the spine has an accuracy of only 31% (167,174).

Modic et al. (114) reported a sensitivity of 96%, a specificity of 92%, and an accuracy of 94% for MRI in diagnosing spinal infections. In a study of 27 patients with pyogenic vertebral osteomyelitis, MRI accurately detected abnormalities in all patients; radiography did so only in 48%, CT in 65%, technetium bone scan in 71%, and gallium scan in 86%. The most consistent finding on MRI was increased signal intensity, particularly on T2-weighted images (Fig. 150.6).

T1-weighted MR images show characteristic findings of disc-space narrowing, low signal intensity in the marrow of at least two adjacent vertebrae, subligamentous or epidural soft-tissue masses, and erosion of cortical bone (152). T2-weighted images demonstrate narrowed discs with variable signal changes, abnormal high signal intensity in the marrow of at least two adjacent vertebrae, high-signal subligamentous or epidural masses, and cortical bony erosion. MRI demonstrates disc sparing in patients with tuberculous spondylitis, as well as the extraosseous soft-tissue extensions.

Gadolinium enhancement of MRI is useful in distinguishing epidural abscesses from the adjacent compressed thecal sac, as well as identifying a paraspinal mass most likely to yield a positive percutaneous biopsy (125,142). Gadolinium contrast also helps distinguish active infection from an infection that has adequately responded to antibiotic therapy (125).

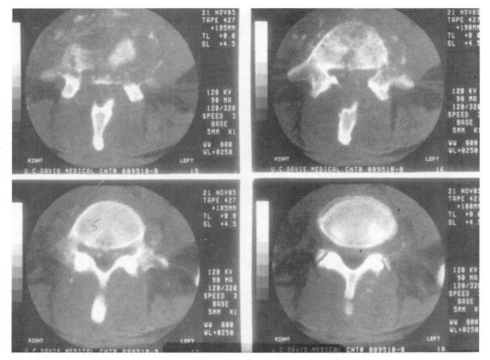

Figure 150.5. CT of an L4-5 infection gives a better picture of the actual bony loss. The cut in the upper right hand corner shows virtually no anterior bony support; the spine is expected to be unstable. This is the same patient described in Figure 150.3. The vertebral angulation can be appreciated on the original lateral x-ray (Fig. 150.3*B*).

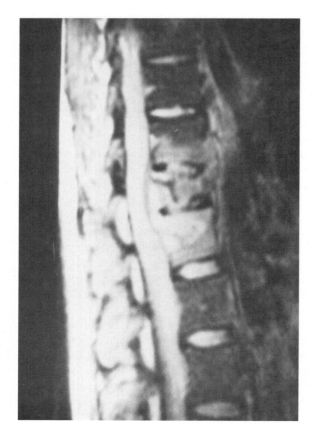

Figure 150.6. MRI provides a means for earlier diagnosis of vertebral osteomyelitis. This T2-weighted image shows increased signal uptake in the involved vertebral bodies. In addition, it yields information about the amount of soft-tissue and spinal cord involvement.

BIOPSY

If the diagnosis is still in question after the above examinations, the differential diagnosis will usually include infection, primary neoplasm, and metastatic involvement of the spine. Tissue from a biopsy is required to differentiate these entities. If the diagnosis is not in question but the causative organism has not been identified, aspiration or biopsy for culture is still required. For the cervical spine, we recommend an anterior approach with a formal operative exposure to avoid the high risk of inadvertently perforating neck structures with a biopsy needle if a percutaneous technique is used. Biopsy samples of the posterior cervical elements may be obtained percutaneously, although formal open exposure facilitates visualization. In the thoracic and lumbar spine, we recommend a posterior CT-guide needle biopsy technique. If additional tissue is required, a Craig needle biopsy can be performed under regional or general anesthesia (Fig. 150.7).

Obviously, the chances of obtaining positive culture results are increased if a patient has not been treated with antibiotics before the biopsy. If a patient's condition permits, discontinue antibiotic therapy for 2 weeks and then proceed with biopsy and culture. Although the clinical

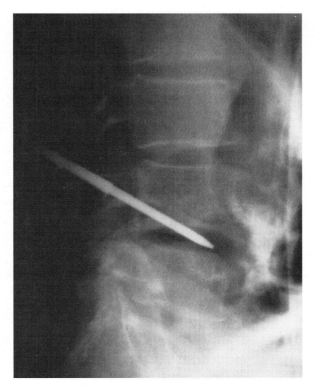

Figure 150.7. A radiograph demonstrates a Craig needle in the L4-5 disc space. Usually, a needle of this size can be used percutaneously in the lumbar spine. In the cervical spine, open techniques are safer. In the thoracic spine, a CT-guided needle biopsy or an open procedure is safer.

presentation and the corroborating radiographic evidence and histology from a biopsy can confirm the presence of infection, culture results are required to prescribe a specific antibiotic regimen. Histology is adequate to diagnose tuberculosis and most fungal infections.

DISEASE-SPECIFIC TREATMENT

Pyogenic Infections

The treatment of most infections of the spine include intravenous antibiotics, rest, and spinal immobilization. In pediatric discitis, this is the treatment of choice. Generally, a regimen of 6 weeks of an intravenous antibiotic followed by 6 weeks of an oral antibiotic is suggested (Table 150.2). Some recommend continuing antibiotic treatment until 3 months after the ESR has returned to normal (163). This presumes that a patient is responding well to treatment and that the response is followed by monitoring the ESR weekly, WBC counts daily (initially) and then every third day, daily temperature reading, and complaints of pain. A Hickman catheter or other long-term indwelling intravenous catheter allows outpatient administration of intravenous antibiotics. We prefer to discontinue antibiotics when a patient is afebrile, pain has nearly resolved, and the ESR is normal. When back pain improves, we allow patients to ambulate in a custom-made thoracolumbar sacral orthosis or, occasionally, in an off-the-shelf brace.

Indications for Surgery

If 2–3 weeks of immobilization and an intravenous antibiotic produce no abatement of fever or decrease in the ESR or WBC count, then consider a thorough anterior debridement and strut grafting (Fig. 150.8). Other indications for surgical intervention include the following:

Large abscess, for which an intravenous antibiotic is usually ineffective
    Neurologic compromise, particularly if it is progressive
    Progressive kyphosis with osseous involvement
    Failure to obtain bacterial cultures by needle biopsy

Neurologic deficits from mechanical failure of the anterior column, which results in kyphosis, are best treated by anterior debridement and mechanical reconstruction with strut grafting (26,46,48,100,105,110). Although several bones may be used for strut grafting, including rib and fibula, tricortical iliac crest autograft is preferred. The cortical portion provides immediate stability, and early union is enhanced by the cancellous component. Before debridement, we recommend a 2-week course of an intravenous antibiotic, if possible, to decrease purulence and surrounding inflammation (153).

Laminectomy for the treatment of spinal infection has been condemned because of its resultant complications

Table 150.2. Intravenous Antibiotics of Choice for Some of the More Common Organisms Causing Pyogenic Infections of the Spine

| Organism | Antibiotic | | |
	1st choice	2nd choice	Oral agent
Staphylococcus aureus	Penicillinase-resistant penicillins (nafcillin, oxacillin)	Cefazolin[a] Vancomycin[a] Ceftriaxone[a]	Cephalexin Cefuroxime axetil Dicloxacillin
Escherichia coli	Gentamicin or cephalosporin	Trimethoprim/ sulfamethoxazole	Trimethoprim/ sulfamethoxazole Ciprofloxacin
Pseudomonas aeruginosa	Tobramycin	Gentamicin Amikacin Ceftazidime Aztreonam Mezlocillin, ticarcillin, or azlocillin[b]	Ciprofloxacin
Staphylococcus epidermidis	Vancomycin	Imipenem	Trimethoprim/ sulfamethoxazole (if sensitive)
β-hemolytic streptococcus	Penicillin G	Cefazolin	Phenoxymethylpenicillin
Enterococci (group D Streptococcus)	Ampicillin plus gentamicin	Vancomycin plus gentamicin	Ampicillin
Bacteroides spp.	Metronidazole	Ampicillin/sulbactam	Metronidazole Amoxicillin/clavulanic acid Clindamycin
Enterobacter spp.	Gentamicin	Tobramycin Amikacin	Ciprofloxacin Trimethoprim/ sulfamethoxazole (if sensitive)
Klebsiella spp.	Cefazolin or ceftizoxime	Gentamicin	Cephalexin Cefixime
Pasteurella multocida	Penicillin G	Tetracycline	Penicillin V
Proteus mirabilis	Ampicillin	Trimethoprim/ sulfamethoxazole	Ampicillin
Serratia marcescens	Gentamicin or amikacin	Third-generation cephalosporins	Ciprofloxacin Trimethoprim/ sulfamethoxazole (if sensitive)

[a] Preferential use for outpatient intravenous antibiotic therapy.
[b] Never used as the single primary drug of therapy, but used for synergy with an aminoglycoside.

(86). The infection decreases the mechanical strength of the anterior and middle bony columns. A laminectomy then destabilizes the remaining (bony–ligamentous) posterior column, adding to instability and increasing the potential for progressive kyphosis. Laminectomy may be appropriate in treating an isolated epidural abscess (29). In this setting, early aggressive laminectomy may be the treatment of choice, permitting decompression and evacuation of the epidural abscess, in conjunction with appropriate antibiotic therapy (68,130).

Several investigators have reported successful anterior bone grafting in the face of infection (26,48,105,110). Safran et al. (131) reported good success with combined same-day simultaneous and sequential anterior decompression and posterior spinal instrumentation. In addition, Hopf et al. (74) recommended anterior debridement

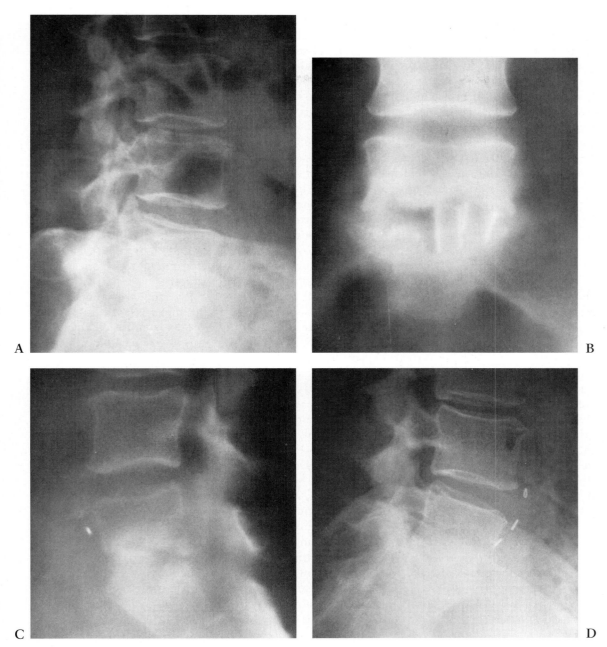

Figure 150.8.   **A:** Lateral radiograph shows disc-space narrowing of L5-S1 due to *Escherichia coli* infection. Antibiotics failed to lower the ESR, and the patient continued to have pain. Anteroposterior (**B**) and lateral (**C**) radiographs show the site after surgical debridement and strut grafting. Two bicortical iliac grafts fill the debrided area of the vertebral bodies. **D:** One year after surgery, the L5–S1 disc space is fused. The patient has no back pain symptoms.

and anterior instrumentation as a single-stage procedure. Rath et al. (127) demonstrated success with posterolateral debridement of the infection and posterior instrumentation and autograft, which represents an alternative way to treat osteomyelitis and disc-space infection. Percutaneous drainage combined with percutaneous placement of pedi-

cle screws for an external fixator has also been used by Jeanneret and Mageral (78). Fusion with bone grafting and instrumentation should be added if a large laminectomy involving multiple segments is performed. This is especially true in children, in whom spinal growth will lead to a progressive kyphotic deformity if fusion is not performed.

Conclusion

Bone grafting and instrumentation in the face of infection is usually successful when performed under the coverage of intravenous antibiotics. The decision to proceed with this major surgery in the face of infection is based on what is best for a patient in the context of a surgeon's abilities and available support services. Anterior debridement and strut grafting followed by posterior instrumentation and grafting work best in our hands and others (59). If one or more vertebral bodies are to be resected to gain adequate anterior decompression and strut grafting, we recommend subsequent posterior stabilization with instrumentation to provide immediate mechanical stability and protection for the neural elements. A spanning segmented instrumentation construct is appropriate (Fig. 150.9).

GRANULOMATOUS INFECTIONS

Historical Background

In the past, tuberculosis was treated by rest, by encouraging patients to spend time in the fresh air, and by relying on patients' natural recuperative powers (67,80). Abscesses were drained when necessary, and the vertebral column was debrided if the patient became paraplegic. In 1895, Menard (113) decompressed an abscess surrounding the spinal cord and was delighted to find that the patient recovered neurologically. This led him and other surgeons to decompress the spinal cord through a variety of posterolateral and anterolateral approaches (17,139). The combination of rest, fusion, and debridement allowed the paraspinal abscesses to regress spontaneously (81). Some patients, however, demonstrated progressive bony destruction, paralysis, and spread of the disease.

Antituberculous drugs changed the surgical approach to spinal tuberculosis. With drugs as the only treatment, patients could be cured not only of active disease but also of paralysis (170). Operative treatment was reserved for failure of drug therapy, recrudescence of disease, Pott's paraplegia that did not resolve after 4–6 weeks of treatment, progressive or worsening paraplegia, or the development of spinal cord involvement or other complications. In 94% of patients without neurologic compromise, clinical healing of the lesion occurred without surgery (154). However, with neurologic involvement, only 38% recovered completely with drug treatment alone, while 69% had complete recovery after surgical decompression.

Martin (109) studied the results of treatment before and after the development of antituberculous drugs and with and without surgical fusion. Of 227 adult patients treated without antibiotics or surgery, bony ankylosis occurred within an average of 5.7 years. Children treated without antibiotics or surgery took even longer to stabilize, requiring on average 9 years to bony ankylosis. Patients treated nonoperatively with antibiotics experienced fusion in 4.9 years. Martin's impression was that antibiot-

ics and surgical fusion produced a more stable spine within a shorter time; he reported a 96.2% fusion rate.

In a later study of patients with Pott's paraplegia (120 of the 740 patients in his total series), Martin (108) found that antibiotics improved patients' general condition and made the surgery safer. It did not, in his opinion, prevent paraplegia or promote recovery from it. He found that 24 (48%) of 50 patients recovered with antibiotics alone, while 60% of patients who underwent surgical decompression recovered. He suggested that an early surgery might prevent or abort the onset of paralysis.

Guirguis (60) reported on 60 patients with Pott's paraplegia, one half of whom were operated on and the other one half treated conservatively. He found better results in the surgically treated patients, with 28 (93%) of 30 patients showing improvement and many being completely cured of any neurologic compromise. Many patients were relieved of their painful flexor spasms.

Neville and Davis (119) also studied patients treated with or without surgery, with emphasis on the fusion rate. In the nonsurgical group, 50% had autofusion at an average of 15.2 months. The surgical group had a fusion rate of 92%.

Arct (7) found that patients older than 60 years of age in Poland could tolerate and benefit from surgical fusion. Of 133 patients, 61 had conservative treatment, while 72 underwent surgical decompression with or without fusion. Only 13 of the conservatively treated patients returned to their regular lifestyle; none could return to work as a farmer or laborer. Of the surgically treated patients, 41 (57%) of 72 had complete clinical and radiographic recovery; 21 patients returned to agricultural work.

In summary, the medical treatment of tuberculosis has been highly effective in controlling bony tuberculosis and even curing it. The newer drugs have been more effective in preventing recurrence of disease due to resistant organisms. However, for at least the first 6 months of chemotherapy, further bony destruction and collapse may occur, causing increased vertebral angulation and cord compression. This is particularly true if a significant amount of kyphotic angulation is already present when drug therapy is started. Without chemotherapy, there will be progressive thinning of the intervertebral space, atrophy of osseous tissue, and decalcification, which can persist for an average of 2–3 years (61). In properly selected patients, medical treatment is adequate and can be expected to yield a relatively high rate (up to 79% in one series) of solid bony fusion (88).

Current Medical Recommendations

Current therapeutic regimen recommended for treating acute tuberculosis of the spine includes the following:

Rifampin: adults, 600 mg daily in a single oral dose 1 hour before or 2 hours after a meal; children, 10–20 mg/kg per day (not to exceed 600 mg)

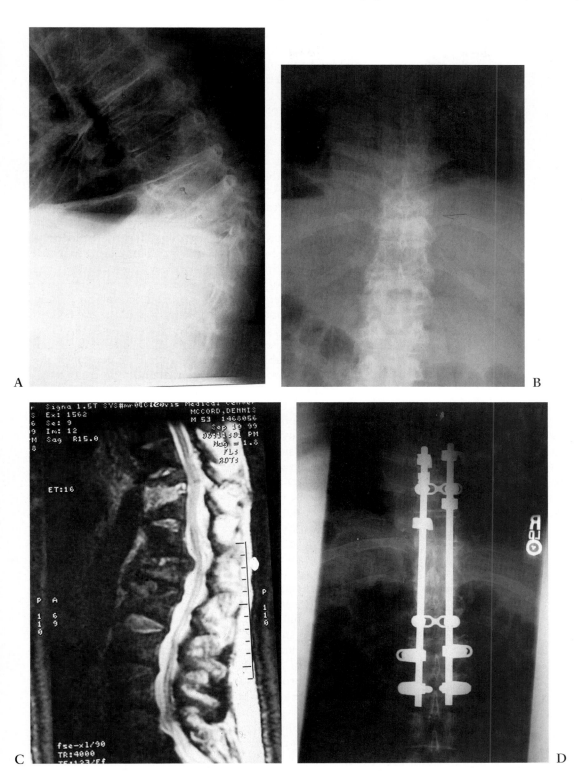

Figure 150.9. A 52-year-old white man had a history of weight loss, fevers, chills, and progressive loss of lower extremity function over 8 months. He presented to the emergency department with weakness in both lower extremities. He had an obvious kyphotic deformity with pain at the apex of the kyphosis as seen on lateral (**A**) and AP (**B**) radiographs, and MRI (**C**). Anterior debridement of T-10 and T-11 vertebral bodies was performed, with subsequent anterior strut grafting with autogenous iliac crest bone graft. Posterior segmental instrumentation and fusion were performed the same day as seen on AP(**D**) and lateral (**E**) radiographs. Intraoperative cultures revealed *S. aureus*, and the patient underwent long-term intravenous antibiotic treatment. He recovered and walked without any assistive devices.

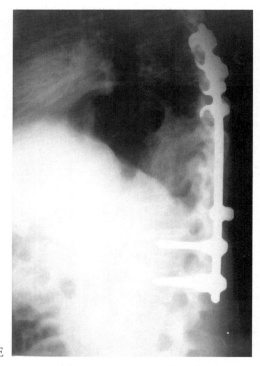

E

Figure 150.9.   (continued)

Isoniazid: adults, 5 mg/kg orally (up to 300 mg per day) in a single dose

Ethambutol: adults only, 15 mg/kg orally in a single dose

Pyrazinamide: 20 mg/kg

Rifampin, isoniazid, and pyrazinamide are each given for 12 months. A four-drug regimen for 12 months or a three-drug regimen for 18 months is appropriate for eradicating difficult infections (115). Initiate antibiotics at least 2 weeks before surgery and, if possible, continue them postoperatively. In cases of acute paraplegia requiring emergency decompression, begin antibiotics before spinal surgery.

Surgical Management

Although antibiotics can medically treat Pott's disease, most orthopaedic surgeons continue to favor surgical debridement. Hodgson et al. (71) proposed that debridement be done as soon as possible after the diagnosis is established for the following reasons:

In the early stages of the disease, extirpation of the infected focus is easier, and fusion without deformity is possible.

Secondary deformities occur as the disease progresses, impairing the patient's cardiopulmonary function.

The patient's general condition improves markedly after evacuation of the abscess.

The patient requires less extended hospitalization and can return to work earlier, often within 4–6 months.

Late recurrence of the disease is less common.

Rapid progression of the abscess along the spine is prevented.

Surgical exploration of the tuberculous lesion is the only way to ensure that the disease is indeed active or healed.

Hodgson et al. (69) also confirmed that tuberculosis can penetrate the covering of the spinal cord (dura), causing irreversible paraplegia; therefore, they felt an urgent need for surgical drainage to prevent this complication. In their hands, early anterior debridement and fusion of the spine resulted in 4% mortality, but the fusion rate was 93% and 26 of 35 patients with paraplegia recovered complete function. There was a close correlation between the duration of neurologic symptoms before operation and the time required to recover from paraplegia (69). In tuberculosis, bone grafting is safe, even in the presence of drainage (4,5).

While anterior decompression and fusion of the spinal column is reliable and effective in treating neurologically compromised patients, posterior laminectomy is not effective and may lead to neurologic deterioration (15). Infectious destruction is usually anterior, causing the involved vertebral body to collapse and angulate into kyphosis. Laminectomy destabilizes the spine further and aggravates this progression into kyphosis. Hence, there is no question as to the superiority of the anterior approach (8,45).

In children, Bailey et al. (8) noted that anterior tuberculous disease was almost always more widespread than demonstrated on radiographs. Even late decompression, when symptoms have been present for an extended period, can produce neurologic recovery. Bone grafting leads to an acceptable risk of fusion in both children and adults (4,79,85).

In the immature spine, there may be progressive kyphosis despite a solid fusion (50), as continuing growth in the posterior spine may create further deformity (79). Schulitz et al. (138) studied anterior fusion, anterior debridement, and combined anterior and posterior fusion in children followed for at least 10 years. Anterior fusion alone had the worst prognosis in terms of progression of kyphosis. Combined anterior and posterior fusion decreased the incidence of kyphosis. On the other hand, Upadhyay et al. (156–160) showed that a short anterior spinal arthrodesis done at a early age was not associated with progression of deformity during growth and development from disproportionate posterior spinal growth. Therefore, they did not recommend a posterior fusion to stop posterior growth. They also reported that patients who had reduction of kyphosis at the time of the fusion showed a difference only at the sixth month of follow-up, compared with patients who had only debridement. At final follow-up, however, they found no difference in kyphosis between the groups and stressed the importance of achieving complete reduction and fusion to prevent kyphosis. In summary, our preferred approach to the treatment of children is a combined anterior and posterior fusion when multiple levels of radical debridement are required; we use the anterior approach only when only a short fusion is necessary.

In a long-term controlled trial comparing radical debridement and anterior fusion, simple debridement, and medical treatment alone, the Medical Research Council showed radical debridement and fusion to be superior in the following ways (31,32,50,150):

Anterior bony fusion occurs earlier and in a higher percentage of patients (70% versus 20% and 26% at 5-year follow-up).

Kyphotic angulation was less common at 5 years.

At 10 years, kyphotic angulation increased further in the simple-debridement group, whereas it actually decreased in the radical-debridement and fusion group.

Others have agreed with this philosophy, although none has had the experience or stated the case so eloquently as the group from Hong Kong (25,51,70,71,79,85,89,90, 144,147,169,175,176). While the surgery is technically demanding and risky, the alternative seems to be worse. Yau and Hodgson (175) reported on the penetration of the lung by vertebral abscesses and on irreversible paraplegia from tuberculous infection passing through the dura and directly involving the spinal cord (61,69).

The bony destruction, collapse, and angulation that can occur while under medical treatment are undesirable and preventable (91). Adding internal fixation to the treatment of tuberculosis of the spine diminishes the incidence of kyphosis and pain, reduces the incidence of bedsores, pulmonary infections, and recurrence rates and shortens hospital stay (73). Moon et al. (116,117) described similar findings in which anterior debridement and posterior fixation provided early fusion, prevented progression of kyphosis, and achieved correction of kyphosis. Other authors have suggested using anterior instrumentation routinely at the time of debridement (74,93). Therefore, if proper facilities and expertise for surgical drainage and grafting of the infected vertebral column are available, surgical fusion and stabilization are indicated (14,25,28, 57,87,101,116,129,160). Nonoperative treatment with antibiotics and orthotic support continues to be an option for patients without significant destruction and kyphosis (125).

Even though anterior instrumentation has successfully been used for pyogenic and granulomatous infections, we have not routinely used it. Anterior instrumentation may be used in these situations if immediate stability is needed or posterior instrumentation cannot be performed in a timely manner.

Even late cases with severe kyphotic deformity can be candidates for surgery. Spinal osteotomy, halo–pelvic dis-

traction, and anterior and posterior surgery have been used to correct these deformities (176). Although the complication rate associated with halo–pelvic traction and the multiple surgical procedures was high, the average amount of correction was 28.3% in 30 patients; more important, further progression of the deformity was halted. Halo–pelvic traction is still a viable technique and sometimes safer than immediate correction with anterior and posterior osteotomies. In these cases, a modest correction of the spinal deformity balanced with prevention of further progression is the goal.

In the cervical spine, Lifeso (99) refined the staging of atlantoaxial tuberculosis, describing three stages with progressive bone destruction. In stage I, there is minimal bony destruction, and a transoral biopsy and decompression can be used to surgically treat the infection, followed by halo orthosis. In stage II, there is minimal bony destruction, but anterior displacement of C-1 and C-2 is present. For this, he advised transoral biopsy and decompression followed by reduction with a halo orthosis and a posterior surgical fusion of C1–2. In stage III, marked bony destruction with displacement of C-1 and C-2 occurs. For this stage, an anterior decompression is performed, followed by halo-traction reduction and posterior fusion from the occiput to C-2 or C-3. We endorse this step-by-step approach as a practical way to approach this difficult problem.

In the lower cervical spine, Hsu and Leong (75) found a high incidence of neurologic compromise and recommended anterior decompression and fusion in all cases of tuberculosis of the cervical spine (see Chapter 151). Other authors have reported similarly on lower cervical spine tuberculosis, noting a high incidence of neurologic compromise requiring surgical treatment with bone grafting and anterior plating combined with antibiotic treatment (102,104).

Conclusion

The major anatomic feature characteristic of all granulomatous diseases is destruction of the anterior column. This is the area that usually needs to be drained or, if weakened by bony destruction, supported by grafting. In most cases, posterior procedures are supplemental to the anterior operation. For Pott's paraplegia, the preferred procedure is anterolateral decompression. Arthrodesis of the spine is usually necessary to support the weakened anterior column. Strut grafting is difficult through a costotransversectomy, so anterolateral decompression, debridement, and fusion are best accomplished through this approach. Posterior decompression further weakens the spinal column and can cause further collapse and neurologic deterioration (106). We prefer anterior decompression and strut grafting followed by a posterior stabilization procedure (Fig. 150.10). We debride infected and weakened bone and reconstruct the anterior column with rigid bone strut

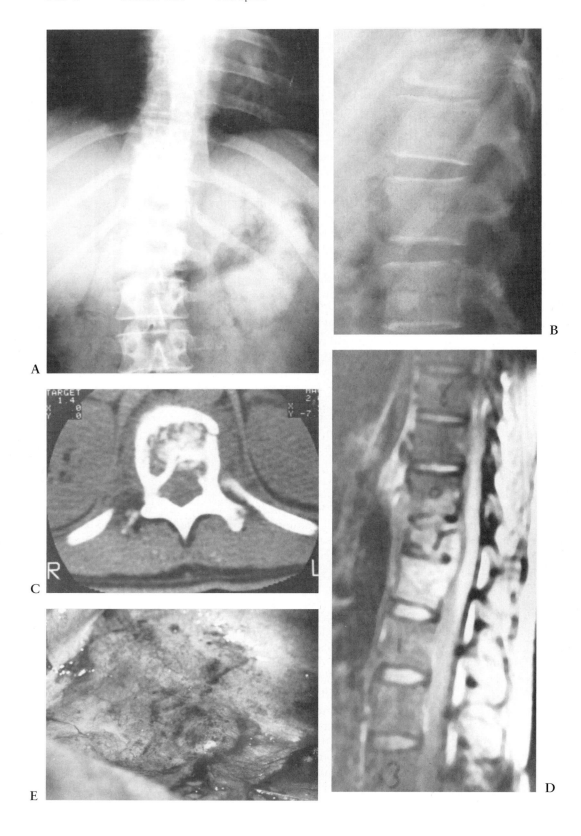

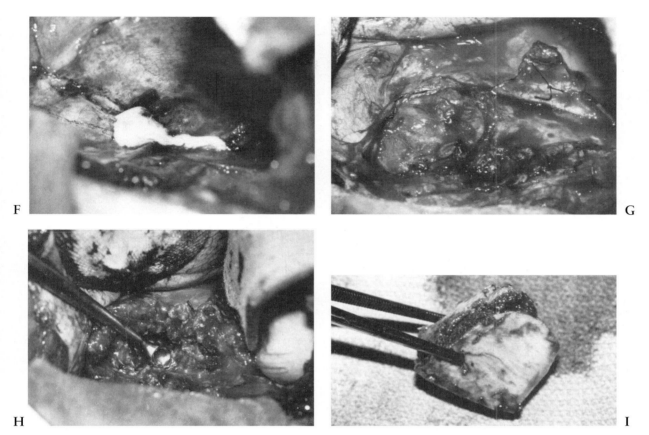

F

G

H

I

Figure 150.10. Anteroposterior (**A**) and lateral (**B**) radiographs from a 30-year-old baker who had back pain after stepping into a hole. He had an ESR of 120 mm/h, a positive PPD with 10 mm of induration, and a negative coccidioidin titer. The lateral film demonstrates loss of height of the T-11 body and endplate destruction. **C:** CT demonstrates destruction of the vertebral body with extension posteriorly into the neural canal. **D:** MRI reveals the amount of vertebral destruction and compression of the spinal cord. Because of the amount of vertebral body involvement, it was elected to debride and strut-graft this lesion anteriorly and to fuse and stabilize the spine with instrumentation posteriorly. **E:** An anterolateral thoracic approach through the tenth rib was used to expose the T-11 vertebra. This photograph demonstrates the abscess over the vertebral body expanding the parietal pleura. The aorta lies just anterior to the spinal column. **F:** The abscess is incised along the posterolateral border of the spinal column parallel to it. Gross purulence exudes from the incision. **G:** A second incision is made perpendicular to the first from posterior to anterior, forming a T, and the corners can be elevated off the vertebral body and anchored anteriorly with skip sutures. Later, these flaps can then be used as closure over the grafted area. The segmental vessels to the vertebral bodies have been ligated. **H:** The necrotic bone and abscess material are removed by curettage or drilling with a high-speed burr. The involved bone, disc, and other debris are removed until good bleeding bone is located at each end of the lesion. If decompression of the spinal cord or cauda equina is needed, it is done at this time. The amount of material removed can be impressive. **I:** Bicortical bone can be removed from the ilium. This should be done with a separate draping and surgical setup so as not to contaminate the graft site. The graft is measured before it is cut to ensure an adequate length to strut the defect. *(continued)*

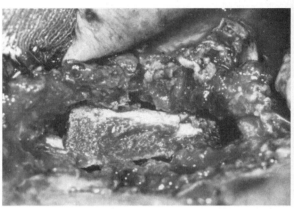
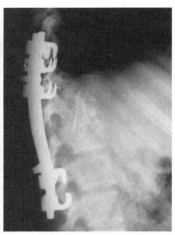

J   K

Figure 150.10.   (continued) **J:** The strut is impacted into the defect created by the debridement. The table, which had previously been flexed to provide access to the chest, is now
straightened, locking the graft in place. If an acute kyphosis is present, additional strut grafts
may be needed to bridge it completely. These are placed more anteriorly and should also be
implanted into the bony portion of the vertebra. **K:** A postoperative lateral radiograph shows
the iliac strut graft to span the infected level extending into the vertebrae above and below.
Cotrel-Dubousset instrumentation extends an additional level above and below the T-11 vertebra. A posterior fusion supplements this instrumentation. The patient was ambulatory and
taking tuberculosis medication when he left the hospital 2 weeks after the second surgery. He
will continue his medication for 1 year after surgery.

grafting, which we then augment by posterior instrumentation using a neutralization construct and fusion.

Atypical Mycobacterial Infections

Atypical mycobacterial disease usually occurs in the extremities, but cases of spinal involvement have been reported. Diagnosis depends on identification of acid-fast
bacilli, as granuloma formation is not necessarily a feature
of the disease (106,133,137). In the presence of a persistent inflammatory process, ask about a history of contact
with shellfish and other sea life, gardening, or trauma.
Surgical excision of the infected focus and antibiotic administration are the mainstays of therapy (54,133).

FUNGAL INFECTIONS

Coccidioidomycosis

Coccidioidomycosis is caused by *Coccidioides immitis,*
the most infectious of all fungi capable of producing systemic disease. The localized form is usually benign, but the
disseminated form is progressive and potentially lethal.
Of those with disseminated disease, 20% have osseous
lesions. The fungus is endemic to the southwestern United
States, Central America, and parts of South America. It
is particularly prevalent in central California, where it carries the name San Joaquin Valley fever (171). Although the
disease occurs in all ages, it is most prevalent in individuals

25–55 years of age, and dissemination is greater in men.
Disseminated disease is 10 times more common in blacks
than whites and is of even greater hazard to Filipinos
(171).

The organisms enter the body via the respiratory tract
and are spread hematogenously. If respiratory symptoms
and fever develop in a patient in an endemic region and
last longer than 1 month, disseminated disease should be
suspected. In an endemic area, 50% to 84% of the population will have a positive coccidioidin skin test. It takes
3–6 weeks for an exposed patient to test positive. Because
of anergy, the test is unreliable when systemic disease is
present. A serologic complement fixation titer of 1:64 or
higher is thought to be diagnostic of disseminated disease
(154).

Most bone lesions are lytic in nature and indiscrimi-
nately involve the vertebrae and other bony elements of
the spine (Fig. 150.11). Often, multiple spinal lesions are
found. Although the discs are spared, paraspinal masses
are seen with contiguous rib involvement (35). Treatment
with amphotericin B or fluconazole (Diflucan) is recommended (39,133). Indications for surgical procedures are
similar to those recommended for tuberculosis.

Blastomycosis

Blastomycosis (North American) is caused by *Blastomyces
dermatitidis,* a fungus causing chronic systemic infection

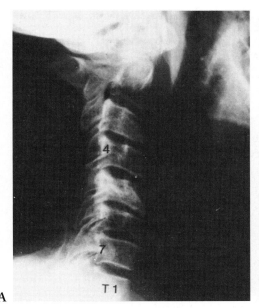
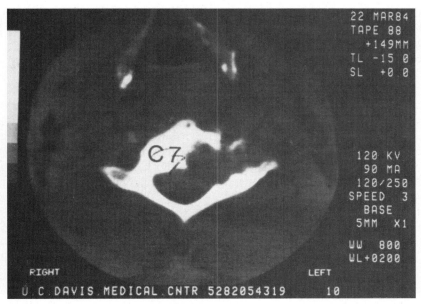

A   **B**

Figure 150.11.   Coccidioidomycosis can occur anywhere in the spine. In this case, the body and left lateral mass of the C-7 vertebra are destroyed. It is not as clearly seen on the lateral radiograph (**A**), but CT reveals the amount of vertebral destruction (**B**). During anterior debridement and strut grafting, the vertebral artery was identified. This 40-year-old man preoperatively received large amounts of amphotericin b with little effect on the bone disease.

that is respiratory in origin but capable of dissemination. It is endemic in the southeastern and midwestern United States. Men are affected nine times more often than women; all ages may be affected, although there is a higher frequency in the third and fourth decades.

The disease usually begins as a mild respiratory infection, but as it disseminates hematogenously, generalized symptoms of fever, night sweats, anorexia, and weight loss develop. Skin tests are often negative early in the disease, but a culture of the skin or lesion will reveal budding yeast cells. Serologic tests may show a high titer only to *Histoplasma capsulatum.*

Osteomyelitis is common in disseminated blastomycosis, and it has a greater tendency than coccidioidomycosis for fistula formation and erosion into joints. The disc cartilage is usually involved early, and large paravertebral masses involving ribs may be seen. Hilar adenopathy may be noted on the chest radiograph, as in tuberculosis (56). Treatment for blastomycosis is oral ketoconazole (Nizoral) or itraconazole (Sporanox), but amphotericin B may be needed in immunocompromised patients. Indications for surgery and the procedures are similar to those for tuberculosis.

Cryptococcosis
Cryptococcosis, caused by *Cryptococcus neoformans,* is a chronic systemic fungal disease originating in the respiratory tract. It may affect all ages, but is most prevalent between 40 and 60 years of age and is twice as common in men. Cryptococcosis is commonly seen in patients with leukemia, Hodgkin's disease, or sarcoidosis in whom central nervous system findings develop. The pulmonary disease is rarely symptomatic. Spread is by the hematogenous route and often results in a cryptococcal meningitis, with 10% of disseminated cases involving bone. The bony lesions are heralded by pain, swelling, and progressive loss of spine motion (34).

Blood, spinal fluid culture, or cultures from bony lesions may reveal the organism. India ink capsule stain is helpful, especially in spinal fluid specimens. Cryptococcal antibodies may be measured, and some authors believe that their presence indicates a good prognosis. Radiographically, the findings are indistinguishable from coccidioidomycosis (34).

Similar to all the fungal diseases, cryptococcosis is treated medically with amphotericin B or fluconazole plus flucytosine (Ancobon) (79). Guidelines for surgery are similar to those for tuberculosis.

Brucellosis
Brucellosis is a systemic infectious disease caused by small, nonmotile, non-spore-forming, gram-negative rods of the genus *Brucella.* Farm animals are primary sources of infection, but many other animals may harbor the bacteria (172). Human infection occurs primarily from ingestion of improperly prepared animal tissues or products or from

skin wound contamination from infected animal tissues. Infection via inoculation of the conjunctiva has been demonstrated, and there is some evidence that inhalation of aerosols containing bacteria can lead to the disease (11, 12).

Brucellar infections are often asymptomatic. Initial infection leads to immunity in about 90% of cases (12,172). Men are affected more often than women, probably because of a higher rate of occupational exposure. Initial symptoms may include fever, sweats, weakness, weight loss, headache, myalgia, lymphadenopathy, and hepatosplenomegaly. Late complications are multisystemic and may include septic arthritis, central nervous system involvement, osteomyelitis, and spine involvement (172). Of patients with spinal involvement, about 12% will have spinal cord compromise.

Brucellae can be cultured from the blood during a bacteremic episode and from involved lymph nodes or granulomas later in the course of the disease. The organisms are dangerous to laboratory personnel, and any suspected materials should be clearly identified (172). The *Brucella* agglutination test is quite reliable, and about 97% of infected patients will become positive within 3 weeks of exposure. Brucellosis is a reportable disease.

Radiographic changes to the spine occur relatively late in the course of the disease and are similar to but less severe than those seen in tuberculosis (11,172). A paravertebral abscess usually is not present, as in tuberculosis, and the spinal involvement usually is in the lumbar area (11,172).

The mainstay of treatment for brucellosis is antibiotic therapy, usually with doxycycline and rifampin, for at least 6 weeks. Surgical intervention is usually limited to a biopsy to obtain a tissue diagnosis. Occasionally, stabilization of the spine or decompression of the cord may be necessary. The indications and techniques are identical to those proposed for treatment of the tuberculous spine. Brucellosis is a completely curable infection. The primary pitfall is a delay in diagnosis of more than 1 month, which can lead to multisystem involvement with severe sequelae (11,12,172).

Aspergillosis

Aspergillosis is a rare form of fungal spinal osteomyelitis (Fig. 150.12) (49,77,140,141,143). It is most common in immunosuppressed patients but has also been reported in cases of postoperative disc-space infection and after invasive monitoring (17,21,76,77,143,146). The radiographic appearance is not pathognomonic but is distinctive, generally demonstrating dense reactive new bone, a small lytic region, and the absence of sequestration. Histologic diagnosis is usually made with a potassium hydroxide preparation. Recommended treatment is amphotericin B alone or together with itraconazole; rifampin may be added (42, 94). Surgery is recommended in accordance with the previ-

ously outlined guidelines for tuberculosis (40,88,133, 136).

Candidiasis

Along with aspergillosis, candidal infections are becoming increasingly common, primarily in the settings of immune compromise or secondary overgrowth following antibiotic usage (44,52,55,67,82,120,146). Systemic candidiasis may be diagnosed with positive sputum, urine, or blood cultures. Medical treatment is amphotericin B or fluconazole, and surgery is indicated within the guidelines described for tuberculosis.

Actinomycosis

Actinomycosis is often confused with fungal infection (33). However, the cause is an anaerobic, gram-positive, branching, filamentous bacterium. In actinomycosis, granulomatous suppurative lesions form and often develop sinus tracts, particularly in the head and neck region (79,136). The infection can be treated medically with penicillin (133). The need for surgery is determined in accordance with the previously delineated recommendations for spinal stabilization.

POSTOPERATIVE SPINAL INFECTIONS

Infection after spinal surgery is a significant complication. Postoperative infection following disc penetration is most likely due to direct inoculation (37,38,122,177). Therefore, the routine use of prophylactic antibiotics is recommended whenever the intervertebral disc is entered (including procedures such as minor discography) or other spinal surgery is undertaken (122). Infection rates increase with the extent or complexity of spinal surgery. The lowest rates (0.7% to 0.8%) are reported with intervertebral disc surgery without fusion (37). For patients undergoing spine fusion without instrumentation, the rates range from 0.9% to 6%. The highest rates are reported with the use of spinal instrumentation (0.5% to 15%); the average is about 8% (149).

Postoperative Discitis

Postoperative discitis has decreased with the use of microsurgical techniques, probably because of decreased soft-tissue injury (37). Patients with discitis will usually be pain-free for 1–2 weeks after surgery, and then progressively increasing low-back pain develops. This may be accompanied by temperature elevation, an increased ESR, elevated CRP and WBC counts, increasingly tender paravertebral musculature, increasing muscle spasm, and decreased lumbosacral range of motion. The neurologic status usually does not change from the immediate postoperative examination. Plain radiographs are rarely definitive in this period, but may demonstrate disc-space

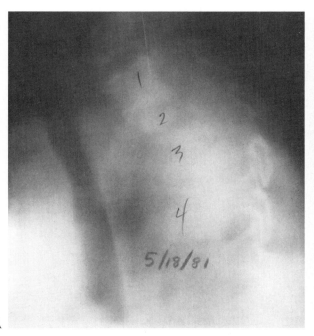
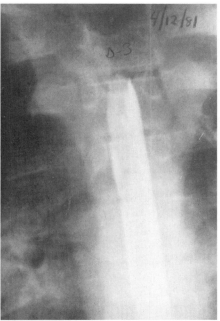

A   B

Figure 150.12.   Aspergillosis can infect the spine in immunocompromised patients, including those with acquired immunodeficiency syndrome (AIDS) or AIDS-related complex, intravenous drug abusers, or patients receiving cancer chemotherapy. This and other unusual organisms (e.g., *Candida*) are appearing with increasing frequency. This young man had aspergillosis that destroyed the T-2 and T-4 vertebral bodies with acute collapse and angulation. **A:** Tomography demonstrates the amount of destruction and angular deformity. **B:** Myelography reveals a blockage of the spinal cord canal created by granulation tissue and the deformity. The patient was paraplegic and required anterior debridement and posterior stabilization. There was complete recovery of neurologic function after anterior decompression.

narrowing and evidence of endplate involvement by 2–3 weeks after the onset of infection. Nucleotide bone scan will be positive because of the surgery, and so are not useful in differentiating infection. If the presentation is delayed, MRI may demonstrate the characteristic findings of a spinal infection (Fig. 150.13). The definitive procedure for accurate diagnosis of postoperative discitis is CT-guide neddle biopsy followed by culture of the organism from the disc space (Fig. 150.14).

With the organism identified, an appropriate antibiotic can be given; most patients can be successfully treated with an intravenous antibiotic, bed rest or immobilization in a brace, and serial monitoring of the ESR and CRP level. We follow the guidelines for surgery discussed previously for primary infection of the disc space if medical treatment fails.

Postoperative Infections with Spinal Implants

A multicenter study by Thalgott et al. (149) resulted in a classification of patients with spinal instrumentation and postoperative infections into three groups on the basis of a clinical staging system for adult osteomyelitis developed by Cierny. Group 1 patients had a single-organism infection, either superficial or deep; group 2 had multiple-organism deep infections; and group 3 had multiple organisms with myonecrosis. Host response was also ranked into three classes: Class A included patients with normal systemic defenses and normal metabolic capabilities and vascularity; class B patients demonstrated local or multiple systemic diseases, including cigarette smoking; and class C patients were immunocompromised or severely malnourished.

Group 1 patients could generally be treated with a single irrigation and debridement, and closure over suction drainage tubes without the use of inflow irrigation (43). Group 2 patients required an average of three irrigations and debridements and had a higher percentage of resolution of the infection when a closed inflow–outflow suction irrigation system was used (53). Group 3 patients were difficult to manage and tended to have a poor outcome. Patients with diminished host defenses (classes B and C) demonstrated an increased risk for postoperative wound infection.

Metallic implants were generally left in place for spinal

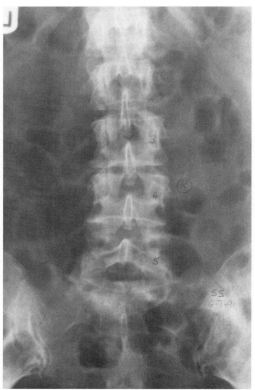
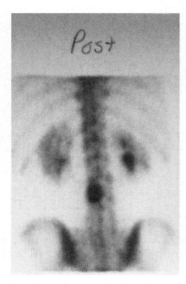
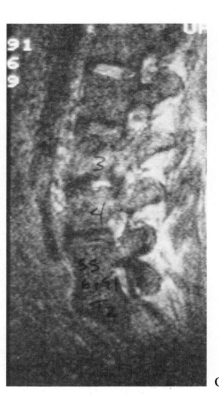

A,B   C

Figure 150.13.   **A:** Back pain and spasms developed in this patient 8 months after a percutaneous discectomy of the L3-4 disc. Percussion at the level of the discectomy produced severe,
localized pain. The ESR was 120 mm/h. This anteroposterior radiograph shows only slight
disc-space narrowing. **B:** Tc 99m bone scan demonstrates increased uptake at the level of the
previous discectomy. This is much too intense to be due to postoperative changes. **C:** T2-
weighted MRI shows increased signal uptake in the L3-4 disc space, indicative of infection.
A Craig needle biopsy confirmed the diagnosis of disc-space infection; *S. aureus* was cultured.
The patient recovered after 6 weeks of immobilization in a body jacket and intravenous
antibiotic treatment.

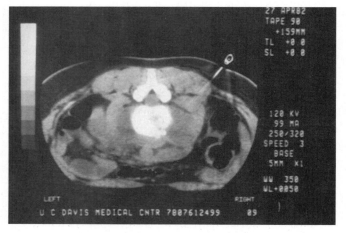

Figure 150.14.   CT shows a needle being directed into a paravertebral abscess surrounding an infected vertebra.

stability during treatment. Bone graft, if loose, grossly infected, and surrounded by purulence, should be debrided;
otherwise the bone graft can be left in place.

Delayed infections following posterior spinal instrumentation have been reported at an average of 25 months
after surgery (128). It is not entirely clear whether this
drainage and infection are due to primary inoculation
with low-virulence organisms or prominence of implants
causing formation of bursal sacs that become infected secondarily. *Propionibacterium* species, *S. epidermidis*, and
Micrococcus species have been found to be the organisms
most responsible for causing these late infections. Treatment requires removal of the implants, debridement, and
intravenous antibiotics.

The most important aspect of treating postoperative
infections is to be aggressive in irrigating and debriding
such wounds, rather than treating them with antibiotics
alone. Multiple debridements may be necessary to achieve
formation of granulation tissue before primary closure can

be performed. Wounds that have gross purulence or failed closure may be managed with dressing changes and healing by secondary intention. At times, latissimus dorsi or rotational flaps may be needed to obtain coverage. In our experience, suction–irrigation and multiple debridements have worked well in treating most infections postoperatively. Antibiotic beads placed at the time of each debridement have also shown promise in terms of adding a concentrated antibiotic locally to the infection.

EPIDURAL ABSCESS

Epidural abscess is a potentially devastating condition. Patients complain of local pain, tenderness over the spine, generalized malaise, and fever. The symptoms may be highly variable in immunocompromised patients. Heusner (66) described four phases of neurologic involvement from epidural abscess. In early phases I and II, there is localized pain with the development of radicular pain and early neurologic changes, such as diminished reflexes. In phase III, progressive neurologic symptoms occur, including evidence of upper motor neuron impairment such as hyperflexia. Motor weakness may eventually develop, with impaired bowel and bladder function. Finally, in phase IV, complete paralysis develops. Epidural abscesses may occur from either metastatic seeding or direct extension (20,66). Spinal cord dysfunction is probably due to a combination of mechanical compression and anterior spinal artery thrombosis, which can cause ischemia and direct infection of the cord (20,66). Multiple reports have described many conditions that can lead to an epidural abscess, including intravenous drug abuse, lumbar puncture, and urinary tract and upper respiratory tract infections (9,13,36,92). Unfortunately, the diagnosis is frequently delayed (9). The ESR will be elevated, and blood cultures may be positive. MRI is the best tool for diagnosing epidural abscess. Radionuclide studies (technetium or gallium scan) may not be helpful.

Differential diagnosis includes metastatic disease to the epidural space and abscess in the subdural space, which is rare. Only 45% of the patients with an epidural abscess are infected by *S. aureus* (41). Gram-negative rods, anaerobes, mycobacteria, and fungi are responsible for the remaining 55%.

Treatment should be emergent. Start intravenous antibiotics immediately. A penicillinase-resistant penicillin or vancomycin will provide coverage for *S. aureus,* and an aminoglycoside for other suspected organisms, until the Gram stain and culture results are available (84). Posterior compressive lesions should be treated with surgical drainage by laminectomy, with maintenance of mechanical stability by preservation of the facets. The wound may be closed over drains or packed open in cases in which there is gross purulence. If an epidural abscess occurs anteriorly, particularly with a disc-space infection with extension into the epidural space, anterior debridement and decompression of the anterior epidural space are necessary.

Although management of epidural abscess with intravenous antibiotics alone without surgery has been reported, the risk of progression of neurologic compromise is high (16,30,98). The current treatment of choice for patients with cord compromise is surgical debridement and antibiotics. In patients without neurologic involvement who are poor surgical candidates, antibiotics may be used initially, with monitoring of neurologic status. Surgery may be necessary if significant neurologic findings develop.

DRAINAGE AND DEBRIDEMENT OF SPINAL ABSCESSES

LUMBAR SPINE

Abscesses secondary to tuberculosis or fungal disease may present as masses that can be palpated externally. Pyogenic abscesses rarely reach this extent without proving lethal. In the lumbar spine, an abscess will generally follow the course of the psoas muscle, although it can also appear as a paravertebral mass. An abscess that dissects along the psoas may extend below Poupart's ligament and present on the anteromedial surface of the thigh (adductor region) or in the gluteal region. Occasionally, an abscess will appear over the crest of the ilium in Petit's triangle.

Paravertebral Abscess
- To drain a paravertebral mass posteriorly, make an incision 4–8 cm lateral to the vertebral spinous processes in a line parallel to the spine.
- Use a Cobb elevator or even finger dissection to bluntly dissect around the erector spinae muscles until the transverse processes of the vertebrae are reached.
- Usually, the abscess is entered immediately. If not, puncture the thoracolumbar fascia that separates the quadratus lumborum muscle from the erector group.
- Locate the abscess by working under the transverse process, and then debride and drain it (173). Send purulent material and tissue for Gram stain, culture, sensitivities, and histology.
- After drainage, close the tissues in layers over a drain, or pack the wound open. This is determined by the local conditions and surgeon preference (71,85).

Psoas Abscess
Posterior Approach Psoas abscesses are extraperitoneal and can be drained posterolaterally through Petit's triangle or anteriorly beneath Poupart's ligament. Petit's triangle is bordered by the lateral margin of the latissimus dorsi muscle, the medial border of the external oblique abdominal muscle, and inferiorly by the crest of the ilium.

- Make an incision 2.5 cm above the crest of the ilium and parallel to it. Begin the incision lateral to the erector spinae muscle group.
- Bluntly dissect through the internal oblique abdominal muscle to gain access to the abscess cavity.
- The incision may be also made directly over the iliac crest, in which case detach the internal and external oblique abdominal muscles from the ilium and expose its inner surface.
- Palpate the abscess extraperitoneally, and then open and drain it.
- Manage the wound as described above.

Anterior Approach
- Make an incision from the anterosuperior iliac spine extending distally and medially for about 6 cm roughly parallel to the inguinal ligament.
- Identify the sartorius muscle, and carry the dissection medial to it to the level of the anteroinferior iliac spine. Protect the femoral nerve, artery, and vein, which lie just medial to this dissection.
- Identify the abscess on the medial surface of the wing of the ilium under Poupart's ligament (173). If the psoas abscess presents medially in the adductor region of the thigh, drain it through a Ludloff approach.
- For the Ludloff approach, make a longitudinal incision on the medial aspect of the thigh, starting 2–3 cm below the pubic tubercle. Develop the interval between the gracilis and adductor longus muscles.

- Develop a plane between the adductor longus and brevis muscles anteriorly and the gracilis and adductor magnus muscles posteriorly.
- Protect the posterior branch of the obturator nerve and the neurovascular bundle to the gracilis.
- The psoas muscle, attaching to the lesser trochanter, and the floor of the hip joint are located in the base of the wound.
- Drain the abscess through this wound (106).

THORACIC SPINE

Abscess Drainage via Costotransversectomy
In the thoracic spine, abscesses are frequently drained through a costotransversectomy approach (Fig. 150.15).

- Make a midline spinal incision extending over two or three spinous processes.
- Reflect the muscle and soft tissues away from the spinous processes and the vertebral laminae on the side of the abscess.
- Widely expose the middle transverse process, and resect it at its base.
- Reflect the periosteum from the contiguous rib, and resect the medial portion of the rib by dividing it 5 cm lateral to the tip of the transverse process. Do not enter the pleural cavity.
- Follow the rib medially, and enter the abscess by bluntly

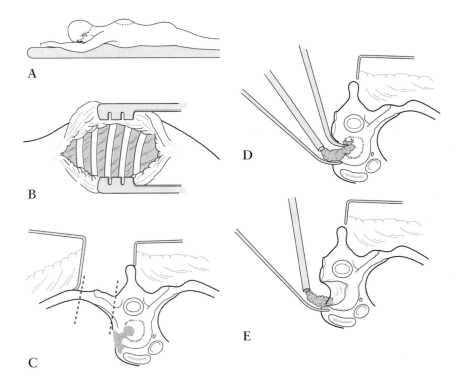

Figure 150.15. **A:** Incision for a costotransversectomy (as described by Capner). With the patient in the prone position, make a curved incision 10 cm above the lesion, curving 7.5 cm laterally and ending 10 cm below. **B:** Reflect the skin and fascial layers medially as a flap. **C:** Remove a portion of the rib and transverse process of the vertebra over the abscess cavity. Expose the ribs and transverse processes of several vertebrae. **D:** The lateral surface of the abscess can be elevated free by working anterior and lateral to the vertebral body, usually without entering the pleural cavity. Curet and debride the abscess as well as possible. **E:** Decompression of the canal is possible if the pedicle and posterior surface of the vertebral body are removed. All debris is curetted and suctioned out of the cavity. It is difficult to insert a strut graft with this approach.

dissecting down the lateral side of the pedicle close to the vertebral body.

■ Remove more than one transverse process and rib, if necessary, to completely debride the abscess.

■ The neurovascular bundles between the ribs must be dissected free, ligated, and sacrificed (24).

Seddon (139) described a similar approach using a semicircular incision lateral to the spine that starts superior to the kyphotic deformity and ends inferior to it.

■ Elevate the skin flap and muscles medially to expose the medial 8 cm of three or more ribs and their transverse processes.

■ Subperiosteally resect the rib judged to be in the center of the abscess, being careful to stay outside the pleura.

■ Remove at least 7 cm of the medial rib in an adult, freeing the medial end with a periosteal elevator.

■ When the rib is teased free, pus should pour out of the gap created.

■ Explore and debride the abscess cavity. Remove the necrotic material and any sequestered bone, and thoroughly irrigate the cavity.

Debridement and Arthrodesis

In addition to evacuating the necrotic debris of a granulomatous infection, many authors recommend immediate arthrodesis of the spine. This requires a more extensive approach than for simple drainage. When neurologic compromise is present, the spinal cord or cauda equina may have to be decompressed by removing additional bone or soft tissue. This is usually the result of bony collapse with the development of an acute gibbus.

Anterior surgical approaches to the thoracic and lumbar spine are described in Chapter 138. The removal of diseased tissue is the same in all areas of the spine.

■ Remove the debris, pus, sequestered bone, and disc, using curets and pituitary rongeurs. Some of this material can be removed with a large sucker tip.

■ Remove the tissue across the entire breadth of the vertebral body.

■ Remove diseased bone or areas where graft will be inserted, using double-action rongeurs, a drill, or an osteotome.

■ Expose the spinal canal for the entire length of the diseased area, decompressing the neural elements. Granulation tissue, fibrous tissue, or the posterior longitudinal ligament may require sharp incision to expose the dura mater.

■ Remove the disc at each end of the cavity to expose the endplates of the vertebrae above and below.

■ Scrape the cartilage off the endplates, revealing bleeding cancellous bone.

■ Place the strut graft into the endplates, keying the grafts into mortises made with a drill or curet to prevent dis-

lodgement. The strut graft should correct the deformity as much as possible and hold the vertebrae apart.

■ The strut grafts should be strong yet osteogenic in nature; autologous cortical or bicortical iliac crest graft is ideal, but the area to be grafted may be too large for the iliac grafts available. Longer struts can be obtained from the fibula or ribs. These should be supplemented with iliac bone because the fibula is strong but mostly cortical bone and the rib is osteogenic but relatively weak and will fail if stressed.

■ The best source of bone is the patient's own ilium, but cadaver bank bone is a good second alternative, especially when a long segment of bone is needed.

■ In the thoracic and lumbar spine, we usually supplement anterior struts with a second-stage posterior instrumentation and fusion. With this technique, there is less chance of graft dislodgement anteriorly. Anterior instrumentation may also be used successfully if immediate stability is needed and posterior fixation cannot be done in a timely manner.

Anterior Decompression and Fusion

Thoracic Spine, C7 to T4

■ Place the patient in a left lateral position on a regular operating table with the right shoulder flexed to 120° and placed on an arm rest.

■ Stand on the spinal side of the patient, tilting the table toward you to afford better visualization.

■ Approach the upper thoracic spine through a right thoracotomy, using the bed of the third rib. If significant kyphosis is present, a costotransversectomy might be better.

   ■ Make a curved incision around the medial and inferior aspects of the scapula. After dividing the parascapular muscles, retract the scapula forward and upward.

   ■ Excise the third rib, and enter the pleural cavity through its bed. To improve visualization, cut the insertion of the scalenus posterior muscle and remove the second rib. The level is decided by following the rib head into the vertebral body. The third rib head articulates with the junction between the T-2 and T-3 vertebral bodies (71).

If more cervical vertebrae are involved, a sternum-splitting operation may be indicated. The procedure is an extension of the exposure for the cervicothoracic junction.

■ Extend the incision in the midline down the sternum to the xiphoid process.

■ Clear the anterior mediastinal tissues by blunt dissection behind the manubrium, working distally from the suprasternal notch. Work proximally from the xiphoid process in the same manner.

■ Divide the sternum with an oscillating saw, and retract the two halves laterally. With this approach, the vessels and midline structures can be retracted more widely.

- Mobilize the recurrent laryngeal nerve so that it will lie obliquely across the operative field. Protect it during the procedure with a moist sponge to prevent paralysis of the vocal cords.
- Identify the vertebral artery behind the carotid sheath. The artery passes upward and laterally to enter the foramen in the C-6 vertebra.
- Approach the spine from the right because the innominate artery on that side takes off from the aorta at a lower level than the left subclavian vessels. In addition, the left innominate vein runs obliquely and distally to join the right innominate vein. The thoracic duct is also avoided.
- Anterior access to the distal cervical and proximal thoracic vertebrae is fairly good when the vessels are retracted.
- After decompression and any stabilization are complete, insert a suction drain, and close the sternum with stainless-steel wire or staples. If the pleura was opened, drain the chest with a large chest tube attached to underwater suction for at least 48 hours (85).

Approach to Lower Thoracic Spine   The chest may be opened from either the left or the right side. In early disease without kyphosis, the right side is best because fewer important structures are present. In more severe or chronic disease when kyphosis is present, the left side is preferable because the vena cava or aorta can become incorporated in the abscess wall. The side of the larger abscess or lung penetration may also determine the side of approach.

- Use a bean bag to hold the patient in the lateral decubitus position, and flex the table at the level of the lesion to facilitate exposure.
- Make an incision along the rib to be excised. It should be two levels higher than the lesion. Additional ribs can be removed for better exposure. Divide muscle layers in line with the incision, and resect the rib subperiosteally.
- Enter the pleural cavity and divide the adhesions (if present), freeing the lung as completely as possible. If thick adhesions between the lung and the abscess are present, portions of the lung inevitably will be left adherent to the abscess cavity in order to mobilize the lung and gain exposure. Open the lung abscess, and remove any caseous material (60). Close the cavity with absorbable suture. A thoracic surgeon often performs this portion of the procedure.
- After the parietal pleura covering the abscess is exposed, mobilize the aorta so that an interval is developed between the two. Ligate and cut the segmental intercostal vessels traversing this segment. If severe kyphosis exists, the aorta will be acutely angulated and the segmentals bunched together at the apex of the curve. Take great care in developing the plane between

the vertebral body and aorta: Adhesions can compromise the integrity of the aortic wall.

- After the aorta is mobilized and protected, open the abscess with a T-shaped incision. Make the transverse portion of the T on the anterior portion of the vertebral body parallel to the aorta. Retract the triangular flaps created by the T incision, and attach them by stay sutures to the muscles at the wound edges. Work from proximal and distal to the mid portion of the kyphosis, particularly if cord compression is present.
- Radically excise all bony sequestra, sequestered disc, granulation tissue, and avascular bone.
- The posterior longitudinal ligament forms the posterior limit of the abscess cavity and is just anterior to the spinal cord. Carefully, incise the ligament and remove it with pituitary rongeurs. Allow the dura to slide or prolapse forward into the area vacated by the debridement.
- Debride the bone until bleeding cancellous bone surfaces are exposed. Cut or drill slots into the exposed cancellous bone of the end vertebrae.
- Apply posterior pressure on the kyphosis to open the interval so that it can be measured with a caliper. Place several ribs or an iliac bicortical graft into the slots, and gently impact the graft into place.
- Release the posterior pressure on the spine, and the grafts will be firmly held in compression. It is wise to supplement the impacted bone with additional struts, although these will not be under compression. Usually, five to six ribs or two bicortical iliac crest grafts can be fitted into the thoracic spine (71,85).
- Complete closure of the abscess cavity flaps is unnecessary. In Hong Kong, streptomycin, 1 g, and isoniazid, 200 mg, are placed in the abscess cavity before closure (Figs. 150.10 and 150.16) (71).

Posterior Procedures for Combined Approaches and Reconstruction   If debridement has required the use of a strut graft, usually a second-stage posterior procedure is planned to provide immediate stability, to support the strut anteriorly, and to prevent later collapse and angulation. In the cervical spine, we use a posterior wiring technique; in the thoracolumbar spine, we most often use segmental instrumentation. In both cases, we combine the instrumentation with a posterolateral spinal fusion. In the cervical spine, the levels of the instrumentation extend from the first good vertebra superiorly to the first good vertebra inferiorly. In the thoracolumbar spine, it is important to include vertebrae at least two levels above and below the resected vertebral bodies.

After patients begin to recover, mobilize them, using external immobilization. Use a halo orthosis vest to control motion in the cervical spine and a polypropylene fitted body jacket for the thoracolumbar area. Continue exter-

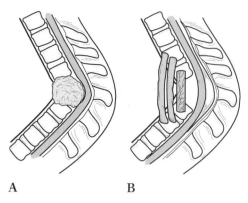

A   **B**

Figure 150.16. **A:** An anterior thoracolumbar approach is best for thoracic or lumbar involvement. With the patient in the lateral decubitus position, make an incision over the rib just superior to the apex of the kyphosis. The rib can be removed for use as a strut graft. Remove the tuberculous debris, devascularized disc, and avascular vertebral body by curettage or use of a power burr. **B:** If the cord is compressed, completely expose it anteriorly to remove any pressure. Place strut grafts of bicortical ilium and rib or fibula to bridge the angular kyphosis from good vertebrae to good vertebrae. Sometimes, correction of the kyphosis can be obtained during the grafting procedure. This anterior fusion will need posterior instrumentation to stabilize the spine and keep the anterior strut grafts from displacing.

nal immobilization for 3 months in the cervical spine and up to 6 months in the thoracolumbar spine. The patient may get out of bed as soon as the external immobilization device is applied and may ambulate, if not paraplegic, as early as tolerated.

Use radiographs and tomograms to confirm graft incorporation and consolidation of the fusion. The vertebral column is also monitored for any angulation or vertebral collapse during the later stages of recovery. Good nutrition and antibiotics complete the treatment program.

◤ PITFALLS AND COMPLICATIONS

The following complications are specific to the treatment of infections.

INTRAOPERATIVE COMPLICATIONS

The lungs can be penetrated during thoracotomy procedures. This is usually of no special concern and can be ignored, unless there is a significant air leak. This will generally scar and seal in time. Use a chest tube if a pneumothorax develops.

The dura can be opened accidentally during the decompression. Always try to close the rent. If closure is unsuccessful, a spinal fluid fistula may result. These eventually heal but may persist for up to 3–4 months.

Injury to the sympathetic nerves in the cervical region will produce Horner's syndrome, which usually is only temporary. In the lumbar area, the extremity of the operated side will be warmer. This too will usually resolve with time.

If there is excessive retroperitoneal scarring, the ureter can be cut accidentally. If so, this must be recognized and a reanastomosis performed at once. If you suspect preoperatively that the ureter might be involved in the abscess, place a stent into the ureter on the side being operated on. This will make the ureter easier to palpate and therefore less likely to be cut. A stent with a fiberoptic light can even allow the ureter to be visualized among the debris and bleeding as the abscess is incised and cleaned out.

Occasionally, the vena cava, aorta, or a common iliac vessel is cut or torn during mobilization of the great vessels. This is most likely to occur at the lumbosacral junction, where the main structure preventing access and mobilization of the common iliac vessels is the iliolumbar vein. Locate this vessel before it is torn. If it cannot be safely moved, ligate and cut it. If the vena cava or aorta is injured, do an immediate vascular repair. Usually, a stitch or two will control the problem, but occasionally a friable vena cava will be impossible to repair and will need to be ligated.

EARLY POSTOPERATIVE COMPLICATIONS

After anterior or even posterior spinal surgery in the thoracolumbar or lumbar area, a paralytic ileus is common. Patients should not be fed until bowel sounds are actively present, and they have noticed some flatus. Even oral fluids, if given too early, can aggravate the ileus and prolong final recovery.

Chest complications are also common, particularly after a thoracotomy. The most common is atelectasis, which will respond to deep breathing, coughing, and use of the inspirometer. However, if left untreated, this can develop into pneumonia. If a chest tube is improperly placed or if it becomes blocked, pleural effusion or hemothorax can occur with lung collapse and subsequent pneumonia.

The most catastrophic complication is deterioration of neurologic status after anterior decompression. This is probably the result of excessive trauma to the already jeopardized spinal cord, particularly if the paraparesis is of long duration and the surgical approach is difficult. It is likely to resolve because the spinal cord in Pott's paraplegia is resilient and can withstand a great deal of trauma without permanent damage. On the other hand, if worsening of paraplegia is caused by spasm of or injury to the anterior spinal artery, then the prognosis for recovery is bleak. There is no good way to know which condition is causing the problem, and treatment for either condition is not very effective. If arterial spasm is suspected, administer intravenous methylprednisolone. Image the strut-grafted area with radiography or CT, or both, to ensure that a graft has not slipped posteriorly into the spinal cord. If this is suspected, reoperate and reinsert the graft into a firm bony bed so that it will not impinge on the cord. Hematoma or abscess is unlikely to cause compression of the spinal cord, because most of the abscess has been removed and the area around the debridement cannot contain the hematoma.

LATE COMPLICATIONS

If the inserted grafts are reabsorbed, usually the infection is not being sufficiently controlled by the antibiotic. This is usually evident 6–12 weeks after surgery, and culture and sensitivity reports will help in modifying the drug regimen. Usually, the grafts need not be replaced, but if destruction is severe, reoperation should be considered.

Long grafts, particularly fibula, are subject to late fracture. Fractures occur 12–18 months after surgery, when the bone is weakened by resorption and replacement by new bone. These resemble stress fractures and will heal with immobilization and rest. Fracture of the graft is best recognized with tomography in the sagittal (lateral) plane.

In 7% to 8% of patients, the spinal fusion will fail. If this is thought to be secondary to persistent infection, it must be dealt with medically. When further spinal collapse and increase in kyphosis occur, restabilization of the vertebral column is required. If the disease is judged to be quiescent, the kyphotic angle is stable, and the patient is asymptomatic, a nonunion can be ignored. If symptoms do occur, a revision posterolateral fusion with instrumentation can be performed.

REFERENCES

Each reference is categorized according to the following scheme: *, classic article; #, review article; !, basic research article; and +, clinical results/outcome study.

+ 1. Abbey D, Rosea S. Diagnosis of Vertebral Osteomyelitis in a Community Hospital by Using CT. *Arch Intern Med* 1989;149:2029.
+ 2. Abdel-Magid R, Korb H. Epidural Abscess after Spinal Anesthesia: A Favorable Outcome. *Neurosurgery* 1990; 27:310.
+ 3. Adatepe M, Powell O, Isaacs G, et al. Hematogenous Pyogenic Vertebral Osteomyelitis: Diagnostic Value of Radionuclide Bone Imaging. *J Nucl Med* 1986;27:1680.
+ 4. Allen A, Stevenson A. The Results of Combined Drug Therapy and Early Fusion in Bone Tuberculosis. *J Bone Joint Surg Am* 1957;39:32.
+ 5. Allen A, Stevenson A. A 10-year Follow-up of Combined Drug Therapy and Early Fusion in Bone Tuberculosis. *J Bone Joint Surg Am* 1967;49:1001.
+ 6. Amir J, Shockelford P. *Kingella kingae* Intervertebral Disk Infection. *J Clin Microbiol* 1991;29:1083.
+ 7. Arct W. Operative Treatment of Tuberculosis of the Spine in Old People. *J Bone Joint Surg Am* 1968;50:255.
* 8. Bailey J, Gabriel M, Hodgson A, Shin J. Tuberculosis of the Spine in Children. *J Bone Joint Surg Am* 1972;54:1633.
+ 9. Baker A, Ojemann R, Swartz M, Richardson E. Spinal Epidural Abscess. *N Engl J Med* 1975;293:463.
* 10. Batson O. The Vertebral Vein System as a Mechanism for the Spread of Metastases. *Am J Roentgenol Radium Ther* 1942;48:75.
# 11. Bennett J. Brucellosis. In: Wyngaarden J, South L, eds. *Cecil Textbook of Medicine*. Philadelphia: WB Saunders, 1985:1614.
# 12. Benson D. Orthopaedic Disorders: The Spine and Neck. In: Gershwin M, Robbins D, eds. *Musculoskeletal Diseases of Children*. New York: Grune & Stratton, 1983:494.
+ 13. Bergman I, Wald E, Meyer J, Painter M. Epidural Abscess and Vertebral Osteomyelitis Following Serial Lumbar Punctures. *Pediatrics* 1983;72:476.
# 14. Boachie-Adjei O, Squillante R. Tuberculosis of the Spine. *Orthop Clin North Am* 1996;27:95.
+ 15. Bohlman H, Freehafer A, Dejak J. The Results of Treatment of Acute Injuries of the Upper Thoracic Spine with Paralysis. *J Bone Joint Surg Am* 1985;67:360.
+ 16. Bouchez B, Arnott G, Delfosse J. Acute Spinal Epidural Abscess. *J Neurology* 1985;231:343.
+ 17. Brandt S, Thompson R. Mycotic Pseudoaneurysm of an Aortic Bypass Graft and Contiguous Vertebral Osteomyelitis Due to *Aspergillus fumigatus*. *Am J Med* 1985;79:259.
+ 18. Brant-Zawadzki M, Burke V, Jeffrey R. CT in the Evaluation of Spine Infection. *Spine* 1983;8:358.
+ 19. Brelt R, Nade S. *Pseudomonas* Osteomyelitis of the Spine: Report of a Case Not Associated with Drug Abuse. *Aust N Z J Surg* 1987;57:871.
+ 20. Browder J, Meyers R. Infections of the Spinal Epidural Space: An Aspect of Vertebral Osteomyelitis. *Am J Surg* 1937;37:4.
+ 21. Brown D, Musher D. Hematogenously Acquired *Aspergillus* Vertebral Osteomyelitis in Seeming Immunocompetent Drug Addicts. *West J Med* 1987;147:84.
+ 21a. Bruschwein DA, Brown ML, McLeod RA. Gallium Scintigraphy in the Evaluation of Disk-Space Infections: Concise Communication. *J Nucl Med* 1980;21:925.
+ 22. Cabezudo M, Olabe J, Bacci F. Infection of the Intervertebral Disc Space after Placement of a Percutaneous Lumboperitoneal Shunt for Benign Intracranial Hypertension. *Neurosurgery* 1990;26:1005.
+ 23. Cahill D, Love L, Rechtine D. Pyogenic Osteomyelitis of the Spine in the Elderly. *J Neurosurg* 1991;74:878.

+ 24. Capener N. The Evolution of Lateral Rachitomy. *J Bone Joint Surg Br* 1957;36:173.

+ 25. Chahal A, Jyoti S. The Radical Treatment of Tuberculosis of the Spine. *Int Orthop* 1980;4:93.

+ 26. Chan K, Leung P, Lee S, et al. Pyogenic Osteomyelitis of the Spine: A Review of 16 Consecutive Cases. *J Spinal Disord* 1988;1:224.

+ 27. Chan S, Leung S. Spinal Epidural Abscess Following Steroid Injection for Sciatica: Case Report. *Spine* 1989;14:106.

+ 28. Chen W, Chen C, Shih C. Surgical Treatment of Tuberculous Spondylitis: 50 Patients Followed for 2–8 Years. *Acta Orthop Scand* 1995;66:137.

+ 29. Clark R, Carlisle J, Valainis G. *Streptococcus pneumoniae* Endocarditis Presenting as an Epidural Abscess. *Rev Infect Dis* 1989;11:338.

+ 30. Colle I, Peeters P, Le Roy I, et al. Epidural Abscess: Case Report and Review of the Literature. *Acta Clin Belg* 1996;51:412.

* 31. A Controlled Trial of Ambulant Out-patient Treatment and In-patient Rest in Bed in the Management of Tuberculosis of the Spine in Young Korean Patients on Standard Chemotherapy: A Study in Masan, Korea. First Report of the Medical Research Council Working Party on Tuberculosis of the Spine. *J Bone Joint Surg Br* 1973;55:678.

* 32. A Controlled Trial of Anterior Spinal Fusion and Debridement in the Surgical Management of Tuberculosis of the Spine in Patients on Standard Chemotherapy: A Study in Hong Kong. Fourth Report of the Medical Research Council Working Party on Tuberculosis of the Spine. *J Brit Surg* 1974;61:853.

+ 33. Cope V. Actinomycosis of Bone with Special Reference to Infection of Vertebral Column. *J Bone Joint Surg Br* 1951;33:205.

+ 34. Cowan N. Cryptococcosis of Bone: Cost Report and Review of the Literature. *Clin Orthop* 1969;66:174.

+ 35. Dalinka M, Dinnenberg S, Greendyke W, Hopkins R. Roentgenographic Features of Osseous Coccidioidomycosis and Differential Diagnosis. *J Bone Joint Surg Am* 1971;53:1157.

36. Danner R, Hartman B. Update of Spinal Epidural Abscess: 35 Cases and Review of the Literature. *Rev Infect Dis* 1987;9:265.

+ 37. Dauch W. Infection of the Intervertebral Space Following Conventional and Microsurgical Operation on the Herniated Lumbar Intervertebral Disc: A Controlled Clinical Trail. *Acta Neurochir (Wien)* 1986;82:43.

+ 38. Deeb ZL, Schimel S, Daffner R, et al. Intervertebral Diskspace Infection after Chymopapain Injection. *AJR* 1985;144:671.

+ 39. DeFelice R, Galgian J, Campbell S, et al. Ketoconazole Treatment of Nonprimary Coccidioidomycosis. *Am J Med* 1982;72:681.

+ 40. Dehring D, Tucker R. Treatment of Invasive Aspergillosis with Intrathecal Ketoconazole. *Am J Med* 1985;86:791.

+ 41. Del Curling OJ, Gower D, McWhorter J. Changing Concepts in Spinal Epidural Abscess: A Report of 29 Cases. *Neurosurgery* 1990;27:185.

+ 42. Denning D, Tucker R, Hanson L, Stevens D. Treatment of Invasive Aspergillosis with Itraconazole. *Am J Med* 1989;86:791.

+ 43. Dernbach P, Gomez H, Hahn J. Primary Closure of Infected Spinal Wounds. *Neurosurgery* 1990;26:707.

44. Edwards J, Lehrer R, Stiehm E. Severe Candida Infections: Clinical Perspective, Immune Defense Mechanisms and Current Concepts of Therapy. *Ann Intern Med* 1978;89:91.

+ 45. Eismont F, Bohlman H, Soni P, et al. Pyogenic and Fungal Vertebral Osteomyelitis with Paralysis. *J Bone Joint Surg Am* 1983;65:19.

+ 46. Emery S, Chan D, Woodward H. Treatment of Hematogenous Pyogenic Vertebral Osteomyelitis with Anterior Debridement and Primary Bone Grafting. *Spine* 1989;14:284.

+ 47. Endress C, Guyot D, Fata J, Salciccioli G. Cervical Osteomyelitis Due to Intravenous Heroin Use: Radiologic Findings in 14 Patients. *AJR* 1990;155:333.

+ 48. Fang D, Cheung K, Dos Remedios I, et al. Pyogenic Vertebral Osteomyelitis: Treatment by Anterior Spinal Debridement and Fusion. *J Spinal Disord* 1994;7:173.

+ 49. Ferris B, Jones J. Paraplegia Due to Aspergillosis. *J Bone Joint Surg Br* 1985;67:800.

* 50. Five-year Assessments of Controlled Trials of Ambulatory Treatment, Debridement and Anterior Spinal Fusion in the Management of Tuberculosis of the Spine: Studies in Bulawayo (Rhodesia) and Hong Kong. Sixth Report of the Medical Research Council. *J Bone Joint Surg Br* 1978;60:163.

+ 51. Fountain S, Shu L, Yau A, Hodgson A. Progressive Kyphosis Following Solid Anterior Spine Fusion in Children with Tuberculosis of the Spine. *J Bone Joint Surg Am* 1975;57:1104.

+ 52. Friedman B, Simon G. Candida Vertebral Osteomyelitis: Report of Three Cases and Review of the Literature. *Diagn Microbiol Infect Dis* 1987;8:31.

+ 53. Garrido E, Rosenwasser R. Experience with the Suction-Irrigation Technique in the Management of Spinal Epidural Infection. *Neurosurgery* 183;12:678.

+ 54. Garvey T, Eismont F. Tuberculous and Fungal Osteomyelitis of the Spine. *Semin Spine Surg* 1990;2:295.

+ 55. Gather J, Harris R, Garland B, et al. Candida Osteomyelitis: Report of Five Cases and Review of the Literature. *Am J Med* 1987;82:927.

+ 56. Gehweiler J, Capp M, Chick E. Observations on the Roentgen Patterns in Blastomycosis of Bone. *AJR* 1970;108:497.

+ 57. Ghobadi F, Potenza A, Dibenedetto A. Spinal Tuberculosis: Treatment by Debridement and Anterior Spine Fusion. *N Y State J Med* 1975;75:1527.

+ 58. Golimbu C, Firooznia H, Rafil M. CT of Osteomyelitis of the Spine. *AJR* 1984;142:159.

+ 59. Graziano G, Sidhu K. Salvage Reconstruction in Acute and Late Sequelae from Pyogenic Thoracolumbar Infection. *J Spinal Disord* 1993;6:199.

+ 60. Guirguis A. Pott's Paraplegia. *J Bone Joint Surg Br* 1967;49:658.

+ 61. Guri J. Pyogenic Osteomyelitis of the Spine. *J Bone Joint Surg Am* 1946;28:29.

+ 62. Haase D, Martin R, Marrie T. Radionuclide Imaging in Pyogenic Vertebral Osteomyelitis. *Clin Nucl Med* 1980; 5:533.

+ 63. Hadden W, Swanson A. Spinal Infection Caused by Acupuncture Mimicking a Prolapsed Intervertebral Disc: A Case Report. *J Bone Joint Surg Am* 1982;64:624.

+ 64. Hales D, Duffy K, Dawson E, Delamarter A. Lumbar Osteomyelitis and Epidural and Paraspinous Abscesses: Case Report of an Unusual Source of Contamination from a Gunshot Wound to the Abdomen. *Spine* 1991; 16:380.

+ 65. Harries T, Licktman D, Swafford A. Pyogenic Vertebral Osteomyelitis Complicating Abdominal Stab Wounds. *J Trauma* 1981;21:75.

+ 66. Heusner A. Nontuberculous Spinal Epidural Infections. *N Engl J Med* 1948;239:845.

+ 67. Hirschmann J, Everett E. Candida Vertebral Osteomyelitis. *J Bone Joint Surg Am* 1976;58:573.

+ 68. Hlavin M, Kaminski J, Ross J, Ganz E. Spinal Epidural Abscess: A 10-year Perspective. *Neurosurgery* 1990;27: 177.

* 69. Hodgson A, Skinsnes O, Leong C. The Pathogenesis of Pott's Paraplegia. *J Bone Joint Surg Am* 1967;42:295.

* 70. Hodgson A, Stock F. Anterior Spine Fusion for the Treatment of Tuberculosis of the Spine. *J Bone Joint Surg Am* 1960;42:295.

* 71. Hodgson A, Stock F, Fang H, Ong G. Anterior Spinal Fusion: The Operative Approach and Pathological Findings in 412 Patients with Pott's Disease of the Spine. *Br J Surg* 1960;48:172.

+ 72. Hoffer F, Strand R, Gebhardt M. Percutaneous Biopsy of Pyogenic Infection of the Spine in Children. *J Pediatr Orthop* 1988;8:442.

+ 73. Hong Z, Zisheng W, Jianziong S, et al. Application of Internal Fixation in the Treatment of Tuberculosis of the Spine. *Chin Med Sci J* 1994;9:179.

+ 74. Hopf C, Meurer A, Eysel P, Rompe J. Operative Treatment of Spondylodiscitis: What is the Most Effective Approach. *Neurosurg Rev* 1998;21:217.

+ 75. Hsu L, Leong J. Tuberculosis of the Lower Cervical Spine (C-2 to C-7). *J Bone Joint Surg Br* 1984;66:1.

+ 76. Ingwer I, McLeish D. *Aspergillus fumigatus* Epidural Abscess in a Renal Transplant Recipient. *Arch Intern Med* 1978;138:153.

+ 77. Jack K, Rhame F. Aspergillus Osteomyelitis: Report of Four Cases and Review of the Literature. *Am J Med* 1982;73:296.

+ 78. Jeanneret B, Mageral F. Treatment of Osteomyelitis of the Spine Using Percutaneous Suction/Irrigation and Percutaneous External Spinal Fixation. *J Spinal Disord* 1994;7:185.

+ 79. Johnson R, Hillman J, Southwick W. The Importance of Direct Attack upon Lesions of the Vertebral Bodies, Particularly in Pott's Disease. *J Bone Joint Surg Am* 1953;35:17.

80. Jones A. The Influence of Hugh Owen Thomas on the Evolution of Skeletal Tuberculosis. *J Bone Joint Surg Br* 1953;35:309.

+ 81. Karlen A. Early Drainage of Paraspinal Tuberculosis Abscess in Children. *J Bone Joint Surg Br* 1959;41:491.

+ 82. Kashimoto T, Kitagawa H, Kachi H. *Candida tropicalis* Vertebral Osteomyelitis and Discitis: Case Report. *Spine* 1986;11:57.

+ 83. Kattapuram S, Phillips W, Boyd R. CT in Pyogenic Osteomyelitis of the Spine. *AJR* 1983;140:1199.

+ 84. Kaufman D, Kaplan J, Litman N. Infectious Agents in Spinal Epidural Abscesses. *Neurology* 1980;30:844.

+ 85. Kemp H, Jackson J, Cook J. Anterior Fusion of the Spine for Infective Lesions in Adults. *J Bone Joint Surg Br* 1973;55:715.

+ 86. Kemp H, Jackson J, Shaw N. Laminectomy in Paraplegia Due to Infection Spondylosis. *Br J Surg* 1974;61:66.

+ 87. Khan M. The Place of Anterior Spinal Fusion in Treatment of Tuberculosis of the Spine. *Clin Orthop* 1964; 35:139.

+ 88. King D, Mayo K. Infective Lesions of the Vertebral Column. *Clin Orthop* 1973;96:248.

+ 89. Kirkaldy-Willis W, Thomas T. Anterior Approaches in the Diagnosis and Treatment of Infections of the Vertebral Bodies. *J Bone Joint Surg Am* 1965;47:87.

+ 90. Kondo E, Yamada K. End Results of Focal Debridement in Bone and Joint Tuberculosis and its Indications. *J Bone Joint Surg Am* 1957;39:27.

+ 91. Konstam P, Blesovsy A. The Ambulant Treatment of Spinal Tuberculosis. *Br J Surg* 1962;50:26.

+ 92. Koppel B, Tuchman A, Mangiardi J, et al. Epidural Spinal Infection in Intravenous Drug Abusers. *Arch Neurol* 1988;45:1331.

+ 93. Korkusuz F, Islam C, Korkusuz Z. Prevention of Postoperative Late Kyphosis in Pott's Disease by Anterior Decompression and Intervertebral Grafting. *World J Surg* 1997;21:524.

+ 94. Korovessis P, Repanti M, Katsardis T, Stamatakis M. Anterior Decompression and Fusion for Aspergillus Osteomyelitis of the Lumbar Spine Associated with Paraparesis. *Spine* 1994;19:2715.

+ 95. Larde D, Mathieu D, Frija J, et al. Vertebral Osteomyelitis: Disk Hypodensity on CT. *AJR* 1982;139:963.

+ 96. Larsson S, Thelander U, Friberg S. C-reactive Protein (CRP) Levels after Elective Orthopaedic Surgery. *Clin Orthop* 1992;275:237.

+ 97. Leibert E, Schluger N, Bonk S, Rom W. Spinal Tuberculosis in Patients with Human Immunodeficiency Virus Infection: Clinical Presentation, Therapy and Outcome. *Tuber Lung Dis* 1996;77:329.

+ 98. Leys D, Lesoin F, Viaud C, et al. Decreased Morbidity from Acute Bacterial Spinal Epidural Abscesses Using Computed Tomography and Nonsurgical Treatment in Selected Patients. *Ann Neurol* 1985;17:350.

+ 99. Lifeso R. Atlanto-axial Tuberculosis in Adults. *J Bone Joint Surg Br* 1987;69:183.

+ 100. Lifeso R. Pyogenic Spinal Sepsis in Adults. *Spine* 1990; 15:1265.

+ 101. Lifeso R, Weaver P, Harder E. Tuberculous Spondylitis in Adults. *J Bone Joint Surg Am* 1985;67:1405.

+ 102. Loembe P. Tuberculosis of the Lower Cervical Spine (C3-C7) in Adults: Diagnostic and Surgical Aspects. *Acta Neurochir (Wien)* 1994;131:125.

+ 103. Lowe J, Kaplan L, Liebergall M, Floman Y. Serratia Osteomyelitis Causing Neurological Deterioration after

Spine Fracture: A Report of Two Cases. *J Bone Joint Surg Br* 1989;71:256.

+ 104. Lukhele M. Tuberculosis of the Cervical Spine. *S Afr Med J* 1996;86:553.

+ 105. Malawski S, Lukawski S. Pyogenic Infection of the Spine. *Clin Orthop* 1991;272:58.

+ 106. Marchevsky A, Damslar B, Green S. The Clinicopathological Spectrum of Non-tuberculous Mycobacterial Osteoarticular Infections. *J Bone Joint Surg Am* 1985;67:925.

+ 107. Markus H, Allison S. *Staphylococcus aureus* Meningitis from Osteomyelitis of the Spine. *Postgrad Med* 1989;65:941.

+ 108. Martin N. Pott's Paraplegia: A Report of 120 Cases. *J Bone Joint Surg Br* 1971;53:596.

+ 109. Martin N. Tuberculosis of the Spine: A Study of the Results of Treatment during the Last 25 Years. *J Bone Joint Surg Br* 1970;52:613.

+ 110. Matsui J, Hirano N, Sakaguchi Y. Vertebral Osteomyelitis: An Analysis of 38 Surgically Treated Cases. *Eur Spine J* 1998;7:50.

+ 111. McGahan J, Dublin A. Evaluation of Spinal Infections by Plain Radiographs, CT, Intrathecal Metrizamide, and CT-guided Biopsy. *Diagn Imaging Clin Med* 1985;54:11.

+ 112. McGrath HJ, McCormick C, Carey M. Pyogenic Cervical Osteomyelitis Presenting as a Massive Prevertebral Abscess in a Patient with Rheumatoid Arthritis. *Am J Med* 1988;84:363.

* 113. Menard V. *Etude Practique sur le Mal de Pott*. Paris: Masson et Cie, 1900.

+ 114. Modic M, Feiglin D, Piraino D. Vertebral Osteomyelitis: Assessment Using MR. *Radiology* 1985;157:157.

+ 115. Moon M. Tuberculosis of the Spine: Controversies and a New Challenge. *Spine* 1997;22:1791.

+ 116. Moon M, Ha K, Sun D, et al. Pott's Paraplegia: 67 Cases. *Clin Orthop* 1996;323:122.

+ 117. Moon M, Woo Y, Lee K, et al. Posterior Instrumentation and Anterior Interbody Fusion for Tuberculous Kyphosis of Dorsal and Lumbar Spines. *Spine* 1995;20:1910.

+ 118. Myllynen P, Klossner O. Pyogenic Vertebral Osteomyelitis as a Complication of an Abdominal Stab Wound. *Ann Chir Gynaecol* 1982;71:344.

+ 119. Neville C, Davis W. Is Surgical Fusion Still Desirable in Spinal Tuberculosis? *Clin Orthop* 1971;75:179.

+ 120. Noble H, Kyne E. Candida Osteomyelitis and Arthritis from Hyperalimentation Therapy. *J Bone Joint Surg Am* 1974;56:825.

+ 121. Osenbach R, Hitchon P, Menezes A. Diagnosis and Management of Pyogenic Vertebral Osteomyelitis in Adults. *Surg Neurol* 1990;33:266.

+ 122. Osti O, Fraser R. Discitis after Discography: The Role of Prophylactic Antibiotics. *J Bone Joint Surg Br* 1990;72:271.

+ 123. Patzakis M, Rao S, Wilkins J, et al. Analysis of 61 Cases of Vertebral Osteomyelitis. *Clin Orthop* 1991;264:178.

+ 124. Pinckney L, Currarino G, Highgenboten C. Osteomyelitis of the Cervical Spine Following Dental Extraction. *Radiology* 1980;135:335.

+ 125. Post M, Sze F, Quencer R, et al. Gadolinium-enhanced MR in Spinal Infection. *J Comput Assist Tomogr* 1990;14:721.

+ 126. Ratcliffe J. Anatomic Basis for the Pathogenesis and Radiologic Features of Vertebral Osteomyelitis and its Differentiation from Childhood Discitis: A Microarteriographic Investigation. *Acta Radiol Diagn* 1985;26:137.

+ 127. Rath S, Neff U, Schneider O, Richter H. Neurosurgical Management of Thoracic and Lumbar Vertebral Osteomyelitis and Discitis in Adults: A Review of 43 Consecutive Surgically Treated Patients. *Neurosurgery* 1996;38:926.

+ 128. Richards B. Delayed Infections Following Posterior Spinal Instrumentation for the Treatment of Idiopathic Scoliosis. *J Bone Joint Surg Am* 1995;77:524.

+ 129. Richardson J, Campbell D, Grover F, et al. Transthoracic Approach for Pott's Disease. *Ann Thorac Surg* 1976;21:552.

+ 130. Rockney R, Ryan R, Knuckey N. Spinal Epidural Abscess: An Infectious Emergency Case Report and Review. *Clin Pediatr* 1989;28:332.

+ 131. Safran O, Rand N, Kaplan L, et al. Sequential or Simultaneous, Same-day Anterior Decompression and Posterior Stabilization in the Management of Vertebral Osteomyelitis of the Lumbar Spine. *Spine* 1998;23:1885.

132. Sapico F, Montgomerie J. Vertebral Osteomyelitis. *Infect Dis Clin North Am* 1990;4:539.

+ 133. Savonia M. An Overview of Antibiotics Useful in the Treatment of Bacterial, Mycobacterial, and Fungal Osteomyelitis. *Semin Spine Surg* 1990;2:309.

+ 134. Schlaeffer F, Mikolich D, Mates S. Technetium (Tc-99m) Diphosphonate Bone Scan: False-normal Findings in Elderly Patients with Hematogenous Vertebral Osteomyelitis. *Arch Intern Med* 1987;147:2024.

+ 135. Schofferman L, Schofferman J, Zucherman J. Occult Infections Causing Persistent Low-back Pain. *Spine* 1989;14:417.

136. Schroeder S, Krupp M, Tierney L Jr, eds. *Current Medical Diagnosis and Treatment*. Norwalk, CT: Appleton & Lange, 1989.

+ 137. Schulak D, Rayhack J, Lippert F. The Erythrocyte Sedimentation Rate in Orthopedic Patients. *Clin Orthop* 1982;167:197.

+ 138. Schulitz K, Kothe R, Leong J, Wehling P. Growth Changes of Solidly Fused Kyphotic Bloc after Surgery for Tuberculosis: Comparison of Four Procedures. *Spine* 1997;22:1150.

* 139. Seddon J. Pott's Paraplegia and its Operative Treatment. *J Bone Joint Surg Br* 1953;35:487.

+ 140. Seligson R, Rippon J, Lerner S. *Aspergillus terreus* Osteomyelitis. *Arch Intern Med* 1977;137:918.

+ 141. Seris J, Ono H. Aspergillosis Presenting as Spinal Cord Compression. *J Neurosurg* 1972;36:221.

+ 142. Sharif H. Role of MR Imaging in the Management of Spinal Infections. *AJR* 1992;158:1333.

+ 143. Shaw F, Warthen H. Aspergillosis of Bone. *South Med J* 1963;29:1070.

+ 144. Shaw T, Thomas T. Surgical Treatment of Chronic Infective Lesions of the Spine. *Br Med J* 1963;1:162.

+ 145. Silverthorn K, Gillespie W. Pyogenic Spinal Osteomyelitis: A Review of 61 Cases. *N Z Med J* 1986;99:62.

+ 146. Simpson M, Nerz W, Kurlinski J. Opportunistic Mycotic

Osteomyelitis: Bone Infections Due to Aspergillosis and *Candida* Species. *Medicine* 1977;56:475.

+147. Stern W, Balch R. Surgical Aspects of Nonspecific Inflammatory and Suppurative Disease of the Vertebral Column. *Am J Surg* 1966;112:314.

+148. Tami T, Burkus J, Strom C. Cervical Osteomyelitis: An Unusual Complication of Tonsillectomy. *Arch Otolaryngol Head Neck Surg* 1987;113:992.

+149. Thalgott J, Cotler H, Sasso R, et al. Postoperative Infections in Spinal Implants: Classification and Analysis—A Multicenter Study. *Spine* 1991;16:981.

+150. A 10-year Assessment of a Controlled Trial Comparing Debridement and Anterior Fusion in the Management of Tuberculosis of the Spine in Patients in Standard Chemotherapy in Hong Kong. Eighth Report of the Medical Research Council. *J Bone Joint Surg Br* 1982; 64:393.

+151. Thelander U, Larsson S. Quantitation of C-reactive Protein Levels and Erythrocyte Sedimentation Rate after Spinal Surgery. *Spine* 1992;17:400.

+152. Thrush A, Enzmann D. MRI of Infectious Spondylitis. *Am J Neuroradiol* 1990;11:1171.

+153. Thurston A, Gillespie W. *Torulopsis glabrata* Osteomyelitis of the Spine: A Case Report and Review of the Literature. *Aust N Z J Surg* 1981;51:374.

+154. Tuli S. Results of Treatment of Spinal Tuberculosis by "Middle Path" Regime. *J Bone Joint Surg Br* 1975;57: 13.

+155. Tuli S, Srivastava T, Varma B, Sinha G. Tuberculosis of the Spine. *Acta Orthop Scand* 1967;38:445.

+156. Upadhyay S, Saji M, Sell P, et al. The Effect of Age on the Change in Deformity after Anterior Debridement Surgery for Tuberculosis of the Spine. *Spine* 1996;21: 2356.

+157. Upadhyay S, Saji M, Sell P, et al. Longitudinal Changes in Spinal Deformity after Anterior Spinal Surgery for Tuberculosis of the Spine in Adults: A Comparative Analysis between Radical and Debridement Surgery. *Spine* 1994;19:542.

+158. Upadhyay S, Saji M, Sell P, et al. Spinal Deformity after Childhood Surgery for Tuberculosis of the Spine: A Comparison of Radical Surgery and Debridement. *J Bone Joint Surg Br* 1994;76:91.

+159. Upadhyay S, Saji M, Sell P, Yau A. The Effect of Age on the Change in Deformity after Radical Resection and Anterior Arthrodesis for Tuberculosis of the Spine. *J Bone Joint Surg Am* 1994;76:701.

+160. Upadhyay S, Sell P, Saji M, et al. Surgical Management of Spinal Tuberculosis in Adults: Hong Kong Operation Compared with Debridement Surgery for Short- and Long-term Outcome of Deformity. *Clin Orthop* 1994; 302:173.

+161. Van Lom J, Kellerhouse L, Pathria M. Infection versus Tumor in the Spine: Criteria for Distinction with CT. *Radiology* 1988;166:851.

162. Vincent K, Benson D. Differential Diagnosis and Conservative Treatment of Infectious Disease. In: Frymoyer J, ed. *The Adult Spine: Principles and Practice.* New York: Raven Press, 1991.

+163. Vincent K, Benson D, Voegeli T. Factors in the Diagnosis of Adult Pyogenic Vertebral Osteomyelitis. *Orthop Trans* 1988;12:523.

+164. Waters R, Adkins R. The Effects of Removal of Bullet Fragments Retained in the Spinal Canal: A Collaborative Study by the National Spinal Cord Injury Model System. *Spine* 1991;16:934.

+165. Wayne D, Muizelaar P. Acute Lumbosacral Epidural Abscess after Percutaneous Transluminal Angioplasty. *Am J Med* 1989;87:478.

+166. Wenningsted-Torgard K, Heyn J, Willumsen L. Spondylitis Following Epidural Morphine: A Case Report. *Acta Anaesthesiol Scand* 1982;26:649.

+167. Whalen JL, Brown ML, McLeod R, Fitzgerald RJ Jr. Limitations of Indium Leukocyte Imaging for the Diagnosis of Spine Infections. *Spine* 1991;16:193.

+168. Wiley A, Trueta J. The Vascular Anatomy of the Spine and its Relationship to Pyogenic Vertebral Osteomyelitis. *J Bone Joint Surg Br* 1959;41:796.

+169. Wiltberger B. Resection of Vertebral Bodies and Bone Grafting for Chronic Osteomyelitis of the Spine. *J Bone Joint Surg Am* 1952;34:215.

+170. Wimmer C, Ogon M, Sterzinger W, et al. Conservative Treatment of Tuberculous Spondylitis: A Long-term Follow-up Study. *J Spinal Disord* 1997;10:417.

+171. Winter W, Larson R, Hoenggar M, et al. Coccidioidal Arthritis and its Treatment. *J Bone Joint Surg Am* 1975; 57:1152.

+172. Wise R. Brucellosis in the United States. *JAMA* 1980; 244:2318.

173. Wood G. Infections of the Spine. In: Crenshaw A, ed. *Campbell's Operative Orthopaedics.* St Louis, MO: Mosby, 1987:1323.

+174. Wukich D, Van Dam B, Abreu S. Preoperative Indium-labeled White Blood Cell Scintigraphy in Suspected Osteomyelitis of the Axial Skeleton. *Spine* 1988;13: 1168.

+175. Yau A, Hodgson AR. Penetration of the Lung by the Paravertebral Abscess in Tuberculosis of the Spine. *J Bone Joint Surg Am* 1968;50:243.

* 176. Yau A, Hsu L, O'Brien J, Hodgson A. Tuberculous Kyphosis: Correction with Spinal Osteotomy, Halo Pelvic Distraction, and Anterior and Posterior Fusion. *J Bone Joint Surg Am* 1974;56:1419.

+177. Zeiger HJ, Zampella E. Intervertebral Disc Infection after Lumbar Chemonucleolysis: Report of a Case. *Neurosurgery* 1986;18:616.

+178. Zigler J, Bohlman H, Robinson R, et al. Pyogenic Osteomyelitis of the Occiput, the Atlas, and the Axis: A Report of Five Cases. *J Bone Joint Surg Am* 1987;69: 1069.

CHAPTER 151
TUMORS AND INFECTIONS OF THE CERVICAL SPINE

Kamshad Raiszadeh and Behrooz A. Akbarnia

This chapter focuses on the surgical management of destructive lesions of the cervical spine. For cervical tumors, the indications and techniques for biopsy are reviewed, followed by the exposure and reconstruction of destructive lesions. Tumor classification and details on the various tumors are presented in Chapters 126 to 130. Many of the general principles of spinal tumors are covered in Chapter 152, Tumors of the Thoracic and Lumbar Spine. This chapter focuses solely on the management of these tumors in the cervical spine. Similarly, the general principles of management of bone infection are covered in Chapters 132 and 133, and the details of the various types of infections are covered in Chapter 150. In this chapter, we focus on the management of cervical infections. The evaluation of osteomyelitis and epidural abscess are reviewed, followed by a discussion of the outcome of different treatments.

K. Raiszadeh: Clinical Instructor, University of California–San Diego School of Medicine, Department of Orthopaedics, San Diego Center for Spinal Disorders, San Diego, California, 92123.

B. A. Akbarnia: Clinical Professor, University of California—San Diego School of Medicine, Department of Orthopaedics, San Diego Center for Spinal Disorders, San Diego, California, 92123.

CERVICAL TUMORS

DIAGNOSTIC EVALUATION

In the preoperative workup for tumors of the cervical spine, the surgeon should first determine the oncologic stage and evaluate for local and systemic disease. The Enneking system of staging for musculoskeletal neoplasms (see Chapter 126) has been adapted to neoplasms of the axial skeleton (4). As with extremity neoplasms, spinal tumors are staged according to histologic grade, compartmental location, and the presence or absence of metastases. There is a major difference between surgical staging of spinal neoplasms compared with neoplasms of long bones; the Weinstein-Boriani-Biagini (WBB) classification addresses the unique anatomy of the spine (25). In the transverse plane, the vertebra is divided into 12 zones, numbered 1 to 12 clockwise starting on the left half of the spinous process. The layers are further divided from paravertebral extraosseous to dura, denoted as layers A through E, with a further layer F for the vertebral artery canal (Fig. 151.1). Recording the spinal segments involved defines the longitudinal extent of tumor involvement. A simpler method of categorizing the level of involvement

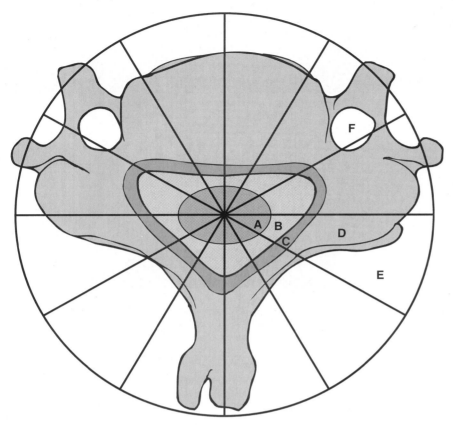

Figure 151.1. Weinstein-Boriani-Biagini classification–surgical staging of spinal neoplasms. There is a major difference between surgical staging of spinal neoplasms compared with neoplasms of long bones. **A:** Intradural. **B:** Epidural. **C:** Involving bony canal. **D:** Intraosseous. **E:** Paravertebral, extraosseous. **F:** Vertebral artery canal.

is to divide the vertebral body into four zones, I through IV. Tumor extension is designated as A, B, and C for interosseous, extraosseous, and distant tumor spread, respectively (Fig. 151.2). This classification is helpful because the zones of tumor involvement correspond to the surgical approach: tumors involving zones I and II are usually resected and, if necessary, stabilized posteriorly. Zone III lesions are usually approached anteriorly. Zone IV lesions that require a complete or *en bloc* excision must be managed through a combined anterior and posterior approach. Zone IIIB lesions should be carefully analyzed preoperatively to anticipate possible invasion of or adherence to critical neural elements, esophagus, or trachea. The general workup of tumors of the cervical spine and the different tumor types are covered in Chapter 152.

Long-term survival and decreased recurrence rates in patients with primary spinal malignancy correlate significantly with tumor type and the extent of the initial surgical procedure. Hart et al. (25) and Boriani et al. (4) showed decreased recurrence rates of giant cell tumor and chordoma, respectively, using the WBB and the Enneking surgical staging systems with *en bloc* excision performed at a tertiary referral center. Although they have not been specifically studied, it is reasonable to extrapolate the results obtained in other areas of the spine to cervical tumors.

The incidence and presentation of cervical disease is different from other regions, however. The reported frequency of cervical metastatic disease is much less than thoracic or lumbar metastases. Also, the presentation of cervical metastatic disease differs from metastatic disease at the thoracic and lumbar levels (49). A review of the natural history shows the average life expectancy to be 14.7 months after cervical metastatic disease is diagnosed (52). Pain with cervical metastatic disease is more frequent (93%), whereas neurologic deficit is less frequent than when disease is present at the thoracic or lumbar levels (5–14% cervical versus 50% thoraco-lumbar) (52,53). The prevalence of upper cervical neurologic deficit is lower than that of the lower cervical spine, possibly related to the wider canal in the upper region.

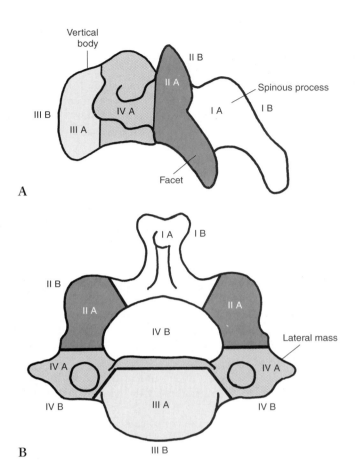

Figure 151.2. Cervical spine tumor staging system, modified from the thoracolumbar staging system of Weinstein and McLain. The vertebral body is divided into zones I to IV. Zones I and II: lamina, facets, and pedicle. Zone III: vertebral body. Zone IV: epidural space, dural contents, and posterior vertebral body and annulus. **A:** Interosseous. **B:** Extraosseous. **C:** Designates distant metastatic spread, not shown. (Modified from McLain RF, Weinstein JN. Tumors of the Spine. *Seminars in Spine Surgery* 1990;2:157.)

BIOPSY AND ASPIRATION

Conditions such as osteoid osteoma and osteoblastoma can be diagnosed solely on the basis of the radiologic workup of plain radiographs and computed tomography (CT) scans. By recognizing the benign or inactive lesions that, by their self-limiting nature, do not require biopsy, an unnecessary procedure can be avoided. Also, in cases such as spinal metastases from a known primary carcinoma, no biopsy is necessary. A similar situation involves the patient with multiple myeloma and spinal involvement with impending or actual cord compression. In patients with multiple myeloma, the laboratory tests provide the diagnosis. Because the myelomas are sensitive to radiation therapy, proceeding directly with radiation rather than performing a biopsy or other surgery is most appropriate.

If the benign or malignant nature of a spinal neoplasm is uncertain, one must make a definitive diagnosis with a complete workup and a biopsy or aspiration. It is important to realize, however, that planning the biopsy should be the last step, after appropriate staging and other workup. The benefit of performing the biopsy at the end of the staging and evaluation are

- Unnecessary biopsy can be avoided (e.g., multiple myeloma)
- Other more accessible sites may be found for biopsy (e.g., a metastatic lesion)
- Prebiopsy embolization can be performed, if necessary (e.g., renal cell metastasis or other vascular lesion).

The biopsy, although seemingly simple, is a difficult procedure with possible complications that can change the course of treatment and significantly alter the treatment outcome (40). *The orthopaedist who is responsible for the definitive treatment and subsequent care should be responsible for performing the initial biopsy.* The recommendations regarding performance of biopsies, either open or percutaneous, are

- Place the biopsy tract where it will be fully removed at the time of definitive treatment. This may not be possible during anterior biopsies.
- Ensure minimal tissue contamination by avoiding excessive dissection of tissue planes.
- Obtain adequate tissue for diagnosis (may require confirmation by frozen section).
- Maintain adequate hemostasis.
- Use drains only through the wound or in proximity so that the track is removed with the definitive resection. The drain can provide a track along which malignant cells can pass, which may increase the margin necessary for subsequent resection.

An adequate amount of tissue must be obtained regardless of whether an aspiration, needle biopsy, or open biopsy is performed. Coexistent infection and tumor have been reported (16); therefore, we recommend routine microbiologic culture. Biopsy techniques include percutaneous (aspiration, fine-needle, or large-bore), open incisional biopsy, or excisional biopsy. When normal marrow elements are present, aspiration effectively rules out metastatic malignancy. Needle aspiration and fine-needle biopsy, however, provide only a small specimen and, therefore, introduce a sampling error. Simple aspiration or fine-needle biopsy should be used predominantly in the cervical spine to rule out infection, confirm suspected metastatic disease, or diagnose recurrence of a known lesion. Because aspiration biopsy may fail to provide definitive diagnosis in up to 20% of cases (6), large-needle or open biopsy is often necessary.

For lesions in the posterior aspect of the cervical spine, large-needle trocar biopsy is relatively easy to perform under CT guidance. If a benign lesion such as osteoid osteoma or osteoblastoma is suspected, however, open biopsy followed by excision often provides the easiest solution. We also do not favor routine needle or trocar biopsy of suspected aneurysmal bone cysts. Most of these lesions, when well-demonstrated radiologically, are typical and do not require biopsy. Some lesions can have a clinical and radiographic appearance similar to that of a malignant tumor and, in fact, may also contain malignant portions; therefore, a gross pathologic specimen may be needed for diagnosis. Additionally, the small amount of tissue obtained with needle or trocar biopsy often creates confusion in the diagnosis or may not include the pre-existing lesion (50). Open biopsy with curettage or excision, or both, on the other hand, provides the entire lesion for pathologic examination. Furthermore, there have been reports that extradural bleeding of aneurysmal bone cysts of the spine following needle biopsy cause neurologic deficit (26). Finally, because open excisional biopsy can cure the condition, there seems to be little justification for needle or trocar biopsy, which may be negative and possibly risky (1).

Biopsy of anterior lesions is performed either laterally or anterolaterally following the standard surgical approach (see the discussion of surgical approaches, later). It is often not possible to entirely excise the biopsy tract with anterolateral and lateral biopsies due to the multiple tissue planes in the anterior neck and the presence of the carotid sheath. Avoid transverse posterior skin incisions. Plan the incision so that it will not compromise subsequent surgical procedures.

For planning the management of suspected metastatic disease, divide the cervical spine into three regions: the upper cervical vertebral bodies (C1–C3), the lower cervical vertebral bodies (C4–C7), and the posterior elements and posterior epidural space. Biopsies of the C1–C3 vertebral bodies can be performed through a transoral approach, with the patient under general nasotracheal anesthesia, or through a high lateral approach. The C4–C7 vertebral bodies can be accessed through a lateral or anterolateral approach (see the discussion of surgical approaches, later) or with open biopsy. Closed biopsy techniques of the cervical spine are technically demanding and often fraught with neurologic and vascular complications. If metastasis is suspected and the lesion is extensive enough to require surgical stabilization, we recommend an open biopsy to confirm the diagnosis by immediate frozen section, followed with a definitive surgical procedure. A fine-needle biopsy is possible under CT guidance, especially if surgical reconstruction is not deemed necessary.

TREATMENT OF CERVICAL TUMORS

An individualized approach is necessary, focusing on the concurrent goals of relief of pain, and the maintenance of spinal stability and neurologic integrity.

Benign Tumors

For benign cervical tumors, these general principles are relevant:

- Differentiate "latent" or "active" (i.e., stage 1 or 2 based on the Musculoskeletal Tumor Society surgical staging system) from "aggressive" or stage 3 lesions.
- Treat stage 1 or 2 lesions with intralesional curettage.
  - Precisely localize the tumor.
  - Protect structural and neurologic integrity.
  - In children, perform a posterior arthrodesis if performing a laminectomy.
- Treat stage 3 lesions with marginal or *en bloc* excision.
  - Be prepared for excessive bleeding.
    - Control bony bleeding with liberal application of bone wax and Gelfoam.
    - Preoperative embolization may be helpful to avoid excessive bleeding, especially in the case of aneurysmal bone cysts.
    - Be prepared to ligate or bypass the vertebral artery if necessary.
    - Perform preoperative angiography to assess collateral blood flow.
    - Consider packing the wound and embolizing the tumor or the vertebral artery if uncontrolled bleeding is encountered.
  - If the anterior part of the vertebra is severely involved, perform a posterior stabilization first to establish stability.

Certain tumors, such as osteoid osteoma and osteoblastoma, are common in children and have a predilection for the posterior elements. For characteristic osteoid osteoma and small osteoblastomas, excisional biopsy and intralesional curettage is sufficient treatment. The key to operative management is precise localization of the osteoid osteoma before surgery. If the lesion is located in the lamina, remove the posterior cortex of the lamina using a power drill to expose the nidus. While removing the nidus, take care not to damage the dura, because the anterior cortex is usually thin.

Larger lesions such as osteoblastomas can involve the soft tissue as well as the vertebral body and, similar to giant cell tumors and aneurysmal bone cysts (ABCs), have the potential for local recurrence. Because of the size and expansile nature of these tumors, surgical excision is more radical and often leads to spinal instability, necessitating spinal fusion. "Active" stage 2 lesions are positive on a bone scan and have a well-marginated sclerotic border. These lesions can be treated by curettage and have a low local recurrence rate (5% to 10%) (3). The "aggressive" stage 3 lesions are surrounded by a large pseudocapsule, which can be observed on a contrast-enhanced CT scan. Intralesional curettage has been associated with a 20% rate of local recurrence (36). Although *en bloc* excision is the treatment of choice, owing to anatomic restraints in the cervical spine, selected stage 3 benign tumors can be treated by incisional biopsy and frozen section confirmation of tumor type, followed at the same surgery with marginal excision.

En bloc excision in the cervical spine is a challenge and, owing to the increased surgical risks, should be reserved for the aggressive stage 3 lesion or recurrent tumors.

- Dissect the tumor outside its wall, leaving some of the soft tissue attached to the thin wall.
- If the tumor is next to the dura, dissect the wall with a Freer elevator, taking care not to compress the spinal cord.
- Be prepared to ligate or bypass the vertebral artery, if necessary.
- If a significant part of the esophagus is encased in tumor, an esophagectomy and gastric pull-up or colon interposition is indicated (8).

Radiation therapy may be considered as adjuvant therapy in the case of ABCs but is generally discouraged because of the potential for cord damage, induced sarcoma, and growth retardation (5). Low-dose radiotherapy may be considered for the well-circumscribed recurrent ABC lesion. Embolization may be effective for decreasing vascularity and making surgical resection and decompression less morbid, and may eliminate symptoms from expansive hemangioma.

After removing the larger posterior benign lesions, consider reconstructing the potentially destabilized spine. The extent of this destabilization depends on the age of the patient as well as the amount of posterior element resection. In children, laminectomy frequently results in secondary kyphosis that is difficult to correct. Therefore, in skeletally immature children, perform a posterior arthrodesis traversing the extent of the laminectomy (37). In the adult, when resection of any part of the lateral mass or pedicle is necessary, simultaneously arthrodese and instrument the affected levels using the remaining posterior spinal elements. Harvest an autologous graft through a separate incision, using a separate setup to avoid cross-contamination of the donor site.

Primary Malignant Tumors

Surgical treatment of primary cervical malignancies is predicated on the tumor type and the extent of local and systemic spread. Avoid surgery for primary malignant spinal tumors unless there is a good chance the surgery can offer significant palliation or a cure. Marginal or intralesional resection of the tumor, followed by radiation therapy, is an appropriate palliative approach to an intermediate-grade osteosarcoma with soft-tissue involvement. A wide resection for a low-grade chondrosarcoma in the vertebral body represents an attempt to cure by surgery alone.

The treatments for solitary plasmacytoma and multiple myeloma should necessarily be somewhat different owing to their different prognoses, although they are a continuum of the same disease and most cases of solitary plasmacytoma progress to multiple myeloma. Radiation is the initial treatment of choice in either case. Prophylactic laminectomy and stabilization before radiotherapy can be used if cord compromise or spinal instability is present. In the rare instance of a cervical solitary plasmacytoma, prognosis is enhanced by surgical excision reducing the tumor burden. In such cases, perform an intralesional excision and stabilization, followed by radiation therapy.

Chordomas pose a difficult problem owing to their high local recurrence rates and the difficulty in accessing this lesion in the cervical spine. Unlike sacral chordomas, in which sacral nerve roots can be sacrificed, cervical chordomas often involve the clivus and upper cervical spine, in which, at best, only decompression and marginal excision is possible. Often, the only option for surgical treatment is posterior stabilization and fusion, followed by anterior intralesional or marginal excision and decompression.

Metastatic Tumors

In the adult population, metastatic tumors are the most common tumors in the cervical spine with a predilection for the anterior column. In the cervical spine, the weight-bearing axis falls at or posterior to the vertebral body, and the articular processes support the weight of the skull. For this reason, destruction of the vertebral body results in some loss of vertebral body height, but kyphotic deformity is uncommon. Instability is also an uncommon. Destruction of the lateral masses as well as the vertebral body must occur to permit rotatory instability. Except for extensive lysis in one or more contiguous bodies, or the involvement of the spinous process of C-2, where the nuchal fascia inserts, metastatic involvement of the upper cervical spine rarely results in kyphosis or true flexion instability (49).

In the upper cervical spine, the prevalence of neurologic deficit is much lower owing to the space available for the cord. The development of neurologic deficit here is usually due to extension of the tumor rather than to angular kyphosis. The sudden onset or rapid progression of neurologic deficit is usually due to a vascular accident rather than vertebral collapse and usually has a poor prognosis. Reporting on all locations of spinal tumors, Harrington (23) noted 62% of initially paraplegic patients regained enough neurologic function to ambulate after surgical intervention, but patients with rapid paraplegia exhibited a poor prognosis for recovery.

Appropriate treatment is selected dependent on life expectancy, type of tumor, location of tumor (accessibility), radiosensitivity, degree of instability, and neurologic status of the patient. Because the primary goal is to improve the patient's quality of life, thoroughly consider the patient's personal preference and family situation. Metastasis of lung carcinoma has a 7- to 9-month mean survival time, whereas breast carcinoma has a survival exceeding 30 months. Consider embolization of tumors with hemorrhagic tendencies, such as renal and thyroid. Treat radiosensitive tumors such as lymphoma, myeloma, and prostate with nonoperative management: Radiate with doses up to 4,000 cGy as long as there is no instability, neurologic threat, or significant deformity. Doses in excess of 5,000 cGy may cause acute or chronic radiation myelitis. Radiation therapy is compatible with internal fixation devices and methacrylate but may cause failure of supporting bone graft struts. Radiation therapy alone is rarely effective in relieving a well-established neural deficit, especially in the presence of a collapsed vertebral body and bony impingement.

With normal neurologic function, consider surgery when there is severe pain, instability, or impending kyphotic collapse, or when the tumor is known to be radioresistant. Tumors with greater than 50% involvement of the vertebral body and greater than 50% destruction of the ipsilateral middle and posterior columns require prophylactic surgical stabilization. Kyphotic deformity and amount of subluxation should also be considered, but the assessment of instability is still somewhat subjective. The goal of surgery is to prevent neurologic compromise, but severe neurologic deficit is not a contraindication for surgery.

Location of the tumor is a major consideration for treatment with immobilization versus early radiation therapy versus surgery.

- Treat patients with tumors in the posterior C-2 arch with early radiation therapy so that progressive kyphosis does not develop.
- For destruction of the lateral mass of C-1, perform an occiput to C-3 fusion with adjunctive radiation therapy because rotatory instability is common (49).
- For destruction of the dens with instability, perform a C1–C2 fusion. If cord compression is impending, remove the arch of C-1 and perform an occiput to C-3 fusion.
- In the lower cervical spine, consider early combined anterior and posterior stabilization owing to the difficulty of fixation and the increased stress at the cervicothoracic junction.

Plan surgery so that it is appropriate for the tumor's stage and extent. Determine what anatomic structures may need to be sacrificed to perform the resection. Sacrifice of one vertebral artery can be tolerated if cure is a reasonable goal, but obtain a preoperative angiogram to assess collateral flow. If the cervical esophagus or a significant part of the thoracic esophagus is involved by tumor, total esophagectomy and gastric pull-up or colon interposition can be performed (8).

The results of surgery for cervical spine metastasis have shown a high rate of pain relief (94% to 95%), motor recovery (64% to 92%), and ambulation (87%). The results of surgery are usually maintained until the terminal stage, with local recurrences in 30% (2,48). In an elderly population with a mean age of 73, a mortality rate of 16% was reported within 7 days after surgery (60).

EXPOSURE, EXCISION, AND RECONSTRUCTION OF CERVICAL DESTRUCTIVE LESIONS

Anterior Approaches

The different incisions for the anterior approaches are shown in Figure 151.3 and are discussed in detail in Chapter 138. The different techniques employ three separate

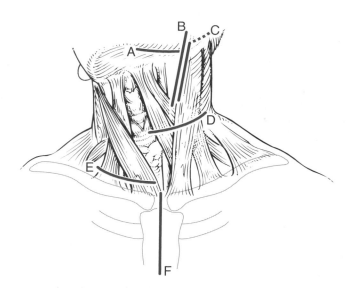

Figure 151.3. Incisions for the anterior approaches to the spine. **A:** Submandibular approach, described by McAfee et al. (43). This approach is retropharyngeal and prevascular (medial to carotid sheath). The incision is 1 cm below the jaw. **B:** Extension of the prevascular approach. This approach is a cephalad extension of the standard anterolateral approach to the midcervical spine, and when it is combined with the submandibular approach, it allows direct exposure from the tip of the clivus and can be extended caudal to the lower cervical spine. **C:** Retrovascular, lateral approach (lateral and posterior to carotid sheath), popularized by Whitesides and Kelly (64). This approach allows direct exposure of one side or the other only at the level of the C1–C2 articulation. **D:** Standard anterolateral approach to the midcervical spine, medial to the carotid sheath. **E:** Exposure to lower cervical spine, which may require clavicular osteotomy for cervicothoracic exposure. **F:** Sternal splitting approach to the cervicothoracic spine.

deep paths to the cervical spine: transpharyngeal, lateral and posterior to the carotid sheath, or anterior to the carotid sheath.

Exposure for Upper Cervical Anterior Lesions The upper cervical spine can be approached through the transoral approach. Routine tracheostomy is necessary only if a tongue or mandible-splitting approach is used. See Chapter 138 for a detailed description. The standard transoral approach can be used for exposure of C1–C2 (Fig. 151.4*A*), and this can be enlarged by the tongue-splitting (Fig. 151.4*B*) or transmandibular (Fig. 151.4*C*) approach, for decompression from the level of the clivus to C-4 (31). If division of the soft palate becomes necessary (only during extensile approaches), it is incised on one side of the midline to avoid the uvula. This approach allows for tumor resection, but the risk of sepsis makes placing implants impractical.

The upper cervical spine can be alternatively approached through the submandibular approach, which is prevascular and retropharyngeal (incision: Fig. 151.3*A*; deep dissection: Fig. 151.5*A*). This approach is a cephalad extension of the standard approach to the midcervical spine (34,43).

■ Make a transverse incision 1 cm below the jaw line, which can be extended into a longitudinal incision if more extensile exposure is needed (Fig. 151.3*A* and *B*).

■ Recruit the assistance of a head and neck surgeon familiar with radical neck dissections to decrease the incidence of complications.

■ Develop the interval medial to the sternocleidomastoid by preserving the mandibular branch of the facial nerve and by dividing the submandibular salivary gland and the vascular leashes of the superior thyroid, lingual, and facial arteries.

■ Keep the patient intubated at least overnight due to the upper pharyngeal edema common with this approach.

This approach permits extensile exposure of the anterior cervical spine. The visualization is similar to that obtained by the transmucosal route. This approach allows decompression up to the clivus and reconstruction of the anterior column with strut graft and internal fixation. We prefer this prevascular extraoral approach to the upper cervical spine owing to the excellent extensile exposure and decreased risk of infection compared with those of the transpharyngeal approach, especially if instrumentation is used. There is a reported 40% incidence of mostly transient palsies of the marginal mandibular branch of the facial nerve (34).

A third approach is the retrovascular, lateral approach popularized by Whitesides and Kelly (incision: Fig. 151.3*C*; deep dissection: Fig. 151.5*B*) (64). Owing to the restriction in mobilizing the carotid sheath, this approach allows direct exposure of one side or the other only at

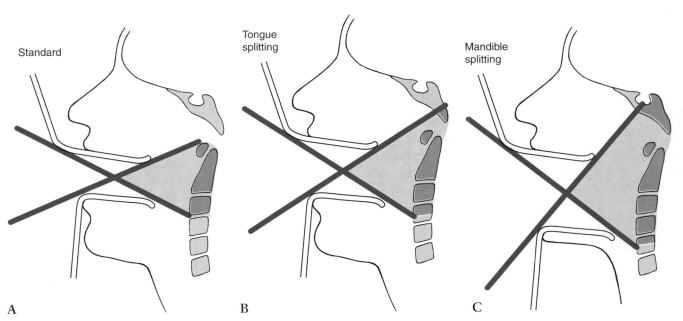

A ⸱ Standard   **B** ⸱ Tongue splitting   **C** ⸱ Mandible splitting

Figure 151.4. Transpharyngeal approaches. **A:** Standard transoral approach: can expose tip of odontoid to C-2. **B:** Tongue-splitting approach: can expose tip of clivus to C-3. **C:** Mandible-splitting approach: can expose clivus to C-4.

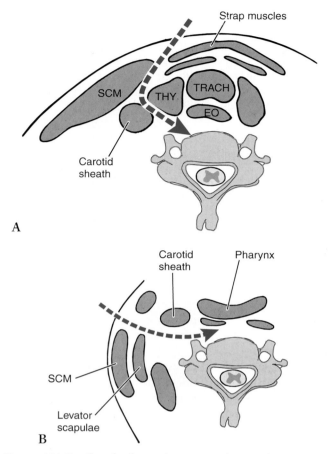

A

B

Figure 151.5. Standard anterior approaches to the spine. **A:** Anterolaterally: medial to the carotid sheath. **B:** Lateral: lateral to the carotid sheath.

the level of the C1–C2 articulation and, therefore, is best suited for fusion and even instrumentation but not decompression. Lans (34) reported on 10 cases of C1–C2 arthrodesis through this bilateral, lateral approach first described by Barbour, with instrumentation using bilateral transarticular screws.

Exposure for Midcervical Anterior Lesions   Corpectomy and stabilization through the standard anterior prevascular approach (see Chapter 138) is usually the surgical treatment of choice for lesions from C-3 to C-7. Rarely, if a lateral biopsy was obtained and the goal of surgery was a wide margin with excision of the biopsy tract, the exposure would need to begin from the lateral approach and proceed posterior to the neurovascular bundle (22).

Exposure for Cervicothoracic Anterior Lesions   Inferior extension of the exposure in the cervical spine may be limited by the diameter of the thoracic inlet, the height of the clavicles and manubrium anteriorly, and the extent of

cervicothoracic kyphosis. Obtain a preoperative radiograph to compare the upper margin of the clavicles and manubrium with the level of the vertebral body. If clearance of the clavicle and manubrium is not possible, we prefer the sternal splitting approach (62) to clavicular osteotomy (33). The sternal splitting approach is very familiar to cardiothoracic surgeons (only the superior portion of the sternum needs to be split) and can be easily extended into the neck. This allows an extensile approach to the cervicothoracic junction, and the exposure can be further enhanced by ligation of the brachiocephalic vein. Such ligation produces significant edema in the upper extremity.

Reconstruction of Anterior Lesions   In the cervical spine, the resultant corpectomy defect can be replaced in several ways. In patients with benign lesions, or lesions with which there is long life expectancy, we prefer to use autograft or allograft struts to replace the anterior defect, followed by anterior instrumentation. If massive resection of the vertebral bodies is necessary at multiple levels, we perform posterior stabilization before anterior resection and reconstruction. The different scenarios for upper cervical, midcervical, and lower cervical reconstructions are shown in Figures 151.6, 151.7, and 151.8.

In the case of giant cell tumor and other aggressive stage 3 lesions, some advocate use of methylmethacrylate (PMMA) anteriorly, with or without posterior arthrodesis or plating (36). Similar to its use in the extremities, PMMA has the advantage of immediate stability, local control due to the heat of polymerization, and rapid recognition of early recurrence. Despite the advantages of PMMA, we recommend reconstruction with autograft or allograft to provide a biologic reconstruction in these patients who usually have a long life expectancy. The benefits of a biologic reconstruction must be weighed against the risk of failure if radiation is used. Use of titanium or carbon fiber cages is controversial, and recognition of early recurrence with use of titanium is more difficult. Postoperative radiation therapy may be used if resection is incomplete, and in these cases, we would recommend use of PMMA.

For metastatic disease, when survival is anticipated to be less than 6 to 12 months, we use PMMA combined with metal implants to give immediate stable fixation (25). Radiation therapy can be used with PMMA without fear of impacting the healing of bone graft. Stabilization of the spine with PMMA can be fraught with major complications, however (42). Take care to avoid spinal cord injury, which can be caused by direct mass effect or by heat generated from the exothermic reaction of cement solidification.

■ Protect the cord with Gelfoam, wire mesh, silicon sheets, or various plastics positioned anterior to the dura.

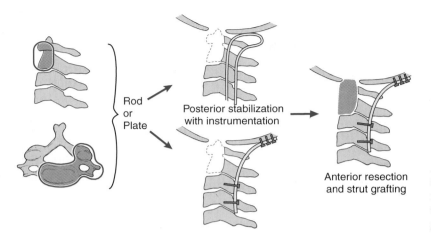

Figure 151.6. Scenario for upper cervical reconstruction. For extensive destruction of C1–C2, perform a posterior stabilization first with instrumentation, with next-stage anterior resection and strut grafting as needed.

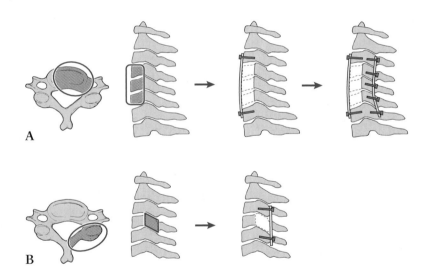

Figure 151.7. Scenario for midcervical reconstruction. **A:** For extensive anterior destruction and fixed kyphosis in the midcervical spine, perform anterior decompression, strut grafting, and instrumentation, followed by posterior instrumentation. Perform the posterior instrumentation can be performed first if there is no significant deformity or if there is severe instability. **B:** For posterior destruction of the facets, perform a posterior-only reconstruction with plating or wiring.

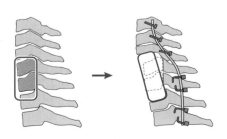

Figure 151.8. Scenario for cervicothoracic reconstruction. For extensive cervicothoracic destruction, perform a posterior stabilization followed by anterior reconstruction.

■ As the cement begins to harden, irrigate with cooled saline to reduce its temperature. When multiple level corpectomies are performed, most authors agree that anterior plating is best (24,35).

■ Do not use PMMA alone for anterior fixation. The average length of time to failure of PMMA fixation anteriorly used alone was 194 days (42).

■ Perform posterior fixation for cases of multiple level corpectomies. In cases of massive anterior instability without rigid kyphosis, we recommend posterior fixation before anterior resection. Owing to different anatomy, the upper, mid-, and lower cervical spine require different strategies for stabilization and fixation (Figs. 151.6, 151.7, and 151.8, respectively).

Posterior Approach and Stabilization

The posterior approach may be preferred in the upper cervical spine or the cervicothoracic junction owing to the difficulties inherent in anterior approach and stabilization in these areas. Laminectomy alone is contraindicated in the presence of anterior compression and kyphosis. If the posterior elements can be left intact, then standard wiring techniques can be used. In the case of a laminectomy, lateral mass plates may be used for stabilization. Special techniques are available for occipitocervical and cervicothoracic instrumentation.

Options for occipitocervical instrumentation are

• Use of a contoured rod with wires for occipital and cervical laminar fixation (Fig. 151.9).

• Plating with use of lateral mass screws in the cervical spine and screws in the occiput
• Combination of the above-mentioned techniques

Options for cervicothoracic instrumentation are

• Use of rods and wires if posterior elements are intact.
• Use of a one-piece plate and rod combination with screws in the cervical lateral masses and hooks in the thoracic spine (Acromed/DePuy/Johnson and Johnson, Rahnam, MA) (Fig. 151.10A).
• Use of a two-piece cervical plate with cervical lateral mass screws and thoracic rod using thoracic hooks or pedicle screw (Danek, Memphis, TN, or Acromed/DePuy/Johnson and Johnson, Rahnam, MA)
• Use of two different diameter rods spanning the cervical and thoracic spine segments, affixed separately to cervical lateral mass screws and thoracic screws or hooks and connected by rod-to-rod connectors (Synthes, Paoli, PA) or (Acromed/DePuy/Johnson and Johnson, Rahnam, MA) (Fig. 151.10B).

The use of methacrylate for posterior stabilization should be condemned unless it is used to augment the lateral mass screws. We do not recommend augmentation of lateral mass screws with PMMA if the anterior cortex has been breached due to risk of vertebral artery injury. In cases in which the patient's life expectancy is more than 2 years (plasmacytoma or breast carcinoma), or in cases in which global instability exists where anterior stabilization alone is insufficient, a combined anterior and posterior approach should be used.

Occipitocervical fixation

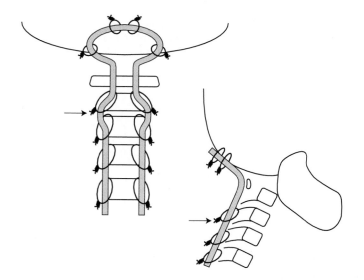

Figure 151.9. Preferred method for occipitocervical instrumentation. Use a contoured rod as shown. Wiring to the occiput is performed through four drill holes through the occiput and passage of the two superior-most wires. The next set of wires are inserted from two occipital drill holes through the foramen magnum. A total of six occipital drill holes are necessary. After wiring of the lamina, the loop resists settling (arrow).

One piece plate-rod combination

Two piece rod combination

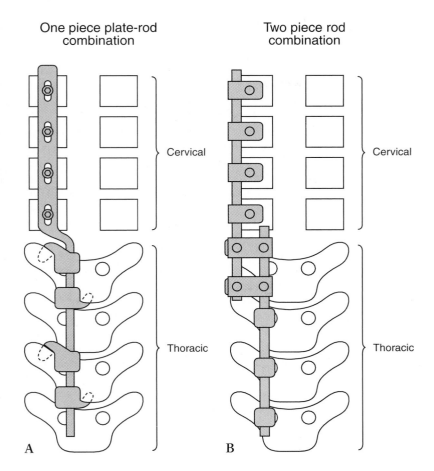

Figure 151.10. Options for cervicothoracic fixation. **A:** Use of a one-piece plate and rod combination. Lateral mass screws in the cervical spine and hooks in the thoracic spine. **B:** Use of two different diameter rods—the cervical rod affixed to the cervical spine via lateral mass screws, and the thoracic rod affixed via thoracic screws or hooks. Use rod-to-rod connectors to attach the two rods together.

INFECTION

VERTEBRAL OSTEOMYELITIS

Diagnostic Evaluation

Infections can be classified as hematogenous or contiguous and postoperative. See Chapter 150 for a general discussion of infections of the spine. Hematogenous spine infections are less common in the cervical spine than in the thoracic or lumbar spines, but they do have a predilection for the anterior compartment of the spine. The most common complaint of patients with cervical infections is neck pain (18). Because of the nonspecific nature of cervical infections, delayed diagnosis is common. Radionuclide studies can detect spinal infection before plain films can and have the advantage of revealing other foci of infection, which occur in 4% of cases (46). Gallium scans have been shown to detect infection earlier in the course of the disease than technetium scans, and they are more useful for following the response to treatment (47). Gallium scans become normal during the resolution of the infection, whereas technetium scans remain positive for many months after the disease has resolved. Single-photon emission computed tomography (SPECT) allows the advantage of three-dimensional localization with higher sensitivity as compared with planar technetium scintigraphy or gallium scintigraphy (17). Indium scans are not helpful owing to their low sensitivity (17%) (63).

When cervical infection is suspected, gadolinium-enhanced MRI is the modality of choice. MRI has 96% sensitivity, 93% specificity, and 94% accuracy in detecting vertebral osteomyelitis and becomes positive at about the same time as the gallium scan (46). Eismont (14) noted some degree of neurologic deficit in 80% of patients with cervical osteomyelitis, and the MRI can also help identify the site and extent of compression.

Despite the accuracy of MRI, the diagnosis is confirmed by bacteriologic or histologic examination of tissue or an aspirate. The only circumstances in which a diagnosis can be made without tissue biopsy are in pediatric discitis (rare in the cervical spine) and when there is a positive blood culture with a patient who has typical signs and symptoms of spinal infection.

Biopsy and Aspiration

A definite diagnosis of the infection is possible with a closed-needle biopsy in 68% to 86% of cases (9,44). In the cervical spine, open biopsy is often performed as part of the definitive surgical procedure.

Treatment

Hematogenous Vertebral Osteomyelitis and Disk-Space Infection   The goals of treatment are to

- Establish diagnosis
- Relieve pain
- Prevent or reverse neurologic deficit
- Establish or maintain spinal stability
- Eradicate infection

Cervical discitis or osteomyelitis can be treated with external immobilization and appropriate antibiotics if there is no abscess formation, neurologic deficit, or vertebral collapse and instability. Associated conditions that compromise wound healing or immune response should be managed aggressively. Bring diabetes or other systemic diseases under control, and address proper nutrition and reversal of hypoxia and metabolic deficits. Compared with thoracic and lumbar spine infections, infections of the cervical spine have a higher risk of complications and surgical treatment is often required in addition to antibiotic therapy.

- Choose the antibiotic according to culture and sensitivity results.
- Withhold antibiotics in cases in which a biopsy is done, in case a second biopsy is required.
- In patients who have systemic toxicity or neurologic deficit, start maximum-dose broad-spectrum bacteriocidal antibiotics as soon as biopsy is obtained.
- If the patient does not respond clinically to antibiotics, or the sedimentation rate does not decrease to one half or two thirds by completion of treatment, perform a repeat biopsy.
- Immobilize patients for pain control and to prevent deformity or deterioration of neurologic status.

Surgical indications include the following:

- The need for tissue and bacteriologic diagnosis
- To drain an abscess that is clinically significant (fevers or sepsis)
- Cases refractory to nonoperative treatment
- Presence of neurologic deficit
- Prevention or correction of spinal deformity or instability

In nearly all cases of hematogenous cervical osteomyelitis, if surgery is deemed to be necessary, a solely anterior surgical approach with discectomy and debridement of pus and strut grafting from healthy bone above to below is sufficient. Laminectomy is contraindicated except for the rare case of associated posterior epidural abscess. If there is evidence of epidural extension, excise the posterior longitudinal ligament to ensure decompression and removal of infected tissue.

Autogenous bone grafting after vertebral body resection in the presence of active infection has been shown to be safe and effective (44). Iliac bone is preferable to that of the fibula because it has more cancellous bone. Revascularization of cortical graft may not be complete even after 1 year (57). Experience has shown that instrumentation and even allograft may also be placed anteriorly in situations of active infection, as long as adequate debridement has been performed back to healthy, bleeding bone (55,57). Dietze et al. (13) reported no recurrence of cervical infection with a 37-month follow-up after debridement and use of allograft and instrumentation, but they presented information on only five patients. In cases of significant kyphosis, or to avoid halo immobilization, the anterior strut graft can be safely followed by second-stage posterior instrumentation.

Infections involving the midcervical spine can be addressed with standard surgical approaches. The occipitocervical junction is difficult to treat owing to anatomic and mechanical constraints. Upper cervical osteomyelitis is rare but generally requires fusion because of associated instability. Stabilization of the upper cervical spine should be performed in cases of instability as defined by traction or flexion-extension radiographs, odontoid and transverse ligament resection or destruction, or clivus and odontoid resection or destruction in the presence of basilar invagination. The principle of debridement to healthy bone still applies. For high cervical infections that require drainage owing to abscess formation or cord compression, we recommend a transoral drainage and posterior stabilization. Many authors recommend posterior stabilization due to the nonsterile environment of the posterior pharynx and devitalized bone (21,39). Zigler et al. (65) described five patients with pyogenic osteomyelitis of the occipitocervical region treated by operation and antibiotics. The options used were anterior debridement and occipitocervical fusion, transoral drainage, posterior occipitocervical fusion, and posterior C1–C2 fusion; and all five patients recovered. The surgical procedure must be individualized in each case according to the degree of bony destruction and instability.

Treatment of Posterior Infection   Most posterior infections result from previous surgery. Treat by irrigation, debridement, and administration of culture-specific intravenous antibiotics. If more than 50% of the facet joint is resected during debridement (very rare), then perform a fusion. Autogenous bone graft placed in a thoroughly debrided bed will usually result in a successful arthrodesis because of the abundant blood supply. We recommend a halo brace for immobilization after debridement of posterior infection and bone grafting. Stabilization with bone screws and plate or wire techniques is possible in spite of the infection, but the use of posterior cervical instrumentation in the presence of active infection is controversial. The length of time of administration of postoperative intravenous antibiotics will depend on the causative organism, but they should be given for at least 6 weeks; however, 4-week courses have been reported with good results (12).

Outcome of Treatment

Cervical infections have a higher rate of spontaneous fusion compared with thoracic and lumbar infections. Almost all cases of cervical infection that can be treated nonoperatively fuse spontaneously (45), as compared with only 50% of all patients with thoracic and lumbar vertebral osteomyelitis treated nonoperatively (19). Human immunodeficiency virus (HIV) status (27) and intravenous drug abuse (59) do not appear to affect the neurologic outcome of patients with spinal infections adversely. Infants with vertebral osteomyelitis (15), elderly patients, and those with underlying disease (58) have a high recurrence rate and a poorer prognosis. Factors that predispose to paralysis include increased age, a subaxial level of infection, and a concomitant disease (diabetes or rheumatoid arthritis) (14). Relapse of infection occurs in up to 25% of cases but is much less common when antibiotics are administered for more than 4 weeks (14,58).

Eismont et al. (14) found that the prognosis for patients with paralysis from cervical spine infection is better with an anterior surgical procedure than with the posterior approach; three of seven patients deteriorated and four remained unchanged after laminectomy. Stone et al. (61) reported that all surgical patients with myelopathy and radiculopathy achieved solid fusion, and at final follow-up, they were ambulatory and neurologically intact. When doubt exists regarding the reversibility of a spinal cord lesion, perform a decompression. Recovery from paralysis has been noted in patients who underwent decompression as late as 5 months after the onset of weakness (47).

EPIDURAL ABSCESS

Diagnosis

Epidural abscess is rare but potentially devastating. In a series of 25 epidural infections, the cervical spine was noted to be involved in 13. Three were multifocal (cervical and thoracic) (54). Cervical epidural abscess may occur via hematogenous spread from a remote location or from a contiguous focus of vertebral osteomyelitis, or by direct inoculation at the time of operation or injection.

The peak incidence of spinal epidural abscess is in the sixth and seventh decade of life, and there is a high incidence in patients who are intravenous drug abusers, so comorbid conditions may impair immunocompetence (29). Even though most epidural abscesses are seen after invasive processes that violate the epidural space, there are reports of multifocal abscesses when systemic infection is the cause of the abscess (7).

Anatomically, the epidural space is not a uniform space (10). Some areas are filled with fat and veins, and others are in direct contact with bone or ligament, creating individual metameric segments. In the cervical spine, except for a space dorsal to the origin of the spinal nerves, the epidural space is mostly a potential space. Individual metamers are septated, preventing free communication between the anterior and posterior epidural space (30). Because the majority of epidural abscesses from hematogenous spread are located posteriorly (29), they do not involve the anterior epidural space or circumferentially surround the thecal sac. Conversely, postsurgical cases or cases associated with discitis or vertebral osteomyelitis not only involve the anterior epidural space but may be circumferential because of the common postsurgical disruption of normal anatomic septations (41).

To diagnose epidural abscess, MRI with contrast is the modality of choice. False-negative results may occur with nonenhanced MRI, especially with extensive abscesses that do not have a discrete proximal or distal extent (20). Concomitant meningitis may also cause signal changes in the abscess that may be similar to infected cerebral spinal fluid, resulting in a false-negative magnetic resonance imaging MRI scan (51). Myelography and CT are sensitive for confirming the presence and extent of an extradural compressive lesion but should be avoided if epidural abscess is suspected because dural puncture risks spreading the infection to the intrathecal compartment. There is also a small but real risk of causing an acute neurologic deterioration owing to resultant spinal coning if lumbar puncture is performed caudal to a spinal block (41). Owing to the frequently rapid evolution of the disease process and associated illnesses, the mortality rate is as high as 20% (29). In cases in which MRI is not readily available, CT with myelography should be performed because, despite the increased risk, confirmation of the diagnosis should not be delayed.

Treatment

Management of spinal epidural abscess is based on the clinical condition of the patient. Medical management is often successful in the treatment of lumbar epidural abscess, but cervical epidural abscess presents an increased risk to the spinal cord. Indications for nonoperative treatment of spinal epidural abscess are

- Poor surgical candidates due to severe concomitant medical problems
- Patients with abscess involving a considerable length of the spinal canal (cervical to lumbar) and who have epiduritis but a normal neurologic examination
- Patients with normal spinal cord or cauda equina function

■ Patients with complete paralysis for more than 3 days (38)

Medical treatment involves 8 to 12 weeks of intravenous antibiotics. Close monitoring with hospitalization and numerous MRIs is needed. The disadvantages of medical treatment are that neurologic deterioration can be precipitous, and once present, the deficits may be irreversible. We recommend aggressive surgical management of cervical epidural abscesses. When surgical drainage is performed and osteomyelitis is not present, shorter courses of intravenous antibiotics (less than 4 weeks) have been successful (11).

When epidural abscesses are located posteriorly, laminectomy is the most effective approach for decompression. The extent of the exposure is determined by the operative findings. If purulent material is found (acute infection), a limited approach can be used (see case example, Fig. 151.11). In chronic infection, dense granulation tissue is present; decompress the full extent of the abscess. Stabilization is usually not necessary.

Anterior epidural infections are usually associated with

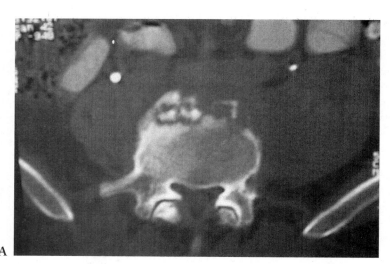

A

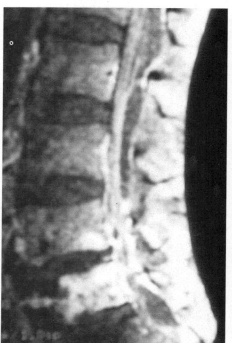

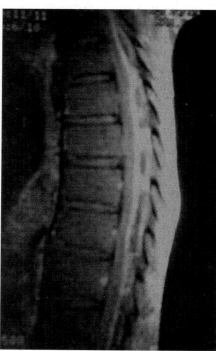

B,C

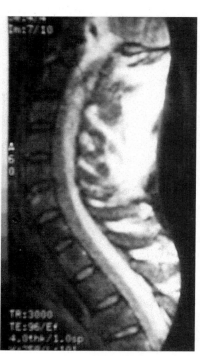

D

Figure 151.11.   A case of epidural abscess formation leading to severe cervical spinal cord impingement. A 45-year-old homeless patient with increasing low back pain for months, fevers, and chills. The patient failed to seek treatment and finally presented with severe progressive neurologic deficit and respiratory difficulties. **A:** Lumbar spine CT scan showing anterior sequestra. **B:** Lumbar MRI showing vertebral osteomyelitis and massive epidural abscess. **C:** Thoracic MRI showing massive posterior epidural abscess involving at least 50% of spinal canal. **D:** Cervical MRI showing massive posterior epidural abscess with almost 75% involvement of the spinal canal at the level of C-2. The probable start of the infection was lumbar discitis and vertebral osteomyelitis that progressed to epidural extension and eventual marked spinal cord compression. Treatment was limited cervical laminectomy. After the cervical laminectomy, the patient was placed in Trendelenberg position, with massive drainage of the thoracic and lumbar pus. Postoperatively, the patient had significant but partial neurologic recovery. The patient was lost to follow-up.

discitis or osteomyelitis and should be approached anteriorly (29). If the patient has discitis, osteomyelitis, and instability, anterior debridement and reconstruction can be carried out without formal excision of the granulation tissue formed by the abscess. Incise the posterior longitudinal ligament to allow evacuation of purulent material. If cord compression is symptomatic, complete exposure of the granulating abscess is necessary to allow excision of this dense, tenacious material from the thecal sack. Extreme caution is advised.

- Remove necrotic disc and endplate material, and resect diseased bone back to healthy, bleeding vertebral bone. If only the endplate and less than half of the body remain at any level, resect the remnant and extend to the next disc space.
- Use a micropituitary and small curet to fenestrate the posterior longitudinal ligament (PLL) laterally. Use small Kerrison rongeur to expand the window, and resect a portion of posterior vertebral rim.
- If there are no signs of cord compression, drain any purulent material, gently irrigate, and proceed with stabilization. If there are signs of cord compromise, carefully resect the posterior vertebral cortex and PLL over the length of the lesion to provide full decompression.
- If the thickened granulation tissue is to be removed from the surface of the cord, magnification is necessary.
- Carefully develop the interval between the abscess and thecal sack with Roton dissectors and a nerve hook.
- Monitor spinal cord function constantly.
- Once the mass is debulked and cultures obtained, irrigate with antibiotic solution and stabilize the resected segment with an autograft strut.
- Stabilize in a halo. Do not use implants in the presence of deep infection.

Outcomes of Treatment of Epidural Infection

As previously stated, the prognosis for patients with cervical epidural abscess is not as favorable as that for thoracic and lumbar infections. The mortality rate with cervical abscess was reported to be as high as 38% despite aggressive treatment, and the neurologic deficits were more severe and refractory to treatment (20). Diabetes, HIV infection (20,33), and vertebral osteomyelitis (28) are associated conditions that carry a poor prognosis. Reporting on predominantly cervical and cervicothoracic epidural abscesses, Redekop and Del Maestro (54) reported a 20% mortality rate, and only 56% retained or recovered ambulation. They attribute the high morbidity and mortality rates to delay in diagnosis and treatment, which has been shown to be a factor in all epidural abscesses. Reporting on all locations of epidural abscesses, no patients with paralysis for longer than 36 hours recovered significant neurologic function (22,28,29), and only 40% of patients who initially had less than antigravity strength were even-

tually ambulatory and continent despite surgical intervention within 36 hours (56). If rapid acute progressive paraplegia occurs within the first 12 hours, prognosis is poor, presumably secondary to spinal cord infarction rather than mechanical compression (33).

REFERENCES

Each reference is categorized according to the following scheme: *, classic article; #, review article; !, basic research article; and +, clinical results/outcome study.

1. Akbarnia BA, Merenda JT. Benign Tumors of the Spine. In: *Spine: State of the Art Reviews,* Vol 10, No 1. Philadelphia: Hanley & Belfus, 1996.

+ 2. Atanasiu JP, Badatcheff F, Pidhorz L. Metastatic Lesions of the Cervical Spine. A Retrospective Analysis of 20 Cases. *Spine* 1993;18:1279.

3. Boriani S, Capanna Donati D, Levine A. Osteoblastoma of the Spine. *Clin Orthop* 1992;278:37.

4. Boriani S, Chevalley F, Weinstein JN, et al. Spine Update: Primary Bone Tumors of the Spine: Terminology and Surgical Staging. *Spine* 1997;22:1036.

+ 5. Capanna R, Albisinni U, Picci P, et al. Aneurysmal Bone Cyst of the Spine. *J Bone Joint Surg [Am]* 1985;67:527.

+ 6. Carson HJ, Castelli MJ, Reyes CV, Gattuso P. Fine-needle Aspiration Biopsy of Vertebral Body Lesions: Cytologic, Pathologic, and Clinical Correlations of 57 Cases. *Diagn Cytopathol* 1994;11:348.

+ 7. Chow GH, Gebhard JS, Brown CW. Multifocal Metachronous Epidural Abscesses of the Spine. A Case Report. *Spine* 1996;21:1094.

+ 8. Coleman JJ. Reconstruction of the Pharynx and Cervical Esophagus. *Semin Surg Oncol* 1995;3:208.

9. Currier BL, Heller JG, Eismont FJ. Cervical Spinal Infections. In: *The Cervical Spine,* 3rd ed. The Cervical Spine Research Society Editorial Committee. Philadelphia: Lippincott-Raven, 1998.

+ 10. Dandy WE. Abscesses and Inflammatory Tumors in the Spinal Epidural Space (So-called Pachymeningitis Externa). *Arch Surg* 1926;13:477.

11. Danner RL, Hartman BJ Update of Spinal Epidural Abscess: 35 Cases and Review of the Literature. *Rev Infect Dis* 1987;9:265.

+ 12. Del Curling O Jr, Grower DJ, McWhorter JM. Changing Concepts in Spinal Epidural Abscess: A Report of 29 Cases. *Neurosurgery* 1990;27:185.

13. Dietze DD Jr, Fessler RG, Jacob RP. Primary Reconstruction for Spinal Infections. *J Neurosurg* 1997;86: 981.

* 14. Eismont FJ, Bohlman HH, Soni PL, et al. Pyogenic and Fungal Vertebral Osteomyelitis with Paralysis. *J Bone Joint Surg [Am]* 1983;65:19.

+ 15. Eismont FJ, Bohlman HH, Soni PL, et al. Vertebral Osteomyelitis in Infants. *J Bone Joint Surg [Br]* 1982;64: 32.

+ 16. Eismont FJ, Green BA, Brown MD, Ghandour-

Mnaymneh L. Coexistent Infection and Tumor of the Spine. A Report of Three Cases. *J Bone Joint Surg [Am]* 1987;69:452.

+ 17. Feiglan D, Modic M, Piraino D, et al. Evaluation of MRI and Nuclear Medicine in Spinal Infection—a Reappraisal. *J Nucl Med* 1985;26:672.

18. Forsythe M, Rothman RH: New Concepts in the Diagnosis and Treatment of Infections of the Cervical Spine. *Orthop Clin North Am* 1978;9:1039.

* 19. Frederickson B, Yuan H, Orlans R. Management and Outcome of Pyogenic Vertebral Osteomyelitis. *Clin Orthop* 1978;131:160.

* 20. Gardner RD, Cammisa FP, Eismont FJ, Green B. Nongranulomatous Spinal Epidural Abscesses. *Orthop Trans* 1989;13:562.

* 21. Ghanayem AJ, Zdeblick TA. Cervical Spine Infections. *Orthop Clin North Am* 1996;27:53.

+ 22. Hakin RN, Burt AA, Cook JB. Acute Spinal Epidural Abscess. *Paraplegia* 1979;17:330.

+ 23. Harrington KD. Current Concepts Review—Metastatic Disease of the Spine. *J Bone Joint Surg [Am]* 1986;68:1110.

+ 24. Harrington KD. The Use of Methylmethacrylate for Vertebral Body Replacement and Anterior Stabilization of Pathological Fracture Dislocations of the Spine due to Metastatic Disease. *J Bone Joint Surg* 1981;63A:36.

* 25. Hart RA, Boriani S, Biagini R, et al. A System for Surgical Staging and Management of Spine Tumors. A Clinical Outcome Study of Giant Cell Tumors of the Spine. *Spine* 1997;22:1773.

26. Hay MC, Patterson D, Taylor TKF. Aneurysmal Bone Cysts of the Spine. *J Bone Joint Surg* 1978;60A:406.

+ 27. Heary RF, Hunt CD, Krieger AJ, Vaid C. HIV Status Does Not Affect Microbiologic Spectrum or Neurologic Outcome in Spinal Infections. *Surg Neurol* 1994;42:417.

28. Heusner AP. Nontuberculosis Spinal Epidural Infections. *N Engl J Med* 1948;239:845.

29. Hlavin ML, Kaminski HJ, Ross JS, Ganz E. Spinal Epidural Abscess: A 10-year Prospective. *Neurosurgery* 1990;27:177.

! 30. Hogan QH: Lumbar Epidural Anatomy: A New Look by Cryomicrotome Section. *Anesthesiology* 1991;75:767.

+ 31. Honma G, Murota K, Shiba R, Hidemaru K. Mandible and Tongue-splitting Approach for Giant Cell Tumor of Axis. *Spine* 1989;14:1204.

+ 32. Koppel BS, Tuchman AJ, Mangiardi JR. Epidural Spinal Infection in Intravenous Drug Abusers. *Arch Neurol* 1988;45:1331.

+ 33. Kurz L, Pursel S, Herkowitz H. Modified Anterior Approach to the Cervicothoracic Junction. *Spine* 1991;16(suppl):2.

+ 34. Laus M, Pignatti G, Malaguti MC, et al. Anterior Extraoral Surgery to the Upper Cervical Spine. *Spine* 1996;21:1687.

35. Levine AM. Operative Techniques for Treatment of Metastatic Disease of the Spine. *Semin Spine Surg* 1990;2:21.

36. Levine AM, Boriani S. Benign Tumors of the Cervical Spine, 3rd ed. The Cervical Spine Research Society Editorial Committee. Philadelphia: Lippincott-Raven, 1998:621.

* 37. Levine AM, Boriani S, Donati D, Campanacci M. Benign Tumors of the Cervical Spine. *Spine* 1992;17:S399.

+ 38. Leys D, Lesion F, Viaud C, et al. Decreased Morbidity from Acute Bacterial Spinal Epidural Abscesses Using Computed Tomography and Nonsurgical Treatment in Selected Patients. *Ann Neurol* 1985;17:350.

* 39. Manasse AM, Van Gilder JC. Transoral-transpharyngeal Approach to the Anterior Craniocervical Junction. *J Neurosurg* 1988;69:895.

* 40. Mankin HJ, Mankin CJ, Simon MA. The Hazards of the Biopsy, Revisited. *J Bone Joint Surg [Am]* 1996;78:656.

41. Martin RJ, Yuan HA. Neurosurgical Care of Spinal Epidural, Subdural, and Intramedullary Abscesses and Arachnoiditis. *Orthop Clin North Am* 1996;27:125.

* 42. McAfee PC, Bohlman HH, Ducker T, Eismont FJ. Failure of Stabilization of the Spine with Methacrylate. A Retrospective Analysis of Twenty-four Cases. *J Bone Joint Surg [Am]* 1986;68:1145.

* 43. McAfee PC, Bohlman HH, Riley LH, et al. The Anterior Retropharyngeal Approach to the Upper Part of the Cervical Spine. *J Bone Joint Surg [Am]* 1987;69:1371.

+ 44. McGuire RA, Eismont FJ. The Fate of Autogenous Bone Graft in Surgically Treated Pyogenic Vetebral Osteomyelitis. *J Spinal Disord* 1994;7:206.

+ 45. Messer HD, Litvinoff J. Pyogenic Cervical Osteomyelitis. Chondro-osteomyelitis of the Cervical Spine Frequently Associated with Parenteral Drug Use. *Arch Neurol* 1976;33:571.

+ 46. Modic MT, Feiglin DH, Piraino DW. Vertebral Osteomyelitis: Assessment Using MR. *Radiology* 1985;157:157.

! 47. Norris S, Ehrlich MG, McKusick K. Early Diagnosis of Disk-space Infection with 67Ga in an Experimental Model. *Clin Orthop* 1979;144:293.

+ 48. Ono K, Yonenobu K, Ebara S, et al. Prosthetic Replacement Surgery for Cervical Spine Metastasis. *Spine* 1988;13:817.

49. Phillips E, Levine AM. Metastatic Lesions of the Upper Cervical Spine. *Spine* 1989;14:1071.

50. Pollack MR, Seiman LP. Aneurysmal Bone Cyst in the Pediatric Spine. *Orthop Grand Rounds* 1986;3:2.

+ 51. Post MJD, Quencer RM, Montalvo BM, et al. Spinal Infection: Evaluation with MR Imaging and Intraoperative US. *Radiology* 1988;169:765.

* 52. Rao S, Badani K. Cervical Metastases. *J Bone Joint Surg* 1994;53A:5511.

53. Rao S, Davis RF. *Cervical Spine Metastases*, 3rd ed. The Cervical Spine Research Society Editorial Committee. Philadelphia: Lippincott-Raven, 1998:603.

54. Redekop GJ, Del Maestro RF. Diagnosis and Management of Spinal Epidural Abscess. *Can J Neurol Sci* 1992;19:180.

+ 55. Redfern RM, Miles J, Banks AJ, et al. Stabilization of the Infected Spine. *J Neurol Neurosurg Psychiatry* 1988;51:803.

+ 56. Rigamonti D, Liem L, Wolf AL, et al. Epidural Abscess in the Cervical Spine. *Mt Sinai J Med* 1994;61:357.

\# 57. Rothman-Simeone XX. Infections, 4th ed. In: Herkowitz et al. *The Spine*. Philadelphia: W. B. Saunders Co., 1999: 1224. Infections chapter 1207-1258. Tumors p1171-1206.

+ 58. Sapico FL, Montgomerie JZ. Pyogenic Vertebral Osteomyelitis: Report of Nine Cases and Review of the Literature. *Rev Infect Dis* 1979;1:754.

+ 59. Sapico FL, Montgomerie JZ. Vertebral Osteomyelitis in Intravenous Drug Abusers: Report of Three Cases and Review of the Literature. *Rev Infect Dis* 1980;2:196.

+ 60. Seifert V, van Krieken FM, Bao SD, et al. Microsurgery of the Cervical Spine in Elderly Patients. Part 2: Surgery of Malignant Tumorous Disease. *Acta Neurochir (Wien)* 1994;131:241.

\# 61. Stone JL, Cybulski GR, Rodriguez J, et al. Anterior Cervical Debridement and Strut-grafting for Osteomyelitis of the Cervical Spine. *J Neurosurg* 1989;70:879.

+ 62. Sundaresan N, Shah J, Feghall J. The Trans-sternal Approach to the Upper Thoracic Vertebra. *Am J Surg* 1984; 198:473.

+ 63. Whalen JL, Brown ML, McLeod R, Fitzgerald RH Jr. Limitations of Indium Leukocyte Imaging for Diagnosis of Spine Infections. *Spine* 1991;16:193.

* 64. Whitesides TE Jr, Kelly RP. Lateral Approach to the Upper Cervical Spine for Anterior Fusion. *South Med J* 1966;59:879.

+ 65. Zigler JE, Bohlman HH, Robinson RA, et al. Pyogenic Osteomyelitis of the Occiput, the Atlas, and the Axis: A Report of Five Cases. *J Bone Joint Surg [Am]* 1987;69: 1069.

CHAPTER 152
TUMORS OF THE SPINE

Robert F. McLain

Appropriate, timely surgical treatment can increase survival and improve the quality of life for many patients with spinal column tumors. The goals of treatment are pain relief, improved function, and the best possible chance of local control and cure of the disease. Aggressive surgical approaches, combined with improved adjuvant therapy, now offer good short-term and long-term outcomes for many lesions previously thought untreatable or unresectable.

DIAGNOSIS

INCIDENCE AND PRESENTATION

Spinal column tumors, malignant and benign, occur in all age groups and at all levels of the spine. Primary tumors can arise from any of the hard or soft tissues of the spinal column, or they can extend directly to the spinal column from contiguous paraspinal lesions. Metastatic tumors, which migrate from distant sites by either lymphatic or hematogenous routes, account for 97% of all spinal column tumors.

Spinal metastases are common among patients with adenocarcinoma. Between 50% and 70% of all patients with carcinoma develop skeletal metastases during the course of their disease, as do 85% of women with breast cancer (9,25,34). The spine is the most common site for these metastases. The most common metastatic lesions are adenocarcinomas from the following:

- Lung
- Breast
- Prostate
- Kidney
- Gastrointestinal tract
- Thyroid

Certain primary tumors, such as chordoma, osteoblastoma, and plasmacytoma, show a preference for the spinal column, but they represent a small proportion of all spinal lesions.

Because of the preponderance of metastatic disease, spinal lesions in all age groups are more likely to be malignant than benign. This is particularly true in adult pa-

R. F. McLain: Department of Orthopaedics, The Cleveland Clinic Foundation, Cleveland, Ohio, 44195.

tients, where an increasing incidence of metastatic disease, an increased risk of systemic diseases such as myeloma and lymphoma, and a greater likelihood of having a malignant primary tumor combine to present a particularly grim prognosis. Seventy percent of primary spine tumors in patients over 25 are malignant, compared with only 30% in patients under 21 years of age (73).

Both primary and metastatic malignancies tend to originate in the vertebral body, involving one or both pedicles. The vertebral body contains most of the bone, hematogenous marrow, and cartilage from which primary lesions arise, and the notochordal rests that give rise to chordoma. Most of the *hematogenous* marrow is also contained in the bodies. Finally, retrograde flow through the venous drainage of the spinal column (Batson's plexus) permits tumor cells from the abdominal cavity to seed the vertebral bodies directly (29). Lesions of the posterior elements are more commonly benign.

PRESENTING SYMPTOMS

Back pain is common and nonspecific, and it is ubiquitous in the age group most at risk for spinal tumors. Whereas idiopathic back pain is typically mechanical, activity related, and self-limiting, neoplastic pain is more often

- progressive and unrelenting,
- unrelated to activity and unresponsive to rest,
- well localized to the spinal segment involved,
- reproduced by palpation or percussion over the involved area,
- and more severe or disturbing at night.

Pain and neurologic dysfunction are the most common presenting symptoms and usually arise from one of the following causes:

- Pathologic fracture
- Expansion of the vertebral cortex and surrounding tissues by tumor
- Compression or invasion of nerve roots
- Segmental instability
- Spinal cord compression

Rapid progression of pain or neurologic symptoms occurs with more aggressive, malignant tumors, whereas symptoms that progress over years are typical of slow-growing and often benign processes. Spine tumor patients most often present with pain. Common presenting symptoms occur as follows:

- Eighty-five percent of spine tumor patients present with pain.
- Back pain is the only symptom in 30%.
- Leg pain is the only symptom in 10%.
- Twenty-eight percent present with a combination of pain and neurologic deficit.

- Forty-two percent of all patients have a neurologic deficit at presentation.
- Sixteen percent have a mass or deformity.
- Spinal tumor is an incidental finding in 2% of patients.

Although radicular symptoms may simulate herniated nucleus pulposis, symptoms from lumbar and sacral neoplasms do not respond to rest and recumbency, and they tend to progress relentlessly (62).

Spinal deformity is rarely associated with spinal neoplasia, except when vertebral collapse results in severe kyphosis. Osteoid osteoma and osteoblastoma may produce a scoliosis that is typically painful, with localized pain, muscle spasm, and limited motion. Deformities associated with tumors may come on suddenly and progress rapidly. Unless addressed early on, these curves will become structural and difficult to manage (35). If the primary lesion is addressed in a timely manner, the curve will often resolve with observation or bracing. However, if the deformity is allowed to persist, surgical correction may be necessary (50).

To make the diagnosis before neurologic symptoms arise, the physician must be alert to any patient with persistent, nonmechanical back pain, age- or activity-related risk factors, or, particularly, a previous history of malignancy (23). Although neurologic injury is rarely the first sign of a spinal neoplasm, it may be present in as many as half of patients by the time they seek medical attention, and they may be recognized in more than 70% by the time a diagnosis is made.

The basic workup of any spine tumor includes the following:

- Complete blood cell count (CBC), differential, sedimentation rate, urinalysis, electrolytes, calcium, and basic chemistry panel
- Serum and urine protein electrophoresis; if positive, bone survey and bone marrow aspirate
- Renal ultrasound or abdominal computed tomography (CT)
- Chest CT
- Bone scan
- Physical exam: breasts, prostate, rectal, stool guaiac, thyroid

EVALUATION

IMAGING

Plain Roentgenograms
Standard anteroposterior and lateral roentgenograms of the spine still represent the most practical first study for

patients with suspected spinal tumor. Good-quality stud-ies of the symptomatic spinal segment may be sufficient to define the characteristic changes of bone destruction and tumor expansion, and they may establish a specific diagnosis in some tumor types. Plain roentgenograms will demonstrate abnormalities in 80% to 90% of patients with a spinal neoplasm (73,74). Even when the precise tumor type cannot be identified, the benign or malignant nature of the lesion can often be implied from the pattern of bone destruction (Fig. 152.1*A,B*).

Nuclear Scans

Technetium bone scans screen for bony turnover that can detect the presence of tumors before they become apparent

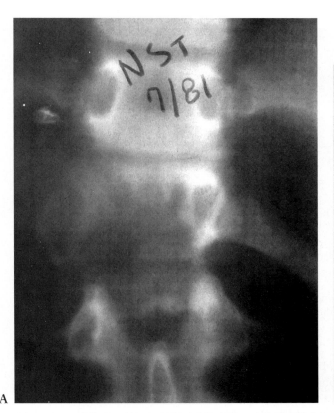

A

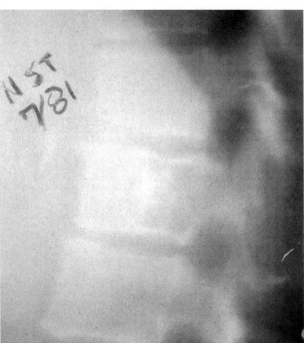

B

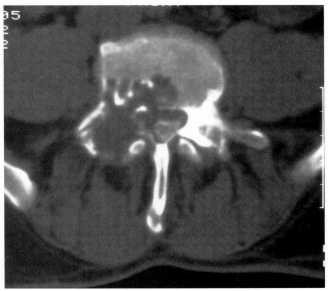

C

Figure 152.1. The 35-year-old patient in (**A**) and (**B**) has giant cell tumor of the T-12 vertebral body. AP (**A**) radiograph shows a classic "winking owl" sign, suggesting destruction of the left pedicle by tumor. The lateral view (**B**) shows a rarified vertebral body with a geographic pattern of bony replacement. In a patient with metastatic renal carcinoma, CT demonstrates bony destruc-tion and expansion of the anterior vertebral cortex (**C**). *(con-tinued)*

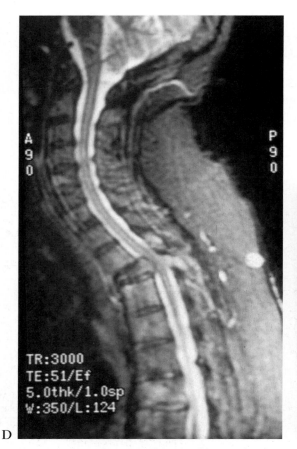

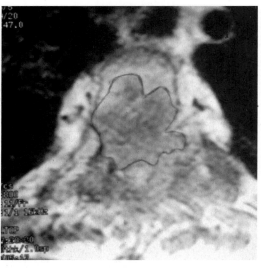

Figure 152.1. *(continued)* Sagittal (**D**) and transverse (**E**) MRIs showing vertebral destruction, collapse, and cord compression caused by a breast metastasis to the T-3 vertebral body.

on plain films. Because roentgenographic evidence of bony destruction is not apparent until after 30% to 50% of the trabecular bone has been demineralized or destroyed, bone scans are far more sensitive for picking up early involvement (17).

Computed Tomography

Computed tomography may provide diagnostic information on small tumor foci early in their development, before extensive bony destruction or intramedullary extension has occurred, and before cortical erosion has advanced to the point of impending fracture. CT is time consuming and not suitable for screening large segments of the spine. Once the suspected lesion is identified on plain films or bone scan, however, CT provides unsurpassed imaging of the bony architecture (Fig. 152.1C). It may also demonstrate characteristic features of soft-tissue calcification or trabecular remodeling, which may be pathognomonic for some types of tumors.

Magnetic Resonance Imaging

Magnetic resonance imaging (MRI) is noninvasive, safe, and readily available to most patients. It provides mul-

tiplanar images of large segments of the spine and surrounding tissues and can be used to screen for disseminated disease. MRI delineates soft-tissue extension from other processes, and newer techniques can accurately differentiate tumor from hematoma, edema, and inflammation (Fig. 152.1D,E). MRI directly images the spinal cord, cauda equina, and nerve roots without the aid of intrathecal contrast (24). It can reveal invasion of paravertebral structures better than either CT or myelography, and with gadolinium enhancement it can differentiate osteoporotic compression fractures from metastatic disease (13). Characteristics of tumors on MRI are (a) convex posterior cortex, (b) epidural mass, (c) low-intensity T1 signal, (d) high or inhomogenous T2 signal intensity, (e) high-intensity signal after gadolinium injection (13,69).

Myelography

Previously the gold standard for spinal imaging, this test has been largely replaced by MRI. When MRI cannot be done, myelography with postmyelogram CT may provide the same information.

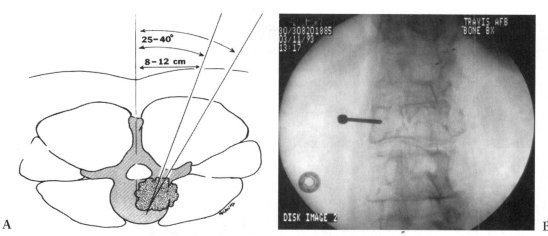

Figure 152.2.   **A:** Percutaneous needle biopsy of the thoracolumbar spine is performed through a posterior, percutaneous route. The needle is positioned 8–12 cm lateral of the midline at the level of the documented lesion. By advancing the needle at a 30° to 45° angle, under fluoroscopic control, the posterolateral aspect of the vertebral body is targeted. **B:** Alternatively, a small posterior exposure is made over the documented lesion, and a burr is used to take down the cortex overlying the pedicle. A Craig needle or a small curet is then passed down the pedicle to harvest bone and tumor from the vertebral body.

BIOPSY

There are three basic approaches to biopsy, each with advantages and disadvantages:

1. Percutaneous needle or trocar biopsy allows aspiration and removal of fine tissue fragments; the advantages are that needle biopsy is minimally invasive and uses local anesthetic. It is most suitable for lesions that are easily differentiated. Because samples are small, they are difficult to read, and they are frequently not diagnostic. When the differential diagnosis is limited to lesions that are easily distinguished histologically, needle biopsy is ideal (Fig. 152.2).

2. Open, incisional biopsy provides moderate-size specimens showing cellular architecture and marginal tissue. It provides diagnostic tissue and may be done just prior to formal excision when used with frozen section. Place the incision so it can be excised with the definitive procedure. Carry out the incisional biopsy as the last step in tumor staging, just before or at the time of definitive resection. The incision must be longitudinal, never transverse. Handle the tissues gently, and provide meticulous hemostasis to prevent tumor spread. Take a section of tissue large enough to allow histologic and ultrastructural analysis as well as immunologic staining from the margin of the lesion (central sections may be necrotic). Take the specimen with a sharp scalpel and be careful not to crush or distort the tissue during harvest. Avoid using electrocautery on the biopsy specimen itself.

3. Open, excisional biopsy includes removal of all tumor tissue at the time of biopsy. It provides complete treatment of local disease. Few tumors are suitable, however; the surgeon must already have a good idea of the diagnosis to plan appropriate excision.

HINTS AND TRICKS

Because of the possibility of catastrophic hemorrhage, renal cell metastases must be approached more cautiously than most other tumors, although metastatic thyroid, melanoma, and some breast lesions may also be highly vascular (67). An abdominal ultrasound or CT will reveal the primary renal lesion before the surgeon performs a biopsy that may lead to uncontrollable bleeding. Preoperative angiography will reveal the extensive neovasculature often associated with these tumors, allowing embolization of abnormal vessels and nonessential segmental arteries.

TUMOR TYPES

PRIMARY TUMORS

Primary tumors make up less than 3% of all spinal lesions. Survival rates are most directly, but not entirely, related to tumor type; some low-grade lesions may permit a long survival despite their malignant nature, whereas some histologically benign lesions may prove lethal because of their location in the spine.

BENIGN PRIMARY TUMORS

Osteochondroma

Vertebral involvement occurs in approximately 7% of osteochondromas, but symptomatic lesions are rare. Eighty percent of symptomatic osteochondromas occur in the cervicothoracic spine, above T-6 (41). MRI demonstrates the radiolucent cartilage cap, which usually causes spinal cord compression. Excision of the tumor, *en bloc* or piecemeal, provides reliable neurologic recovery with little risk of recurrence. Enchondromas rarely produce any symptoms but may prove a diagnostic dilemma when encountered incidentally. Enchondromas develop a well-defined, benign-appearing cortical margin, but calcific stippling of the lesion may suggest chondrosarcoma, prompting an excisional biopsy (46).

Osteoid Osteoma and Osteoblastoma

Osteoid osteoma and osteoblastoma are benign neoplastic lesions frequently found in the spine, originating in or from the posterior vertebral elements (35,43). Symptoms in the spine are similar to extremity lesions (see Chapter 127), except for the occasional development of a painful scoliosis.

Because osteoid osteoma is often obscured by the overlying shadows of the vertebral body, it is most readily localized by bone scan. Excision of the lesion reliably and immediately relieves the patient's pain. The key to successful treatment is accurate localization of the tumor nidus, confirmed by directed CT of the area. Osteoblastoma is considerably larger than the 2 cm osteoid osteoma; it is characterized by the expansion of the overlying cortical bone and a thin rim of reactive bone among the trabeculae. When complete excision of the osteoblastoma is not feasible, curettage and bone grafting may provide an acceptable long-term result (27,43). Scoliosis related to these lesions is often flexible and will usually improve or resolve after the lesion is removed. Instrumentation and fusion of the curve may be required if the scoliosis has been present for a long period and has become structural. Corrective surgery may be planned after the patient has recovered from the tumor surgery and has had a chance to improve spontaneously.

Hemangiomas

Magnetic resonance imaging shows that vertebral hemangiomas are common, occurring in approximately 10% of all adults. Fortunately, only a small proportion are ever symptomatic. Reports of deformity or pain associated with hemangioma are rare, and surgeons should hesitate before attributing mechanical or chronic pain symptoms to these lesions. Asymptomatic hemangiomas rarely develop into symptomatic ones, and follow-up is unnecessary (19). Plain radiographs typically show vertical striations indicative of thickened trabeculae within the involved vertebral body, and CT usually demonstrates these same trabeculae dotting the region of the lesion. These lesions often respond to radiotherapy or vascular embolization alone. If vertebral collapse or neural compression occurs, surgical decompression and reconstruction through an anterior approach are indicated.

Giant Cell Tumor

Because of the tendency of giant cell tumors to recur, these histologically benign lesions may behave in a far more malignant fashion in the spinal column, resulting in significant mortality as well as morbidity (45,70). Usually seen in the third or fourth decade of life, the tumors appear lucent on plain radiographs, with marginal sclerosis and a geographic pattern of bone destruction. These slow-growing tumors are usually anterior and may expand the surrounding cortical bone as they grow. Some authors have suggested that spinal tumors are less aggressive than extremity lesions (15,56), whereas others have acknowledged the aggressive nature of the tumor in this vulnerable region and have recommended adjuvant irradiation (55) or cryotherapy (42) for local control.

Because of the tendency of giant cell tumors to recur locally, CT and MR imaging are particularly important in planning an operation that will provide as wide a margin as possible. Complete excision is the key to eradicating these tumors (Fig. 152.3). Anterior/posterior vertebrectomy with an *en bloc* excision, followed by a combined reconstruction, limits the likelihood of recurrence and allows the most rapid return to function.

Eosinophilic Granuloma

Eosinophilic granuloma is a benign, self-limiting lesion commonly seen in children under the age of 10 years. Vertebral involvement occurs in approximately 15% of all cases and can be associated with any of three syndromes: isolated eosinophilic granuloma, Hand-Schüller-Christian disease, and Letterer-Siwe disease. The classic radiographic presentation is caused by near-complete collapse of the vertebral body, resulting in a vertebra plana, or "coin" lesion (57). Although classic, this appearance is not pathognomonic, and a similar picture can result from either infection or Ewing's sarcoma (51). Once a definitive diagnosis is established, usually by trocar biopsy, the patient may be effectively treated by bracing and observation. Although radiotherapy has been advocated in the past, it can be avoided in most patients.

When neurologic symptoms of eosinophilic granuloma are present, either with or without vertebral collapse, the established course of biopsy followed by irradiation and immobilization remains the most widely accepted (26).

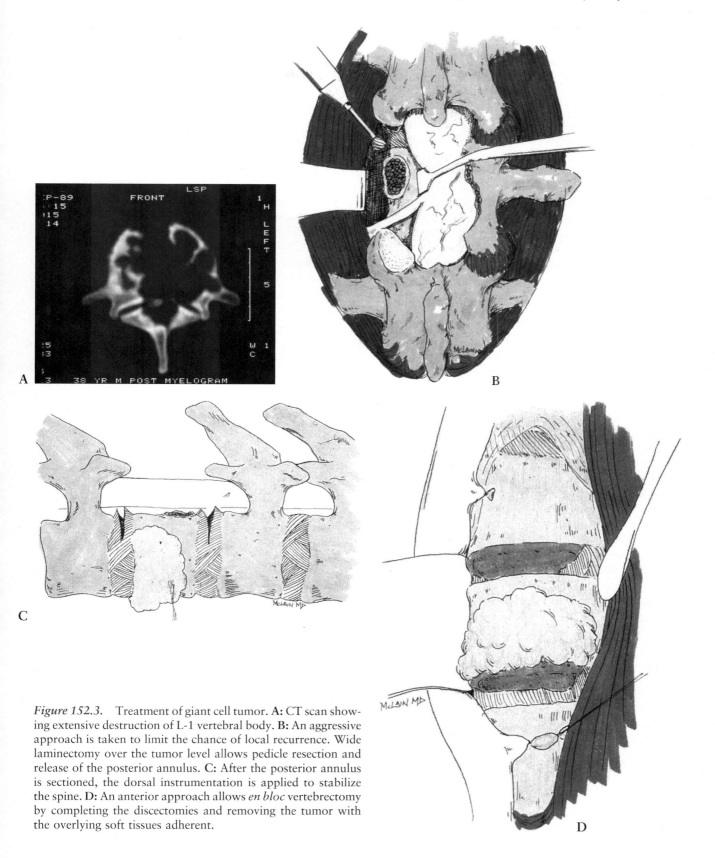

Figure 152.3. Treatment of giant cell tumor. **A:** CT scan showing extensive destruction of L-1 vertebral body. **B:** An aggressive approach is taken to limit the chance of local recurrence. Wide laminectomy over the tumor level allows pedicle resection and release of the posterior annulus. **C:** After the posterior annulus is sectioned, the dorsal instrumentation is applied to stabilize the spine. **D:** An anterior approach allows *en bloc* vertebrectomy by completing the discectomies and removing the tumor with the overlying soft tissues adherent.

Recovery of neurologic function is usually excellent, and some reconstitution of vertebral height is seen in most young patients.

Aneurysmal Bone Cyst

Aneurysmal bone cysts (ABCs) rarely involve the spinal column. When they do, they usually involve the posterior elements and are most commonly seen in the lumbar spine. Radiographs demonstrate an expansile lesion with an osteolytic cavity that may extend across segmental levels to involve two or even three adjacent vertebrae. The cortex is often eggshell thin and blown out, and the cyst contains numerous strands of bone which give the "bubbly" appearance typical of ABCs. Curettage usually eradicates the lesion, and recurrences, which do not tend to invade vital structures, may be successfully treated by repeated curettage or excision (32).

MALIGNANT PRIMARY TUMORS

Chordoma

Chordoma is a relatively rare lesion arising exclusively in the axial skeleton, most often in the spine and sacrum. The tumor is derived from rests of notochordal tissue residing in the skull base, sacrococcygeal region, and the vertebral segments in between (49). The tumor is characterized by slow but relentless local progression. It metastasizes late, but it has an aggressive tendency to recur at the surgical site, which makes it highly lethal. Although uncommon in children, chordomas are more histologically variable and more clinically aggressive in this age group than in adults (11). Because of their insidious development, chordomas can reach remarkable size before they are recognized. Patients may present after months or even years of progressive pain, sitting intolerance, urinary obstruction, and constipation. Sacrococcygeal tumors are easily detected on rectal examination as firm, fixed lesions displacing the posterior rectal wall.

Surgical resection is the only curative procedure for chordomas. A wide margin is crucial to local control because these lesions are generally unresponsive to radiotherapy and chemotherapy. Whereas only 5% of patients with spinal chordoma develop metastases, nearly 70% will die of their disease, reflecting the seriousness of local tumor extension (3). Intralesional resection is associated with a high rate of local recurrence (82%) and a high mortality (71%) (7). Carry out biopsy of a suspected chordoma through a posterior approach, after all other staging studies are done. Never biopsy a sacral lesion through the rectal vault; violation of the rectal wall necessitates colectomy.

Osteosarcoma

Osteosarcoma of the spine remains an ominous disease—the median survival following diagnosis has ranged from 6 to 18 months, irrespective of surgical approach (1,58,65). When effective local control can be obtained surgically, survival is comparable to that of extremity lesions; fewer than half of all spine patients achieve complete local excision, however (2).

Spinal osteosarcoma usually arises in the vertebral body. Radiographs reveal cortical destruction, soft-tissue calcification, and periosteal reaction. The paraspinal soft-tissue mass may be extensive and may encase or invest the great vessels or other contiguous structures. Intraspinal extension of the soft-tissue mass may result in either cord or cauda equina compression.

Even though cure of osteosarcoma remains elusive, more aggressive treatment protocols have improved overall survival. By combining current adjuvant therapy with extensive anterior/posterior resections, surgeons have provided patients with improved local control, neurologic function, and improved survivals (65,73).

Chondrosarcoma

Approximately 10% of chondrosarcomas arise in the spinal column or sacrum. Resistant to both radiotherapy and chemotherapy, these tumors are slow growing, locally invasive, and difficult to eradicate from the spinal column. Although survival may be prolonged in spite of residual disease, the final prognosis for patients with spinal chondrosarcoma is poor.

Radiographically, chondrosarcoma is characterized by a prominent soft-tissue mass stippled with flocculent calcifications (33). CT and MR imaging are crucial to determining soft-tissue extensions and the potential for surgical resection. Although long-term survivals are occasionally associated with intralesional resection, a wide margin is the most reliable means of local control and cure (59,63).

Ewing's Sarcoma

Ewing's sarcoma may arise in the spine as a primary or a metastatic lesion. Approximately 3.5% of Ewing's lesions are thought to arise in the spinal column primarily. These tumors produce a permeative destructive pattern that can be difficult to discern on plain radiographs, so that the first radiographic finding may be vertebral collapse and vertebra planum (51). Intraspinal extension may produce neurologic symptoms before bony involvement becomes apparent on plain radiographs. MRI will demonstrate the lesion and its extension, as well as showing occasional epidural metastasis that do not involve bone.

Effective therapy for Ewing's sarcoma revolves around a program of multiagent chemotherapy and high-dose radiotherapy. Surgical treatment is indicated to decompress neurologic structures and stabilize the spinal column. Thoracic and thoracolumbar laminectomies should be instrumented to prevent kyphosis (28). Although the prognosis is generally worse than for extremity lesions, encouraging disease-free survival rates have been obtained using current multimodality regimens (28,36).

Solitary Plasmacytoma

Solitary plasmacytoma and multiple myeloma represent two ends to the continuum of B-cell lymphoproliferative diseases. Multiple myeloma is rapidly progressive and highly lethal, requiring little more than supportive care for spinal involvement. Solitary plasmacytoma may remain localized for years before eventually disseminating. Prolonged survival is possible if local control can be obtained (44).

Solitary plasmacytomas make up only 3% of all plasma cell neoplasms. Whereas spinal involvement in multiple myeloma is associated with a poor 1-year survival rate, patients with solitary plasmacytoma of the spine have a 60% 5-year survival rate (44,71). Although most, if not all, of these lesions will eventually degenerate into disseminated multiple myeloma with a rapidly lethal course, survivals of 20 years or more have been reported.

Plasmacytoma and myeloma are radiosensitive tumors. Surgical treatment is indicated to stabilize the spine and reduce mechanical pain and to decompress neurologic elements in patients with rapidly progressive symptoms. Surgery is also warranted for those patients with recurrent disease or tumors that have not responded to radiotherapy (Fig. 152.4). Follow-up with MRI and serum protein electrophoresis provides the earliest indication of recurrence or dissemination.

Lymphoma

Lymphoma may occur as an isolated lesion or as a focal manifestation of a disseminated disease. As with plasmacytoma, surgical treatment is an adjuvant to systemic therapy and radiotherapy. Surgical decompression is indicated to decompress cord, cauda equina, or nerve root injured by tumor extension or pathologic fracture, and to stabilize damaged spinal segments.

METASTATIC DISEASE

The vertebral column is predisposed to metastatic disease by its vascular anatomy, its architecture, and its proximity to common sources of disease. The venous drainage of the spine is contiguous with that of the thoracic and abdominal viscera. Retrograde venous flow provides a variety of tumors access to the vertebral body. There, metastatic emboli settle and implant in the capillary end-loops adjacent to the vertebral endplates. The red marrow of the vertebral body provides a physiologically favorable environment for tumor cell proliferation. The vertebral trabecular bone has a rich blood supply, with few barriers to tumor extension; once established, the tumor can grow for some time before it becomes clinically apparent.

Almost any neoplastic process can establish skeletal metastases; however, certain tumors are particularly adept at reaching and surviving in the trabecular environment (Table 152.1). Breast, lung, prostate, and lymphoreticular disease account for approximately 60% of all spinal column metastases requiring treatment. Whether a tumor requires surgical treatment is determined by the behavior of the primary lesion and the metastasis. Patients with breast, prostate, renal, thyroid, or gastrointestinal carcinoma may experience extended survivals with current adjuvant protocols, despite established metastases. Patients with multiple myeloma or pulmonary carcinoma typically deteriorate and die soon after metastasis. Breast, prostate, and renal carcinomas tend to establish spinal metastases early in the disease process, whereas gastrointestinal carcinomas typically seed the liver and lungs first. Hence, patients with breast, prostate, and renal carcinoma tend to live long enough for their spinal metastases to become a specific threat to function and quality of life, while patients with lung carcinoma and myeloma will often die before the spinal metastasis needs more than palliation, and patients with gastrointestinal carcinoma are often more directly affected by their visceral metastases than their skeletal disease.

PEDIATRIC TUMORS

Metastatic disease is the most common malignancy of the spine in children; neuroblastoma accounts for nearly one third of all pediatric spinal tumors (20,39). Ewing's sarcoma is the most common primary malignancy, but it is still more often a metastasis than a primary lesion (73). However, 70% of primary pediatric tumors are benign.

Neuroblastoma

Neuroblastoma is an aggressive malignancy that may spread to the spine either by vascular dissemination or by contiguous spread from the primary lesion. Treated with a combination of chemotherapy, radiotherapy, and surgical excision, patients with these tumors have a poor prognosis overall. Those patients that do survive are at high risk of developing a progressive spinal deformity as a result of either rib resection or hemibody irradiation (21,52).

Leukemia

Leukemic infiltrates may occasionally present as the initial finding in a patient with systemic disease. Most of these patients will have back pain, and some may have vertebral collapse at the time of presentation (53). Nonspecific complaints of muscular aches and pains, lethargy, fatigue, and fever, as well as findings of anemia, should prompt a search for the underlying disease. Radiographs are not characteristic: They may show vertebral collapse, focal lytic changes, or sclerotic, geographic lesions, or they may

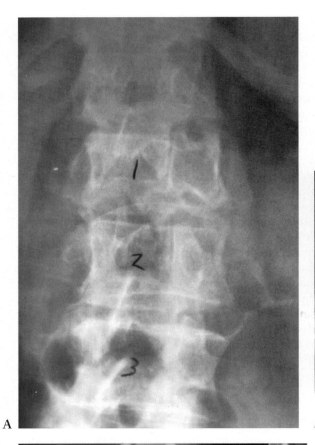

A

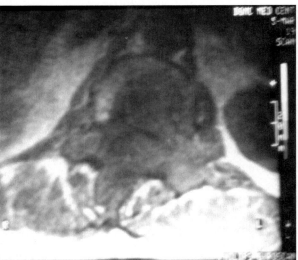

B

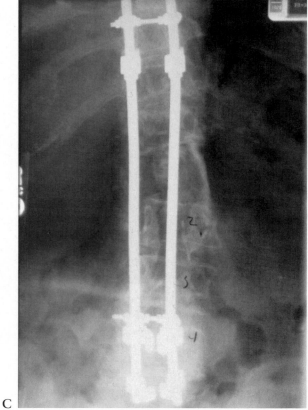

C

Figure 152.4. **A:** AP radiograph of a 68-year-old woman with solitary plasmacytoma of the T-12 vertebra, refractory to radiotherapy. **B:** MRI shows the extent of the tumor. **C:** Complete anterior/posterior excision was followed by anterior tricortical graft and long segmental instrumentation posteriorly. She was disease free for 5 years before recurrence and dissemination occurred.

Table 152.1. *Trabecular Carcinomas*

Carcinoma	Percent (%) of All Spinal Metastases
Breast	21
Pulmonary	14
Prostate	7.5
Renal	5.5
Gastrointestinal	5.0
Thyroid	2.5

be entirely normal. Bone scan may also be equivocal, but MRI will reliably demonstrate the infiltrate (10).

TREATMENT

The correct treatment of any tumor depends on a number of factors unique to the individual patient:

- Is the tumor benign or malignant? Primary or metastatic?
- Is the patient systemically ill, or fit?
- Is the tumor slow growing, locally aggressive, or widely disseminated?

- Is there any neurologic compromise?
- Is there a fracture or instability?

The surgeon cannot reliably offer the patient the best treatment until these questions have been answered. See the algorithms for diagnostic workup (Fig. 152.5) and treatment and reconstruction (Fig. 152.6).

There is a broad spectrum of medical therapies available to treat spinal tumors, ranging from observation to total spondylectomy (Table 152.2). Both undertreatment and overtreatment can lead to trouble.

A radical margin cannot be achieved in the spinal column because any break in the vertebral ring violates the osseous "compartment." The necessary cuts through the bony ring could expose normal tissues to contamination even in well-circumscribed tumors. Hemorrhage from the cut bone can carry tumor cells throughout the field, reducing the chance for local control. Once the tumor has extended beyond the vertebral cortex, even a marginal excision may be difficult to obtain. A tumor that adheres to or invades the dura or aorta may prove difficult or impossible to resect, and a tumor that involves the vena cava is usually unresectable. In these cases, the risks of attempting a wide resection with vascular or dural grafting must be weighed against those of following up a marginal excision with adjuvant radiation.

INDICATIONS FOR SURGERY

Patients with extensive metastases from a previously documented primary, or with peripheral metastases that can

Table 152.2. *Medical Therapies to Treat Spinal Tumors*

Therapy	Indication
Observation	Indolent and clearly *benign tumors*—hemangioma, osteochondroma, bone island, or infarct
Radiotherapy	*Metastatic lesions* from a known radiosensitive primary; disseminated myeloma, breast carcinoma
Chemotherapy	*Metastatic lesions* from a known chemosensitive primary tumor—thyroid; usually with radiotherapy
Intralesional excision, curettage	*Benign tumors* with limited potential for local recurrence—aneurysmal bone cyst, osteoblastoma; and *metastatic lesions* where local control will be obtained through radiotherapy
Marginal excision (with or without adjuvant cryotherapy or radiotherapy)	*Locally aggressive benign lesions*—giant cell tumor; *primary and metastatic lesions* sensitive to radiotherapy—solitary plasmacytoma, breast and prostate metastases; and low-grade malignancies—soft-tissue chondrosarcoma
Wide excision (modified)	All *primary malignancies* without known metastases—osteosarcoma, chondrosarcoma, chordoma; *solitary metastases* with likelihood of prolonged survival—breast, prostate, renal carcinoma; locally aggressive benign tumors—giant cell tumor

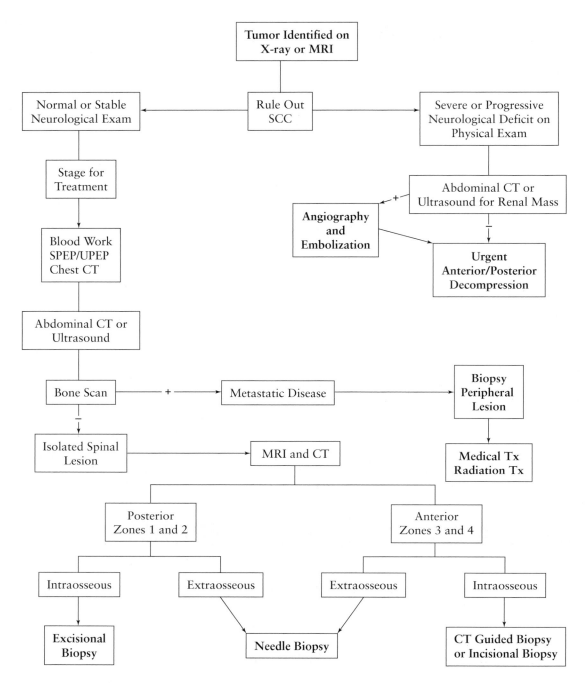

Figure 152.5.   Diagnostic workup algorithm for spinal tumor. *SCC*, spinal cord compression;
SPEP, serum protein electrophoresis; *UPEP*, urine protein electrophoresis; *TX*, treatment;
Zones, see Figure 152.7.

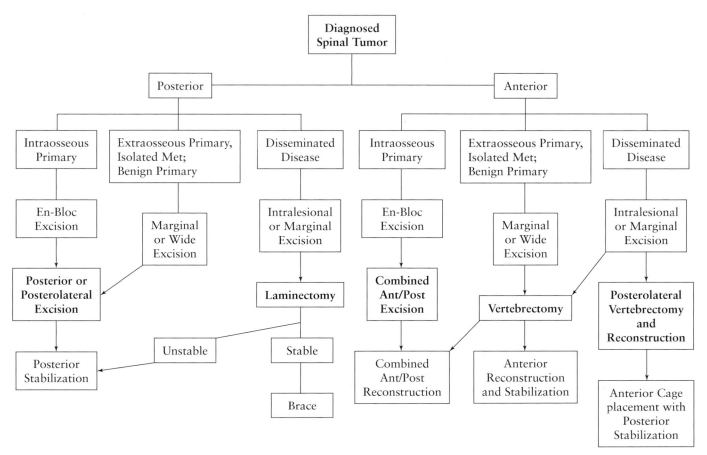

Figure 152.6. Treatment and reconstruction algorithm for spinal tumor. *Met,* metastasis.

be easily biopsied, may not require any spinal surgery. Unless there is neurologic impingement or mechanical instability, radiation or chemotherapy can retard tumor progression and control the spinal lesion.

Principal indications for surgical treatment include the following:

- Inability to obtain a tissue diagnosis by other methods
- Neurologic compression due to pathologic fracture or bony impingement
- Mechanical instability, with severe pain or impending neurologic injury
- Tumor progression despite, or following, radiotherapy
- Known radioresistant tumor
- Primary malignant tumor
- Resectable solitary metastasis in patient with potential long-term survival

If the tumor is resistant to radiation therapy, or if the patient suffers from neurologic compromise, spinal instability, or collapse, surgical treatment will be needed following biopsy. Three issues must be considered in de-

veloping a surgical plan—first, the proper margin of resection (of primary concern in locally aggressive and malignant primary tumors); second, the need for neurologic decompression; and third, the means of reconstruction.

Resection

Numerous studies show that the ability to completely resect the primary lesion significantly improves patient survival (4,58,63,73). Even in metastatic lesions, a complete resection can confer improved survival and quality of life (66). In locally aggressive tumors, resect the anterior and posterior longitudinal ligaments, vertebral body, adjacent discs, and the overlying dura, if necessary, to avoid leaving residual tumor behind. It is sometimes necessary to sacrifice one or more nerve roots to provide a suitable margin of excision.

Plan the surgical approach and resection margins using Weinstein's staging system (72), which divides the vertebral body into four zones and three grades of tumor extension (Fig. 152.7):

- Tumors in zones 1, 2, and 3 involve the posterior ele-

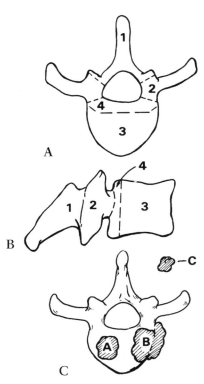

Figure 152.7. Tumor staging. Axial (**A**) and lateral (**B**) views of vertebral body showing four zones of tumor involvement. **C**: Grade A represents intraosseous spread; grade B, extraosseous extension; and grade C, distant metastasis.

ments, pedicle and transverse process, and anterior vertebral body, respectively.

- Zone 4 lesions involve the posterior portion of the vertebral body and that portion of the cortex just anterior to the spinal cord or neural elements.
- To address any lesion involving zone 4, the surgeon must cross zone 3 and must release the vertebra from the pedicles, resecting zones 1 and 2 as well.
- Zone 4 lesions frequently require a subtotal or total vertebrectomy to obtain a clean margin. This assumes that the tumor is still intraosseous (grade A), without extraosseous spread (grade B), or distant metastases (grade C).

Computed tomography and MRI provide most of the information needed for staging, with bone scan and serologies added to determine metastatic status. Pay particular attention to the possibility of extraosseous extension—Grade B lesions may prove unresectable if vital structures are directly invested by tumor. The decision to attempt a wide resection in these lesions must be weighed against the risks of vascular or neurologic injury. In some cases, the most prudent approach may be to accept a marginal or intralesional margin, supplementing local treatment with adjuvant radiotherapy or cryotherapy.

Choose the proper surgical approach for the tumor type and location:

- Zone 1 lesions are best approached through a standard posterior incision, with the extent of the incision based on the extent of the soft-tissue mass, if any.
- Zone 2 lesions require a posterolateral approach (Fig. 152.8). The laminectomy and bone resection necessary for tumor excision generally results in some degree of segmental instability, and posterior instrumentation and fusion is usually necessary.
- Zone 3 lesions can often be addressed through an anterior approach alone.
- 3A lesions can be adequately resected at any level of the spine, but 3B lesions may present different challenges at different levels. Depending on the extent of resection, a formal reconstruction may or may not be necessary.
- Zone 4 lesions require a combined surgical approach if a marginal or wide margin is to be obtained. Zones 1, 2, and/or 3 must be crossed to gain access to the zone 4 lesion, and more than one zone is usually involved with the tumor.
- Complete resection of the vertebral body requires separating the posterior structures (zones 1 and 2) from the anterior structures (zones 3 and 4), at the junction between the pedicles and the vertebral body (Fig. 152.9).

The standard approach to vertebrectomy combines a midline posterior incision with either a retroperitoneal, a thoracoabdominal, or a transthoracic approach to the anterior vertebral body. An alternative approach is to extend the posterior dissection around the side of the vertebral body, completing the vertebrectomy through a pos-

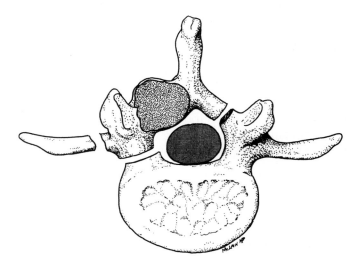

Figure 152.8. Resection of zone 2 lesion. Posterolateral approach allows access to uninvolved lamina on contralateral side along with uninvolved ipsilateral pedicle. A marginal margin is obtainable if the pedicle is free of tumor.

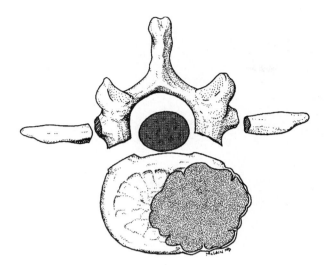

Figure 152.9. A zone 4 lesion *en bloc* excision of the involved thoracolumbar vertebra.

terolateral resection (18). If at least one pedicle is uninvolved, a wide margin is possible (6). Complete vertebrectomy requires both anterior and posterior stabilization, but experience has shown that this aggressive surgical approach does improve patient survival and neurologic function even when cure cannot be obtained (66).

For sacral lesions, a high sacral amputation is the procedure of choice (64). This combined anterior/posterior sacral approach provides improved outcome with surprisingly little long-term morbidity; as long as the S-2 nerve roots are spared bilaterally, or S-2 and S-3 are retained unilaterally, bowel and bladder function are usually unharmed (22,54). In more proximal tumors, these roots must be sacrificed to obtain local control and a reasonable likelihood of survival.

Decompression

As many as 20% of all patients with disseminated carcinoma develop symptomatic spinal cord compression (12, 60). To prevent permanent neurologic injury, the surgeon must recognize and treat spinal cord compression early in its development. Compression may result when an enlarging soft-tissue mass encroaches on cord or nerve roots, or when a pathologic fracture results in retropulsion of bone fragments into the canal, vertebral collapse, or kyphosis. Soft-tissue metastasis to the meninges or epidural space may directly compress neural elements (5,30).

Patients often complain of persistent and progressive back pain, radicular symptoms or "girdle" pain, lower extremity weakness, sensory loss, and bowel or bladder dysfunction. Acute spinal cord compression typically results from rapid tumor growth or pathologic fracture caused by extensive bony destruction. Early treatment is crucial:

- Patients with rapidly progressive paralysis have a poor prognosis for recovery compared to those who develop symptoms over a prolonged period.
- In ambulatory patients, 60% to 95% will retain that function after treatment.
- Only 35% to 65% of paraparetic patients will walk independently after treatment.
- Less than 30% of paraplegic patients will regain ambulation after either surgical or medical treatment (31,38).

Radiotherapy remains the most appropriate treatment for most patients with spinal column metastases. Different tumor types exhibit different levels of radiosensitivity, however, and different clones of the same primary tumor may behave differently as well:

- Prostatic and lymphoreticular neoplasms are typically radiosensitive, and satisfactory local control can be gained through postoperative radiotherapy, even after an intralesional resection (68).
- Gastrointestinal and renal neoplasms, on the other hand, are often unresponsive to irradiation.
- A number of primary tumors (e.g., chondrosarcoma, chordoma) are not radiosensitive, and, consequently, neurologic compromise resulting from these lesions is best treated by operative methods.

The best results are obtained when the surgical approach is properly matched to the compressive lesion: anterior decompression for anterior tumors and posterior decompression for posterior lesions. Using the wrong approach (e.g., laminectomy for anterior compression) provides little benefit and increases complications. For example, laminectomy has shown no added benefit relative to radiation alone in treating anterior spinal lesions, and it can compound problems by introducing or increasing segmental instability in the compromised segment (23,30). Overall, decompressive laminectomy provides neurologic improvement in only 33% of cases, and an overall satisfactory outcome (maintenance of ambulation and sphincter control) in 37% (45). By comparison, anterior decompression results in 79% improvement and 80% satisfactory outcome in similar patients (Fig. 152.10).

Reconstruction

Spinal instrumentation and fusion are often needed after tumor resection to restore stability, prevent progressive deformity, and facilitate graft incorporation and fusion. The surgeon must choose an instrumentation construct that (a) can meet the mechanical demands it will face following tumor resection, (b) can compensate for loss of bony elements due to resection or laminectomy, and (c) will permit postoperative imaging with CT and MRI. Key principles to reconstruction are the following:

- Restore or augment the anterior weight-bearing column to prevent vertebral collapse and kyphosis.

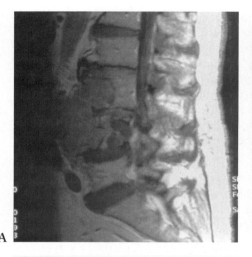

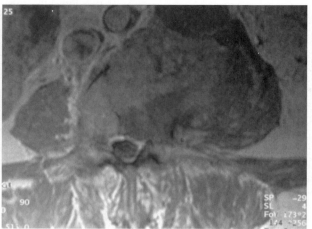

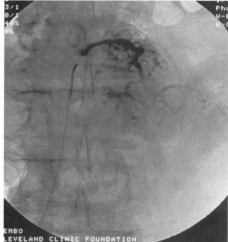

Figure 152.10. Anterior vertebrectomy for metastatic disease. Sagittal (**A**) and axial (**B**) MRIs demonstrating extent of an isolated renal cell metastasis involving both L-3 and L-4 vertebral bodies. The lesion probably seeded in one vertebral body, then spread contiguously to the adjacent level. **C:** Angiography prior to surgery shows blush of neovasculature in the tumor mass just prior to embolization. *(continued)*

- Use posterior instrumentation to provide a tension-band effect after laminectomy, to compensate for lost muscular attachments, and to prevent progressive kyphosis.
- Combine anterior and posterior constructs to restore axial, sagittal, and torsional stability after vertebrectomy.
- Anticipate disease progression—extend fixation over longer segments, maximize fixation points, and combine anterior and posterior constructs to ensure construct survival.
- Anticipate patient survival—strive for spinal fusion in patients likely to live more than 3 to 6 months.

Posterior Instrumentation

Distraction instrumentation (Harrington rods) can be combined with sublaminar or Drummond wires to provide segmental fixation in the thoracic spine, but they do not contour well to the lumbar spine and they tend to flatten the normal lumbar lordosis, resulting in a painful lumbar deformity. These systems are inexpensive and are adequate to stabilize thoracic compression fractures or laminectomies. They are not the best choice for cases with extensive bone destruction, however. Rod breakage and hook pullout are common, particularly when applied to patients with combined anterior and middle column insufficiency. These systems are vulnerable to fatigue failure, particularly in tumor patients where perioperative irradiation and systemic disease increase the risk of delayed union, and nonunion.

Luque rods, used in conjunction with sublaminar wires, provide better fixation than the Harrington system in soft bone (14,16). The Luque rods–sublaminar wire system has been used successfully in treating degenerative and neoplastic disease of the cervical, thoracic, and lumbar spine. The system has good stability in torsion and flexion but cannot resist pure axial loads—the sublaminar wires are free to slide down the rod, allowing the instrumented segment to collapse considerably along the axis of the rods.

Newer segmental instrumentation systems are versatile

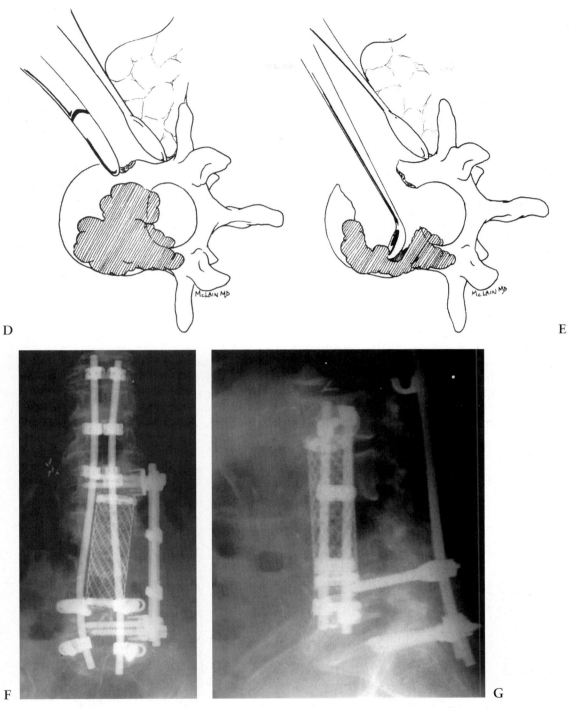

D

E

F

G

Figure 152.10. *(continued)* **D:** Anterior decompression of radiosensitive tumors begins by resecting the normal bone exposed during the anterior approach, then excising the tumor tissue in as few pieces as can be managed, moving quickly to limit blood loss. **E:** After removal of the bulk of involved vertebra, meticulous dissection is carried out to remove retropulsed fragments and extruded tumor from in front of the thecal sac, and to curet away all gross tumor from the resection margins. AP (**F**) and lateral (**G**) radiographic views, 2 years postoperative. After resection, the anterior column is reconstructed with a strut or cage. The titanium cage selected here is packed with autograft bone because successful treatment may provide this patient with several years of life. An anterior construct stabilizes the spine until the posterior reconstruction, using segmental instrumentation, can be performed.

and resilient. They allow the surgeon to neutralize the overall length of the spine while either compressing or distracting the intercalary segments involved in the reconstruction. Hook and screw fixation at multiple levels improves fixation strength, and pedicle screws allow fixation to levels where posterior elements have been removed. These systems have superior torsional and sagittal strength and are widely available in titanium, improving postoperative imaging capabilities. These versatile systems also allow the surgeon to address multiple levels of vertebral involvement, restoring normal thoracic kyphosis and lumbar lordosis in the same construct.

Pedicle screw fixation is particularly helpful in patients who have undergone previous laminectomy. They allow the surgeon to minimize the number of segments instrumented, limiting the need to extend fusions to additional levels for support. Combined with an anterior strut, screw-and-rod and screw-and-plate constructs provide sufficient axial, torsional, and sagittal rigidity to allow the surgeon to instrument only two motion segments when treating primary and metastatic lesions of the thoracolumbar spine (47). Screw failure can be expected, however, if the anterior weight-bearing column is incompetent and is not reconstructed (48).

Pedicle screws are most useful in the thoracolumbar and lumbar regions, where pedicles are relatively large and the spinal cord is not at risk. They may prove useful for lower thoracic lesions, as well, by securely anchoring the caudal end of a longer thoracolumbar construct. Use in the thoracic spine is more limited, although some authors have found that screw fixation is an important alternative in patients with extensive laminectomies. Screw-and-plate constructs can be used in the upper thoracic spine to stabilize the cervicothoracic junction, to treat laminectomized segments, and to limit the bulk of instrumentation placed under thin, irradiated soft tissues (Fig. 152.11).

Anterior column reconstruction may be necessary in addition to posterior procedures, or as the primary treatment in some patients. Posterior instrumentation alone cannot provide adequate stability in all cases. When posterior decompression is superimposed on anterior and middle column vertebral collapse, the resulting instability can be severe (16), and untreated anterior column deficiency leads to pedicle screw fatigue and breakage (47,48). Moreover, there is a significant incidence of wound complications associated with posterior surgery. These patients are often systemically ill. Many have undergone regional radiation therapy, have lost muscle mass and subcutaneous fat, and have impaired healing potential. Wound dehiscence, infection, and skin problems are common enough to prompt many surgeons to consider anterior reconstruction as their primary avenue of treatment.

If vertebrectomy is performed, the axial weight-bearing column must be reconstructed. Depending on the situation, the surgeon can chose from bone, methylmethacrylate, or a variety of prosthetic struts (Table 152.3).

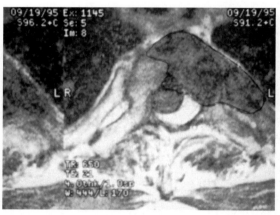
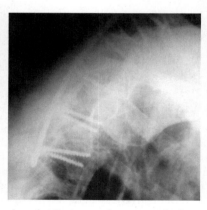
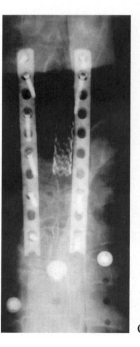

A,B   C

Figure 152.11.   **A:** MRI of T_2 metastasis. **B,C:** Lateral and AP views of screw and plate construct for upper thoracic spine. An alternative to rod-and-hook constructs, low-profile plates may be useful in patients with absent or incompetent posterior elements, or those with tenuous skin following irradiation.

Table 152.3. *Choice of Struts or Spacers for Reconstruction of Anterior Spinal Tumors*

Expected survival	Strut or spacer	Considerations
<3 mo	Polymethylmethacrylate (PMMA)	Only for patients with very limited life expectancy is PMMA without bone graft indicated. Functions well as spacer but has no biological fixation
3–6 mo	Prosthetic cage, with PMMA, *or*	Provides immediate axial stability with no risk of late collapse; subsidence can occur; can be contoured to fit any defect; no graft site morbidity
3–6 mo	Allograft fibula or tricortical graft	Some potential for incorporation but typically slow in irradiated tissue; may collapse late in course due to remodeling
>6 mo	Prosthetic cage, with autograft, *or*	Provides immediate axial stability without risk of late collapse; subsidence can occur; can be contoured to fit any defect; reduced graft site morbidity
>6 mo	Autograft fibula or tricortical graft, *or*	Maximum potential for incorporation; at risk for collapse during remodeling; graft site morbidity is considerable; may contain micrometastatic disease
>12 mo	Strut graft or cage with anterior spinal instrumentation	Anterior instrumentation markedly increases torsional and sagittal stiffness of construct. May eliminate need for posterior procedure; technically demanding

Polymethylmethacrylate (PMMA) is frequently used to reconstruct the vertebral column in metastatic disease. It is resilient in compression, but because it has no potential for biological incorporation it has a tendency to loosen and extrude over time.

- Incorporate longitudinal Steinmann pins into the PMMA mass and drive them proximally and distally into the adjacent vertebrae to anchor the spacer and improve its bending resistance (Fig. 152.12). Alternatively, insert Harrington distraction rods or Knodt rods into the vertebrectomy site to distract the defect and anchor the PMMA mass (61).
- Countersink the rod ends into the opposing endplates and distract to restore alignment.
- Apply PMMA in its dough phase to fill the defect.
- Place a Silastic or Gelfoam dam in front of the dura to protect the spinal cord from compression or thermal injury, and wash the PMMA mass constantly with cool saline during polymerization.

A tricortical strut graft or titanium cage with morcelized autograft is favored in the treatment of benign or slow-growing tumors in patients whose survival is likely to be measured in years, and similarly in malignant primaries, where successful treatment will result in prolonged survival.

- Cut tricortical struts from the anterior superior iliac crest, measuring 5–10 mm longer than the defect to be filled. Cut graft with a saw, not an osteotome.

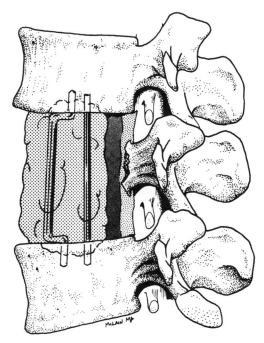

Figure 152.12. Reconstruction of the anterior column with polymethylmethacrylate.

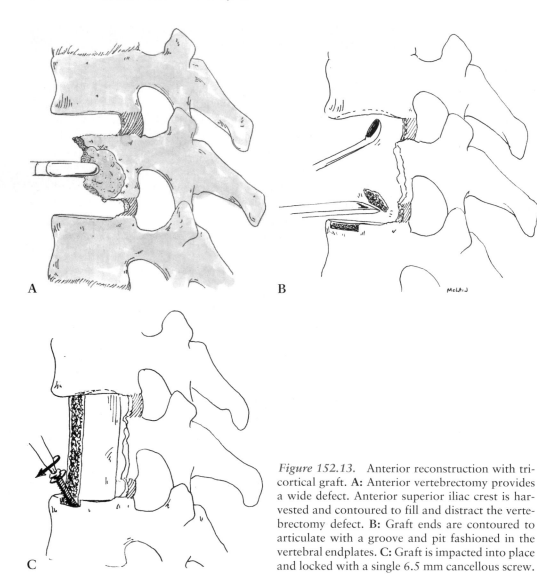

Figure 152.13. Anterior reconstruction with tri-cortical graft. **A:** Anterior vertebrectomy provides a wide defect. Anterior superior iliac crest is harvested and contoured to fill and distract the vertebrectomy defect. **B:** Graft ends are contoured to articulate with a groove and pit fashioned in the vertebral endplates. **C:** Graft is impacted into place and locked with a single 6.5 mm cancellous screw.

- Key the graft into the vertebral endplates to prevent displacement when the patient is mobilized (Fig. 152.13).
- To prevent displacement, drive a single 6.5 mm cancellous interference screw into the vertebral endplate just lateral to the graft. This will keep the graft from slipping back out through the keyhole defect.

Titanium cages can be used to supplement either methylmethacrylate or autograft reconstructions.

- Impact the cage into the vertebrectomy defect.
- Sagittal compressive forces will tend to hold the cage in place until anterior or posterior instrumentation can be added.
- Do not penetrate the endplates during cage placement. Do not "key" the cage into place.
- If fusion is intended, pack the cage full of morcelized

autograft bone before placing it into the defect. After inserting the cage, place more graft anteriorly to augment the fusion.
- Because the cage provides little torsional rigidity on its own, apply an anterior fixation system to stabilize the spinal construct.

TREATMENT OF METASTATIC SPINAL TUMORS

When conservative therapy fails to control metastatic disease, the physician must determine whether surgery is likely to improve the patient's function, quality of life, or longevity. In cases of severe pain, segmental instability, or neurologic compromise, operative intervention may be indicated.

Patients with an asymptomatic or minimally symptomatic spinal metastasis often do not require surgery. Patients who may require surgery include those with known radioresistant tumors, solitary metastasis with potential for wide resection, unknown tumor type despite systemic workup and needle biopsy, bony compression of neural elements, and mechanical instability and bone destruction.

Patients with mechanical instability and no neurologic deficit need treatment to restore stability and function.

- Treat patients with mechanical instability and neck or back pain with bracing and irradiation, unless other factors dictate surgery.
- Consider surgical reconstruction once bony destruction is advanced.
- If the tumor is radiosensitive, stabilize the spine with posterior instrumentation and control tumor growth with adjuvant radiotherapy.
- If the tumor is not radiosensitive, or if bony destruction is advanced, perform an anterior/posterior or posterolateral decompression and stabilization, and mobilize the patient early.
- If the patient presents with a solitary metastasis from a tumor with potential long-term survival (breast, colon, prostate, kidney), consider a combined procedure to obtain a wide excision of the lesion. Treat the tumor in the same way as a primary malignancy.

Once the neural elements are involved, the need for direct decompression becomes the primary indication for surgery.

- If the tumor is radiosensitive and neural progression is gradual, radiotherapy is the initial treatment of choice. If progression is rapid, unresponsive to radiotherapy, or secondary to bony as opposed to soft-tissue encroachment, decompress the cord or roots through the most direct approach.
- Use the posterior surgical approach in the cervical spine, above the level of C-3.
- Below C-3, the posterior approach should be limited to lesions of the dorsal elements. Address lesions of the vertebral body successfully through the appropriate anterior approach.
- As an alternative in lesions of the thoracic spine, use a costotransversectomy or transpedicular technique to access the vertebral body and decompress the anterior aspect of the spinal cord (37,38), (Fig. 152.14).

Although some authors have been dissatisfied with the decompression allowed through the posterolateral approach (8), the quality of both the decompression and the reconstruction can be improved by employing endoscopic control (Fig. 152.15).

TREATMENT OF BENIGN TUMORS

The principal reasons for operating on benign tumors are to treat pain and to prevent local tumor expansion. Intralesional excisions are adequate in many tumor types (e.g., aneurysmal bone cyst, osteoblastoma) and should be carried out through the most direct approach with the least disruption of normal vertebral elements.

- Treat locally aggressive (aggressive benign and low-grade malignant) tumors rigorously, ensuring a clear margin wherever possible. Because recurrent tumors are more difficult to eradicate than primary lesions, these locally aggressive lesions may become unresectable if not adequately addressed in the first place.
- Resect giant cell tumors *en bloc* when possible, and check the bone margins for residual tumor.
- Repeat curetments if necessary to obtain a clean margin, and consider adjuvant cryotherapy or postoperative radiotherapy to ensure a clean tumor bed (42,55).
- As an alternative to the traditional anterior/posterior approach, consider a posterolateral dissection and vertebrectomy through a T posterior incision (18).

TREATMENT OF PRIMARY MALIGNANT TUMORS

In primary malignancies, the principal goal of surgical treatment is local control of the disease. Plan the approach and resection to give the best chance of an adequate resection margin with the least disruption of vertebral stability.

- Approach dorsal tumors through a longitudinal posterior approach, incorporating any previous biopsy wound in the incision.
- Take care not to enter the soft-tissue mass of the tumor, either surgically or with retractors or rakes.
- Excise a cuff of normal muscle tissue with the tumor.
- Perform a laminectomy above and below the involved level and cut through uninvolved lamina or pedicle to isolate and resect the involved elements.
- Remove the tumor *en bloc* and stabilize the spine with a posterior instrumentation construct.

For anterior column tumors, combine an anterior and posterior approach to provide the widest possible margin for local control.

- Embolize the lesion preoperatively to limit blood loss during the procedure.
- Resect the posterior elements and posterior disc first to allow the vertebral body to be removed *en bloc* through an anterior approach.
- Use a transthoracic or retroperitoneal approach to reach the tumor from the front.
- Excise the adjacent discs back to the posterior longitudinal ligament, and remove all anterior soft tissues with

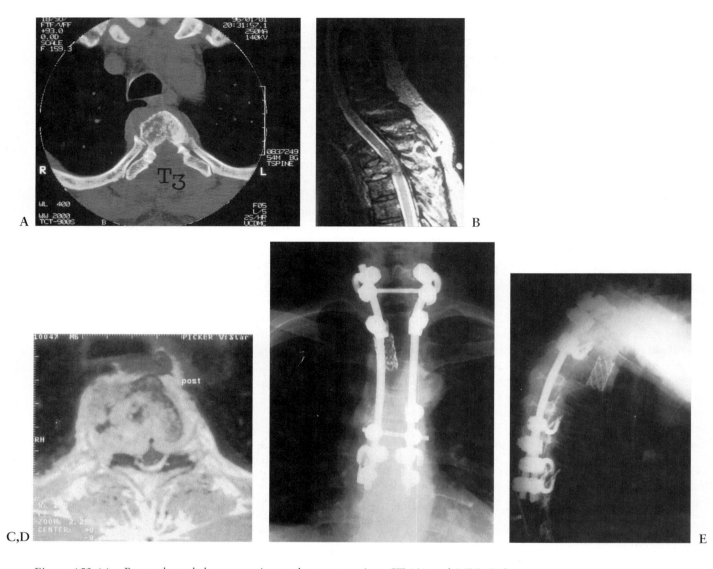

Figure 152.14. Posterolateral decompression and reconstruction. CT (**A**) and MRI (**B,C**) images of a 65-year-old man with T-3 solitary plasmacytoma, cord compression, and incomplete paraplegia. **D,E:** Endoscopically assisted posterolateral approach allowed complete vertebrectomy and spinal cord decompression. Titanium cage reconstruction and posterior instrumentation through the single dorsal incision provided immediate stability as seen on AP(**D**) and lateral (**E**) radiographs. Complete neurologic recovery was facilitated by rapid mobilization and rehabilitation.

the body, developing a plane between the great vessels and the anterior longitudinal ligament.

- Separate adherent tumor from the dura using a Freer elevator as the body is excised. Excise any involved dura and patch the defect with a fascial graft to improve local control.
- Stabilize the spine posteriorly with a segmental system at the time of posterior release.
- Restore the anterior weight-bearing column, filling the vertebrectomy defect with tricortical or fibular graft, or with a prosthetic cage.

- Use anterior plate fixation to augment overall stability.

Once extensive collapse has occurred, as in vertebra plana, a clear surgical margin is not possible, and local control is dependent on adjuvant therapy.

- Perform an intralesional resection of the vertebral body to debulk the tumor and prepare the vertebrectomy site for anterior reconstruction (40,44).
- Provide an adequate axial strut even when part of the involved vertebra can be retained, because progressive

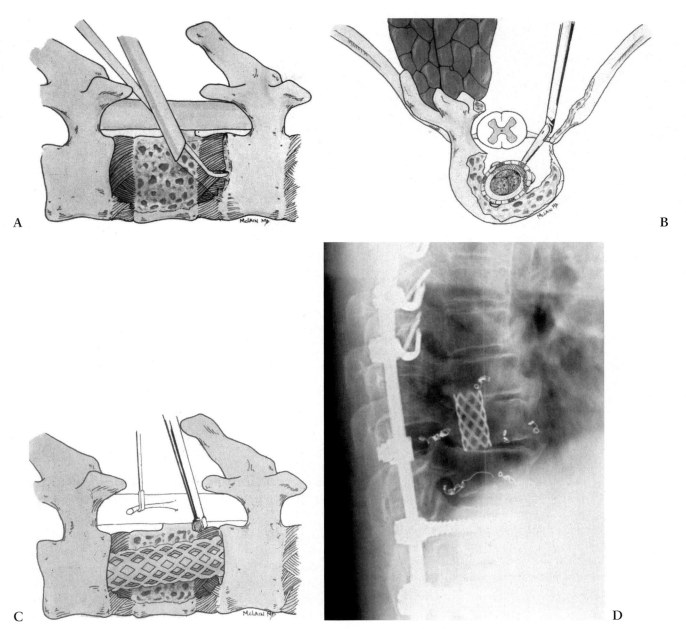

Figure 152.15.   Endoscopically assisted posterolateral vertebrectomy. **A:** After laminectomy and pedicle resection, the posterolateral aspect of the vertebral body and tumor mass are cavitated with pituitaries and curets. The endoscope is then used to visualize the undersurface of the cord, the endplates, and the far pedicle. Complete decompression can be confirmed without manipulating the neural tissues. **B,C:** Once the endplates are prepared, an appropriately sized cage, packed with autograft bone or PMMA, is introduced into the defect between the ipsilateral nerve roots and impacted into place. The endoscope confirms a safe interval between the cage and thecal sack before posterior instrumentation is applied. **D:** Lateral radiograph of a patient with metastatic adenocarcinoma treated with posterolateral decompression and reconstruction.

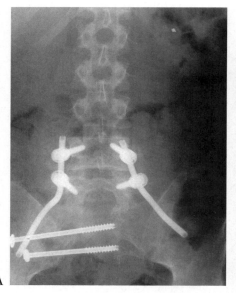 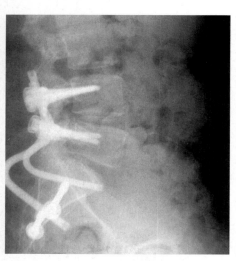

A   B

Figure 152.16. AP (**A**) and lateral (**B**) radiographs after resection and reconstruction of sacral metastasis. Patient with destructive lesion of the sacral ala, presenting with pain and weakness. Posterior intralesional resection was followed by reconstruction of the ala with a bicortical iliac autograft contoured to fill the defect and transfixed with transiliac screws. Lumbosacral stability was provided with a short pedicle construct using Galveston-type fixation into the pelvis. This construct is suitable for limited resections such as this, or for more extensive tumors requiring sacrectomy and prosthetic reconstruction.

collapse can occur despite successful radiotherapy, leading to intractable pain and potential neural injury.

- In radioresistant tumors such as chondrosarcoma or chordoma, make every effort to obtain a clear surgical margin.

Lesions of the sacrum present a particular therapeutic and reconstructive dilemma. A chordoma involving the distal sacrum requires a partial sacral amputation through a combined anterior and posterior approach, sacrificing whatever nerve roots exit the involved segment. For higher sacral lesions, more roots will need to be sacrificed. If the S-2 roots can be spared bilaterally, or if S-2 and S-3 roots are spared on one side, bowel and bladder function should be retained (22). Reconstruction following sacral amputation is most challenging when one or both of the sacroiliac joints is involved (Fig. 152.16).

Patients presenting with a primary spinal tumor and neurologic deficit generally have one of three problems: a pathologic fracture, which may either retropulse bone fragments into the spinal canal or produce kyphosis; extraosseous extension through the posterior vertebral cortex, producing direct compression of the neural elements; or direct extension of the tumor involving one or more nerve roots.

- In every case, the resection margins are likely to be contaminated, and adjuvant therapy is the key to eventual outcome.

- Resect any nerve roots directly involved by tumor along with the primary mass.
- Adherence to or investment of the dura or great vessels is an ominous finding. Consider nonoperative or palliative modalities in these cases.

Once metastasis has occurred, the patient's survival becomes dependent on systemic therapy. Local control is still important to prevent neurologic compromise and pain, but the impetus toward more aggressive and potentially dangerous procedures is reduced. Reconstruct the involved segments carefully, however, addressing both anterior and posterior columns to ensure that late collapse, kyphosis, and pain will not occur.

 AUTHOR'S PERSPECTIVE

Improved medical and adjuvant therapies continue to enhance cancer survival in patients with both primary and metastatic disease. As patients live longer, metastatic lesions will pose a greater threat to independence and survival, and musculoskeletal lesions will require treatment that provides pain relief and protects function for years rather than months. It is no longer acceptable to assume that the patient with spinal metastasis is near death and beyond help; benign neglect is not benign, and it is neither fiscally or ethically conscionable. Vertebrectomy, considered a radical procedure in the past, is coming to be seen as the conservative approach to tumor management in many situations. Advanced technologies have made aggressive surgery less invasive and dangerous, and improved instrumentation has all but eliminated the prolonged immobilization associated with spinal reconstruction. Appropriate surgical management can have an immediate and dramatic impact on patient function and survival, and it should never be dismissed without consideration.

REFERENCES

Each reference is categorized according to the following scheme: *, classic article; #, review article; !, basic research article; and +, clinical results/outcome study.

\# 1. Barwick KW, Huvos AG, Smith J. Primary Osteogenic Sarcoma of the Vertebral Column. *Cancer* 1980;46:595.

\+ 2. Bielack SS, Wulff B, Delling G, et al. Osteosarcoma of the Trunk Treated by Multimodality Therapy: Experience of the Cooperative Osteosarcoma Study Group. *Med Pediatr Oncol* 1995;24:6.

\+ 3. Bjornsson J, Wold LE, Ebersold MJ, Laws ER. Chordoma of the Mobile Spine. A Clinicopathological Analysis of 40 Patients. *Cancer* 1993;71:735.

\# 4. Bohlman HH, Sachs BL, Carter JR, et al. Primary Neoplasms of the Cervical Spine. *J Bone Joint Surg Am* 1986; 68:483.

* 5. Boland PJ, Lane JM, Sundaresan N. Metastatic Disease of the Spine. *Clin Orthop* 1982;169:95.

\+ 6. Boriani S, Biagini R, De Lure F, et al. En-bloc Resections of Bone Tumors of the Thoracolumbar Spine. A Preliminary Report on 29 Patients. *Spine* 1996;21:1927.

\+ 7. Boriani S, Chevalley F, Weinstein JN, et al. Chordoma of the Spine above the Sacrum: Treatment and Outcome in 21 Cases. *Spine* 1996;21:1569.

\+ 8. Bridwell KH, Jenny AB, Saul T, et al. Posterior Segmental Spinal Instrumentation (PSSI) with Posterior Decompression and Debulking for Metastatic Thoracic and Lumbar Spinal Disease. *Spine* 1988;13:1383.

* 9. Clain A. Secondary Malignant Disease of Bone. *Br J Cancer* 1965;19:15.

\+ 10. Clausen N, Gotze H, Pedersen A, et al. Skeletal Scintigraphy and Radiography at Onset of Acute Lymphocytic Leukemia in Children. *Med Pediatr Oncol* 1983;11:291.

\+ 11. Coffin CM, Swanson PE, Wick MR, Dehner LP. Chordoma in Childhood and Adolescence. A Clinicopathological Analysis of 12 Cases. *Arch Pathol Lab Med* 1993;117:927.

* 12. Constans JP, Divitiis E, Donzelli R, et al. Spinal Metastases with Neurological Manifestations: Review of 600 Cases. *J Neurosurg* 1983;59:111.

\# 13. Cuenod CA, Laredo JD, Chevret S, et al. Acute Vertebral Fracture due to Osteoporosis vs. Malignancy: Appearance on Unenhanced and Gadolinium-enhanced MR Images. *Radiology* 1996;199:541.

\+ 14. Cybulski GR, Von Roenn KA, D'Angelo CM, DeWald RL. Luque Rod Stabilization for Metastatic Disease of the Spine. *Surg Neurol* 1987;28:277.

* 15. Dahlin DC. Giant-Cell Tumor of Vertebrae above the Sacrum. *Cancer* 1977;39:1350.

\+ 16. DeWald RL, Bridwell KH, Prodromas C, Rodts MF. Reconstructive Spinal Surgery as Palliation for Metastatic Malignancies of the Spine. *Spine* 1985;10(1):21.

\! 17. Edelstyn GA, Gillespie PJ, Grebell ES. The Radiologic Demonstration of Osseous Metastases: Experimental Observations. *Clin Radiol* 1967;18:158.

\+ 18. Fidler MW. Radical Resection of Vertebral Body Tumors: A Surgical Technique Used in Ten Cases. *J Bone Joint Surg Br* 1994;76:765.

\# 19. Fox MW, Onofrio BM. The Natural History and Management of Symptomatic and Asymptomatic Vertebral Hemangiomas. *J Neurosurg* 1993;78:36.

\# 20. Fraser RD, Paterson DC, Simpson DA. Orthopaedic Aspects of Spinal Tumours in Children. *J Bone Joint Surg Br* 1977;59:143.

\# 21. Freiberg AA, Graziano GP, Loder RT, Hensinger RN. Metastatic Vertebral Disease in Children. *J Pediatr Orthop* 1993;13:148.

\+ 22. Gennari L, Azzarelli A, Quagliuolo V. A Posterior Approach for the Excision of Sacral Chordoma. *J Bone Joint Surg Br* 1987;69:565.

* 23. Gilbert RW, Kim JH, Posner JB. Epidural Spinal Cord Compression from Metastatic Tumor: Diagnosis and Treatment. *Ann Neurol* 1978;3:40.

\# 24. Godersky JC, Smoker WRK, Knutzon R. Use of Magnetic Resonance Imaging in the Evaluation of Metastatic Spinal Disease. *Neurosurgery* 1987;21:676.

\# 25. Graham WD. Metastatic Cancer to Bone. In: *Bone Tumours*. London: Butterworths, 1966:94.

\+ 26. Green NE, Robertson WW, Kilroy AW. Eosinophilic Granuloma of the Spine with Associated Neural Deficit. *J Bone Joint Surg Am* 1980;62:1198.

\+ 27. Griffin JB. Benign Osteoblastoma of the Thoracic Spine. *J Bone Joint Surg Am* 1978;60:833.

\+ 28. Grubb MR, Currier BL, Pritchard DJ, Ebersold MJ. Primary Ewing's sarcoma of the Spine. *Spine* 1994;19:309.

\! 29. Harada M, Shimizu A, Nakamura Y, Nemoto R. Role of the Vertebral Venous System in Metastatic Spread of Cancer Cells to the Bone. *Adv Exp Med Biol* 1992;324:83.

\# 30. Harrington KD. Current Concepts Review: Metastatic Disease of the Spine. *J Bone Joint Surg Am* 1986;68:1110.

\+ 31. Harrington KD. Anterior Decompression and Stabilization of the Spine as a Treatment for Vertebral Collapse and Spinal Cord Compression from Metastatic Malignancy. *Clin Orthop* 1988;233:177.

\+ 32. Hay MC, Paterson D, Taylor TKF. Aneurysmal Bone Cysts of the Spine. *J Bone Joint Surg Br* 1978;60:406.

\+ 33. Hermann G, Sacher M, Lanzieri CF, et al. Chondrosarcoma of the Spine: An Unusual Radiographic Presentation. *Skeletal Radiol* 1985;14:178.

34. Jaffe HL. *Tumors and Tumorous Conditions of the Bones and Joints*. Philadelphia: Lea and Febiger, 1958.

* 35. Keim HA, Reina EG. Osteoid-Osteoma as a Cause of Scoliosis. *J Bone Joint Surg Am* 1975;57:159.

+ 36. Kornberg M. Primary Ewing's Sarcoma of the Spine. *Spine* 1986;11:54.

* 37. Kostuik JP. Anterior Spinal Cord Decompression for Lesions of the Thoracic and Lumbar Spine, Techniques, New Methods of Internal Fixation, Results. *Spine* 1983; 8:512.

+ 38. Kostuik JP, Errico TJ, Gleason TF, Errico CC. Spinal Stabilization of Vertebral Column Tumors. *Spine* 1988; 13:250.

+ 39. Leeson MC, Makley JT, Carter JR. Metastatic Skeletal Disease in the Pediatric Population. *J Pediatr Orthop* 1985;5:261.

+ 40. Loftus CM, Michelsen CB, Rapoport F, Antunes JL. Management of Plasmacytomas of the Spine. *Neurosurgery* 1983;13:30.

+ 41. Malat J, Virapongse C, Levine A. Solitary Osteochondroma of the Spine. *Spine* 1986;11:625.

+ 42. Marcove RC, Sheth DS, Brien EW, et al. Conservative Surgery for Giant Cell Tumors of the Sacrum: The Role of Cryosurgery as a Supplement to Curettage and Partial Resection. *Cancer* 1994;74:1253.

* 43. Marsh BW, Bonfiglio M, Brady LP, Enneking WF. Benign Osteoblastoma: Range of Manifestations. *J Bone Joint Surg Am* 1975;57:1.

+ 44. McLain RF, Weinstein JN. Solitary Plasmacytomas of the Spine: A Review of 84 Cases. *J Spinal Disord* 1989; 2:69.

* 45. McLain RF, Weinstein JN. Tumors of the Spine. *Semin Spine Surg* 1990;2:157.

+ 46. McLain RF, Weinstein JN. An Unusual Presentation of a Schmorl's Node. Report of a Case. *Spine* 1990;15: 247.

+ 47. McLain RF, Kabins M, Weinstein JN. VSP Stabilization of Lumbar Neoplasms: Technical Considerations and Complications. *J Spinal Disord* 1991;4:359.

* 48. McLain RF, Sparling E, Benson DR. Failure of Short Segment Pedicle Instrumentation in Thoracolumbar Fractures: Complications of Cotrel-Dubousset Instrumentation. *J Bone Joint Surg Am* 1993;75:162.

49. Mindell ER. Current Concepts Review: Chordoma. *J Bone Joint Surg Am* 1981;63:501.

* 50. Pettine KA, Klassen RA. Osteoid-Osteoma and Osteoblastoma of the Spine. *J Bone Joint Surg Am* 1986;68: 354.

+ 51. Poulsen JO, Jensen JT, Tommesen P. Ewing's Sarcoma Simulating Vertebra Plana. *Acta Orthop Scand* 1975;46: 211.

+ 52. Rate WR, Butler MS, Robertson WW Jr, D'Angio GJ. Late Orthopaedic Effects in Children with Wilm's Tumor Treated with Abdominal Irradiation. *Med Pediatr Oncol* 1991;19:265.

53. Rogalsky RJ, Black GB, Reed MH. Orthopaedic Manifestations of Leukemia in Children. *J Bone Joint Surg Am* 1986;68:494.

+ 54. Samson IR, Springfield DS, Suit HD, Mankin HJ. Operative Treatment of Sacrococcygeal Chordoma. A Review of Twenty-One Cases. *J Bone Joint Surg* 1993;75:1476.

+ 55. Sanjay BK, Sim FH, Unni KK, et al. Giant Cell Tumor of the Spine. *J Bone Joint Surg Br* 1993;75:148.

+ 56. Savini R, Gherlinzoni F, Morandi M, et al. Surgical Treatment of Giant-Cell Tumor of the Spine. *J Bone Joint Surg Am* 1983;65:1283.

* 57. Sherk HH, Nicholson JT, Nixon JE. Vertebra Plana and Eosinophilic Granuloma of the Cervical Spine in Children. *Spine* 1978;3:116.

* 58. Shives TC, Dahlin DC, Sim FH, et al. Osteosarcoma of the Spine. *J Bone Joint Surg Am* 1986;68:660.

* 59. Shives TC, McLeod RA, Unni KK, Schray MF. Chondrosarcoma of the Spine. *J Bone Joint Surg Am* 1989;71: 1158.

+ 60. Siegal T, Siegal T. Current Considerations in the Management of Neoplastic Spinal Cord Compression. *Spine* 1988;14:223.

* 61. Siegal T, Tiqva P, Siegal T. Vertebral Body Resection for Epidural Compression by Malignant Tumors. *J Bone Joint Surg Am* 1985;67:375.

* 62. Sim FH, Dahlin DC, Stauffer RN, Laws ER. Primary Bone Tumors Simulating Lumbar Disc Syndrome. *Spine* 1977;2:65.

+ 63. Stener B. Total Spondylectomy in Chondrosarcoma Arising from the Seventh Thoracic Vertebra. *J Bone Joint Surg Br* 1971;53:288.

+ 64. Stener B, Gunterberg B. High Amputation of the Sacrum for Extirpation of Tumors. *Spine* 1978;3:351.

+ 65. Sundaresan N, Rosen G, Huvos AG, Krol G. Combined Treatment of Osteosarcoma of the Spine. *Neurosurgery* 1988;23:714.

+ 66. Sundaresan N, Sachdev VP, Holland JF, et al. Surgical Treatment of Spinal Cord Compression from Epidural Metastasis. *J Clin Oncol* 1995;13:2330.

+ 67. Sundaresan N, Scher H, DiGiacinto GV, et al. Surgical Treatment of Spinal Cord Compression in Kidney Cancer. *J Clin Oncol* 1986;4:1851.

+ 68. Tomita T, Galicich JH, Sundaresan N. Radiation Therapy for Spinal Epidural Metastases with Complete Block. *Acta Radiol Oncol* 1983;22:135.

+ 69. Traill Z, Richards MA, Moore NR. Magnetic Resonance Imaging of Metastatic Bone Disease. *Clin Orthop* 1995; 312:76.

+ 70. Turcotte R, Sim FH, Unni KK. Giant Cell Tumor of the Sacrum. *Clin Orthop* 1993;291:215.

* 71. Valderrama JAF, Bullough PG. Solitary Myeloma of the Spine. *J Bone Joint Surg Br* 1988;50:82.

+ 72. Weinstein JN. Surgical Approach to Spine Tumors. *Orthopaedics* 1989;12:897.

* 73. Weinstein JN, McLain RF. Primary Tumors of the Spine. *Spine* 1987;12:843.

+ 74. Wong DA, Fornasier VL, MacNab I. Spinal Metastases: The Obvious, the Occult, and the Impostors. *Spine* 1990; 15:1.

CHAPTER 153

SURGERY OF THE SPINE IN ANKYLOSING SPONDYLITIS

Edward H. Simmons

Ankylosing spondylitis and rheumatoid arthritis, although commonly considered together, are two distinct diseases. Ankylosing spondylitis has often been described as "rheumatoid" spondylitis, but it is a different disease with a different serology. It is more common in men than in women and has a predilection for the spine and major joints; rheumatoid arthritis is more common in women and tends to affect smaller joints and the joints of the appendicular skeleton (10,15,16). Clinical manifestations of ankylosing spondylitis occur in 0.2% to 0.3% of the general population.

In ankylosing spondylitis, the major clinical problems of the spine are gross fixed deformities. In rheumatoid arthritis the spine is subject to local destruction and instability. Atlantoaxial subluxation and dislocation may occur in both diseases, however.

E. H. Simmons: Buffalo, New York, 14201.

ATLANTOAXIAL INSTABILITY

Recognizing atlantoaxial instability in patients with rheumatoid arthritis and ankylosing spondylitis requires careful clinical monitoring. Rheumatoid disease is discussed in greater detail in Chapter 154. In ankylosing spondylitis, a solid column of bone below may place excessive stress at the craniocervical junction. With the attritional effects of inflammation of the transverse ligament and associated hyperemia on its bony attachments, atlantoaxial subluxation and dislocation may occur. With subluxation, the joint may subsequently stabilize in the subluxated position without significant symptoms.

Consider the possibility of significant instability when planning surgery on any patient who might undergo neck manipulation, either by the anesthesiologist or during the surgery itself. Obtain routine flexion and extension lateral radiographs of the cervical spine before performing any such procedures.

POSTERIOR ARTHRODESIS OF C1–C2

Surgical stabilization is justified when there is gross symptomatic atlantoaxial instability and the patient is at risk. Stabilization can be effectively achieved by a Gallie-type posterior atlantoaxial arthrodesis (12,19,22,23,25).

■ Shape a modified H graft from the iliac crest and contour it to fit over the posterior arches of C-1 and C-2, astride the spinous process of C-2.

■ Pass a single piece of 22-gauge stainless-steel wire infe-rior to the spinous process of C-2 and through the interspinous ligament of C2–C3. Carry the ends of the wire upward posteriorly to the graft around a notch in its upper border and under the arch of C-1 on each side of the graft.

■ Tie the wire ends posteriorly over the graft, fixing it into position and pulling back the arch of C-1 into alignment with the arch of C-2 (Fig. 153.1). Some form of wire tightener is needed, such as that developed by Harris (8). The wire tightener grasps the wire, allowing tension to be applied, so that a knot

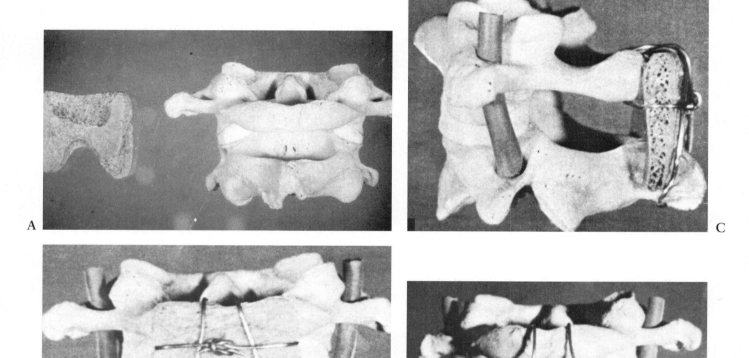

Figure 153.1. **A:** Skeletal model showing deep cancellous surface of Gallie modified H-graft, which is contoured from the posterior iliac crest to fit over the posterior arches of C-1 and C-2, sitting astride the spinous process of C-2. **B:** Posterior view showing the graft in position with cortical surface superficially. Pass the Gallie wire through the interspinous ligament of C2–C3 below the spinous process of C-2, upward over the graft on each side. Bring it out below the arch of C-1 laterally and tie it firmly posteriorly. **C:** Lateral view showing the position of the modified H-graft, with the wire pulling back the C-1 vertebra into a normal relationship with the odontoid. The inferior portion of the wire passes below the spinous process of C-2 through the interspinous ligament of C2–C3, which should be preserved during exposure and wiring because it assists in maintaining the wire in position until it is tightened. **D:** Posterior view of model showing the configuration of the wire without the graft in position.

can be tied firmly in the narrow confines of the wound with only gentle manual pressure (discussed in more detail in Chapter 154).

TRANSORAL DECOMPRESSION

In the few instances when the odontoid is causing major anterior pressure that cannot be reduced, transoral resection of the odontoid may be required. This procedure is more hazardous than posterior decompression and stabilization; if the instability is recognized earlier, the procedure will be less frequently required. Transoral surgery is reserved for patients with significant anterior compression.

Two different types of abnormality can be differentiated: In the first, basilar invagination is present without gross instability, and in the second there is additional atlantoaxial instability and luxation. Posterior column involvement also may be evident in the second type, caused by posterior compression of the spinal cord by the posterior arch of C-1, which slides anteriorly.

Pure basilar invagination with narrowing of the anterior cerebellomedullary cistern is the primary indication for transoral decompression. Decompression may involve the removal of not only the odontoid process, but also the body of C-2 and the space-occupying portion of the clivus. In cases of pure atlantoaxial instability, a stable posterior atlantoaxial arthrodesis is preferred. Results of primary anterior decompression combined with simultaneous anterior fusion are not encouraging, and it would appear preferable to perform a posterior fusion as a secondary procedure following a primary anterior decompression.

Before surgery, identify and clear any evidence of oral infection or dental sepsis. Obtain nasal, oral, and pharyngeal swabs for bacterial culture and sensitivity, and administer the most appropriate antibiotic combination before surgery, intravenously during surgery, and in the immediate postoperative period.

Operative Technique

■ Position the patient supine for surgery, with the neck extended. Lateral radiographic control is necessary. Some recommend routine tracheostomy and endotracheal anesthesia (6). However, the endotracheal tube is not an obstacle at surgery, and in some ways it is best to leave the airway intact.

■ In patients who do not have a tracheostomy, place a gastric tube for postoperative nutrition, with normal oral nutrition beginning 7–8 days after surgery. If tracheostomy is indicated, perform it at the beginning of the operation with ventilation continued through a cuffed tracheal tube.

■ After preparation of the oral cavity, introduce a Whitehead retractor and depress the tongue. Pack off the nasopharynx and hypopharynx.

■ The procedure can usually be done without division of the soft palate. Fold the soft palate back on itself and

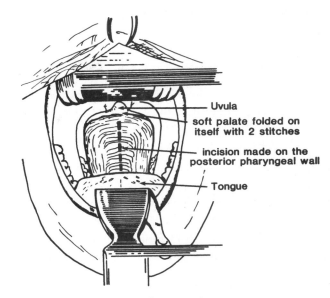

Figure 153.2. Diagram of transoral exposure. Use two stay sutures to fold the soft palate on itself and keep it in position. Incise the posterior pharyngeal wall vertically.

suture it to the junction of the hard and soft palates to expose the lower portion of the nasopharynx. Release these sutures at the end of the procedure (Fig. 153.2).

■ If division of the soft palate is considered necessary, incise it on one side of the midline to avoid the uvula, and retract the flaps laterally (Fig. 153.3).

■ Palpate the posterior pharyngeal wall to locate the prominence of the anterior tubercle of the atlas. In atlantoaxial dislocation, it is quite evident.

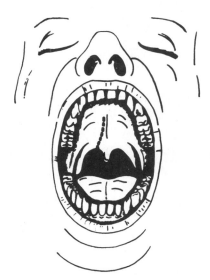

Figure 153.3. Exposure showing incision of the soft palate on one side, avoiding the uvula.

- Make a 2-inch midline incision from the lower portion of the clivus to the lower portion of C-2.
- Center the incision one finger breadth below the anterior tubercle of the atlas.
- Carry the incision down to bone.
- Strip the soft tissues laterally to the outer margin of the lateral masses of the atlas and axis. The soft tissues may be anchored with retraction stay sutures.
- Expose the anterior arch of the atlas and the body of the axis.
- Remove the anterior arch of the atlas with sharp rongeurs and expose the odontoid (Fig. 153.4).
- Remove the odontoid process with a high-speed drill and a diamond burr.

Removal of the odontoid process, which is displaced upward and projects backward, is the most complicated part of the surgery.

- Carefully and gently free the odontoid of its soft-tissue attachments, using sharp dissection as necessary.
- If resection of the odontoid is difficult because of its elevation and the angle of approach, commence the resection in the central part of the body of the axis.
- Remove the lower portion of the clivus (anterior margin of the foramen magnum) only when necessary; when it is required, I recommend a diamond burr and upward-cutting bone forceps.
- If lateral fusion of the C1–C2 joint is to be attempted, clear the articular cartilage from the joints and wedge iliac grafts between the lateral masses.
- Close the posterior pharyngeal wall.

Some authors recommend a multilayer closure involving the anterior ligament, the buccopharyngeal fascia and constrictor muscles, and the pharyngeal mucosa. Many, however, recommend a loose, single-layer closure because it allows wound secretions to drain more easily and it has technical advantages (6,7,14). Defer oral feedings 6–7 days to allow adequate healing; introduce liquids before solids. See Chapters 138 and 154.

ATLANTO-OCCIPITAL DISABILITY

Occasionally in ankylosing spondylitis, severe disability may arise from destructive changes at the atlanto-occipital joint. Destructive changes may produce intractable pain associated with minimal persisting motion, justifying surgical stabilization. On occasion, subluxation or even rotatory deformity can occur, which may warrant gradual reduction with halo traction followed by stabilization with occipitocervical fusion.

OCCIPITOCERVICAL FUSION

I prefer to use double-cortical and cancellous onlay iliac grafts fixed to the base of the skull and the upper cervical spine, reinforced by multiple cancellous bone grafts. The onlay grafts are contoured to fit over the posterior arches of the upper cervical vertebrae (usually down to C-4), the cancellous surface of the graft being contoured to fit over the posterior arches.

- Apply a cranial halo preoperatively to support the head during surgery.
- Position the patient supine and prepare and drape the neck well up onto the head and to the ears.
- Hold the grafts firmly against the skull and fix them directly to the posterior arches of the cervical vertebrae using transfixing threaded Compere wires. Drive these wires percutaneously from the side of the neck, through the graft on one side of the spine, then through the base of the spinous process, and then through the graft on the opposite side. Cut the wire free on the side of its entrance in the wound lateral to the graft.
- Before the grafts are fixed to the upper cervical spine, pass a wire through drill holes in the skull to fix the grafts against the skull, which has been denuded; then pass it around the ends of the threaded Compere wires for fixation to the skull and to fix the grafts to the posterior arches of the cervical spine.

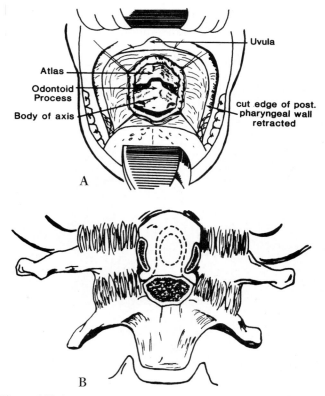

Figure 153.4.   **A:** Anterior exposure of the atlas and axis with the soft tissues stripped laterally. **B:** Excision of the anterior arch of the atlas allowing exposure of the odontoid.

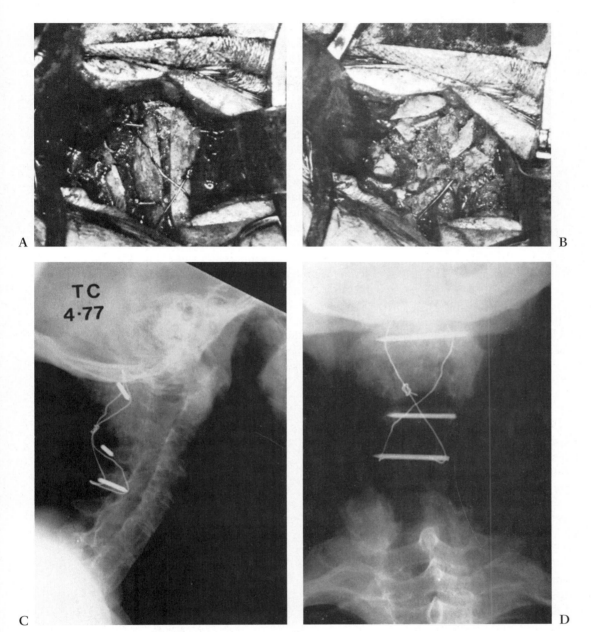

Figure 153.5. Occipitocervical Fusion: **A:** Posterior operative view showing double onlay cortical and cancellous iliac grafts. **B:** Operative view showing additional onlay cancellous bone grafts, which reinforce the main grafts and extend from the cervical spine to the skull. **C:** Postoperative lateral radiograph showing a solid fusion extending from the occiput to the cervical spine. The wiring passes through the skull. Compere wires fix onlay grafts to the posterior arches of the cervical spine. **D:** Postoperative anteroposterior radiograph demonstrating the configuration of the wire loop, Compere wires, and grafts.

- Reinforce the main grafts with cancellous strips laterally on both sides and superiorly against the skull (Fig. 153.5).
- Postoperative immobilization in a well-fitted halo cast is essential to protect the area of fusion from abnormal stress (5).

SPONDYLODISCITIS

Erosion and sclerosis of bone adjacent to the sacroiliac joints is a typical radiographic feature of ankylosing spondylitis. This erosive, sclerotic process may occasionally extend into the intervertebral disc and adjacent bone, and

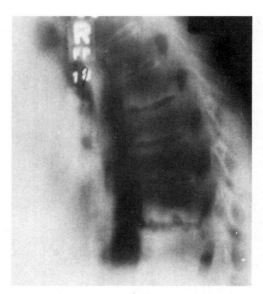

Figure 153.6. Lateral radiograph showing the typical lesion of spondylodiscitis in the lower thoracic spine (the most frequent location). Erosive sclerotic changes involve the vertebral end-plates adjacent to the disc space.

it is then called spondylodiscitis. Such lesions were first reported by Andersson in 1937 (2).

Two opposing views exist as to the nature of these lesions. The first view is that spondylodiscitis is an inflammatory process affecting the intervertebral disc and surrounding bone. Detailed assessment and biopsy specimens support this view. The second, less commonly held view is that spondylodiscitis is secondary to trauma with excessive forces localized at one intervertebral segment, resulting in mechanical destruction and a functional pseudarthrosis.

The radiographic appearance is fairly typical (Fig. 153.6). The erosive process widens the disc space, breaking down the subchondral bony plates. The surrounding bone becomes sclerotic and radiodense. The prominence of either erosion or sclerosis varies. Spondylodiscitis has a reported incidence of 5% to 6% in ankylosing spondylitis (9,17,18). Most of the lesions develop in the lower thoracic spine. A little more than half the lesions are discovered on routine radiographic studies and are asymptomatic (9). About half the patients with spondylodiscitis present with back pain.

The lesion generally follows a benign course and usually responds to conservative management. Surgical stabilization may occasionally be required for intractable pain, particularly when there is an associated fracture or disruption of the posterior fused spine resulting from loss of bony substance anteriorly. If the lesion presents with intractable pain and no deformity, as in the mid-thoracic spine, then anterior resection and strut grafting may be

indicated. The involved disc space and adjacent eroded bone are resected, and fibular or iliac strut grafts are fixed into the defect in a keystone fashion (24). Supplemental rib and iliac grafts are added as necessary.

When the lesion is painful, it is most often in the lower thoracic spine—an area subject to shear stress—with increasing deformity shifting the weight-bearing line anterior to the lesion, causing further erosion and increasing pain. In my experience, successful handling of this lesion requires correction of the overall spinal deformity. In my experience with more than 20 patients with this problem, the lesion has healed following resection–extension osteotomy of the mid-lumbar spine, shifting the weight-bearing line posteriorly, and changing the direction of the area of spondylodiscitis to horizontal, thus converting the shear force to a compression force (Fig. 153.7). This outcome is preferable to multiple anterior and posterior procedures, which have a higher failure rate when the overall deformity is not corrected, and which do not alleviate the shear stress.

The incidence of spondylodiscitis may be greater than previously suggested. In my review of 124 patients referred for surgical correction of spinal deformity for

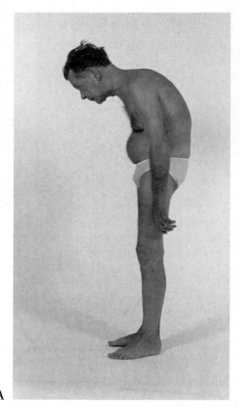

A

Figure 153.7. **A:** A 58-year-old man had severely painful spondylodiscitis at T12–L1, which resulted in an increasing flexion deformity of the thoracolumbar spine. *(continued)*

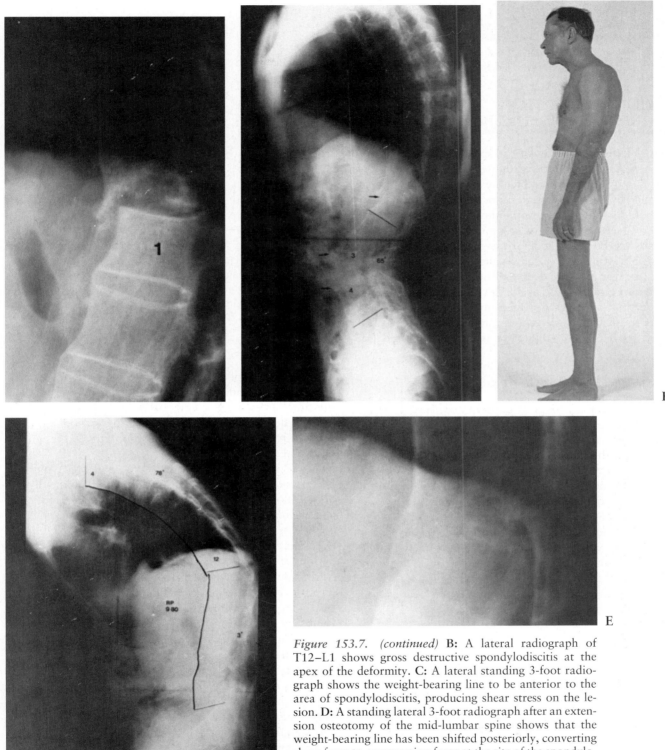

Figure 153.7. (continued) **B:** A lateral radiograph of T12–L1 shows gross destructive spondylodiscitis at the apex of the deformity. **C:** A lateral standing 3-foot radiograph shows the weight-bearing line to be anterior to the area of spondylodiscitis, producing shear stress on the lesion. **D:** A standing lateral 3-foot radiograph after an extension osteotomy of the mid-lumbar spine shows that the weight-bearing line has been shifted posteriorly, converting shear force to compression force at the site of the spondylodiscitis. **E:** A lateral radiograph at T12–L1, 4 months after surgery, shows spontaneous healing of the area of spondylodiscitis as a result of the conversion of shear stress to compression. **F:** The patient following healing of the osteotomy and area of spondylodiscitis. The extension osteotomy of his lumbar spine corrected his deformity and allowed spontaneous healing of the spondylodiscitis.

whom radiographs of the entire spine were available for study, 28 (23%) were found to have spondylodiscitis. When the lesion was in the area of the deformity and contributed to it, correction of the deformity resulted in fusion at the site of the spondylodiscitis (20,21).

FLEXION (KYPHOTIC) DEFORMITIES OF THE SPINE

Severe flexion deformities of the spine may occur in patients suffering from Marie-Strümpell spondylitis or ankylosing spondylitis associated with psoriasis. Prevention of deformity by early recognition and appropriate medical care should be the aim. Despite improvements in medical care, however, patients still present with gross disability from advanced kyphotic deformity of the trunk.

The indications for surgical correction vary with the extent of deformity, the degree of functional impairment, the general condition and age of the patient, the feasibility of correction, and, perhaps most important, the willingness of the patient to accept the risks and undergo the reconstructive and rehabilitative measures required for correction.

CLINICAL ASSESSMENT

If any major correction is to be obtained, surgery must address the area of involvement. For example, a patient with apparent spinal deformity actually may have a major deformity in the hip joints. If a hip flexion deformity is the cause of the patient's malalignment, then it should be corrected through surgery on the hip joints. Also, accurate assessment and measurement of any deformity are required to gauge the results of treatment. The most effective and reliable measure of a spine flexion deformity is the chin-brow-to-vertical angle. It is a measure of the angle formed by a line from the brow to the chin through the vertical, when the patient stands with the hips and knees fully extended, and the neck in its neutral or fixed position (Fig. 153.8).

KYPHOTIC DEFORMITY OF THE LUMBAR SPINE

Kyphotic deformity of the lumbar spine was the first type of deformity corrected surgically in arthritic disease, as reported by Smith-Peterson et al. in 1945 (26). The initial procedure was done under general anesthesia with the patient lying prone. Difficulties with the prone position were later avoided by performing the surgery with the patient on the side, as recommended by Adams (1).

Some have recommended a two-stage or double-exposure procedure with surgical division of the longitudinal ligament anteriorly. I do not find it necessary: Correction can be achieved through the posterior approach alone.

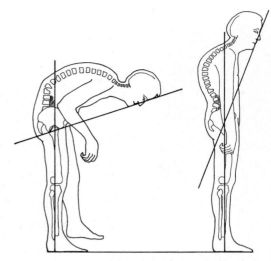

Figure 153.8. Technique for measuring the degree of flexion deformity of the spine in ankylosing spondylitis. The chin-brow-to-vertical angle is measured from the brow to the chin to the vertical, with the patient standing with hips and knees extended and the neck in its fixed or neutral position.

A major complication of lumbar osteotomy is gastric dilatation and abdominal ileus. As the spine is extended, the superior mesenteric artery is stretched over the third part of the duodenum, predisposing to gastric dilatation. A nasogastric tube must be in position after surgery until intestinal motility is established.

A review of the literature until 1969 indicated a mortality rate of 8% to 10% with this procedure; some degree of neurologic deficit, including paraplegia, occurred in up to 30% of patients. Two thirds of the deaths were related to the use of general anesthesia. As a result, I used my experience in cervical osteotomy, as well as the recommendations of others, to perform surgical correction of lumbar flexion deformity with a resection–extension osteotomy under local anesthesia. From the 1970s to the early 1990s, I used this method in a series now totaling 100 patients. Generally, correction under local anesthesia has proved to be a safe, reliable, and practical procedure (19,21,23). The main advantage of local anesthesia is that it allows a critical assessment of the patient's neurologic and vital functions throughout the operation.

Over the past 10 years, there have been substantial improvements in anesthesia, including fiberoptic intubation and spinal cord monitoring. The risks of surgery under general anesthesia have decreased; therefore, today I use general anesthesia following the strict guidelines that will be discussed later.

Resection–Extension Osteotomy at L3–L4
The primary deformity of patients selected for lumbar extension osteotomy is in the lumbar spine and loss of lum-

bar lordosis. There may be some associated increase in thoracic kyphosis, which can be balanced by overcorrecting the lumbar deformity so that the chin-brow-to-vertical angle will be normal. This angle is measured and transposed to a lateral radiograph of the lumbar spine, placing the apex of the angle at the posterior longitudinal ligament over the L3-4 disc space. The L3–L4 level is selected for correction because it is the center of the lumbar lordosis and is below the spinal cord. The L4–L5 level is used only on rare occasions.

Do a careful preoperative evaluation, including medical assessment, pulmonary function tests, and electrocardiography. Instruct the patient in deep breathing and extremity exercises, which will be used postoperatively. Psychological preparation includes explaining to the patient the procedure and the importance of awake intubation and positioning, prior to inducing general anesthesia. Make plaster molds of the upper and lower halves of the body before surgery. The upper half extends from the waist up, supporting the chest and head; the lower half extends from the waist to the knees. These shells are used for support when the patient is turned prone after the correction is done. The molds protect the face and allow the anesthesiologist to administer oxygen by face mask through the opening in the shell (Fig. 153.9).

In planning the osteotomy, it is important to know whether the patient has normal spinal canal dimensions.

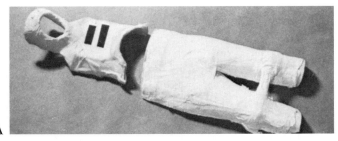

A

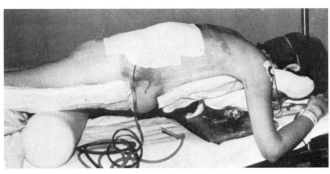

B

Figure 153.9. **A:** Cephalad and caudad anterior molds. The cephalad mold supports the head and has an opening for the face. **B:** Postoperative view. After correction of deformity, the patient is supported in the prone position by the anterior molds with a jack below the upper mold. Note the restoration of lordosis with correction of the flexion deformity.

If the patient has a canal of normal or above-average size, then less bone may be removed posteriorly with closer approximation of the laminae. However, if the canal dimensions are fairly small (less than 20 mm on the anteroposterior diameter) or in the stenotic range, then considerably more caution must be taken to ensure that the posterior decompression is generous, particularly superiorly. In this situation, it is best to leave the central laminectomy area open significantly above and below to avoid any compression from postoperative edema, buckling of the dura, or minimal translation. Some indication of adequate canal size may be noted on a lateral view of the spine; patients with large foramina and long pedicles have a greater canal size than those in whom the foramina appear small and the pedicles short. If a narrow canal is suspected, make accurate computed tomography (CT) canal measurements.

My method is based on the original technique by Smith-Petersen et al. (26). They described a posterior wedge resection of the mid-lumbar spine in a V fashion. This resection was carried superiorly and laterally through the superior facet of the vertebra above and the inferior facet of the vertebra below in an oblique fashion. More bone was resected superiorly than inferiorly. The oblique plane of the osteotomy was designed to produce overlap of the posterior elements following correction, in an effort to prevent displacement. Since the deformity was corrected by manipulation of the spine after the posterior resection was completed, the anteriorly longitudinal ligament was fractured. This technique is the basis for the procedure described next.

- Have your neuromonitoring technician apply the spinal cord monitoring electrodes and confirm that the spinal cord monitoring is satisfactory.
- Have the anesthesiologist intubate the patient while he is awake and lying on the gurney on which he was brought into the operating room. When the endotracheal tube is in position, ask the patient to stand (with assistance) and transfer to a suitable spinal OR table with his knees and hips flexed. Adjust the supports to provide comfortable positing for his head, chest, and pelvis, avoiding any strain on his neck. Ask him to give an OK signal with his hand when he is comfortable, and then induce general anesthesia (28).
- Compared to our previous use of local anesthesia only, general anesthesia makes the posterior bony resection easier to perform. It is much easier to undercut the pedicles above and below the area of resection, and a more complete decompression of the L-3 nerve roots is possible.
- Prepare and drape the back.
- The general anesthesia can be augmented by infiltration of the skin and the paravertebral muscles with 0.5% bupivacaine with 1:200,000 epinephrine. This will re-

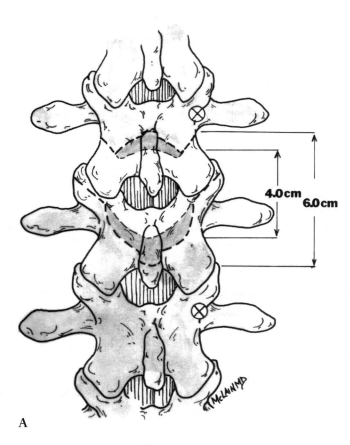

A

Figure 153.10. Resection-Extension Osteotomy, L3–4: **A:** The osteotomy is planned to completely decompress the thecal sack in the midline, with symmetrical lateral resections extending cranially and laterally. Pedicle screw insertion sites are identified, and screws may be placed prior to osteotomy. **B:** Following decompression, the Smith-Peterson osteotomy provides two wedges of posterior bone that will lock together when the spine is placed in extension. Relieve the undersurface of the lamina to prevent impingement as the spine is extended into its reduced position. **C:** Closure of the osteotomy by extension of the spine. Pack resected bone and autograft posterolaterally over the transverse processes and dorsal cortex of the osteotomy. Place the fixation rods into the screws and compress the osteotomy site, locking the wedges together to ensure stability and reliable arthrodesis.

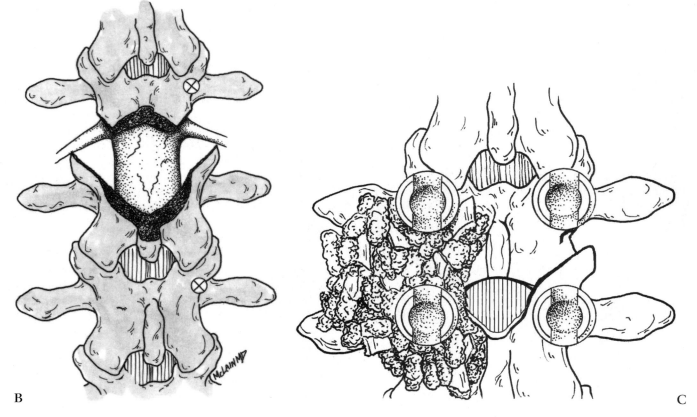

B

C

duce somewhat the level of general anesthesia required and provides some hemostasis.

■ Make a midline exposure and confirm the proposed L3–L4 osteotomy site radiographically with towel clips placed on the base of the spinous processes at the level of the laminae of L-3 and L-4.

■ I now routinely use pedicle screw fixation; therefore the next step is the insertion of the pedicle screws prior to the performance of the osteotomy. The number of levels of fixation required depends on bony quality, but usually I place screws in the pedicles of L-1, L-2, L-3, as well as L5 and S-1 (Fig. 153.10*A*).

■ Next, perform a V-shaped wedge resection osteotomy at the interlaminar space, as recommended by Smith-Petersen et al. (26), resecting the ossified ligamentum flavum and adjacent laminae.

■ Extend the resection upward and laterally on each side through the fused posterior joints at L3–L4. The amount of bone to be removed posteriorly is measured from the radiograph at the level of the tips of the spinous processes, the laminae, the posterior aspect of the posterior joints, and inside the canal at the level of the pedicles. The obliquity of this resection allows locking of the vertebrae following correction.

■ Remove the spinous processes in small strips to be used for grafting. Remove the bone with bone cutters and rongeurs.

■ A power burr may be a useful tool for cutting slowly through the fused posterior elements toward the spinal canal, which is opened. The ossified ligamentum flavum is harder and denser than the vertebral elements.

■ Protect the dura with cotton patties. In many instances, the dura is atrophic and occasionally it may adhere to the laminae, making separation difficult.

■ Completely expose the dural sac laterally on each side to the level of the pedicles.

■ Undercut the laminae above and below to avoid impingement on the dura following extension. Undercut the pedicles to avoid any impingement on the third lumbar nerve roots following extension.

■ Remove bone from each side symmetrically, to allow symmetrical closure of the defect (Fig. 153.10*B*).

■ When the osteotomy is completed, correct the kyphotic deformity by extending the hips with the adjustments of the spine table. This will produce an anterior osteoclasis and an opening wedge anteriorly with closure of the posterior osteotomy. Perform this maneuver gently and carefully, constantly watching the neuromonitoring for any evidence of compromise of neurologic function, and close the osteotomy down to obtain good posterior bone apposition (Fig. 153.10*C*).

■ Full correction must be obtained with the weight-bearing line shifted posterior to the osteotomy site, so that gravity will maintain and increase the correction as it heals; it will also stimulate bone formation across the osteotomy sites of the resected posterior fusion masses (Fig. 153.11).

■ Complete the stabilization by fixing the rods to the ped-

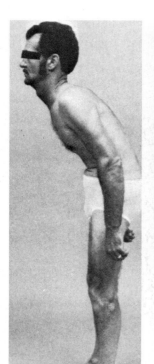
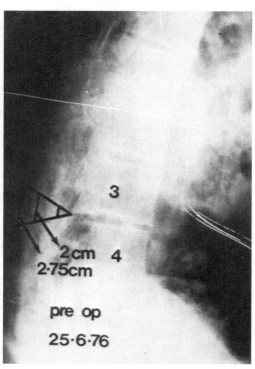

A,B

Figure 153.11. **A:** Lateral view of a patient standing with hips and knees extended. This patient still had mobility of his cervical spine and was compensating with the neck hyperextended. When the neck was in the neutral or comfortable position, he had a chin-brow-to-vertical angle of 45°. **B:** Lateral radiograph of lumbar spine showing the chin-brow-to-vertical angle superimposed with the apex at the L3-4 disc space. The amount of bone to be resected is indicated at each depth posteriorly. *(continued)*

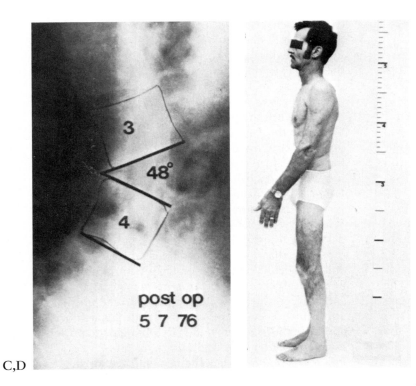

C,D

Figure 153.11. *(continued)* C: Postoperative lateral radiograph following correction under local anesthesia showing the angle of correction obtained after closure of the resected defect posteriorly with an opening osteoclasis at L3-4 of 48°. The weight-bearing line has been shifted posterior to the osteotomy site. D: Postoperative standing lateral radiograph showing complete correction of the deformity after removal of a calculated wedge of bone based on preoperative assessment.

icle screws using TSRH instrumentation (Sofamor-Danek, Memphis, TN).

Initially, I used no internal fixation, as suggested by Smith-Petersen et al. (26), relying on the V-shaped configuration of the osteotomy to provide locking and reasonable stability. The patients were kept recumbent for 6 weeks, followed by ambulation in a Minerva plaster cast (19,21,23). Subsequently, I used internal wire loop fixation for additional stability and comfort in the early postoperative interval. Before the advent of pedicle screw fixation, I used a Luque rectangle with posterior segmental instrumentation and Drummond buttons and wires. The advantage of internal fixation with segmental instrumentation was that it decreased the risk of translation and allowed earlier postoperative mobilization (Fig. 153.12). I now prefer pedicle screw and rod fixation with the decompression technique just described, as it allows easier and more liberal decompression; the rigid internal fixation decreases the risk of displacement and allows easier and quicker mobilization of the patients, who seem to have less postoperative pain. The disadvantages of pedicle screw and rod fixation are increased operating time, and increased risk of neurologic injury from improper insertion of bone screws because of the altered anatomy of the pedicles. Overall, however, I feel that the advantages outweigh the disadvantages, as illustrated by the patient in Figure 153.13.

■ Strip the spine further lateral to the osteotomy site, ex-

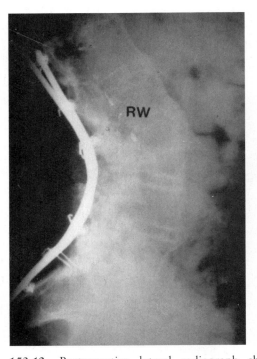

Figure 153.12. Postoperative lateral radiograph showing Luque instrumentation in position using Drummond buttons and wires, which add stability to the osteotomy. A rectangle is usually used and is bent to the desired angle of correction at the time of insertion. The use of Drummond buttons avoids the necessity to invade the spinal canal, the insertion being done under local anesthesia.

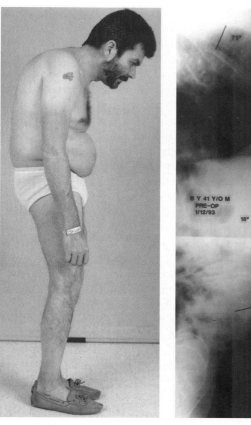
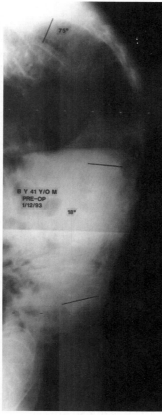
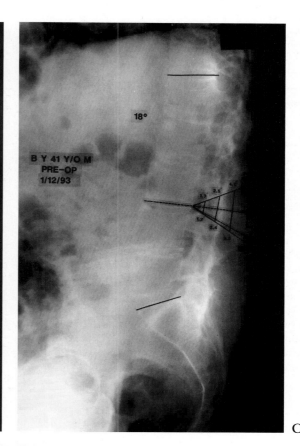

A,B

C

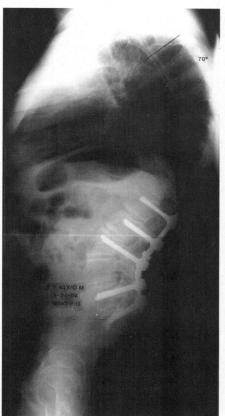
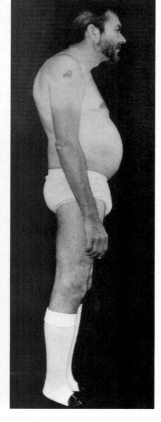

D,E

Figure 153.13. **A:** This 41-year-old man with a 21-year history of ankylosing spondylitis has had a major kyphotic deformity for 10 years, with a chin-brow-to-vertical angle measuring 55°. He has been unable to work for about 6 years. **B:** Lateral standing 3-foot radiograph of the spine shows a thoracic kyphosis of 75° and a decreased lumbar lordosis of 18°. The weight-bearing line is well anterior to the mid-lumbar spine. **C:** Preoperative lateral radiograph of the lumbar spine shows the planned resection/osteotomy of 50° to 55° located at L3–L4. **D:** This lateral standing 3-foot radiograph, taken 16 months postoperatively, shows the healed lumbar osteotomy with pedicle screw fixation and rods in place. The lumbar lordosis now measures 74°; the thoracic kyphosis is approximately 70° and the spine is in balance. The weight-bearing line is posterior to the osteotomy site. **E:** The patient 16 months after surgery. He returned to a normal lifestyle. (From White AH, Schofferman JA. *Spine Care: Operative Treatment,* vol.2. Philadelphia: Mosby, 1995:1678, with permission.)

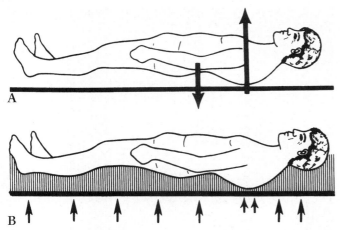

Figure 153.14. **A:** Lateral diagrammatic view showing the contour of the corrected spine when lying supine unsupported. The posteriorly projecting thoracic hump bears most of the weight, with less support on the lumbar spine and the spine below the osteotomy. As a result, the rigid thoracic hump tends to be displaced forward and the lumbar spine posteriorly. **B:** With the patient supine in a well-molded, rigid shell, equal support is created throughout the spine, with elimination of any uneven contact forces that would tend toward displacement.

posing the transverse processes of L-3 and L-4. Divide the autogenous bone removed during the resection into equal portions and place it posterolaterally on both sides, creating an adequate fusion mass.

■ Close the wound with suction drainage.
■ When the patient is still prone after wound closure, apply a well-molded posterior plastic shell, before transfer to a Roto-rest bed. The shell must be rigid and the contour of the spine must be maintained with adequate support under the pelvis, so that the rounded hump of the thoracic spine is not pushed forward in relation to the lumbar spine as the patient rests in the supine position (Fig. 153.14). The posterior shell is necessary to support the patient adequately when the Roto-rest trap door is removed for use of a bedpan.

Postoperative Care   Continue nasogastric suction until the patient is expelling flatus. About 7–10 days after surgery, when the patient is comfortable, he is lifted to an orthopaedic table in the posterior shell. Partly suspend the patient by the lower portion of the shell while the upper portion and sides are trimmed away, and then immobilize him in a well-molded plaster jacket. Take care in transferring and supporting him during application of the jacket, to avoid any loss of position.

Results and Complications   This technique, with Luque instrumentation and performed under local anesthesia, was used in 100 patients between 1969 and 1993 without

major intraoperative difficulty. Satisfactory correction was achieved, with restoration of normal functional alignment. There were no major respiratory complications and there was no pneumonitis in the series. Three nonunions occurred, one in a patient without internal fixation who subsequently responded to posterior instrumentation and fusion. In one patient, the fusion site appeared to be united, but a fracture of the osteotomy site was sustained in an automobile accident, requiring anterior strut-grafting. In a third patient who had severe osteopenia, union was not achieved and subsequent anterior strut-grafting with allograft and autogenous bone was performed.

One female patient who was on oral contraceptives suffered a sudden fatal pulmonary embolism 15 days after surgery, at which time she had been ambulatory in a plaster jacket. Eight patients developed L-3 root or cauda equina compression within 2 to 14 days after surgery; all except two compressions occurred in patients in whom internal fixation with segmental instrumentation was not used. In one of these, the compression was thought to be vascular in nature—he was an obese patient (about 300 pounds) who developed vena caval compression from thrombosis with neural venous stasis.

Management problems contributing to other cases of compression included patients slipping during the course of turning on a Circoelectric frame, the removal of the trap door on a Roto-rest bed with the patient not supported in a posterior shell, and in one patient, manipulation on a table for cast application. In most of these, estimates of canal dimension had not been done and in retrospect were probably on the low side. In most of these patients, the osteoclasis occurred through the body of L-2 rather than through the disc space, and this would appear to be a risk factor.

In certain instances when the ossification at the disc is considerably greater than at the vertebral body, selected preliminary anterior L3–L4 disc division might be considered, but I have not done this. Patients who presented with these problems were promptly reexplored and further decompression was carried out (usually superiorly), with the spine stabilized by internal fixation in the form of Luque instrumentation and Drummond buttons. On the whole, this prompt treatment allowed satisfactory recovery.

In my experience, if the correction is complete and the weight-bearing line is shifted posterior to the osteotomy site, fusion will occur with a 97% success rate and the correction will be maintained. Our results using pedicle screw fixation under general anesthesia are equally good.

Resection–extension osteotomy of the lumbar spine is a reasonably safe, practical, and reliable procedure in this high-risk type of patient. This technique allows a greater degree of correction of purely lumbar spinal deformity, in that it produces more hyperextension at the osteotomy site than can be obtained with multiple anterior and posterior osteotomies using compression instrumentation (either

Harrington or Zielke) of the thoracolumbar spine. The range of osteotomy correction in our patients was from 40° to 104° (average, 56°). The preoperative chin-brow-to-vertical angle varied from 35° to 134° (the latter was in a patient with associated hip deformity), with an average of 60°. The postoperative chin-brow-to-vertical angle ranged from −5° to +15°, with an average of +15° (Fig. 153.11).

Alternative Approach to Lumbar Osteotomy and Stabilization

The technique presented in this section was contributed by Dr. Isadore Lieberman.

The "eggshell" closing wedge osteotomy is an alternative to the opening wedge technique just described. In this approach, carry out the dorsal osteotomy and decompression as described, but complete the anterior correction through the posterior approach by removing the vertebral pedicles, and by decancellating and collapsing the vertebral body to correct the sagittal alignment. Then stabilize corrected segments with a pedicle screw fixation construct.

- Position the patient prone as described, and use the routine midline longitudinal dorsal approach to the thoracic and thoracolumbar spine.
- Begin by removing the spinous processes and laminae over the L2–L3 interspace, cutting a wedge-shaped defect posteriorly.
- Isolate and remove the pedicles and transverse processes of L-2, carefully resecting the pedicles until they are flush with the back of the vertebral body.
- Working through the pedicles, use curets and pituitary rongeurs to break up and remove the cancellous bone from within the vertebral body.
- Use curved curets or a burr to remove cancellous bone from between the pedicles and along the dorsal cortex of the body.
- Take care not to breach the anterior cortical wall.
- Place pedicle screws at adjacent levels before attempting the final correction.
- Use a blunt impactor to fracture the posterolateral cortex of the body, then score the dorsal cortex with an osteotome and implode it into the vertebral body cavity, away from the thecal sack.
- Slowly hyperextend the operating table, or bring the patient's legs into extension to collapse the dorsal aspect of the vertebral body and close the dorsal osteotomy.
- Instrument the spine from L-4 to the thoracic spine and graft for fusion (Fig. 153.15).
- Place the patient in a molded thoracolumbosacral orthosis for 4–6 months after surgery.

KYPHOTIC DEFORMITY OF THE THORACIC SPINE

A degree of thoracic kyphosis is common in spinal deformity associated with ankylosing spondylitis. It is much less common for the only deformity or primary deformity to be in the thoracic region, requiring the correction to be confined to that area.

Patients with thoracic kyphosis can be classified into two groups (19,21,23). In the first group, the main or primary deformity is in the thoracic spine, but in addition there is a loss of lumbar lordosis. If the thoracic kyphosis is mild or moderate and the lumbar spine rigid and flattened, the overall deformity can be satisfactorily corrected by a compensatory osteotomy in the midlumbar spine. With sufficient extension of the lumbar spine, the thoracic kyphosis can be compensated for with restoration of spinal balance and a normal chin-brow-to-vertical angle.

Patients in the second group have thoracic kyphosis with normal or exaggerated cervical and lumbar lordosis. These patients require correction of the primary thoracic deformity. It is impossible to do this safely with a single major angular correction. Correction of purely thoracic deformity requires multiple anterior and posterior intervertebral osteotomies, instrumentation, and grafting.

Patients who have thoracic kyphosis with normal cervical and lumbar lordosis can be further subdivided into two subgroups, depending on the rigidity of the thoracic spine. In the first subgroup, with incomplete ossification of the thoracic spine or extensive areas of destructive spondylodiscitis, preliminary correction can be obtained by halo-dependent traction; this is followed by multiple posterior resection osteotomies and compression instrumentation with second-stage anterior resection of the areas of spondylodiscitis and the disc spaces, with supportive strut-grafting (Fig. 153.16).

The second and more common subgroup involves patients with rigid thoracic kyphosis and relatively complete ossification. These patients require a first-stage anterior transthoracic procedure.

Correction of Thoracic Kyphosis

- Approach the thoracic spine through a right-sided thoracotomy with removal of the rib at the level of the apex of the deformity in the midaxillary line.
- Reflect the pleura and resect the ossified disc spaces completely from right to left, anterior to the posterior longitudinal ligament. Thoroughly curet the disc spaces and pack them with autogenous bone, using portions of the removed rib supplemented by iliac crest bone where necessary.
- Apply halo-dependent traction after surgery.
- Perform the second-stage procedure about 7–10 days later using a posterior approach. Perform multiple V-shaped resection osteotomies at each level, resecting the

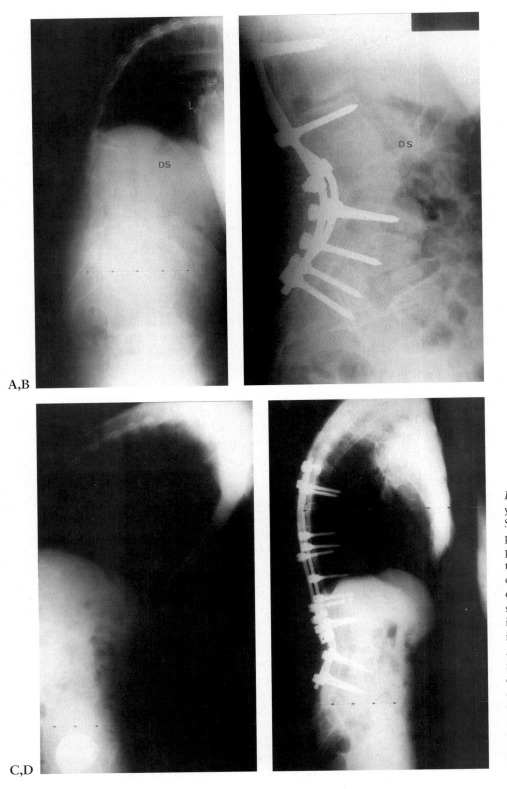

A,B

C,D

Figure 153.15.   **A:** Lateral view of a 50-year-old man with multilevel deformity. Severe cervical deformity was corrected prior to treating the thoracolumbar kyphosis. He also suffered from a persistent thoracolumbar pseudarthrosis. An L-2 decancellation and pedicle reduction osteotomy was carried out, fully correcting sagittal balance. **B:** Posterior segmental instrumentation and grafting provided immediate stability and a solid fusion. **C:** A 58-year-old man with severe, fixed deformity, localized primarily to the thoracolumbar junction. **D:** After "eggshell" osteotomy of L-2, posterior instrumentation was extended from the upper thoracic segments to L-5. Sagittal correction was excellent and well maintained. The patient's visual horizon was restored to normal.

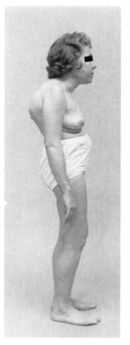
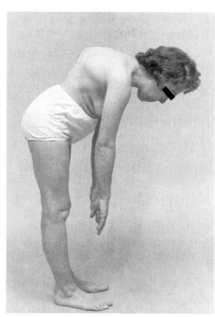
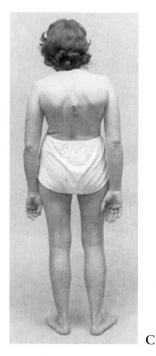

A,B   **C**

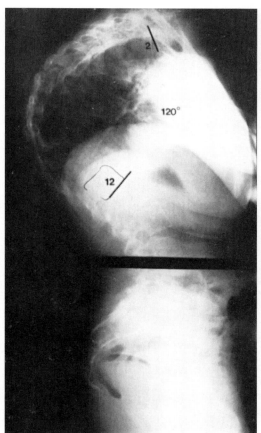
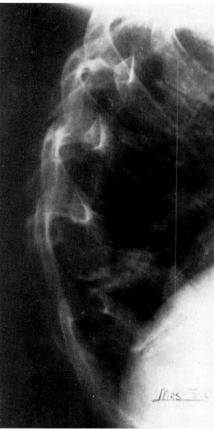

D,E

Figure 153.16. **A:** Lateral view of a 32-year-old woman with severe kyphosis confined to the thoracic region, associated with ankylosing spondylitis and steroid therapy. Patient had lost 6 inches in height, and her ribs impinged against the pelvis. **B:** Lateral bending view showing angular kyphotic deformity. **C:** Posterior view showing impending skin breakdown. **D:** Standing lateral radiograph showing thoracic kyphosis of 120° with increased lumbar lordosis. **E:** Lateral radiograph showing destructive spondylodiscitis at the apex of the thoracic deformity, indicating that it is likely to be flexible. The patient was treated with halo-dependent traction to reduce the main deformity, followed by posterior joint resections with bilateral Harrington compression instrumentation and fusion. *(continued)*

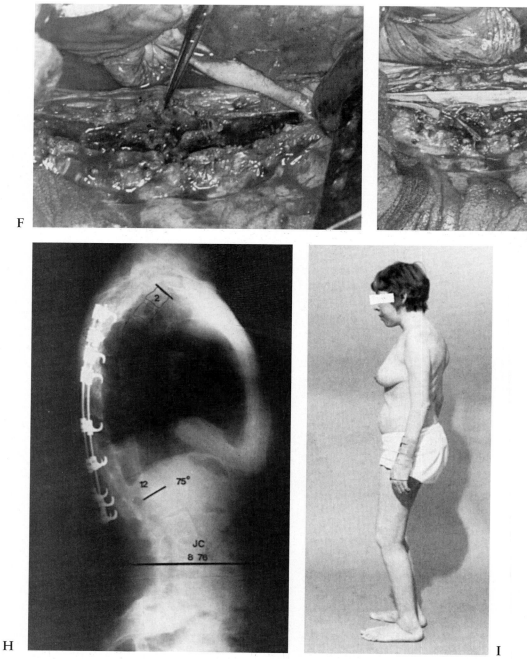

Figure 153.16.   (continued) **F:** Operative view at second-stage anterior procedure (following previous posterior instrumentation) showing resection of areas of spondylodiscitis with a trough prepared from T-6 to T-11 for a fibular strut graft. **G:** Operative view showing the fibular strut graft locked into the spine from T-6 to T-11 with onlay rib grafts. **H:** Postoperative standing lateral radiograph showing posterior Harrington compression instrumentation with fibular strut grafts supporting the spine anteriorly. **I:** Postoperative standing lateral view of the patient showing correction of the deformity. She had regained 5 inches in height.

ossified ligamentum flavum and adjacent portions of the laminae upward and outward on each side through the intervertebral foramen, removing enough bone to allow adequate correction following closure.

■ Apply bilateral segmental compression instrumentation, gradually closing the osteotomy sites and correcting the deformity (Fig. 153.17).

HINTS AND TRICKS

- Perform multiple osteotomies in the thoracic region so that correction at any one level is minimal, yet the cumulative effect allows substantial improvement.
- Anterior and posterior osteotomies with interval traction produce some of the correction while the patient is awake, reducing neurologic risk.
- Place the posterior instrumentation using spinal cord monitoring to allow reasonable correction in a critical area with greater safety.
- The technique of multiple, two-stage anterior and posterior osteotomies with posterior instrumentation is the obvious choice for primary thoracic deformity with a normal cervical and lumbar lordosis.
- Resection–extension osteotomy of the mid-lumbar spine is ideal for purely lumbar kyphosis with a normal or reduced thoracic kyphosis.

Despite the feasibility, multiple anterior and posterior osteotomies under general anesthesia in two procedures are more hazardous than a single-stage extension correction of the lumbar spine under local anesthesia. Tracheostomy, with its attendant problems, may be required in the management of patients with kyphotic deformity. However, where the primary deformity is thoracic with a normal lordosis above and below, these risks must be accepted if the deformity is to be corrected.

Although Harrington, Zielke, and Cotrel-Dubousset instrumentation systems have been used in the past, current segmental instrumentation systems offer more reliable correction and fixation. I favor the TSRH system, which provides a variety of pedicle-screw fixation options that allow the surgeon to tailor the instrumentation construct to the individual. Other systems are available that provide similar features. The surgeon should be well versed in the technical features of any selected instrumentation before undertaking this sort of reconstruction.

- In kyphosis procedures, place pedicle screws above and below the selected level before performing the osteotomy.

- Use fluoroscopy or plain radiography to confirm position and alignment during placement. I use spinal cord monitoring in all patients done under general anesthesia, and I stimulate the screws to confirm safe placement during instrumentation.
- After the osteotomy is completed, extend the patient's hips until the osteoclasis occurs, then place contoured fixation rods into the screws and fix them in place.
- Pack milled bone graft along the lateral gutters and across the osteotomy site. Place a well-molded plaster shell over the patient's back before rolling him off the operating table. This will prevent excessive pressure over the dorsal kyphosis in the immediate postoperative period, and it will be converted to a plaster cast when abdominal distension resolves.

KYPHOTIC DEFORMITY OF THE CERVICAL SPINE

In a few patients with ankylosing spondylitis, flexion deformity of the spine occurs primarily in the cervical region. This deformity can be severely disabling, with restriction of the field of vision, and it may progress to the point where it interferes with opening of the mouth. Surgical correction is fraught with hazard. Anecdotal reports of isolated attempts to correct this deformity under general anesthesia indicate a high rate of disastrous complications including death.

For the few severely afflicted patients with this type of deformity, it is important that the surgeon clearly understand the principles related to its possible correction and its indications. Over the past 30 years, I have routinely used a technique of correction under local anesthesia that has allowed a consistent, satisfactory, and somewhat dramatic correction with relative safety (3–5,7).

Diagnosis of Fracture

Not all patients with a "chin-on-chest" deformity in ankylosing spondylitis require cervical osteotomy, as the underlying problem is fracture. Those who present with a recent onset of a painful flexion deformity often do not require osteotomy, as, again, an underlying problem is fracture. In fact, any patient with ankylosing spondylitis whose spinal alignment has been relatively unchanged over time and who has had little pain, who then experiences painful, progressive flexion deformity after minor trauma, has a fracture of the cervical spine until proven otherwise. The fracture is usually at the base of the neck at the cervicothoracic junction. Unfortunately, the pain is often attributed to the patient's disease.

A fracture of the spine in ankylosing spondylitis resembles a fracture of an osteoporotic tubular bone, with a transverse shear pattern. The fracture is difficult to recog-

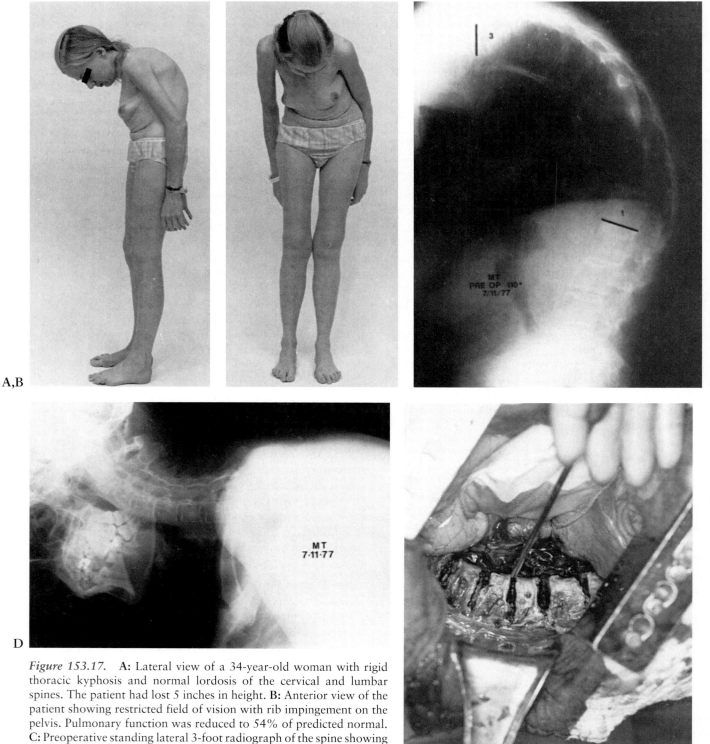

A,B

C

D

MT
7-11-77

E

Figure 153.17.   **A:** Lateral view of a 34-year-old woman with rigid thoracic kyphosis and normal lordosis of the cervical and lumbar spines. The patient had lost 5 inches in height. **B:** Anterior view of the patient showing restricted field of vision with rib impingement on the pelvis. Pulmonary function was reduced to 54% of predicted normal. **C:** Preoperative standing lateral 3-foot radiograph of the spine showing thoracic kyphosis of 110° with normal lumbar lordosis. **D:** Lateral radiograph of the cervical spine showing normal or increased cervical lordosis. **E:** Operative view showing anterior transthoracic resection of the ossified disc spaces completely through, from one side to the other. *(continued)*

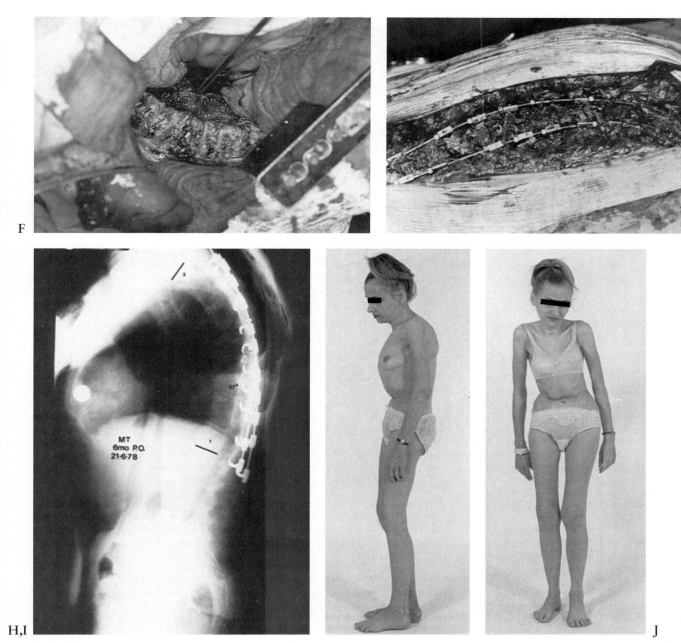

Figure 153.17. *(continued)* **F:** Operative view showing rib grafting of resected ossified disc spaces. **G:** Operative view showing multiple posterior V-shaped osteotomies, which were followed by bilateral posterior Harrington compression instrumentation with fusion. The ossified ligamentum flavum has been resected at each level, passing upward and laterally through the fused posterior joints. The margins are undercut before the compression instrumentation was performed. **H:** Postoperative lateral standing 3-foot radiograph showing correction of major deformity with restoration of normal spinal alignment. **I:** Postoperative lateral view of patient showing correction of the thoracic kyphosis with the ribs being lifted out of the pelvis. **J:** Postoperative anterior view of the patient showing restoration of normal field of vision.

nize radiographically, being obscured by the shoulders, and it may vary in its location from C-6 to T-2, although most commonly it is in the area of C-7 or T-1.

The fracture undergoes gradual erosion, causing compression and collapse anteriorly, with the chin approaching the chest. The patient is aware that the position of the head varies during the day, being more elevated on waking in the morning and dropping more toward the chest after being ambulatory during the day. The patient may hold the head with the hands to ease the distress.

It is important to diagnose this fracture using lateral tomography at the cervicothoracic junction. Patients with this fracture do not require cervical osteotomy. Apply a cranial halo and initiate traction along the line of the deformed neck. Then slowly restore normal alignment under careful observation until the head is restored to its normal functional position. It is usually possible to obtain a fairly normal chin-brow-to-vertical angle, after which place the patient in a well-molded halo cast for 4 months. The halo cast is essential: A halo vest does not provide adequate immobilization.

The craniocervical junction is the other area of the cervical spine where lesions may occur that cause painful flexion deformities. Destructive arthritis at the atlanto-occipital joint may cause the patient to flex the neck at this joint with the chin held downward, while the lateral radiograph of the cervical spine shows a relatively normal lordosis. Correct this by graduated halo traction to restore a normal chin-brow-to-vertical angle, followed by posterior stabilization, usually with occipitocervical fusion and, where necessary, excision of the posterior fragmented arch of C-1.

Cervical Osteotomy under Local Anesthesia

Unrecognized and untreated fractures at the base of the cervical spine ultimately heal, at which time the pain disappears, leaving the patient with a painless, fixed flexion deformity. At this stage, osteotomy is required for correction.

Of those patients for whom I have performed cervical osteotomy, 36% have shown evidence of previous cervical fracture. In 31%, the fracture contributed significantly to the spinal deformity. In only 15% of those who presented with evidence of fracture had the fracture been diagnosed previously. This experience underscores the fact that early recognition of the fracture and adequate immobilization are essential if the risk of further deformity is to be avoided.

Preoperative Considerations   Determine the amount of bone to be resected from preoperative radiographs. Measure the chin-brow-to-vertical angle and transpose it to a lateral radiograph of the cervical spine with the apex of the angle at the posterior margin of the C7–T1 disc space. A lateral tomogram probably will be necessary to show this clearly. Center the angle over the posterior arch of C-7. The amount of bone to be resected is determined from the radiograph with the angle superimposed over the spinous processes, the laminae, the posterior margin of the facet joints, and the posterior margin of the spinal canal at the level of the pedicles. The lines of resection are beveled upward at the superior margin and downward at the inferior margin. Following correction, the two surfaces will be parallel and in apposition.

One or two days before surgery, fit the patient with a rigid plaster or fiberglass body jacket incorporating the supports for the halo unit. The jacket must be rigid and made of a material that will not soften with body heat. It must be very skillfully contoured to the patient's trunk so that it cannot slide up or down. It must be molded under the rib cage and the sides of the chest to prevent it from going upward, and over the pelvis and iliac crests to prevent it from moving distally.

A commercial plastic halo jacket is inadequate for the postoperative immobilization required for these patients. In most instances, because the spine is completely solid above and below the area of osteotomy, a flexible jacket creates excessive forces that tend to cause movement at the osteotomy site with almost any activity. If the patient is not rigidly immobilized, he will have extreme distress when trying to get in or out of bed or to move about. Excessive mobility can even result in some neurologic compromise with irritation of the C-8 nerve root. Apply the jacket and test it carefully with the patient up and about to make certain that it is well contoured and secure; do this far enough before the surgery that there is time to make any necessary adjustments. Fit a halo to the skull preoperatively under local anesthesia in a stable position, below the maximum circumference of the skull.

Operative Technique   As Urist (27) has recommended, perform the operation under local anesthesia with the patient in the sitting position. Use a dental-type chair, so that the patient can be placed in a recumbent position if necessary. Having the patient awake avoids any major anesthetic hazards, and allows accurate monitoring of neurologic and other vital functions. The patient can assist with anatomic localization of the level during the decompression by indicating at any time any paresthesias or discomfort along the distribution of a cervical nerve root: This ability is of real value in confirming the location of the C-8 nerve root canal and the level of the root.

Perform the excision posteriorly with subsequent fracturing and extension of the spine at the cervicothoracic junction. The preferred level for correction is between C-7 and T-1 (Fig. 153.18), because, as Mason et al. (11) and Urist (27) have indicated, this interspace is more receptive to surgical treatment than any other level of the cervical region. The advantages are many:

- The spinal canal is relatively wide.
- The cervical cord and C-8 nerve root have reasonable mobility in this area.
- Any weakness caused by compromise of the C-8 nerve root results in less disability than with other roots.
- The vertebral artery and veins usually pass in front of the transverse process of C-7 and enter the transverse foramen at the sixth vertebra.
- The position of these vessels above the level of T-1 protects them from injury during osteotomy at the C7–T1 level (Fig. 153.19).

Use diazepam for preoperative sedation, with the exposure carried out posteriorly under local infiltration (1% lidocaine and epinephrine 1:200,000). Use fentanyl for supplementary analgesia during the procedure.

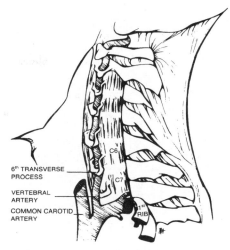

Figure 153.19. Lateral anatomic diagram showing the normal passage of the vertebral arteries and veins in front of the transverse process of the seventh vertebra, entering the transverse foramen at the sixth vertebra. (Simmons EH. Surgery of the Spine in Rheumatoid Arthritis and Ankylosing Spondylitis. In: Cruess RL, Mitchell NS, eds. *Surgery of Rheumatoid Arthritis.* Philadelphia: Lippincott, 1971, with permission.)

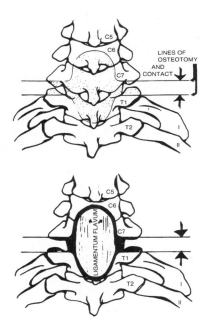

Figure 153.18. Diagrammatic posterior view of the area of resection for cervical osteotomy. Bevel the margins of the resection of the lateral fused joints slightly away from each other extending posteriorly, so that after correction the two surfaces are parallel and in apposition. Undercut the pedicles significantly to avoid impingement on the C-8 nerve roots. Bevel the midline resection on its deep surface above and below to avoid impingement against the dura after extension correction. (From Simmons EH. Surgery of the Spine in Rheumatoid Arthritis and Ankylosing Spondylitis. In: Cruess RL, Mitchell NS, eds. *Surgery of Rheumatoid Arthritis.* Philadelphia: Lippincott, 1971, with permission.)

■ Identify the last bifid spinous process, which is usually C-6. Compare the architecture of the lower cervical spinous processes using a lateral radiograph of the cervical spine. If you encounter any difficulty in anatomic localization, obtain radiographic confirmation of the level.

■ Remove the C-7 spinous process, the inferior spine of C-6, and the superior spine of T-1 in strips and preserve them for grafting. Remove the entire posterior arch of C-7 along with the inferior half of the arch of C-6 and the superior half of the arch of T-1 (Fig. 153.20).

■ Open the spinal canal. Protect the dura and spinal cord with cotton patties.

■ Extend the decompression laterally on each side beyond the lateral margin of the spinal cord to the level of the pedicles. Undercut the laminae above and below the decompression to avoid impingement following extension correction.

■ Identify the C-8 nerve root and pass a curved probe into its canal. The patient may be able to assist in confirmation of the level by indicating the distribution of any paresthesias associated with displacement of the root. Extend the resection through the fused area of the posterior joints of C7–T1, decompressing the C-8 nerve root completely.

■ Expose the inferior aspect of the pedicles of C-7 and the superior aspect of the pedicles of T-1.

■ Cut the pedicles through in a curved fashion away from the C-8 root, leaving a shell to protect the nerve root while the main bone is removed; the shell is removed

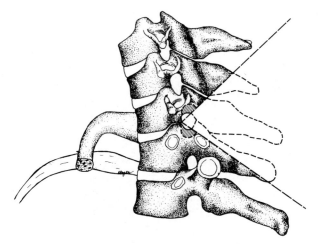

Figure 153.20. Lateral diagrammatic outline of the area of posterior resection at the C7–T1 level. The *shaded areas* represent where the pedicles are undercut to avoid nerve root impingement after extension correction.

at the completion of the nerve root decompression. This is done to undercut the pedicles above and below adequately, so that after the extension correction, there will be a bony recess for the eighth nerve root to avoid impingement or a pincer effect.

■ Follow the nerve root laterally, and remove all bone that could impinge on it.

■ Resect the lateral masses completely through from medial to lateral so that there is no remaining bridge of bone laterally that could interfere with extension correction (Fig. 153.21*A*).

■ Insert the deep closing sutures and a suction drain before the osteoclasis is done.

■ Have the anesthesiologist give supplemental oxygen during the procedure, either by nasal catheter or face mask. The patient is allowed to listen to music from a radio or tape recorder. This is an important part of the anesthetic management, along with a continuing, cheerful conversation between the anesthesiologist or an attendant and the patient. When this is done well, the amount of discomfort or concern expressed by the patient can be minimized.

■ Complete the decompression. The patient is given a small dose of a short-acting barbiturate, such as brevitol.

■ When the anesthesiologist indicates the sedation is effective, extend the neck by grasping the halo firmly and tilting the neck backward. An audible snap may be heard and a physical sense of fracture will be appreciated.

■ Extend the neck until resistance occurs. The lateral

masses can be palpated as they come together posteriorly on each side (Fig. 153.21*B*).

■ The patient is allowed to awaken almost instantly and can confirm normal neurologic function of the extremities.

■ Hold the head firmly in the corrected position while an assistant stabilizes it by connecting the anterior supports for the halo unit to the cast.

■ Avoid overcorrection, particularly in patients with a rigid cervical spine and no compensatory movement at the occipitocervical junction. The final position should effect a compromise for the patient between looking ahead for walking and being able to work at a desk (Fig. 153.22).

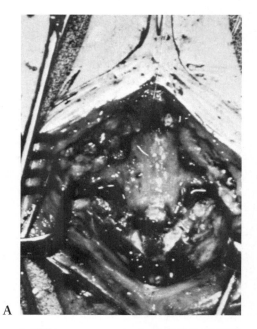

A

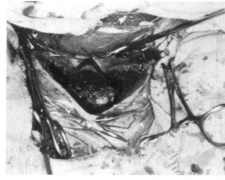

B

Figure 153.21. **A:** Posterior operative view showing midline decompression with resection of lateral masses, decompression of C-8 nerve roots, and undercutting of pedicles. **B:** Posterior operative view of wound after anterior osteoclasis and extension correction. The lateral masses have come together posteriorly on each side. The wound has been transformed from a vertical configuration to a transverse one.

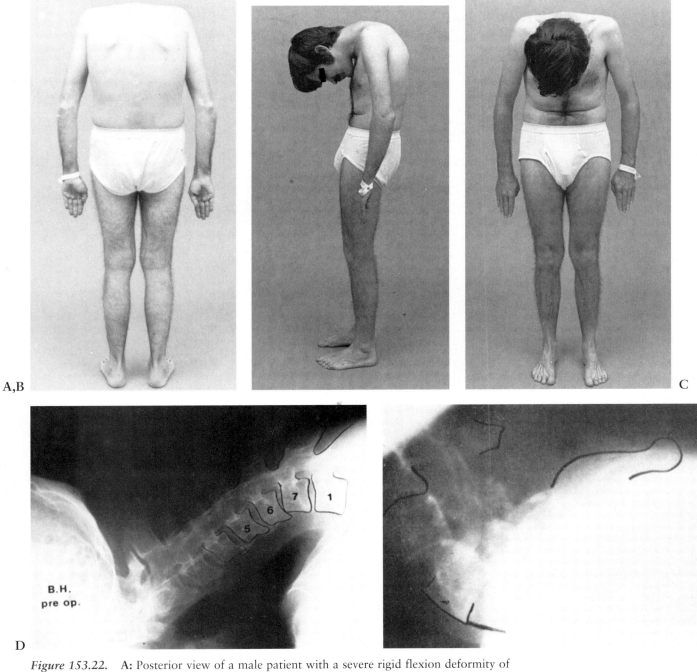

A,B

C

D

E

Figure 153.22. **A:** Posterior view of a male patient with a severe rigid flexion deformity of the cervical spine. His head is not visible from the posterior aspect. **B:** Lateral view of the patient showing marked restriction of the field of vision. His chin is rigidly fixed against his chest, interfering with his ability to open his mouth. **C:** Anterior view showing complete restriction of his field of vision. **D:** Lateral view of the cervical spine showing ossification of posterior joints with previous subluxation of C6–C7. **E:** Postoperative lateral radiograph of the cervical spine showing extension–resection osteotomy correction. *(continued)*

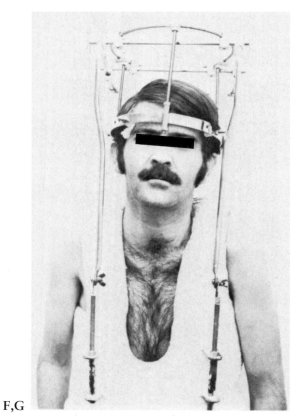
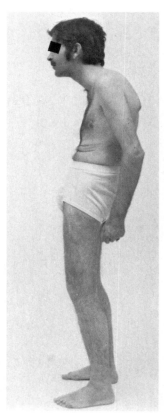
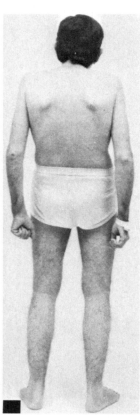

F,G   H

Figure 153.22. (continued) **F:** Postoperative anterior view of the patient in a halo cast, showing return of his normal field of vision. **G:** Postoperative lateral view of the patient after union of the osteotomy, demonstrating return of normal chin-brow-to-vertical angle. **H:** Postoperative posterior view of the patient demonstrating return of normal head–trunk configuration.

- Place the bone that has been removed during the course of the decompression posterolaterally on both sides over the apposed lateral masses; do not place it in the midline over the exposed dura.
- Tie the deep sutures after extension correction, and complete the wound closure.

Excessive force is not required to straighten the neck if there has been an adequate and complete decompression posteriorly. If the spine does not fracture readily, check to be sure there is not a bridge of bone remaining laterally and that the correct level has been operated on.

Although full correction is usually obtained at the initial procedure, correction of a severe deformity is sometimes limited by tightness of the anterior musculature, or by the patient's apprehension that the deformity is going to be overcorrected. In this case, most of the correction can be established at the time of surgery, with further correction added 7–10 days later by adjustment of the halo-jacket. By this time, the soft tissues will have had an opportunity to stretch and the patient will have had an opportunity to assess the amount of correction that has been achieved. With the patient supine under diazepam and fentanyl sedation, the head may be supported by the surgeon, and the attachments for the halo released, and the neck allowed to extend to obtain full correction.

Postoperative Care   Place the patient on a circo-electric bed during the immediate postoperative period. It allows the patient to be brought to a vertical position fairly easily, to stand and walk about and then return to the recumbent position without difficulty. When sufficiently mobile to get in and out of a regular bed, the patient is transferred to a hospital bed with or without a trapeze attachment.

Immobilize the patient in a halo cast for 4 months, then remove the cast and perform careful radiographic studies, including lateral tomography centered at C7–T1. When there is radiographic evidence of union and clinical evidence of stability and no pain, remove the halo. Have the patient wear a skull-occiput-mandibular immobilizer (SOMI) brace for at least 2 more months or until it is certain that there is solid union, clinically and radiographically.

Results and Complications I have used this technique consistently without any major deviations over the past 20 years in a total of 130 patients. The results have been exceedingly satisfactory, with a minimum of complications, considering the nature of the deformity and the associated disease process. Nonunion occurred in four patients (3%). Three of these responded to anterior cervical fusion at the C7–T1 level with an iliac crest graft. The fourth patient required not only anterior cervical fusion, but also posterior segmental instrumentation and fusion to obtain solid union. Transient neurologic complaints occurred in 16 patients, including 13 patients with transient C-8 paresthesias, one with Horner's syndrome, one with mild central cord syndrome 2 weeks after surgery, and one with transient paresis of the ninth and tenth cranial nerves thought to be secondary to traction. All of these cleared spontaneously without treatment. Five other patients had persistent C-8 nerve root deficits; one of these underwent further decompression, with subsequent improvement. All improved with minimal residual signs and no gross functional handicap.

There has been no major permanent injury to the spinal cord. One dramatic intraoperative experience demonstrates the necessity for surgery performed under local anesthesia. A 70-year-old man had a severe flexion deformity accentuated by an unrecognized fracture that had healed in such a way that his chin rested on his chest. On posterior decompression, dense scarring was noted about the dura related to the previous fracture. As the spine was decompressed in the midline, the patient suffered increasing weakness of his lower limbs and had difficulty with speech.

The dura was exceedingly tense with dense scarring about it. In view of this tension, it was split longitudinally down to the arachnoid. As this was done, there was an immediate, dramatic return of neurologic function in the lower extremities, and the patient's speech returned to normal. The operation was continued and as the decompression was being completed on both sides, he again developed weakness of his lower extremities. The remaining exposed dura was split further distally, again with immediate recovery of neurologic function. The operation was completed without any further difficulty and the patient went on to a satisfactory result without neurologic deficit.

This observation is in keeping with McKenzie and Dewar's report (13) describing the results of laminectomy for cord compression associated with kyphoscoliosis. They related the compressive effect of the dura to the kyphosis and recommended that the dura be split both longitudinally and transversely. Surgeons undertaking this type of surgery should be familiar with this recommendation. If this problem should occur during surgery, adequate splitting of the dura should be done longitudinally and transversely. When incising the dura, take care not to violate the arachnoid; cerebrospinal fluid leakage is thus avoided. If leakage should occur, it can be stopped with a sheet of Gelfoam or a free fat graft.

No major intraoperative problems were noted immediately following the osteoclasis. However, a sudden cardiac arrest occurred in one patient toward the end of the decompression. The chair was flattened and the patient responded to resuscitation without late sequelae. The cause of this arrest remains unknown. Air embolism was considered, but aspiration of the heart showed negative for it. Air embolism is a possibility with surgery in the sitting position, and a doplar is now routinely used over the chest and care is taken to control venous bleeding.

One 79-year-old woman suffered a fatal pulmonary embolism 21 days after surgery; her lungs showed multiple previous areas of subclinical embolism. Another patient suffered a fatal pulmonary embolism before the osteotomy was done. Autopsy revealed multiple thrombi in his leg veins, with evidence of previous pulmonary infarctions. Other complications have been related to the age of the patient and associated disease processes, including one nonfatal pulmonary embolism, a perforated peptic ulcer, and myocardial infarction.

Considering the age and medical risk factors of these patients, the results and complication rates compare favorably with any other type of major reconstructive procedure in a similar group of patients with the same disease process. These patients have an increased tendency for peptic ulceration. Considering the lethal nature of any intra-abdominal catastrophe in these patients, who breathe entirely with the diaphragm, I now place all patients routinely on cimetidine.

In this series of patients the average desired angle of correction was 60°. In 15 patients, cervical osteotomy was combined with lumbar osteotomy for major deformity in both areas; the procedures were performed either on separate admissions or during the same hospitalization. When you plan to repair severe deformity in both areas during the same admission, do the cervical osteotomy first, followed by lumbar osteotomy 1–2 weeks later. Both procedures are done under local anesthesia (Fig. 153.23).

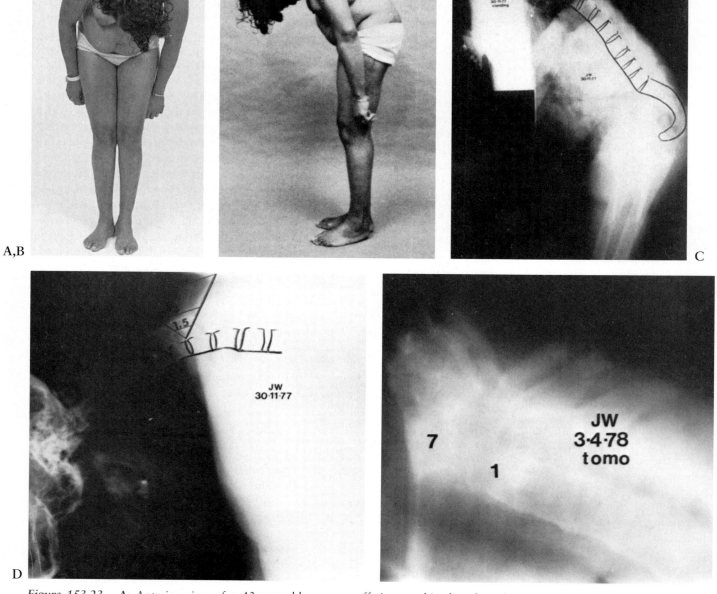

Figure 153.23.   **A:** Anterior view of a 43-year-old woman suffering combined neck and lumbar flexion deformities with severe restriction of field of vision. She had suffered arthritic disease since her teens. **B:** Lateral view demonstrating severe flexion deformity of the cervical spine combined with flexion deformity of the lumbar spine. Patient had undergone total hip replacement arthroplasties with some residual hip flexion deformity. **C:** Composite lateral radiograph showing combined neck and lumbar flexion deformities. **D:** Lateral radiograph of the cervicothoracic spine showing the plan of the extension osteotomy. **E:** Postoperative lateral tomogram showing resection–extension osteotomy at C7–T1. *(continued)*

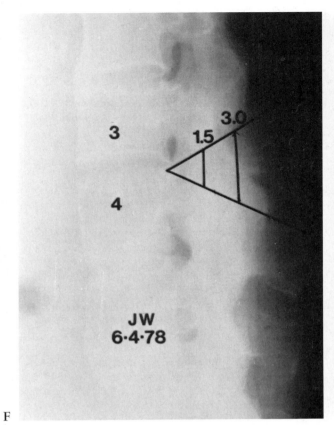

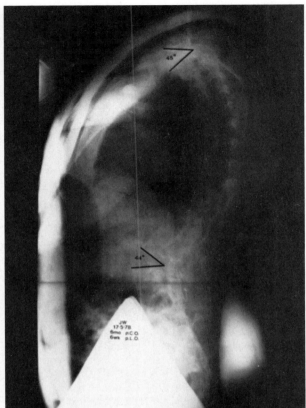

F

G

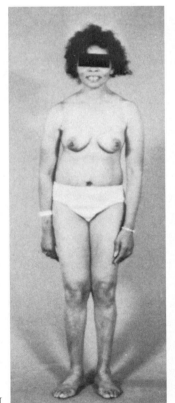

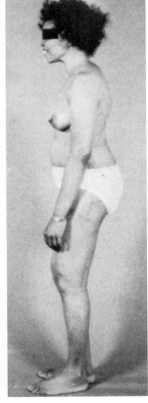

H,I

Figure 153.23. *(continued)* **F:** Planned resection–extension osteotomy of the flattened lumbar spine, which was performed 6 weeks after cervical osteotomy. Both procedures were performed under local anesthesia. **G:** Standing lateral 3-foot radiograph of the spine showing cervical and lumbar extension osteotomies. The weight-bearing line is shifted posterior to the lumbar osteotomy site. **H:** Postoperative anterior view demonstrating normal field of vision. **I:** Postoperative lateral view showing complete correction of spinal deformities with restoration of normal chin-brow-to-vertical angle.

REFERENCES

Each reference is categorized according to the following scheme: *, classic article; #, review article; !, basic research article; and +, clinical results/outcome study.

+ 1. Adams JC. Technique, Dangers and Safeguards in Osteotomy of the Spine. *J Bone Joint Surg Br* 1952;34:226.

* 2. Andersson O. Rontgenbilden vid Spondylarthritis Ankylopoetica. *Nord Med* 1937;14:2000.

3. Bland JH. Rheumatoid Arthritis of the Cervical Spine. *J Rheumatol* 1974;3:319.

+ 4. Conlon PW, Isdale IC, Rose BS. Rheumatoid Arthritis in the Cervical Spine: An Analysis of 333 Cases. *Ann Rheumatol Dis* 1966;25:120.

+ 5. Davey JR, Rorabeck CH, Bailey SI, et al. A Technique of Posterior Cervical Fusion for Instability of the Cervical Spine. *Spine* 1985;10:722.

+ 6. Fang HSY, Ong GB. Direct Approach to the Upper Cervical Spine. *J Bone Joint Surg Am* 1962;44:1588.

+ 7. Gilsbach J. Transoral Operations for Craniospinal Malformations. *Neurosurg Rev* 1983;6:199.

* 8. Harris RI. New Investigations: Instrument for Tightening Knots in Steel Wire. *Lancet* 1944;1:504.

+ 9. Little H, Urowitz MB, Smythe HA, et al. Asymptomatic Spondylodiscitis: An Unusual Feature of Ankylosing Spondylitis. *Arthritis Rheum* 1974;17:487.

+ 10. Martel W, Duff IF, Preston RE, et al. The Cervical Spine and Rheumatoid Arthritis: Correlation of Radiographic Clinical Manifestations (abstr.). *Arthritis Rheum* 1964; 7:326.

+ 11. Mason CC, Cozen L, Adelstein L. Surgical Correction of Flexion Deformity of the Cervical Spine. *Calif Med* 1953;7:244.

+ 12. McGraw RW, Rusch RM. Atlanto-Axial Arthrodesis. *J Bone Joint Surg Br* 1973;55:482.

+ 13. McKenzie KG, Dewar FP. Scoliosis with Paraplegia. *J Bone Joint Surg Br* 1949;31:162.

+ 14. Pasztor E. Transoral Approach for Epidural Cranio-Cervical Pathological Processes. *Adv Tech Stand Neurosurg* 1985;12:125.

+ 15. Pellicci PM, Ranawat CS, Tsarairis P, et al. Progression of Rheumatoid Arthritis of the Cervical Spine. *J Bone Joint Surg Am* 1981;63:342.

+ 16. Ranawat CS, O'Leary P, Pellicci PM, et al. Cervical Spine Fusion in Rheumatoid Arthritis. *J Bone Joint Surg Am* 1979;61:1003.

+ 17. Rosen PS, Graham DC. Ankylosing Spondylitis: A Clinical Review of 128 Cases. *Arch Int Am Rheumatol* 1962; 5:158.

+ 18. Scuhlitz KP. Destruktive Veranderungen an Wirbelkorpern bei der Spondylarthritis Ankylopoetica. *Arch Orthop Unfall Chir* 1968;64:116.

19. Simmons EH. Surgery of Rheumatoid Arthritis. In: *Surgery of the Spine in Rheumatoid Arthritis and Ankylosing Spondylitis*. Philadelphia: Lippincott, 1971.

+ 20. Simmons EH. The Surgical Correction of Flexion Deformity of the Cervical Spine in Ankylosing Spondylitis. *Clin Orthop* 1972;86:132.

+ 21. Simmons EH. Kyphotic Deformity of the Spine in Ankylosing Spondylitis. *Clin Orthop* 1977;128:65.

22. Simmons EH. Alternatives in the Surgical Stabilization of the Upper Cervical Spine. In: Tator CH, ed. *Early Management of Acute Spinal Cord Injury*. New York: Raven Press, 1982.

23. Simmons EH. Surgery of the Spine in Rheumatoid Arthritis and Ankylosing Spondylitis. In: Evarts CM, ed. *Surgery of the Musculoskeletal System*, vol. 2. New York: Churchill-Livingstone, 1983.

+ 24. Simmons EH, Bhalla SK. Anterior Cervical Discectomy and Fusion (Keystone Technique). *J Bone Joint Surg Br* 1969;51:225.

+ 25. Simmons EH, Fielding JW. Atlanto-Axial Arthrodesis. *J Bone Joint Surg Am* 1967;49:1022.

* 26. Smith-Petersen MN, Larson CB, Aufranc OE. Osteotomy of the Spine for Correction of Flexion Deformity in Rheumatoid Arthritis. *J Bone Joint Surg* 1945;27:1.

* 27. Urist MR. Osteotomy of the Cervical Spine: Report of a Case of Ankylosing Rheumatoid Spondylitis. *J Bone Joint Surg Am* 1958;40:833.

+ 28. Wills DG. Anesthetic Management of Posterior Lumbar Osteotomy. *Can Anesth Soc J* 1985;83:248.

## CHAPTER 154

RHEUMATOID ARTHRITIS OF THE CERVICAL SPINE

Robert A. Hart and Charles R. Clark

Rheumatoid involvement of the articulations of the cervical spine is extremely common among patients with rheumatoid arthritis. Estimates of frequency vary. Conlon et al. (16) documented radiographic changes in the cervical spine for 85% (283 of 333) of patients with classic rheumatoid arthritis. While the majority of such patients do not develop significant neurologic deficits, identification of those at high risk of neurologic compromise remains a difficult clinical problem.

The three primary patterns of instability due to rheumatoid involvement of the cervical spine are referred to as atlantoaxial instability, cranial settling, and subaxial instability. Clinically relevant radiographic measurements associated with the risk of neurologic compromise have been described for these instability patterns (4). In addi-

tion, advanced radiographic techniques such as magnetic resonance imaging (MRI) allow a more precise determination of spinal cord compression.

Surgical indications have historically included significant neurologic compromise, intractable pain, or both. As the concept of impending neurologic compromise has been defined, the selection of patients at risk for neurologic injury for surgical stabilization has also improved. Given the uncertainty of recovery once significant neurologic deficits are present, early stabilization of the unstable rheumatoid spine appears to improve the outcome for these patients. In addition, continued developments of surgical and anesthetic techniques have facilitated their management.

PATHOPHYSIOLOGY

The involvement of synovial articulations by rheumatoid arthritis is well described. The response to immune com-

R. A. Hart: Department of Orthopaedic Surgery, Division of Spine Surgery, Oregon Health Sciences University, Portland, Oregon, 97201.
C. R. Clark: Departments of Orthopaedic Surgery and Bioengineering, University of Iowa Hospitals and Clinics, Iowa City, Iowa, 52242.

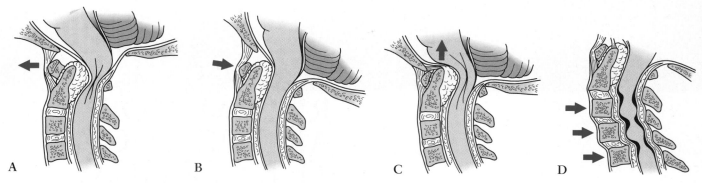

Figure 154.1. Patterns of cervical spine instability due to rheumatoid arthritis. **A,B:** Atlantoaxial instability. **C:** Cranial settling. **D:** Subaxial instability.

plex (IgG and antibodies to IgG) deposits in the articular cartilage and synovium of involved joints includes proliferation of fibrovascular tissue, known as pannus. Examination of these tissues shows the presence of chronic and acute-phase inflammatory cells, including lymphocytes, plasma cells, and macrophages. The persistent inflammation leads to cartilage loss and bony erosion, as well as ligamentous laxity. In addition, the rheumatoid disease process per se leads to diffuse osteopenia. Chronic steroid use may contribute to these ligamentous and osseous changes as well.

The cervical spine is susceptible to involvement with rheumatoid arthritis because of the large number of articulations and their significant mobility. The subaxial facet joints and intervertebral discs as well as the ligaments and bursae of the cervical spine are all potential locations of involvement (10,25). The most common clinical involvement, however, includes the atlanto-occipital, the atlantoaxial, the periodontoidal, and the zygoapophyseal (facet) joints.

Historically, the patterns of instability described in rheumatoid patients are anterior atlantoaxial instability, cranial settling, and subaxial instability (Fig. 154.1) (16, 43,54). In addition to these patterns, other observed instability types have included posterior instability of the atlas, subaxial dislocation, and rotation and lateral subluxation of the atlas (5,26,42,45–46,50,57,60).

The primary concern with all patterns of cervical involvement is the development of neurologic compromise due to compression of the spinal cord and nerve roots. This compression can arise as a dynamic phenomenon due to the instability, or it can be secondary to a mass effect caused by fixed vertebral subluxations or pannus formation. In addition, deficits can arise that are attributable to compromise of vascular supply at the level of either the anterior and posterior spinal arteries or the vertebral arteries themselves (19,21,56).

Patterns of neurologic involvement can include radiculopathy, myelopathy, and cranial nerve compromise. The most common radicular complaint is suboccipital headache due to irritation of the second cervical nerve root by atlantoaxial degeneration or instability (14,43). Radiculopathy can also produce motor weakness due to disc collapse or instability in the subaxial spine. The symptoms of myelopathy are hyperreflexia and spasticity, with or without motor weakness. The Ranawat classification of neurologic compromise has been widely used in published reports of rheumatoid patients. Normal patients are considered grade I, patients with paresthesias and hyperreflexia but without motor weakness are grade II, and patients who demonstrate motor weakness constitute grade III. Grade IIIA describes ambulatory patients, and grade IIIB is used for nonambulatory patients (43).

Motor compromise resulting from spinal cord involvement may be asymmetric, and it may show greater involvement of the upper extremities. Cruciate paralysis (of Bell) develops in some patients, with a striking lack of weakness in the lower extremities but profound involvement of the upper extremities due to medullary compression at the pyramidal decussation of upper extremity motor fibers (3, 65). Cranial nerves, particularly the lower cranial nerves such as cranial nerve IX (involving the gag reflex), can also be compromised, especially in patients with cranial settling. Finally, respiratory paralysis may also occur with upper cervical involvement, sometimes with fatal results (16).

DIAGNOSTIC EVALUATION

Neurologic examination of patients with rheumatoid arthritis can be notoriously difficult because of the effects of extremity contracture, deformity, pain, and inflammation, as well as weakness from muscle wasting and mechanical loss of function. A high index of suspicion in patients complaining of neck and occipital pain or new extremity weakness or loss of function is therefore important. Descriptions of an electric shock sensation with head and neck motion (Lhermitte's sign) should also arouse suspicion.

Begin diagnostic imaging with cervical spine plain radiographs, including an open-mouth odontoid view and lateral flexion–extension views. These films may disclose osteopenia, erosion of the atlantoaxial and subaxial facet joints, or erosion of the odontoid process itself. While plain radiographs do not directly demonstrate synovial pannus or spinal cord compression, much indirect information may be gained, such as the presence of bony instability.

Atlantoaxial instability is measured from lateral flexion–extension cervical spine radiographs. Historically, instability was measured as the change in the anterior atlantodental interval (AADI) (Fig. 154.2). Posterior displacement greater than 3 mm of the dens relative to the anterior ring of the atlas is considered abnormal. Displacement ranging from 6 to 10 mm has been considered an indication for surgery, even in patients without neurologic abnormalities (14,15,27,43,51).

A better radiographic measurement for predicting spinal cord compromise due to atlantoaxial instability is the posterior atlantodental interval (PADI). Also referred to as the space available to the cord, the PADI is measured from the posterior aspect of the dens to the anterior edge of the posterior ring of the atlas, along the transverse axis of the ring of the atlas (Fig. 154.2). Boden et al. (4) demonstrated that a PADI of less than 14 mm correlated with a significant risk of neurologic impairment, and that the PADI was a better predictor of not only the development of neurologic compromise but also the potential for neurologic recovery.

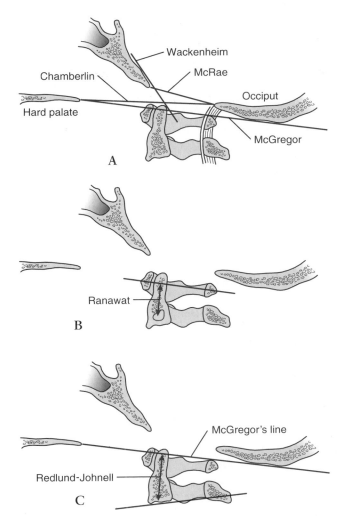

Figure 154.3. Measures of cranial settling. **A:** Radiographic landmarks of the craniocervical junction. Chamberlain's line extends from the posterior foramen magnum to the hard palate. Wackenheim's line is a tangent to the cranial surface of the clivus. McGregor's line extends from the lowest point of the occiput to the hard palate. McRae's line extends between the basion and the posterior edge of the foramen magnum. **B:** Ranawat's measure of cranial settling extends from the center of the pedicle of the second cervical vertebra to the transverse plane of the ring of the atlas. **C:** The Redlund-Johnell method measures the distance from the base of the axis to McGregor's line.

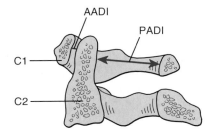

Figure 154.2. Measures of atlantoaxial instability. The anterior atlantodental interval (AADI) measures mobility between the anterior ring of C-1 and the dens. The posterior atlantodental interval (PADI) also measures this mobility but also directly measures the space available to the spinal cord. The PADI has been shown to more accurately predict neurologic impairment than the AADI.

Numerous landmarks for measurement of cranial settling have been described (Fig. 154.3A). Chamberlain's line runs from the posterior foramen magnum to the hard palate. Wackenheim's line is drawn tangent to the cranial surface of the clivus. McGregor's line runs from the lowest point of the occiput to the hard palate. McRae's line extends between the basion and the posterior edge of the foramen magnum. For the projection of the dens above

McGregor's line, 4.5 mm is considered the upper limit of normal (12,20).

Ranawat et al. (43) proposed a measurement from the center of the pedicle of the second cervical vertebra to the transverse axis of the ring of the atlas (Fig. 154.3B). They found normative values for this distance of 17 mm in men and 15 mm in women. This measurement has the advantage that visualization of the dens and skull base is not required.

Redlund-Johnell and Patterson (46) measured the distance from the base of the axis to McGregor's line (Fig. 154.3C). Less than 34 mm in men or 29 mm in women indicates cranial settling. The Sakaguchi-Kauppi method involves determination of the station of the medial aspect of the superior facet of the axis relative to the anterior ring of the atlas. These authors (29) felt that their method was easier to apply than the Redlund-Johnell method, and that it had the advantage of not relying on visualization of the skull base or odontoid tip.

Computerized tomography (CT) evaluation of the cervical spine provides excellent detail of the bony structures. Erosion of the dens and facet joints is much better demonstrated on CT images than on plain radiographs (6). In addition, fractures of the dens may be diagnosed with this modality.

Sagittal reconstructions based on CT scans are important not only diagnostically, but also in some cases for surgical planning. Posterior atlantoaxial arthrodesis using transarticular screws requires sufficient width of the cervical two-vertebral isthmus to allow passage of a 3.5 mm screw (35). In addition, sclerosis and erosion of the posterior ring of the atlas may result in insufficient bone stock for arthrodesis with conventional atlantoaxial wiring techniques and thereby require atlantoaxial screw fixation or extension of the arthrodesis to the occiput (14). There can be problems even with these techniques, however, when there is significant bone loss.

Magnetic resonance imaging has become the best imaging modality for evaluation of neurologic compression; use it to evaluate any patient who has neurologic weakness or spasticity (7,30,31). MRI provides enhanced definition of soft tissues and can demonstrate spinal cord compression from pannus at the atlantodental articulation. Recently, use of dynamic flexion–extension MRI views has been recommended for preoperative planning in patients with neurologic compromise (34). Patients for whom neurologic compression is not relieved by maximal reduction of the atlantodental articulation may be candidates for posterior decompression either by removal of the posterior rim of the foramen magnum and laminectomy of the atlas, or by anterior resection of the odontoid.

Sensory impairment in patients with rheumatoid arthritis has been demonstrated with somatosensory evoked potentials and cutaneous electric stimulation, both peripherally and in the trigeminal nerve distribution (58). While such techniques may confirm neurologic impairment, they are not widely used by orthopaedic surgeons or neurosurgeons for diagnosis or treatment planning, although they may have expanded roles in the future.

NATURAL HISTORY

It is clear that as a direct result of cervical spinal instability, some patients with rheumatoid arthritis develop severe neurologic impairment with profound motor deficits, occasionally leading to respiratory paralysis and death. It is also clear that once neurologic deficits develop, there is no universally successful means of regaining lost function. Unfortunately, our understanding of which factors predict neurologic progression remains incomplete (12).

Several investigations of the natural history of rheumatoid involvement of the cervical spine have been reported (16,40,43,51,52,55,62,63). Conlon et al. (16) provided an early estimate of the incidence of cervical instability among an unselected group of 333 rheumatoid patients. Plain radiographs disclosed atlantoaxial subluxation in 84 (25%) of their patients, while an additional 23 (7%) demonstrated subaxial subluxation. Although cervical instability was statistically correlated with the severity of peripheral disease, no correlation was found with duration of disease or use of steroid medications. Although 23 patients (7%) demonstrated symptoms of spasticity, the authors did not feel that these findings correlated with the presence of cervical instability.

Smith et al. (55) reviewed 130 rheumatoid arthritis patients with significant atlantoaxial instability but without neurologic compromise at the time of initial radiographs. They reevaluated 84 surviving patients an average of 7.8 years after the initial examination. Four patients (3%) had developed spinal cord compromise, while an additional six (5%) described symptoms of transient weakness. Of the 84 (74%) surviving patients, 62 had been maintained on chronic oral steroid medication, which appeared to correlate with radiographic progression of instability. No effect of cervical instability on long-term survival could be demonstrated.

Winfield et al. (62,63) followed 100 patients prospectively with annual flexion–extension radiographs. Over an average of 7 years' follow-up, they documented that 12 patients (12%) developed atlantoaxial instability, 8% developed subaxial instability, and 3% developed cranial settling. All the patients who developed instability demonstrated onset of subluxations within 2 years of diagnosis with rheumatoid arthritis. By an average of 9 years and 5 months' follow-up, one patient had developed myelopathy and two had undergone posterior cervical fusion for severe occipital headache (3%). These authors also demonstrated a significant correlation between the presence of severe peripheral erosive disease and cervical spine involvement.

Santavirta et al. (51) described the progression of symptoms in 16 patients with 8 mm or greater atlantodental instability or cranial settling. They compared disease progression in these patients with a group of 18 surgically treated patients with a comparable degree of radiographic instability but more significant neurologic symptoms. Although this was not a randomized study, they found that none of the operatively treated group had worsening of their neurologic status, and 8 of 14 (57%) who had had preoperative neurologic deficits showed improvement. Postoperative complications were relatively minor. In the nonoperatively treated group, however, 7 of 14 surviving patients (50%) suffered neurologic worsening. A further report on this patient group documented progression of cranial settling in 12 untreated patients, three of whom developed neurologic progression (52).

Pellici et al. reported prospective data on 106 rheumatoid arthritis patients with initial complaints of cervical pain over a 5-year period (40). They noted neurologic progression in 27 of 85 surviving patients (36%) and ra-

diographic progression in 60 (80%). Seven patients had undergone surgical intervention by the end of the study secondary to severe neurologic involvement. Only two patients underwent spontaneous fusion of the atlantoaxial articulation, one of whom subsequently developed subaxial subluxations (Fig. 154.4). They also found that patients without radiographic changes at the time of their initial complaints did not develop significant instability over the 5 years of the study.

Boden et al. (4) described 73 patients followed for an average of 7 years, 42 of whom (58%) developed neurologic compromise. These authors demonstrated the importance of the PADI as a predictor for neurologic injury (Fig. 154.2). They noted that a reduction of the PADI below 14 mm, or a reduction of the spinal canal diameter below 14 mm in the subaxial cervical spine, was correlated with an increased prevalence of nonrecoverable neurologic deficit. They also demonstrated an increased risk of neurologic deficit in patients with atlantoaxial subluxation combined with cranial projection of the odontoid of 5 mm or greater above McGregor's line.

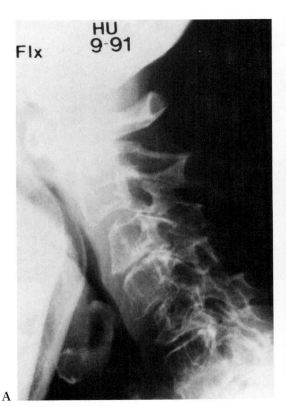
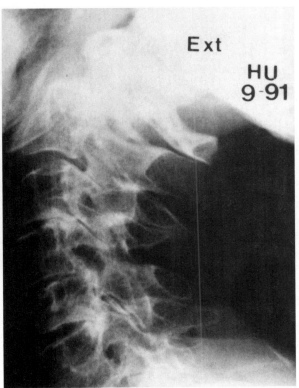

A

B

Figure 154.4.   An adverse natural history. **A,B:** Flexion–extension lateral radiographs obtained in 1991 demonstrate significant atlantoaxial instability, although the patient was neurologically normal. Significant erosion of the dens was already present, allowing posterior displacement of the ring of C-1 in extension. *(continued)*

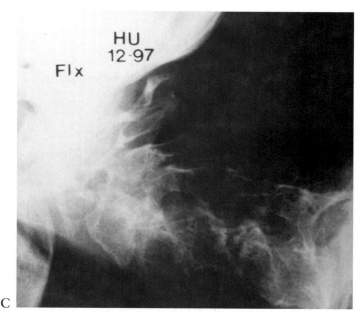

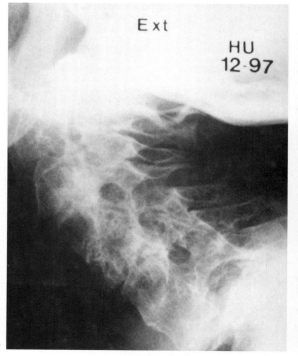

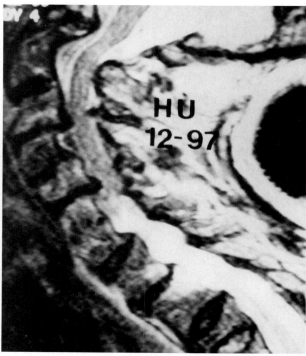

Figure 154.4. *(continued)* **C,D:** Six years later, a fixed posterior subluxation of C-1 has developed. Subaxial subluxation is also present. The patient at this time was quadriparetic and unable to ambulate (Ranawat IIIB). **E:** A sagittal view from an MRI scan demonstrates cord compression at both the atlantoaxial and subaxial levels. This patient would likely have benefited from an atlantoaxial arthrodesis at an earlier stage.

PERIOPERATIVE MANAGEMENT

Medical management of rheumatoid arthritis continues to improve. Many patients are now maintained on methotrexate or other nonsteroid medical regimens, with steroid use limited to short-duration bursts for flares of the rheumatoid disease. The effect of this shift in treatment patterns on the progression of cervical instability is not known.

Patients with rheumatoid arthritis who are scheduled for other operative procedures requiring general anesthetic should undergo cervical radiographic evaluation with dynamic flexion–extension lateral views. Patients with neck pain but without significant instability can be treated with pain medication and a cervical orthosis. While orthotics may provide symptomatic relief, they neither slow the disease process nor provide significant additional stability, and these patients should be followed for possible progression of their disease (1).

Airway and pulmonary management is a significant concern in surgical patients with rheumatoid arthritis. Patients undergoing multiple-level anterior cervical spine procedures and those with severe neurologic compromise should be considered for elective tracheostomy (27). If a tracheostomy is not likely to be necessary, patients may need to remain intubated postoperatively for an additional period of time. All other rheumatoid patients should be considered for fiberoptic intubation (14). This a good practice for all neurologically vulnerable patients, and a reduction in postoperative airway complications in rheumatoid patients undergoing fiberoptic intubation has been demonstrated (59).

Preoperative skull traction has been recommended for patients with cranial settling or subluxations that do not reduce on voluntary flexion–extension lateral radiographs. Traction for 24–48 hours has proven useful, with most reductions occurring within this time (38). Extended periods of traction probably do not improve reduction and should generally be avoided because of the preexisting physical weakness of many patients with rheumatoid arthritis and the rapid physical deterioration that occurs with extended bed rest. Halo-wheelchair traction provides traction while allowing the patient to be upright.

Postoperative immobilization must be tailored to the individual patient's needs. Historically, several means of immobilization have been used ranging from skull traction or a halo cast to a cervicothoracic or hard cervical orthosis (14,16,27,43,66). Halo-bracing is generally well tolerated by rheumatoid patients, perhaps because of their lower physical demands. The advantages of reducing the risks of hardware failure and nonunion in this patient population probably outweighs the easier mobility afforded by less aggressive bracing.

Evaluate the patient's suitability for cervical spine surgery before deciding on a specific surgical plan; pay attention to the patient's activity level, expectations, and overall health status. Preoperative evaluation should include pulmonary, cardiac, and renal testing. Patients with longstanding, severe neurologic injury and patients with limited pulmonary or cardiac reserve should be considered for nonoperative management.

OPERATIVE TREATMENT AND RESULTS

ATLANTOAXIAL ARTHRODESIS

Indications for atlantoaxial arthrodesis include neurologic compromise demonstrated by spasticity or motor weakness (Ranawat II or III), impending neurologic compromise as demonstrated by spinal cord compression on MRI or a PADI of 14 mm or less on plain films, and intractable occipital headache with demonstrated atlantoaxial degeneration or instability. If preoperative reduction in cranial traction is insufficient to allow spinal cord decompression, consider a laminectomy of the atlas, and enlargement of the foramen magnum as well, which usually requires extension of the arthrodesis to the occiput.

A number of methods of posterior atlantoaxial arthrodesis have been described. Historically, posterior wiring techniques have been very successful in other patient populations but have had significant nonunion rates in patients with rheumatoid arthritis. In addition, atlantoaxial wiring techniques require availability of the posterior ring of the atlas. Recently, the technique of transarticular screw fixation has improved fusion rates and can be performed with laminectomy of the posterior ring of the atlas. Risks of neurologic and vascular injury with this technique are still being evaluated, however, and it should not be used when reduction of the atlantoaxial facet joints cannot be achieved. A CT scan with sagittal reconstructions to evaluate the position of the vertebral arteries is a prerequisite for this technique.

Brooks and Jenkins (8) described their wedge compression method of bone grafting and sublaminar wiring as an alternative to Gallie's (22) midline wiring and demonstrated fusion in 12 of 13 patients (Fig. 154.5*A,B*). They had less success in patients with rheumatoid arthritis, however, describing one patient who developed nonunion and a second who suffered an intraoperative fracture and required extension of the arthrodesis to the occiput. Clark et al. (14) modified this technique by using a single, larger piece of corticocancellous bone graft (Fig. 154.5*C*). They reported a bony fusion rate of 75% in a series of 20 patients with rheumatoid arthritis, with an additional two patients achieving stable fibrous union (Fig. 154.6).

Bryan et al. (9) described the use of polymethylmethacrylate (PMMA) as part of a longer arthrodesis construct

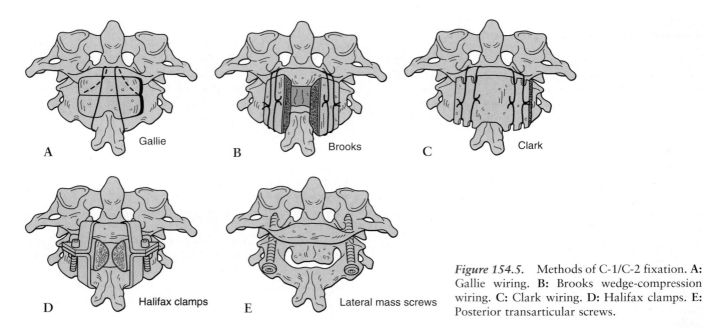

A Gallie   **B** Brooks   **C** Clark

D Halifax clamps   **E** Lateral mass screws

Figure 154.5. Methods of C-1/C-2 fixation. **A:** Gallie wiring. **B:** Brooks wedge-compression wiring. **C:** Clark wiring. **D:** Halifax clamps. **E:** Posterior transarticular screws.

from the atlas to the subaxial spine in a series of five patients with either prior nonunions (two patients) or combined atlantoaxial and subaxial subluxations (three patients). Two of these patients progressed to nonunion, and a third patient developed a wound infection and fistula. Because of this higher incidence of wound problems, as well as reports of bone lysis, PMMA is no longer recommended as a supplement to cervical fixation (37).

Moskovich and Crockard (39) described results with an interlaminar clamp in a series of 25 patients (Fig. 154.5D). While the overall fusion rate in this series was 80% (20 of 25), the rate for rheumatoid arthritis patients was only 73% (11 of 15). This technique thus seems to offer little improvement over wiring techniques with respect to fusion rate, although it may be neurologically safer than sublaminar wires for patients with severe stenosis.

Since Magerl and Seemann (36) described posterior transarticular screw placement for atlantoaxial stabilization and arthrodesis, this technique has been given increasing attention (Fig. 154.5E). Grob et al. (24) described their experience with transarticular 3.5 mm screws supplemented with midline wiring in a series of 161 patients, including 51 with rheumatoid arthritis. They achieved a 99.4% fusion rate at an average of 24 months. Although no symptomatic vertebral artery injuries were reported, there were five postoperative deaths, three in patients undergoing simultaneous transoral odontoid resection.

The issue of injury to the vertebral arteries or other structures due to screw malposition continues to be evaluated. Madawi et al. (35) reported an 87% fusion rate in

61 patients (37 rheumatoid patients) using transarticular screw fixation. They reported that 14% of screws were malpositioned with an 8% (5 of 61) rate of vertebral artery injury, although only one patient was symptomatic. These authors also described anatomic measurements on 25 cadaverous C-2 vertebrae, demonstrating an insufficient diameter of the pars interarticularis to accommodate a 3.5 mm screw in 20% of individuals. Recently published survey data from 847 neurosurgeons regarding 1,318 patients treated with transarticular screws revealed a rate of vertebral artery injury of 4.1%. Most arterial injuries were asymptomatic, however, with only 0.2% of all patients suffering a neurologic deficit (64).

While surgeons have gained substantial experience with the transarticular atlantoaxial screw technique (64), the risk of vertebral artery injury in rheumatoid patients has not been fully evaluated. This risk is probably somewhat higher than in the nonrheumatoid population because of the tortuous anatomy of the vertebral artery that can develop with rheumatoid arthritis, as well as the difficulty of reducing the atlantoaxial facets in some patients, complicating appropriate screw trajectory.

While transarticular screw fixation seems to offer a higher rate of arthrodesis, further documentation of outcome in rheumatoid patients is needed. Despite a lower mechanical rigidity compared with transarticular screw fixation, wiring techniques are still appropriate in many patients because they offer a reduced risk of neurologic and vascular complications, particularly when reduction of the atlantoaxial articulation cannot be obtained, or when the isthmus is smaller than 3.5 mm in diameter (53).

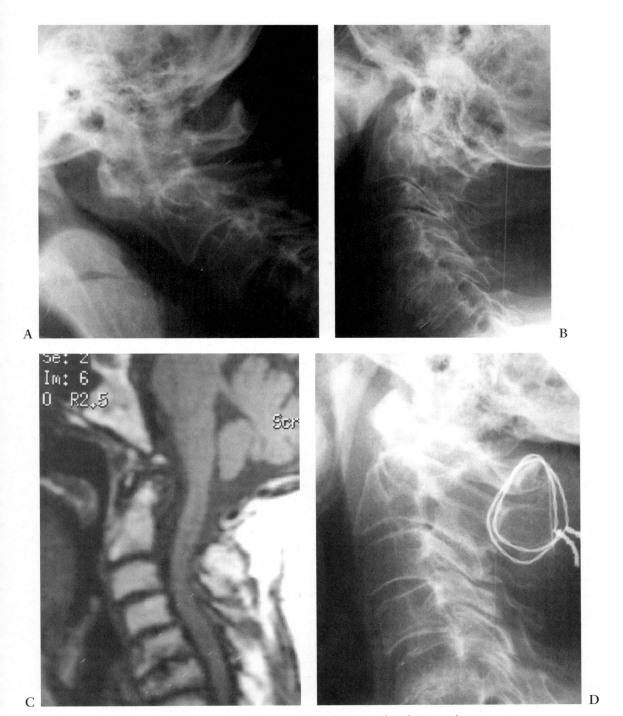

Figure 154.6. This female patient had longstanding rheumatoid arthritis with new-onset long-tract signs without motor weakness (Ranawat II). **A,B:** Flexion–extension lateral radiographs demonstrate significant atlantoaxial instability with full reduction in extension. **C:** MRI in extension demonstrates resolution of neurologic compression with reduction of the atlantoaxial articulation. **D:** Following posterior wiring and fusion, solid arthrodesis occurred with resolution of myelopathic symptoms.

OCCIPITOCERVICAL ARTHRODESIS

Indications for including the occiput in a posterior cervical arthrodesis include cranial settling with current or impending neurologic compromise, inability to obtain fusion to the posterior ring of the atlas due either to insufficient bone stock or to the need for a laminectomy, nonunion from a prior atlantoaxial arthrodesis, and severe involvement in patients with combined atlantoaxial and subaxial instability. While inclusion of the occiput in the arthrodesis further reduces neck motion over an isolated atlantoaxial fusion, incorporating the occiput affords strong fixation, allowing a variety of constructs for stabilization.

As with atlantoaxial arthrodesis, wiring techniques have historically provided acceptable results in a large number of patients. De Groote et al. (18) described results in 14 rheumatoid arthritis patients using an H-graft and a wiring technique based on the method of Robinson and Southwick (47). They obtained fusion in 11 patients, and none of the three patients with nonunion required revision surgery during the follow-up period.

Wertheim and Bohlman (61) described a three-wire technique [also derived from Robinson and Southwick (47)] using a spinous process wire at C-2, a looped sublaminar wire at C-1, and a wire through the inion along with structural corticocancellous bone grafting posteriorly. In a series of 13 patients, eight of whom had rheumatoid arthritis, they achieved a 100% fusion rate with all patients with preoperative neurologic deficits showing improvement. Clark et al. (11,14) described a six-wire technique using paired lateral sublaminar wires at the atlas and axis (Fig. 154.7A). This method can still be used when a laminectomy of the atlas has been performed.

McAfee et al. reported on 37 patients, 20 of whom had rheumatoid arthritis. They had an 85% fusion rate (33 of 37 patients). They noted that when reduction of cranial settling was achieved and maintained, patients had a significantly better prognosis for neurologic recovery than when reduction was not possible (93% versus 40%). Only two patients underwent a late anterior odontoid resection due to persistent compression and neurologic deficits; both eventually recovered normal neurologic function.

Ransford et al. (44) described occipitocervical fixation with a contoured, threaded Steinmann pin and sublaminar wiring along with laminectomy of the atlas and foramen magnum enlargement in a series of three patients (Fig. 154.7B). Although none of the patients had rheumatoid arthritis, the authors recognized the potential application to this population. Itoh et al. (28) described 13 rheumatoid patients treated with this technique, fusing an average of 5.9 cervical levels. Ten of these patients had cranial settling, and 12 had subaxial involvement. Of 8 patients with moderate or severe myelopathy, 7 (88%) had significant postoperative neurologic improvement. Twelve of 13 patients (92%) went on to solid arthrodesis. All patients had relief of occipital pain.

Apostolides et al. (2) reported results with this technique in 39 patients, 12 of whom had rheumatoid arthritis. Five of the 12 rheumatoid patients (42%) had cranial settling, while 4 (33%) had prior nonunions. Four patients (33%) underwent foramen magnum enlargement and laminectomy of the atlas, while 5 (42%) underwent transoral resection of the odontoid. Ten of these patients (83%) went on to solid arthrodesis, with 2 developing stable fibrous union. None of these patients suffered hardware failure. All 10 patients with preoperative myelopathy showed improvement, although 9 (90%) demonstrated persistent deficits to varying degrees.

Occipitocervical plating has gained popularity in recent years (Fig. 154.7C). Like transarticular screw fixation for atlantoaxial arthrodesis, this technique was developed in Europe but is increasingly used in the United States as well. The advantages claimed for occipitocervical plating include avoiding entry into the spinal canal and reducing the number of caudal segments required to obtain rigid

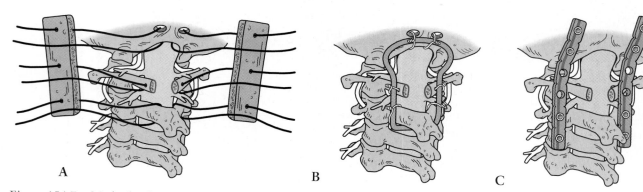

Figure 154.7.   Methods of occipitocervical stabilization. **A:** Clark wiring. **B:** Ransford loop. **C:** Occipitocervical plating.

fixation. An early report by Grob et al. (23) described this technique in 14 patients, seven of whom had rheumatoid arthritis. Using a Y-shaped plate with a single arm for cranial fixation and including transarticular atlantoaxial screws as part of their construct, they reported fusion in all patients.

Smith et al. (54) described preliminary results in 14 patients using bilateral, contoured steel pelvic 3.5 mm reconstruction plates. They used a pedicle screw at the C-2 vertebra in place of transarticular screws. Five of these patients had rheumatoid arthritis, and the arthrodesis extended an average of 4.6 cervical levels. Fusion was reportedly obtained in all patients. While these early results are promising, long-term follow-up of these patients to evaluate for instability caudal to the arthrodesis is needed.

As in instrumentation for atlantoaxial arthrodesis, these techniques require training and experience prior to routine use. The specific risks of neurologic or vertebral artery injury during lateral mass or atlas pedicle screw placement have not been documented in rheumatoid arthritis patients, where marked distortion of the anatomy can occur. A CT scan to determine the course of the vertebral arteries is advised. While these techniques offer the potential to improve fusion rates and reduce postoperative immobilization, the long-term effects of these constructs on adjacent motion segments is also unknown.

SUBAXIAL ARTHRODESIS

Posterior arthrodesis with or without laminectomy is indicated for patients with subaxial instability or fixed subluxation with impending or actual neurologic compromise. As with atlantoaxial instability, a measurement of the space available to the cord on a lateral radiograph of 14 mm or less indicates that the spinal cord is at risk of compromise. Patients with subaxial instability who also have atlantoaxial instability or cranial settling often require treatment of these combined instability patterns by a single operation (4).

Less has been reported about treatment of isolated subaxial rheumatoid spine problems than of upper cervical spine involvement. Ranawat et al. (43) discussed posterior arthrodesis in six patients with subaxial subluxations. Three of these patients underwent arthrodesis to the occiput due either to coexisting atlantoaxial instability or cranial settling. All patients had significant pain relief and three (50%) had improvement of myelopathic symptoms. Less-satisfactory results occurred in five patients treated with anterior surgery; no patient achieved neurologic improvement, because of graft collapse and dislodgement. These authors felt that anterior surgery was contraindicated in patients with rheumatoid arthritis because of the mechanically insufficient, osteopenic bone of the vertebral bodies (43). In addition, the anterior longitudinal ligament may be one of the last remaining stabilizers in rheumatoid patients, and this ligament is necessarily disrupted during an anterior procedure.

Conaty et al. (15) reported results in seven patients with isolated subaxial involvement treated by posterior fusion without wiring. Two patients underwent laminectomy due to severe neurologic compromise, but neither recovered significant function. Patients were managed postoperatively either in cranial traction or a halo. All six surviving patients went on to solid arthrodesis, with satisfactory results reported in 4 of 7 patients (57%).

Heywood et al. (27) treated seven patients with subaxial instability, four of whom had had preoperative myelopathy. Five patients treated with posterior subaxial bone grafting and wiring went on to solid fusion, with all neurologically compromised patients experiencing significant recovery. No laminectomies were performed in this series. Two patients treated with anterior procedures died postoperatively of pulmonary complications. These authors argued against the need for a laminectomy to obtain neurologic recovery, and they argued for posterior rather than anterior procedures.

Clark et al. (14) reported on 41 rheumatoid patients, seven of whom had posterior subaxial arthrodesis for subaxial instability. They reported no subaxial nonunions with spinous process wiring and bone grafting. Four patients (67%) had clinical improvement of pain complaints, and no patient suffered neurologic worsening. One patient who had undergone an anterior corpectomy and attempted arthrodesis had developed graft subluxation, which necessitated the posterior procedure.

Santavirta et al. (49) reported results in 16 patients with subaxial instability treated with a posterior procedure. Ten patients had myelopathy and seven had severe neck and shoulder pain. All patients underwent posterior wiring and arthrodesis, and patients with myelopathy also underwent laminectomy. Eight patients were treated in postoperative skull traction. All achieved solid fusion, and 90% (9 of 10) with myelopathy recovered. Two perioperative deaths occurred. Three patients developed adjacent segment instability during an average follow-up period of 4.4 years.

Several authors have reported disappointing results for subaxial anterior decompression procedures in patients with rheumatoid arthritis (14,27,43). The reasons for failure seem to be the tendency of the osteoporotic vertebral bodies to collapse around the bone graft, with resulting nonunion, kyphosis, and graft extrusion. In most cases, rheumatoid patients with subaxial instability and osteopenia or combined subaxial and upper cervical involvement should be treated with posterior surgery.

Patients with persistent neurologic deficits and anterior spinal cord compression following posterior fusion may be candidates for anterior decompression and structural bone grafting. In addition, there appears to be a subclass of rheumatoid patients with less severe involvement that can be effectively treated with anterior decompression and arthrodesis procedures. These patients may have fewer peripheral joint deformities, less corticosteroid exposure, greater bone density, and a shorter duration of rheumatoid disease. The radiographic appearance of these patients is similar to that of patients with cervical spondylosis, without significant subaxial or atlantoaxial instability (Fig. 154.8).

ODONTOID RESECTION

Anterior decompression at the level of the odontoid process is sometimes required because of severe cranial settling with persistent neurologic compression despite maximal reduction in skeletal traction. For many patients, decompression can be accomplished at the time of occipitocervical arthrodesis via traction reduction with foramen magnum enlargement and laminectomy of the atlas. For patients who fail to improve despite this treatment or whose compression is so severe that posterior decompression is likely to be inadequate, anterior resection of the odontoid is indicated.

Resection of the odontoid is usually performed through a transoral approach. Crockard et al. (17) performed simultaneous odontoid resection and posterior occipitocervical arthrodesis in 14 patients with rheumatoid arthritis, all of whom had myelopathy with significant weakness. One patient suffered a vertebral artery injury requiring abortion of the procedure. No patient developed a wound infection. These authors argue that this procedure results in faster neurologic recovery and avoids the need to obtain intraoperatively and hold postoperatively an anatomic reduction.

Many authors, however, report good results with only limited use of this procedure (4,14,28,37,43). Postoperative MRI imaging has documented reduction in the periodontoid pannus following solid arthrodesis. In addition, significant numbers of patients have demonstrated good

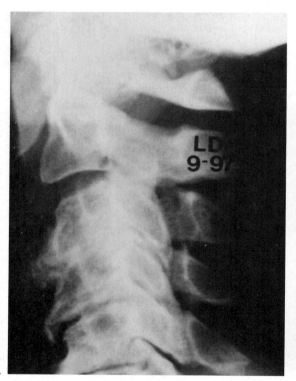

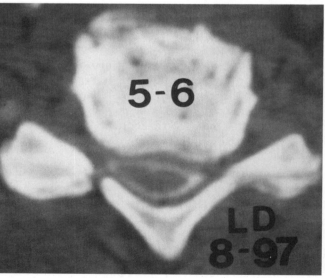

A   B

Figure 154.8.   Subaxial cervical degeneration treated by anterior corpectomy and fusion. **A:** Lateral cervical spine radiograph demonstrates subaxial spondylosis in this 66-year-old man. He had a 20-year history of seropositive rheumatoid arthritis but displayed limited peripheral joint deformity. He was maintained on a combination of methotrexate and a daily dose of 5 mm prednisone. Despite the long history of rheumatoid arthritis, his clinical appearance is more consistent with cervical spondylosis without significant instability. **B:** Postmyelogram CT image through the C-5/C-6 disc level demonstrates significant spinal cord compression. Spasticity without motor weakness was present. The patient had undergone a laminoplasty with subsequent reclosure of the laminae. *(continued)*

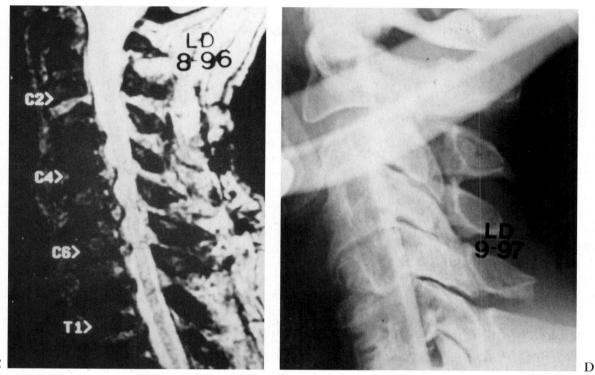

Figure 154.8. *(continued)* **C:** Sagittal MRI demonstrates spinal cord compression at the C-3/C-4, C-4/C-5, C-5/C-6, and C-6/C-7 discs. **D:** This patient underwent anterior corpectomy of C-4, C-5, and C-6 with autologous fibular strut grafting with successful fusion and resolution of his myelopathic symptoms.

neurologic recovery with solid posterior arthrodesis in a reduced position (14,37). Be aware of the fact that the physiologic stress and difficulties of airway management during combined anterior/posterior cervical spine surgery in this population are considerable. Finally, patients who do not fully recover from neurologic deficits following arthrodesis may obtain further neurologic recovery after a delayed anterior odontoid resection (37).

SURGICAL TECHNIQUES

ATLANTOAXIAL WIRING

- After fiberoptic intubation and placement of spinal cord monitoring leads, position the patient prone using tongs or halo traction on a head rest to control the head position. Position the head in sufficient extension to reduce the atlantoaxial articulation, and verify the reduction fluoroscopically prior to preparing and draping. Recheck neurologic status after positioning, either via spinal cord monitoring or a brief wake-up test. Alternatively, position patients while awake to allow continu-

ous neurologic monitoring prior to the induction of general anesthesia.

- Following a midline posterior approach, expose the ring of the atlas; strip only 1.5 cm laterally on either side of the midline to avoid injuring the vertebral arteries.
- Expose the C-2 and C-3 vertebrae to the lateral edge of the C-2 and C-3 facets, avoiding injury to the joint capsules.
- Gently strip the attachments of ligamentum flavum from the cranial and caudal edges of the laminae of both the atlas and the axis vertebrae with a 4-0 curved curet. Pass a threaded 1.5-cm-diameter French-eye needle, blunt end first, sequentially under both laminae, retrieving the leading end with a small needle driver.
- Carefully follow the curvature of the needle during advancement under the laminae to avoid injuring the dura. Repeat this maneuver until a total of four sutures (usually #2 Ticron) are under the laminae of both the atlas and the axis.
- Tie a free end of one of the sutures to the looped end of a 24-gauge wire that has been doubled on itself and twisted to form a single strand. Gently pull this wire into position under the lamina and detach the suture.
- Be careful to avoid significant pressure on the dura dur-

ing positioning of the wire, pulling the wire posteriorly away from the spinal cord with a small nerve hook at the C1-2 interspace.

- Position the wire laterally and repeat this maneuver with the remaining sutures to produce two pairs of sublaminar wires on either side.
- Once the paired sublaminar wires are in place, obtain a thick corticocancellous bone graft from the posterior iliac crest. It should be a plate of cortical bone with the full thickness of cancellous bone remaining underneath, measuring at least 2 by 4 cm.
- Shape the graft on its cancellous surface, removing bone to form a wedge shape, thickest at the center and diminishing toward the cranial and caudal edges.
- Notch the caudal edge of the graft centrally with a rongeur to accommodate the spinous process of the atlas.
- Lightly decorticate the posterior elements of C-1 and C-2 with a burr.
- Once the cancellous side of the graft lies flush against the laminae of the atlas and axis, tighten one wire by twisting with steady posterior tension. Tighten it until it is flush with the cortical surface of the graft throughout its length and the knot just begins to double on itself.
- Alternate sides until all four wires are tight, cutting the ends and tamping them down to the cortical surface of the bone graft.
- Following closure and dressing of the wound, place the patient in a halo brace in neutral flexion–extension to be worn for 12 weeks (Figs. 154.5C and 154.6).

HINTS AND TRICKS

- Do not dissect farther than 1.5 cm lateral to midline at the ring of C-1 to avoid injury to the vertebral arteries.
- Thoroughly free the cranial and caudal attachments of the ligamentum flavum before attempting to pass the free needle. A 4-0 curved curet should pass readily along the cranial and caudal surfaces of the laminae. Do not, however, attempt to pass the curet or any other instrument underneath the laminae.
- Once sutures or wires are in place, clamp free ends with a small hemostat to prevent entanglement.
- Avoid breaking the graft during removal. Thoroughly cut all four sides of the graft with an osteotome, visualizing the end of the osteotome all the way to the end of the cut. Do not lever the graft out until the deep surface of cancellous bone has been completely separated from the deep cortex and the graft moves freely.

POSTERIOR ATLANTOAXIAL TRANSARTICULAR SCREWS

- Place the patient in three-point tongs prior to positioning. Radiolucent tongs with a radiolucent operating table improve fluoroscopic visualization of the atlantoaxial facet joints. Position the patient prone, with the upper cervical spine in slight flexion and the lower cervical spine in extension. This position allows better access to the starting points and better trajectory for screw placement. Check fluoroscopically that the atlantoaxial articulation is reduced and that both facet joints are visible on the anteroposterior (AP) view. Reassess neurologic function after positioning, either by a brief wake-up test or by verification of maintenance of baseline somatosensory evoked potentials. Position patients with marked instability while they are awake to allow continuous neurologic monitoring prior to inducing general anesthesia.
- Use a midline posterior cervical approach. Take care not to expose the occiput, as the fusion mass can unexpectedly extend to areas of exposed bone.
- Achieve the exposure described for the atlantoaxial wiring and extend it cranially from the C-2/C-3 facets along the isthmus of C-2 to expose the C-1/C-2 facet joint. Be careful to remain subperiosteal and to perform the dissection bluntly to avoid injury to the C-2 nerve roots exiting posterior to the C-1/C-2 facets. Place a Penfield 4 elevator gently along the medial wall of the C-2 pedicle and into the C-1/C-2 facet joint to verify orientation.
- Obtaining a sufficiently steep trajectory for screw placement can be very difficult. Start the screw on the medial side of the inferior facet of the axis, aiming for the exposed isthmus cranially.
- Under fluoroscopic or stereotactic guidance, aim for the middle of the C-1/C-2 facet joint on the AP view, and for the anterior ring of the atlas on the lateral view.
- Use a cannulated drill system to allow repositioning of the guide wire until you are satisfied with the orientation and location.
- The thoracic cage can obstruct hand position and block the appropriate trajectory. If it does, a percutaneous incision distally on the back can improve orientation. Use a flexible, cannulated 2.5 mm drill and articulated screwdriver to improve the inclination.
- Place both guide wires prior to drilling and screw placement, to stabilize the articulation during passage of the first screw.
- Tap past the facet joint to improve ease of screw insertion. After cannulated drilling and tapping, place either a solid 3.5 mm or cannulated 4.0 mm screw. Use fully threaded narrow-pitch screws for the best purchase. Screw length should come just to the inferior edge of the anterior C-1 ring on the lateral view.
- If entry into the vertebral artery is suspected, abandon

the procedure on the opposite side to avoid the potential of a bilateral injury.

- Once screws have been placed, augment the construct with a corticocancellous bone graft and wiring following the previous guidelines (Figs. 154.5E, 154.9).

  See Hints and Tricks on the next page.

OCCIPITOCERVICAL WIRING

- Prepare and position the patient as in previous descriptions. Check atlantoaxial reduction radiographically and verify neurologic status once positioning is complete. Prepare and drape well the back of the head, approximately 5 cm cranial to the inion. Use a posterior

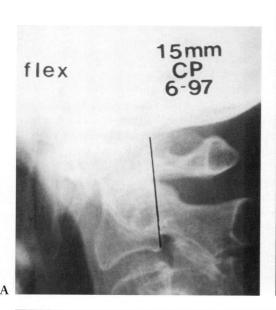

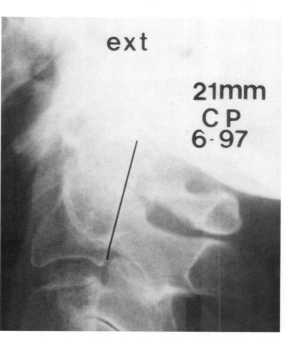

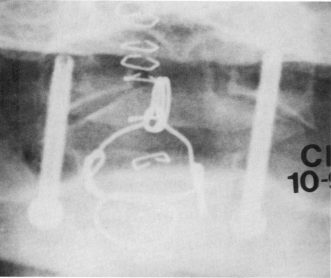

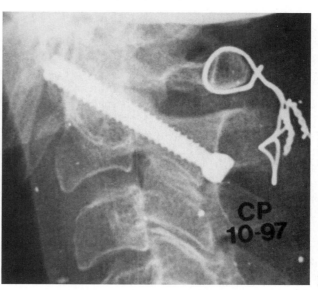

Figure 154.9. This 66-year-old woman had hyperreflexia in upper and lower extremities without weakness or pathologic reflexes. **A,B:** Flexion–extension lateral radiographs demonstrate reduction of the posterior atlantodental interval to 15 mm in flexion. Full reduction occurs with extension. **C,D:** Because of the limited space available to the spinal cord, this patient underwent posterior atlantoaxial arthrodesis with transarticular screw fixation and supplementary wiring. She obtained a solid fusion with no neurologic deterioration.

cervical approach, extending the cranial exposure approximately 1 cm cranial to the inion. Exposure of the posterior ring of the atlas should extend no more than 1.5 cm lateral on either side.

- If a laminectomy of C-1 and foramen magnum enlargement are necessary, do these before preparing for wiring.
- Free the ring of C-1 of ligamentous attachments cranially and caudally with a sharp 4-0 angled curet. If the ring is too thick to remove with a 1 mm Kerrison rongeur, it may be thinned with a burr.
- Start the resection at the lateral limits of the exposure of the laminae first, leaving a floating central fragment to be resected last. This technique reduces the potential pressure against the cord during the laminectomy.
- Enlarge the foramen magnum by thinning the occiput with a burr in a semicircle measuring approximately 5–7 mm. Then resect the remaining inner table piecemeal with a 2 mm Kerrison rongeur to remove the posterior lip of the foramen magnum; always do this to allow safe passage of occipital wires.
- Create two occipital burr holes with a 4 mm carbide burr approximately 1 cm lateral to the inion and approximately 7 mm cranial to the foramen magnum.
- Complete the holes through the inner table with a diamond burr. Elevate the dura off the inner table toward the burr holes and from the foramen magnum with a 4-0 curved curet.
- Pass a looped, double-twisted 24-gauge wire through the holes on both sides using the suture-passing technique previously described.
- If a laminectomy of C-1 has been performed, drill a small hole through the remnant of the lamina on either side, if there is sufficient remaining bone, and pass a single 24-gauge wire through this hole. Otherwise, pass bilateral sublaminar wires at both C-1 and C-2 using a technique similar to that described for atlantoaxial wiring.
- Alternatively, if neurologic compression is present, pass a wire through the spinous process of C-2 by drilling transversely approximately a third of the length up the spinous process from the laminae. Use a 2 mm burr to perforate the cortex on either side of the spinous process and connect those holes with a towel clip. Then pass a 20-gauge wire through the hole, loop it under the spinous process, and pass it a second time. Use a similar method if the fusion is to be extended caudally; we do not use sublaminar wires caudal to C-2.
- As in atlantoaxial arthrodesis, obtain a thick corticocancellous bone graft from the posterior iliac crest. For occipitocervical arthrodesis, harvest a graft measuring approximately 3 by 5 cm.
- Divide the graft lengthwise and place three evenly spaced drill holes in both grafts.
- Lightly decorticate the occiput, C-1 ring (if still present), and C-2 laminae using a carbide burr.
- Thread the more lateral arm of the wire at each level through the corresponding holes, and maneuver the graft down the wires until it is in apposition to the decorticated bone. Bring the second arm of each wire medially around the graft and tighten the wires sequentially as described previously.
- If fixation is secure and bone quality is good, use a skull–occiput–mandibular immobilization (SOMI) or Minerva brace postoperatively. If fixation is compromised because of osteopenic bone, maintain the patient in a halo vest for 6–12 weeks after surgery (Figs. 154.7A, 154.10).

SUBAXIAL ARTHRODESIS

The subaxial arthrodesis in the patient with rheumatoid arthritis is essentially the same as that in cervical trauma and is discussed in Chapter 140.

- Approach the appropriate cervical vertebrae through a midline posterior approach. Place a Gelpy retractor longitudinally in the incision to remove skin folds. For subaxial approaches, obtain a lateral radiograph with a Kocher clamp placed on an exposed spinous process

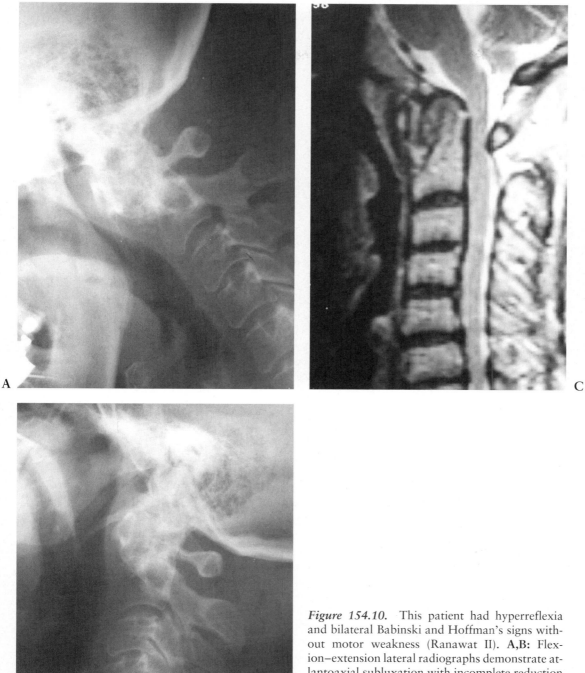

Figure 154.10. This patient had hyperreflexia and bilateral Babinski and Hoffman's signs without motor weakness (Ranawat II). **A,B:** Flexion–extension lateral radiographs demonstrate atlantoaxial subluxation with incomplete reduction in extension. Posterior atlantodental interval (PADI) is 11 mm. Mild cranial settling is also present. **C:** MRI demonstrates persistence of spinal cord compression by the posterior ring of the atlas despite maximal reduction in extension. *(continued)*

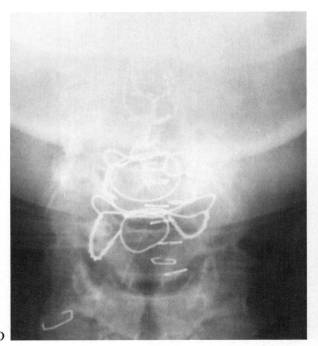
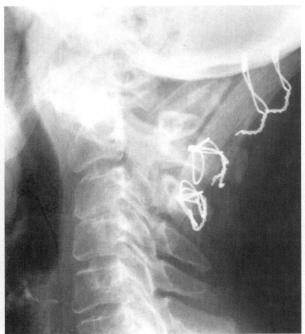

D

E

Figure 154.10.   (continued) **D,E:** This patient underwent occipitocervical arthrodesis with laminectomy of the atlas and foramen magnum enlargement. Spinous process wires were used at C-2 and C-3. The patient obtained solid arthrodesis with resolution of spasticity.

to determine the appropriate spinal level. A triple-wire fixation technique is most widely applicable. If the spinous processes are deficient, use lateral mass plates.

■ Postoperatively, immobilize the patient in a Philadelphia collar for 12 weeks.

HINTS AND TRICKS

- Pay careful attention to staying in the midline during initial dissection. If you can see muscle fibers, the dissection has strayed to one side. Maintaining a midline position will limit bleeding.
- Stabilize the C-2 vertebra with a towel clip or Kocher clamp during dissection of soft tissues to prevent gross movements of the vertebrae.
- Do not use sublaminar wires at C-1 or C-2 if neurologic compression is present. In these cases, perform a careful laminectomy of C-1 and use a spinous process wire at C-2.
- If a spinous process wire is used, gently work the towel clip from side to side until it moves readily through the hole. This technique will allow passage of the transverse wire with relative ease.

PITFALLS AND COMPLICATIONS

Early complications from these procedures include perioperative mortality due to airway compromise, neurologic deterioration, infection and wound problems, hardware and graft failure, and surgical complications such as myocardial infarction, pulmonary embolus, and pulmonary or urinary tract infection. Late complications include nonunion and adjacent segment instability with recurrent neurologic compromise.

Airway and pulmonary complications are always a significant concern after cervical spine surgery. These concerns are magnified in the case of rheumatoid arthritis, because these patients often have decreased pulmonary reserve and difficulties with postoperative mobilization. For these reasons, consider preoperative tracheostomy for patients undergoing anterior corpectomies or dens resection and patients with severe neurologic compromise (14, 27). Alternatively, maintain these patients on a ventilator for several days postoperatively to allow resolution of airway edema. All other patients with rheumatoid arthritis should undergo fiberoptic intubation to reduce postoperative airway complications (59).

Infection and wound healing problems are a significant concern in rheumatoid patients because of the atrophy of their skin and soft tissues, as well as the immunosuppressive effects of their medication regimens. Administer intravenous antibiotics preoperatively, and maintain patients on antibiotics until postoperative drains have been removed. Reduction of foreign material in the wound is also important in obtaining wound healing. While supplementary PMMA was recommended in the past, it has been associated with wound healing problems and is no longer used (9,13,14).

Intraoperative or acute postoperative neurologic deterioration should be a rare occurrence. Interoperative spinal cord monitoring should be used routinely to allow the earliest possible detection of potential spinal cord injury and immediate institution of measures with the potential to reverse neurologic compromise, such as removal of hardware or wires. Obtain a CT scan or MRI on patients in whom deficits develop or worsen postoperatively to rule out an epidural hematoma and bone graft or hardware malposition. Patients with new deficits and radiographic evidence of spinal cord compromise should undergo an emergent wound exploration, and appropriate steps should be taken to reverse the source of the neurologic compression.

The majority of patients with preoperative neurologic deficits experience improvement in function with surgical decompression and solid fusion. The long-term stability of these results, however, has been a concern because of the potential for new subluxations caudal to the original arthrodesis (41). While new subluxations may partly reflect disease progression, they also may be accelerated by the mechanical effect of the adjacent fusion.

Santavirta et al. (48) reported a minimum 10-year follow-up of a series of 38 patients treated with posterior arthrodesis. Nineteen patients died during the follow-up period. Four patients (11%) underwent further arthrodesis for subluxations caudal to the original procedure. Although 12 of 24 patients (50%) undergoing a Gallie (22) atlantoaxial arthrodesis developed nonunion, it did not appear to adversely affect their clinical outcome.

Kraus et al. (32) reported the incidence of caudal subluxations of 79 patients treated with either occipitocervical (24 patients) or atlantoaxial (55 patients) arthrodesis. They found that patients undergoing occipitocervical arthrodesis experienced a higher and more rapid rate of caudal subluxation requiring revision surgery. Of the patients with occipital arthrodesis, 36% developed subaxial subluxation in an average of 2.6 years, compared with 5.5% of the patients undergoing atlantoaxial arthrodesis in an average of 9 years postoperatively.

Krieg et al. (33) performed a minimum 7-year follow-up of the 41 patients originally studied by Clark et al. (12, 14). Thirteen patients (32%) had died by the time of the later follow-up. Eighteen patients underwent clinical and radiographic evaluation, and nine were interviewed. None of these 27 patients had had clinical or radiographic deterioration over the length of the follow-up.

Nonunion has also been a significant problem for rheumatoid patients following arthrodesis. Overall rates of nonunion have ranged from 8% to 50% in various series of posterior cervical arthrodesis in patients who have rheumatoid arthritis (8,14,27,28,41,43,48,49). In series of patients with mixed diagnoses treated with uniform surgical procedures, rates of nonunion are somewhat higher for rheumatoid patients than for patients with other diagnoses (2,8,35,37,39,61). While new technology may ultimately improve patient outcomes, adherence to proven surgical techniques such as use of structural corticocancellous autograft, good apposition of graft to bony surfaces, and appropriate postoperative bracing lead to good results for the majority of patients.

 ## AUTHORS' PERSPECTIVE

It is worthwhile to identify patients with rheumatoid arthritis who are at risk of developing neurologic injury, as recovery of neurologic function once deficits develop is uncertain and often incomplete. New imaging modalities, as well as means of interpretation of plain radiographs, allow more accurate selection of patients at risk for neurologic injury. While new techniques of internal stabilization should improve rates of achieving solid arthrodesis, an assessment of the risks of these techniques in rheumatoid patients is needed. The long-term effect of such fixation on adjacent motion segments is not known. The primary determinants of satisfactory outcomes remain careful patient selection, appropriate choice of surgical procedures, and adherence to the principles and techniques of neurologic decompression and spinal arthrodesis.

REFERENCES

Each reference is categorized according to the following scheme: *, classic article; #, review article; !, basic research article; and +, clinical results/outcome study.

+ 1. Althoff B, Goldie I. Cervical Collars in Rheumatoid atlantoaxial Subluxation: A Radiographic Comparison. *Ann Rheum Dis* 1980;39:485.

+ 2. Apostolides P, Dickman C, Golfinos J, et al. Threaded Steinmann Pin Fusion of the Craniovertebral Junction. *Spine* 1996;21:1630.

* 3. Bell H. Paralysis of Both Arms from Injury of the Upper Portion of the Pyramidal Decussation: "Cruciate Paralysis." *J Neurosurg* 1970;33:376.

* 4. Boden S, Dodge L, Bohlman H, Rechtine G. Rheumatoid Arthritis of the Cervical Spine. *J Bone Joint Surg Am* 1993;75:1282.

+ 5. Bogduk N, Major G, Carter J. Lateral Subluxation of

the Atlas in Rheumatoid Arthritis: A Case Report and Post-mortem Study. *Ann Rheum Dis* 1984;43:341.

+ 6. Braunstein E, Weissman B, Seltzer S, et al. Arthritis and Rheumatism. *Arthritis Rheum* 1984;27:26.

+ 7. Breedveld F, Algra P, Vielvoye C, Cats A. Magnetic Resonance Imaging in the Evaluation of Patients with Rheumatoid Arthritis and Subluxations of the Cervical Spine. *Arthritis Rheum* 1987;30:624.

* 8. Brooks A, Jenkins E. Atlantoaxial Arthrodesis by the Wedge Compression Method. *J Bone Joint Surg Am* 1978;60:279.

+ 9. Bryan W, Inglis A, Sculco T, Ranawat C. Methylmethacrylate Stabilization for Enhancement of Posterior Cervical Arthrodesis in Rheumatoid Arthritis. *J Bone Joint Surg* 1982;64:1045.

+ 10. Bywaters E. Rheumatoid and Other Diseases of the Cervical Interspinous Bursae, and Changes in the Spinous Processes. *Ann Rheum Dis* 1982;41:360.

11. Clark C. Occipitocervical Fusion for the Unstable Rheumatoid Neck. *Orthopaedics* 1989;12:469.

12. Clark C. Rheumatoid Involvement of the Cervical Spine: An Overview. *Spine* 1994;19:2257.

13. Clark C, Boden S. Rheumatoid Arthritis of the Cervical Spine. In: Clark C, ed. *The Cervical Spine*. Philadelphia: Lippincott-Raven, 1998:693.

* 14. Clark C, Goetz D, Menezes A. Arthrodesis of the Cervical Spine in Rheumatoid Arthritis. *J Bone Joint Surg Am* 1989;71:381.

+ 15. Conaty J, Mongan E, California D. Cervical Fusion in Rheumatoid Arthritis. *J Bone Joint Surg* 1981;63:1218.

* 16. Conlon P, Isdale I, Rose B. Rheumatoid Arthritis of the Cervical Spine. *Ann Rheum Dis* 1966;25:120.

+ 17. Crockard H, Poxo J, Ransford A, et al. Transoral Decompression and Posterior Fusion for Rheumatoid Atlantoaxial Subluxation. *J Bone Joint Surg Br* 1986;68:350.

+ 18. De Groote W, Vercauteren M, Uyttendaele D. Occipitocervical Fusion in Rheumatoid Arthritis. *Acta Orthop Belg* 1981;47:685.

+ 19. Delamarter R, Bohlman H. Postmortem Osseous and Neuropathologic Analysis of the Rheumatoid Cervical Spine. *Spine* 1994;19:2267.

+ 20. El-Khoury G, Wener M, Menezes A, et al. Cranial Settling in Rheumatoid Arthritis. *Diagn Radiol* 1980;137:637.

+ 21. Fedele F, Ho G Jr, Dorman B. Pseudoaneurysm of the Vertebral Artery: A Complication of Rheumatoid Cervical Spine Disease. *Arthritis Rheum* 1986;29:136.

* 22. Gallie W. Fractures and Dislocations of the Cervical Spine. *Am J Surg* 1939;46:495.

+ 23. Grob D, Dvorak J, Panjabi M, et al. Posterior Occipitocervical Fusion. *Spine* 1991;16:S17.

+ 24. Grob D, Jeanneret B, Aebi M, Markwalder T. Atlantoaxial Fusion with Transarticular Screw Fixation. *J Bone Joint Surg Br* 1991;73:972.

+ 25. Halla J, Fallahi S. Cervical Discovertebral Destruction, Subaxial Subluxation, and Myelopathy in a Patient with Rheumatoid Arthritis. *Arthritis Rheum* 1981;944.

+ 26. Halla J, Fallahi S, Hardin J. Nonreducible Rotational Head Tilt and Lateral Mass Collapse. *Arthritis Rheum* 1982;25:1316.

+ 27. Heywood A, Learmonth I, Thomas M. Cervical Spine Instability in Rheumatoid Arthritis. *J Bone Joint Surg* 1988;70:702.

+ 28. Itoh T, Tsuji H, Katoh Y, et al. Occipitocervical Fusion Reinforced by Luque's Segmental Spinal Instrumentation for Rheumatoid Diseases. *Spine* 1988;13:1234.

+ 29. Kauppi M, Sakaguchi M, Konttinen Y, Hamalainen M. A New Method of Screening for Vertical atlantoaxial Dislocation. *J Rheumatol* 1990;17:167.

+ 30. Kawaida H, Sakour T, Morizono Y, Yoshikuni N. Magnetic Resonance Imaging of Upper Cervical Disorders in Rheumatoid Arthritis. *Spine* 1989;14:1144.

+ 31. Kinnunen EKM, Ketonen L, Sepponen R, et al. Low-field MRI in the Evaluation of Rheumatoid Cervical Spine. Comparison with Neurological Findings and Routine Plain Radiography. *Clin Exp Rheumatol* 1990;8:365.

+ 32. Kraus D, Peppelman W, Agarwal A, et al. Incidence of Subaxial Subluxation in Patients with Generalized Rheumatoid Arthritis Who Have Had Previous Occipital Cervical Fusions. *Spine* 1991;16:S486.

+ 33. Krieg J, Clark C, Goetz D. Cervical Spine Arthrodesis in Rheumatoid Arthritis: A Long-Term Follow-Up. *Yale J Biol Med* 1993;66:257.

+ 34. Krodel A, Refior H, Westermann S. The Importance of Functional Magnetic Resonance Imaging (MRI) in the Planning of Stabilizing Operations on the Cervical Spine in Rheumatoid Patients. *Arch Orthop Trauma Surg* 1989;109:30.

+ 35. Madawi A, Casey A, Solanki G, et al. Radiological and Anatomical Evaluation of the atlantoaxial Transarticular Screw Fixation Technique. *J Neurosurg* 1997;86:961.

+ 36. Magerl F, Seemann P. Stable Posterior Fusion of the Atlas and Axis by Transarticular Screw Fixation. In: Kehr P, Weidner A, eds. *Cerv Spine* Wien: Springer-Verlag, 1986;322.

+ 37. McAfee P, Cassidy J, Davis R, et al. Fusion of the Occiput to the Upper Cervical Spine: A Review of 37 Cases. *Spine* 1991;16:S490.

+ 38. Meijers KAE CA, Kremer HPH, Luyendijk W, et al. Cervical Myelopathy in Rheumatoid Arthritis. *Clin Exp Rheumatol* 1984;2:239.

+ 39. Moskovich R, Crockard H. Atlantoaxial Arthrodesis Using Interlaminar Clamps: An Improved Technique. *Spine* 1992;17:261.

* 40. Pellicci P, Ranawat C, Tsairis P, Bryan W. A Prospective Study of the Progression of Rheumatoid Arthritis of the Cervical Spine. *J Bone Joint Surg Am* 1981;63:342.

+ 41. Peppelman W, Kraus D, Donaldson W, Agarwal A. Cervical Spine Surgery in Rheumatoid Arthritis: Improvement of Neurologic Deficit After Cervical Spine Fusion. *Spine* 1993;18:2375.

* 42. Rana NA, Hancock DO, Taylor AR, Hill AGS. Upward Translocation of the Dens in Rheumatoid Arthritis. *J Bone Joint Surg Am* 1973;55:471.

* 43. Ranawat C, O'Leary P, Pellicci P, et al. Cervical Spine Fusion in Rheumatoid Arthritis. *J Bone Joint Surg Am* 1979;61:1003.

+ 44. Ransford A, Crockard H, Pozo J, et al. Craniocervical Instability Treated by Contoured Loop Fixation. *J Bone Joint Surg Br* 1986;68:173.

+ 45. Redlund-Johnell I. Subaxial Caudal Dislocation of the Cervical Spine in Rheumatoid Arthritis. *Neuroradiology* 1984;26:407.

* 46. Redlund-Johnell I, Pettersson H. Vertical Dislocation of the C1 and C2 Vertebrae in Rheumatoid Arthritis. *Acta Radiol Diagn* 1983;25:133.

47. Robinson R, Southwick W. Surgical Approaches to the Cervical Spine. *Instr Course Lect* 1960;299.

+ 48. Santavirta S, Konttinen Y, Laasonen E, et al. Ten-year Results of Operations for Rheumatoid Cervical Spine Disorders. *J Bone Joint Surg Br* 1991;73:116.

+ 49. Santavirta S, Konttinen Y, Sandelin J, Slatis P. Operations for the Unstable Cervical Spine in Rheumatoid Arthritis. *Acta Orthop Scand* 1990;61:106.

+ 50. Santavirta S, Sandelin J, Slatis P. Posterior Atlantoaxial Subluxation in Rheumatoid Arthritis. *Acta Orthop Scand* 1985;56:298.

+ 51. Santavirta S, Slatis P, Kankaanpaa U, et al. Treatment of the Cervical Spine in Rheumatoid Arthritis. *J Bone Joint Surg Am* 1988;70A:658.

+ 52. Slatis P, Santavirta S, Sandelin J, Konttinen Y. Cranial Subluxation of the Odontoid Process in Rheumatoid Arthritis. *J Bone Joint Surg Am* 1989;71:189.

! 53. Smith M, Kotzar G, Yoo J, Bohlman H. A Biomechanical Analysis of atlantoaxial Stabilization Methods Using a Bovine Model: C1/C2 Fixation Analysis. *Clin Orthop* 1993;290:285.

+ 54. Smith M, Anderson P, Grady M. Occipitocervical Arthrodesis Using Contoured Plate Fixation. *Spine* 1993; 18:1984.

+ 55. Smith P, Benn R, Sharp J. Natural History of Rheumatoid Cervical Luxations. *Ann Rheum Dis* 1972;31:431.

+ 56. Snelling J, Pickard J, Wood S, Prouse P. Case Report: Reversible Cortical Blindness as a Complication of Rheumatoid Arthritis of the Cervical Spine. *Br J Rheumatol* 1990;29:228.

+ 57. Teigland J, Magnaes B. Rheumatoid Backward Dislocation of the Atlas with Compression of the Spinal Cord. *Scand J Rheumatol* 1980;9:253.

+ 58. Toolanen G, Knibestol M, Larsson S, Landman K. Somatosensory Evoked Potentials (SSEPs) in Rheumatoid Cervical Subluxation. *Scand J Rheumatol* 1987;16:17.

+ 59. Wattenmaker I, Concepcion M, Hibberd P, Lipson S. Upper-Airway Obstruction and Perioperative Management of the Airway in Patients Managed with Posterior Operations on the Cervical Spine for Rheumatoid Arthritis. *J Bone Joint Surg Am* 1994;76:360.

+ 60. Weiner S, Bassett L, Spiegel T. Superior, Posterior, and Lateral Displacement of C1 in Rheumatoid Arthritis. *Arthritis Rheum* 1982;25:1378.

+ 61. Wertheim S, Bohlman H. Occipitocervical Fusion. *J Bone Joint Surg Am* 1987;69:833.

+ 62. Winfield J, Cooke D, Brook A, Corbett M. A Prospective Study of the Radiological Changes in the Cervical Spine in early Rheumatoid Disease. *J Rheum Dis* 1981;40: 109.

+ 63. Winfield J, Young A, Williams P, Corbett M. Prospective Study of the Radiological Changes in Hands, Feet and Cervical Spine in Adult Rheumatoid Disease. *Ann Rheum Dis* 1983;42:613.

+ 64. Wright N, Lauryssen C. Vertebral Artery Injury in C1-2 Transarticular Screw Fixation: Results of a Survey of the AANS/CNS Section on Disorders of the Spine and Peripheral Nerves. *J Neurosurg* 1998;88:634.

65. Zeidman S, Duckler T. Rheumatoid Arthritis. *Spine* 1994;19:2259.

+ 66. Zoma A, Sturrock R, Fisher W, et al. Surgical Stabilization of the Rheumatoid Cervical Spine. *J Bone Joint Surg Am* 1987;69:8.

## CHAPTER 155

ANTERIOR APPROACH TO SCOLIOSIS

We wish to thank Drs. Alan Moskowitz, Randal Betz, and Marc Asher for their technical contributions to this chapter.

Jesse Butler and Michael F. Schafer

HISTORICAL BACKGROUND

Scoliosis is a complex three-dimensional deformity characterized by coronal, sagittal, and horizontal plane deviation. Although posterior spinal fusion and instrumentation can be used for most patients, there are many situations in which the anterior approach is necessary. With recent advances in thoracoscopic techniques, the indications for anterior surgery may be expanded (46). The deformity surgeon must, therefore, be aware of the anterior surgical options available.

Although Compere reported the resection of a hemivertebra by the anterior approach in 1932 (4), anterior surgery for the treatment of spinal conditions started with Hodgson, who reported the results of anterior spinal de-

compression and fusion for tuberculosis of the spine in 1956 (13,14). Dwyer expanded the technique developed by Hodgson to approach the convex side of a scoliosis curve (9,10). During the past 30 years, spinal surgeons have become facile with the anterior or combined anterior and posterior approaches.

INDICATIONS

Indications for an anterior approach include certain cases of idiopathic, congenital, neuromuscular, and adult scoliosis. The neuromuscular curves include those caused by cerebral palsy, myelomeningocoele (MM), muscular dystrophy, polio, trauma, Friedrich's ataxia, and syringomyelia. The combination of curve magnitude, rigidity, spasticity, and paralysis frequently necessitates combined anterior and posterior spinal fusion.

The spinal deformities associated with neuromuscular disease are often progressive and disabling. The indica-

J. Butler: Department of Orthopaedic Surgery, Our Lady of Resurrection Spine Center, Chicago, Illinois, 60646.
M. F. Schafer: Department of Orthopaedic Surgery, Northwestern University Medical School, Chicago, Illinois, 60611.

tions for surgery are at times controversial in severely involved children, and complications are frequent. Patients with impending skin compromise due to pelvic obliquity or kyphosis, poor sitting balance with muscular fatigue and pain, loss of upper extremity function due to using their arms to support and elevate the trunk, and progressive deterioration of pulmonary function are strong indications for surgery (39). Attempts to delay surgery with bracing until adequate trunk height is obtained are a common dilemma in the preadolescents with significant deformity. Absolute Cobb angular measurements for which surgery is indicated range from 40° to 60°. Issues regarding age, medical comorbidity, and family acceptance make rigid guidelines difficult to implement.

When combined anterior and posterior fusion is indicated, same-day sequential surgery usually is performed. The anterior approach allows more correction by excising the discs and ligaments (5), increases fusion rates, prevents crankshafting in immature spines (8,20,21), decompresses the spinal cord, and provides exposure for internal thoracoplasty (40). This is followed by posterior instrumentation and fusion. Powell et al. (36) compared the results between staged and same-day surgery. They found less blood loss, shorter hospital stays, and reduced cost with same-day surgery. Ferguson et al. (11) reviewed the results of same-day surgery in patients with neuromuscular scoliosis. The overall complication rate was reduced from 124% to 88%. The number of patients without any complications in this high-risk group increased from 35% to 63%.

The indications for anterior instrumentation have changed since the second edition of this book. The Dwyer and Zielke instrumentations are no longer used in our practice. Anterior instrumentation is used now for structural support as well as for deformity correction. In select cases of idiopathic scoliosis, anterior instrumentation may be all that is necessary. Valuable motion segments may be preserved in the lumbar spine when fusing with anterior instrumentation.

PREOPERATIVE PLANNING

The initial step in preparing the patient for an anterior procedure is a thorough history and physical examination. For all cases, obtain an appropriate medical consultation prior to surgical intervention. A complete examination of the chest, abdomen, back, and lower extremities is important. Assess spinal balance, as this aides in determining fusion level. For example, a lumbar scoliosis with an associated rigid thoracic kyphosis must be fused across both curves to prevent decompensation and progression of the thoracic deformity.

Carefully evaluate neuromuscular patients for asymetric muscle strength, rapid curve progression, increasing motor weakness, or cavus foot deformity. Evaluate with magnetic resonance imaging (MRI) to look for an intraspinal lesion or tethered cord (37). Do a myelogram only in cases that are difficult to interpret. An assessment of pelvic obliquity and hip joint contracture is vital if the fusion is to be carried into the lumbosacral region. At times, a release of hip flexion contracture may be required to decrease excessive lumbar lordosis prior to spine surgery.

A complete radiographic assessment includes standing or sitting 14 × 36 films in the posteroanterior and lateral planes. Supine side bending films determine the curve flexibility and assist in determining the fusion endpoint. Image the lumbosacral junction to detect an occult spondylolisthesis. Preoperative MRI is not necessary for idiopathic adolescent (48) and adult deformity.

Pulmonary function studies are mandatory. This helps determine which group of patients will require respiratory assistance in the perioperative period. Forced vital capacity (FVC) values less than 40% of predicted values, and small children with recurrent upper respiratory infections should be evaluated closely (16). In idiopathic scoliosis, little effect on the FVC occurs until curves approach 60° to 100°. However, patients with spinal muscular atrophy or muscular dystrophy have marked reductions in FVC to less than 50% with curves of only 30° (39).

We obtain preoperative lower extremity somatosensory evoked potential exams to establish a baseline with which comparison can be made intraoperatively. Theoretically, detecting early subtle changes in evoked potential can enhance the safety of the procedure.

Congenital curves require a detailed evaluation by multiple disciplines. A careful history should elicit any urologic, cardiac, musculoskeletal, or neurologic anomalies. Approximately one third of these patients have urologic abnormalities, and 10% possess cardiac malformations (24). Evaluation of the genitourinary system with an intravenous pyelogram or ultrasound can detect anomalies, which may need treatment prior to spinal surgery.

Perioperative nutritional assessment is important to minimize infection and wound healing problems (1). Mandelbaum's review (28) of staged anterior and posterior surgery noted that all infectious complications but one occurred in malnourished patients. A serum albumin over 3.5 g/dl and total lymphocyte count of more than 1,500/μl are acceptable. The normalization of nutritional parameters following combined spinal surgery correlates with the length of fusion according to Lenke et al. (22). Shorter fusions required approximately 6 weeks, and longer fusions about 12 weeks before nutritional parameters normalized when perioperative hyperalimentation was not used.

We use intravenous hyperalimentation in all of our patients undergoing combined anterior and posterior procedures. We place a central line at surgery and continue hyperalimentation until the postoperative ileus resolves and the patient's appetite returns. We have found a decrease in hospital stay and perioperative morbidity with this regimen.

We encourage the preoperative donation of autologous blood (6,31). Autologous donation does not compromise nutritional status, nor does it increase complication rates or the need for postoperative transfusions. The blood lost during surgery in these patients is more dilute, since their hematocrit at the time of surgery is lower. Homologous blood donation causes immunosuppression and places the patient at risk for transmission of viral diseases.

While intraoperative autologous transfusion (IAT) is used in our institution, there are recent studies that question its utility (41–43) in selected populations. There are significant costs for equipment and technicians, and the salvaged blood has a low hematocrit. There is no definitive evidence that IAT reduces the need for postoperative transfusion in select populations. However, for our combined procedures to correct scoliosis and kyphosis, IAT is used. We feel that this decreases the amount of homologous blood required for the surgery.

SELECTION OF LEVELS TO BE FUSED

IDIOPATHIC SCOLIOSIS

The majority of cases will be approached posteriorly, but for certain lumbar and thoracolumbar curves we use the anterior approach. Anterior instrumentation systems provide better correction of rotation, as forces are exerted directly through the vertebral body and disc spaces. When an anterior approach is selected, fewer levels are fused, which may prevent the future development of low-back pain. The Dwyer system was one of the first used this way (9,10). The lower pseudarthrosis rates and improved sagittal contour fueled the transition to solid rod systems such as Isola, the Texas Scottish Rite Hospital system (TSRH), and Kaneda.

The patients selected should have a lumbar or thoracolumbar curve of 60° or less, with a flexible thoracic deformity that reduces to less than 20° on supine bending films. The number of levels to be fused depends on whether the curve apex is at the disc or the vertebral body level. When the apex lies at the disc, two levels above and below are fused. If the apex is at the body, then one body above and below the apical vertebra is fused.

Hall et al. (12) noted similar correction of coronal deformity when comparing their results using the Dwyer, Zielke, and TSRH systems. The TSRH system produced less segmental kyphosis. There was only one pseud-

arthrosis in their series of 18 cases with TSRH. This was successfully salvaged with a posterior fusion.

PARALYTIC SCOLIOSIS

While the etiologies of paralytic scoliosis are diverse, there are many common features. The curves tend to occur early, progress rapidly, involve the entire spine, and result in pelvic obliquity, and they progress in adulthood (39). A combined anterior and posterior procedure is often utilized with fusion from T2 to the pelvis.

The criteria for anterior release are based on curve flexibility and leveling of the pelvis on side-bending films. When the pelvis becomes level on side-bending films, an anterior release is not necessary. However, when lumbar rigidity precludes correction to less than 30°, the anterior discectomy and bone grafting is performed prior to the posterior procedure.

We have modified our technique from combined anterior and posterior instrumentation (Dwyer anterior and Luque-Galveston posterior) to anterior release with segmental fixation posteriorly with either Isola (DePuy Acromed, Warsaw, IN) or CD Horizon (Sofamor Danek, Memphis, TN) instrumentation. This change emphasizes the role of the anterior procedure in mobilizing a rigid deformity, establishing lumbar lordosis, and improving fusion rates and overall sagittal balance. Recently, we have utilized titanium cages anteriorly to improve sagittal contour prior to the posterior procedure. This prevents loss of lordosis from graft settling that may be seen with the use of autograft or allograft alone. Pelvic fixation varies with the patients' anatomy, but an iliac post is most commonly used. The iliac post, placed between the inner and outer tables of the ilium, increases the rigidity of the fixation.

MYELOMENINGOCOELE

The treatment of scoliosis in the MM population is complex and complications are frequent (see Chapter 157). As the level of neurologic compromise rises, so does the incidence of spinal deformity (25,37), approaching 100% in thoracic-level patients. Nearly 60% of L4 level patients have scoliosis. The overall goal of surgery is to achieve a vertical torso centered over a level pelvis. Therefore, most patients require a fusion from T2 to the sacrum (Fig. 155.1).

From 1980 to the early 1990s, we followed all anterior instrumentation and fusions with the Dwyer technique with a supplemental posterior fusion to the sacrum with Luque instrumentation. This technique allowed excellent coronal and sagittal correction. We had only one pseudarthrosis with this technique and it was associated with persistent infection necessitating early removal of the posterior hardware.

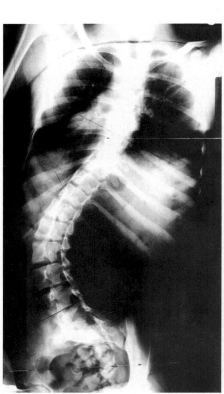
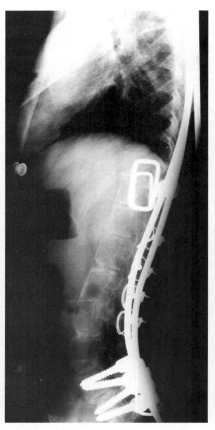
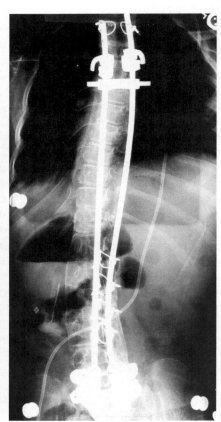

A,B   **C**

Figure 155.1.   **A:** Preoperative AP view of a child with myelomeningocoele and a curve of 58°. A combined anterior release and posterior fusion with Cotrel-Dubousset rods, pedicle screws, and Luque wires was utilized. Postoperative lateral (**B**) and AP (**C**) views show excellent correction of coronal and sagittal deformities. A solid fusion is evident at 1-year follow-up. (Courtesy of John Sarwark.)

Currently, we perform anterior discectomy and fusion followed by posterior Isola instrumentation with iliac post fixation in the pelvis. The fusion rates have remained acceptable with this modification. The real benefit has been the improved sagittal balance obtained from the anterior mobilization followed by posterior deformity correction and fusion. Segmental fixation posteriorly combines hooks, sublaminar wires, and pedicle screws.

We have not used isolated anterior instrumentation for MM patients because of reported high complication and revision rates (25,44). The kyphosis caused by some anterior instrumentation is only exacerbated in this population. Anterior instrumentation also reduces the sagittal correction obtained by posterior techniques.

CEREBRAL PALSY

There is controversy over the treatment of scoliosis in cerebral palsy (CP) patients. As the magnitude of neurologic involvement increases, the severity of the curve increases (27,38,39). Ambulatory patients with CP have approximately half the rate of significant deformity that nonambulators have. Curve progression into adulthood is known to occur; therefore, maintenance of ambulation through aggressive physical therapy and close follow-up is necessary.

There is often not one right answer for the CP patient. The risks and benefits of surgery should be thoroughly discussed with the parents. When there is any prospect of functional benefit to the patient, surgery is recommended. It is difficult to judge the true benefit for those with severe cognitive impairment, seizure disorder, and malnutrition.

The curves frequently are quite large and rigid. Therefore, fusion is required from the upper thoracic spine to the pelvis. The anterior procedure releases the rigid structures, which enhances posterior correction and fusion. If pelvic obliquity is not significant (i.e., it corrects on side-bending films), then fusion may be carried down to L4 or L5.

CONGENITAL HEMIVERTEBRA

Treatment of a congenital hemivertebra depends on whether the hemivertebra is segmented, semisegmented, or incarcerated. The fully segmented variety is the most common and produces the greatest deformity. In growing patients, use an anterior and posterior approach to perform a hemiepiphysiodesis, where obliteration of the convex endplates will halt spinal growth on the convexity and allow concave growth to correct the deformity (47). Thompson et al. (45) reported their results of convex epiphysiodesis for hemivertebra. The operative objectives were to prevent the development of severe deformity and allow growth of the remaining concave epiphysis to correct scoliosis. They found the procedure to be safe, and it yielded some correction in 76% of their patients and slowed progression in the remaining patients. The greatest correction was obtained in the lumbar spine of the youngest patients in their series.

Hemivertebral excision is an alternative treatment. The technique has been described for lumbosacral hemivertebra with severe coronal plane imbalance. Callahan et al. (3) reported the results of hemivertebral excision in 10 patients. Nine of 10 were excised in a single stage from T12 to L3. The procedure was safe and effective with a curve correction of 67% obtained. Greatest correction was obtained in the younger patients (under 4 years old).

ADULT SCOLIOSIS

One of the major concerns in the treatment of adult scoliosis is the high rate of complications, particularly pseudarthrosis. In a review of 62 adult cases, a 16.7% incidence of pseudarthrosis was present among patients undergoing posterior spinal fusion with Harrington rod instrumentation (34).

To minimize pseudarthrosis and improve correction, we treat all thoracolumbar or lumbar structural curves greater than 65° by combined anterior discectomy and fusion, followed by posterior spinal fusion with Cotrel-Dubousset (CD) instrumentation. This aggressive approach is indicated because these curves are stiff and there is little correction with posterior instrumentation and fusion alone. The anterior discectomy and fusion, followed by posterior instrumentation and fusion, results in a better correction of the curve and a more balanced spine, and it enhances the fusion rate (Fig. 155.2).

In adult curves of less than 65° that are located in either the thoracolumbar or the lumbar area, an anterior approach using anterior CD instrumentation is performed. If a curve has an associated kyphosis of the thoracolumbar or lumbar spine, we have used titanium cages to correct sagittal alignment. The cage size is selected to restore each disc space to a more lordotic posture.

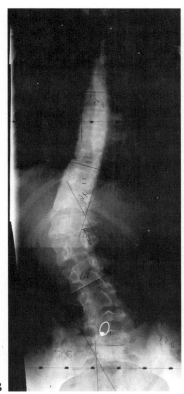 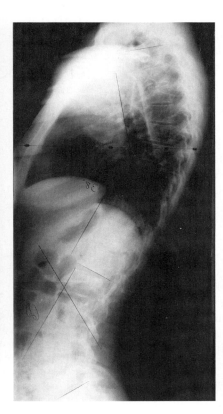

A,B

Figure 155.2. **A:** A 26-year-old woman with an increasing throracolumbar curve and low back pain. **B:** A lateral x-ray reveals a junctional kyphosis from T11 to L1. *(continued)*

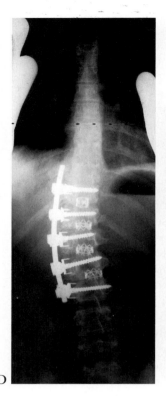
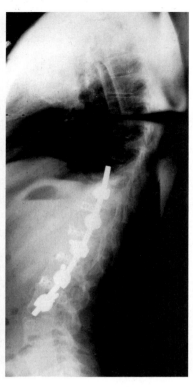

C,D

Figure 155.2. (continued) **C:** The postoperative AP x-ray shows correction of the curve to 20° with titanium cages filled with autogenous bone placed between T11 and L3. **D:** The lateral x-ray demonstrates the restoration of the normal lordosis between T11 and L3.

 SURGICAL TECHNIQUE

- Place the patient in the lateral decubitus position with the table in a flexed position. Move the upper arm forward to rotate the scapula away from the posterior portion of the vertebral column. Place an axillary roll between the patient and the table to minimize pressure on the brachial plexus during the procedure (Fig. 155.3).
- Expose the anterior spine by one of two standard approaches: Approach the thoracic spine through the bed of the convex fifth rib, which provides good visualization of T5 to T12 (Fig. 155.3); or approach the thoracolumbar spine through the bed of the tenth rib. Extend this incision anteriorly to the lateral border of the rectus sheath. The incisional length varies, depending on the number of levels exposed.

The rib to be removed by either the thoracic or thoracolumbar approach is the rib cephalad to the upper-end vertebra in the fusion. For example, if the upper vertebra to be instrumented or fused is T10, then the ninth rib is resected. Once the rib is excised, the pleura is incised to expose the vertebral column. A double lumen endotracheal tube combined with moist laparotomy sponges and a well-contoured malleable retractor allows excellent retraction of the thoracic contents.

- The thoracolumbar approach enters the retroperitoneal space on the convex side of the curve.

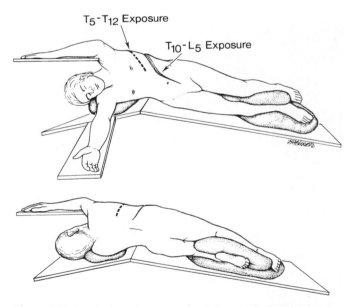

Figure 155.3. **A:** Anterior view of a patient in the lateral decubitus position. A roll is placed under the axilla to minimize the compression of the axillary artery. The *dotted line* represents the skin incision for exposure of T5 to T12. For both exposures, the table is flexed to accentuate the spinal curvature. **B:** The posterior view of the patient showing the position of the arms and the posterior extent of the incisions.

- After removing the appropriate rib, split the costal cartilage along the longitudinal axis. Identify the yellow fatty tissue of the retroperitoneal space immediately beneath the split costal cartilage. Enter the plane by blunt, finger dissection.
- Sweep the peritoneum off the undersurface of the diaphragm and the anterior surface of the psoas muscle to expose the spine. Incise the diaphragm along its peripheral margin from anterior to posterior (Fig. 155.4). Leave 1.5 cm of diaphragm as an edge for reattachment at the conclusion of the procedure. Place stay sutures at 3 cm intervals. If the diaphragm is cut too close to the periphery, muscular contraction may make closure difficult.
- Reflect the pleura and ligate the intercostal vessels in the midportion of the vertebral body to complete the thoracic exposure (Fig. 155.5). Carefully elevate the vessels off of the vertebral body, and double-ligate with suture, then retract the vascular elements from the working field.

The segmental vessels usually join the anterior median longitudinal arterial trunk of the spinal cord and also the posterior lateral longitudinal arterial trunks of the cord. Spinal cord blood supply is not compromised by ligating multiple intercostal vessels as long as this anastomosis is preserved (7).

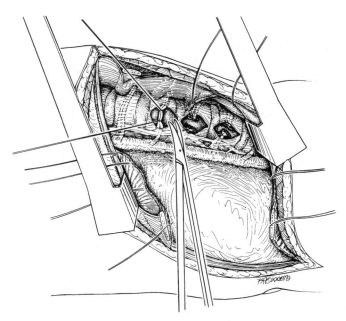

Figure 155.5.   The segmental vessels are ligated at the midportion of the vertebral body.

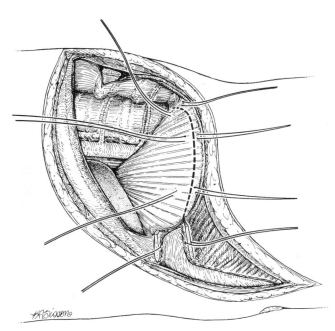

Figure 155.4.   The costal cartilage has been split and marking sutures are placed on both cut ends. The *dotted line* demonstrates the detachment of the peripheral portion of the diaphragm. The diaphragm is detached 0.75 inch from the periphery to facilitate closure.

- Detach the crura of the diaphragm to expose the thoracolumbar spine at L1-2. Detach the origin of the psoas at the L1 vertebral body or reflect it anteriorly. For patients with large psoas muscles, the muscle may be split along its longitudinal axis to expose the spine.

When exposure of the L4 level is required, it is critical that the lumbar segmental vessels arising from the iliac artery and vein be ligated in the middle of the vertebral body. There is also a lumbar segmental vessel from the iliac artery and vein that passes into the pelvis. Identify this vessel carefully so that the iliac artery and vein can be mobilized away from the spine. Inadvertent transection of this vessel is difficult to manage because the vessel retracts into the pelvis. This can lead to extensive hemorrhage.

- Once the spine is completely exposed, place retractors to protect the vascular structures. Place a Chandler elevator on the opposite side of the disc space to be resected.
- Resect the disc back to the posterior longitudinal ligament with a knife and rongeurs (Fig. 155.6). Use a headlight and loupes during this phase of the procedure. Meticulous technique is needed to avoid inadvertently penetrating the ligament, which is closely adherent to the dura and spinal cord. Exposing a broader surface area improves the fusion rate.

HINTS AND TRICKS

- If the posterior longitudinal ligament is inadvertently transected, brisk bleeding may be encountered from the epidural venous plexus. Obtain control by gently packing with thrombin-soaked Gelfoam pledgets. Small dural tears may be sealed in a similar fashion. It is the second-listed author's experience that this local treatment plus curve correction will cause the tear to seal off. Larger tears require closure. Facilitate exposure of the tear by removal of a portion of the vertebral body, and use 6-0 nylon sutures to repair the dural tear.

- On completion of the discectomy, excise the vertebral endplates using a fine osteotome. Take care to remove only the endplate. If too much of the body is removed, the purchase of any form of instrumentation on the vertebra will be compromised.

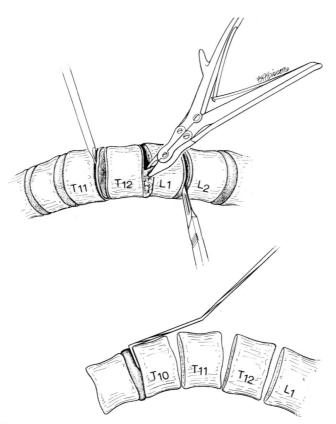

Figure 155.6.   **A:** After exposure of the spinal column, the intervertebral disc is removed thoroughly by means of sharp dissection with a knife and rongeur. The vertebral endplates are removed by using a fine osteotome. **B:** After the disc has been removed at all levels, the staple starter is placed on the superior border of the uppermost vertebra that is to be fused.

SELECTION OF INSTRUMENTATION

Recent technical advances in instrumentation have given the surgeon multiple options for anterior fixation. The anterior surgical options include discectomy and fusion with autograft or threaded/solid rod systems. Personal experience, anatomy and location of the curve, number of levels, patient age, and cost will dictate the specific approach. The indications and contraindications for anterior instrumentation are outlined in Table 155.1. Additional consideration should be given for anterior instrumentation when prominent posterior hardware and crankshaft phenomena are a concern.

The number of levels to be instrumented anteriorly is determined the same way regardless of the instrumentation used. The apex of the curve of concern is determined from the standing radiograph. It is the most laterally displaced portion of the Cobb curve from a line joining the center of the end vertebral bodies as measured by the Cobb method. If the regional apex is a vertebra, further apparent as the single most rotated vertebra, the apex vertebra plus one vertebra above and one below are included in this instrumentation construct. As the scoliosis reaches 55° or greater, it is generally necessary to add two vertebrae above and two vertebrae below the end vertebra. If the regional apex is a disc, further apparent because of similar adjacent vertebral rotation, then two vertebrae above and two vertebrae below are added. In addition, the first caudal disc space that shows reversal of coronal plane angulation on a convex bending radiograph can usually be excluded.

The following sections describe the specific surgical techniques for insertion of a threaded rod system [Zielke (Osteotech, Inc., Eatontown, NJ)] and two solid rod systems (DePuy Motech and Isola).

Table 155.1. Indications and Contraindications for Anterior Instrumentation	
Indications	*Contraindications*
Thoracolumbar and lumbar curves	Need to extend fusion to L5
Compensatory thoracic curve is flexible.	Severe curves > 75°F
Lordosis across segment to be fused	Kyphosis across fusion segment
Strong vertebral bodies	Osteoporotic bodies
Minimize fusion levels	

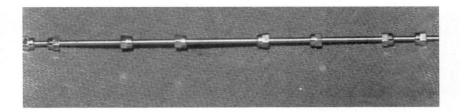

Figure 155.7. The threaded Zielke rod with associated locking nuts. (Courtesy of Daniel Benson, M.D.)

ZIELKE INSTRUMENTATION

Zielke instrumentation utilizes a threaded rod and vertebral body screws to correct deformity (Fig. 155.7).

■ Insert the instrumentation after exposure of the anterior spine has been completed. Place appropriate-size screws across the vertebral bodies (Fig. 155.8) by measuring the width of the vertebral body, and selecting the appropriate-length screw to allow several threads to protrude from the opposite cortex. Place the screw as posterior as possible in the vertebral body.

■ Following appropriate placement of the screws (Fig. 155.9), place a threaded rod in the screw heads, beginning at the apex; working proximally and distally, compress the convexity (Fig. 155.10).

■ Prior to any significant compression across the apex, place the derotator bar (Fig. 155.11). This consists of a metal bar that is fitted to the ends of the rod. and a tension screw that is placed between the apex of the rod and the bar. Tightening the tension screw affords some increase in lordosis of the spine, which may be further increased by rotating the bar (Fig. 155.12). This is seen intraoperatively by an opening anteriorly of the disc spaces.

■ Place rib graft anteriorly to facilitate fusion and maintain adequate lumbar lordosis. Then achieve compression by tightening the hex nuts.

Results

The Zielke procedure is an accepted treatment for coronal correction of scoliosis. The rate of curve correction varies between 60% and 80%, with adolescents achieving the higher rate of correction. In an early report that looked at the correction of this instrumentation, 19 patients were evaluated with an average success rate of 77% for the thoracolumbar curve and 92% correction in the lumbar curve (49). These results have been duplicated in many studies (15,30,35). In a report that stratified results obtained by Zielke, Dwyer, and Harrington rod instrumentation, the Zielke appeared to have the highest rate of correction (26).

The adult population does not fare as well as the adolescents. Kaneda reported a correction rate of 59%, with all developing a pseudarthrosis. The literature suggests that loss of correction occurs between surgical intervention and later follow-up. In one report, 18 patients who had an initial mean correction of 82% in the lower curve found the rate dropped to 63% at follow-up. The same

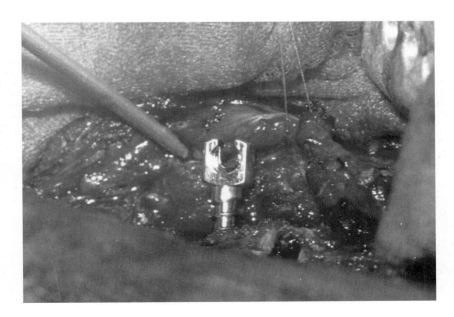

Figure 155.8. The slotted screw head for the insertion of the Zielke rod. (Courtesy of Daniel Benson, M.D.)

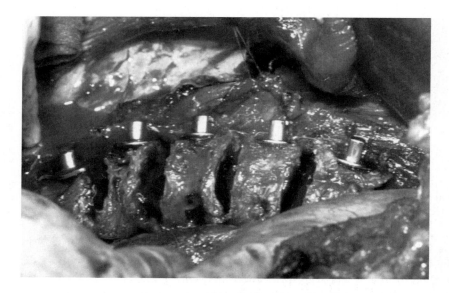

Figure 155.9. The spine has been exposed and all the Zielke screws are in place. (Courtesy of Daniel Benson, M.D.)

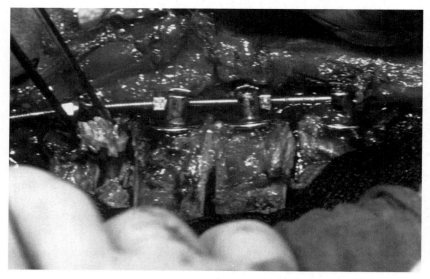

Figure 155.10. The compression force has been applied to the convex side of the curve, and resected rib for the graft is placed into the intervertebral disc space. (Courtesy of Daniel Benson, M.D.)

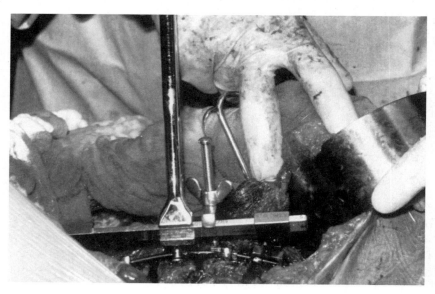

Figure 155.11. The derotation bar has been applied to the Zielke rod. (Courtesy of Daniel Benson, M.D.)

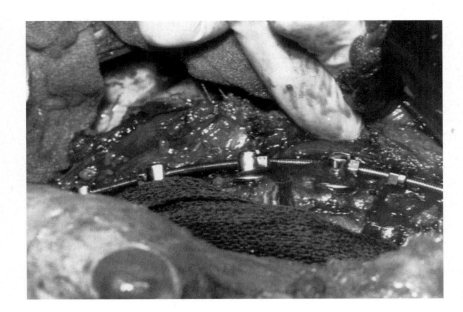

Figure 155.12. The Zielke rod has been inserted and all hex nuts tightened. This provides the curve correction. (Courtesy of Daniel Benson, M.D.)

trend was found in the correction rates associated with the upper curve, with a loss from 33% to 18% at follow-up. Rotational correction was also reduced from 66% to 56%. This loss of correction is likely the result of a lack of stiffness of the threaded rod.

The Zielke instrumentation tends to produce kyphosis with an average loss of lordosis of 8° to 10° over the instrumented segments. Many studies (17,23,32) have documented the occurrence of this increased kyphosis, but none have shown it to affect the surgical outcome. This, however, can be reduced with appropriate anterior column support by structural grafts such as femoral rings, and threaded or titanium cages.

DEPUY MOTECH

The anterior instrumentation developed by DePuy Motech uses a solid rod connected to vertebral screws.

■ Place the patient in the lateral decubitus position and make a single skin incision paralleling the eighth rib. Mobilize and detach the serratus anterior muscle. Make an incision in the intercostal space at T4 or T5 for instrumentation of the T5 vertebra. Make a second incision between the intercostal space three or four ribs distally (i.e., to T8 or T9) for instrumentation of T12 (Fig. 155.13).

■ If the preoperative analysis suggests that a thoracoplasty is necessary for cosmetic reasons, perform it at this stage. A rib approximately 2 cm in length is removed as far posteriorly as possible between the two intercostal space entrances. If there is a very significant rib hump, then the entire posterior 2 cm of rib is removed from each of the vertebrae to be instrumented.

Rib resections better mobilize the chest wall, making the discectomies and instrumentation less difficult to perform.

■ Facilitate exposure of the disc space, especially near the proximal vertebrae, by removing the rib head covering the disc space. Insert the vertebral body staples in approximately the same anatomic position in each vertebral body. Position these as far posteriorly as possible to prevent penetration of the spinal canal with the staple prongs.

■ In the most proximal vertebrae, insert the most proximal staple so that the screw can be placed eccentrically into the vertebral body. Insert the screw from posterior

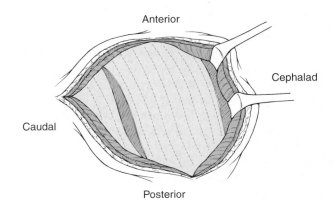

Figure 155.13. Incisions made at the intercostal space at T4 or T5, and between the intercostal spaces at approximately three to four ribs distally. (Redrawn from Moss Miami 4.0 mm Anterior System Surgical Technique: Anterior Treatment of Thoracic Idiopathic Scoliosis. DePuy Motech, Warsaw, Indiana, 1997.)

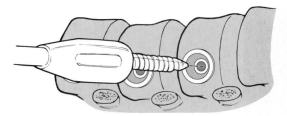

Figure 155.14. Proximal screw placed in inferior aspect of vertebral body. (Redrawn from Moss Miami 4.0 mm Anterior System Surgical Technique: Anterior Treatment of Thoracic Idiopathic Scoliosis. DePuy Motech, Warsaw, Indiana, 1997.)

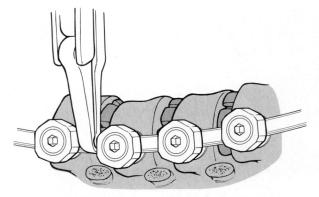

Figure 155.15. Rotating the rod into a normal sagittal plane. (Redrawn from Moss Miami 4.0 mm Anterior System Surgical Technique: Anterior Treatment of Thoracic Idiopathic Scoliosis. DePuy Motech, Warsaw, Indiana, 1997.)

to anterior, as with the other screws. This superior eccentric placement adds strength by putting the screw threads against the superior endplate of the vertebral body. Place an identical staple in the most inferior vertebral body so that the screw is in the inferior aspect of that vertebral body (Fig. 155.14).

■ Use an awl to make a hole for the insertion of the screws. When the screws are positioned, it is important that they penetrate the concave side of the vertebral body.

■ Perform bone grafting before rod insertion. Begin distally, and wedge the disc space open and pack the interspaces. It is important to pack the discs between T10 and L2 firmly with bone graft. A structural type of anterior support may be needed to help ensure maintenance of the sagittal correction. When grafting the apical vertebrae, consider the original sagittal contour. If the starting sagittal profile is lordotic or hypokyphotic, only a small amount of graft can be inserted into the disc at the apex of the curve, to allow kyphosis to occur during compression with instrumentation.

■ Measure the appropriate length of the rod from the proximal to the distal screw. Add ¼ inch (i.e., ⅛ inch for each end), and cut the rod. Bend the rod to parallel the anatomically correct kyphosis–lordosis of the area of the spine needing instrumentation. Insert the rod so that the kyphosis is used to accommodate the scoliosis that is still present. It is important to remember to straighten out the table if it has been bent to facilitate the thoracotomy and disc exposure. When applying the nuts, it is easier to start at the top three nuts and then work toward the distal end.

■ After inserting the inner setscrews and outer nuts, the rods should be loose. The spine can be corrected by rotating the rod into a normal sagittal plane (Fig. 155.15). Correction can be facilitated by the anesthesiologist pulling on the lower arm and by the surgeon pressing on the apex of the curvature. With the rod rotated into an anatomically correct position, tighten both the inner and outer apical nuts. At this point, a

decision has to be made about the anticipated coronal correction that is needed. If there is a structural upper thoracic curve, only a modest correction can be obtained in the main thoracic curve equal to the correction seen on the bending films of the upper thoracic curve. If there is no residual structural curve, then near-complete reduction of the curve can be obtained.

■ Obtain correction by using a compressor on each screw. Gradually compress each screw toward the apex. This needs to be done slowly and sequentially. After it has been completed, perform the final tightening in both the inner setscrews and the outer nuts. It is important to be cautious during this final tightening, especially in the end vertebrae. Torquing the screw could translate the screw out of the vertebral body. It is recommended that you use the rod stabilizer device that goes over the

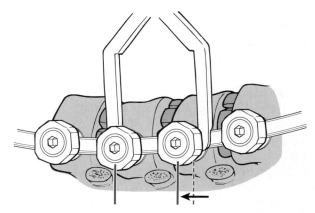

Figure 155.16. Screws are gradually compressed toward the apex. (Redrawn from Moss Miami 4.0 mm Anterior System Surgical Technique: Anterior Treatment of Thoracic Idiopathic Scoliosis. DePuy Motech, Warsaw, Indiana, 1997.)

rod and provides neutralizing forces while tightening the inner setscrews and outer nuts (Fig. 155.16).

Figure 155.17 shows the results obtained with this instrumentation. Preoperative side-bending films of a thoracic curve show excellent flexibility. The postoperative anteroposterior (AP) and lateral films show near-complete correction.

ANTERIOR ISOLA INSTRUMENTATION

- Expose the anterior spine as previously described.
- Place the end screws first from posterior to anterior, horizontal to the frontal plane of the vertebral body and paralleling the apex. Start the hole with an awl and continue with the 5.5 mm tap. Tap the vertebra until

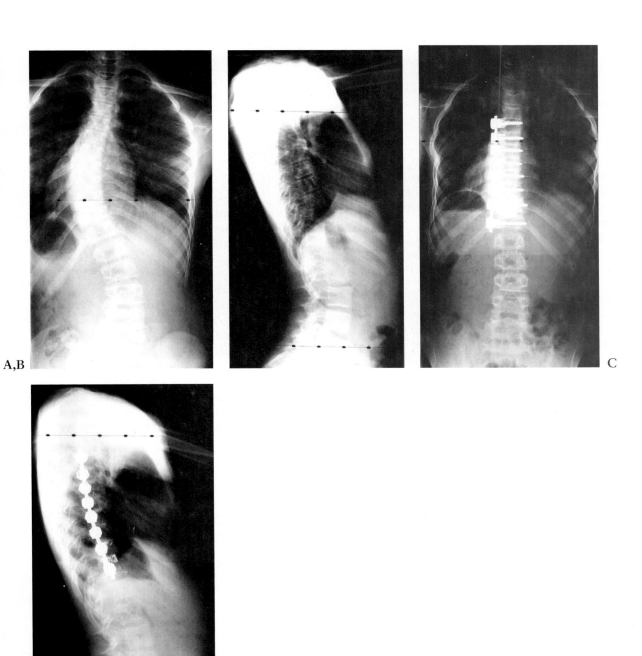

Figure 155.17. The preoperative AP (**A**) and lateral (**B**) views of a child with a thoracic scoliosis. The postoperative films (**C,D**) show near complete correction of the coronal and sagittal deformities. The cage is used to prevent kyphosis at the thoracolumbar junction.

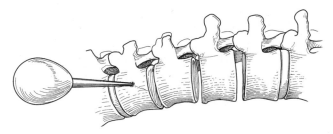

Figure 155.18. Following a thorough 360° discectomy in which the posterior longitudinal ligament is exposed, placement of the upper vertebral screw site is begun with an awl, which is positioned at the furthest lateral waist of the vertebral body. (Redrawn from Asher MA. *Surgical Technique for Anterior Segmental Instrumentation of Thoracolumbar and Lumbar Scoliosis Using the Anterior Isola Spinal System.* AcroMed Corp., Cleveland, OH, 1996.)

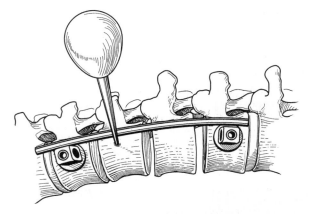

Figure 155.20. Rod is cut and contoured. Intermediate screws should be placed very slightly posterior on the waist of the body. (Redrawn from Asher MA. *Surgical Technique for Anterior Segmental Instrumentation of Thoracolumbar and Lumbar Scoliosis Using the Anterior Isola Spinal System.* AcroMed Corp., Cleveland, OH, 1996.)

the tip just exits the far side of the cortex (Fig. 155.18). Insert a ballpoint probe to make sure that the far side of the cortex has been exited. Tap the first third of the hole with a 7 mm tap and insert a 7 mm closed-top screw with washer (Fig. 155.19).

■ Use a staple, and place it prior to the insertion of the screw. Insert the screw to maximum torque. The screw should protrude through the far cortex by at least one to two threads.

■ Repeat the same process at the lower-end vertebra. After the superior and inferior vertebrae have been instrumented with the staple and screws, cut the rod and contour it so that it fits through both the superior and inferior screws (Fig. 155.20). Add about 1 cm to each side of the rod to ensure that the rod passes completely through the end screws. After the rod has been cut to length and contoured, it is used as a guide for placement of the intermediate screws.

■ Insert open-ended screws and staples at the intervening levels. Insert the rod into the superior and inferior

screws and drop into the intermediate screws (Fig. 155.21). Place caps on the intermediate screws. After placing the caps, rotate the rod approximately 180° to obtain both a coronal and a sagittal correction (Fig. 155.22).

■ Secure the rod by tightening one of the intermediate setscrews. After the rod has been rotated, a Cobb elevator can be placed into the vertebral space to pry open the previously concave side of the curve (Fig. 155.23). At this point, some distraction may actually be applied between the screw connector bodies to further open the space. Completely fill the disc spaces with bone graft.

■ Compress the vertebral screws in order to compress the disc spaces. This is done sequentially, starting from the top to the second screw (Fig. 155.24). The second

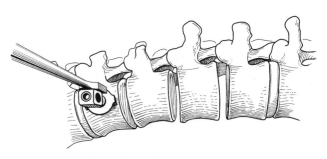

Figure 155.19. Insertion of a 7 mm closed-top screw with washer. A staple may be used if desired. (Redrawn from Asher MA. *Surgical Technique for Anterior Segmental Instrumentation of Thoracolumbar and Lumbar Scoliosis Using the Anterior Isola Spinal System.* AcroMed Corp., Cleveland, OH, 1996.)

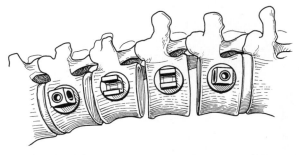

Figure 155.21. The middle screws are 7.0 mm in diameter and should protrude through the far cortex of the body by one to three turns. (Redrawn from Asher MA. *Surgical Technique for Anterior Segmental Instrumentation of Thoracolumbar and Lumbar Scoliosis Using the Anterior Isola Spinal System.* AcroMed Corp., Cleveland, OH, 1996.)

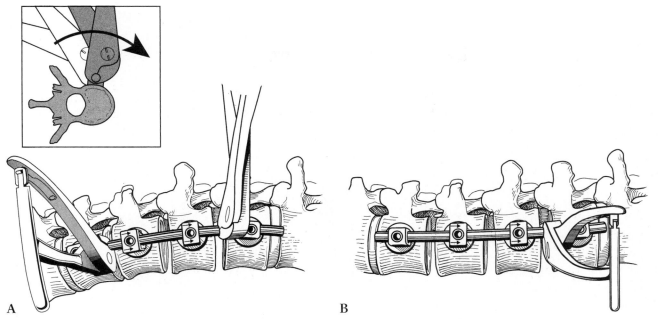

A   B

Figure 155.22. **A:** The rod is rotated to place the sagittal plane contour of the rod (**B**) in the true sagittal plane. (Redrawn from Asher MA. *Surgical Technique for Anterior Segmental Instrumentation of Thoracolumbar and Lumbar Scoliosis Using the Anterior Isola Spinal System.* AcroMed Corp., Cleveland, OH, 1996.)

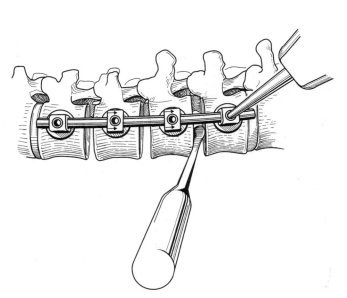

Figure 155.23. Disc space is restored utilizing a Cobb elevator. (Redrawn from Asher MA. *Surgical Technique for Anterior Segmental Instrumentation of Thoracolumbar and Lumbar Scoliosis Using the Anterior Isola Spinal System.* AcroMed Corp., Cleveland, OH, 1996.)

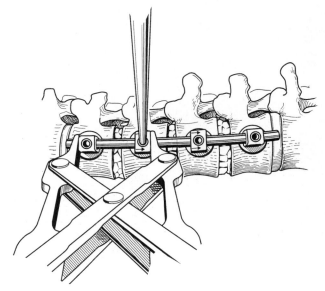

Figure 155.24. Disc spaces are compressed to provide anterior column load sharing. (Redrawn from Asher MA. *Surgical Technique for Anterior Segmental Instrumentation of Thoracolumbar and Lumbar Scoliosis Using the Anterior Isola Spinal System.* AcroMed Corp., Cleveland, OH, 1996.)

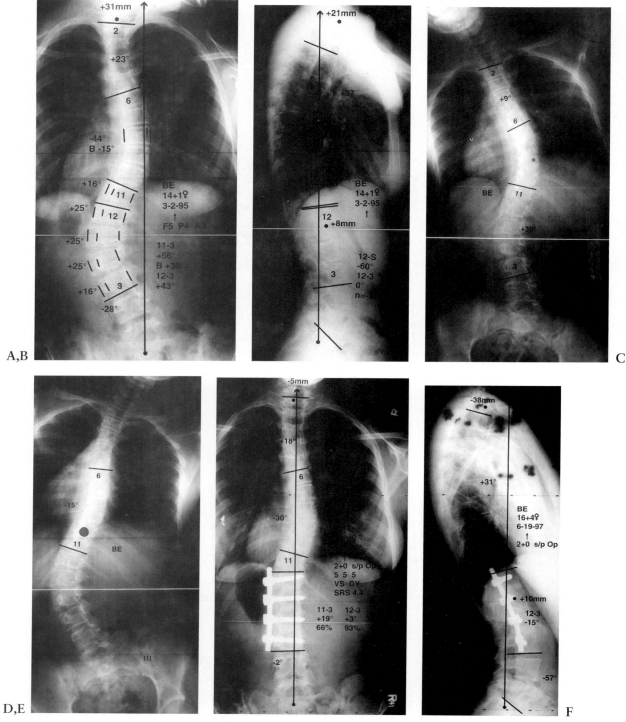

Figure 155.25.   This 14-year-old girl has left thoracolumbar major and right thoracic compensatory scoliosis. Standing frontal plane (**A**) and sagittal plane (**B**) radiographs show imbalance to the left in the coronal plane, and in the sagittal plane flattening of the upper lumbar spine. On the left bend x-ray, there is not a clear opening of the disc space above the lower Cobb (**C**). On the right bend (**D**), the upper scoliosis corrects from 44° to 15°. Two-year postoperative radiographs (**E,F**) show restoration of coronal balance and a well-healed fusion with normal sagittal plane alignment. The standing postoperative posteroanterior radiograph (**E**) shows instrumentation from T12 to L3, the upper end vertebra level having been left out to allow for compensation. The sagittal plane angulation has been restored (**F**).

compression occurs between the bottom and the next upper screw. The final compression is applied across the apical vertebra.

■ Close the wound over a chest tube as previously described. A sample case is illustrated in Fig. 155.25.

POSTOPERATIVE CARE

Monitor all patients in an intensive care unit postoperatively. Carefully monitor hemodynamic parameters such as hemoglobin and hematocrit, platelets, blood coagulation, electrolytes including calcium and magnesium, and urinary output. Record chest tube and drain outputs. Obtain daily chest radiographs until the chest tube is discontinued, usually by the third postoperative day. The goal of respiratory care is to prevent atelectasis and wean the patient from the ventilator safely and as soon as possible.

Mobilize the patient to a chair once extubated. The patient may ambulate when the chest tube is removed. Apply a custom-molded underarm thoracolumbar spine orthosis (TLSO) to all patients; this is worn full time for 6 months. Strongly stress walking to improve aerobic conditioning and an overall sense of well-being. Formal physical therapy is not required except for gait training.

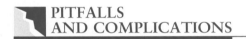

PITFALLS AND COMPLICATIONS

INSTRUMENTATION

Significant compressive forces are generated by all instrumentation systems, and vertebral fracture can occur. Apply corrective force slowly over time to allow the viscoelastic characteristics of the spine to work. Patients with osteoporosis require even more care while tensioning instrumentation. Advanced osteoporosis is a contraindication to anterior instrumentation.

Hardware pullout is another potential complication. Bicortical fixation significantly improves fixation strength and should be attempted at each level. Many systems utilize screw–staple or screw–washer combinations that maximize stability. When pullout does occur, it is usually at the proximal or distal end of the instrumented levels. Augmentation with methylmethacrylate can be utilized, or the level may need to be bypassed.

MEDICAL

Perioperative medical complications are classified as major when they significantly alter the expected course of recovery, or minor when there is no delay in expected recovery. McDonnell et al. (29) reviewed complications of anterior spine procedures. They noted that pulmonary (37%) and thoracostomy tube (14%) complications were the most common of the major complications. Genitourinary complications were present in 11.6% of all patients and made up 42% of the minor complications.

Certain diagnostic groups are at higher risk for complications. The neuromuscular, adult, and congenital scoliosis groups had overall complication rates of 52%, 41%, and 36%, respectively (29). Patient age is also a significant factor contributing to perioperative morbidity. McDonnell et al. (29) found that the complications increased with patient age and were highest in the 61- to 85-year age group.

Prolonged operative time, dilutional anemia, and hypothermia can produce a severe coagulopathy. Careful monitoring of only the hemoglobin during surgery is not adequate. The prothrombin and partial thromboplastin times and platelet counts must also be monitored in these procedures. The administration of fresh frozen plasma and platelets may at times be required. Arrangements with the hematology lab to provide a quick turnaround on coagulation profiles can be critically important.

NEUROVASCULAR

Vascular compromise of the spinal cord after the ligation of multiple segmental vessels is rare. Take care to avoid the foraminal region where the vascular anastomosis of the cord lies. The aorta and vena cava need to be carefully protected. Reported rates of injury in 447 cases of anterior spine procedures are low, with McDonnell et al. (29) reporting no great vessel injuries in 447 cases.

Spinal cord injury may result from overcorrection of deformity. Animal studies have confirmed that spinal cord injury can result from distraction or compression of the spine. While mechanical disruption does not typically occur, infarcts or hemorrhages can result from aggressive deformity correction. Bridwell et al. (2) reported their incidence of major neurologic deficits after adult and pediatric deformity surgery: Four cases were identified in 1,153 patients. All these cases were similar in that anterior and posterior procedures were performed on the same day for large deformity with the ligation of segmental vessels on one side, and intraoperative or perioperative hypotension placing the mean arterial pressure below 50 mm Hg for at least 15 minutes.

Mechanical damage to the cord may be the result of misdirected vertebral body screws. Taking care to place the screws parallel to the posterior longitudinal ligament can avoid canal penetration. If misdirection occurs, revise the screw or bypass the level.

Postoperative blindness is a rare but devastating complication after spine surgery. Myers et al. (33) reviewed 37 cases of postoperative visual loss. Significant risk factors were intraoperative hypotension, prone positioning, anemia, and prolonged operative time. They noted that "the lowest intraoperative blood pressure averaged 77 mm Hg, with an average of 260 minutes spent below 75% of the baseline preoperative pressure." The cause of blindness was ischemic optic neuropathy in 19 and retinal artery occlusion in seven. Improvement was obtained in only five patients who had partial loss of vision initially. Mayfield tongs may be of benefit in reducing facial pressure when the patient is placed prone for posterior surgery.

REFERENCES

Each reference is categorized according to the following scheme: *, classic article; #, review article; !, basic research article; and +, clinical results/outcome study.

\# 1. Boachie-Adjei O. Implications of Malnutrition in the Surgical Patient. In: Bridwell KH, DeWald RL, eds. *Textbook of Spinal Surgery*. Philadelphia: JB Lippincott, 1997:101.

! 2. Bridwell KH, Lenke LC, Baldus C, Blanke K. Major Intraoperative Neurologic Deficits in Pediatric and Adult Spinal Deformity Patients—Incidence and Etiology at One Institution. *Proceedings of the Scoliosis Research Society*, 1996.

! 3. Callahan BC, Georgopoulos G, Eilert RE. Hemivertebral Excision for Congenital Scoliosis. *J Pediatr Orthop* 1997;17:96.

* 4. Compere EL. Excision of Hemivertebrae for Correction of Congenital Scoliosis. *J Bone Joint Surg* 1932;14:555.

* 5. Denis F. Anterior Surgery in Scoliosis. *Clin Orthop* 1994;300:38.

! 6. Dick J, Boachie-Adjei O, Wilson M. One Stage vs. Two Stage Anterior and Posterior Spinal Reconstruction in Adults. *Spine* 1992;18(S):310.

* 7. Dommissee GF. The Blood Supply of the Spinal Cord. *J Bone Joint Surg Br* 1974;56:225.

* 8. Dubousset J, Herring JA, Shufflebarger H. The Crankshaft Phenomenon. *J Pediatr Orthop* 1989;9:541.

* 9. Dwyer AF, Newton NC, Sherwood AA. An Anterior Approach to Scoliosis: A Preliminary Report. *Clin Orthop* 1969;62:192.

! 10. Dwyer AF, Schafer MF. Anterior Approach to Scoliosis: Results of Treatment in Fifty-One Cases. *J Bone Joint Surg Br* 1974;56:218.

! 11. Ferguson RL, Hansen MM, Nicholas DA, Allen BL. Same-Day vs. Staged Anterior-Posterior Spinal Surgery in a Neuromuscular Scoliosis Population: The Evaluation of Medical Complications. *J Pediatr Orthop* 1996;16:293.

\# 12. Hall JE, Millis MB, Snyder BD. Short Segment Anterior Instrumentation for Scoliosis. In: Bridwell KH, DeWald RL, eds. *Textbook of Spinal Surgery*. Philadelphia: JB Lippincott, 1997:665.

* 13. Hodgson AR, Stock FE. Anterior Spine Fusion. *Br J Surg* 1956;44:266.

* 14. Hodgson AR, Stock FE, Fang HSY, Ang GB. Anterior Spine Fusion. *Br J Surg* 1960;48:172.

* 15. Kaneda K, Fujiya N, Satoh S. Results with Zielke Instrumentation for Idiopathic Thoracolumbar and Lumbar Scoliosis. *Clin Orthop* 1986;205:195.

\# 16. Kemp JS. Pulmonary Function Testing. In: Bridwell KH, DeWald RL, eds. *Textbook of Spinal Surgery*. Philadelphia: JB Lippincott, 1997:101.

* 17. Kostuik JP, Carl AL, Ferron S. Anterior Zielke Instrumentation for Spinal Deformity in Adults. *J Bone Joint Surg Am* 1989;51:898.

! 18. Kostuik JP, Maurais GR, Richardson WJ, et al. Combined Single Stage Anterior and Posterior Osteotomy for Correction of Iatrogenic Lumbar Kyphosis. *Spine* 1988;13:257.

! 19. Lagrone MO, Bradford DS, Moe JH, et al. Treatment of Symptomatic Flatback after Spinal Fusion. *J Bone Joint Surg* 1988;70:569.

! 20. Lapinsky AS, Richards BS. Preventing the Crankshaft Phenomenon by Combining Anterior Fusion with Posterior Instrumentation. *Spine* 1995;20:1392.

! 21. Lee CS, Nachemson AL. The Crankshaft Phenomenon after Posterior Harrington Fusion in Skeletally Immature Patients with Thoracic or Thoracolumbar Idiopathic Scoliosis Followed to Maturity. *Spine* 1997;22:58.

! 22. Lenke LG, Bridwell KH, Blanke K, Baldus C. Prospective Analysis of Nutritional Status Normalization Following Spinal Surgery. *Spine* 1995;20:1359.

! 23. Lowe TG, Peters JD. Anterior Spinal Fusion with Zielke Instrumentation for Idiopathic Scoliosis. *Spine* 1993;18:423.

\# 24. Lubicky JP. Congenital Scoliosis. In: Bridwell KH, DeWald RL, eds. *Textbook of Spinal Surgery*. Philadelphia: JB Lippincott, 1997:345.

\# 25. Lubicky JP. Spinal Deformity in Myelomeningocele. In: Bridwell KH, DeWald RL, eds. *Textbook of Spinal Surgery*. Philadelphia: JB Lippincott, 1997:903.

! 26. Luk KD, Leong JC, Reyes FL, Hsu LC. The Comparative Results of Treatment in Idiopathic Thoracolumbar and Lumbar Scoliosis Using the Harrington, Dwyer and Zielke Instrumentation. *Spine* 1989;14:275.

! 27. Madigan RR, Wallace, SL. Scoliosis in Institutionalized Cerebral Palsy Population. *Spine* 1981;6:583.

! 28. Mandelbaum BR, Tolo VT, McAfee PC, Burest P. Nutritional Deficiencies after Staged Anterior and Posterior Spinal Reconstructive Surgery. *Clin Orthop* 1988;234:5.

! 29. McDonnell MF, Glassman SD, Dimar JR, et al. Perioperative Complications of Anterior Procedures on the Spine. *J Bone Joint Surg* 1996;78:839.

! 30. Moe JH, Purcell GA, Bradford DS. Zielke Instrumentation (VDS) for the Correction of Spinal Curvature. *Clin Orthop* 1983;180:133.

! 31. Moran MM, Kroon D, Tredwell SJ, Wadsworth LD. The Role of Autologous Blood Transfusion in Adolescents Undergoing Spinal Surgery. *Spine* 1995;20:532.

! 32. Moskowitz A, Trommanhauser S. Surgical and Clinical Results of Scoliosis Surgery Using Zielke Instrumentation. *Spine* 1993;18:244.

! 33. Myers MA, Hamilton SR, Wagner TA. Postoperative Blindness after Spine Surgery: An Analysis of 37 Cases. *Proceedings of the Scoliosis Research Society*, 1996.

34. Nuber GW, Schafer MF. Surgical Management of Adult Scoliosis. *Clin Orthop* 1986;208:228.

* 35. Ogiela DM, Chan DP. Ventral Derotation Spondylodesis. *Spine* 1986;11:18.

! 36. Powell ET, Krengel WF, King HA, Lagrone MO. Comparison of Same-Day Sequential Anterior and Posterior Spinal Fusion with Delayed Two-Stage Anterior and Posterior Spinal Fusion. *Spine* 1994;19:1256.

! 37. Rodgers WB, Frim DM, Emans JB. Surgery of the Spine in Myelodysplasia. *Clin Orthop* 1997;338:19.

! 38. Rosenthal RK, Levine OB, McCarver CL. The Occurrence of Scoliosis in Cerebral Palsy. *Dev Med Child Neurol* 1974;16:664.

39. Shook, J.E, Lubicky, J.P. Paralytic Scoliosis. In: Bridwell KH, DeWald RL, eds. *Textbook of Spinal Surgery*. Philadelphia: JB Lippincott, 1997:839.

! 40. Shufflebarger HL, Smiley K, Roth HJ. Internal Thoracoplasty. *Spine* 1994;19:840.

! 41. Siller TA, Dickson JH, Erwin WE. Efficacy and Cost Considerations of Intraoperative Autologous Transfusion in Spinal Fusion for Idiopathic Scoliosis with Predeposited Blood. *Spine* 1996;21:848.

! 42. Simpson MB, Georgopoulos G, Eilert RE. Intraoperative Blood Salvage in Children and Young Adults Undergoing Spinal Surgery with Predeposited Autologous Blood: Efficacy and Cost Effectiveness. *J Pediatr Orthop* 1993; 13:777.

! 43. Solomon MD, Rutledge ML, Kane LE, Yawn DH. Cost Comparison of Intraoperative Autologous versus Homologous Transfusion. *Transfusion* 1988;28:378.

! 44. Stark A, Saraste H. Anterior Fusion Insufficient for Scoliosis in Myelomeningocele. *Acta Orthop Scand* 1993; 64:22.

! 45. Thompson AG, Marks DS, Sayampanathan S, Piggott H. Long-Term Results of Combined Anterior and Posterior Convex Epiphsiodesis for Congenital Scoliosis Due to Hemivertebrae. *Spine* 1995;20:1380.

* 46. Waisman M, Saute M. Thoracoscopic Spine Release before Posterior Instrumentation in Scoliosis. *Clin Orthop* 1997;336:130.

! 47. Winter RB, Lonstein JE, Denis FE, Roscoe HS. Convex Growth Arrest for Progressive Congenital Scoliosis Due to Hemivertebrae. *J Pediatr Orthop* 1988;8:633.

! 48. Winter RB, Lonstein JE, Heithoff KB, Kirkham JA. Magnetic Resonance Imaging Evaluation of the Adolescent Patient with Idiopathic Scoliosis before Spinal Instrumentation and Fusion. *Spine* 1997;22:855.

* 49. Zielke K, Stunkat R, Beaujean F. Ventrale Derotations Spondylodese. *Arch Orthop Unfallchir* 1976;85:257.

CHAPTER 156

POSTERIOR SURGERY FOR SCOLIOSIS

Howard A. King

PRINCIPLES OF POSTERIOR TECHNIQUES

The principles of achieving a solid arthrodesis and a stable, balanced spine tend to be overshadowed by the marketing of new implant systems. With the development of each new system comes the promise of "perfect results with no complications." The belief that more hardware is better has shifted our focus away from the concepts of precise planning and selection of fusion levels, meticulous operative technique, and careful postoperative management. New implant systems can and should be added to our armamentarium of scoliosis management, but scientific study is mandatory, and the tried and proven principles must not be forgotten.

Posterior techniques are effective for managing scoliosis associated with a wide variety of disease processes (Table 156.1). Establish the exact diagnosis in each patient whenever possible. An understanding of the natural history and the type of curve pattern that might develop is necessary to determine the appropriate approach for the treatment of idiopathic scoliosis; a patient with congenital scoliosis requires still another approach during evaluation and treatment.

INDICATIONS FOR SURGERY

The indications for surgical treatment vary, depending on the underlying diagnosis, curve magnitude and progression, the patient's age and health, and the surgeon's skill and judgment. All variables must be carefully considered

H. A. King: St. Luke's Regional Medical Center, Boise, Idaho 83712.

Table 156.1.   Etiology of Scoliosis: Conditions for Which Posterior Techniques Are Useful

Idiopathic scoliosis	Collagen disorders
Infantile	Marfan syndrome
Juvenile	Ehlers-Danlos syndrome
Adolescent	
Adult	Infections
Neuromuscular	Tumors
Upper motor neuron	Vertebral column
Cerebral palsy	Spinal cord
Spinocerebellar degeneration	
Charcot-Marie-Tooth	Trauma
Friedreich's ataxia	Fracture
Syringomyelia	Surgical
Viral myelitis	Postlaminectomy
Trauma	Postthoracic procedure
Spinal cord tumor	Irradiation
Lower motor neuron disorders	
Poliomyelitis	Osteochondrodystrophies
Spinal muscle atrophy	Dwarfing syndromes
Myopathy	Mucopolysaccaridoses
Muscular dystrophy	Spondyloepiphyseal dysplasia
Arthrogryposis	Other
Congenital hypotonia	
	Metabolic disorders
Congenital	Rickets
Failure of formation	Osteogenesis imperfecta
Failure of segmentation	Others
Neurofibromatosis	Congenital heart disease
	Congenital limb deficiency

before rendering a surgical decision. In general, there are four indications for surgical treatment in idiopathic or congenital scoliosis: severe curves, unacceptable curve progression, pain, and unacceptable cosmesis (Table 156.2).

Table 156.2.   Indications for Surgery for Idiopathic Scoliosis

Unacceptable curve progression

Unacceptable curve magnitude
   Greater than 50° if skeletally mature
   Greater than 40° if skeletally immature

Failure of bracing to control progression if curve magnitude meets above criteria

Intolerable Pain

Unacceptable cosmesis

Loss of neurologic function

Curves of greater than 65° reduce total lung capacity (8,14,39,55). Therefore, large or progressive curves should be corrected and stabilized. Winter et al. (61,62) reported on the role that thoracic lordosis plays in decreasing pulmonary function and recommended screening and treatment in severe cases. In patients with thoracic lordosis, surgery may be necessary even though the coronal curve may not appear large enough to warrant it.

Collis and Ponseti (14) have shown that curves greater than 50° tend to progress even after skeletal maturity. There is a correlation between age, Risser sign, and curve magnitude as prognostic indications for progression (34, 54). In young patients without evidence of menarche, a Risser sign of 1 or less, and a curve of 40° or more, orthotics management is less effective and surgery might be indicated. On the other hand, there are times when combined thoracic and lumbar curves exceed 45° to 50° in magnitude but show no loss of pulmonary function, are cosmetically acceptable, and remain stable. These curves might be best managed by observation. All patients are different, so determine treatment on an individual basis.

Pain is rarely associated with idiopathic scoliosis in the adolescent group. If a patient complains of pain, a thor-

Table 156.3. Indications for Surgery for Neuromuscular Scoliosis

Unacceptable curve progression

Unacceptable curve magnitude
  More than 40°–50°

Failure of bracing to control progression of the curve

Intolerable pain

Unacceptable loss of function
  Impaired ambulation
  Loss of or impaired sitting balance

ough investigation to rule out organic causes must be undertaken. Adults with untreated curves, especially large curves, may have disabling pain that can be relieved by surgical treatment (30,43,48,51,57).

An unacceptable cosmetic appearance may be an indication for surgical treatment. Severe trunk decompensation or rotation may be a reason for surgery, but that decision must be made by the patient and family. Scoliosis surgery is a major undertaking: Careful thought must be given if the only indication is cosmesis. Rib deformity may not be corrected by correcting the curve, and improving the deformity always leaves a surgical scar.

In neuromuscular conditions, the indications for surgery are similar to those for idiopathic or congenital problems (Table 156.3). In patients who are marginal ambulators or wheelchair bound, progressive spinal curvatures may compromise ambulation or sitting balance. In wheelchair-bound patients, listing to the side because of a decompensated spine necessitates increased use of the upper extremities to achieve support and balance, which severely impairs overall function. In patients with poor sensation, progressive scoliosis tends to create pelvic obliquity, with subsequent asymmetric pressure-loading on the buttocks and eventual skin breakdown.

PREOPERATIVE PLANNING

Careful preoperative evaluation and planning are integral to the overall success of spinal surgery. Attention to detail at this phase is essential for a smooth perioperative course. Document a careful history and physical examination of the patient. The neurologic evaluation is especially important in patients with congenital or neurologic conditions. Any abnormal findings will necessitate further evaluation with electromyography, myelogram, computed tomography (CT), or magnetic resonance imaging (MRI). In the physical examination of the spine, note rotational promi-

nences, the amount of decompensation of the spine, and any evidence of defects or cutaneous abnormalities along the midline. Cutaneous abnormalities such as hair patches, nevi, dermal sinuses, and lipomas are frequently associated with intraspinal pathology (19,27,61). Myelography or MRI may be indicated to rule out disease in or about the spinal cord.

RADIOLOGIC EVALUATION

Magnetic resonance imaging is a relatively recent advance for evaluating the spinal column and its contents. This noninvasive tool has been valuable in diagnosing syringomyelia and other spinal cord anomalies. However, the three-dimensional nature of scoliosis can make clear imaging difficult. A close working relationship with the radiologist is necessary so that specific problems may be more carefully evaluated. (See Chapter 4 on imaging modalities.)

Myelography is indicated when abnormal neurologic findings are present on the physical examination, when spinal dysraphism is expected, and when MRI has proven inadequate or equivocal. Water-soluble dyes are preferred whenever possible because they can be used in conjunction with CT and are useful in conditions in which the neurologic deficits are not consistent with the known diagnosis.

Begin preoperative radiographic evaluation with upright posteroanterior and lateral radiographs of the spine. Measure the curve by the Cobb method (12). Look for rotation and any evidence of congenital anomalies, tumors, or bony abnormalities. The Nash and Moe classification of rotation is useful in determining structural curvatures and selecting fusion levels (29). The lateral radiograph shows curvatures in the sagittal plane and the possible coexistence of lumbosacral spondylolisthesis. Supine right and left side-bending films demonstrate curve flexibility and give a good indication of the amount of correction that can be anticipated from surgery (29). In severe deformities, bending films help in deciding whether to perform anterior procedures. For patients with severe rigid curves, it may be desirable to consider anterior releases or wedge resection before the posterior procedure. (See Chapter 155 for the anterior approach to scoliosis.) This allows better mobility of the spine and may decrease the pseudarthrosis rate. When excessive kyphosis or lordosis is noted, take lateral flexion and extension views. In patients with paralytic scoliosis, a supine view in maximum traction including the pelvis is useful to determine the amount of curve flexibility and what type of correction of pelvic obliquity might be expected.

Other diagnostic modalities may be necessary, depending on the clinical setting. In adolescent patients with scoliosis and back pain, perform technetium polyphosphate bone imaging to rule out tumor or inflammatory causes.

Keim and Reina (28) have reported osteoid osteoma as a cause of painful scoliosis.

LABORATORY STUDIES

Preoperatively, obtain a complete blood count, urinalysis, and electrolyte values in patients who are otherwise healthy. Any major medical problem might necessitate further studies. In patients with neuromuscular conditions or with severe scoliosis, obtain a preoperative electrocardiogram. Electrocardiography is also indicated in adults undergoing corrective spinal surgery. In patients with known cardiomyopathy, congenital heart disease, or cor pulmonale, obtain anesthesia, pulmonary, and cardiology consultations before surgery. For patients with severe debilitating health problems, careful preoperative evaluation and management by an appropriate team of physicians, surgeons, and paraprofessionals ensures an easier and smoother postoperative course.

PULMONARY EVALUATION

Vital capacity and total lung capacity are decreased in patients with scoliosis (8,18,38,60). The amount of decrease seems to correlate with the degree of curvature (39, 60). Neuromuscular conditions tend to compound the loss of vital capacity from the scoliosis (17). For most patients, however, the decreased pulmonary function does not play a major role in the perioperative course. Therefore, routine preoperative pulmonary function studies are unnecessary.

Pulmonary function studies and arterial blood gases are indicated in patients with cor pulmonale, severe curves, thoracic lordosis, neuromuscular conditions, or a history of pulmonary problems. A 40% or greater loss of vital capacity and maximum breathing capacity increases the risk of postoperative complications (60). In patients with recurrent pneumonia and bronchitis secondary to scoliosis, a complicated postoperative course must be anticipated; pulmonary studies are helpful in these patients.

A trial of halo traction may be indicated in patients with severe lung disease or cor pulmonale. This trial of traction will establish the operability of a patient's curve. Any increase in cardiac or pulmonary compromise in halo traction is a contraindication for surgery (9).

The use of preoperative casting, traction, and other modalities to make the curve more mobile (or limber) or to obtain preliminary correction has been advocated in the past. There are now few indications for these methods because they add little if any correction to the spine. With rare exception, they have limited applicability.

SELECTION OF FUSION LEVELS

Proper selection of fusion levels is one of the most important aspects of the preoperative planning. An inadequate length of fusion will lead to progression of the curve above or below the fusion (lengthening or "adding on" to the curve). This may eventually lead to loss of spine balance. A fusion that is too long, however, unnecessarily immobilizes the spine. A careful review of curve patterns and preoperative side-bending radiographs is valuable in defining the primary and compensatory curves. In general, the primary curve should be fused and the compensatory curves should be left unfused. For idiopathic scoliosis, fusion levels should include all vertebrae that are measured as a part of the primary curve (9,11,16,47).

When pelvic obliquity is present in neuromuscular scoliosis, understanding the curve pattern will help avoid a common pitfall: not incorporating the sacrum into the fusion. An oblique sacrum and pelvis must be considered as part of the curvature and should be included in the instrumentation and fusion.

Idiopathic Scoliosis

The selection of fusion levels is controversial in combined thoracic and lumbar idiopathic scoliosis. It is generally accepted that the fusion should include all vertebrae that are a part of the measured curve. In thoracic scoliosis, Harrington (24,25) suggests fusion from one level above the curve to two levels below, as long as the inferior level falls within the "stable zone." Moe (44,45,47) and Goldstein (20–22) stressed the importance of extending the fusion from the neutrally rotated vertebra superiorly to the neutral vertebra inferiorly. Moe advocates thoracic fusion for combined thoracic and lumbar curves when the lumbar curve is more flexible on preoperative side-bending radiographs.

In 1983, King et al. (29) reported the long-term results of the Twin Cities Scoliosis Center's management of thoracic and combined thoracic and lumbar scoliosis. A category of curve types and criteria for selection of fusion levels were established. In addition, the results of this work support the concept of selective fusion of the thoracic spine in selected cases. These authors were able to identify five different thoracic curve patterns (Table 156.4). Type I curves are managed by fusion to L-4. In curve types II through V, a selective thoracic fusion can be performed if the lowest level of the fusion is centered over the sacrum (Figs. 156.1–156.5). The lowest level of the fusion is established by drawing a line parallel to the iliac wings. A vertical line is then drawn perpendicular to the pelvic line centered on the sacrum. (It is important that any limb-length inequality be compensated for when the radiographs are taken.) The lowest vertebra most closely bisected by this line is called the stable vertebra (Fig. 156.6). Ending the fusion at the stable vertebra gives uniformly good results.

In most curves, this method produces a fusion area that is substantially shorter than the standard T4–L4 fusion previously recommended. King et al. (29) concluded that

Table 156.4. *Thoracic Scoliosis Curve Patterns*

Type I
 Combined thoracic and lumbar
 Lumbar curve larger than the thoracic curve
 Thoracic curve more flexible than the lumbar curve on
   side-bending radiographs

Type II
 Thoracic curve larger than the lumbar curve
 Lumbar curve more flexible than the thoracic curve on
   side-bending radiographs

Type III
 Thoracic curves when the lumbar curve does not cross
   the midline

Type IV
 Long thoracic curve when L-5 is centered over the sacrum but L-4 tilts into the lumbar curve

Type V
 Double thoracic curve with T-1 tilted into the concavity
   of the upper curve
 The upper curve structural on side-bending radiographs

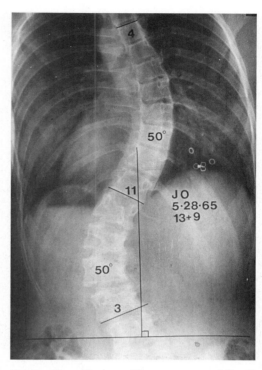

Figure 156.2. Type II curve. The center sacral line has been created. The stable vertebra is T-12.

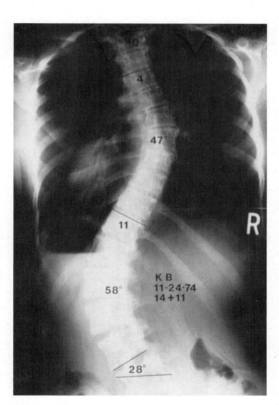

Figure 156.1. Type I curve. (From King HA, Moe JH, Bradford DS, Winter RB. The Selection of Fusion Levels in Thoracic Idiopathic Scoliosis. *J Bone Joint Surg Am* 1983;65:1302, with permission.)

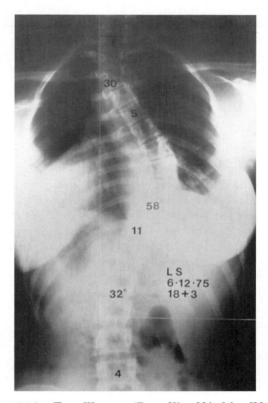

Figure 156.3. Type III curve. (From King HA, Moe JH, Bradford DS, Winter RB. The Selection of Fusion Levels in Thoracic Idiopathic Scoliosis. *J Bone Joint Surg Am* 1983;65:1302, with permission.)

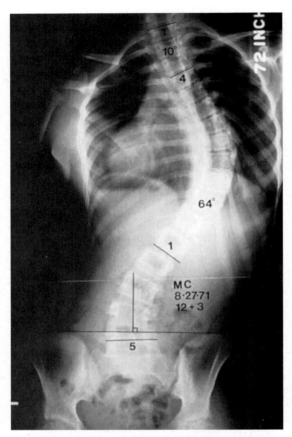

Figure 156.4. Type IV curve. (From King HA, Moe JH, Bradford DS, Winter RB. The Selection of Fusion Levels in Thoracic Idiopathic Scoliosis. *J Bone Joint Surg Am* 1983;65:1302, with permission.)

spondylolysis or spondylolisthesis is present, fusion using the criteria just outlined can be safely performed (9).

Neuromuscular Scoliosis

In many neuromuscular conditions (e.g., Friedreich's ataxia, Charcot-Marie-Tooth disease, and ambulators with cerebral palsy), the curve patterns are similar to idiopathic scoliosis. In those instances, fusion levels may be chosen as just described for idiopathic curves. Analysis of the lateral roentgenograms is important to avoid stopping the fusion at the apex of a kyphosis.

In the more common neuromuscular curve where pelvic obliquity is noted, the sacrum and pelvis must be considered part of the scoliosis. This situation is most frequently seen in cerebral palsy, myelomeningocele, muscular dystrophy, spinal muscle atrophy, and scoliosis secondary to spinal cord injury. If the sacrum and pelvis are not included in the instrumentation and fusion, progressive pelvic obliquity and loss of sitting balance result. If there is doubt about extending the fusion to the pelvis in a neuromuscular curve, err on the side of extending the fusion.

selective thoracic fusion can give good long-term results with balanced stable spines. When the fusion falls short of the stable vertebra, the curves tend to progress, adding vertebrae to the measured curve, and occasionally an additional surgical procedure is needed to extend the fusion. Fusing beyond the stable vertebrae, especially in type II curves, tends to aggravate the lumbar curve and also removes additional valuable motion segments.

Aaro and Ohlen (1) and Chochran et al. (13) have clearly detailed the complications of fusion that extend into the lumbar spine. Harrington rod fusions flatten the lumbar spine, and fusions to L-4 and L-5 carry a higher incidence of back pain on long-term follow-up. In their report, 62% were fused to L-4, and 82% were fused to L-5. (1). Be aware of compensatory curves and avoid extensive fusion when possible. In idiopathic scoliosis, avoid fusion to L-4. Rarely, if ever, is fusion to L-5 indicated. Fusion to the sacrum is not indicated in adolescents. However, if symptomatic spondylolisthesis is present, lumbosacral fusion might be indicated. When an asymptomatic

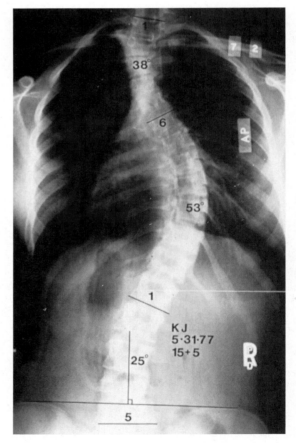

Figure 156.5. Type V curve. (From King HA, Moe JH, Bradford DS, Winter RB. The Selection of Fusion Levels in Thoracic Idiopathic Scoliosis. *J Bone Joint Surg Am* 1983;65:1302, with permission.)

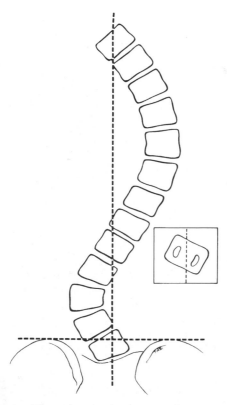

Figure 156.6. The technique for creating the center sacral line to establish the stable vertebra.

In the nonambulator with pelvic obliquity, a short fusion invariably leads to curve progression. When the sacrum is included in the fusion, lumbar lordosis must be maintained. A flat lumbar spine leads to poor sitting balance, and to skin breakdown in patients with insensate skin.

The superior level of fusion is more controversial. In patients with idiopathic patterns, the rules are similar to idiopathic curves. In wheelchair-bound patients, the superior extension of the instrumentation and fusion should be carried high into the thoracic spine, usually to T-2 or T-3. The underlying problem is poor muscle tone or muscle imbalance. Failure to extend the fusion proximally will lead to the development of deformity above the fusion. A progressive kyphosis above a short lumbar fusion inevitably leads to loss of sitting balance and risks potential skin breakdown.

Congenital Scoliosis

When congenital scoliosis has progressed and surgical treatment is contemplated, carefully analyze the curves in the coronal and sagittal planes. Preoperative MRI or myelography is warranted. Use side-bending films to analyze compensatory curve flexibility. Much as in the patient with idiopathic scoliosis, the fusion must be balanced over the center of gravity, and compensatory motion must be

preserved. I tend to follow guidelines similar to those given previously in the section on idiopathic scoliosis. In congenital scoliosis, curves are variable, so exact guidelines are difficult to define. Carefully analyze primary and compensatory curves and adhere to the principles of balancing the fusion mass over the center of gravity and fusing selectively, and you will generally obtain a good result. (See Chapter 158 for further details on congenital conditions of the spine.)

◢ SURGICAL TECHNIQUES

POSTERIOR SPINAL FUSION

The primary goal of spinal arthrodesis is to establish an environment favorable for bone maturation and union. For the surgery, a four-poster frame (a variation of the Hall-Relton frame) allows the abdomen to fall free, thereby decreasing intra-abdominal and venous pressure.

- Position the patient prone on the frame, avoiding pressure on the brachial plexus and ulnar nerves. Pad the knees and ankles. When fusion to the lumbar spine or sacrum is planned, position the patient with the hips extended to maintain normal lumbar lordosis.
- Prepare and drape the back for an extensive surgical exposure.
- Make a straight incision and infiltrate the skin with 1:500,000 epinephrine in normal saline to help control bleeding.
- Use self-retaining retractors for exposure. The pressure from the retractors also helps reduce the capillary bleeding.
- Use electrocoagulation to control all bleeders.
- Initiate the subperiosteal exposure of the spine with a sharp Cobb elevator.

It is absolutely mandatory that the elevators, curets, gouges, and osteotomes be sharp and well maintained. Avoid excessive force at all times around the spine! Sharp instruments make gentle surgery possible.

- Use the Cobb elevator to dissect the soft tissues from the spinous processes, lamina, and facets out to the tips of the transverse processes. Control bleeding with electrocautery and sponge packs.
- Place a metallic marker on a spinous process and obtain an intraoperative radiograph to document the position on the spine. It is amazingly easy to become confused about the proper spine level without radiographic control.
- Place Adson self-retaining retractors deep into the wound and clear the facet joints of ligaments and capsules. Sharp curets facilitate adequate clearing of the soft tissues.
- Roll and pack gauze sponges along the areas that have

been exposed. Gentle pressure, along with meticulous electrocoagulation, will maintain a dry field. Good-quality bone and instrument work are impossible in a bloody operative field.

- Bone bleeding can also be controlled with bone wax and Gelfoam patties soaked with topical thrombin.
- Blood loss is best reduced by meticulous operative technique and controlled hypotension by an anesthesiologist experienced in hypotensive anesthesia. (See Chapter 7 for more details.)
- When you have adequate exposure of the spine and hemostasis, obtain a bone graft from the posterior iliac crest if autologous bone is to be used for fusion. Either use a separate incision over the iliac crest or, if the primary surgical incision is to be carried down to the lumbar spine, the same surgical incision can be used. A subperiosteal exposure of the iliac crest is preferred. (For many neuromuscular conditions and for spina bifida, I have had excellent results using cadaver bone.)
- With a Capner gouge or air-driven impact osteotome, take cortical and cancellous strips of bone from the outer table and the underlying cancellous bone. Harvest a generous amount of bone and carefully store it in saline or cover it with a blood-soaked sponge. (See Chapter 9 for bone-graft harvesting techniques.)
- Control graft-site bleeding with bone wax.
- Fuse the facet joints as a standard procedure, regardless of the instrumentation system used. The long-term success of any fusion depends on a solid arthrodesis, and it is the combination of techniques and instrumentation that will accomplish this.
- In the thoracic spine, use a Capner gouge to remove a generous portion of the inferior facets on both the concave and convex sides of the curve.
- With a curet, remove the visible cartilage. Then use the gouge to decorticate the superior portion of the junction of the transverse process and the facet. Pack a generous piece of cancellous bone into the facet with the Moe bone impactor (Fig. 156.7).
- In the lumbar spine, the facet joints can be excised using a straight ¼-inch Lambotte osteotome or a Lexcel rongeur. It is important to see the joint and remove the articular cartilage completely (Fig. 156.8). Then pack a piece of cancellous bone into place with the Moe impactor.
- After the facets have been excised and the bone grafts placed, remove the spinous processes. Complete decortication of the spine with either a sharp, curved gouge or with an air-driven impact osteotome. Use extreme caution here, because open lamina or instrument sites are present and may be entered by the gouge. Pack the bone graft obtained by decortication of the spinous processes and iliac crest along the decorticated spine.

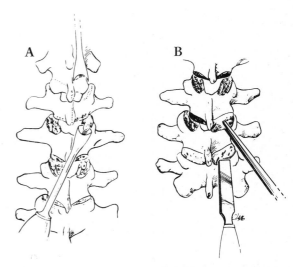

Figure 156.7. The techniques used for excising the thoracic joint (**A**) and packing with cancellous bone (**B**).

RESECTION OF THE RIB HUMP

In patients with large, unsightly rib humps, rib resections can be performed through the same surgical incision.

- Develop a skin and subcutaneous flap on the affected side to the posterior axillary line.
- Subperiosteally dissect each rib and then cut it with a rib cutter medially and as far laterally as possible. Steel

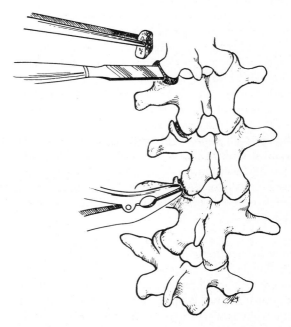

Figure 156.8. The technique used for excising lumbar facets and packing with cancellous bone plugs.

(56) has reported excellent cosmetic results with this technique.

- The ribs supply abundant bone graft and make a separate iliac exposure unnecessary.
- Take care to avoid entering the pleural cavity. If the pleural cavity is entered, place a chest tube and connect it to a closed water-seal suction system.
- Close the wound using a running 0 Vicryl (Ethicon) suture for the fascia.
- Prior to closure of the wound, I routinely place a suction drainage system. Place the tubing on the fascia, not next to the cancellous bone, to avoid excessive drainage of blood and to prevent clogging of the drain by the bone.
- Close the subcutaneous tissue with a 2-0 Vicryl suture and the skin with a running subcuticular 3-0 Vicryl suture. The latter makes a good cosmetic closure and avoids the cross-hatching of interrupted sutures. Relieve skin tension with adhesive skin tapes and apply a bulky pressure dressing.

INSTRUMENTATION SYSTEM

Recent years have brought many new spinal instrumentation systems to the forefront, and more and better systems will undoubtedly be developed. Evaluate each system on its own merits (Table 156.5). One system will probably not solve every problem, so you must be facile and knowledgeable in the use of many systems.

As implant systems have come onto the market, the most successful seem to have similar characteristics. They generally have a broad range of applicability and usually combine options for the use of hooks, screws, and wires. Most combine open and closed hooks for ease of use. It is important that the implant profile is such that it is not prominent in thin patients.

Harrington Instrumentation

The Harrington instrumentation system was the gold standard in the treatment of idiopathic scoliosis for many years. New implant systems using dual rods and multiple points of fixation with hooks, wires, and screws have replaced the Harrington system. Most systems have moved away from simple distraction and have evolved into a more three-dimensional technique using translation, counter torsion, and limited distraction.

Instrumentation without Fusion

When the patient's curve is difficult or impossible to manage with braces or orthoses, and spinal growth is desirable, instrumentation without fusion can be performed (15,35–37,40,46). The technique is useful in small children with infantile idiopathic scoliosis and in patients with selected neuromuscular conditions in whom curve control and spinal growth are necessary.

The surgical technique is similar to standard instrumentation technique, varying with the patient's size and bone stock.

- Use standard positioning, preparation, draping, and incision as described previously, but expose the spine only at the proximal and distal hook sites. Do not expose the remainder of the spine.
- Confirm proper levels by radiography.
- I prefer to use one of the new multi-hooks and rod systems for the implant system. I originally used the Harrington system, but it allowed for simple distraction only and could not accommodate more than one hook at the top and one at the bottom of the instrumented levels. I currently prefer the ISOLA system (DePuy Acromed, Raynham, MA) because of its low profile and adaptability for difficult problems.
- Create a claw configuration at the top of the curve and use a down-going hook at the inferior end of the curve. A claw can also be created on the inferior end of the curve, if desired. This will add extra stability (Figs. 156.9, 156.10).

Table 156.5. *Harrington Instrumentation System and Variations*

	Cobb correction	Rotation correction	Stability	Safety	Ease of use	Cost	Postoperative immobilization
Harrington	+ +	+	+ +	+ + +	+ + + +	+ + + +	+
Harrington sublaminar wire	+ +	+	+ + +	+ +	+ +	+ + + +	+ +
Luque	+ +	+	+ + +	+ +	+ +	+ + + +	+ +
Cotrel-Dubousset	+ +	+	+ + +	+ +	+	+	+ + +
3-D rod, wire, hook system	+ + +	+ +	+ + +	+ +	+	+	+ + +

+, least; + +, average; + + +, above average; + + + +, most.

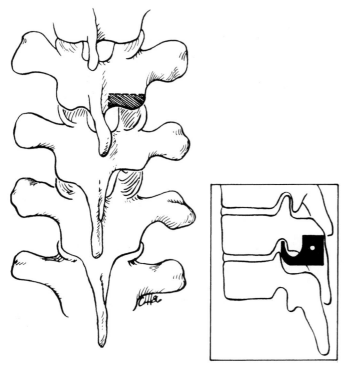

Figure 156.9. Create hook sites in the thoracic spine by excising a portion of the inferior facet.

- It is possible to use concave and convex rods to enhance correction and control of the curve.
- Thread the rods beneath the skin and through the subcutaneous tissues in the middle of the curve, and avoid subperiosteal stripping, which risks spontaneous fusion.
- Use two rod segments connected by an axial connector (i.e., a rod sleeve into which both rods fit and are held in place with screw fixation). Axial connectors allow

you to return to the site in 6–9 months and lengthen the rods without having to open the entire incision. Such lengthening can often be done as an outpatient procedure.
- It is also possible to merely leave the rods long on either end. This allows extra length for subsequent lengthenings and avoids the need of axial or side-by-side connectors.

In very young patients with very small and soft bones, expose the superior and inferior hook sites and place bone graft at these areas. This will create a localized fusion that can be used for hook placement 4–6 months later, at which time these "platforms" can be used to establish claw constructs as previously described.

Postoperative Care   After subcutaneous rodding, keep the patients in a postoperative orthosis. Lengthening is generally necessary every 6–9 months and can be continued until adequate growth has been achieved. At that time, the definitive spinal fusion and instrumentation can be completed.

Luque Instrumentation
Luque has described a procedure combining segmental instrumentation and rodding but no fusion (35–37,53). Theoretically, this avoids the need for postoperative immobilization. Luque has clearly shown that subperiosteal dissection alone does not alter spinal growth. However, this is a procedure with many complications. I prefer a modification of the Moe (15) and Marchetti (40) techniques of rodding without fusion.

The concept of segmental spine instrumentation was introduced by Eduardo Luque in 1975 (36,37). He originally developed the technique by augmenting standard Harrington rods with segmental sublaminar wires, then modified it to use dual smooth L-shaped rods with sublaminar wires and spinal fusion.

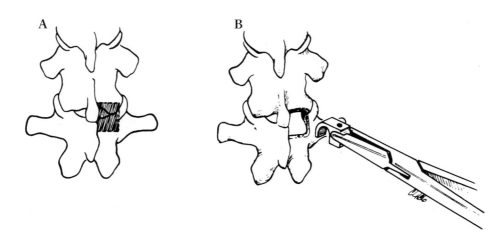

Figure 156.10.   **A:** Position of the laminar Harrington hook. **B:** The Cotrel-Dubousset laminar hooks are positioned with similar technique.

I use many of Luque's original concepts but have adapted newer approaches combined with sublaminar wire fixation. The technique is excellent for neuromuscular scoliosis, in patients with soft bone, and in patients where fusion to the sacrum may be necessary. When fusion to the sacrum is indicated, I combine the modified Luque technique with Galveston pelvic fixation as described by Allen and Ferguson (2). I also use pedicle screw fixation in the sacrum, and I may also use pelvic screws instead of the contoured smooth rod for pelvic fixation. The addition of sacral screws has been invaluable in obtaining sacral fixation. The conventional L-shaped rod with Galveston fixation does not obtain sacral purchase. It really bypasses the sacrum, crosses the sacroiliac joint, and obtains fixation in the iliac wings. This has some obvious disadvantages; however, the fixation to the pelvis combined with screw fixation in the sacrum seems to give the best purchase and best control of the lumbosacral junction.

The Luque technique begins with the standard positioning, preparation, and surgical exposure as described earlier in this chapter.

- Excise the facets at each level and the ligamentum flavum with a Lexcel rongeur. Kerrison rongeurs can be used to complete removal of the ligamentum flavum.
- Loop a 16-gauge wire and pass it carefully under the lamina at each level to be fused. The diameter of the curve in the wire should be about the same width of the lamina, so that as the wire passes, it will smoothly pass under the lamina and then come out over the superior edge of the next lamina (Figs. 156.11, 156.12).
- Grasp the wire with a needle holder and pull it through. Maintain constant upward force, which keeps the wire taut against the undersurface of the lamina and avoids downward movement toward the spinal cord.
- Wire management is very important to avoid deep wire penetration into the spinal canal. I prefer the technique described by Yngve et al. (65) (Fig. 156.11).
- As the wire comes up, tighten it down over the lamina.
- After positioning the rod, cut the loop on the wire, creating two separate wires at each level (Fig. 156.11C). The wires can then be sequentially tightened, bringing the spine to the rod. This technique decreases the amount of wire handling and tends to keep the operative field easier to manage.

I have recently changed my technique for the superior portion of the rod. Luque described using wires at all levels, including the top of the rod. However, on occasion a junctional kyphosis can develop at the superior end of the fusion because of the removal of the ligamentum flavum and posterior interspinous ligaments. I now use open hooks at the top two levels to create a claw construct.

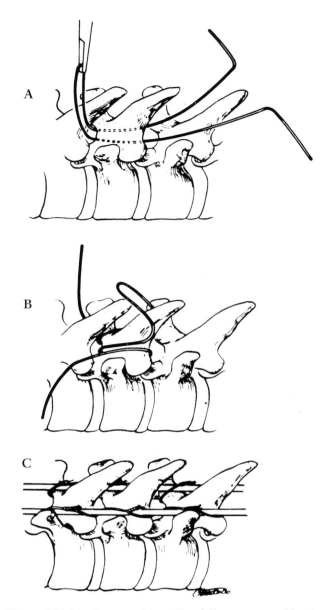

Figure 156.11. Luque wiring; Carefully manage sublaminar wires. A looped wire may be cut to create two wires. **A:** Carefully pass a looped wire beneath the lamina from inferior to superior, avoiding impingement on the spinal cord or roots. **B:** Centralize the wire and place a strand of wire on each side of the spinous process. **C:** Cut the loop of the wire and secure it around the rods on each side.

- Place a supra-laminar hook or transverse process hook from cephalad to caudad.
- Place the up-going hook at the level of the down-going hook, or at the level below (Fig. 156.13).
- Excise the inferior facet with a ¼-inch osteotome. Remove the cartilage with a sharp curet and position an open hook.

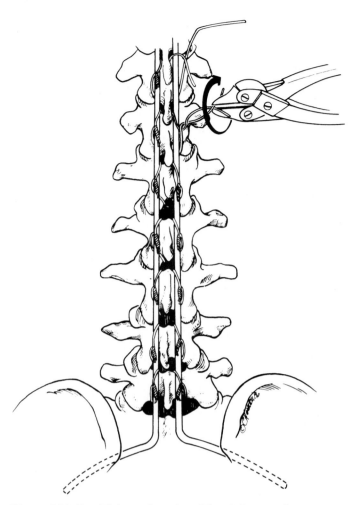

Figure 156.12.   Tighten the wires. The Galveston fixation is positioned between the inner and outer tables just below the posterior superior iliac spine and above the greater sciatic notch. See text for details.

- As the rod is brought close to the spine by wire tightening, the rod will come into the open hooks and then can be secured with hook caps (Figs. 156.14, 156.15).

The choice of system is generally decided by the surgeon's own personal preference. At the inferior level of the sacrum, use sacral screw fixation in addition to the Galveston or pelvic screw fixation. The sacral screws link the ilium and the sacrum and help reduce the amount of stress on the pelvis. I have noted significantly less bone absorption around the pelvic posts with the addition of sacral screw fixation, especially in patients with neuromuscular scoliosis and soft bone.

The screws are usually situated in the sacral pedicle just below and lateral to the L5–S1 facet.

- Identify the pedicle and probe it with the gear shift probe.

- Confirm the placement with a ball-tipped pedicle probe and lateral roentgenogram.
- I generally use bicortical purchase.
- Tap for the screw, and again probe, and then position a screw of the appropriate length and diameter.
- Confirm screw placement with a roentgenogram or fluoroscopic image.
- Once the screws have been placed, attach them to the rod using slotted connectors. If the angle is difficult to accommodate with rod contouring, use a variable-angle slotted connector.

When the fusion is continued to the pelvis, I tend to favor the Galveston technique or the use of an iliac bolt,

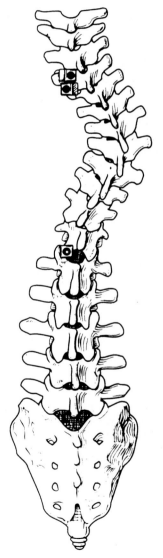

Figure 156.13.   Create anchor sites at the superior curve and inferiorly at the stable vertebra in thoracic types II, III, IV, and V curves. See text for details. (By permission of Dr. Marc Asher.)

which can be attached to the rod by a slotted connector. I generally expose both iliac wings through the midline incision. Adequate exposure is necessary to visualize the greater sciatic notches bilaterally. The entry point for the **L** portion of the rod is usually just below the posterior superior iliac spine (PSIS).

- Make a hole in the superior border of the posterior ileum just below the PSIS with a ³⁄₁₆- or ¼-inch drill, depending on the size of the rod chosen.
- Insert the rod between the tables of the ileum so that it lies 1–1.5 cm above the greater sciatic notch. The length of the rod or screw is usually 6–8 cm, depending on the size of the patient.

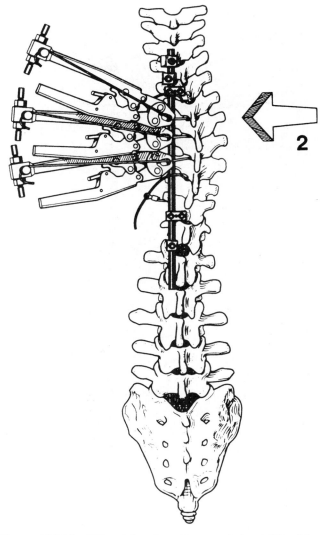

Figure 156.15. Wire tightening. (By permission of Dr. Marc Asher.) See text for details.

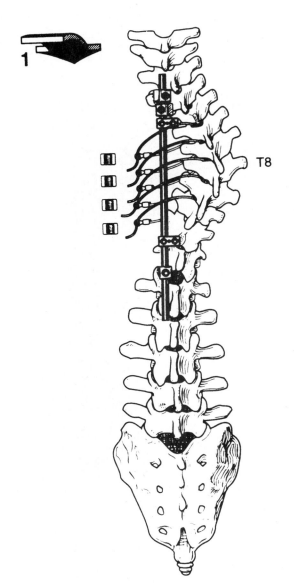

Figure 156.14. Place sublaminar wires at the apex to help create translation forces. See text for details. (By permission of Dr. Marc Asher.)

- Rod contour is important to correct the deformity and maintain normal sagittal balance. I generally use a malleable template to help establish the appropriate bend. The rods are then contoured using the Cotrel-Dubousset French bender and the Asher ISOLA bending irons.
- After appropriate bending, position the rods and sequentially tighten and secure the wires (Figs. 156.16–156.18).
- After the hardware is secured and all wires are tightened, decorticate the remaining exposed transverse processes and lamina using gouges and rongeurs. Take great care to avoid penetrating the open laminotomies.
- Carefully pack autogenous iliac bone or banked bone around the decorticated spine.

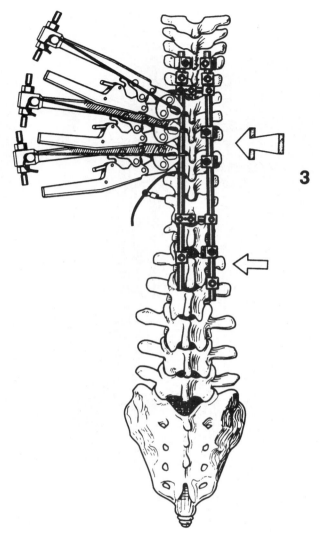

compression and derotation of the spine. Their system consisted of a series of open and closed hooks and a knurled rod with a diamond-patterned surface. It allowed the two rods to be connected by cross-links, increasing the overall stability of the system. Cotrel and Dubousset stressed the importance of maintaining and creating normal sagittal contours. Their system of rotation and Luque's concept of translation were the first efforts to move away from the old concept of pure distraction and move toward an attempt to obtain three-dimensional spine correction. As the popularity of the Cotrel-Dubousset system grew, others started to develop their own implant systems. Most of the new systems have been based on the concept of flexibility in use and the ability to fix to the spine with multiple points of fixation. Most use hooks, wires, and screws, in combination, as the means

3

Figure 156.16.   Place a convex rod to create a countertorsion force. (By permission of Dr. Marc Asher.) See text for details.

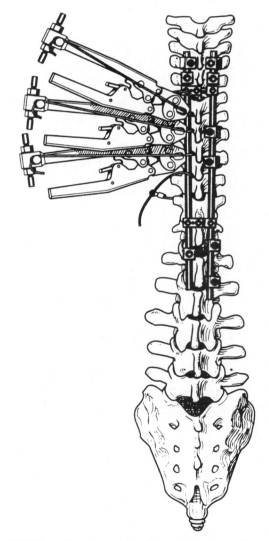

■ Close the wound using a drain above the fascia as described previously.

Although some surgeons (2,35–37) feel that no postoperative immobilization is necessary, Herndon et al. (26) reported a 10% pseudarthrosis rate when no postoperative bracing was used, and a near-zero incidence with bracing. In my experience, a custom-molded, bivalved, polypropylene brace prevents loss of correction and makes most patients more comfortable and more mobile postoperatively.

Multi-Hooks and Rod Systems
Historical Background   In 1981, Yves Cotrel and Jean Dubousset of France introduced a spine implant system that combined segmental fixation with distraction

Figure 156.17.   Complete tightening of the wires. (By permission of Dr. Marc Asher.) See text for details.

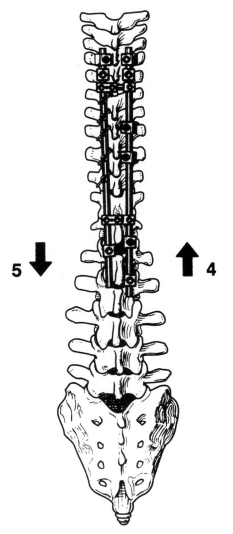

5 ⬇   ⬆ 4

Figure 156.18.   Application of concave distraction and convex compression complete the instrumentation sequence. See text for details. (By permission of Dr. Marc Asher.)

of spine fixation. Virtually all of the systems, when used properly, will give good spine correction and excellent results.

The new multi-hooks and rod systems are complicated, and their application is complex. When first using these systems, obtain hands-on training with surgeons who are experienced with them.

Because these new systems use multiple hooks, screws, and wires to rigidly stabilize the cross-linked dual rods, the need for bracing is diminished, which is a huge advantage for the patient. Bracing is occasionally used for patients who have soft bone or for whom compliance is questionable. I have used bracing to control an unfused lumbar curve, surgically treating the thoracic curve and using bracing to control the unfused segment. The criteria for

discontinuing the use of a brace are those used in a standard brace program.

The selection of fusion levels using the new systems has been controversial. I select fusion levels based on the criteria established by King et al. (29). Early in the Cotrel-Dubousset experience, there were numerous reports of lumbar curve decompensation after selective thoracic fusion (10,33,41). These problems had not been noted in series reporting the use of Harrington instrumentation. Cotrel and Dubousset have proposed that instrumentation levels should include all sagittally abnormal zones, create rotational neutralization, and finish in the Harrington stable zone. This frequently necessitates fusion into the upper lumbar spine. Thompson et al. (58) and Wood et al. (63, 64) have reported data suggesting that overrotation of the thoracic curve locks the transitional thoracolumbar rotation segments, making it impossible for the lumbar curve to balance the thoracic spine. This situation leads to a shift of the thoracic curve to the left and frequently causes progression of the lumbar curve. Richards et al. (52) and Benson et al. (7) have shown that large curves and less flexible lumbar curves are more likely to decompensate with standard Cotrel-Dubousset techniques. Richards et al. believe that in thoracic curves greater than 60°, with a lumbar component greater than 45°, lumbar decompensation may occur with selective thoracic fusion (52). They suggested fusion of both curves when the thoracic and lumbar curves are large.

In 1949, Von Lackum and Miller (59) advised caution when correcting the primary curve. They stated that the primary curve must not be corrected beyond the compensatory curve's ability to correct and balance the spine. It is important to realize that these words were written prior to the advent of internal fixation; with advanced corrective devices they are more timely than ever! Massey et al. (42) have reported on their series of fusions using Cotrel-Dubousset instrumentation and fusing to levels selected according to King's criteria. They found no problems with lumbar decompensation as long as no attempt was made to overcorrect the thoracic spine. Previous implant systems have not provided the powerful corrective forces that the newer systems offer. We may have temporarily lost sight of the importance of spinal stability and balance. Our patients are not as concerned about the number of degrees of correction as they are about the appearance of a balanced stable spine. We must remember the wisdom of Von Lackum and Miller (59).

Recent work by Asher and others has advanced our concept of scoliosis correction. Asher has done extensive three-dimensional studies to better understand and explain the findings noted in idiopathic scoliosis. In a report of his three-dimensional studies of the scoliosis deformity, Asher and Cook (5) found that in progressive curves the apex vertebra tends to displace laterally and posteriorly, and that the spine tends to collapse toward the midcoronal plane as the curve progresses. This was consistent with Pedriolle and Vidal's (50) concept of the evolution of scoliosis in the transverse plane. Asher believes that this fits well with the engineer's concept of scoliosis as a geometrical torsion or a property of a helical line. This is in distinction to a mechanical torsion in which two objects immediately adjacent to each other are rotated on each other. It is Asher's idea that scoliosis develops as a series of imperfect torsions. He notes that the apical vertebra did not always torque posteriorly in thoracolumbar curves. He believes that there are many reasons for these findings, including rib cage constraints, soft tissues, and asymmetry of motion segments (3–6).

It is my belief that correction of scoliosis should include translation and countertorsion if we hope to correct the true complex scoliosis deformity described by Asher. I have tended to drift away from the derotation maneuver described by Cotrel and Dubousset because of the problems seen with lumbar decompensation in type II curves and the intuitive notion that the derotation movement is done in the same counterclockwise motion that scoliosis tends to develop in.

The rules of selective fusion have changed little from the days of Harrington instrumentation. I still use the concept of selective fusion in thoracic curve patterns to avoid unnecessary fusion of the lumbar spine. The fusion should end at the stable vertebra unless that vertebra is at the apex of a kyphosis. If the stable vertebra is located at the apex of those segments, variation of standard hook-and-wire patterns may be applied in compression across the kyphotic segments to correct the abnormal segment (23).

Thorough preoperative planning is essential to ensure a smooth operation (it helps avoid confusion for the surgeons and nursing staff) and a good result. One may choose to label the hook-and-wire sites on the preoperative roentgenogram, or know in advance where sites might be most appropriate. The predetermined hook sites, however, may need to be altered in response to findings during surgery.

Operative Technique   For the standard right thoracic curve, I use a basic hook-and-wire placement, which is useful in types II, III, IV, and V curves. The type V curve differs only in that the upper stiff thoracic curve must also be instrumented and fused to avoid an objectionable shoulder asymmetry. I generally choose the upper level of instrumentation as the upper level mea-

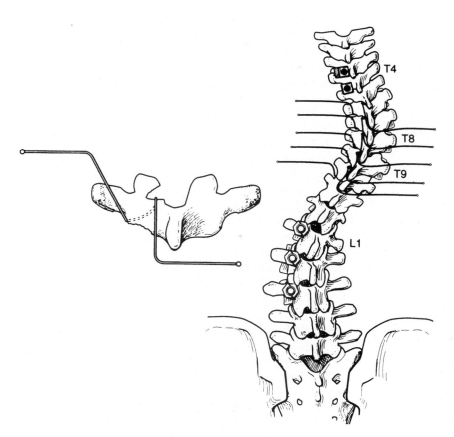

Figure 156.19.   Type I thoracic and lumbar curve screw foundation wire fixation on thoracic cavity. See text for details. (By permission of Dr. Marc Asher.)

sured by the Cobb method, or a level that is closest to the midline (Fig. 156.6). The upper level of instrumentation is generally T-3 or T-4. I currently use the ISOLA system, which uses open and closed hooks, wire, and screw fixation.

■ Prepare the upper facets on both sides of the superior vertebra by removing 4 mm of the inferior facet with a ¼-inch osteotome. Remove the cartilage with a curet.
■ Position an appropriate-size hook in the up-going position (Fig. 156.9). The hook should have a nice snug fit, and the throat of the hook should allow adequate room around the facet.
■ On both sides of the upper vertebra, create a "claw" by placing a closed hook on a holder, placing the foot of the hook on the superior edge of the transverse process, and allowing the hook to slide around the process (Fig. 156.19). This should give firm fixation on the vertebra.
■ I generally use an intermediate up-going pedicle hook on the concave side of the curve, one or two levels below the upper end vertebra. This hook is positioned in a similar manner.
■ On the convex side at the apical vertebra, create another claw to assist in the countertorsion movement with the second rod.
■ Position the inferior hook on the concave side after a limited laminotomy is created. It is important that the laminotomy be large enough to position the hook, but small enough to prevent deep penetration of the hook into the spinal canal.
■ I generally use a closed hook with an appropriate radius to just fit around the lamina (Fig. 156.10).

Some surgeons have started to use screw fixation on the inferior end vertebra for right thoracic curves. I have experience with this technique in types III and IV curves but have not used it in type II curves because the lower thoracic pedicles in adolescents tend to be quite small. The lumbar pedicles, however, can be quite large and adequate for screw placement. The advantages of screw fixation are the secure purchase and the translational control that can be achieved.

■ At this point in the procedure, segmentally secure the apical three or four vertebra with sublaminar wires or cables. I use the same technique described in the Luque fixation section (Fig. 156.19).
■ After the wires have been passed, excise the concave facets and graft bone.
■ Fashion and contour an appropriate length of rod using French and tube benders. (A malleable template is useful to obtain rod length and contour.)
■ Feed the rod up through the upper hooks and then ro-

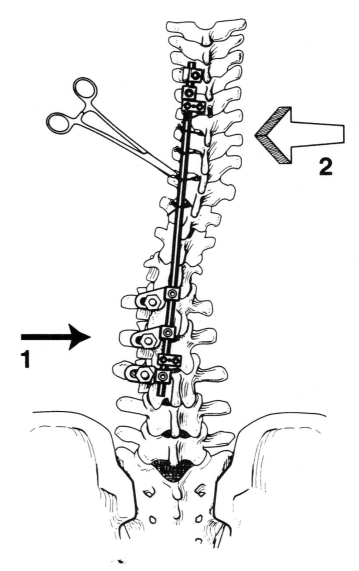

Figure 156.20. Thoracic concave rod placement wire tightening. See text for details. (By permission of Dr. Marc Asher.)

tate into the appropriate plane (Fig. 156.20). Then feed the rod down into the inferior hook.
■ The upper claw can then be secured with the compression device and the setscrews tightened (Fig. 156.21).
■ Sequentially tighten the wires or cables, translating the spine toward the rod (Fig. 156.22).
■ I generally favor wires because of their low cost and ease of use. Braided cables are an alternative.
■ After the wires have been tightened, complete distraction and secure all setscrews.
■ Position the convex rod after facets have been excised and bone grafted (Fig. 156.22).
■ Pass the rod through the upper hooks, place the intermediate hooks on the rod, and bring the positioned rod

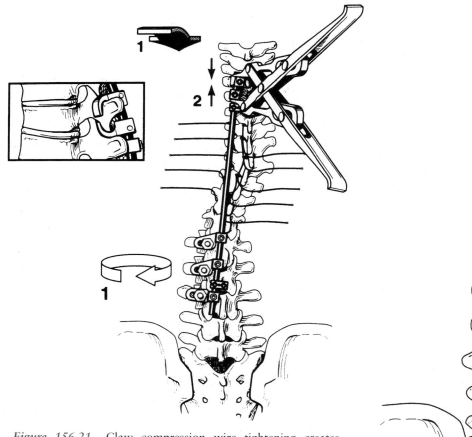

Figure 156.21. Claw compression wire tightening creates translation of the thoracic spine, and rod rotation creates countertorsion in the lumbar spine. See text for details. (By permission of Dr. Marc Asher.)

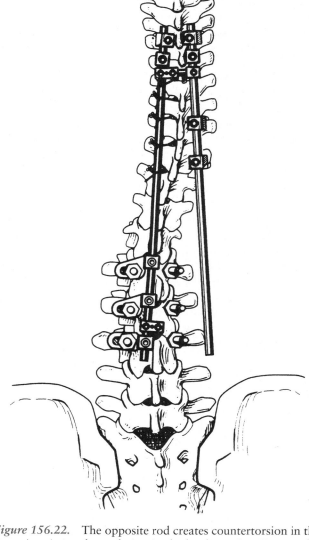

Figure 156.22. The opposite rod creates countertorsion in the thoracic spine and translation in the lumbar spine. See text for details. (By permission of Dr. Marc Asher.)

down to the spine. The positioning of the rod serves as a countertorsion movement and tends to push the spine out of rotation and toward the midline (Fig. 156.23).

- Place an upward-directed hook under the inferior lamina and advance the rod to engage the hook.
- After the rod is positioned, apply compressive forces to complete the sequence. The sublaminar wires can be retightened; revisit and tighten all setscrews a final time.
- I use cross links to create a rectangle and increase the strength of the system (Fig 156.24).

Avoid overcorrection of the instrumented curve. The lumbar curve must be able to accommodate the corrected thoracic curve. Type II curves require particular care and caution. Overcorrection of the thoracic curve can lead to lumbar curve decompensation. I have had minimal problems with lumbar curve decompensation using the translation and countertorsion technique. It seems to cause far

fewer problems than the old derotation technique that was based on the techniques of Cotrel and Dubousset. Particularly in the type II curves, we use instrumentation and fusion to treat the main thoracic curve, and then a thoracolumbosacral orthosis (TLSO) to treat the unfused lumbar curve. This has been an effective technique for young patients with a Risser sign of 0 to 2 where growth is anticipated and possible progression of the lumbar curve might be expected.

The double thoracic and lumbar type I curves can be treated with a technique different from that used for thoracic scoliosis curve types. In type I curves, fuse both thoracic and lumbar curves, choosing the upper level of fusion

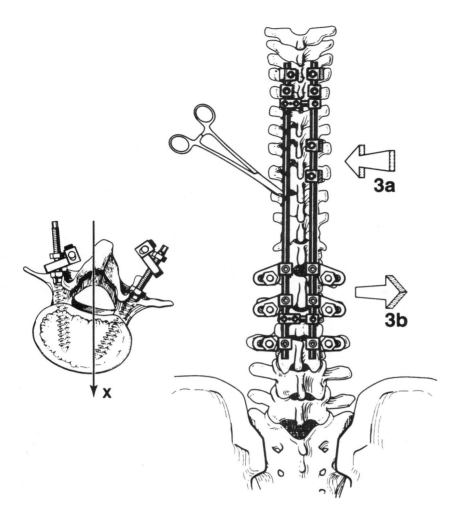

3a

3b

X

Figure 156.23. Rod sequence is completed. The screws allow a solid inferior anchor and move corrective forces anteriorly into the vertebral body. See text for details. (By permission of Dr. Marc Asher.)

as for the type II to IV curve patterns. (Figs. 156.25 to 156.30 show typical cases.)

- First, create bilateral claws at the upper level of the fusion, and place a claw or up-going hook at the apex of the thoracic curve.
- At the inferior level of the thoracic curve, place a down-going hook; it is usually preferred to use an open hook at this level.
- On the convex side of the lumbar curve, screw fixation is preferable to hooks, as it seems to give a better base for correction and avoids possible hardware displacement.
- The thoracic curve is generally managed with sublaminar wires.
- Place the concave thoracic and convex lumbar rod first.
- Before tightening the setscrew, rotate the rod counterclockwise. This rotation movement does not change the thoracic curve much, but it does effectively translate and countertorque the lumbar curve.

- Place the second rod and anchor it superiorly with hooks.
- Use an up-going hook at the thoracolumbar junction.
- Use sublaminar wires on the concavity of the lumbar curve, and generally use screws at the last two or three levels.
- Place the second rod with wires or screws in the lumbar curve.
- Use compression along the convexity of the thoracic curve and distraction along the concave lumbar curve.
- Apply transverse connectors and retighten all setscrews.

It is important to be aware of sagittal plane alignment. When fusions must be extended into the lumbar spine, maintain the normal lordosis to avoid the creation of flatback syndrome.

The postoperative program is similar to that of other techniques. Where poor bone or inadequate fixation has

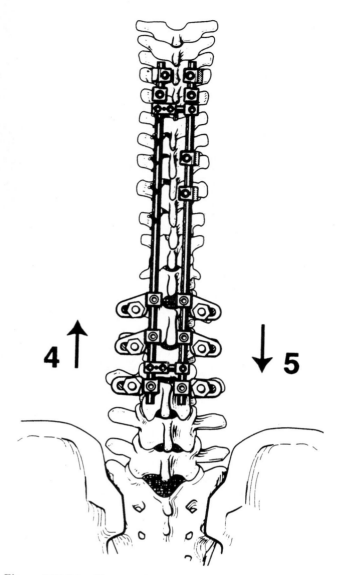

4 ↑   ↓ **5**

Figure 156.24. Compression and distraction are completed. See text for details. (By permission of Dr. Marc Asher.)

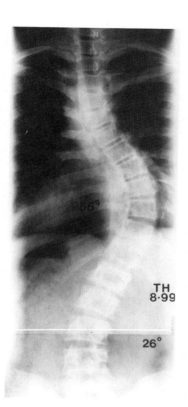

Figure 156.25. Preoperative AP radiograph of the right thoracic curve.

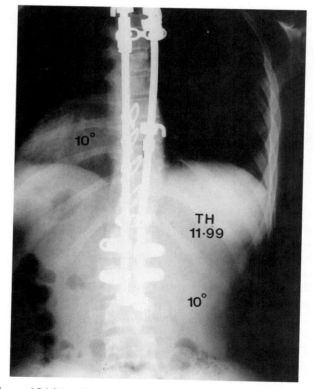

Figure 156.26. Postoperative AP radiograph of the right thoracic curve.

been encountered, a bivalved TLSO brace is used. For patients in whom firm fixation is achieved, no postoperative immobilization is required. Mobilize patients on the first or second postoperative day. Encourage them to start walking early, and let them return to school when comfortable. Generally, hold them out of sports for 6–9 months.

The ISOLA system has proven to be a very flexible system that can be applied to many spine problems. Evolution of implant systems is inevitable, and with each new change we are better able to manage more complex deformities.

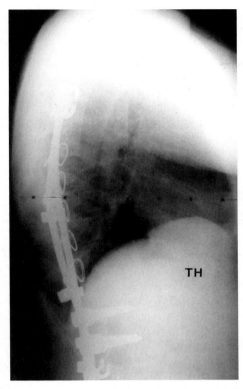

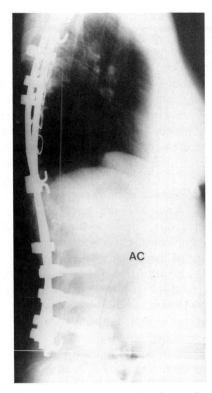

Figure 156.27. Postoperative lateral radiograph of the right thoracic curve.

Figure 156.29. Postoperative lateral radiograph of type I thoracic and lumbar curves.

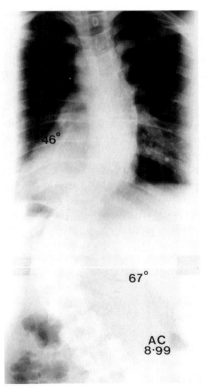

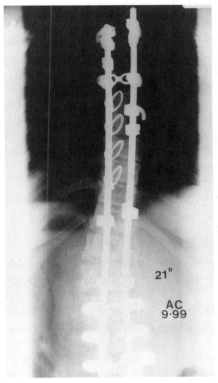

Figure 156.28. Preoperative AP radiograph of type I thoracic and lumbar curves.

Figure 156.30. Postoperative AP radiograph of type I thoracic and lumbar curves.

POSTOPERATIVE MANAGEMENT

Postoperative management is extremely important. Careful attention to detail is as necessary for this phase as it is for the preoperative planning and the surgical procedure.

After surgery, manage patients in a conventional hospital bed (rather than turning frames or other rotating beds), as patient acceptance and nursing familiarity make this an excellent choice. Use foam pad and sheepskins to facilitate skin care. In the immediate postoperative period, log-roll the patient every 1–2 hours to prevent skin sores, improve ventilation, and reduce pulmonary complications.

During the initial 48-hour postoperative period, administer intravenous fluids and limit oral intake. Avoid early oral feeding because postoperative ileus is common. An aggressive pulmonary care program with frequent coughing, deep breathing, and the use of an incentive spirometer is a standard part of the postoperative program. For patients with reduced pulmonary capacity, a respiratory therapist can be called in to use suction and a more aggressive pulmonary program.

Provide postoperative support of the spine with a plastic bivalved body jacket. It is easy to use and is equally well tolerated by patients with idiopathic scoliosis and those with a wide variety of neuromuscular conditions. If patient compliance is questionable, a more standard Risser cast can be used successfully. A cervicothoracolumbosacral orthosis (CTLSO) is helpful when instrumentation is carried into the high thoracic spine. In patients with neuromuscular curves or when instrumentation high into the thoracic spine necessitates immobilization, a sternal-occipital-mandibular immobilization (SOMI) device can be added to a bivalved jacket. Maintain postoperative immobilization for 4–6 months. The removable jackets make postoperative hygiene and skin care much easier; allow compliant patients to shower without the brace after the first few weeks. The multi-hooks and rod systems require no postoperative immobilization.

During the early postoperative period, encourage patients to increase their aerobic activities by walking, gradually increasing to several miles per day after the first 2 weeks. Their endurance and normal physiologic functions improve more rapidly with a regular walking program.

A patient with idiopathic scoliosis may resume noncontact sports after the first month if wearing a postoperative orthosis. For a patient with a multi-hooks and rod system, noncontact sports are not allowed for 3–4 months unless the patient is wearing a body jacket.

Obtain radiographs of the spine before the patient is discharged from the hospital. This set of films establishes the amount of correction and confirms adequate positioning of the hardware. Virtually all hardware pullout occurs in the early postoperative period. Have the patient return 3–4 weeks after discharge for posteroanterior and lateral radiographs to confirm curve stability and hardware position. Take subsequent films at 3 and 6 months. Also take oblique radiographs at the 6-month visit to check the maturity and integrity of the spinal arthrodesis. If the fusion is questionable or unclear on standard radiographs, obtain tomograms. If poor incorporation of the graft is noted, additional immobilization or augmentation of the fusion with additional bone graft may be necessary.

PITFALLS AND COMPLICATIONS

Unfortunately, major surgical procedures have the potential for complications. Many can be avoided by careful planning and surgical execution. Others, however, occur despite the best efforts.

BLOOD LOSS

The best way to avoid complications from blood transfusion is to minimize intraoperative blood loss. Proper positioning, hypotensive anesthesia, and careful surgical technique are the cornerstones of minimizing blood loss. I have used preoperative autologous blood donations for about 5 years. Preoperative donations can begin 3–4 weeks before surgery. Iron supplementation is helpful to maintain adequate red blood cell production. With a good autologous blood program, banked blood can generally be avoided. The risks of human immunodeficiency virus (HIV) transmission from bank blood are low, but they can be eliminated with an autotransfusion plan. In cases where blood loss is expected to be high (e.g., in osteotomy or reconstructive procedures), another cost-effective and safe way to reduce the need for blood transfusion is intraoperative blood salvage with a cell-saver.

If major intraoperative blood loss is encountered, immediate hematologic workup, even during the procedure, is mandatory. Transfusion of platelets and appropriate clotting factors can be lifesaving. Fortunately, in my experience, major blood loss is rare if attention to detail is observed.

SPINAL CORD INJURY

Spinal cord injury is one of the most feared complications in treating scoliosis. The neurologic injury may occur from direct trauma to the cord by instruments, hooks, or sublaminar wires, or by stretch of the spinal cord. Stretch of the spinal cord is presumed to cause vascular compromise that leads to neurologic loss. Certain techniques seem to carry more risks. The 1997 Morbidity and Mortality Report (available from the Scoliosis Research Society) reported an incidence of spinal cord injury during adolescent idiopathic scoliosis surgery of 0.28%. There did not seem to be a correlation based on the type of implant used. A 0.14% incidence of nerve root injury was also noted.

Excessive traction on the spinal cord can occur during correction of scoliosis. This is most frequently seen in large rigid curves but can occur with the manipulation and correction of any curve. Congenital scoliosis carries a higher risk of neurologic injury; these curves tend to be rigid and may be associated with cord tethering by bone spurs, fibrous bands, or a tight filum terminale. As discussed earlier, we recommend the use of MRI prior to the surgical treatment of congenital curves.

The advent of the wake-up test gave spine surgeons a way to assess neurologic function after instrumentation and before sending the patient to the recovery room. In this test, the patient is momentarily awakened from anesthesia and asked to move her toes. Lack of volitional movement calls for careful examination of the procedure and elimination of any potential cause of neurologic impairment. Because of the anesthetic medication, the patient usually neither recalls the wake-up test nor mentions that she felt pain during the procedure. I usually use electronic spinal cord monitoring with sensory evoked potentials (SEP) during surgery. This gives continuous readouts of cord function without waking the patient, with the risks of extubation and the increased bleeding that occur when the blood pressure rises during wake-up. I had false-positive readings during my early experience with SEP, so the wake-up test was used to confirm that no neurologic deficits were present. With added experience and the use of multiple recording sites (epidural, scalp, and cervical), the SEP has proved to be reliable, and it is most helpful during long, involved reconstruction procedures.

Electronic monitoring necessitates careful coordination with the anesthesia staff, because many of the popular anesthetic agents interfere with accurate monitoring. If a neurologic deficit is noted during or after surgery, reduce the traction force on the spine. This usually necessitates releasing distraction and may require hardware removal. If a severe neurologic deficit is noted in the recovery room or after surgery, immediately return the patient to the operating room for wound exploration and probable hardware removal. Laminectomy is not usually indicated unless an epidural hematoma is identified or bone is encroaching on the cord. If early sublaminar wire removal is indicated, the technique should be that of cutting one end of the wire close to the lamina, grasping the other end, and pulling straight up. The work of Nicastro et al. (49) shows this to be least likely to cause the wire to push down into the spinal cord.

WOUND INFECTION

With careful technique and the use of intraoperative and postoperative antibiotics, postoperative wound infection should be 1% or less. If an early infection occurs, prompt wound debridement is indicated, and a successful spinal correction and fusion can be salvaged.

- Obtain blood cultures before surgery.
- Take the patient to the operating room, where, under anesthesia, the skin is prepared and draped, and the entire wound is opened. Do not disrupt the hardware and bone graft.
- Obtain cultures.
- Carefully debride the hematoma and nonviable tissue, followed by irrigation with antibiotic solution. Leave the bone graft intact.
- Generally, avoid large retention sutures.
- Close the wound in layers over suction irrigation tubes that are left in for 3–5 days.
- Administer appropriate intravenous antibiotics for 7–10 days; then, if antibiotic sensitivity allows, change to an oral agent for an additional 6 weeks.

DURAL TEARS

If, during the process of passing sublaminar wires or placing hardware, a dural tear is noted by the leakage of clear cerebrospinal fluid, repair it immediately. Patients fare better with early repair than with later repairs of chronic leaks. Perform a limited laminotomy, or laminectomy if necessary, to expose the dural tear. Once the extent of the tear is identified, repair by careful suturing with a fine, nontraumatic needle and 5-0 or 6-0 nylon. If large tears are noted, it may be necessary to perform a fascial graft. the lumbodorsal fascia is a good source for a patch graft. Keep patients with this complication at bed rest for several days after repair.

FLATBACK SYNDROME

The loss of normal lumbar lordosis is a major long-term problem (1,31,32). It creates an unsightly cosmetic deformity and leads to back pain. This flattening of the lumbar spine is associated with instrumentation of the lumbar spine and can be created by using noncontoured Harrington rods (15). The best way to prevent this iatrogenic problem is to avoid fusion of the lumbar spine when possible. As described earlier in this chapter, selective thoracic fusion is the best way to maintain lumbar motion. When fusion into the lumbar spine is necessary, position the patient on the operating table to maintain lordosis and contour the rods. When fusion to the sacrum is indicated, the Luque rods with Galveston pelvic fixation and sacral screws are the best means of creating or maintaining lumbar lordosis.

PSEUDARTHROSIS

Successful completion of a scoliosis procedure is based on obtaining a solid fusion. After 4–6 months, perform an evaluation for a solid arthrodesis. Take oblique views and carefully review the films for lucent lines in the fusion mass. If broken hardware is noted, a pseudarthrosis is highly likely.

When there is hardware breakage or when oblique radiographs demonstrate a pseudarthrosis, open and explore the entire wound. The pseudarthrosis may be covered by a fine layer of bone. Therefore, careful evaluation is mandatory. The pseudarthrosis is generally difficult to expose and will show motion when stressed. Freshen the bone with a gouge, and instrument the pseudarthrosis with a heavy Harrington compression system. The multihooks and rod system can also be used to apply compression. Apply generous quantities of local and iliac bone graft to complete the procedure. I immobilize the patient for 4–6 months in a bivalved body jacket. Lumbosacral pseudarthroses that have failed repeated attempts at repair may be best managed by an additional anterior fusion. It is mandatory that solid arthrodesis be achieved if you hope to obtain a stable balanced spine.

◢ AUTHOR'S PERSPECTIVE

The surgical management of scoliosis requires careful preoperative evaluation and planning. Curve types and patterns must be carefully identified to select fusion levels. Spinal fusion and instrumentation techniques are demanding and should be carefully performed. The surgeon should have hands-on experience with these systems before initiating the procedure. The keys to success are attention to detail and skillful surgical execution. The new implant systems seem to offer better correction and more options in treatment, but they do not replace the need for good fusion techniques.

REFERENCES

Each reference is categorized according to the following scheme: *, classic article; #, review article; !, basic research article; and +, clinical results/outcome study.

+ 1. Aaro S, Ohlen G. The Effect of Harrington Instrumentation on the Sagittal Configuration and Mobility of the Spine in Scoliosis. *Spine* 1983;8:570.

2. Allen BL, Ferguson RL. Basic Considerations in Pelvic Fixation Cases. In: Luque ER, ed. *Segmental Spinal Instrumentation*. Thorofare, NJ: Slack, 1984:185.

3. Asher MA. ISOLA Spinal Instrumentation System for Scoliosis. In: Bridwell KH, DeWald RL, eds. *The Textbook of Spinal Surgery*. Philadelphia: Lippincott, 1996:569.

+ 4. Asher MA, Cook L. Adolescent Idiopathic Scoliosis Transverse Plane Evolution. In: D'Amico M, Merrill A, Santambrogio GC, eds. *Three Dimensional Analysis of Spine Deformities*. Amsterdam: IOS Press, 1995:353.

+ 5. Asher MA, Cook L. The Transverse Plane Evolution of the Most Common Adolescent Idiopathic Scoliosis Deformities. A Cross-Sectional Study of 181 Patients. *Spine* 1995;20:1386.

6. Asher MA, Strippgen WE, Heinig CF, Carson WL. ISOLA Spinal Instrumentation: Emphasizing Application during the First Two Decades of Life. In: Weinstein SC, ed. *The Pediatric Spine: Principles and Practice*. New York: Raven Press, 1999:1619.

+ 7. Benson L, Ibrahim K, Goldberg B, Harris G. Coronal Balance in Cotrel-Dubousset Instrumentation: Compensation vs. Decompensation. Presented at the Scoliosis Research Society Annual Meeting, Honolulu, September, 1990.

+ 8. Bergofsky EH, Turino GH, Fishman AP. Cardiorespiratory Failure in Kyphosciolosis. *Medicine* 1959;38:263.

9. Bradford DS, Moe JH, Winter RB. Scoliosis and Kyphosis. In: Rothman RH, Simeone FA, eds. *The Spine*, 2nd ed. Philadelphia: Saunders, 1982.

+ 10. Bridwell KH, McAllister JW, Betz RR, et al. Coronal Decompensation Produced by Cotrel-Dubousset "Derotation" Maneuver for Idiopathic Right Thoracic Scoliosis. *Spine* 1991;16:769.

+ 11. Butte FL. Scoliosis Treated by the Wedging Jacket. Selection of the Area to be Fused. *J Bone Surg* 1983;20:1.

* 12. Cobb JR. Outline for the Study of Scoliosis. *Instr Course Lect* 1948;5.

+ 13. Cochran T, Irstam L, Nachemson A. Long Term Anatomic and Fuctional Changes in Patients with Adolescent Idiopathic Scoliosis Treated by Harrington Rod Fusion. *Spine* 1983;8:576.

+ 14. Collis DK, Ponseti IV. Long Term Followup of Patients with Idiopathic Scoliosis Not Treated Surgically. *J Bone Joint Surg Am* 1969;51:425.

+ 15. Cummine J, Winter R, Grobler C, et al. Harrington Instrumentation without Fusion Combined with Milwaukee Brace for Difficult Scoliosis Problems in Young Children. *Orthop Trans* 1979;3:59.

* 16. Ferguson AB. The Study and Treatment of Scoliosis. *South Med J* 1930;23:116.

* 17. Flagstad AE, Kollman S. Vital Capacity and Muscle Study in One Hundred Cases of Scoliosis. *J Bone Joint Surg* 1928;10:724.

+ 18. Gazioglu K, Goldstein LH, Femi-Pearse D, Yu PN. Pulmonary Function in Idiopathic Scoliosis: Comparitive Evaluation Before and After Orthopaedic Correction. *J Bone Joint Surg Am* 1968;50:1391.

+ 19. Gillespie R, Faithfull DK, Roth A, Hall JE. Intraspinal Anomalies in Congenital Scoliosis. *Clin Orthop* 1973; 93:103.

+ 20. Goldstein LA. Surgical Management of Scoliosis. *Clin Orthop* 1964;35:95.

+ 21. Goldstein LA. Surgical Management of Scoliosis. *J Bone Joint Surg Am* 1966;48:167.

+ 22. Goldstein LA. Surgical Management of Scoliosis. *Clin Orthop* 1971;77:32.

+ 23. Hammill GL, Lenke LG, Bridwell KH, et al. The Use of Pedicle Screw Fixation to Improve Correction in the Lumbar Spine of Patients with Idiopathic Scoliosis: Is It Warranted? *Spine* 1996;21:1241.

* 24. Harrington PR. Treatment of Scoliosis: Correction and Internal Fixation by Spine Instrumentation. *J Bone Joint Surg Am* 1962;44:591.

* 25. Harrington PR. Technical Details in Relation to the Successful Use of Instrumentation in Scoliosis. *Orthop Clin North Am* 1972;3:49.

+ 26. Herndon W, Sullivan JA, Gross R, et al. Segmental Spinal Instrumentation: Critical Appraisal. *Orthop Trans* 1986;10:492.

+ 27. Hood RW, Riseborough EJ, Nehme AM, et al. Diastematomyelia and Structural Spinal Deformities. *J Bone Joint Surg Am* 1980;62:520.

+ 28. Keim HA, Reina EG. Osteoid Osteoma as a Cause of scoliosis. *J Bone Joint Surg Am* 1975;57:159.

+ 29. King HA, Moe JH, Bradford DS, Winter RB. The Selection of Fusion Levels in Thoracic Idiopathic Scoliosis. *J Bone Joint Surg Am* 1983;65:1302.

+ 30. Kostuik JP, Israel J, Hall JE. Scoliosis Surgery in Adults. *Clin Orthop* 1973;93:225.

+ 31. LaGrone MO. Loss of Lumbar Lordosis. A Complication of Spinal Fusion for Scoliosis. *Orthop Clin North Am* 1988;19:383.

+ 32. LaGrone MO, Bradford DS, Moe JH, et al. Treatment of Symptomatic Flatback after Spinal Fusion. *J Bone Joint Surg Am* 1988;70:569.

+ 33. Lenke LG, Bridwell KH, Blanke K. Preventing Decompensation in King Type II Curves Treated with Cotrel-Dubousset Instrumentation. *Spine* 1992;17:S274.

+ 34. Lonstein JE, Carlson JM. The Prediction of Curve Progression in Untreated Idiopathic Scoliosis during Growth. *J Bone Joint Surg Am* 1984;66:1061.

+ 35. Luque ER. Paralytic Scoliosis in Growing Children. *Clin Orthop* 1982;163:202.

* 36. Luque ER, Cardosa AM. Segmental Correction of Scoliosis with Rigid Internal Fixation. *Orthop Trans* 1977; 1:136.

* 37. Luque ER, Cardosa AM. Treatment of Scoliosis without Arthrodesis or External Support. *Orthop Trans* 1977;1: 37.

+ 38. Makley JT, Herndon CH, Inkley S, et al. Pulmonary Function in Paralytic and Non-Paralytic Scoliosis Before and After Treatment. A Study of Sixty-Three Cases. *J Bone Joint Surg Am* 1968;50:1379.

+ 39. Mankin HJ, Graham JJ, Schack J. Cardiopulmonary Function in Mild and Moderate Idiopathic Scoliosis. *J Bone Joint Surg Am* 1964;46:53.

40. Marchetti PG. Harrington Rods. In: Bradford DS, Hensinger RH, eds. *The Pediatric Spine.* New York: Thieme, 1985;426.

+ 41. Mason DE, Carango P. Spinal Decompensation in Cotrel-Dubousset Instrumentation. *Spine* 1991;16: 5394.

+ 42. Massey TB, Winter RB, Lonstein JE, Denis F. Selection of Fusion Levels with Special Reference to Coronal and Sagittal Balance in Right Thoracic Adolescent Idiopathic Scoliosis Using Cotrel-Dubousset Instrumentation. Presented at Scoliosis Research Society Annual Meeting, Honolulu, September, 1990.

43. Micheli LJ, Riseborough EJ, Hall JE. Scoliosis in the Adult. *Orthop Rev* 1977;6:27.

* 44. Moe JH. A Critical Analysis of Methods of Fusion for Scoliosis. An Evaluation of Two Hundred and Sixty-Six Patients. *J Bone Joint Surg Am* 1958;40:529.

+ 45. Moe JH. Methods of Correction and Surgical Techniques in Scoliosis. *Orthop Clin North Am* 1972;3: 17.

+ 46. Moe JH, Sundberg B, Gustilo R. A Clinical Study of Spine Fusions in the Growing Child. *J Bone Joint Surg Br* 1964;46:784.

47. Moe JH, Winter RB, Bradford DH, Lonstein JE. Scoliosis and Other Spinal Deformities. Philadelphia: W.B. Saunders, 1978.

* 48. Nachemson A. A Long Term Followup Study of Non-Treated Scoliosis. *Acta Orthop Scand* 1968;39:466.

! 49. Nicastro JF, Hartjen CA, Traina J, Lancster JN. Intraspinal Pathways Taken by Sublaminal Wires during Removal. An Experimenatl Study. *J Bone Joint Surg Am* 1986;68:1206.

+ 50. Pedriolle R, Vidal J. Morphology of Scoliosis. Three Dimensional Evolution. *Orthopaedics* 1987;10:909.

* 51. Ponder RC, Dickson JH, Harrington PR, Erwin WE. Results of Harrington Instrumentation and Fusion in the Adult Scoliosis Patient. *J Bone Joint Surg Am* 1975;57: 797.

+ 52. Richards BS, Burch JG, Herring JA, et al. Frontal Plane and Sagittal Plane Balance Following Cotrel-Dubousset Instrumentation for Idiopathic Scoliosis. *Spine* 1989;14: 733.

+ 53. Rinsky LA, Gamble JG, Bleck EE. Segmentation Instrumentation without Fusion in Children with Progressive Scoliosis. *J Pediatr Orthop* 1985;5:687.

* 54. Risser JC. The Iliac Apophysis. An Invaluable Sign in the Management of Scoliosis. *Clin Orthop* 1958;11:111.

+ 55. Shannon DC, Riseborough EJ, Valeca LM, Kazemi H. The Distribution of Abnormal Lung Function in Kyphoscoliosis. *J Bone Joint Surg Am* 1970;52:131.

+ 56. Steel HH. Rib Resection and Spine Fusion in Correction of Convex Deformity in Scoliosis. *J Bone Joint Surg Am* 1983;65:920.

+ 57. Swank S, Lonstein JE, Moe JH, et al. Surgical Treatment of Adult Scoliosis. *J Bone Joint Surg Am* 1981;63: 268.

+ 58. Thompson JB, Transfeldt EE, Bradford DS, et al. Decompensation after Cotrel-Dubousset Instrumentation of Idiopathic Scoliosis. *Spine* 1990;15:927.

+ 59. Von Lackum WH, Miller JP. Critical Observation of the Results in the Operative Treatment of Scoliosis. *J Bone Joint Surg Am* 1949;31:102.

+ 60. Westgate HD. Pulmonary Function in Thoracic Scoliosis Before and After Corrective Surgery. *Minn Med* 1970; 53:839.

+ 61. Winter RB, Lipscomb PR. Back Pain in Children. *Minn Med* 1978;61:141.

+ 62. Winter RB, Lovell WW, Moe JH. Excessive Thoracic Lordosis and Loss of Pulmonary Function in Patients with Idiopathic Scoliosis. *J Bone Joint Surg Am* 1975; 57:972.

+ 63. Wood KB, Olesweski JM, Schendel MJ, et al. Rotational Changes of the Vertebral Pelvic Axis after Sublaminar Instrumention in Adolescent Idiopathic Scoliosis. *Spine* 1997;22:51.

+ 64. Wood KB, Transfeldt EE, Ogilvie JW, et al. Rotational Changes of the Vertebral-Pelvic Axis Following Cotrel-Dubousset Instrumentation. *Spine* 1991;16:5401.

+ 65. Yngve DA, Burke SW, Price C, Riddick MF. Sublaminar Wiring. *J Pediatr Orthop* 1986;6:605.

CHAPTER 157

SPINAL SURGERY FOR MYELO-MENINGOCELE

Thomas E. Kuivila

Myelomeningocele is a serious and complex congenital abnormality associated with a host of problems that cross several disciplines of medicine and rehabilitation. Of the problems presenting to pediatric orthopaedic surgeons, none is as daunting, complex, and fraught with pitfalls as the management of the associated spinal deformities. In addition to the kyphotic, lordotic, or scoliotic deformities typically faced by spinal-deformity surgeons, patients with myelomeningocele bring the added challenge of a markedly abnormal anatomy marked by the absence of a significant portion of the posterior spinal elements. Additionally, these structures are frequently smaller, the bone is more osteopenic, the skin, muscle, and fascia available for coverage of hardware are frequently poor, and significant additional medical problems frequently coexist (13). A solid grounding in the treatment of idiopathic spinal deformities is therefore a prerequisite to embarking on the management of patients with myelomeningocele (6,34).

Orthopaedic care for patients with spina bifida should not exist in a vacuum. More than perhaps any other condition with which orthopaedists are concerned, myelomeningocele should be managed by a team of pediatric specialists. In addition to an orthopaedic surgeon, a pediatric neurosurgeon, a urologist, a neurologist, and a physiatrist must be allied with a health care team consisting of occupational and physical therapy, social workers, and nutritionists. As patient demands on each of these individuals is fairly high, most major pediatric centers employ specialty clinics, where the specialists convene on individual patients, rather than each specialist seeing patients individually. Once thought to be a chronic and stable condition, myelomeningocele is now known to be condition that changes throughout life (8). It is therefore necessary for patients to be followed well into their adult years.

While the focus of this chapter is the surgical management of spinal deformities, readers need to be ever mindful

T. E. Kuivila: Department of Orthopaedic Surgery, The Cleveland Clinic Foundation, Cleveland, Ohio 44195.

of the associated conditions and the need to manage the spine within the larger framework just discussed.

PATHOPHYSIOLOGY

The mechanism by which myelomeningocele occurs embryologically is unknown. Two major theories exist, and both have their proponents. Von Recklinghausen, who initially described the condition, felt that the abnormality was due to a failure of closure of the neural canal. The opposing theory is that a closed neural tube ruptures, exposing the neural elements (16). This theory was initially advanced by Morgagni (33). A long discussion of the points that make both theories at least histologically plausible is beyond the scope of this chapter; suffice it to say that a certain modicum of evidence exists for both viewpoints. The abnormality resulting in the formation of a myelomeningocele occurs very early in gestation—most likely at the third to fourth week after conception. In many cases, the defect is present before a woman recognizes that she is pregnant.

While there is no agreement on the embryologic process that causes the formation of a myelomeningocele, many risk factors have been identified that markedly increase the incidence of this birth defect. Use of the the antiseizure medication valproic acid (Depakene) during pregnancy has been demonstrated to markedly increase the risk of myelomeningocele (9). As valproic acid can alter serum folate levels, this adds credence to the work of Yates et al. (45), who showed an association between the incidence of neural tube defects and depressed red cell folate levels. In their study, the diminished folate levels could not be entirely attributed to decreased dietary intake, suggesting that an inborn error of folate metabolism existed. This study was subsequently supported by Seller and Nevin (40), who noted a decreased incidence of myelomeningocele and other neural tube defects when adequate vitamin and folate supplementation began before conception. These studies led to the general dietary recommendation that all women of childbearing age consume a minimum of 1.0 μg of folic acid daily (9). Many foods are being supplemented with folic acid in direct response to this work.

The gold standard for the prenatal diagnosis of myelomeningocele remains the amniotic fluid level of alpha-fetoprotein (AFP) obtained through amniocentesis. A high concentration of AFP within the amniotic fluid, which is usually sequestered within the cerebrospinal fluid (CSF) of the fetus, is pathognomonic for an open or otherwise compromised neural canal. Most centers continue to use serum AFP levels to screen expectant mothers. While high AFP concentrations have a relatively high correlation with neural tube defects, the sensitivity and specificity of this test is only about 80% (1). Prenatal diagnosis is most useful because it is important to plan for delivery at a tertiary care facility, where neurosurgical and neurosurgical intensive care unit support is available; it is also important because it is believed that elective cesarean section may result in neural function at one to two levels higher than otherwise.

PRINCIPLES OF TREATMENT

The management of a child born with myelomeningocele begins with closure of the defect, typically by a neurosurgeon, within the first 12–24 hours of life. Without treatment, such children will typically die. Several series of untreated children reported in the 1970s demonstrated mortality rates in the range of 90% to 100% (20,23). The cause of death in untreated infants is bacterial meningoventriculitis. Those who survive meningoventriculitis have higher levels of paralysis, more profound mental retardation, and frequently uncontrolled hydrocephalus, leading to additional problems. Therapeutic nihilism was frequently practiced in the United States 40 years ago because of the difficulty in treating many of the sequelae of myelomeningocele. However, with advances in orthopaedic, neurologic, and urologic care, myelomeningocele is very treatable. It has therefore become the standard of care in the United States to perform early sac closure and ventriculoperitoneal shunting in infants with myelomeningocele.

Positioning of the patient after sac closure is very important to protect the fragile soft tissues overlying the repair. Additionally, this period of prone recumbency is advantageous in positioning the hips to avoid subluxation or dislocation.

It is possible, though unusual, for a neurosurgeon to require the services of an orthopaedist when performing the initial shunt closure. Occasionally, the child will be born with a severe gibbous deformity that will necessitate a two- to three-level kyphectomy to facilitate closure.

PATIENT ASSESSMENT

As with the management of any spinal deformity, take a careful history and perform a thorough physical examination. Do not immediately focus on the spinal deformity. It is important relative to surgical indications, as well as other prognostic factors, to know about the general health of the child. Inquire about the patient's mental functioning, school attendance, and level of socialization, as well as the activities of daily living that the patient is able to perform. The presence or absence of hydrocephalus or a shunt is prognostic relative to overall intellectual function (Fig. 157.1) (18). Inquire about the patient's urologic status and bowel function. Knowledge of the status of these

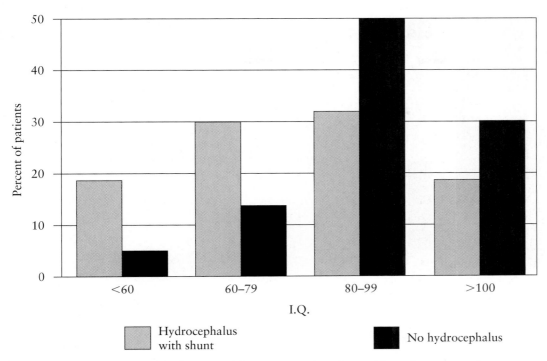

Figure 157.1.   Average I.Q. as a function of shunt presence in patients with myelomeningocele.

matters is yet another reason why a multidisciplinary clinic is so valuable. Finally, it is important to have a good understanding of parents' perceptions and patients' needs, desires, and expectations regarding eventual ambulation and the use of ambulatory aids.

As far as the spine is concerned, determine the level of neurologic function, the perception of patients and caregivers regarding spinal curvature progression, and any symptoms or problems directly related to the curve, including pain, skin breakdown, loss of balance, difficulty with breathing, or changes in gastrointestinal (GI) or genitourinary (GU) function. It is also important to inquire about previous trials of bracing and spinal surgery.

An increasingly common finding in patients with myelomeningocele is sensitivity to latex. It is mandatory to ask a dermatologist to test patients for latex allergy in the preoperative period. Use a latex-free protocol in surgery and in the postoperative period, even with nonallergic patients. Allergic reactions to latex have become a significant health problem for patients and health care professionals over the last 5 years. It is believed that 50% of spina bifida patients in the United States have evidence of severe allergy to latex. As many as 5% to 10% of myelomeningocele patients may have a potentially life-threatening form of this allergy (3,11). The allergen causing the hypersensitivity response is a component of the latex substance itself, and therefore only strict avoidance of latex contact is effective (42). Immediate hypersensitivity reactions to latex

have been reported through several different routes of exposure. Deaths have been reported after mucous membrane exposure and infusion through latex-containing intravenous lines (3,11). Intraoperative anaphylactic reactions have been reported simply after the opening of latex gloves in the operating suite. It is believed that patients with myelodysplasia are at increased risk for latex allergy due to the multiple contacts that they have had with the substance (11), although some feel that there is a yet unknown reason for their proclivity to an allergic response.

As improved non-latex-containing operative and patient care materials become available, inadvertent exposure to latex will become less and less common. The Joint Commission for the Accreditation of Hospital and Healthcare Organizations currently requires that all patients be asked specifically about a history of latex sensitivity at their initial outpatient or inpatient visit. All hospitals should have policies and procedures in place regarding bed assignment and room preparation and strict protocols for direct patient care activities in a nonlatex environment. It behooves the surgeon and operative team, however, to doubly reinforce this concept in the operating room and with the ancillary staff.

Next, perform a detailed physical examination. Examine the extremities, paying special attention to the neurologic examination. Whereas the lower extremities are typically the sites of major neurologic compromise, conditions

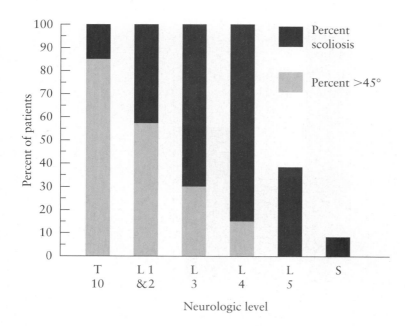

Figure 157.2. The incidence and the severity of scoliosis depend on the level of neurologic compromise.

such as hydromyelia or syringomyelia may also compromise strength and sensation in the upper extremities. Careful neurologic examination to identify the specific level of neurologic involvement is important as a predictor of both ambulatory ability and the likelihood of curve progression (Fig. 157.2). It must be kept in mind that the neurologic pattern may differ from one extremity to the other, even (in rare cases) nearly to the point of having one normal extremity and near-total paralysis of the other extremity, a condition known as hemimyelodysplasia (29).

In addition to observing the general curvature of the spine (lordosis, kyphosis, scoliosis), examine the spine to assess flexibility and balance. Additionally, assess the quality and the condition of the skin throughout the torso. This is important not only for wound coverage and closure but also for any postoperative casting or bracing that may be anticipated. While radiographic studies will convey a good deal of information regarding the underlying bony structure, careful and thorough palpation of the spine for the presence or absence of bony elements can immeasurably add to one's understanding of the deformity.

RADIOLOGIC EVALUATION

Plain radiographs, preferably standing or sitting in the posteroanterior (PA) and lateral projections and supine bending films, are essential for preoperative planning. Magnetic resonance imaging (MRI) of the spine, as well as spiral computed tomography (CT) with three-dimensional (3D) reconstruction, adds to one's ability to understand the nuances of the curve, note congenital elements and

dysplastic features, and undertake rigorous preoperative planning. There is no aspect of spinal surgery where the adage "failure to plan is a plan for failure" better applies than in myelosurgery.

Ultrasound may be useful in the very immature, minimally ossified spine and in areas where there is no bone overlying the neural elements. For the most part, myelography has been replaced by MRI.

PRINCIPLES AND INDICATIONS FOR SURGICAL TREATMENT

The orthopaedic management of myelomeningocele centers around three major goals:

To maximize patients' abilities and maintain the stability and range of motion of the spine and extremities

To provide for locomotion either by wheelchair or by ambulation with or without braces and orthotics, depending on the level of neurologic involvement

To prevent deterioration of neurologic function

As previously noted, myelomeningocele is a condition in which neurologic change can be expected. The observation of diminished extremity function frequently leads to the diagnosis of subtle neurologic deterioration.

The specific goal in the management of the myelomeningocele spinal deformity is to maintain or achieve a well balanced spine (Fig. 157.3). Spinal balance is important for compensated sitting, as well as standing. A well supported spine (12) allows free use of the upper extremities,

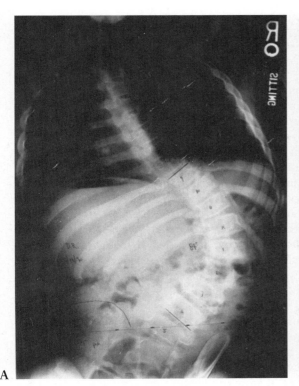
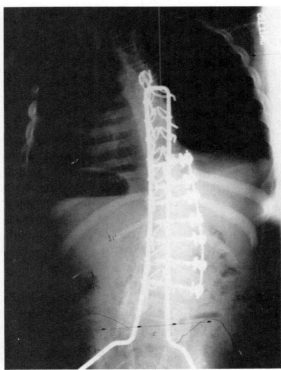

Figure 157.3. **A:** A 13-year-old boy with a thoracic-level myelomeningocele. He had a severe, progressive right thoracolumbar paralytic curve of 84° and significant pelvic obliquity of 21°. Staged anterior and posterior procedures 1 week apart were necessary to correct the rigid spinal deformity and pelvic obliquity. The combination of an anterior Zielke procedure followed by posterior instrumentation and fusion with a Luque rod with Galveston pelvic fixation provided adequate correction of his deformities (**B**).

and balanced seating pressure diminishes the likelihood of skin breakdown in insensate areas.

As with any spinal deformity, the three options for management include observation, bracing, and surgery. However, unlike idiopathic adolescent spinal deformities, there is no "routine" management for the myelodysplastic spine. Patient size and age, level of curve involvement, coexisting hemivertebrae, and wildly variant anatomy make a highly individualized treatment plan mandatory. However, certain rules do apply and are useful to bear in mind.

Because of coexistent muscle paralysis, scoliosis in patients with spina bifida tends to progress faster and more relentlessly than in idiopathic scoliosis. When scoliosis is simply being observed, this option is generally chosen not so much because of the low-level magnitude of the curve but because the patient either may not be of appropriate size for definitive surgery or may have a curve that is not amenable to orthotic management.

Orthotic treatment of scoliosis should be considered a temporary measure, intended to allow further spinal growth and patient maturation before definitive operative management. Many potential problems exist with bracing the paralytic spine. First, the brace exerts pressure on insensate or sensory-impaired skin, which can result in decubitus ulcers, particularly over the bony prominences of the spine and the edges of the rib cage and pelvis. Second, the degree of compression necessary to maintain control of the curve will frequently compromise an already restricted pulmonary capacity and definitely impair an already compromised ability to be mobile. Any orthotic must be custom-made and requires very careful fitting and supervised wear. Insensate skin can break down very quickly, and children must be introduced to the orthotic slowly, beginning with 1 hour at a time. Inspect the skin carefully after removal of the orthosis. Increase the wearing time slowly over 3–4 weeks until the patient is wearing it throughout the waking hours. Remember that night- and nap-time brace wear is not as beneficial in slowing the progression in the paralytic spine as it is in the idiopathic spine.

Although spinal deformities develop in 75% of children with spina bifida (7), most are not present at birth. Deformities usually appear by age 5 years and, in most cases, are fully developed by 10 years of age (25,37). Congenital deformities (unsegmented bars and hemivertebrae, and combinations thereof) can coexist. These will be noted at birth and tend to require surgery at an earlier age than the paralytic deformity (2). Despite the high percentage of spinal deformities, one cannot be complacent regarding the exact cause of any given curve. As in any spinal deformity, investigation is necessary to determine whether there is an underlying correctable cause for the disorder, and therefore MRI and CT are useful in evaluating the spine for hydromyelia, a tethered spinal cord, or ventricular porencephaly, which can contribute to the deformity (8).

SURGICAL GOALS

The goal of surgery is to provide a stable, well balanced spine with the head centered over a nonoblique pelvis, allowing good balance and affording patients the use of both hands. Those with collapsing deformities, who must push up with their hands to support themselves or to maintain good pulmonary or GI function, are severely hindered in their ability to perform activities of daily living (27).

SURGICAL DECISION MAKING

As a general rule, curves that progress beyond 50° require surgery. It is assumed that most children with myelomeningocele, who will eventually require spinal surgery, will have curves greater than 50° well before skeletal maturity. Whereas it is preferable to wait until age 10–12 years for instrumented fusion, one will occasionally need to intervene at an earlier age to prevent irretrievable progression. As with surgery for other medically "delicate" patients, such as those with muscular dystrophy, optimization of general medical health at the time of surgery is important. Before surgery, any hydrocephalus should be well controlled, and shunts, if in place, should function normally. Ideally, the urinary tract should be free of any obstruction, ureteral reflux managed, and the urine sterile. In many cases, of course, obtaining sterile urine is temporary at best, and in these instances, the known colonizing bacteria should be suppressed with appropriate antibiotic prophylaxis. Failure to control bacteria in the urinary tract can lead to an inordinately high infection rate (2). Finally, the condition of the skin generally and in the operative area, in particular, must be at its best. Whenever the potential for the introduction of infection into the fusion through skin contaminants is high, it is advisable to do appropriate plastic surgical reconstruction first. This will often require tissue expansion, midline scar excision, and closure. After the new area is well healed, definitive spinal surgery can then proceed with less risk of infection.

PREOPERATIVE PLANNING AND MANAGEMENT

IMAGING

The explosion in technology over the past decade has greatly enhanced the ability to image the deformed spine, immeasurably improving preoperative planning. Despite these advances, however, plain radiographs (standing or sitting PA and lateral views and supine bending films) are critical for initial planning. These images will demonstrate the existing spinal alignment, head and shoulder balance, and pelvic obliquity. Bending films assess the degree of correction that may be possible. Keep in mind that the bone in the paralytic spine is likely not to be as strong as in the idiopathic spine and may not tolerate attempts to restore true anatomic alignment.

Bone scans are generally not required, although they are useful in diagnosing a preexistent underlying osteomyelitis, which would be a short-term contraindication for instrumented fusion. Patients with chronic skin breakdown over the deformity or a history of prolonged drainage may have chronic osteomyelitis. Bone infection must be eradicated before correction of the deformity.

In the evaluation of the bony anatomy, CT is most useful when 3D reconstructions are performed. Spiral CT data can be manipulated into excellent 3D images, and this minimizes the amount of radiation to which patients are exposed. 3D reconstructions allow virtual spinal visualization and can be useful when placement angles of hooks or pedicular screws are being planned.

It has been said that all patients with myelomeningocele who underwent a surgical closure after birth have by definition a degree of cord tethering (21). In some patients, the tethering is a major factor in scoliosis progression. In addition to demonstrating significant tethering, MRI will show any other cord abnormalities that may be present, including syringomyelia and hydromyelia, which may need correction before a definitive spinal fusion. MRI will also demonstrate the degree of Arnold–Chiari malformation and any change from baseline.

SURGICAL PRINCIPLES

In no area of orthopaedic surgery is preoperative planning more important than in the paralytic spinal deformity. Be prepared for the following:

Patients as a rule are smaller.
The deformities are more severe and more rigid.
Bone is osteopenic.
Spinal elements in the involved area are altogether absent.
Patients' underlying medical condition is frequently more precarious then expected.
Arrangements may need to be made to have special

instrumentation and additional bone-grafting products available.

Most patients with spina bifida require combined anterior and posterior spinal instrumentation combined with fusion that includes the sacrum.

- Start the fusion typically two levels above the end of the curve, and extend to the sacrum or pelvis (25,34).
- The most common technical error is to perform too short a fusion that necessitates later revision for progressive imbalance.
- Wait until age 10–12 years if the curve magnitude is moderate.
- It is better to accept some permanent truncal shortening than to let a curve progress beyond 70° to 80°.
- The majority of patients with myelodysplasia have a small, underdeveloped, osteopenic pelvis. Plan to use allograft bone and other bone-graft extenders for the primary grafting material.

As these typically are lengthy procedures, controlling blood loss intraoperatively is critical (17).

- Use subcutaneous epinephrine (1:400,000–500,000) and a Bovie electrocautery, a bipolar coagulator, and in some cases an argon laser to maintain a dry operative field. Employ hypotensive anesthesia judiciously to minimize uncontrolled blood loss.
- Remember that one of the most important factors related to complications and blood loss is the prevention of hypothermia (24).
- Use blood and intravenous fluid warmers, as well as warming blankets, to maintain normothermia. Simply turning the room temperature up to 85° will not have the desired effect.
- Intraoperative salvage of blood with a cell saver is useful because the volume of blood in these patients as a result of their size is frequently not enough for salvage by conventional means. Use of state-of-the-art processing units and intraoperative plasmapheresis is an exciting new concept for intraoperative cell salvage that requires markedly less volume of salvaged cells to be useful.

A surgeon managing the spinal deformity of myelomeningocele must deal with the issue of deficient bone stock on two levels. First, is a congenital deficiency of the posterior elements that provides limited sites for traditional sublaminar wires or hooks. Secure the rods to the spine at these levels with a cable or a wire encircling the pedicle through the neural foramen; otherwise do not instrument these levels. Where soft-tissue coverage is adequate, the newer, smaller pedicle screw systems appear to be an excellent means of securing these levels of the spine to the rod. Remember that the majority of pull-out strength with a pedicle screw is within the pedicle itself. The screw should be optimally sized to the pedicle and need not extend far-

ther than 50% of the way through the vertebral body. Be fully familiar with the available instrumentation, and arrange to have a wide array of screw sizes and lengths available on the day of surgery.

The second problem with deficient bone stock is the availability of autogenous graft. Portions of both iliac crests, the ribs, and portions of the spinous processes were once the only bone available. With modern bone banking technology and the availability of graft extenders, the use of autogenous graft is now typically not advised unless a patient is unusually robust; commercially available graft extenders include Grafton (Grafton Corporation, Edison, NJ), a demineralized bone matrix; Coralene (Interpore International, Irvine, CA), and Osteoset pellets (Wright Medical Products, Arlington, TN). Additional products on the horizon will make the issue of deficient autogenous graft a moot point.

Postoperative infection is one of most serious and devastating complications that may follow instrumented spinal fusion in this patient population. At our institution, dual-coverage antibiotics (a first-generation cephalosporin and an aminoglycoside) are typically given for 48–72 hours postoperatively.

- Prolong antibiotic coverage if drains remain in place or significant drainage persists.
- A potential for later infection is present if systemic urosepsis occurs or if the soft tissue overlying the instrumentation breaks down.
- Use all available means of obtaining thick, well vascularized flaps to cover the spinal instrumentation, particularly in the lumbar region, where the overlying tissue is typically most atrophic and poorly vascularized.
- Stage procedures in instances where the scarred area has had repeated episodes of breakdown or the scar is in particularly poor repair.
- Excise nonviable scar initially, and mobilize flaps to bring new, healthy skin to the midline.
- As simple flap mobilization may not be possible, consider placing tissue-expansion bladders on either side of the midline to create new skin.
- Then resect the midline scar, bring the new expanded skin together in the midline, and allow the wound to heal for 4–6 weeks before the definitive procedure.

Much has changed in spinal instrumentation since the 1982 paper by Osebold et al. (34), for whom the best results for spinal fusion in these patients involved combined anterior and posterior instrumentation. They noted that the anterior–posterior approach gave the best degree of correction, best maintenance of correction, and best correction of pelvic obliquity. The instrumentation in this series was with Harrington rods and either the Dwyer or Zielke device anteriorly. These three systems have long since passed out of favor, but the concept of a 360° fusion still makes sense from the standpoint of maximal rigidity and stability. However, with improved posterior segmental instrumentation, a separate anterior approach is not always necessary.

Permanent wheelchair users usually require fusion to the pelvis. One problem with fusion to the pelvis is the historically high rate of pseudarthrosis (10,14,15,34). The development by Allen and Ferguson (2) of the Galveston technique, in which Luque rods are inserted into the iliac wing, was a significant advance in pelvic fixation. Their first reported series in 1979 demonstrated that the technique, although not foolproof, was a major improvement over previous attempts to fix the rod to the sacrum.

The chief problem with this technique is that the pelvis, particularly in nonambulators, tends to be osteopenic and hypoplastic. Rods can migrate within the bone and can break out through the thin cortex anteriorly or posteriorly. The other frequent problem is the difficulty in securing adequate fixation in the lower lumbar spine, where the posterior elements are absent (10). No study has yet been published in which pedicular hooks were used at the lower lumbar levels along with the Galveston technique; however, one would expect that problems with iliac wing breakage would be less common.

A modification of the Luque-Galveston technique has been described by Dunn (14,19). In this technique, the rod is contoured to fit just anterior to the sacral ala or passed through a window in the superior aspect of the ala down into the sacrum itself, paralleling the sacroiliac joint rather than going into the ilium. Our experience with the latter intraosseous modification suggests that rod pull-out by fracture of the posterior sacral cortex is a major drawback.

Another technique for securing the long spinal construct to the pelvis employs an intrailiac bolt or a long pedicle screw inserted in the same manner as the end of the rod in the Luque-Galveston technique. The rod is then appropriately contoured and attached to the screw or bolt in the same fashion as the screw would otherwise be attached to a rod. The advantage of this technique is that the rod–screw construct may be inserted in a "modular" fashion. The screw has a greater initial pull-out strength than the smooth end of a contoured rod. Studies have not shown a long-term benefit from this construct relative to improved lumbosacral fusion. It is, however, easier for surgeons to place. Be certain that the screw–rod interface is sufficiently tight, as any modular system can disengage over time.

SCOLIOSIS

Scoliosis is the most common spinal deformity in myelomeningocele, afflicting 80% of patients (27,38). The risk of scoliosis is higher with progressively higher levels of neurologic involvement (Fig. 157.2). As previously noted, typical management usually involves anterior and poste-

rior fusion (32). With improved segmental fixation, a patient who is beginning to show signs of skeletal maturity or in whom the triradiate cartilage of the acetabulum has closed (39), may not require additional anterior fixation. However, when the anterior procedure is performed, it is done first and consists of anterior release or discectomy and fusion, anterior release with strut grafting, or, most commonly, anterior fusion and correction with CD Horizon, CD Hopf (Sofamor-Danek, Medtronic-Sofamor-Danek, Memphis, TN), or Kaneda (Johnson & Johnson, Depuy-Acromed, Raytham, MA) style instrumentation.

Anterior Lumbar Fusion

■ After induction of general anesthesia, place the patient in the lateral decubitus position with the convexity of the lumbar curve placed upward. Place the apex of the curve at the break in the operating table so that the table can be gently flexed, with the head and foot portion lower than the middle. A deflatable bean bag, with or without kidney rests, maintains excellent positioning of the patient. Carefully pad all bony prominences, and ensure that the Bovie pad is not over a minimally protected bony prominence. Perform a wide field preparation of the skin. If an adhesive surgical drape is not utilized over the entire surgical field, seal the edges of the drapes.

■ Enter the thorax one or two levels above the superiormost vertebrae to be instrumented. Utilizing two levels above will facilitate placing the uppermost screw in its best position, parallel to the end plates.

■ If not experienced in using the Bovie cautery for all cutting beyond the dermal level, use subcutaneous epinephrine to secure hemostasis.

■ A needle-tip Bovie unit is particularly useful for the subcutaneous dissection.

■ Start the incision proximally, approximately a hand's-breadth from the midline over the rib in question, and extend along the rib to the costochondral junction. Then curve the incision gently distally, following the lateral edge of the rectus sheath.

■ The distal extent of the incision will depend on whether the instrumentation is to be carried down to the L-3 or L-4 level. It is exceedingly difficult and perhaps dangerous to attempt to get to the L-5 level through this approach.

■ Carry the incision down proximally to the periosteum of the rib, and incise it longitudinally.

■ Expose the rib subperiosteally without violating the chest cavity. When the rib is freed, disarticulate it from its chondral end, and with blunt finger dissection remove it entirely from its vertebral articulation.

■ Place a ringed lap sponge into the proximalmost portion of the wound to maintain hemostasis.

■ Incise the costal cartilage longitudinally with a knife, and find the extraperitoneal plane immediately beneath with blunt finger dissection. The key to this exposure is developing the correct retroperitoneal plane. Open the rib bed longitudinally to enter the chest, and use a self-retaining chest retractor to spread the ribs.

■ Carry the incision distally under direct vision, taking care to not transect the external oblique, internal oblique, and transverse abdominal muscles other than through their tendinous condensations at the lateral aspect of the rectus sheath.

■ Take down the diaphragm from the chest wall from the site of the chondral split, working posteriorly toward the diaphragmatic crus. The diaphragm may be taken off the chest wall nearly flush, as some surgeons prefer, or, more typically, with a 1–1.5 cm cuff left, which is useful for reapproximation at closure.

■ Place marking sutures of alternating colors every 3–4 cm to facilitate a more anatomic closure.

■ After the diaphragm has been taken down to the vertebral body or the crus and the distal extent of the abdominal portion is complete, use a self-retaining retractor system, such as a laparotomy retractor (Omnitract, Omnitract Surgical, Minneapolis, MN), to maintain broad exposure.

■ Incise the pleura over the thoracic levels to be instrumented, and using a Kidner sponge, elevate the pleura generously toward the opposite side of the vertebral body and equally generously back over the heads of the ribs. Taking time at this point to mobilize the good pleura will facilitate covering the upper end of the hardware construct at the end of the procedure.

■ If instrumentation is placed, then gently and carefully isolate, ligate, and tease the vertebral segmental vessels from the vertebral body with a Kidner-type sponge.

■ Vessels may be ligated with suture or with vascular clips. Clips should be made of titanium, and use of an automatic clip loader will speed the process. The vessels are readily and easily exposed to the level of L-1, beyond which they are obscured by the psoas musculature.

■ Be careful of the nearby genitofemoral and ilioinguinal nerves.

■ Pay close attention to the tributaries of the thoracic duct, as well as the sympathetic chain. If a portion of the lymphatic chain is inadvertently cut, chylous spillage will be evident; the two duct ends may be ligated without complication.

■ After ligating the segmental arteries, remove the intervertebral discs.

■ Use a long handled #15 blade to incise the annulus as near the endplate as possible.

■ Resect the annulus as fully as possible, except posteriorly, where a portion is frequently left adherent to the posterior longitudinal ligament.

■ The endplates are generally thick and are easily removed with a large curet within the intervertebral space. Pay particular attention not to stray through the fairly soft subchondral bone into the vertebral body itself (Fig. 157.4).

■ As each discectomy is performed, pack the intervertebral space with thrombin-soaked Surgicel to provide hemostasis.

■ When the desired degree of release has been achieved, place the vertebral screws across the vertebral bodies. The dual-screw systems available (CD-Horizon) and the Kaneda anterior scoliosis system (KASS) demonstrate improved pull-out strength compared with single-screw systems (Fig. 157.5) (32). However, the small myelodysplastic spine may not always accommodate two screws. The choice of whether to use a one- or two-screw vertebral construct is an essential part of the preoperative planning.

■ If possible, place screws with bicortical fixation to maximize pull-out strength.

■ After placement of the screws in each vertebral body, contour a flexible template rod to the spinal deformity.

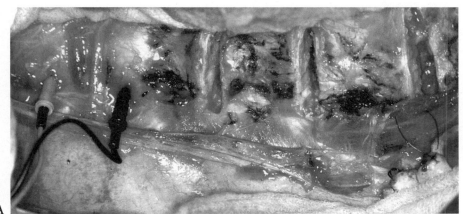

A

Figure 157.4. Anterior discectomy technique. **A:** Intraoperative photograph demonstrates the anterior lumbar discectomies. Note the motor-potential monitoring electrodes to the left. This patient had some distal motor sparing. *(continues)*

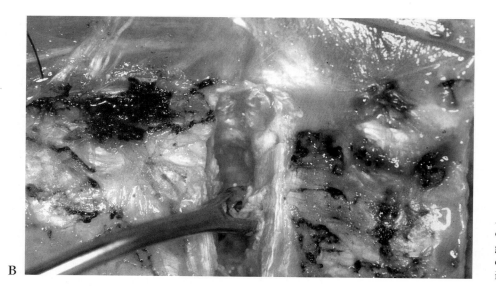

B

Figure 157.4. (continued) **B:** A uterine curet may be useful to remove the cartilaginous endplate. Care needs to be exercised in endplate removal, as the underlying bone is frequently very soft.

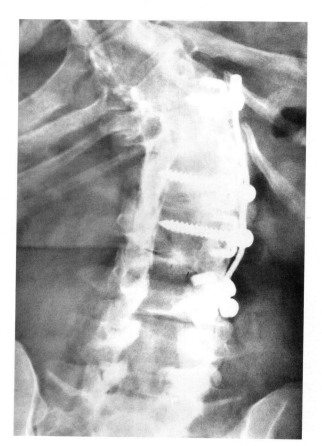

Figure 157.5. PA radiograph of the lumbar spine after Dwyer instrumentation. The lumbar component is well fused despite hardware pull-out. However, note the decompensation at the thoracolumbar junction secondary to "fusing too short."

- Cut and carefully contour an appropriate-length implantable rod to match the curvature of the template rod.
- After fixing the rod to the vertebral screws, reinflate the vacuum bean bag to soften it and make the table surface flat.
- Now, slowly and gently rotate the rod anteriorly to convert the scoliotic curve into a gentle lumbar curve. When 90° of rotation has been achieved, lock the rod into position.
- Sequentially, beginning from the center, gently distract the intervertebral disc spaces, remove the thrombin-soaked Surgicel, and pack the disc space with bone graft. Use the excised rib and additional allograft cancellous bone as needed. Pack the disc space completely and tightly, and then gently compress the disc.
- Fill each vertebral level with bone graft so that at completion of the grafting, the spine appears as though arthrodesis has already occurred. Leaving large segments of unfilled disc space will increase the likelihood of fibrous union or nonunion, which can lead to hardware failure (6,15,31).
- Allow the reflected psoas musculature to overlie the distal construct, and close the pleura superiorly with a running 2-0 absorbable suture attached to a tapered needle; the use of a cutting needle will result in excessive tearing of the pleura. Reattach the diaphragm either in layers or in a single layer, depending on your preference. Alternate #1 Vicryl and Ethibond sutures for a very strong and secure diaphragmatic closure. Place an appropriate-size chest tube in the anterior axillary line, and tubularize the rib bed to facilitate regrowth of the rib. Close the remainder of the wound in layers. Typi-

cally, no drain other than the chest tube is needed. If the anterior–posterior fusion is to be staged, do the posterior procedure in 7 days. However, there is no reason why the procedure must be staged, provided it is safe to proceed with several hours of additional anesthesia. Blood loss from the anterior approach can be kept to a reasonable amount—usually less than 150 ml.

An advantage to same-day anterior–posterior surgery is that the nutritional status of any patient is usually at its best at the time of the first surgery (4,35). It is therefore advisable, whenever possible, to do anterior and posterior surgery under the same anesthetic.

Posterior Spinal Fusion

Use the prone position. Depending on the patient's size, the surgeon's preference, and associated contractures and deformities, any of several positioning devices is appropriate. I believe that the four-post frame is the most useful for smaller adolescents. Once again, it is extremely important to carefully pad all bony prominences, as skin slough at the chest and anterior iliac wings is a significant potential pitfall from prolonged prone positioning.

Preoperative evaluation of the scarred, closed dural sac is mandatory. If the original scar remains in place, take meticulous care to keep the flap edges as thick as possible. Do not use subcutaneous epinephrine in this scarred area because of the increased risk of postoperative skin slough.

- After positioning the patient in the prone position, make a straight midline incision as for any posterior spinal approach.
- As the distal anatomy is often quite difficult, approach the abnormal anatomy from areas of normal anatomy demonstrated cephalad.
- As the paraspinal musculature is stripped from the posterior elements, maintain good hemostasis and use Bovie cautery for the majority of soft-tissue cutting.
- To avoid the midline scarred area, use an inverted-Y incision. With this approach, one entirely avoids the midline sac area, and the midline lumbar area is not undermined at all. This allows good exposure of the transverse processes and pedicles but avoids entering the dural sac, which increases the likelihood of wound breakdown or infection. Be prepared for a small skin slough at the junction of the Y, and be careful that the distal limbs of the Y portion are far enough apart to allow adequate collateral blood flow to this "island" flap.
- When the spine has been subperiosteally exposed to the transverse processes throughout the length of the incision, facilitate further lateral exposure at the caudal end by transecting the paraspinal muscles in an L-type fashion.
  - Contour the appropriate-length rods to maintain the sagittal curves, especially the lumbar lordosis.
  - The degree of contouring toward the scoliosis will

depend on the degree of correction that can be obtained once the rod is in place. Gentle pressure on the spine from two persons will allow fairly accurately prediction of what curvature correction will be possible.

- Affix the upper end of the rod to the spine with a sublaminar hook or sublaminar wires or cables. Sublaminar cables have the advantage of being more flexible; however, they are clearly more expensive, and retightening a cable once crimped is generally not possible unless a second crimp device has been added first. If one desires to maintain an all-titanium construct, however, cables may be the only option (Fig. 157.6).
- Pass the sublaminar wires or cables in the usual fashion in the normal part of the spine and around the remaining pedicle through the neural foramen in the bifid portion of the spine.

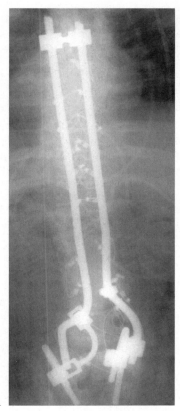

A

Figure 157.6. PA (**A**) view of a patient who initially underwent pelvic fixation with insertion of rod ends into the sacral ala. Approximately 2 weeks postoperatively, the rod ends displaced dorsally through the bone. Revision surgery utilized a construct with a separate rod placed anterior to the ala and attached posteriorly with Texas Scottish Rite Hospital links (TSRH, Medtronic-Sofamor-Danek, Inc., Memphis, TN). The patient did well after the revision. (See Figure 157.11 for clinical photos.)
(continues)

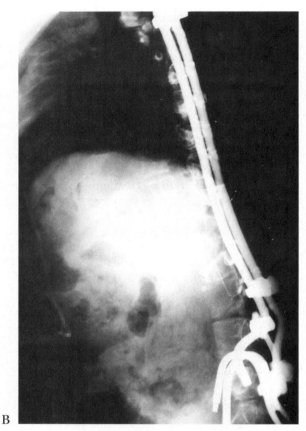

B

Figure 157.6. *(continued)* Lateral (**B**) view of a patient who initially underwent pelvic fixation with insertion of rod ends into the sacral ala. Approximately 2 weeks postoperatively, the rod ends displaced dorsally through the bone. Revision surgery utilized a construct with a separate rod placed anterior to the ala and attached posteriorly with Texas Scottish Rite Hospital links (TSRH, Medtronic-Sofamor-Danek, Inc., Memphis, TN). The patient did well after the revision. (See Figure 157.11 for clinical photos.)

- Pedicle screws can be used where the posterior elements are deficient, as noted previously.
- Fixation to the pelvis, also previously discussed, is based on surgeon preference and bony anatomy. The traditional one-piece Luque "unit" rod is technically demanding, but fortunately alternatives exist. The one-piece bilateral rod may be cut and then reconnected with any of several rod cross-links available on the market. The overall stability will not be compromised by this technique (Fig. 157.7). Additionally, there may even be cases in which the surgeon may wish to use two rods on each side connected by rod-to-rod connectors.
- After completion of the instrumentation, carefully decorticate the spine before applying the bone graft. If the soft tissue has been satisfactorily removed from the bone, this may be sufficient for the myelodysplastic

spine. Meticulous decortication, as done in idiopathic scoliosis, runs the risk of further weakening already weak bone, which results in lamina fracture and wire pull-through. The experienced surgeon will need to straddle this fine line between risk of hardware failure and potential for nonunion.

Again, while the tendency in idiopathic scoliosis surgery is to allow patients to be free of bracing or an orthosis postoperatively, such is not the case in the myelodysplastic spine. There is much greater risk for hardware failure, and most surgeons place patients into a custom-made bivalved underarm body jacket 5–7 days after surgery. It should be worn for 9–15 months after surgery (34). Whereas bracing has significant pitfalls in attempting to *improve* a curve, the likelihood of skin problems with a postoperative brace that is simply *holding* position is much less. However, do advise the family that skin problems can still occur. It is important that an experienced orthotist make these braces.

Many patients with scoliosis have a congenital compo-

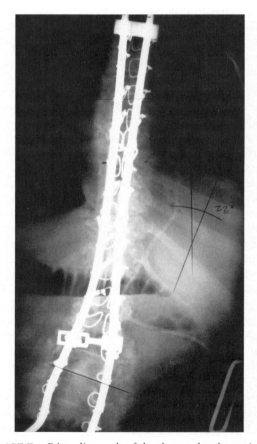

Figure 157.7. PA radiograph of the thoracolumbar spine demonstrates a segmental sublaminar fixation utilizing flexible stainless steel cables. Cross-links are required to maintain rod–rod stability. Fixation to the pelvis (not seen here) is by the Galveston technique.

nent to their curve. Congenital curves are best addressed early and are most frequently treated by *in situ* fusion of the congenital curve. Resection of hemivertebrae is rarely indicated, except in the lower-lumbar regions, most typically at L-5. A hemiepiphysiodesis will occasionally allow the contralateral portion of the spine to grow and actually provide some correction. However, in the majority of patients, epiphysiodesis serves to stop all growth, and significant improvement is never realized.

Many myelodysplasia clinics have patients with 100° + curves that have progressed relentlessly to this point through the desire of the family to refrain from surgery or by fear that early surgery will result in too much truncal shortening. Surgeons must be aggressive about treating the progressive and significant curve, even in a patient with 6–8 years of growth remaining. It is better to have a short trunk than to end up with a severe curve and loss of function. The subcutaneous "growth" rod remains an excellent short-term way of slowing some curve progression. The growth rod is similar to the concept developed for juvenile idiopathic curves, but in the myelodysplastic spine, it frequently requires additional points of skeletal fixation. The Luque trolley, utilizing loose sublaminar wires and no bone graft, was introduced in an attempt to maintain position until formal fusion (36). The chief problem with it is the difficulty in getting the spine to truly "slide." This may still be worth a try if it is the only alternative to fusing a spine prematurely, and has been shown of greater utility when combined with short-segment epiphysiodesis (36).

KYPHOSIS

Significant structural lumbar kyphosis occurs in approximately 15% of patients with myelomeningocele (30). Operative management of collapsing kyphosis routinely requires an anterior and posterior approach, and unlike the typical anterior procedure, these frequently require some additional posterior-element resection so that the kyphotic component can be corrected toward a more anatomic configuration.

Normal lumbar lordosis rarely develops in children with a mid- to upper-level lumbar meningocele. The absence of the posterior elements and overlying musculature, combined with tight hamstrings rocking the pelvis posteriorly, creates a hypolordotic, if not kyphotic, lumbar spine. In severe cases, the kyphosis becomes profound, and in some the lumbar spine will virtually fold over on itself, creating a near 180° gibbous deformity (Fig. 157.8). Lumbar kyphosis is more disabling than scoliosis in many respects because the forward-flexed lumbar spine creates a relatively hypokyphotic thoracic spine. Such spines are not mechanically stable, and patients must prop themselves up on their hands. This creates problems with pulmonary function, as well as with GI and GU tract motility

in the long-term. In addition, by constantly having to prop themselves up with their hands, patients are unable to function well in activities of daily living.

Lumbar kyphosis is often present at birth and may be significant very early on. Bracing is very difficult because of the very prominent bone underlying poor skin (5).

There are two broad categories of lumbar kyphosis. The more common type is a rigid kyphotic deformity, usually with the apex at the L1-2 level. This is associated with a rigid compensatory lower-thoracic lordosis. The other, less common, less severe kyphosis is typically less rigid and has no proximal lordosis (19). Indications for correcting lumbar kyphosis include recurrent skin ulcerations over the prominence, difficulty with wheelchair fitting, progressive pulmonary, GI, or GU problems, and difficulties with activities of daily living secondary to the forward-flexed posture (5). Surgical reconstruction (26,43), a major undertaking, should accomplish three goals, according to Lindseth and Slezer (22): It should (a) straighten and stabilize the spine for better sitting posture, (b) markedly diminish the prominence of the kyphos, and (c) increase the overall height of the abdominal cavity.

Sharrard (41) was the first to describe resection of vertebral bodies in the management of this condition. His 1968 study demonstrated good correction, but follow-up studies have demonstrated that simple excision of the apex leads to an unacceptable recurrence rate of the initial kyphosis (22). Lindseth and Slezer (22) showed that excision of one or two vertebrae proximal to the apex of the kyphosis both realigned the lumbar spine to the proximal thoracic portion and improved long-term results.

Kyphectomy is generally done at birth, in 2–5-year-olds, or most commonly in young adolescents. A one- to two-vertebral-level kyphectomy may be required at birth for the very rare situation in which skin closure is not possible. For the 2–5-year-old group, in whom the gibbus is a problem, a procedure has been described in which the proximal segment of the gibbus is resected and the remaining lumbar spine is brought into apposition with the thoracic spine and held with a single-level wiring of one pedicle to the other (Fig. 157.9) (22). No fusion or other instrumentation is necessary in these young, usually quite lightweight patients who then wear a pantaloon cast or brace for 6 months followed by an additional 6 months of underarm bracing. The advantage of doing this procedure earlier rather than later stems from the fact that only one level is fused and the remainder of the lumbar and thoracic vertebral bodies continue to grow. The majority of these patients will likely require additional surgery in the long term, but the benefits tend to outweigh this minor drawback. The Luque trolley, as noted previously, has also been utilized for kyphotic deformities (36). I prefer to wait until a child is 10–12 years of age before proceeding with a multisegmented instrumentation.

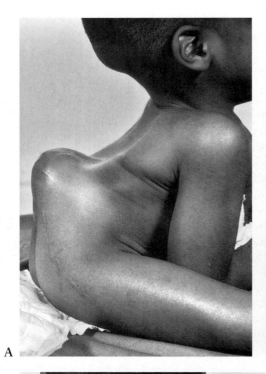

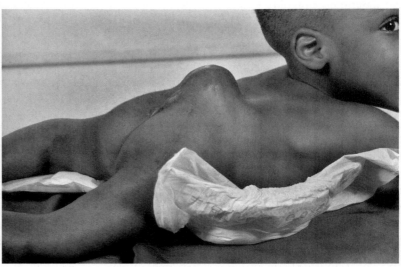

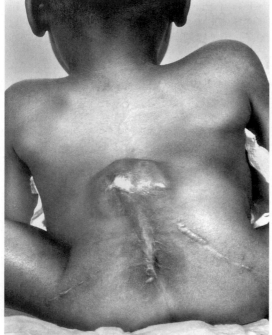

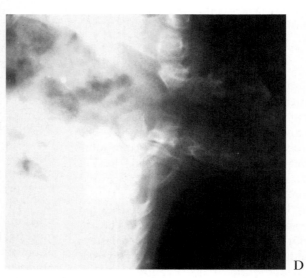

Figure 157.8.   A 4-year-old boy with a 180° gibbus. **A:** Lateral sitting view demonstrates the problems with a significant gibbus. There is limited upper-extremity mobility, as the elbows support much of his weight. **B:** A recumbent view demonstrates no appreciable mobility of the gibbous segment. **C:** Note the extensive scarring in the midline and the fragility of the skin overlying the gibbus. **D:** Lateral radiograph shows the hairpin bony deformity.

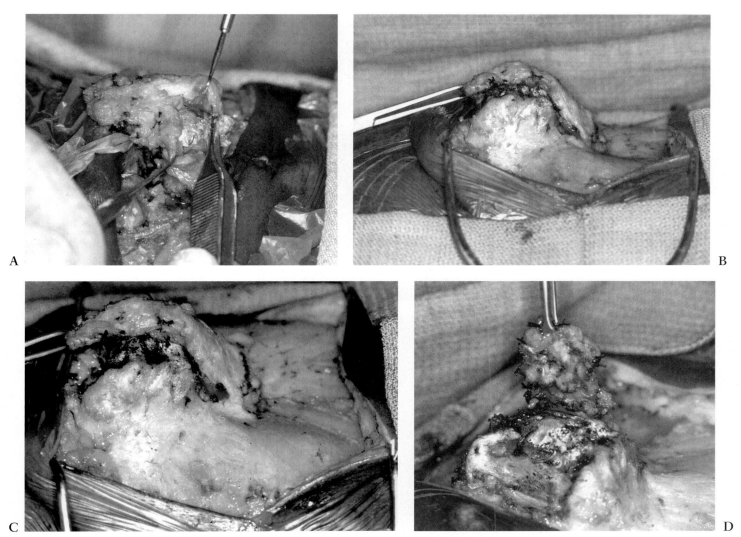

Figure 157.9.   Intraoperative photographs of the patient in Figure 157.8. **A:** In a patient undergoing a gibbus resection in whom significant growth remains, the spine is opposed after resection with single-level wiring of one pedicle to the other. Note the transverse incision. Here, the dural sac is being freed from the posterior aspect of the bony canal. **B,C:** Nonfunctional nerve roots are ligated. **D:** The dural sac is carefully elevated in a subperiosteal manner. *(continues)*

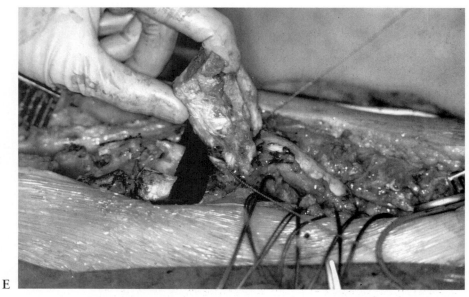

E

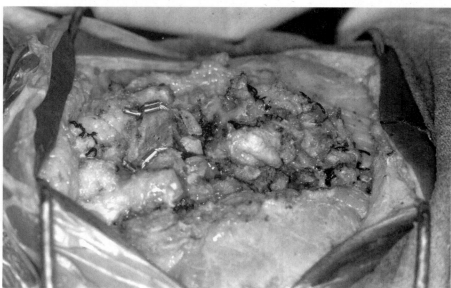

F

*Figure 157.9.   (continued)*E: While the sac is retracted cephalad, a Gigli saw is used to resect the superior portion of the gibbus. F: The vertebral bodies have been opposed and cabled together.

Lumbar Kyphectomy

Kyphectomy in a 10–12-year-old patient typically involves the same technique in which the superior portion of the apex is resected and the lumbar and thoracic segments are joined back together with an accompanying segmental instrumentation construct extending from the pelvis to the upper-lumbar spine (Figs. 157.10 and 157.11). In contrast to the approach in 2–5-year-old patients, in whom a transverse incision works very nicely, use a traditional longitudinal incision for this procedure. Start in the midline from the more normal upper-thoracic spine and extend downward to the sacrum. The dura is typically just beneath the skin, and care must be exercised as the dissection proceeds from the midline laterally to leave the dura intact and the overlying skin as thick as possible. It is very easy to violate the dural sac. Promptly close any durotomy.

■ While dissecting laterally after exposing the posterior elements, elevate the dural sac from the spinal canal to expose the posterior aspects of the vertebral bodies. This is done after distal transection of the dura. (These

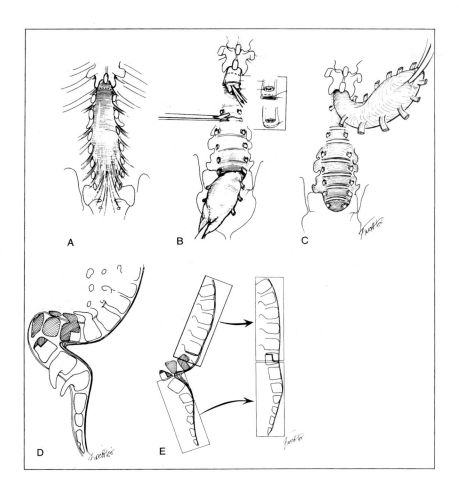

Figure 157.10.   **A:** A typical total spina bifida of the lumbar spine as seen in congenital lumbar kyphosis. The *dotted line* shows the level of dural transection. **B:** The nonfunctional cord is transected, and the dura is sutured distal to the cord transection. The central canal of the cord must be left open to communicate with the subdural space. The nerve roots are transected at each foramen. The discs are removed from behind. **C:** An alternative technique is distal detachment of the neural sac and progressive upward dissection with division of the nerve roots at the level of the foramina. The sac is usually not entered, and the cord does not have to be transected. The risk of acute hydrocephalus is reduced, and the sac is laid down over the instrumentation to provide better coverage. **D:** A typical rigid myelomeningocele kyphosis. The *hatched area* represents the vertebrae to be resected, usually those between the apex of the kyphosis and the apex of the lordosis. **E:** The general principle is to relate the distal segment (sacrum and lower-lumbar vertebrae) to the proximal segment (thorax) so that the two are in a stable vertical relationship. The anterior longitudinal ligament is preserved as the hinge on which the segments are aligned. (From Bradford DS, Lonstein JE, Moe JH, et al. *Moe's Textbook of Scoliosis and Other Spinal Deformities.* Philadelphia: WB Saunders, 1987:322, with permission.)

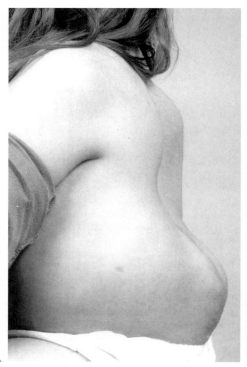
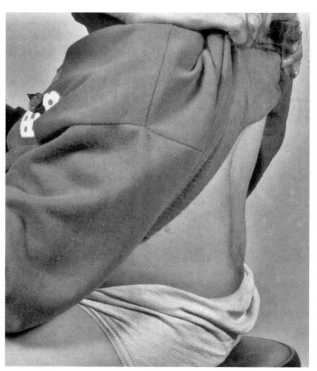

A   B

Figure 157.11.   Pre- (**A**) and postoperative (**B**) photographs show a 12-year-old girl who underwent kyphectomy and thoracolumbar instrumented fusion. Note the improved sitting balance and the better contour for seating. (The same patient is the subject as Figure 157.6.)

patients typically have a functioning level at L-1 or higher.)

■ Typically, when the dura is transected at the sacral level, the spinal cord itself, even in cases of significant tethering, is well proximal. Take extreme care when closing this dural transection not to ligate any element of the cord itself, as this can result in sudden increased CSF pressure that will cause profound intraoperative hypotension and possibly death. The central canal often functions as a major CSF conduit when there are poorly functioning ventricles (18,44).

■ Cut the nerve roots at each level, and ligate them to prevent CSF leakage. (The roots may be ligated, as there is no CSF circulation within the nerve roots themselves.)

■ After these have been ligated, elevate the sac, from distal to proximal, off the posterior aspect of the vertebral bodies (Fig. 157.9D).

■ Avoid significant blood loss by taking care to stop the bleeding from the numerous venous sinuses lying within the canal. Bovie electrocautery is useful for extraosseous bleeding, and bone wax packed into the interstices is useful for bone bleeding.

■ After the sac has been mobilized anteriorly and the

stump is closed without evidence of leakage, turn your attention to the kyphotic segment. With the nerve roots gone, gently elevate the structures on either side of the transverse processes subperiosteally, and proceed anteriorly back toward the midline. This dissection generally proceeds quite easily if one takes time and care to stay, if not subperiosteal, immediately supraperiosteal. Remember that the aorta and vena cava are in this soft-tissue mass that you are dissecting off the anterior portion of the vertebral body and these vessels could be injured by any sharp transgression into the mass.

■ After the spine is circumferentially freed (Fig. 157.9E), determine the segments for excision. It is always better to start with a fewer number than your preoperative template led you to believe.

■ Typically, two to three vertebral bodies must be removed to realign the spine in a reasonable configuration.

■ After the appropriate vertebral segments are resected *en bloc* (Fig. 157.9E), the proximal and distal portions will still be prominent. Use gentle finger pressure to approximate the two ends, which can then be approximated with pedicle-to-pedicle wire or cable, following with an overlying construct of hooks, wires, cables, or pedicle screws (Fig. 157.9F). Pelvic fixation may be of the Galveston type in the manner described by Dunn (14) or the variation described by McCarthy et al. (28).

■ After instrumentation is completed, allow the dural sac to fall back into its original position, and close the wound in routine fashion. Some authors advise against using a suction drain because it may increase the potential for CSF leak in their view.

Note that before you allow the dural sac to lay back down over the lumbar spine, several intravertebral discs will be exposed. This represents an excellent opportunity to perform a posterior lumbar interbody fusion (PLIF) and obviate a second stage of fusion to be performed later from the front. Obviously, in certain situations, a formal anterior fusion may be needed, but with several levels of PLIF in a patient who is unlikely to crankshaft, a second-stage anterior procedure is not always necessary.

Begin mobilizing patients by 1 week after surgery after fabrication of a custom bivalved underarm body jacket, which is worn for 12–18 months after surgery.

POSTOPERATIVE CARE AND REHABILITATION

Scoliosis correction and kyphectomy are extensive operations in children with multiple medical problems. Blood loss can be high, anesthesia times are long, and a postoperative pediatric intensive care unit is therefore mandatory. Many patients will remain intubated for 24 hours, and some will require short-term ventilatory support. Aggressive blood replacement therapy is indicated, and good urinary output must be maintained. As these patients are at higher risk for postoperative infection, maintain a longer period of prophylactic antibiotic therapy (often 5–7 days after surgery), and at the very least prescribe one dose beyond the point when all drains and central lines are removed. Use an aminoglycoside together with a cephalosporin to adequately cover the gram-negative organisms associated with chronic GU tract colonization and infection.

Other authors have advocated the use of total parenteral nutrition for patients undergoing staged procedures whose nutritional status is poor. This is certainly an option if the anterior–posterior fusion cannot be accomplished under one anesthetic. While monitoring of somatosensory-evoked potentials is typically not used intraoperatively, postoperative clinical neurologic monitoring is extremely important, especially in patients who have a history of hydrocephalus and a working shunt.

After patients have been medically stabilized, it is imperative to mobilize them as quickly as possible. However, do not place a patient in a sitting or standing position until the custom orthosis is available. A good relationship with the orthotist will facilitate obtaining a brace with 24°

to 48° postoperatively. Early mobilization helps prevent muscle atrophy and acute postoperative osteopenia. There is typically no reason or indication for prolonged bed rest after surgery.

Physical skills, which these patients have slowly gained, are rapidly lost after surgery, and physical therapy is exceedingly important to regaining their preoperative level of function. Whereas the surgery should improve sitting and standing balance, there is definitely a risk for marginal ambulators to become wheelchair-bound, particularly after fusion to the pelvis. This functional loss frequently occurs in patients with myelomeningocele in the early teenage years, but this possibility or eventuality should be discussed and well understood by patients and families before the surgical procedure. As socialization of these patients is of high importance as well, they should be allowed to return to their school setting as soon as they are ready—usually at about 4 weeks after surgery.

PITFALLS AND COMPLICATIONS

The surgical management of spinal deformity in myelodysplasia is difficult because of the severity of the deformity, the abnormal anatomy, and the multiple medical problems with which patients present. The first caveat therefore regarding this sort of spine surgery is that it is not for the casual spinal surgeon. Even in the best of hands, the postoperative complication rate is high. Without an experienced surgical team and an experienced surgeon in charge, the results can be disastrous.

Whereas any spinal deformity in any patient should be approached on an individual case-by-case basis, patients with myelomeningocele, perhaps even more so, cannot be treated in assembly-line or cookbook fashion. While the newer instrumentation may make it somewhat less necessary to combine anterior with posterior fusion, one must be careful not to neglect to perform both when both are necessary. It can be difficult to achieve a good, solid fusion if the posterior elements do not lend themselves to good bone-rod fixation or the exposed areas are too sparse to achieve a good fusion mass.

As these procedures are not cookbook in their design, the surgeon must be willing and able to compromise, devise, create, and improvise intraoperatively. Routine surgery always needs a flexible plan. Surgery of this nature requires not only plans A and B but plans C, D, and E, as well.

One of the most common technical errors is to attempt to preserve distal-lumbar motion segments and to "fuse too short" (6). Whereas maintaining lumbar motion is desirable in virtually any other spinal surgery, it is a significant mistake to leave the L5-S1 junction mobile in the paralytic spine. Not only will this area degenerate and cause pain over time in some patients, but it will almost certainly be unstable and can result in a junctional kyphosis or hyperlordosis in the paralytic spine. Similarly, stopping the fusion too short proximally can allow the upper portion of the thoracic spine to develop forward kyphosis, which will cause postural difficulties.

Never perform a unilateral fusion. The amount of bone stock present is rarely sufficient to provide significant stability by fusion of only one side of the spine.

Infection, the second most common postoperative complication, rears its ugly head in up to 25% of cases (34). As previously noted, prophylaxis with two antibiotics is considered the standard of care. It is very difficult to achieve true urine sterility in most patients, but if the organisms can be suppressed to the colonization level, postoperative sepsis secondary to GU contamination is less likely. Infection secondary to hematoma and dead-space and wound breakdown secondary to poor skin is best addressed preoperatively, as previously noted. The two best options for preventing deep infection because of skin problems include using an inverted-Y incision or doing a two-stage tissue expansion, as previously outlined.

Pseudarthrosis has been a common problem in the past. With the availability of bank bone graft and bone-graft extenders, the pseudarthrosis rate should decline in future studies. However, it is important to realize that bone must fuse to bone and therefore meticulous preparation of the bone graft bed is a requirement.

Instrumentation failure is also a common problem both intraoperatively and in the early postoperative period. Its cause is rarely metal breakage, but rather rod, hook, or wire pull-out from osteopenic bone. Addressing calcium balance and osteopenia preoperatively can be of use. One must be careful about being overly aggressive in tightening wires and distracting hooks. Despite adequate segmental fixation, the postoperative brace is still key in the postoperative management. Late instrumentation failure (wire or rod breakage) must be considered a pseudarthrosis until proven otherwise. Again, meticulous attention to bone grafting technique will minimize the pseudarthrosis rate.

Sometimes, even when the most extreme care has been exercised in providing postoperative hardware coverage, a sore will form over a prominent portion of the hardware. Once this covering is violated to the point where the metal is observable from the outside, securing a sterile environment is virtually impossible until all metal has been removed. If the wound becomes colonized and infected, significant long-term complications can ensue, resulting in difficult-to-treat chronic deep infections. If spinal osteomyelitis occurs, I have used debridement, long-term parenteral antibiotics, free-flap coverage to provide improved blood supply, and even hyperbaric oxygen to manage this most difficult problem.

REFERENCES

Each reference is categorized according to the following scheme: *, classic article; #, review article; !, basic research article; and +, clinical results/outcome study.

+ 1. Alan LD, Donald I, Gibson AA, et al. Amniotic Fluid Alpha-fetoprotein in the Antenatal Diagnosis of Spina Bifida. *Lancet* 1973;2:522.

2. Allen B, Ferguson R. Operative Treatment of Myelomeningocoele Spinal Deformities. *Orthop Clin North Am* 1979;10:845.

+ 3. American Academy of Allergy and Immunology: Task Force Report on Allergic Reactions to Latex. *J Allergy Clin Immunol* 1993;92:16.

+ 4. Banta J, Park SM. Improvement in Pulmonary Function in Patients Having Combined Anterior and Posterior Spine Fusion for Myelomeningocoele Scoliosis. *Spine* 1983;8:766.

+ 5. Banta JV, Hamanda JS. Natural History of the Kyphotic Deformity in Myelomeningocele. *J Bone Joint Surg Am* 1976;58:279.

6. Bradford DS, Lonstein JE, Moe JH, et al. *Moe's Textbook of Scoliosis and Other Spinal Deformities*, 3rd ed. Philadelphia: WB Saunders, 1995.

7. Brown HP. Management of Spinal Deformity in Myelomeningocele. *Orthop Clin North Am* 1978;9:391.

+ 8. Bunch WH, Sharff TB, Dvonch VM. Progressive Neurological Loss in Myelomeningocele Patients. *Orthop Trans* 1983;7:185.

+ 9. Centers for Disease Control and Prevention. Recommendations for the Use of Folic Acid to Reduce the Number of Cases of Spina Bifida and Other Neural Tube Defects. *MMWR* 1992;41(RR-14):1.

+ 10. Dickens DVR. The Surgery of Scoliosis and Spina Bifida. *J Bone Joint Surg Br* 1979;61:386.

11. Dormans JP, Templeton JJ, Edmonds Cl, et al. Intraoperative Anaphylaxis Due to Exposure to Latex (Natural Rubber) in Children. *J Bone Joint Surg Am* 1994;76:1688.

! 12. Drennan JC. The Role of Muscles in the Development of Human Lumbar Kyphosis. *Dev Med Child Neurol* 1970;12:33.

+ 13. Drummond DS, Moreau M, Cruess RL. The Results and Complications of Surgery for the Paralytic Hip and Spine in Myelomeningocoele. *J Bone Joint Surg Br* 1980;62:49.

+ 14. Dunn HK. Kyphosis of Myelodysplasia: Operative Treatment Based on Physiology. *Orthop Trans* 1983;7:19.

* 15. Dwyer AF, Newton MD, Sherwood AA. An Anterior Approach to Scoliosis. *Clin Orthop* 1969;62:192.

+ 16. Gardner WJ. Myelocele: Rupture of the Neural Tube? *Clin Neurosurg* 1968;15:57.

17. Hack HP, Zielke K, Harms J. Spinal Instrumentation and Monitoring. In: Bradford DS, Hensinger RM, eds. *The Pediatric Spine*. New York: Thieme, 1985.

+ 18. Hall PV, Lindseth RE, Campbell RL, et al. Scoliosis and Hydrocephalus in Myelocele Patients: The Effects of Ventricular Shunting. *J Neurosurg* 1979;50:174.

+ 19. Heydemann JS, Gillespie R. Management of Myelomeningocele Kyphosis in the Older Child by Kyphectomy and Segmental Spinal Instrumentation. *Spine* 1987;12: 37.

+ 20. Hide DW, Williams HP, Ellis HL. The Outlook for the Child with a Myelomeningocele for Whom Early Surgery was Considered Inadvisable. *Dev Med Child Neruol* 1972;14:304.

+ 21. Hull WJ, Moe JH, Winter RB. Spinal Deformity in Myelomeningocoele: Natural History, Evaluation, and Treatment. *J Bone Joint Surg Am* 1974;56:1767.

+ 22. Lindseth RE, Slezer L. Vertebral Excision for Kyphosis in Children with Myelomeningocele. *J Bone Joint Surg Am* 1979;61:699.

+ 23. Lorber J. Selective Treatment of Myelomeningocele: To Treat or Not to Treat? *Pediatrics* 1974;53:307.

+ 24. Matan AJ, Smith JT, Dunn HK. Risk Factors Associated with Anterior Surgery of the Thoracic Spine. Presented at the Pediatric Orthopaedic Society of North America Annual Meeting, Cleveland, Ohio, May 1998.

25. Mayfield JK. Spine Deformity in Myelomeningocele. In: Bradford DS, Hensinger RM, eds. *The Pediatric Spine*. New York: Thieme, 1985.

+ 26. Mayfield JK. Severe Spine Deformity in Myelodysplasia and Sacral Agenesis: An Aggressive Surgical Approach. *Spine* 1981;6:498.

+ 27. Mazur J, Menelaus MB, Dickens DR, et al. Efficacy of Surgical Management for Scoliosis in Myelomeningocele: Correction of Deformity and Alteration of Functional Status. *J Pediatr Orthop* 1986;6:568.

+ 28. McCarthy RE, Dunn J, McCullough FL. Luque Fixation to the Sacral Ala Using the Dunn-McCarthy Method. *Spine* 1989;14:281.

+ 29. McGuire CD, Winter RB, Mayfield JK, Erickson DL. Hemimyelodysplasia: A Report of Ten Cases. *J Pediatr Orthop* 1982;2:9.

+ 30. McMaster MJ. The Long-term Results of Kyphectomy and Spinal Stabilization in Children with Myelomeningocele. *Spine* 1988;13:417.

+ 31. McMaster MJ. Anterior and Posterior Instrumentation and Fusion of Thoracolumbar Scoliosis Due to Myelomeningocele. *J Bone Joint Surg Br* 1987;69:20.

+ 32. Moe JH, Purcell GA, Bradford DS. Zielke Instrumentation (VDS) for the Correction of Spinal Curvature. *Clin Orthop* 1983;180:133.

! 33. Morgagni JB. *The Seats and Causes of Diseases Investigated by Anatomy,* vol 3. London: A Millar & T Cadell, 1979.

+ 34. Osebold WR, Mayfield JK, Winter RB, Moe JH. Surgical Treatment of Paralytic Scoliosis Associated with Myelomeningocele. *J Bone Joint Surg Am* 1982;64:841.

+ 35. Powell ET, Krengel WF, King HA. Comparison of Same-day Sequential Anterior and Posterior Spinal Fusion with Delayed Two-stage Anterior and Posterior Spinal Fusion. *Spine* 1994;19:1256.

+ 36. Pratt RK, Webb JK, Burwell RB, Cummings SL. Luque Trolley and Convex Epiphysiodesis in the Management of Infantile and Juvenile Idiopathic Scoliosis. *Spine* 1999; 24:1538.

37. Raycroft JE, Curtis BH. Spinal Curvature in Myelomeningocele: Natural History and Etiology. In: *American Academy of Orthopaedic Surgeons: Symposium on Myelomeningocele*. St. Louis, MO: Mosby, 1972.

+ 38. Samuelsson L, Eklof O. Scoliosis in Myelomeningocele. *Acta Orthop Scand* 1988;59:122.

* 39. Sanders JO, Nerring JA, Browne RH. Posterior Arthrodesis and Instrumentation in the Immature (Risser Grade-0) Spine in Idiopathic Scoliosis. *J Bone Joint Surg Am* 1995;77:39.

+ 40. Seller MD, Nevin NC. Periconceptional Vitamin Supplementation and the Prevention of Neural Tube Defects in South-east England and North Ireland. *J Med Genet* 1984;21:325.

+ 41. Sharrard WJ. Spinal Osteotomy for Congenital Kyphosis in Myelomeningocele. *J Bone Joint Surg Br* 1968;50: 466.

+ 42. Tosi LL, Slater JE, Shaer C, Mostello LA. Latex Allergy in Spina Bifida Patients: Prevalence and Surgical Implications. *J Pediatr Orthop* 1993;13:709.

+ 43. Warner WC Jr, Fackler CD. Comparison of Two Instrumentation Techniques in Treatment of Lumbar Kyphosis in Myelodysplasia. *J Pediatr Orthop* 1993;13:704.

+ 44. Winston K, Hall J, Johnson D, Micheli L. Acute Elevation of Intracranial Pressure Following Transection of Non-functional Spinal Cord. *Clin Orthop* 1977;128:41.

+ 45. Yates JR, Ferguson-Smith MA, Shenkin A, et al. Is Disordered Folate Metabolism the Basis for the Genetic Predisposition to Neural Tube Defects? *Clin Genet* 1987;31: 279.

CHAPTER 158

SPINAL SURGERY IN CONGENITAL SYNDROMES

Paul D. Sponseller

The development of the spine may be upset by abnormalities of connective tissue, muscle balance, or ossification. Although a congenital syndrome is by definition present at birth, an associated spinal deformity in most cases is not. It may develop with growth as a result of bone dysplasia, a connective tissue disorder, or miscellaneous chromosomal abnormalities. The orthopaedic surgeon must understand the natural history of these growth disturbances to determine when, as well as how, to intervene. Three factors should always be kept in mind when evaluating the patient with a congenital syndrome: (a) coexisting medical problems, (b) characteristics of bone shape and quality, and (c) the effect of the syndrome on the neural elements.

P. D. Sponseller: Department of Pediatric Orthopaedics, Johns Hopkins Hospital School of Medicine, Baltimore, Maryland, 21287.

CERVICAL SPINE ABNORMALITIES

The cervical spine in many congenital syndromes is vulnerable to deformity, stenosis, and, most important, instability. The surgical team must rule out or characterize the potentially unstable cervical spine before general anesthesia is administered or any skeletal surgery is performed. Plain film radiography with or without flexion–extension may be helpful. Table 158.1 lists characteristic cervical spine problems in most common congenital syndromes.

ODONTOID HYPOPLASIA/ ATLANTOAXIAL INSTABILITY

The term *hypoplastic odontoid* generally refers to an odontoid process that does not extend to the midportion of the ring of the atlas. It may be seen in numerous condi-

Table 158.1.   *Characteristic Cervical Spine Problems in Common Congenital Syndromes*

Condition	Deformity	Anomaly	Instability	Stenosis	Special features
Achondroplasia	Thoracolumbar kyphosis; 75% resolve by age 2–3 years	—	—	Foramen pan-spinal increases	Frequent weakness due to DJD as adult
Diastrophic dysplasia	Midcervical kyphosis; T-L scoliosis; kyphosis	Spina bifida occulta (C) T-L vertebral fusion	—	Lumbar; rare	Moderate cervical kyphosis may resolve scoliosis; usually rigid
Metatrophic dysplasia	T-L kyphosis; scoliosis	Odontoid hypoplasia	C1–C2 rotatory or AP	Upper	Coexisting restrictive lung disorder
SED congenita	T-L kyphosis; scoliosis	Odontoid hypoplasia	C1–C2	—	—
Kneist syndrome	T-L scoliosis	Odontoid hypoplasia	C1–C2	—	—
Morquio syndrome	T-L kyphosis	Odontoid hypoplasia	C1–C2	—	—
Hurler syndrome	T-L kyphosis; scoliosis		C1–C2	—	Most live 1–2 decades
Osteogenesis imperfecta	T-L kyphosis; scoliosis	—	—	—	Scoliosis related to overall severity
Neurofibromatosis	Cervical kyphosis; nondystrophic scoliosis; dystrophic kyphoscoliosis	—	C1–2 rotation, C2–3 subluxation	—	Intracanal tumor, meningocele, rib may penetrate foramina
Larsen syndrome	Cervical kyphosis	Cervical spondylolisthesis	Chronic mid-cervical	—	—
Down syndrome	—	Odontoid hypoplasia; os odontoideum, spina bifida	Occiput–C1 C1–C2	—	—
Marfan syndrome	Kyphosis; scoliosis; spondylolisthesis	—	—	—	Dural extasia

DJD, degenerative joint disease; T, thoracic; C, cervical; L, lumbar; SED, spondyloepiphyseal dysplasia.

tions; the most common are skeletal dysplasia and Down syndrome (21,31,35). Odontoid hypoplasia may also be an idiopathic occurrence. In extreme cases, the dens may be essentially absent (*aplasia*). The majority of these cases of odontoid hypoplasia are the result of skeletal dysplasias. Another condition that exhibits similar clinical symptoms is *transverse ligament insufficiency*, which may be caused by ligamentous laxity or damage to the ligament.

Finally, a number of patients have an *os odontoideum*, a chronic condition in which the odontoid is present only as a small ossicle, not united to the body of the axis. Although os odontoideum was long presumed to be a congenital lesion, more recent evidence suggests that most cases may be the result of unrecognized fracture of the odontoid.

Patients with any of these four problems share a variety

of symptoms: (a) They may show signs and symptoms of neck instability, manifested by the muscles' response to guard it: neck pain and spasm, torticollis, or headache. These symptoms appear most often after activity or a fall. (b) Neurologic symptoms involving the long cervical tracts may be present, such as developmental delay, hyporeflexia or hyperreflexia, and weakness. (c) Finally, cerebrovascular symptoms may prevail, from ischemia to stroke involving the posterior circulation. Plain radiographs are helpful in establishing the diagnosis, and computed tomography (CT) can usually demonstrate the pathology clearly, if needed.

Plain films that include lateral views in flexion and extension will help to quantify the instability. The normal space available for the cord at this level should be at least 13 mm, and the translation of the ring of the atlas should be less than 5 mm. Magnetic resonance imaging (MRI) may be helpful to demonstrate cord impingement, but this can often be deduced from plain films and clinical exam alone.

If radiography reveals signs of instability beyond a critical limit (more than 5–8 mm of translation on flexion/extension films), stenosis, or neurologic signs, surgical fusion of C-1 to C-2 is indicated (24). Reduction to a neutral position is the goal; if this cannot be accomplished, decompression may also be required.

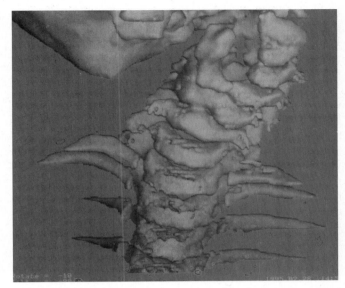

Figure 158.1. Torticollis in a young child, in this case due to three consecutive hemivertebrae in the upper cervical spine. In infants, computed tomograms provide superior visualization compared with plain films, because of the baby's large head, difficulty positioning, and the complexity of the case. Treatment was by realignment with distraction of the concave side and derotation in a halo-vest, followed by fusion.

CERVICAL STENOSIS

When cervical stenosis is seen in children, the diagnosis is usually achondroplasia, Klippel-Feil syndrome (36), or idiopathic congenital cervical stenosis. Signs and symptoms include those of acute compression (numbness and tingling in the extremities, acute weakness) or chronic myelopathy with developmental delay, spasticity, weakness, and muscle atrophy. In the teenage athlete with idiopathic cervical stenosis, transient quadriparesis is a common presenting phenomenon, with forced hyperextension in the presence of a narrowed spinal canal (41). Fortunately, this symptom tends to resolve rapidly if there is no vertebral subluxation or dislocation. In the child with achondroplasia, the greatest degree of stenosis occurs at the foramen magnum, causing failure to meet developmental milestones and a tendency to develop sleep apnea. Clinically significant stenosis of the remainder of the cervical spine in the person with achondroplasia generally develops only in adulthood, if at all.

Certain other skeletal dysplasias (such as spondyloepiphyseal dysplasia and mucopolysaccharidoses) may produce localized stenosis of the ring of the axis as well as atlantoaxial instability; these can cause additive damage to the cord. On lateral radiographs, cervical stenosis should be suspected if the distance from the posterior laminar line to the posterior vertebral body line is less than 80% of the width of the vertebral bodies (Pavlov's ratio)

(41). Also, the distance from the posterior laminar line to the line of the facets is diminished (Fig. 158.1). In patients with Klippel-Feil syndrome, this finding may be missed because attention is drawn to the vertebral fusions. The stenosis is made more problematic if there are large blocks of fusion with just a few motion segments.

Patients with known cervical stenosis should be counseled to avoid contact sports, especially those that produce forcible flexion or extension of the cervical spine, such as wrestling and playing lineman in American football. Surgical decompression of the lower cervical spine is generally best avoided, as it could produce a region of decreased stability adjacent to further stenosis. Localized decompression and fusion may be carried out if indicated. Patients with congenital stenosis of the upper cervical spine may require decompression. If this is so, fusion should be considered if there is associated instability or if the decompression involves more than two segments, in order to prevent development of localized kyphosis.

CERVICAL SPINA BIFIDA

Occult defects in the cervical spine occur primarily in two congenital syndromes: Larsen syndrome and diastrophic dysplasia. Larsen syndrome is characterized by multiple joint dislocations, foot deformities, and an accessory calcaneal apophysis. In one series, more than half the patients had cervical spina bifida and resultant kyphosis (22). In diastrophic dysplasia, diastrophic patients are often born with significantly short stature, rigid clubfeet, joint contractures, and a closed cervical spina bifida, although the incidence of kyphosis is not as high.

The presence of spina bifida in the cervical region indicates a deficiency of posterior ligamentous support (interspinous ligament, ligamentum flavum) as well as of posterior muscle control. This may be a reason for the development and progression of kyphosis. In addition, the vertebral bodies in the region are hypoplastic and may be rounded or wedge shaped. The kyphosis may progress as the child becomes upright. Initially, the physical features of kyphosis are not externally evident, except for a slight loss of the normal cervical lordosis. There are no external clues to the presence of bifid cervical laminae. Therefore, a high index of suspicion must be maintained for these conditions.

Patients may exhibit myelopathy, which may be difficult to detect in children with severe skeletal deformities. Signs such as muscle weakness, failure to achieve normal milestones, and hyperreflexia or clonus may be seen. Endotracheal intubation for other surgical procedures in the presence of this kyphosis may worsen the neurologic condition if not done by knowledgeable persons. In some patients with diastrophic dysplasia, a mild cervical kyphosis may improve spontaneously with time (18). Observation may be indicated if there are no established signs of neurologic compromise. Bracing, however, does not seem to be feasible or warranted. In Larsen syndrome, progression is more likely (22).

Posterior Fusion

The optimal treatment is an early posterior fusion, which may function as a tether and allow spontaneous correction of the deformity.

- Perform fusion early in the patient with Larsen syndrome, before the kyphosis exceeds 50° and becomes rigid. Consider fusion in patients with diastrophic dysplasia who do not improve over the first several years of life, or whose deformity or neurologic condition worsens.
- Perform posterior fusion over the levels involved in the kyphosis, using autogenous bone graft from the iliac crest or the tibial metaphysis.
- Use a halo-vest or halo-cast to control the head and prevent the kyphosis from worsening during incorporation of the fusion. For mild deformities, a Minerva-type cast or orthosis is also an option. Order them in advance of the procedure.
- Take care in exposing the spine, because of the open laminae.
- Dissect the muscles off only the extent of the spine intended for fusion, since extension of the fusion to adjacent exposed levels is a risk. Confirm levels radiographically.
- Decorticate the spine gently and perform a bone graft.

Instrumentation of the spine is not possible for patients of a very young age. Some degree of correction in the halo-vest may be possible by a combination of three maneuvers: (a) positioning the head in slight extension and posterior translation, (b) securing the shoulder straps of the vest so that they are snug (but not too tight), to maintain the length of the cervical spine rather than allowing it to settle, and (c) placing a padded sling behind the apex of the kyphosis, which is attached to the bars of the halo-vest, to prevent the kyphosis from settling posteriorly. When this is done, the tension of the strap must be checked periodically to be certain that there is not too much pressure on the skin.

If the deformity is severe or there is significant neurologic compromise, an anterior decompression and strut graft may be needed in addition to the posterior fusion. The spine should be immobilized for a minimum of 3 months, and continuity of the fusion mass should be demonstrated radiographically at the end of this period to prevent loss of position due to a pseudarthrosis.

Congenital fusion of the cervical spine, or Klippel-Feil syndrome, may occur with congenital upper or lower thoracic or lumbar fusion, or it may be present as an isolated finding. It has been classified into three types: *Type I* involves fusion of cervical and upper thoracic vertebrae, *type II* involves isolated fusions of the cervical spine, and *type III* refers to cervical fusions associated with lower thoracic or upper lumbar fusion (36). Surgery is almost never required for the cervical anomaly itself.

The main significance of the diagnosis is to encourage a search for other anomalies both within and outside the spine, such as Sprengel deformity, hearing impairment, spina bifida, and associated scoliosis. Scoliosis is most common in types I and III. Progressive congenital cervical scoliosis is rare and usually involves the cervicothoracic junction. Monitor young children with this finding closely, since the shoulder tilt it produces may be highly deforming. Perform surgery if progression of more than 10° is seen. A posterior fusion *in situ* is the gold standard for this region.

Scoliosis of the upper cervical spine is quite rare and usually presents as torticollis, which must be differentiated from muscular torticollis, Grisel syndrome, ocular disturbance, and abnormalities of the brainstem and cord. Other causes of fusion in a young child include juvenile rheumatoid arthritis, as well as residua of infection in the region. The upper cervical spine may be very hard to image in children under age 5; it is frequently necessary to obtain a multiplanar CT or an MRI under sedation. If a vertebral anomaly is seen that is deforming, surgery may be indicated (Fig. 158.1).

HINTS AND TRICKS

- Achieve a degree of correction of the head tilt by applying a halo-vest and gradually adjusting the head position using the uprights.
- Any malrotation may be improved by using bilateral rotation with Ilizarov turnbuckles attached to the halo (15).
- Once an acceptable head position is achieved, carry out fusion.
- If more than two levels are fused, consider an anterior epiphyseodesis as well, to prevent progressive lordosis with growth.

OPERATIVE TECHNIQUES

Because in many congenital syndromes, age and bone quality affect halo application and upper cervical fusion, these techniques deserve special consideration (10).

Halo Application

Check the halo size and shape in advance, and modify it if there is plagiocephaly or cranial disproportion (14). Also, if there is risk of positional neurologic damage in children too young to cooperate with examination, evoked potentials are useful.

- General anesthesia is preferred for halo application, although local anesthesia and sedation are possible.
- Because of the danger of hyperflexion caused in part by children's relatively large head size, elevate the torso or have an assistant hold the head off the end of the table.
- Do not place pins in the thin temporal regions (14).
- In children under 2 years of age, Mubarak et al. (28) recommend placement of six to ten pins at low torque (finger tightness through 2 inch-pounds) in the four traditional regions (Fig. 158.2).) Kopits and Steingass (25) found four pins to be sufficient in most cases, and loads up to 5 inch-pounds to be safe in older children. My experience confirms these findings. At our institution, we use 4 inch-pounds of torque for children up to age 4 years, 6 inch-pounds for those aged 5 to 10, and 8 inch-pounds for those over 10.
- The vest may be custom ordered from a prior cast or from tape measurements, or it may be made of plaster using a special frame. The pins may be retightened on the first or second day after halo placement using intravenous analgesia, but do not retighten after this time. If a pin becomes painful later, it is usually that it has become loose or infected. Try oral antibiotics first if there is no obvious loosening; if there is no relief, replace the pin in an alternative site.

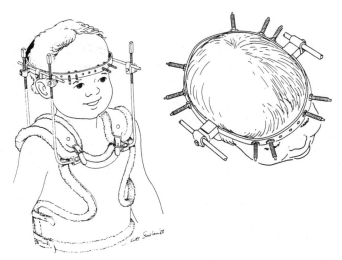

Figure 158.2. A technique of halo application in the infant or child under age 2. The increased number of pins allows decreased torque on each. (Reproduced with permission from Mubarak SJ, Camp JF, Vuletich W, et al. Halo Application in the Infant. *J Pediatr Orthop* 1989;9:612.)

Posterior Cervical Fusion

Many congenital disorders require fusion of the upper cervical spine for deformity or instability. Techniques of fusion are well described elsewhere (in Chapters 139, 140, and 154). Two special aspects require further comment. First, anomalies of the posterior arches are common in several syndromes. Second, in very young children, the posterior elements and occipital cortex may not allow wire fixation of any substantial strength, or the lamina may be resected in cases of stenosis. Study good plain radiographs and, in most cases, CT scans in the areas of planned fusion to rule out spina bifida or anomalies of the arches. If anomalies are present, start dissection from a "normal" area, where depth can safely be established, and proceed up and down over the facets in the deficient areas.

Posterior Occipitocervical Fusion

Koop Technique Koop et al. demonstrated a union rate of greater than 90% for upper cervical fusion in children with halo immobilization, even when grafts are not wired in place (24). This finding is relevant for infants or certain patients with skeletal dysplasia who do not have adequate bone size or quality for wire fixation.

- Apply the halo as described previously for young children.
- Turn the patient prone and affix the halo to a halo-holder. Use spinal cord monitoring during turning and throughout the entire procedure.
- Check a lateral radiograph to confirm proper alignment of the neck.

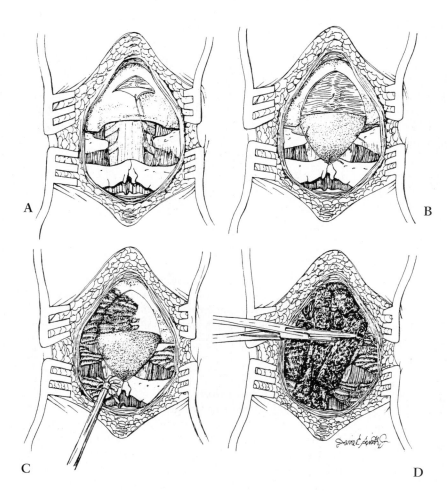

Figure 158.3. Technique of occipitocervical fusion in infants. **A,B:** An occipital periosteal flap is raised and sutured distally. **C,D:** An air drill is used for decortication, and the graft is inserted. (Reproduced with permission from Koop SE, Winter RB, Lonstein JE. The Surgical Treatment of Instability of the Upper Part of the Cervical Spine in Children and Adolescents. *J Bone Joint Surg Am* 1984;66:403.)

- Gently expose the spine, taking care to remain medial to the vertebral arteries at C1–C2.
- Avoid unnecessary exposure of caudal levels, which often leads to unwanted extension of the fusion distally. If a distal level is exposed unintentionally, covering it with bone wax may prevent it from incorporating into the fusion mass.
- After exposure and wide decortication, place autologous bone in the desired areas (Fig. 158.3).
- When fusion to the occiput is desired, use a triangular periosteal flap equal to the distance to C-2. Using a stay suture, dissect the flap, leaving it attached at its base, and suture it to C-1 and C-2. Place the bone graft on top, abutting the decorticated occiput.

The average time in halo until radiographic union is seen is 5 months.

Dormans and Drummond Technique   An alternative technique has been described by Dormans and Drummond for children whose bone is adequate to permit wire fixation (11). Use of autogenous bicortical iliac crest in combination with occipitocervical wires forms a construct that is stable in flexion and extension.

- Perform the halo placement, with positioning and exposure as previously described.
- Fashion a trough in the outer table of the base of the occiput below the inion, at a level so that a graft can be inserted on top of the laminae (Fig. 158.4).
- Make two burr holes through both cortices of the occiput just superior and lateral to the trough.
- Loop a 16- to 18-gauge wire through these holes.
- Make a hole at the base of the most caudal lamina to be fused, and pass a pair of Wisconsin (Drummond) wires through the hole in opposite directions.
- Obtain a corticocancellous autogenous iliac crest graft the width of the laminae and the height of the combined levels to be fused.
- Fashion a notch in the inferior edge to fit around the lowest spinous process, and lay it in place after the Wisconsin wires have been placed.
- Start each Wisconsin wire distally under the graft, then pass it around the graft and over it, across to the spinal wire in the opposite side of the occiput.

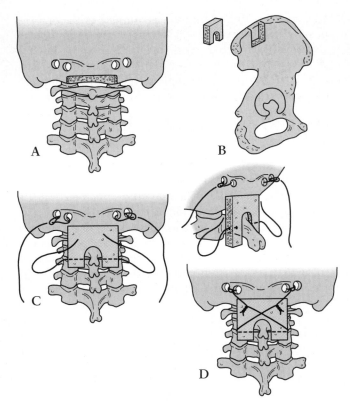

Posterior Atlantoaxial Fusion

For children with intact laminae and an isolated mild to moderate C1–C2 instability, Mah et al. (27) described a modified Gallie method of wiring around the base of the spinous process to preserve strength yet avoid the risks of wire passage under C-2 (Fig. 158.5). It also avoids the risks of cutout or dorsal displacement of the wires, which could otherwise occur in children with standard Gallie technique.

- Position the patient in the standard fashion, with the cervical spine reduced to an optimal position, and the neck draped widely, allowing access to the lateral portion of the neck from both sides.
- Contour a rectangular unicortical iliac crest graft to fit over the C-1 arch and straddle the C-2 spinous process.
- Drill a threaded Steinmann pin percutaneously through the widest portion of the base of the spinous process of C-2 and cut it to leave 1 cm on each side.
- Pass an 18-gauge sublaminar wire under the C-1 arch.
- Place the loop of the wire deep to the Steinmann pin and draw it tightly over the graft, keeping it apposed to the lamina. This placement allows the wire to obtain good cortical purchase around C-2 and prevents dorsal migration.

Figure 158.4. Technique of occipitocervical fusion (Drummond), used for children with slightly better bone density that can support wire fixation. **A:** A trough is made in the base of the occiput, and two burr-holes are made on either side. **B:** A corticocancellous graft is taken from the ilium and shaped to fit the space between the occiput and the second or third cervical vertebra. **C:** Four strands of wire are passed to be ready to twist together: one from each side of the occiput, and one Drummond button-wire from each side of the C-2 or C-3 spinous process. **D:** The wires are twisted together to lock the graft into place. (Redrawn from Dormans JP, Drummond DS, Sutton LN. Occipitocervical Arthrodesis in Children: A New Technique and Analysis of Results. *J Bone Joint Surg Am* 1995;77:1234.)

- Control the extension of the spine by the head position and the size and shape of the graft.
- Tighten the wires and take a lateral radiograph to confirm alignment.
- Place extra bone graft at the upper and lower edges of the main graft.
- Take flexion–extension radiographs about every 4 weeks.
- The halo may be removed after a mean of only 8 weeks with excellent results; have the patient wear a hard collar for 4–6 weeks after the halo is removed.

This technique is also applicable even if laminectomy has been performed at levels above the lowest level to be fused.

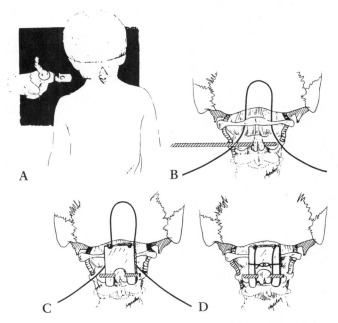

Figure 158.5. Atlantoaxial fusion by the modified Dewar technique. **A:** After C-1 and C-2 are exposed, a threaded Steinmann pin is inserted percutaneously through the base of C-2. **B:** A sublaminar wire is passed under the C-1 arch. **C,D:** The wire is brought over the contoured graft and held under the Steinmann pin. (Reproduced with permission from Mah JY, Thometz J, Emans J, et al. Threaded K-Wire Spinous Process Fixation of the Axis for Modified Gallie Fusion in Children and Adolescents. *J Pediatr Orthop* 1989;9:675.)

■ Add extra cancellous graft. Tie the free ends of the wire transversely over the graft.

Postoperatively, use a soft collar until union, if the translatory instability of the atlantoaxial segment is not too great. A halo-vest may be used at the surgeon's discretion.

Bone Graft

Some bone graft is almost always obtainable from the posterior ileum in children. If the amount is inadequate, such as in an infant with a small pelvis in whom long cortical and cancellous grafts are needed, the grafts may be obtained from one or both tibiae (see Chapter 9).

THORACOLUMBAR ABNORMALITIES

CONGENITAL STENOSIS

Congenital stenosis of the thoracic and lumbar spine is seen mainly in achondroplasia; to a lesser degree, it is seen in other skeletal dysplasias such as hypochondroplasia, diastrophic dysplasia, and spondyloepiphyseal dysplasia. Patients with isolated congenital spinal malformations such as scoliosis and kyphosis also commonly have associated narrowing of the spinal canal in the region. Take this narrowing into account when planning deformity correction and instrumentation.

A rare syndrome of focal, severe congenital stenosis, termed *segmental spinal dysgenesis*, has been described (13). It is usually present at the thoracolumbar junction and may be associated with segmental instability, scoliosis, or kyphosis. In patients with complete neurologic deficit, return has not been seen after decompression and stabilization, but these are indicated in those with preservation of at least some distal neurologic function who have progression or instability.

In addition, there are some young patients without any congenital malformation, who exhibit spinal stenosis that has been made symptomatic by disc protrusion or mild degenerative change. Symptoms include pain and tingling or numbness in the lower extremities more than pain in the back. Standing or walking worsens these symptoms, and rest usually relieves them. Plain films suggest stenosis by virtue of the narrow distance between the posterior laminar line and the posterior vertebral line, but they are less accurate in identification of stenosis in the thoracic and lumbar spine than they are in the cervical spine. MRI more clearly delineates the degree of neurologic compression.

Conservative treatment such as activity modification or a flexion back brace may alleviate symptoms. Hip flexion contractures may need to be addressed, as they increase the obligatory lumbar lordosis. Decompressive laminectomy may be necessary if these measures fail; careful examination and judgment are necessary to determine the extent of unroofing required. Techniques of decompression may involve traditional laminectomy, laminoplasty (enlarging the canal by hinging open the lamina), or fenestration (removal of the stenotic inferior portion of each involved lamina and the medial facets). Further details are discussed in the later section on achondroplasia.

CONGENITAL AND ACQUIRED KYPHOSIS

Congenital kyphosis is less common but has potentially more serious neurologic consequences than congenital scoliosis. The basic types include failure of vertebral formation (type I) and failure of segmentation (type II) (see Chapter 161). If progression is seen, treatment is required. Bracing has no value in halting the increase of the curve.

Surgery is indicated at an early age if any progression at all is discovered. It should take the form of an *in situ* posterior fusion of the level above and the one below the abnormal vertebra in a type I kyphosis, unless it exceeds about 55°. If it exceeds this value, the fusion mass will be under tension and will not effectively halt growth; an anterior epiphyseodesis may be needed as well. A type II kyphosis may be fused posteriorly between the two involved vertebrae, to match the anterior bar; this may be extended one level above and one below in young children if it is desired to achieve some correction with cast and growth.

Postoperative cast immobilization for 3 months is the rule; follow-up should be performed to rule out pseudarthrosis and progression. Undertake osteotomy or vertebrectomy in treatment of congenital kyphosis only if the deformity is severe and is causing neurologic compromise or an unacceptable appearance.

Acquired kyphosis in children is seen most often after laminectomy, especially of the cervicothoracic or thoracolumbar junctions. In congenital syndromes, this situation may occur after decompression of spinal stenosis (in achondroplasia) or of intradural tumors (in neurofibromatosis) (17,19). More detail is given later in the sections on these conditions. It is important to realize that the risk of this phenomenon is greater in children than it is in adults. When there is preexisting kyphosis or vertebral wedging, it becomes even more likely.

Prevention of kyphosis is much easier than later treatment of an established deformity, if it can be anticipated. Limited posterior fusion *in situ* over the region of the junction is usually effective. Another alternative is laminoplasty, which allows many of the interlaminar ligaments to remain intact and may prevent kyphosis from developing.

CONGENITAL SCOLIOSIS

Congenital scoliosis may be an isolated finding, or it may be associated with various syndromes. The most common association is with the VATER syndrome (vertebral anomalies, anal atresia, tracheoesophageal fistula, renal and radial abnormalities). Some physicians include a C for cardiac abnormalities. The vertebral anomalies are the most common component of the VATER syndrome, so orthopaedic surgeons will see most of these children. Other syndromes that include congenital vertebral anomalies are Goldenhar (oculoauriculovertebral) syndrome, myelomeningocele, Klippel-Feil syndrome, and Jarcho-Levin syndrome (spondylothoracic dysplasia).

Although there may be a dimple, a vascular marking, or a patch of hair over the spine in the occasional case of congenital scoliosis, often patients have no external physical findings except for the deformity, which may be mild in early childhood. Early diagnosis usually comes about because of an incidental event such as a radiograph for trauma or a chest film. Vertebral anomalies are frequently seen on ultrasound of fetuses, and concerned parents as well as sonographers often consult the orthopaedist for a prognosis. Isolated hemivertebrae without neural tube defects or other sonographic anomalies typically have a good outcome. The presence of other abnormalities reduces the rate of survival.

Radiographic findings in congenital scoliosis usually include hemivertebra, wedged vertebra, or fusion of vertebrae (bar). Many times there are elements of both in a given curve. The best opportunity to understand the underlying growth abnormality is to study the films of the patient at the youngest possible age; they will show the asymmetries of ossification and allow diagnosis of hemivertebrae and fusion.

If a hemivertebra does not have a growth plate on both surfaces, or if it is "carved into" the adjacent vertebra (incarcerated), it is less likely to produce an increasing curve. Upon diagnosis of congenital scoliosis, do a thorough exam, searching for limb atrophy or other deformities. Chest auscultation should be done, but cardiac imaging is not routinely indicated. However, the genitourinary tract should be visualized at least once by ultrasound or intravenous pyelogram. Some experts recommend a routine MRI on all children with this diagnosis, since at least 25% will show some abnormality such as a Chiari malformation, syrinx, or tether. This is not a well-accepted recommendation, however, as the indications for treating these conditions in the asymptomatic stage are highly debatable. Most surgeons instead prefer to order an MRI only when corrective surgery is planned, or if unexplained progression occurs.

Treatment of congenital scoliosis is largely surgical. There is no documented efficacy of brace treatment. Some curves such as those with a segmented hemivertebra and a contralateral bar have a virtual certainty of progression and should be fused when first seen. All others should be followed during growth with serial radiographs, always comparing them to the first film, rather than to the last prior film.

If progression of more than 5° to 10° is seen, I recommend surgery. There are several surgical options, whose indications depend on the characteristics of the curve, the acceptability of the current deformity, and the likelihood of future increase in the curve. Options include the following:

- Posterior fusion *in situ*
- Anterior and posterior fusion
- Hemiepiphyseal fusion
- Hemivertebral excision
- Spinal osteotomy for correction

Operative Techniques

Posterior Fusion *in Situ*   Posterior fusion *in situ* is the most widely accepted procedure. It is indicated for progressive curves if the deformity is acceptable and the likelihood of anterior crankshaft progression is not high.

- Take care in exposing the spine, since midline laminar defects are sometimes seen in congenital curves.
- Fuse all vertebrae within the curve.
- Some correction may be obtained through bracing if there is flexibility in the curve.
- Postoperatively, immobilize the patient in a cast or brace for 3 to 4 months, when consolidation of the fusion should be demonstrated.

Anterior and Posterior Fusion   If you suspect that significant growth potential also exists anteriorly that could cause a deformity due to the crankshaft phenomenon, perform anterior and posterior fusion.

- Perform the anterior procedure in the traditional open fashion, through a thoracoscopic approach, or by a transpedicular or costotransversectomy approach. See Chapter 155.
- Consider a hemiepiphyseodesis, as a variation on this theme, for young patients' curves with some growth potential on the concave side.
- Fuse the curve anteriorly and posteriorly only on the convexity, to allow for some corrective growth on the concavity. Measurable correction is seen only in children under age 6 at surgery, and the amount of correction rarely exceeds 10° to 20°.
- Hemivertebra excision is now accepted as a safe alternative for curve correction in experienced hands (8) (see the Surgical Techniques section later). It is mostly, although not solely, applicable to anomalies at or below the thoracolumbar junction. Use this technique for curves too large to be fused *in situ*.
- Both anterior and posterior procedures may be performed in the same operative session.
- Spinal osteotomy may be needed to correct large, stiff curves composed of multiple bars, or ones that have

been fused previously. It carries an element of risk and should be performed by experienced surgeons and only for curves that are significantly disabling.

■ In all cases where corrective surgery is planned for congenital deformities, a preoperative MRI of the spinal canal is indicated.

MANAGEMENT OF SPECIFIC SYNDROMES

Down syndrome (trisomy or translocation involving chromosome 21) is commonly associated with cervical abnormalities. Anterior subluxation of C-1 on C-2 of more than 5 mm in flexion is seen in 15% to 20% of patients. Over 4 mm posterior translation of the occiput on C-1 is seen in 60% (29,31). Also seen is increased frequency of os odontoideum, ossiculum terminale, and spina bifida of any upper cervical vertebra (31). Management of the instability is controversial.

Screen all Down syndrome children, and restrict from high-risk sports those with more than 5 mm C1–C2 subluxation. Perform fusion for those with more than 1 cm subluxation, neurologic deficit, or persistent neck pain. In cases to be fused, it may be necessary to extend the fusion to the occiput (42) if there is significant posterior atlanto-occipital translation in extension. Increasing quadriparesis during surgery has been reported in cases of preoperative myelopathy or longstanding displacement. It appears that in such cases there may be chronic degeneration within the cord, rendering it extremely susceptible to insult. In addition, the space available for passing wires is decreased. Reduction, if necessary, should be achieved before surgery with evoked potential monitoring or preoperative awake traction. If significant reduction cannot be achieved but the patient's neurologic condition is acceptable, only a fusion without wires is recommended. Use a CT scan to rule out spina bifida.

SKELETAL DYSPLASIAS

Cervical spine abnormalities are common in many skeletal dysplasias. Odontoid hypoplasia and ligamentous laxity are common in spondyloepiphyseal dysplasia (congenita more than tarda), Morquio syndrome, Kniest syndrome, and metatrophic dysplasia (2,38). It may also be seen in the occasional patient with pseudoachondroplasia. Symptomatic instability frequently results. In addition, cervical stenosis may be seen with metatrophic dysplasia, Maroteaux-Lamy syndrome, or achondroplasia. Obtain neutral, flexion, and extension cervical spine films in all patients with these conditions. Diagnosis of cervical myelopathy is difficult in infants and may be aided by checking motor milestones, and spinal cord monitoring, flexion–extension MRI, and sleep studies. Metatrophic

patients may also have painful torticollis due to rotatory C1–C2 instability (Fig. 158.6).

In contrast to the upper cervical abnormalities seen in other dysplasias, diastrophic dysplasia frequently causes mild cervical kyphosis and spina bifida (19). Surprisingly, many of these kyphoses, especially those that are less than 80°, resolve over time with or without bracing. Quadriplegia has been reported with some larger kyphoses, however, so surgical treatment is indicated for those with progression or neurologic deficit.

If the curve is flexible, correction may be accomplished by postural reduction and posterior fusion. Place the patient in a halo body jacket, and gradually extend the head over several days with serial neurologic examinations. A posterior sling may be added at the apex of the curve. If satisfactory improvement is obtained, identify bifid areas on CT and perform a posterior fusion with a tibial cortical graft. If the kyphosis is rigid, anterior release and strut graft fusion, followed by posterior fusion, are indicated. Apply the halo before the fusion, to protect the strut graft in young patients. The anterior bar of the frame should be removable on the side of the anterior approach.

Larsen syndrome of multiple joint dislocations with flattened facies is occasionally associated with cervical spondylolysis and kyphosis, causing neurologic deficit (22). Screening of the cervical spine is recommended for all patients with this diagnosis. Treatment follows the guidelines given for diastrophic dwarfism. Note, however, that spontaneous resolution has not been documented in this condition, and the posterior arches may also be deficient.

Achondroplasia

In achondroplasia, panspinal developmental stenosis, sagittal deformity, and arthrosis combine to produce compressive neurologic lesions in 30% to 80% of patients. Infantile kyphosis at the thoracolumbar junction, resulting from muscular hypotonia, ligamentous laxity, and a relatively large head, resolves in 75% to 85% of cases but persists or progresses in the remainder, leading to wedging of thoracolumbar vertebrae (19,26,37,40). Wedging may be focal, involving a single vertebra, or gradual, involving multiple levels. Some geneticists feel that it is important to prevent children with achondroplasia from sitting unsupported, and to use hard-backed sitting devices (30). I feel that it is impossible to prevent a child from sitting who is developmentally ready, and that the only effective support is a thoracolumbosacral orthosis. Therefore, it seems prudent to brace all achondroplastic children with significant kyphosis after 2 to 3 years of age.

Correction of kyphosis should be undertaken in the following situations:

• For any curve more than 50° to 60° with focal wedging, in patients over age 5 to 6 years

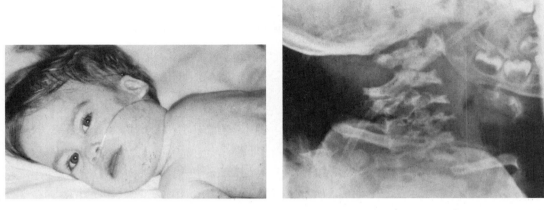

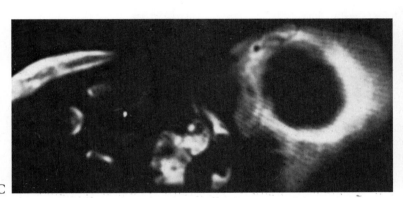

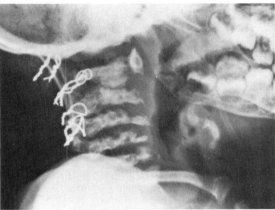

Figure 158.6.   **A:** A 15-month-old child with metatrophic dysplasia and painful torticollis. The head is kept in marked hyperextension. **B:** Lateral roentgenogram shows some anterior C-1 displacement with rotation and stenosis. **C:** CT-myelogram confirms rotational malalignment and stenosis. **D:** Posterior C1–C2 decompression and occiput to C-3 fusion done by the method of Koop. Wires seen are through facets (Southwick type). Tibial graft is used. Unfortunately, the patient died 3 months postoperatively due to the restrictive lung disease associated with metatrophic dysplasia.

- In any patient undergoing laminectomy with a curve over 30° in the thoracolumbar region or 50° in the thoracic region
- For any curve that progresses on its own (37)

Fusion should always be both anterior and posterior because of deformity and small posterior elements, especially after laminectomy. If the kyphosis is sharp and angular, and if neurologic deficit is present, perform a corpectomy with strut graft fusion. Follow with posterior fusion. Both procedures can be done on 1 day if the patient is young, or 1–2 weeks apart in older patients or those requiring extensive laminectomy. Correction of deformity may be either by cast or instrumentation. There is a 25% or greater chance of somatosensory evoked potential or clinical neurologic deterioration when instrumentation is used, although recovery is common (37). This effect is probably caused by instrumentation impinging on a narrowed canal, downward pressure on apical laminae, or stretch of nerve roots in lordotic segments. This risk can be minimized by using cast correction only, with 4–6 months of recumbency. If instrumentation is used, it should include only pedicle screws in the lower thoracic or lumbar region (Fig. 158.7). Stabilization and fusion, rather than significant correction, should be the goals. It is best not to fuse below L-4 in most cases, because mobility is always a problem in patients with achondroplasia. Laminectomies should be done in marginally stenotic levels. Spinal stenosis in achondroplasia is caused by deficient endochondral growth in the neurocentral synchondroses, with decreased sagittal and coronal canal dimensions, increasing in severity caudally. Foramen magnum and cervi-

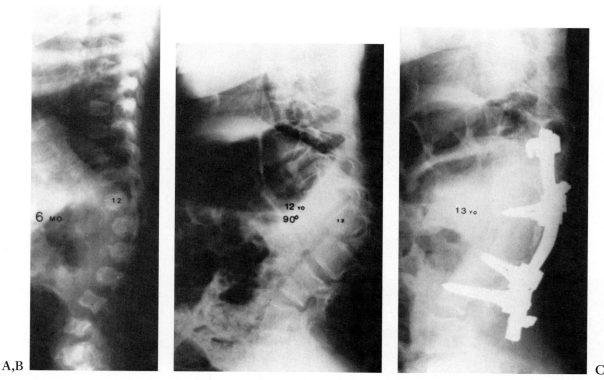

A,B   C

Figure 158.7.   **A:** A 6-month-old girl with achondroplasia, never braced. **B:** The same patient at age 12 with severe 90° wedging of L-2 with early weakness. **C:** One year after anterior decompression and posterior fusion. The patient had an initial postoperative increase in weakness, but recovered fully within 3 months.

cal stenosis may occur in addition to the more common thoracolumbar stenosis.

Degenerative changes or disc bulge may make the narrowing symptomatic. True disc herniations are a distinct minority, however. Symptoms in older teenagers or adults include leg pain while standing or walking, decreased endurance, numbness, and urgency or incontinence. On examination, an upper or lower motor neuron picture may be seen, depending on the level of compression. Evaluation should include CT-myelography, cystometrogram, and postvoid residual. MRI is less helpful because it does not show the bony compressive structures as well. If stenosis symptoms or any neurologic deficit is present, decompressive laminectomy should be done, after ruling out disc herniation (43). Laminectomy should include all involved levels, most commonly T8–S1. The most frequently reported surgical error is insufficient length of laminectomy. Because of the limited canal space, dural tear or cord contusion during decompression is not infrequent.

Diastrophic Dysplasia
In diastrophic dysplasia, scoliosis or kyphosis is extremely common (4,5,18), having been seen in over 70% of patients in the largest reported series. Only 30% of the curves, however, were over 30°. Two curve types are seen: benign and idiopathic-like, and severe, rigid types with kyphosis. The latter are considered by Tolo to be the result of wedged or unsegmented vertebrae like those seen in congenital scoliosis (39). These curves are apparent before age 4, often in infancy.

Try bracing early, for all curves. It is sometimes successful for the gradual idiopathic-like curves. If the curve progresses past 45° despite bracing, consider instrumentation without fusion in young children if there is not too much kyphosis. Tolo and Kopits (39) state that significant growth ceases at age 9–10 in these patients, so fusion at this age, if it is necessary, would have little effect on height. At any point where the curve progresses significantly despite subcutaneous instrumentation, perform fusion, for little of what is lost in progression can be regained.

To arrest progression effectively, add anterior release and fusion if the kyphosis or scoliosis is large or if there is much growth remaining before skeletal maturity. Although the canal is relatively stenotic in the lower lumbar region, hook placement can be done safely (38). The incidence of postoperative neurologic deficit in hook placement was more than 50% in one series (5). The deficit seems to be due to zealous attempts to correct these rigid curves, rather than to the instrumentation itself.

Pseudoachondroplasia

Pseudoachondroplasia is occasionally associated with thoracolumbar kyphosis and hip flexion contractures. Treat the kyphosis by anterior and posterior fusion if severe. Neurologic injury from surgery is less common than in achondroplasia because the canal is larger. Sublaminar instrumentation may be used. If excessive lumbar lordosis is present and flexible, correction of any hip flexion contracture by femoral extension osteotomies should be the first step.

Metatrophic Dysplasia

Metatrophic dysplasia is usually associated with curves that appear early and are difficult to control. The most common pattern is a double major scoliotic curve with a severe junctional kyphosis, which may equal or exceed the scoliosis in magnitude. The curves are rigid, and bracing is poorly tolerated. The kyphosis and poor bone quality contraindicate subcutaneous instrumentation. Definitive spine fusion is frequently necessary at an early age. Restrictive lung disease is common because of short ribs. Consult a pulmonary specialist if you are contemplating anterior fusion or to determine if even posterior fusion will be tolerated. Fusion with cast correction is the most common method used.

Kniest Syndrome

Kniest syndrome and its resultant scoliosis are similar to metatrophic dysplasia but less severe. Rib length is normal, and restrictive lung disease is not as frequent as in metatrophic dysplasia (2).

Mucopolysaccharidoses

Of the mucopolysaccharidoses, kyphosis with or without scoliosis is common in Hurler syndrome. It most often has an apex at the thoracolumbar junction, where wedging of vertebrae and translation may occur. Bracing is warranted, but its efficacy remains unproven. The limited life expectancy of these patients historically has made fusion untenable. With the increasing success of bone marrow transplantation, patients who are longer-term survivors may require treatment by a limited posterior fusion over the kyphotic segment if it is progressive.

Spondyloepiphyseal Dysplasia

Spondyloepiphyseal dysplasia is manifested in the spine by marked platyspondyly and, frequently, thoracic kyphosis and scoliosis (2). Bracing is advised for scoliosis less than 45° or for any increased kyphosis in growing children. In some cases, the kyphosis has been permanently improved by bracing. Scoliosis should be fused if the curve is over 45°. Pseudarthrosis is common after posterior fusion of either kyphosis or scoliosis, resulting in significant loss of correction. Therefore, patients with severe curves may need an anterior as well as a posterior fusion if the curve is rigid, if the patient is adult, or if he has had prior laminectomy.

OSTEOGENESIS IMPERFECTA

Spine deformity in osteogenesis imperfecta correlates with bone involvement (3,16,47) (see Chapter 180). Although many classification systems have been proposed, the radiographic system of Hanscom has been best correlated with spinal involvement (16). Type A patients, those with only bowing of the long bones, have the best bone quality and generally maintain some correction if scoliosis surgery and instrumentation are required. Type B patients, who also have biconcave vertebrae, and type C, who have a trefoil pelvis, have a greater tendency to kyphosis. Type D patients are more severely involved, having also cystic changes in the metaphyses. With these latter three types, less correction is obtainable, and there is more postoperative loss. Type E patients, with absent long-bone cortices, should not be subjected to instrumentation at all.

Brace treatment has little if any role in osteogenesis imperfecta curves except for postoperative protection because of the potential for rib deformation. Posterior fusion should be done for curves of more than 45° in type A, or 35° to 40° in types B through E. Even at a young age, delaying fusion to preserve trunk height should not be a consideration, because the trunk is so short in nonscoliotic adults of these types, let alone those with curves.

In some cases of severe deformity with poor bone stock, carefully applied halo–gravity traction after anterior release may be used to decrease the amount of force that must be applied through the rods. All patients should be evaluated preoperatively for basilar invagination and for pulmonary compromise. Segmental fixation using hooks at as many levels as possible, augmented when necessary by doubled Luque wires, is the preferred technique. The following points should be noted:

- Hooks placed on fragile laminae may be supplemented with methylmethacrylate.
- Pack the methylmethacrylate after the hook is inserted; it should extend to the lamina above and below.
- Preserve the spinous processes at these levels.
- Supplement the fusion with banked bone.
- Bone from other spinous processes is also helpful; these may be relatively large in osteogenesis imperfecta.
- Blood loss is usually greater than in other conditions.
- Use postoperative recumbency and orthoses as the quality of fixation dictates.

ARTHROGRYPOSIS MULTIPLEX CONGENITA

Scoliosis is present in up to one third of patients with the diagnosis of arthrogryposis multiplex congenita. Usually the curve is a long, uncompensated, "paralytic" type. Increased lumbar lordosis may occur, especially with hip flexion contractures. In a sizable minority, congenital anomalies may occur; take care to distinguish these patients from those with multiple pterygium syndrome.

Congenital curves should be treated according to the usual rules. Noncongenital curves can be braced if less than 50°, but fusion should be performed for larger curves. The spine, like the joints, is stiff, and correction is not often great unless the spine is mobilized extensively anteriorly and posteriorly. Bone is osteoporotic and hypervascular. Low lumbar curves with pelvic obliquity should have fixation extended to the pelvis. Where excessive lumbar lordosis is the main problem, patients respond poorly to posterior distraction, and anterior column shortening by multiple partial vertebrectomies is most successful.

NEUROFIBROMATOSIS

Neurofibromatosis is estimated to make up 1% to 2% of a scoliosis clinic population, so its signs should be looked for on all initial examinations (9,44). The diagnosis can be made with the presence of two or more of the criteria from the 1987 Consensus Development Conference of the National Institutes of Health (Table 158.2). In a patient with neurofibromatosis, it is important to make the distinction between dystrophic and nondystrophic curves

Table 158.2.   Relevant Aspects of Neurofibromatosis

Diagnosis: Two or More of NIH Criteria
   Six or more café-au-lait spots >1.5 cm
   Subcutaneous neurofibromas
   Elephantiasis neuromatosa
   Positive biopsy
   Positive family history
   Dystrophic osseous manifestation

Features of Dystrophic Spinal Curve
   Vertebral scalloping
   Spindled ribs or transverse processes
   Paravertebral soft-tissue mass
   Short curve with severe apical rotation
   Foramenal enlargement

Possible Abnormalities of Spinal Canal or Cord
   Dural ectasia
   Meningocele
   Neurofibroma in canal
   Stretch over sharp kyphosis
   Ribs impinging on spinal cord through foramina

NIH, National Institutes of Health.

(44). Nondystrophic curves can be treated with brace or surgery according to guidelines for idiopathic scoliosis. They are in the minority, however, making up 25% to 35% of most series.

Dystrophic curves require more aggressive treatment. Bracing is unsuccessful. Obtain cervical spine films and MRI or a myelogram with CT before surgery. To rule out cervical deformity, which is frequently associated with thoracolumbar deformity, obtain radiographs of the neck before general anesthesia is done or halo traction is applied (46). Abnormalities identified within the canal by MRI or myelogram, such as thinning of laminae, neurofibromas, meningoceles, and rib penetration, have obvious implications for both the technique of the dissection and the choice of fixation levels (6,12,23).

Dystrophic curves more than 35° to 45° should be fused regardless of age because progression may be rapid, and loss of height will be greater if the curve is allowed to progress than if early fusion is accomplished. If the curve is less than 50°, kyphosis less than 60°, and no obvious anterior scalloping or bony involvement is present, posterior fusion alone is indicated (9). Six months postoperatively, obtain oblique films or tomograms, or perform routine reexploration to detect and treat early pseudarthrosis.

Curves with kyphosis over 50°, anterior scalloping or deficiency, or scoliosis more than 50° should have anterior and posterior fusion. Because of potential vertebral body destruction by tumor, anterior surgery has a more important mechanical role in neurofibromatosis than in other conditions. Note the following points:

- Fuse all involved levels.
- If there is significant anterior tumor, use strut grafts of fibula or vascularized rib, and establish good bone continuity with vascularized tissue on the concavity of the curve.
- Halo traction may be used to optimize correction at the time strut grafts are inserted.
- Posteriorly, segmental hook fixation is desirable; increasing rigidity of fixation will increase success of surgery (20).
- Use postoperative bracing if the vertebrae are weakened or the severity or location of the kyphosis is causing excessive strain on end hooks, or if there are not optimum numbers of fixation points above and below the apex (three on each side).

Treatment of neurologic deficit depends on its cause. If it is due to intracanal tumor or rib penetration, decompress it posteriorly and do subsequent fusion according to previous guidelines. If it is due to kyphosis, correct it anteriorly and posteriorly with decompression if focal.

In summary, spinal curvature in neurofibromatosis patients ranks as a major threat to patient welfare. Take all possible care in preoperative planning, surgery, and postoperative follow-up.

MARFAN SYNDROME

Improved cardiovascular management has greatly increased the life expectancy of patients with Marfan syndrome to nearly that of the general population, thereby increasing the importance of appropriate treatment of spinal disorders. Scoliosis of greater than 10° is present in approximately half of these patients. Less than 10%, however, will require a brace or surgery (33). There is no typical curve: In Marfan syndrome, the patient may have any of the curve types seen in idiopathic scoliosis. Sagittal plane deformities are equally common and vary from hyperkyphosis to hypokyphosis. There is a fairly common finding of thoracolumbar kyphosis. Use bracing for the same standard indications as in idiopathic scoliosis; although the success rate is lower, there are cases where the brace has been associated with curve stabilization.

Severe infantile or early juvenile curves are in some cases treated with subcutaneous distraction instrumentation if they are greater than 50° (34). This technique is contraindicated, however, in cases where significant kyphosis exists. The rod should be contoured to match the patient's sagittal profile—that is, not too straight. Dorsal displacement of hooks is a frequent cause of failure of this technique, and it is due in part to inadequate contouring.

Postoperative bracing is mandatory. Despite all of these precautions, the rate of hook cutout or continued progression is significant. If cutout occurs, undertake posterior fusion with or without anterior fusion, depending on curve size and the patient's overall condition.

Curve patterns in adolescents and adults are similar to idiopathic patterns (33). One difference is the tendency to develop moderate thoracolumbar kyphosis and the marked rotational listhesis that sometimes occurs in lumbar curves. Evidence suggests an increased risk of pseudarthrosis in patients with Marfan syndrome, especially in regions of kyphosis at the thoracolumbar junction (7). Anterior release and fusion should be added in such cases (Fig. 158.8) or when curves are large and rigid. Spondylolisthesis of severe degree occurs in approximately 2% of Marfan patients. Check for it on lateral radiographs.

Other features of Marfan syndrome that should be kept in mind include the following: (a) The rate of dural ectasia is high (63%) in the lower lumbar or sacral canal (32) (Fig. 158.9). The dural ectasia is probably another manifestation of the effect of gravity on abnormal connective tissues. The enlarged sac has thin dural walls and may leak or erode laminae; take care with decortication and instrumentation in these areas. (b) Instrumentation of

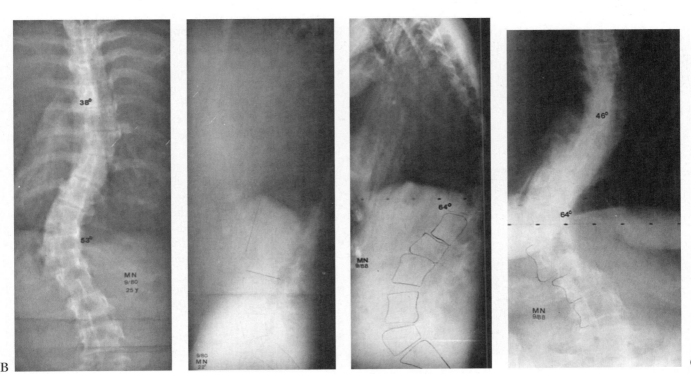

A,B   C,D

Figure 158.8. Progressive kyphoscoliosis in Marfan syndrome. **A,B:** Posteroanterior and lateral films at age 25, with 53° thoracolumbar scoliosis and 22° kyphosis. **C,D:** Repeat films 8 years later (after two pregnancies) show increase of scoliosis to 64° and, especially, of kyphosis to 64°. *(continues)*

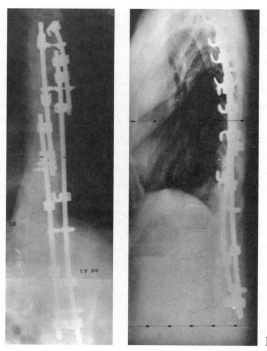

E   **F**

Figure 158.8.   (continued) **E,F:** One year after anterior release and fusion and posterior fusion with Cotrel-Dubousset instrumentation. Note that standard rods were not long enough in this patient; longer rods may be specially ordered.

double curves in these already tall patients may require special ordering of long rods (Fig. 158.8). (c) The patients have implanted cardiovascular devices that must be considered when ordering prophylactic antibiotics or treating a postoperative infection.

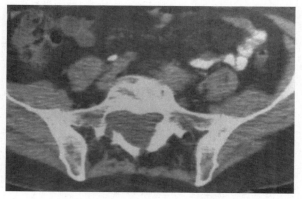

Figure 158.9.   CT scan without contrast shows dural ectasia with foramenal meningocele. This is common in Marfan syndrome, in the lower lumbar spine and sacrum. Exercise care if working inside the canal. Marked thinning of laminae may compromise fixation strength.

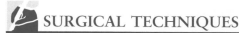

SURGICAL TECHNIQUES

Some authors advocate subcutaneous instrumentation for young patients with considerable growth remaining. I try to avoid subcutaneous instrumentation in almost all cases, because the gains over time are minimal and not worth the time and morbidity.

HEMIEPIPHYSEODESIS FOR CONGENITAL DEFORMITY DUE TO HEMIVERTEBRAE

Hemiepiphyseodesis (Winter technique) is intended not only to prevent progression of a congenital curve but also to allow some correction of the curve with growth (45). It is indicated for patients under about age 6 years who have some growth potential on the concavity of the curve. The advantage of the procedure is that it does not destabilize the spine and does not require internal fixation, even though it is a corrective procedure. The disadvantage is that it does not work for very large curves and is not recommended for curves over 70°. There should be no significant kyphosis or lordosis in the area to be fused. Although the anterior portion of the procedure may be performed endoscopically, the patient must be a satisfactory candidate for a thoracotomy. Take bending films to assess the flexibility of the spine preoperatively. If some correction of the curve is possible, accomplish it in the cast after surgery.

- Place the patient in the lateral position so that both anterior and posterior exposures may be performed without repositioning (Fig. 158.10*B*).
- In the open technique, expose the spine anteriorly through the rib that is one level above the most cranial to be fused.
- Confine dissection primarily to the convexity of the curve, and confirm the levels either by the characteristic shapes of the vertebrae, or by an intraoperative radiograph with markers both anteriorly and posteriorly over the levels to be fused.
- Remove the lateral one third to one half of the disc along with the corresponding portion of the endplates of the vertebrae.
- Obtain bone graft from the morcelized rib or from another source and pack into the disc spaces to promote fusion (Fig. 158.10*C*).
- Make a trough across consecutive vertebrae to allow a bone graft (such as rib) to be placed longitudinally, bridging them.
- Perform posterior exposure at the same time, to be sure that the levels fused in the front and in the back correspond exactly (Fig. 158.10*D*).
- Expose only the convexity of the posterior curve.

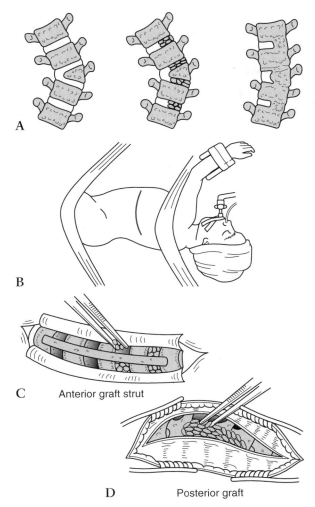

Figure 158.10. Technique of hemiepiphyseodesis for congenital scoliosis. **A:** Concept: The spine is fused anteriorly and posteriorly over the convexity, allowing some correction to occur with growth. **B:** The patient is placed in the mid-lateral position so that anterior and posterior approaches may be made simultaneously. **C:** Anteriorly, 30% to 50% of the disc and endplates are removed and replaced with bone graft; a strut graft is added if available. **D:** Posteriorly, only the convex side of the curve is exposed and grafted over the involved levels. (Redrawn with permission from Winter RB, Lonstein JE, Denis F, de la Rosa HS. Convex Growth Arrest for Progressive Congenital Scoliosis due to Hemivertebrae. *J Pediatr Orthop* 1988;8:633.)

■ Avoid elevating the muscles from the concavity of the curve, to prevent fusion from occurring on this side as well.
■ Verify which levels are the end vertebrae to be fused by palpating the vertebrae from the front and the back simultaneously.
■ If in doubt, pass small Kirschner wires from front to

back at the tip of a transverse process to help confirm levels.
■ Excise the convex facets and decorticate the spine.
■ If additional correction is desired, a level above and below the curve itself may be partially fused as well, to allow further correction with growth.
■ Postoperatively, place the patient in a cast to correct as much of the flexible portion of the deformity as possible. Apply the cast either in the operating room, or a few days after surgery, if there is significant edema or need to have access to the patient. The patient wears the cast, or a cast followed by a brace, for at least 6 months postoperatively. In the series of 13 patients reported by Winter et al. (45), prevention of curve progression was achieved in all but one, and in five of these, curve correction occurred with growth. The mean correction for these five patients was 10° (Fig. 158.11).

HEMIVERTEBRA EXCISION

Excision is indicated for rigid decompensation of the spine due to a hemivertebra. It entails somewhat more risk than a hemiepiphyseodesis because the spinal canal is entered both anteriorly and posteriorly, and the spine is partially destabilized to achieve the correction. A significant degree of correction is possible, however, and the risks are generally acceptable with current techniques in experienced hands (8).

Preoperative assessment may include bending films to determine whether the desired degree of correction can be obtained without vertebral resection. In addition, MRI should be performed in all patients preoperatively because there is an increased frequency of abnormalities within the spinal canal (Chiari malformation, syrinx, diastematomyelia, and fibrous tether), which may predispose the patient to neurologic complications. Hemivertebra excision in the thoracic spine generally entails more neurologic risk as well as less correction, but it is not contraindicated.

Usually, both the anterior and the posterior portions of the procedure are performed in the same surgical session, if possible. Use sensory and motor spinal cord monitoring.

■ Place the patient in the straight lateral position (Fig 158.12).
■ Make a transpleural, transdiaphragmatic, or retroperitoneal anterior approach as dictated by the level of the curve.
■ Identification may be possible by local landmarks as well as by the shape of the vertebrae, but it should be confirmed by a radiograph if there is any question.
■ If segmental arteries are to be ligated in the thoracic spine of a patient with congenital anomalies, some sur-

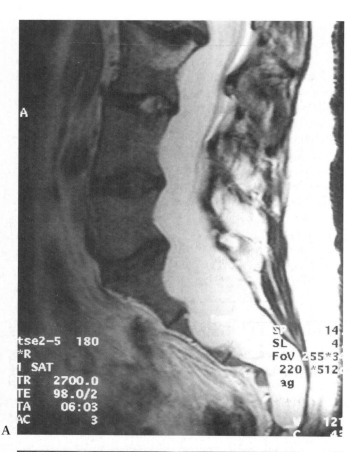

geons recommend placing a "bulldog" vascular clamp on the vessels to occlude flow for 10 minutes, using spinal cord monitoring to be sure that the intended vessels do not provide critical perfusion to the cord (1).

■ Resect the discs above and below the vertebrae first, followed by the body.

■ Leave the posterior portion of the vertebra and the medial cortex of the pedicle intact until last, as their resection may cause epidural bleeding.

■ Place bone graft into the defect, but not so much as to limit the correction.

■ Resect the posterior elements over the corresponding level.

In young patients whose correction is maintained without excessive difficulty, a pantaloon cast may be all that is necessary for correction. However, if the patient's size and bone density are adequate, use internal fixation, which may include a wire for a simple resection, or more rigid and complex fixation. It is the surgeon's judgment whether to perform these procedures in the same position, or whether to turn the patient prone for the posterior fixation. It depends on the complexity of the fixation intended.

The entire extent of the curve should generally be fused. Bone from the resected vertebra and rib usually provides adequate graft. The need for a postoperative brace depends on the security of fixation and the presence of other, noncongenital curves in the spine (Figs. 158.12, 158.13). In the largest recently reported series (21), the mean final correction was 35%, and there were 16% neurologic complications, but only 3% were permanent.

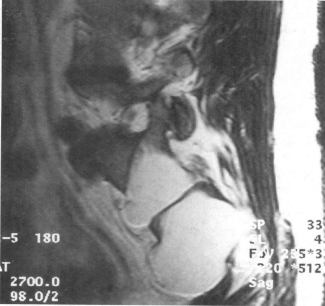

Figure 158.11. Result of convex hemiepiphyseodesis at 6-year follow-up. **A:** Curve measures 27° at age 4, due to unincarcerated hemivertebra with a bar just distal to it on the opposite side. The hemiepiphyseodesis extended two levels above and one level below the hemivertebra. **B:** At age 10½, the curve has corrected itself to 10°.

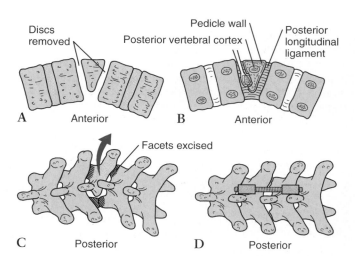

Figure 158.12. Hemivertebra excision. **A:** Remove discs and endplates above and below the hemivertebra. **B:** Curet and remove the hemivertebra. **C:** Resect the corresponding posterior elements. **D:** Complete the correction with posterior compression rod or wire fixation.

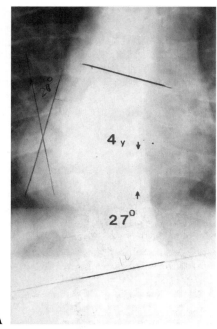

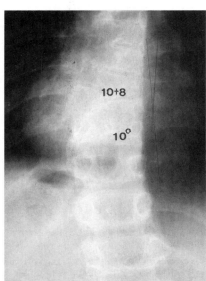

Figure 158.13. Patient with congenital scoliosis due to thoracic hemivertebra, treated with anterior and posterior convex hemi-epiphyseodesis. **A:** At age 4, immediately before surgery, the curve had progressed to 27°. **B:** At 6 years postoperatively, the curve has improved to 10°.

THORACOLUMBAR LAMINOPLASTY VERSUS LAMINECTOMY

Spinal decompression in young people is most commonly indicated for tumor or for stenosis, as in achondroplasia. In both cases, the presence of mild preexisting kyphosis when there is remaining growth increases the risk of pro-

gression postoperatively. This is greatest at the cervicothoracic and thoracolumbar junctions. Progressive kyphosis may be prevented by performing a fusion at the time of decompression, or in some cases by performing a laminoplasty.

To accomplish a safe and effective decompression in achondroplasia, Uematsu et al. recommend a technique that involves minimal use of instruments in the canal (Fig. 158.14) (43). Spinal motor and sensory monitoring is helpful.

■ Position the patient prone, taking care to reverse as much of the increased lumbar lordosis as possible.
■ Make bilateral laminar grooves just medial to the facets, using a high-speed burr.
■ Carry these down to the deep cortex, and gently lift off the laminae.
■ Preserve the facets if possible.
■ Perform the amount of length and width of decompression necessary.
■ A small (#10) rubber catheter should be able to pass centrally into the opening in the canal when the decompression is adequate.
■ Suture paraspinous muscles over the defect.

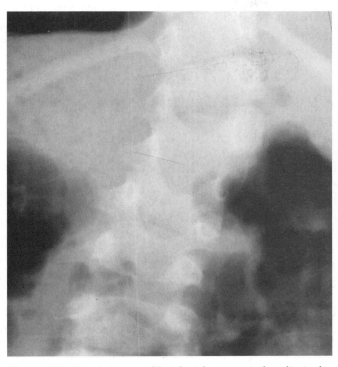

Figure 158.14. A 5-year-old girl with congenital scoliosis due to hemivertebra at <2. She has the VATER association. Her curve has progressed to 45°. Treatment by hemivertebra excision was selected because the hemivertebra is easily accessible and the patient is significantly off-balance. **A:** Preoperatively, the hemivertebra may be easily seen. *(continues)*

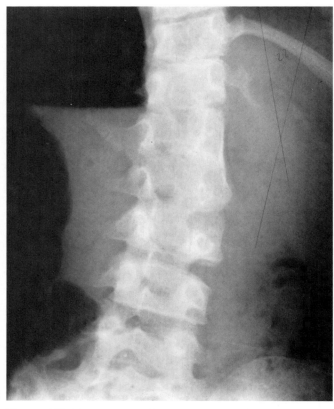

B

Figure 158.14. *(continued)* **B:** Two years after excision and fusion, the patient is in much better balance.

If there is kyphosis more than 30° over the area to be decompressed, posterior (with possible anterior) fusion should be done as described previously. Even if no significant kyphosis is present preoperatively, it should be watched for postoperatively and fused if it develops. If laminoplasty is to be performed, the laminae with interspinous ligaments are elevated in one continuous strip, and reattached at the end with sutures into the adjacent facets, using bony "shims" if needed to elevate the laminae.

REFERENCES

Each reference is categorized according to the following scheme: *, classic article; #, review article; !, basic research article; and +, clinical results/outcome study.

+ 1. Apel DM, Marrero G, King J, et al. Avoiding Paraplegia during Anterior Spine Surgery: The Role of Somatosensory Evoked Potential Monitoring with Temporary Occlusion of Segmental Spinal Arteries. *Spine* 1991; 16(suppl):365.

2. Bassett GS, Scott CI Jr. The Osteochondrodysplasias. In: Morrissy RT, Weinstein SL, eds. *Pediatric Orthopaedics*, 4th ed. Philadelphia: Lippincott-Raven, 1996:203.

+ 3. Benson DR, Newman DC. The Spine and Surgical Treatment in Osteogenesis Imperfecta. *Clin Orthop* 1981; 159:147.

+ 4. Bethem D, Winter RB, Lutter L, et al. Spinal Disorders of Dwarfism. *J Bone Joint Surg Am* 1981;63:1412.

+ 5. Bethem D, Winter RB, Lutter L. Disorders of the Spine in Diastrophic Dwarfism. *J Bone Joint Surg Am* 1980; 62:529.

+ 6. Betz RR, Iorio R, Lombardi AV, et al. Scoliosis Surgery and Neurofibromatosis. *Clin Orthop* 1989;245:53.

+ 7. Birch JG, Herring JA. Spinal Deformity in Marfan Syndrome. *J Pediatr Orthop* 1987;7:546.

+ 8. Bradford DS, Boachie-Adjei O. One-Stage Anterior and Posterior Hemivertebral Resection and Arthrodesis for Congenital Scoliosis. *J Bone Joint Surg Am* 1990;72:536.

+ 9. Crawford AH. Pitfalls of Spinal Deformities Associated with Neurofibromatosis in Children. *Clin Orthop* 1989; 245:29.

+ 10. Dormans JP, Criscitiello AA, Drummond DS, Davidson RS. Complications in Children Managed with Immobilization in a Halo Vest. *J Bone Joint Surg Am* 1995;77: 1370.

+ 11. Dormans JP, Drummond DS, Sutton LN, et al. Occipitocervical Arthrodesis in Children: A New Technique and Analysis of Results. *J Bone Joint Surg Am* 1995;77: 1234.

+ 12. Flood BM, Butt WP, Dickson RA. Rib Penetration of Intervertebral Foraminae in Neurofibromatosis. *Spine* 1986;11:172.

+ 13. Flynn JM, Otsuka NY, Emans JB, e al. Segmental Spinal Dysgenesis: Early Neurologic Deterioration and Treatment. *J Pediatr Orthop* 1997;17:100–104.

+ 14. Garfin SR, Roux R, Botte MJ, et al. Skull Osteology as It Affects Pin Placement. *J Pediatr Orthop* 1986;6:434.

+ 15. Graziano G, Herzenberg JE. Halo Ilizarov Distraction Cast for Correction of Cervical Deformity. Report of Six Cases. *J Bone Joint Surg Am* 1993;75:996.

16. Hanscom DA, Bloom BA. The Spine in Osteogenesis Imperfecta. *Orthop Clin North Am* 1988;19:449.

+ 17. Hensinger RN. Kyphosis Secondary to Skeletal Dysplasias and Metabolic Disease. *Clin Orthop* 1987;128:113.

18. Herring JA. The Spinal Disorders of Diastrophic Dwarfism. *J Bone Joint Surg Am* 1978;60:177.

+ 19. Herring JA. Kyphosis in an Achondroplastic Dwarf. *J Pediatr Orthop* 1982;3:250.

+ 20. Holt RT, Johnson R. Cotrel-Dubousset Instrumentation in Neurofibromatosis Spinal Curves. *Clin Orthop* 1989; 245:19.

+ 21. Holte DC, Winter RB, Lonstein JE, Denis F. Excision of Hemivertebrae and Wedge Resection in the Treatment of Congenital Scoliosis. *J Bone Joint Surg Am* 1995;77: 159.

+ 22. Johnston CE III, Birch JG, Daniels JL. Cervical Kyphosis in Patients Who Have Larsen Syndrome. *J Bone Joint Surg Am* 1996;78:538.

23. Kim HW, Weinstein SL. Spine Update—The Management of Scoliosis in Neurofibromatosis. *Spine* 1997;22: 2770.

+ 24. Koop SE, Winter RB, Lonstein JE. The Surgical Treatment of Instability of the Upper Part of the Cervical Spine in Children and Adolescents. *J Bone Joint Surg Am* 1984; 66:403.

+ 25. Kopits S, Steingass MH. Experience with the Halo Cast in Small Children. *Surg Clin North Am* 1970;50:934.

26. Lonstein JE. Treatment of Kyphosis and Lumbar Stenosis in Achondroplasia. In: Nicoletti B, Kopits SE, Ascani E, McKusick VA, eds. *Human Achondroplasia. Basic Life Science*, 48:283. New York: Plenum Press, 1988.

+ 27. Mah JY, Thometz J, Emans J, et al. Threaded K-Wire Spinous Process Fixation of the Axis for Modified Gallie Fusion in Children and Adolescents. *J Pediatr Orthop* 1989;9:675.

+ 28. Mubarak SJ, Camp JF, Vuletich W, et al. Halo Application in the Infant. *J Pediatr Orthop* 1989;9:612.

+ 29. Nordt JC, Stauffer ES. Sequelae of Atlanto Axial Stabilization in Two Patients with Down's Syndrome. *Spine* 1981;6:437.

+ 30. Pauli RM, Breed A, Horton VK, et al. Prevention of Fixed Angular Kyphosis in Achondroplasia. *J Pediatr Orthop* 1997;17:726.

+ 31. Pueschel SM, Scola FH, Tupper TB, Pezzillo JC. Skeletal Anomalies of the Upper Cervical Spine in Children with Down Syndrome. *J Pediatr Orthop* 1990;10:667.

+ 32. Pyeritz RE, Fishman EK, Bernhardt BA, Siegelman SS. Dural Ectasia Is a Common Feature of the Marfan Syndrome. *Am J Hum Genet* 1988;43:726.

+ 33. Sponseller PD, Hobbs W, Riley LH III, Pyeritz RE. The Thoracolumbar Spine in Marfan Syndrome. *J Bone Joint Surg Am* 1995;77:867.

+ 34. Sponseller PD, Sethi N, Cameron DE, Pyeritz RE. Infantile Scoliosis in Marfan Syndrome. *Spine* 1997;22:509.

+ 35. Svensson O, Aaro S. Cervical Instability in Skeletal Dysplasia. *Acta Orthop Scand* 1988;59:66.

+ 36. Thomsen MN, Schneider U, Weber M, et al. Scoliosis and Congenital Anomalies Associated with Klippel-Feil Syndrome Types I–III. *Spine* 1997;22:396.

37. Tolo VT. Surgical Treatment of Kyphosis in Achondroplasia. In: Nicoletti B, Kopits SE, Ascani E, McKusick VA, eds. *Human Achondroplasia. Basic Life Science*, 48: 257. New York: Plenum Press, 1988.

38. Tolo VT. Spinal Deformity in Short Stature Syndromes. *Instr Course Lect* 1990;39:399.

+ 39. Tolo VT, Kopits SE. Spinal Deformity in Diastrophic Dysplasia. *Orthop Trans* 1983;7:31.

+ 40. Tolo VT, Kopits SE. Surgical Treatment of Thoracolumbar Kyphosis in Achondroplasia. *Orthop Trans* 1988; 12:254.

+ 41. Torg JS, Pavlov H, Genuario SE, et al. Neurapraxia of the Cervical Spinal Cord with Transient Quadriplegia. *J Bone Joint Surg Am* 1986;68:1354.

+ 42. Tredwell SJ, Newman DE, Lockitch G. Instability of the Upper Cervical Spine in Down Syndrome. *J Pediatr Orthop* 1990;10:602.

+ 43. Uematsu S, Wang H, Hurko O, Kopits SE. The Subarachnoid Space in Achondroplastic Spinal Stenosis: The Surgical Implications. In: Nicoletti B, Kopits SE, Ascani E, McKusick VA, eds. *Human Achondroplasia. Basic Life Science*, 48:275. New York: Plenum Press, 1988.

+ 44. Winter RB, Moe JH, Bradford DS, et al. Spine Deformity in Neurofibromatosis. *J Bone Joint Surg Am* 1979;61: 677.

+ 45. Winter RB, Lonstein JE, Denis F, de la Rosa HS. Convex Growth Arrest for Progressive Congenital Scoliosis due to Hemivertebrae. *J Pediatr Orthop* 1988;8:633.

+ 46. Yong-Hing K, Kalamchi A, MacEwen GD. Cervical Spine Abnormalities in Neurofibromatosis. *J Bone Joint Surg Am* 1979;61:695.

+ 47. Yong-Hing K, MacEwen GP. Scoliosis Associated with Osteogenesis Imperfecta. *J Bone Joint Surg Br* 1982;64: 36.

CHAPTER 159

SURGICAL TREATMENT OF ADULT SCOLIOSIS

Robert F. McLain and Isador Lieberman

Adult scoliosis is usually the product of an unarrested adolescent idiopathic curve. It may also develop secondary to progressive degenerative collapse or neuromuscular disease. It may, rarely, be attributable to a progressive idiopathic curve arising after skeletal maturity, in which the curves tend to be more rigid than those seen in adolescence.

Scoliosis in adults brings with it a host of associated problems (pain, neurologic signs and symptoms, progression of deformity, and cosmetic concerns). Postsurgical complications are more common, more severe, and less well tolerated than in younger patients. Even though advances in diagnostic modalities and surgical technique provide for more effective treatment options than in the past, the treatment of adult scoliosis remains one of the most complex and challenging disorders confronting the spinal surgeon.

NATURAL HISTORY

Adolescent idiopathic scoliosis was once believed not to progress past skeletal maturity. It is now well documented that large curves continue to progress into adulthood. Curves less than 30° at the end of growth rarely progress and do not need close observation, but as Weinstein and Ponseti have shown, curves measuring greater than 50° at skeletal maturity are at significant risk for progression (28). Thoracic curves are even more likely to progress than lumbar curves.

Scoliosis arising from degenerative disc disease with asymmetric disc space collapse is distinct from adolescent and adult idiopathic scoliosis. The degenerative scoliosis is commonly a lumbar curve of moderate severity characterized by less rotation at the apex and more lateral listh-

R. F. McLain: Department of Orthopaedics, The Cleveland Clinic Foundation, Cleveland, Ohio, 44195.

I. Lieberman: Department of Orthopaedics, The Cleveland Clinic Foundation, Cleveland, Ohio, 44195.

esis between adjacent segments. Degenerative scoliosis is discussed more fully in Chapter 160.

CLINICAL PRESENTATION

Pain is the most common complaint among adults with scoliosis. The pain tends to be mechanical in nature, worse in the morning and late evening, exacerbated by strenuous activity and certain bending or twisting activities, and characterized by limited sitting tolerance. Pain along the convexity of the curve can also be due to muscle fatigue or scapulothoracic incongruency. With advancing age and curve severity, the pain tends to concentrate in the concavity of the curve. Focal back pain across the concavity may be due to disc degeneration, facet arthrosis, junctional disc degeneration, or segmental instability (30).

Patients with scoliosis experience the same progression of disc degeneration as seen in normal spines, but eccentric loads may accelerate the degenerative process. Distortion of the outer annulus or posterior longitudinal ligament could generate back pain localized to the site of highest compressive load. The degenerating disc may release pain mediators that sensitize local receptors or the nerve root

itself. The asymmetrically loaded facet joints could also be the source of pain in some patients.

Facet arthrosis or subluxation in both the concavity and convexity of the curve can stimulate capsular receptors capable of generating pain. Painful degeneration of the junctional disc may occur at the end of a rigid structural segment, within a flexible compensatory curve, or between opposing curves. In these areas, exaggerated bending forces tend to break down normal restraints and produce instability that may eventually result in coronal or sagittal displacements, abnormal motion, or axial and radicular pain. Radicular pain usually occurs on the concavity of lumbar or thoracolumbar curves, where nerve root compression in the lateral recess or foramen is caused by facet arthrosis and hypertrophy, disc herniation, or a combination of the two (Fig. 159.1). Radicular symptoms may also occur on the convexity when traction and kinking of the nerve root occur as it passes around the pedicle and out of the foramen.

Curve progression is another common presenting complaint. Patients may complain of a loss of height, an increase in rib prominence, or changes in shoulder or waistline symmetry. In general, scoliosis in the adult progresses slowly, in the range of 1° per year (28). More rapid changes in posture may signal a more complex underlying

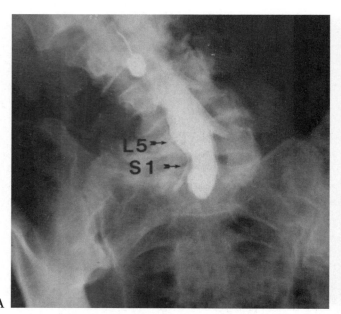
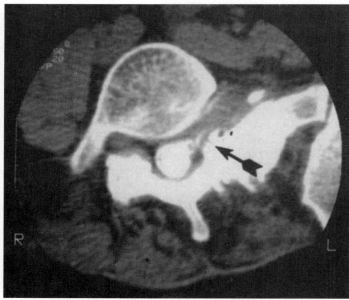

A   B

Figure 159.1.   A 55-year-old woman with a large lumbar curve that was not progressing. She developed radicular pain in her lower left extremity that markedly limited her walking and standing tolerance. Back pain had not changed for years. Myelogram (**A**) and postmyelographic (**B**) CT scan demonstrated nonfilling of left L-5 nerve root and displacement of left S-1 nerve root secondary to facet hypertrophy and subarticular and foraminal stenosis. Limited decompression consisting of left hemilaminotomy, partial medial facetectomy, and internal foraminotomy provided relief of lower extremity radicular pain. The curve has not progressed in over 1 year since surgery.

disorder (i.e., metabolic bone disease, associated neurologic disorders, unrecognized congenital abnormalities) or may simply mean that the patient is losing the ability to compensate for the longstanding deformity.

When compared with progressive adolescent curves, the progressive adult scoliotic spine acts more like a leaning tower of Pisa, in that the rigid spine cannot compensate for curve progression to maintain sagittal or coronal balance. Since the primary curve (thoracic, thoracolumbar, or lumbar) becomes rigid early in the curve's development, it can no longer compensate in the sagittal or coronal plane as the compensatory curve progresses and eventually becomes structural. Frequently, the patient notices progression of coronal and sagittal imbalance as he or she falls farther and farther to one side (Fig. 159.2).

Cosmesis is often a major concern for patients seeking treatment, but many patients are reluctant to raise this issue with their doctors. Rib prominence, changes in the waistline, and lateral postural imbalance all contribute to an undesirable appearance. While the cosmetic aspects of spinal deformity are often downplayed by physicians, they are often extremely important to the patient and should be carefully considered in formulating a treatment plan.

Cardiopulmonary compromise can occur in idiopathic scoliosis but is rarely the main reason the patient seeks treatment. Large thoracic curves (greater than 100°) may cause restrictive pulmonary disease, particularly when the chest is hypokyphotic (3). Although most patients with large curves have pain as their major complaint, the presence of deteriorating pulmonary function is an additional indication for surgical intervention. Key features of cardiopulmonary involvement include

- Measurable losses in pulmonary function that are first noted in curves greater than 60°; significant impairment occurs where curves exceed 100°;
- Direct correlation between curve magnitude and loss of pulmonary capacity;
- Complaints of fatigue and shortness of breath with minor exertion;
- Neuromuscular disease that can amplify pulmonary compromise.

Pulmonary function testing is indicated for any patient with significant signs or symptoms.

Neurologic deficits are uncommon in scoliosis. Spinal cord compression with myelopathy has not been reported in idiopathic scoliosis. Occasionally, patients may have activity-related deficits due to central stenosis. These deficits usually occur in older patients, where degenerative changes have set in on top of the original deformity. Lateral or sagittal translation can cause rapid progression of stenosis symptoms.

INDICATIONS FOR SURGERY

The major indications for surgery in adults with scoliosis are the following:

- Pain, focal or radicular
- Documented curve progression
- Curve greater than 60°
- Severe cosmetic deformity
- Flatback syndrome, sagittal or coronal imbalance
- Vertebral translation or instability due to severe lumbar curve

Once curve progression has been documented, nonsurgical modalities are ineffective in stopping it and surgical treatment should be considered. Because of the high likelihood of progression, patients with thoracic curves measuring 60° or more should generally consider surgical treatment. Patients with lumbar curves of less magnitude may sometimes require surgery because of pain and progression (4).

If pain alone is the indication for surgery, the patient must decide if the symptoms are severe and limiting enough to justify the risks of major surgery. The physician must be certain that the pain is related to a structural spinal problem, since idiopathic back pain is just as common in people with scoliosis as in the general population. Discography may be helpful in determining whether

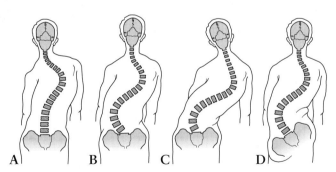

Figure 159.2. Progression and decompensation. **A:** Adult patient with longstanding thoracic curve. The curve is rigid but well balanced in coronal plane. The lumbar compensatory curve is low-grade and supple. **B:** Over time, the lumbar compensatory curve progresses. The ability of the spinal column to compensate is limited by the rigid thoracic curve. Degenerative changes, superimposed on the secondary curve, accelerate the curves' progression. **C:** When the limits of spinal compensation are reached, the progressive lumbar curve begins to throw the thoracic curve out of coronal balance. The patient begins to lean or collapse to one side. Decompensation progresses rapidly because of the mechanical disadvantage, and the apparent deformity becomes dramatically worse in a short time. **D:** The final compensatory mechanism is postural; the patient stands with the left hip flexed and shoulders askew, trying to balance the head over the pelvis.

symptoms of low back pain are related to disc degeneration or junctional problems. The radiographic appearance of the discogram is not important, but the reproduction of the patient's pain pattern during injection is diagnostic (13,26).

PREOPERATIVE PLANNING AND PREPARATION

Before embarking on surgical treatment, clearly define the goals of surgery and the treatment expectations to the patient. The treatment recommendations must be tailored to the patient's specific complaints. In most cases, they represent a combination of pain, neurologic symptoms, curve progression, and cosmesis. When pain is the major complaint, *the pain generator* must be identified and treatment targeted accordingly. The contribution of sagittal and coronal imbalance to pain must be evaluated and treatment planned to include the appropriate realignment procedure. If neurologic symptoms are the major concern, the source of root or cord compression must be identified and treated.

Neurologic symptoms may be addressed through direct posterior decompression or may be alleviated by indirect decompression through curve realignment. When curve progression is the most significant concern, its rate and extent must be documented to provide the correct treatment recommendation—fusion *in situ* or curve correction. If cosmesis is the primary indication for surgery, then the curve flexibility must be evaluated and the most appropriate realignment technique utilized. Thoracoplasty may be needed to correct the rib hump in patients with adult scoliosis.

During preoperative planning, mark radiographs to indicate the location of implants and the application of corrective forces to be used (Fig. 159.3). Side-bending radiographs are crucial to the decision process. Measure bending films to determine the best passive correction obtainable for each curve. Most adult curves can be adequately treated with posterior techniques alone, but larger, more rigid curves are better treated with a combined approach of anterior release and interbody grafting followed by posterior instrumentation and grafting. Anterior release and interbody fusion should be considered when

- The thoracic and thoracolumbar curves do not correct to an angle of less than 50° on lateral-bending radiographs;
- The primary curve cannot be corrected on lateral-bending radiographs to match the corrected compensatory curve (to achieve two balanced curves) (5);
- The patient has a higher than usual risk of pseudarthrosis (neurofibromatosis);

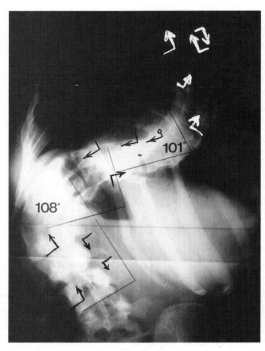

Figure 159.3. Radiograph marked before surgery to indicate types and sites of hook placement in a 24-year-old woman with double major thoracic and lumbar curves.

- L-4 does not reach neutral on maximal side-bending radiographs and the surgeon wants to avoid fusion to L-5 or the sacrum;
- Fusion to the sacrum is necessary.

An L-5–S-1 interbody fusion minimizes the risk of pseudarthrosis in a posterior lumbosacral fusion. In painful curves, discography can ensure that the fusion is not terminated at the level of a symptomatic degenerative disc. If radicular symptoms are prominent, magnetic resonance imaging (MRI) is indicated.

When possible, plan to do anterior and posterior fusions as a single surgical procedure. Preoperative autologous blood donation is routine unless contraindicated. Perform pulmonary function tests, measure nutritional parameters, and do a full medical workup before undertaking a combined procedure. Although a single-stage operation is physically taxing, complications for it are significantly less than for two-stage procedures (19,20). If blood loss during the anterior approach is excessive or the patient is hemodynamically unstable, the posterior procedure may be postponed for 5–7 days. In the interim, maximize pulmonary function, prevent or treat urinary tract or wound infections, and maintain sound nutritional status.

If a severe rigid curve is encountered and maximal correction is the goal, consider a staged procedure incorporating 2 to 3 weeks of halo–femoral traction between the anterior and posterior surgeries. Most adults can tolerate this regimen physically and psychologically. Pin site and skin care must be meticulous. We recommend prophylaxis against deep-vein thrombosis. Initiate physical therapy to encourage deep breathing and extremity range-of-motion exercises. During traction, tilt the head of the bed up 15° to 20°. Attach the halo ring to the bed frame and apply 10–20 pounds of weight to each of the femoral traction pins. The patients may be out of traction for bathing and may be up with a walking or wheelchair traction frame as tolerated.

PRINCIPLES OF SEGMENTAL INSTRUMENTATION

Segmental fixation is the preferred method of internal fixation in adult scoliosis. Greater curve correction and better sagittal plane balance are possible with segmental instrumentation than with traditional Harrington instrumentation. Modern segmental instrumentation systems are based on a longitudinal member to which a variety of hooks, screws, sublaminar wires, or connectors can be attached. Stronger spinal fixation is afforded by multiple fixation points along the rod and by using strategic combinations of screws, sublaminar wires, and hooks to gain firm purchase on the pedicles, laminae, and transverse processes.

Place additional fixation whenever possible to increase implant stability, as adults fuse more slowly than adolescents, and they have stiffer curves and often poorer bone stock. The rate of pseudarthrosis and rod failure with segmental instrumentation is lower than with Harrington instrumentation (18,22,24). In addition, the prolonged postoperative immobilization necessary after Harrington instrumentation is often unnecessary after segmental instrumentation.

The use of pedicle screws in the treatment of scoliosis is controversial and does carry a theoretically greater risk of screw misplacement because of the bony deformity. Pedicle screws do provide superior fixation in adult patients, however, and their use can enhance correction by harnessing the "force nucleus" (junction of pedicle lamina and transverse process), as described by Steffee et al. (23) and others (27). Pedicle screws also allow for parallel, purely axial corrective forces between adjacent segments.

Hooks, by contrast, may produce focal kyphosis or lordosis when distraction or compression forces are applied. Specifically, pure distraction in the lumbar spine can produce a painful flatback syndrome unless multiple hooks are used and rods are carefully contoured to maintain lordosis. Sublaminar wires are most valuable in lateral translation of the spine during correction. They cannot control rotation or axial collapse and as such work best in a combined construct with hooks or screws.

Traditional teaching has been that the fusion should end at the stable vertebra, which is the vertebra intersected by the central sacral line (12) (see chapter 156). With segmental instrumentation, the lower end of the fusion should be the vertebra that becomes level on maximal side-bend radiographs. Patients with a rigid lumbosacral curve who have significant residual tilt of L-4 on bending films, and those with low back pain due to disc degeneration at L-4–L-5 or L-5–S-1, require fusion to the sacrum. Avoid fusion down to L-5 alone, as the incidence of subsequent low back pain is high (6).

Segmental instrumentation systems improve correction of spinal deformity by addressing all three planes of deformity (7):

- Coronal plane deformities can be corrected by longitudinal compression and distraction forces.
- Sagittal plane contours can be restored by properly contouring the rods and avoiding strong distraction forces in the lower lumbar segment.
- Finally, there is limited potential to improve rotational deformity through proper contouring of the rods.

By correcting rotational deformity, the cosmetic results of surgery can be improved, especially with regard to the thoracic rib hump. The cosmetic correction possible in the adult is usually less than what can be achieved in the adolescent, but it can be maximized by a circumferential release of the spine including concave and convex facetectomies. Severe rib-cage deformities may be improved through thoracoplasty, but not without some additional pain and potential morbidity.

Long scoliosis fusions ending at the sacrum have a high rate of pseudarthrosis and fixation failure. For neuromuscular scoliosis, the modified Galveston technique of Allen and Ferguson achieves firm pelvic fixation and a high fusion rate (1). For ambulatory patients, instrumenting across the intact sacroiliac joints is not recommended and sacral fixation is needed. Single-level hook or screw purchase into the sacrum is often inadequate when an extended construct acts as a long lever arm above the sacrum. The two options that can be considered are (a) additional pedicle screws into S-2 and (b) an intrasacral rod technique. Any long construct terminating at the sacrum should be augmented with an L-5–S-1 interbody fusion using either an anterior or a posterolateral technique.

Anterior segmental instrumentation can correct and stabilize a curve until fusion is achieved. The Zielke instrumentation is the prototype, but many useful systems are now available. Double-rod anterior systems have recently been described (11) and appear promising. Anterior instrumentation can be more advantageous than posterior and may even preclude a posterior procedure.

By virtue of their anatomic location, anterior instrumentation systems are better suited to correct deformity in the coronal, sagittal, and axial planes (8,10,14), but they have their limitations. If screws are not properly aligned, anterior instrumentation may produce kyphosis in the thoracolumbar and lumbar spine. Also, instrumentation extending to the low lumbar spine may impinge on the vascular structures.

Placement of the screws must be meticulous to avoid penetration of the spinal canal. Protect the spinal canal by identifying landmarks and bluntly dissecting around the opposite side of the vertebral body. Place a finger at the junction of the transverse process, pedicle, and vertebral body to act as an aiming guide.

With the first-generation anterior implant systems, screw and rod breakage were common. With more modern, robust instrumentation, breakage is far less common, but screw pullout at the proximal or distal end of the construct remains a problem. To prevent this problem, use

a pullout-resistant nut on the opposite side of the vertebral body (16), or extend the instrumentation to other levels to distribute the load.

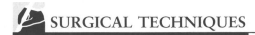

SURGICAL TECHNIQUES

POSTERIOR PROCEDURES

▪ Position the patient on an appropriate spinal frame, ensuring that the abdomen hangs freely and that compression of the inferior vena cava is minimized. If pedicle screws will be needed, use a radiolucent table or frame; otherwise, use either a Wilson frame or longitudinal bolsters. Take care during positioning to make sure that the face is well padded and that there is no

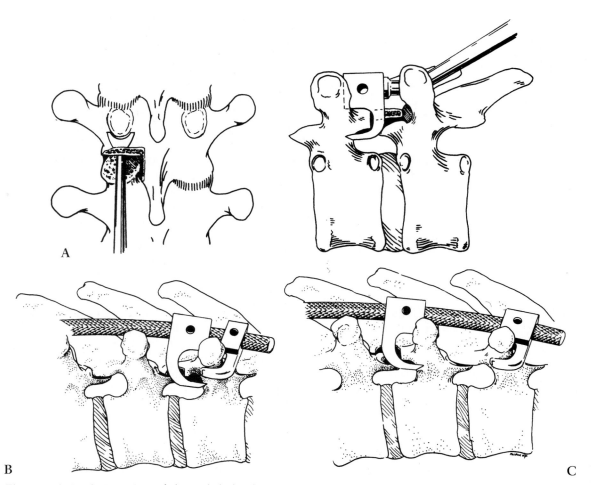

Figure 159.4. **A:** Insertion of the pedicle hook. **B:** Construction of the upper claw. Two forms of transverse-pedicular claws can be used to secure the upper end of the construct. A single-level claw using a transverse process hook and standard pedicle hook is the most common combination. **C:** For longer constructs, a two-level claw may be easier to apply. Use standard closed lumbar lamina and pedicle hooks. Either of these constructs can be substituted for the other when a transverse process is fractured during instrumentation.

pressure on the eyes. Drape the back to provide access to the entire spine and to the iliac crest for graft harvest.

▪ Center a longitudinal midline incision over the apical vertebra. After stripping the paraspinous musculature, expose the spine subperiosteally to the tips of the transverse processes.

▪ Identify levels radiographically by placing a towel clip through the transverse process of the selected vertebra.

▪ After exposing the lamina at the levels to be fused, identify hook and screw sites and prepare them for implant placement. The technique of hook insertion is identical to that performed in adolescent patients (Fig. 159.4).

▪ After excising the inferior facet with a narrow osteotome, remove the articular surface of the underlying superior facet with a straight curet. Locate the pedicle, which lies at the level of the transverse processes, with the pedicle finder. With the finder well seated on the pedicle, the vertebral body can be moved side to side with the finder. If the two do not move as a unit, the purchase is inadequate.

▪ Then insert the pedicle hook, taking care not to split the lamina during placement.

▪ Place additional hooks, if desired, to increase the overall strength of the construct and to distribute forces over a greater number of vertebrae (Fig. 159.5). Extra hooks may be especially helpful in patients with osteoporotic bone (Fig. 159.6).

▪ Although rotational correction is possible in reasonably flexible curves, derotation may not be possible or safe in very stiff curves. Overzealous attempts to derotate or translate vertebral elements may result in fractures of the laminae or pedicles, and possible penetration of implants into the spinal canal (9).

▪ For stiffer curves, gain correction by segmental distraction, along with appropriate sagittal contouring to maintain or correct kyphotic or lordotic segments. Large, rigid thoracic curves may be partially corrected with a short apical rod placed in the concavity, before completing the construct with a long distraction rod. The long rod can then be coupled to the short apical distraction rod, and, after distraction, both can be coupled to the convex rod (Fig. 159.7).

▪ Always crosslink rod constructs to increase the torsional stiffness of the construct (2).

▪ Before completing the instrumentation, excise all facet joints and thoroughly decorticate the exposed spine. Although segmental instrumentation offers rigid fixation, strict adherence to these principles is crucial to obtain a consistent fusion in adult patients. During decortication, preserve the integrity of the laminae and transverse processes on which hooks are to be placed.

▪ We advocate the use of autogenous iliac bone graft, particularly if wide laminectomy has been performed in the lumbar spine, in cases of pseudarthrosis, or with fusion to the sacrum.

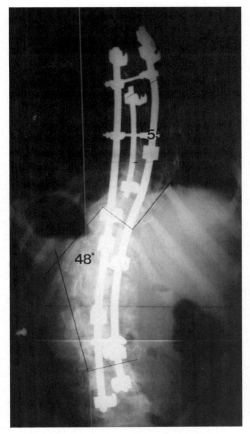

Figure 159.5.   Postoperative radiograph of patient in Figure 159.3, treated with Cotrel-Dubousset segmental instrumentation. This triple-rod technique distributes corrective forces over many spinal segments using multiple fixation hooks. Combined with anterior thoracic and lumbar releases, this approach provided 45% correction of the thoracic curve (101° to 55°) and 55% correction of the lumbar curve (108° to 48°).

▪ Radicular pain resulting from foraminal or lateral recess stenosis often resolves with curve correction and stabilization. Medial facetectomies and foraminotomies, however, may be carried out if there is documented foraminal or lateral recess stenosis consistent with the lower extremity symptoms. If the curve is stable, and not progressive, root compression may be treated with decompression alone. Partial medial facetectomies and foraminotomies may be carried out through a limited laminotomy, taking care to preserve the pars interarticularis and dorsal facet joints.

▪ Achieve posterior releases by performing an osteotomy at each of the rigid periapical segments. Beginning in the midline, open the ligamentum flavum, and then use Kerrison rongeurs to excise the ligamentum flavum. In longstanding deformities, the ligamentum flavum may be ossified and will need to be taken down with a burr

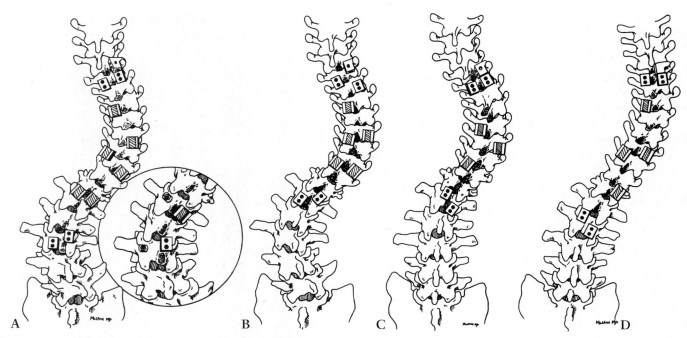

Figure 159.6.   Hook patterns for specific scoliotic curves. **A:** King type I curve—S-shaped curve with lumbar curve that is larger and less flexible than the thoracic. This hook pattern uses the standard thoracic pattern (see type III) but adds hooks distally to allow compression of the lumbar convexity and distraction of the lumbar concavity. (*Inset*) Pedicle screws may be used in the lumbar segment and are most easily placed on the convexity. Distal hooks or screws allow correction of any junctional kyphosis when the curve is corrected. **B:** King type II curve—S-shaped curve in which both thoracic and lumbar curves cross the midline. In this curve, the lumbar curve is more flexible and does not require full instrumentation. Correction of the thoracic curve using a standard thoracic pattern is adequate to provide a satisfactory anteroposterior (AP) contour. Add upper lumbar fixation to help prevent decompensation and to restore sagittal balance. **C:** King type III curve—typical right thoracic curve. Construct other fixation patterns around this one. Instrument the concavity with pedicle hooks at the upper end-vertebra and one level above the apex, and sublaminar hooks downgoing at the lower end-vertebra and one level below the apex. This pattern allows uniform distraction over the concave side, along with some derotation. Provide compression over the convex side with a transverse-pedicular claw at the upper end-vertebra, an open pedicle hook at the level of the apex, and a sublaminar hook under the lamina of the lower end-vertebra. Additional open hooks may be added in patients with poor bone quality. **D:** King type IV curve—long thoracic curve in which lower lumbar vertebrae also tilt into the curve. Instrumentation of this curve is similar to that of type III, with the distal hooks carried to the upper lumbar spine to correct the longer curve. Attempt to spare the lower lumbar segments and allow the patient to compensate spontaneously. If the lumbar deformity is rigid, instrumentation and fusion may have to be extended to the lower lumbar spine.

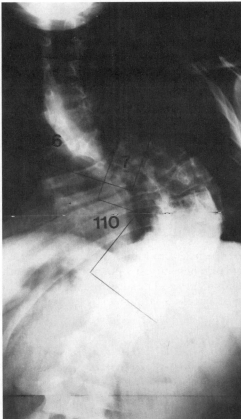
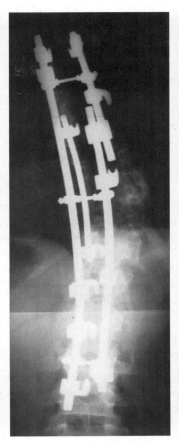
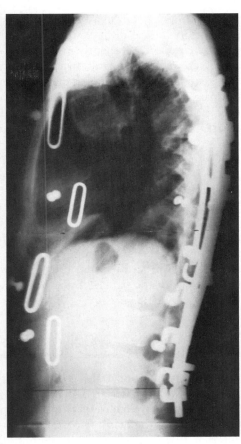

A,B   C

Figure 159.7.   A 28-year-old woman with a stiff King-type V thoracic scoliosis. **A:** Preoperative PA radiograph demonstrates double thoracic curve. Upper curve (apex T-5) measured 76°. Lower curve (apex T-10–T-11) measured 110°. **B:** Following right anterior thoracic release, a short, apical distraction rod used to correct the uppermost curve. A longer rod spanning the convexity of the lower thoracic curve was connected to the first rod in bayonet fashion with a double-barrel "domino." Both these rods combine to make the third member of a triple-rod construct using a short reduction rod at the apex of the lower thoracic curve. **C:** Lateral view shows restoration of thoracic kyphosis and neutral thoracolumbar alignment.

and Kerrison rongeurs. Proceeding laterally on both sides, excise the facets and enter the neural foramen. These osteotomies will significantly increase the mobility of the curve.

ANTERIOR PROCEDURES

■ Treat rigid, high-degree curves by anterior release and interbody grafting before proceeding with posterior instrumentation, correction, and grafting. Carry out the traditional anterior release as described in Chapter 155, with two particular precautions: First, because vascular supply to the cord is less robust in adults, and particularly tenuous in kyphotic segments, exercise caution when approaching those segments anteriorly. It may be wise to preserve segmental vessels in these regions, or

at least to temporarily occlude large segmentals with a vascular clamp and observe for changes in the somatosensory evoked potentials.

■ Second, very rigid curves may require an extensive release, including excision of the posterior longitudinal ligament, before correction can be obtained. In order to shorten the vertebral column (to restore thoracic kyphosis and avoid stretching the neural elements) during correction, partial vertebrectomy may be necessary at apical levels.

■ Anterior instrumentation may improve curve correction and may allow the surgeon to spare lower lumbar segments in some patients with thoracolumbar and lumbar curves. Place vertebral body screws as far posteriorly as possible on the convex side of the spine, traversing each body in an anterolateral direction, slightly away from the canal. In a badly rotated specimen, this orientation can be difficult to obtain. By placing the end-vertebral screws slightly more anterior to the periapical screws, instrumentation and correction will naturally tend to rotate the lumbar curve and restore lumbar lordosis.

- Because the vertebral cortex in the midbody is thin, create the starting hole with a hand-held awl. Bicortical purchase is desirable, particularly at end vertebrae. If posterior pedicle screw instrumentation is planned, place the anterior vertebral body screws below the midpoint of the vertebral body.
- With the advent of endoscopic techniques, thoracotomy and thoracolumbotomy may be avoided and the anterior release and interbody grafting performed in a minimally invasive fashion. Using endoscopy, the anterior and posterior procedures may even be performed simultaneously with the patient in the prone position (17).

POSTOPERATIVE MANAGEMENT

Try to get patients out of bed to a chair the day after surgery, and walking within 3–5 days. If bone quality is good and implant purchase is thought to be secure, no brace is needed. If there is any concern about the security of internal fixation, use a thoracolumbosacral orthosis (TLSO) for 4 to 6 months. Bracing is also commonly used in patients fused to L-3 or L-4, as there is greater stress on the lower lumbar implants. Bracing to neutralize lower lumbar or lumbosacral curves should include a thigh cuff with a drop-lock hinge.

Patients are allowed to sleep and shower without the brace. Walking is recommended from the outset. A walking program, progressing to 1 mile daily, provides regular exercise during fusion consolidation.

PITFALLS AND COMPLICATIONS

Potential complications in the surgical treatment of adult scoliosis are the following:

- Blood-loss-induced anemia
- Pulmonary compromise
- Pseudarthrosis
- Failure of instrumentation
- Flatback syndrome
- Neurologic compromise
- Continued pain
- Infection

PSEUDARTHROSIS AND FAILURE OF INSTRUMENTATION

The complication rate in adults is significantly higher than in adolescents undergoing surgery for scoliosis (21). The most common complication, pseudarthrosis, occurs in 9% to 27% of patients (18,22,24,25). Hook dislodgement and rod fractures have been common, but primarily with Harrington instrumentation.

Although long-term complication rates of segmental instrumentation are not yet known, these will probably be lower than with older systems due to the more rigid fixation. Hook displacement and cutting-out of lumbar hooks have been reported with Cotrel-Dubousset instrumentation (9). "Claw" hook configurations on a single lamina may predispose to lamina fracture, and an inferior claw spanning two laminae is recommended to help prevent pullout. The use of pedicle screws in lower lumbar vertebrae may improve purchase in osteoporotic patients and those with stiff lumbar curves. The surgeon may use multiple pedicle screws or a pedicle–laminar claw for maximum fixation (Fig. 159.8).

FLATBACK SYNDROME

Lumbar flatback syndrome is a known complication of distraction instrumentation, but it has been less trouble-

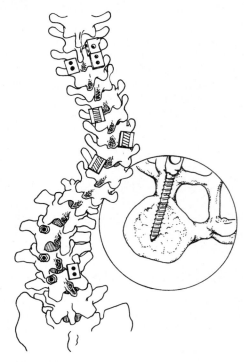

Figure 159.8. Lumbar fixation can be maximized by using pedicle screws in stiff thoracolumbar and lumbar curves. The rotation of the vertebra leaves the convex pedicle oriented in the AP plane, allowing easy placement of screws. Place a sublaminar hook on the concave side to allow distraction.

some since the introduction of segmental systems. This disabling condition causes back pain, forward tilt of the trunk, and severe sagittal imbalance (15). It can be avoided in segmental fixation systems by carefully contouring the rods to the normal lumbar lordosis and avoiding excessive distraction in the lumbar spine. Preventing this complication is critical, as surgical correction of the established condition is fraught with complications and often gives a poor result.

PERSISTENT PAIN

Few patients become completely pain free after spinal fusion, but, if a discreet pain generator has been identified, improvement can generally be expected (18,22). Even though the curve has been stabilized, patients may continue to experience back pain.

NEUROLOGIC COMPROMISE

Intraoperative complications, such as excessive blood loss and neurologic injury, are more common in adults than in adolescents. Neurologic complications with Harrington instrumentation have been uncommon; the risk of spinal cord injury is primarily related to overdistraction of a rigid curve. The same risks are present during distraction using segmental instrumentation and may be magnified by the increased mechanical advantage provided by segmental systems. Attempts to derotate a rigid curve in an osteoporotic spine may cause a concave pedicle hook to fracture the pedicle and penetrate the spinal canal. Gurr and McAfee reported such a case, which resulted in a Brown-Séquard syndrome (9). Rigid curves, especially in the presence of osteoporosis, should be treated with distraction and compression, avoiding derotation or strong translation forces. Remember that the primary goal of surgery in the adult with scoliosis is to stabilize the curve and halt progression; correction is a secondary objective.

Spinal cord monitoring should be used in all cases, as this allows recognition of subtle neurologic changes, permitting the surgeon to take prompt action to reverse them (29).

AUTHORS' PREFERRED TECHNIQUE

There is no routine approach to adult patients with scoliosis; each curve has its own "personality," and each patient presents with his own confounding variables (Fig. 159.9). The presenting complaint, level of deformity, and rigidity of the curves dictate the specifics, but a general approach can be proposed.

■ Release any curve that cannot be reduced to less than

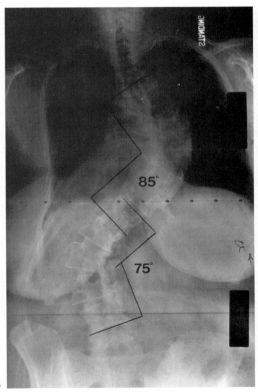 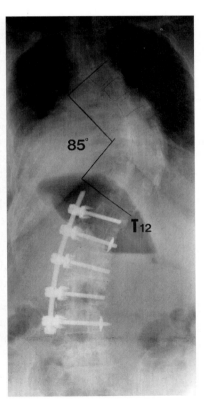

A,B

Figure 159.9. A 46-year-old woman with severe, progressive thoracolumbar scoliosis. **A:** Preoperative PA radiograph demonstrates high-degree thoracic and lumbar curves. Bending films revealed little correction of either curve. Occiput was 4.0 cm left of the central sacral line. **B:** After anterior lumbar release and instrumentation, the lumbar curve was improved but the thoracic curve was no better and out of balance. *(continued)*

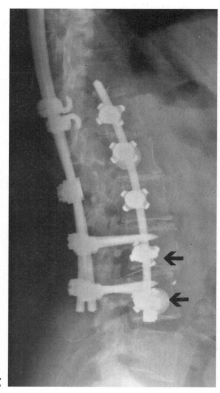
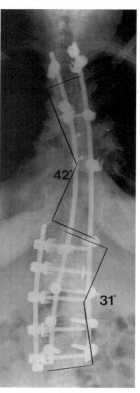

C

D

Figure 159.9.   (continued) C: Thoracic release and posterior instrumentation were performed 7 days later, under one anesthetic. Lateral view shows pedicle screws properly placed in the lumbar pedicles, passing above the vertebral body screws that were placed low in each vertebral body. Thoracolumbar kyphosis has been improved to mild lordosis. Custom-designed pullout nuts (*lower arrow*) improve pullout strength of the vertebral body screws. **D:** Anterior thoracic release, combined with posterior segmental instrumentation, provided 50% correction of the thoracic curve. The combined approach to the lumbar curve provided correction of almost 60%.

50° on bending films anteriorly prior to posterior instrumentation.

■ If both thoracic and lumbar curves must be addressed, carry out the lumbar retroperitoneal approach at the initial operation. Perform an anterior release, interbody fusion, and anterior instrumentation.

■ Give the patient 5–7 days to recover before performing the definitive second procedure.

At the second operation, carry out an anterior thoracic release and full-length posterior instrumentation as staged or simultaneous procedures.

■ In the staged procedure, place the patient in a lateral decubitus position with the curve convexity up. Through the anterior approach, release as many levels as can be reached, removing as much of the concave soft tissues as is necessary to allow motion when pressure is applied to the vertebral body.

■ Once the convex release is completed, lightly pack the morcelized rib into the intervertebral spaces, close the wound, and turn the patient prone on the spinal frame.

■ Perform posterior instrumentation, incorporating all of the thoracic and lumbar curves.

■ Place multiple hooks to correct both coronal and sagittal alignment. Place pedicle screws distally to obtain the most stable foundation for the rest of the construct.

■ Contour the rods to impart more normal thoracic kyphosis and lumbar lordosis, and then lock them into the lumbar screws distally.

■ Sequentially reduce the rods into remaining hooks, taking time to allow viscoelastic forces to dissipate.

For severe curves, the thoracic and lumbar sagittal curves may reflect the existing scoliotic curves, and rod placement may be easier if the rods are placed in an off-axis, rotated position (Fig. 159.10).

■ After loosely affixing the hooks and screws to the rod, apply C-rings to prevent hooks from displacing.

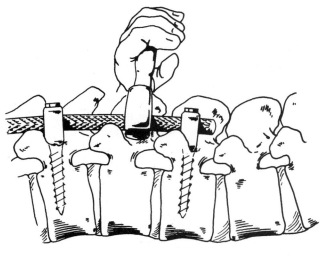

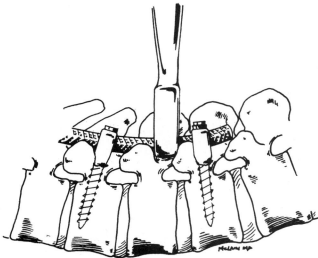

Figure 159.10. Correction of junctional kyphosis is crucial to sagittal plane balance. Derotation of a contoured fixation rod using hooks or pedicle screws allows the surgeon to restore thoracolumbar lordosis and thoracic kyphosis at the time of curve correction.

■ Slowly rotate the rods back into normal orientation, placing the kyphotic and lordotic curves back in the sagittal plane. This "derotation" maneuver simply uses rod contours to apply translational forces to correct the coronal deformity. There is no actual derotation of the vertebrae.

In the simultaneous approach, place the patient prone, and prep anteriorly to the midaxillary line on the side of the concavity. A thoracoscopic approach can then be used to release multiple disc spaces through a few periapical portals. Carry out the posterior instrumentation without changing the patient's position.

AUTHORS' PERSPECTIVE

Adult idiopathic scoliosis is a complex disorder requiring thorough patient evaluation and careful preoperative planning. An accurate assessment of spinal pain and curve progression, and knowledge of the natural history of scoliosis are essential components in formulating an appropriate treatment plan. With more advanced surgical techniques, patients once thought to be untreatable may now be effectively managed. Although surgery is a major undertaking, with a significant complication rate, the results of surgical treatment of adult scoliosis can be extremely gratifying.

REFERENCES

Each reference is categorized according to the following scheme: *, classic article; #, review article; !, basic research article; and +, clinical results/outcome study.

* 1. Allen BL Jr, Ferguson RL. The Galveston Technique for L Rod Instrumentation of the Scoliotic Spine. *Spine* 1982;7:276.
# 2. Ashman RB, Birch JG, Bone LB, et al. Mechanical Testing of Spinal Instrumentation. *Clin Orthop* 1988;227: 113.
* 3. Bjure J, Nachemson A. Nontreated Scoliosis. *Clin Orthop* 1973;93:44.
# 4. Briard JL, Jegou D, Cauchoix J. Adult Lumbar Scoliosis. *Spine* 1979;4:526.
+ 5. Byrd JA, Coles PV, Winter RB, et al. Adult Idiopathic Scoliosis Treated by Anterior and Posterior Spinal Fusion. *J Bone Joint Surg Am* 1987;69:843.
+ 6. Cochran T, Irtam L, Nachemson A. Long-Term Anatomic and Functional Changes in Patients with Adolescent Idiopathic Scoliosis Treated by Harrington Rod Fusion. *Spine* 1983;8:576.
+ 7. Cotrel Y, Dubousset J. A New Technique of Segmental Instrumentation of the Spine. *Orthop Trans* 1985;9:584.
* 8. Giehl JP, Zielke K, Hack HP. Die Ventrale Derotationsspondylodese nach Zielke. *Orthopade* 1989;18:101.
+ 9. Gurr KR, McAfee KC. Cotrel-Dubousset Instrumentation in Adults, A Preliminary Report. *Spine* 1988;13: 510.
+ 10. Kaneda K, Fujiya N, Satoh S. Results of Zielke Instrumentation for Idiopathic Thoracolumbar and Lumbar Scoliosis. *Clin Orthop* 1986;205:195.
+ 11. Kaneda K, Shono Y, Satoh S, Abumi K. Anterior Correction of Thoracic Scoliosis with Kaneda Anterior Spinal System. A Preliminary Report. *Spine* 1997;22:1358.
* 12. King HA, Moe JH, Bradford DS, Winter RB. The Selection of Fusion Levels in Thoracic Idiopathic Scoliosis. *J Bone Joint Surg Am* 1983;65:1302.
# 13. Kostuik JP. Decision-Making in Adult Scoliosis. *Spine* 1979;4:521.

+ 14. Kostuik JP, Carl A, Ferron S. Anterior Zielke Instrumentation for Spinal Deformity in Adults. *J Bone Joint Surg Am* 1989;71:898.

* 15. Lagrone MO, Bradford DS, Moe JH, et al. Treatment of Symptomatic Flat Back after Spinal Fusion. *J Bone Joint Surg Am* 1988;70:569.

! 16. Lieberman IH, Khazim R, Woodside T. Anterior Vertebral Body Screw Pull-out Testing: A Comparison of Zielke, Kaneda, Universal Spine System, and Universal Spine System with Pull-out Resistant Nut. *Spine* 1998;23:908.

+ 17. Lieberman IH, Orr RD, Salo PT, Kraetschmer BG. The Results of Simultaneous Endoscopic Anterior Release and Posterior Instrumentation for Spinal Deformity. Orthopaedic Proceedings. *J Bone Joint Surg Br* 1998;80(supp 1):5.

* 18. Ponder RC, Dickson JH, Harrington PR, Erwin WD. Results of Harrington Instrumentation and Fusion in the Adult Scoliosis Patient. *J Bone Joint Surg Am* 1975;57:797.

+ 19. Schiffman DN, McLain RF, Benson DR. Luque Galveston Instrumentation in Neuromuscular Scoliosis: Surgical and Functional Outcomes. *Proceedings of the Scoliosis Research Society*, 32nd Annual Meeting, St Louis, MO, September 1997.

+ 20. Shufflebarger HL, Grimm JO, Bui V, Thomson JD. Anterior and Posterior Spinal Fusion: Staged versus Same Day Surgery. *Spine* 1991;16:930.

+ 21. Simmons EDJ, Kowalski JM, Simmons EH. The Results of Surgical Treatment for Adult Scoliosis. *Spine* 1993;18:718.

* 22. Sponseller PD, Cohen MS, Nachemson AL, et al. Results of Surgical Treatment of Adults with Idiopathic Scoliosis. *J Bone Joint Surg Am* 1987;69:667.

* 23. Steffee AD, Biscup RS, Sitkowski DJ. Segmental Spine Plates with Pedicle Screw Fixation. A New Internal Fixation Device for Disorders of the Lumbar and Thoracolumbar Spine. *Clin Orthop* 1986;203:45.

+ 24. Swank S, Lonstein JE, Moe JH, et al. Surgical Treatment of Adult Scoliosis: A Review of 222 Cases. *J Bone Joint Surg Am* 1981;63:268.

+ 25. Van Dam DE, Bradford DS, Lonstein JE, et al. Adult Idiopathic Scoliosis Treated by Posterior Spinal Fusion and Harrington Instrumentation. *Spine* 1987;12:32.

! 26. Walsh TR, Weinstein JN, Spratt KF, et al. Lumbar Discography in Normal Subjects. *J Bone Joint Surg Am* 1990;72:1081.

+ 27. Webb JK, Burwell RG, Cole AA, Lieberman I. Posterior Instrumentation in Scoliosis. *Eur Spine J* 1995;4:2.

* 28. Weinstein SL, Ponseti IV. Curve Progression in Idiopathic Scoliosis. *J Bone Joint Surg Am* 1983;65:447.

+ 29. Wilber RG, Thompson GH, Shaffer JW, et al. Postoperative Neurological Deficits in Segmental Spinal Instrumentation. A Study Using Spinal Cord Monitoring. *J Bone Joint Surg Am* 1984;66:1178.

30. Winter RB, Lonstein JE, Dennis F. Pain Patterns in Adult Scoliosis. *Orthop Clin North Am* 1988;19:399.

## CHAPTER 160

SURGICAL MANAGEMENT OF DEGENERATIVE SCOLIOSIS

Serena S. Hu and David S. Bradford

Degenerative scoliosis is a curvature that develops in the adult secondary to degenerative disc disease. It may be difficult in many cases to determine whether scoliosis is arising *de novo* or if patients had mild to moderate degrees of scoliosis that became symptomatic or progressed late in adulthood. The treatment of degenerative scoliosis follows many of the same principles as the treatment of adult idiopathic scoliosis, however, so the distinction in many cases may be moot. This chapter discusses the factors that should be considered in treating patients with this condition.

CLINICAL PRESENTATION

NATURAL HISTORY

Mild to moderate degrees of degenerative scoliosis may not progress, and they may not be symptomatic. With

S. S. Hu and D. S. Bradford: Department of Orthopaedic Surgery, University of California Medical Center, San Francisco, California, 94143.

more advanced disease, axial pain and neurogenic claudication are typical symptoms. As with any degenerative spine disease, facet hypertrophy, diffuse disc bulges, disc degeneration, and narrowing and redundant ligamentum flavum can result in spinal stenosis and produce symptoms of neurogenic claudication and radiculopathy (25). The degree of compression can be aggravated in the presence of lateral listhesis or spondylolisthesis, by traction on the nerve roots.

Lateral listhesis, where slippage of one vertebra upon another occurs in the coronal plane, appears to correlate with a greater risk of curve progression (25,27). Significant lateral listhesis, particularly when it occurs at multiple adjacent levels, can result in significant truncal imbalance with resultant pain and fatigue. In many patients, these symptoms can be managed conservatively with anti-inflammatories, physical therapy, and epidural steroids. With progression of the patient's curvature, however, failure to respond to conservative measures or significant compromise of the patient's quality of life may call for consideration of surgical intervention.

Curve progress is variable, but among those who progress, it has been reported to average 3° a year (25). Risk factors for curve progression include curve magnitude greater than 30°, osteoporosis, and lateral listhesis or rotatory spondylolisthesis (9,14). Prior decompressive surgery, such as a laminectomy, can increase curve progression as well, sometimes secondary to development of a postsurgical fracture of the pars interarticularis and spondylolisthesis. Rapid progression of scoliosis in a patient with a prior laminectomy is highly suspect for a pars fracture, which should be sought in the workup of such a patient.

COMPONENTS OF DEFORMITY

Asymmetric *disc space collapse* can result in spinal deformity, as can rotatory *spondylolisthesis* or lateral listhesis. *Compression fractures* with a lateral wedge component may aggravate or cause development of scoliosis. These patients may have a relative loss of lumbar lordosis as well. Patients with *lateral listhesis* appear to be at greater risk for curve progression (25,27), and, in addition, they are subject to traction on their nerve roots at the involved levels. Asymmetric wear on the facet joints may contribute to facet arthropathy, leading to central or foraminal stenosis. Although most patients present with pain secondary to nerve root compression, others present with weakness. Pain and weakness may be particularly intractable from severe disc space collapse, with or without listhesis, and decreasing space between the adjacent pedicles results in foraminal stenosis. Patients with stenosis secondary to degenerative scoliosis suffer a similar pathophysiology as a cause of their neurogenic claudication—namely, a vascular insufficiency to the neural elements secondary to the stenosis, which is generally worsened by lumbar extension.

Clearly, vascular claudication and neurogenic claudication occur in similar patient populations, and it is important to distinguish the true cause of the patient's leg pain. A careful history, palpation of distal pulses, examination of feet and skin, and, if indicated, referral to a vascular specialist may be needed. In general, neurogenic claudication is improved by forward flexion of the spine, including sitting, and it may be worse going downhill because hyperextension is necessary (see Chapter 147). However, at least some patients with stenosis secondary to degenerative scoliosis have reported that their extremity symptoms are not reliably relieved by forward flexion (11).

CONSERVATIVE MANAGEMENT

Patients with degenerative scoliosis can be managed according to the conditions that cause the most symptoms. For example, the patient with more back pain secondary to the degenerative disease can be managed successfully using nonsteroidal anti-inflammatories, rest, physical therapy, cardiovascular conditioning, and, occasionally, bracing. Patients with neurogenic claudication may respond to any of these measures but may receive relief from epidural cortisone injections. Bracing can be used on occasion for the patient with mild degenerative scoliosis with back pain only. Rigid bracing has not been shown to prevent progression in adults with scoliosis. However, bracing may be a reasonable alternative for a patient who has a degenerative scoliosis with mild to moderate progression, but who is medically unable to tolerate a major reconstructive procedure.

Bracing may need to include a rigid molded thoracolumbar orthosis for more severe scoliosis or kyphosis, or it may simply be a lightweight, corset-type brace for milder curves. However, since symptom improvement is the primary goal, rather than curve control, results with a specific patient will be the final determining factor.

INDICATIONS FOR SURGERY

As for adult idiopathic scoliosis, pain, curve, and neurologic deterioration are the main indications for surgical intervention. In general, bracing in adults is discouraged because it does not halt progression and may result in patient dependence on the brace and associated trunk deconditioning. However, in certain cases, such as an elderly patient who is too ill to tolerate a major surgical procedure, or a patient whose severely osteoporotic bone is too weak to support instrumentation, bracing may slow progression or attenuate the pain symptoms.

Determining whether a patient's back pain can be improved by stabilization and fusion of her degenerative scoliosis can be difficult. Once surgery has been deemed likely to help such a patient, however, choice of the fusion levels requires consideration of curve pattern, sagittal and coronal balance, pain locale, levels needing decompression, and the presence of degenerated or listhetic levels, as well as patient expectations and activity levels. Facet blocks, discography, and nerve root blocks may be helpful in determining symptomatic levels, although their predictive value for fusion surgery has not been proven. Grubb et al. (12) used provocative discography to help determine fusion levels in adult scoliosis patients (degenerative and idiopathic) and felt that this aided them in their surgical planning. However, in their study, all positive discograms were at morphologically abnormal levels, and it is not clear whether they might have included such levels based on radiographic or magnetic resonance imaging (MRI)–determined degenerative levels. Fortunately, fusion for back pain secondary to scoliosis appears more predictable than fusion for back pain secondary to degenerative disc disease without deformity. We do not routinely perform discography in these patients, because it has not proven of benefit in predicting the outcome of fusion surgery.

Patients with degenerative scoliosis and neurogenic claudication should have their stenosis decompressed concurrently with stabilization of the curvature. In most patients, an MRI will give adequate information for localization of stenotic levels; in some patients, however, the lateral deformity or rotatory component precludes clear delineation of the anatomy. In these cases, computed tomography (CT) or myelography is indicated for preoperative planning.

 # SURGICAL TECHNIQUES

DECOMPRESSION

For patients with limited regions of spinal stenosis, neurogenic claudication, and only mild degrees of scoliosis, it may be reasonable to address the compressive symptoms with laminotomy, laminectomy, or foraminotomy as needed. Aggressive decompression can result in curve progression; this isolated procedure should be reserved for milder cases in which limited decompression can be expected to help the patient. Be sure the patient understands the possibility of curve progression and recurrence of symptoms.

FUSION *IN SITU*

For patients with limited disease, a posterior fusion alone may be sufficient. The majority of patients with degenerative scoliosis will require instrumentation and grafting to achieve fusion over multiple segments that require stabilization. Because of the increased pseudarthrosis rate with multiple-level fusions, it is rare to have a patient who can be managed without instrumentation. However, certain older patients, particularly the medically fragile, may better tolerate laminectomy and limited uninstrumented fusion (i.e., at the level where there is a degenerative spondylolisthesis). In some patients, moderate to severe osteoporosis may preclude fixation, but, as with laminectomy alone, there is a risk of curve progression and recurrence of symptoms. Therefore, this approach is limited to patients who clearly understand the limitations of what surgery can accomplish for them and are willing to risk recurrent symptoms. In general, we have not found age or osteopenia to be a contraindication for fusion with instrumentation.

Selection of fusion levels should take into account several factors. The levels that should be fused should include at least the entirety of the symptomatic curve, but often additional levels must be included to address symptomatic degenerative levels and permit maintenance or restoration of coronal and sagittal balance. Generally, preoperative bending films can help predict the amount of correction that can be obtained after exposure, facetectomy, and application of appropriate corrective forces. The end vertebra, particularly distally, should be a vertebra that is level on side bending. Sagittal balance is exceedingly important to consider, particularly because many of these patients have osteoporosis. Most degenerative curves are kyphotic; if the kyphosis is not flexible, a combined anterior–posterior approach may be indicated to achieve sagittal realignment and successful arthrodesis. It is also important not to end the fusion at a kyphotic segment. Many of these patients have lumbar or thoracolumbar curvatures, and including only the major curve often can result in ending the fusion at the mid or lower thoracic spine—in the middle of the kyphosis. Such patients are at considerable risk for development of progressive junctional kyphosis, and in general it is best to include the minor compensatory thoracic curve and end the fusion at the end vertebra of the kyphosis (usually T-4 or T-5).

Only in patients with acceptable bone quality and a nonkyphotic thoracolumbar junction can the fusion safely stop at the thoracolumbar junction. Choosing the distal end vertebra can be difficult in the patient with degenerative scoliosis and low back pain. Deciding whether L-4–L-5 and/or L-5–S-1 is symptomatic is crucial because long fusions to the sacrum generally necessitate combined anterior and posterior surgery and have a higher rate of complications. Not including a symptomatic level will result in limited pain relief, however, and thus it will decrease the success of the surgery. In addition, fusions ending at L-4 or L-5 are at risk for development of symptomatic degeneration below the fusion. This development 5–10 years after the surgery may be acceptable for the older patient, but its occurrence 2 years or so after the surgery is not. Therefore, consider whether a more distal fusion is indicated. Involvement of the lumbosacral region is very common in degenerative scoliosis, and the majority of these patients require combined anterior and posterior spinal fusion to the sacrum.

Considerations for Instrumentation

Segmental instrumentation in the form of variable hook-and-rod systems are preferred for instrumentation of degenerative scoliosis. These systems allow much better correction of coronal and particularly sagittal plane deformity. However, such surgery is technically demanding, and the surgeon must have a clear understanding of the corrective forces that should be applied and how they affect the patient's curvature, coronal balance, sagittal balance, and shoulder obliquity. The following considerations are important:

- Avoid distraction in the lumbar spine to avoid flattening

it. Apply compression across the curve convexity first in the lumbar spine.

- It is rare to be able to perform rod rotation in the patient who has degenerative scoliosis.
- If the patient has significant osteoporosis, and multiple-level laminectomy is not required for coexisting spinal stenosis (see below), consider using sublaminar wires supplemented by hooks and/or pedicle screws at strategic levels (generally the end vertebra of each curve and sometimes the apical vertebra as well). Such wires are quite easy to attach to rods and, for an osteoporotic patient whose trabecular bone has numerous vascular channels, their use can potentially decrease operative time and therefore decrease blood loss.
- Do not affix rods to end vertebrae with sublaminar wires, because wires do not provide axial control of the spine and can allow axial collapse and subsequent junctional kyphosis. Use pedicular fixation or hook combinations at the ends of constructs to decrease the likelihood of this problem.
- To ensure coronal balance, we prefer to obtain intraoperative long radiographs of the entire spine after the correction has been partially or completely performed. Adjustments in the corrective forces can be made at this time if desired.
- Although *in situ* bending to fine-tune the coronal balance can be performed in some adult scoliosis patients, most patients with degenerative scoliosis have osteoporotic bone, and *in situ* bending can result in loss of fixation.

DECOMPRESSION AND FUSION

Many patients with degenerative scoliosis also have spinal stenosis as part of their degenerative process. As part of preoperative planning, evaluate with an MRI or CT/myelogram any patient with degenerative scoliosis who notes leg pain or buttock pain. As previously noted, the MRI is adequate for many patients; with greater degrees of curvature, however, CT/myelography gives better bony detail and permits better understanding of the anatomy in the presence of the curvature. It is important to identify symptomatic levels of stenosis so that decompression can be performed at the time of posterior fusion. In most cases, this can be determined anatomically according to dermatomal levels and nerve root distributions; however, occasionally, selective nerve root injections may be needed to determine which levels with mild to moderate degrees of stenosis are the symptomatic ones.

Once laminectomy has been performed for decompression, pedicle screw instrumentation may be needed to attain fixation. Generally, fusion rates are improved with instrumentation, particularly in patients with conditions such as degenerative scoliosis (13). As with deformity surgery in general, try to visualize the medial wall of the pedicle before screw placement, to correctly account for spinal rotation. This is a simple matter after laminotomy or laminectomy has already been performed. Frazier et al. (8) reported on patients who underwent decompression for spinal stenosis, including 19 who had at least 15° of scoliosis preoperatively. The majority of their patients with scoliosis did not have fusion performed at the time of decompression. They found that a greater degree of preoperative scoliosis was associated with less improvement in back pain. We have not found curve severity to correlate with outcomes of reconstructive surgery in these patients. We do take a more aggressive approach, however, preferring to fuse patients with scoliosis who are undergoing a laminectomy even if the underlying medical condition permits only limited fusion.

Selection of fusion levels and instrumentation guidelines are otherwise as noted in the prior section.

COMBINED ANTERIOR–POSTERIOR TECHNIQUES

If they are fairly healthy, the majority of patients with degenerative scoliosis will require anterior and posterior procedures to achieve fusion, as well as coronal and sagittal balance. There are several indications for combined techniques in this complex patient population.

- Inflexible sagittal-plane imbalance is one of the most common indications for combined surgery. Relative lumbar kyphosis must be corrected to achieve sagittal plane balance. The use of structural allografts facilitates the restoration of lumbar lordosis. We favor femoral allografts, packed with autogenous cancellous graft; Harms-type mesh cages with autograft may also be used. Consideration of the scoliotic deformity is necessary; otherwise, mere placement of the structural grafts on the side of the approach—usually the curve convexity—will limit correction of the scoliosis.
- Degenerative curves of significant magnitude, especially with limited flexibility, may also require combined surgery. Coronal imbalance may also indicate the need for combined surgery.
- Patients who require a long fusion to the sacrum should also have a combined procedure because posterior fusion alone in this setting has a high incidence of failure (4,12). Most of these patients have significant degeneration across the lumbosacral junction, and many also have thoracolumbar kyphosis (which is a contraindication for ending the fusion at the thoracolumbar junction), so combined surgery is frequently indicated.
- In patients who have had failed posterior instrumented fusions, consider combined surgery. We and others (1,10,23) have found iliac fixation in the form of Galveston rods or iliac screws to be useful for achieving distal

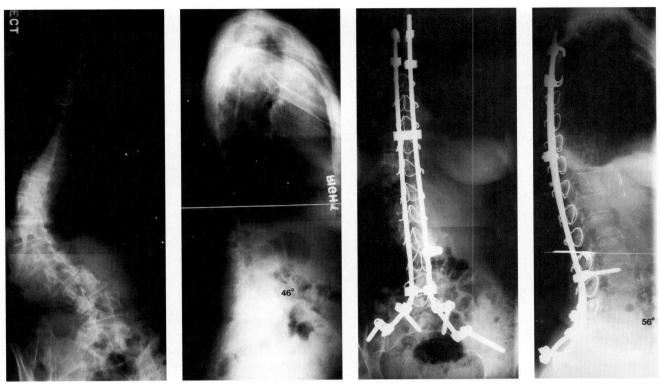

A,B   C,D

Figure 160.1.   This 71-year-old woman was first diagnosed with scoliosis at age 45. In the 5 years previous to presentation at this institution, she developed increasing low back pain and increasing prominence of her right hip. Anteroposterior (**A**) and lateral (**B**) standing radiographs demonstrate degenerative scoliosis with collapsing curve. The patient underwent a staged anterior and posterior spinal fusion, T-5 to the sacrum; the posterior fusion included multiple sublaminar wires and iliac screws. Her postoperative course had some brief episodes of cardiac ectopy and a urinary tract infection. Postoperative radiographs (**C,D**) demonstrate correction of the deformity, with coronal and sagittal balance achieved. At 2-year follow-up, she was doing well, with excellent improvement of her function and marked pain relief.

fixation (Fig. 160.1). For patients with reasonable bone quality, anterior structural allograft at the lumbosacral junction coupled with sacral screws alone that penetrate the anterior cortex may be adequate. Others (2,7,16,17) have used iliosacral screws or intrasacral screws (Jackson technique) for distal fixation.

As with posterior instrumented fusions, segmental fixation is preferred for combined surgery in this patient population. Sublaminar wires may be used as a component of the fixation, but use fixed components (hooks in a claw construct in the mid and upper thoracic spine, pedicle screws at the thoracolumbar junction) at the proximal end of the construct to decrease the risk of junctional kyphosis.

When the patient can tolerate it, perform both procedures under a single anesthetic to lower overall incidence of complications, nutritional depletion, and blood loss (5,21,24). Older patients, particularly those with coexist-

ing medical conditions or significant osteoporosis, may be less able to tolerate the lengthy anesthetic, however. Older patients with significantly osteoporotic bone may experience increased blood loss, which can lead to development of a coagulopathy during a prolonged procedure.

If the combined procedures in these older patients cannot be completed in 8–10 hours, then stage the procedure. The scheduled delay between stages may be 3–7 days, depending on coexisting medical conditions, the age of the patient, and scheduling issues. The occurrence of complications, however, may further delay the second-stage procedure.

Staged spinal surgery can result in nutritional depletion, which may lead to an increased incidence of infection, pneumonia, and urinary tract infection (5,21,24). We have shown that, particularly in the older patient population, use of total parenteral nutrition may decrease the rate of nutritional depletion, which may in turn decrease the risk of complications (15).

Grubb et al. (12) have found an average of 70% reduction of pain in patients fused for painful degenerative scoliosis, which is somewhat less than that seen for patients fused for painful adult idiopathic scoliosis (80% pain relief).

ANTERIOR FUSION WITH FEMORAL RINGS

- Perform a standard thoracoabdominal or retroperitoneal approach on the convexity of the curve to be addressed. Be sure to prep down to the pubic symphysis if L-5–S-1 is to be fused, as is the case in most of these patients.
- Identify segmental vessels and ligate or clip. Sweep the psoas muscle posteriorly, using bipolar cautery to control bleeding. Use blunt but careful dissection to sweep the great vessels forward. The common iliac will need to be mobilized if L-4–L5 or L-5–S-1 is to be exposed. This generally requires ligating the recurrent lumbar vein.
- Incise the disc space with a #11 blade. Use a rongeur to remove loose disc material, and a rongeur or osteotome to remove the osteophyte so that the endplate can be visualized. Peel the disc from the endplate using a Cobb elevator—exercise care in patients with osteoporosis.
- Remove additional disc material with a curved or straight curette, supplementing with a rongeur. A Blount spreader may be used with care to keep the disc space from collapsing in the convexity. The release must extend across to the contralateral annulus. If there is significant kyphosis, divide the anterior longitudinal ligament.
- The distalmost levels generally are in the fractional curve and also are most important for maintaining lordosis. Therefore, placement of the structural allograft should not block correction. If disc spaces in the convexity are to be placed, take care to place them as far toward the concavity as possible; do not place so large a graft that correction is blocked. For disc spaces that are not to receive structural allograft, pack morcelized cancellous bone lightly within, preferably autograft, although allograft can be used.
- Measure the height of the disc space to be filled with allograft. We use femoral shaft pieces cut at the time of surgery to fit the evacuated disc space. (Other surgeons prefer mesh cages.) The graft should be snug but not overly tight; that is, the release should open the disc space, not the graft itself. After confirming the size, fill the marrow cavity of the femoral allograft with rib graft or local bone graft, or morcelized cancellous allograft, and impact gently into place. Forcing an overly large

graft or inadequate release will result in graft breakage (with high risk for pseudarthrosis) or endplate fracture (with increased risk for subsidence).
- Use interference screws to prevent allograft migration. Place a 6.5 mm cancellous screw with a plastic washer lateral to the graft, into the vertebral body. Alternatively, a long enough screw can be placed lateral to the adjacent graft, skewering the graft below, to prevent migration of two allografts. It may be necessary to burr a small impression into the lateral aspect of the adjacent allograft to allow the washer to seat snugly. Although theoretically possible, we have not generally found that these screws impair our ability to place pedicle screws during the posterior instrumentation. Since instituting the use of these interference screws, we have not needed to replace anterior structural allograft.

PITFALLS AND COMPLICATIONS

Technically, surgery in this patient population can be very challenging for the following reasons:

- Osteoporotic bone is nearly always present and its vascular channels can contribute to greater bleeding rates than seen in the patient with normal bone.
- Many of these patients may have chronic hypertension, coronary artery disease, or other vascular conditions that contraindicate or limit the use of controlled hypotension to decrease surgical blood loss.
- One must select fusion levels carefully. Ending the fusion at a kyphotic level can lead to junctional kyphosis.
- Although sublaminar wires may be preferred in many patients because their use spreads corrective forces over many levels, they should not be used at the end vertebra because they do not control the spine in the axial plane; they may also result in junctional kyphosis. Use hooks or screws at the ends of the construct.
- Overcorrection of the curve may lead to truncal imbalance, which, if significant, may require revision surgery.
- Patients who undergo fusion surgery are at risk for developing degeneration above or below the fusion. Consider including severely degenerated adjacent levels to avoid rapid development of this problem. Extending the fusion should be balanced by the consideration of how much surgery should be done on the older, less healthy patient.
- Although osteoporotic patients have not been shown to have a higher rate of pseudarthrosis, poorer fixation due to poor bone quality, combined with autogenous bone graft from a site with more fat infiltration and fewer osteoprogenitor cells, is of concern.

The risk of complications among older patients

undergoing spinal surgery is about 60% (6,12,18,19,22). Although the rate is not significantly greater with increasing age (60–70 years, 70–80 years), there is no doubt that older patients are less able to tolerate complications and recover quickly from them. Keep this in mind when planning the surgery. We have shown that older patients may be more at risk for development of complications such as pneumonia and urinary tract infections, particularly if they are undergoing staged surgery. Consider nutritional supplementation to decrease their risk of nutritional depletion (15). Thromboembolic disease leading to pulmonary embolism occurs more commonly in older patients, particularly after combined anterior and posterior surgery (3). Our current practice is to use elastic stockings and sequential compression boots for prophylaxis of deep venous thrombosis. We remain vigilant in patients who have combined surgery, but we do not routinely anticoagulate these patients.

Although the mortality rate is not known, and most published studies in this patient population include small numbers of patients, we estimate it to be 1% to 5%. Discuss fully the numerous potential risks of spinal surgery with the patient, as well as her family, if desired, when she is offered any spinal surgery.

MINIMALLY INVASIVE TECHNIQUES

Recent advances in minimally invasive surgery have suggested that endoscopic surgery, both thoracoscopy and lumbar endoscopy, may result in lower morbidity and decreased length of hospital stay (20,26). Unfortunately, such techniques are difficult to learn and have not yet been proven to demonstrate comparable fusion rates to that achieved in open procedures. In general, for degenerative scoliosis, the indicated anterior procedure is in the lumbar or lumbosacral spine. Currently, most of the lumbar endoscopic techniques have concentrated on screw-in–type cages, which are not well suited for degenerative scoliosis because of the presence of multiplanar deformity.

 AUTHORS' PERSPECTIVES

Reconstructive surgery in the patient with degenerative scoliosis is complex and requires a thorough understanding of a multitude of factors, including pain sources, coronal and sagittal balance, fusion techniques, indications for decompression, indications for combined anterior and posterior surgery, and instrumentation choices, as well as the potential for complications. With appropriate patient selection, however, and realistic expectations of surgery on the part of both the patient and the surgeon, the majority of patients will have a satisfactory outcome.

REFERENCES

Each reference is categorized according to the following scheme: *, classic article; #, review article; !, basic research article; and +, clinical results/outcome study.

+ 1. Boachie-Adjei O, Dendrinos G, Ogilvie J, et al. Management of Adult Spinal Deformity with Combined Anterior-posterior Arthrodesis and Luque-Galveston Instrumentation. *J Spinal Disorder* 1991;4:131.

! 2. Camp JF, Caudle R, Ashmun RD, Roach J. Immediate Complications of Cotrel-Dubousset Instrumentation to the Sacro-pelvis: A Clinical and Biomechanical Study. *Spine* 1990;15:932.

+ 3. Dearborn J, Hu S, Tribus C, et al. Thromboembolic Complications after Spinal Reconstructive Surgery. *Spine* 1999;24:1471.

+ 4. Devlin V, Boachie-Adjei O, Bradford D, et al. Treatment of Adult Spinal Deformity to the Sacrum Wing: CD Instrumentation. *J Spinal Disord* 1991;4:1.

* 5. Dick J, Boachie-Adjei O, Wilson M. One-stage versus Two-stage Anterior and Posterior Spinal Reconstruction in Adults. *Spine* 1992;17:S310.

6. Dickson J, Mirkovic S, Noble P, et al. Results of Operative Treatment of Idiopathic Scoliosis in Adults. *J Bone Joint Surg Am* 1995;77:513.

+ 7. Farcy J, Rawlins B, Glassman S. Technique and Results of Fixation to the Sacrum with Iliosacral Screws. *Spine* 1992;17:S190.

+ 8. Frazier D, Lipson S, Fossel A, et al. Associations between Spinal Deformity and Outcomes after Decompression for Spinal Stenosis. *Spine* 1997;22:2025.

+ 9. Gillespy T, Gillespy T, Revak C. Progressive Senile Scoliosis: Seven Cases of Increasing Spinal Curves in Elderly Patients. *Skeletal Radiol* 1985;13:280.

! 10. Glazer P, Colliou O, Lotz J, et al. Biomechanical Analysis of Lumbosacral Fixation. *Spine* 1996;21:1211.

+ 11. Grubb S, Lipscomb H, Coonrad R. Degenerative Adult Onset Scoliosis. *Spine* 1988;13:241.

+ 12. Grubb S, Lipscomb H, Suh P. Results of Surgical Treatment of Painful Adult Scoliosis. *Spine* 1994;19:1619.

13. Hanley E. The Indications for Lumbar Spinal Fusion With and Without Instrumentation. *Spine* 1995;20:S143.

+ 14. Healey J, Lane J. Structural Scoliosis in Osteoporotic Women. *Clin Orthop* 1985;195:216.

* 15. Hu S, Fontaine F, Kelley B, et al. Nutritional Depletion in Staged Spinal Reconstructive Surgery: The Effect of Total Parenteral Nutrition. *Spine* 1998;23:1401.

! 16. Jackson RP, McManus AC. The Iliac Buttress: A Computer Tomographic Study of Sacral Anatomy. *Spine* 1993;18:1318.

+ 17. Jackson RP, Ebelke DK, McManus AC. Clinical Results and Standing Radiographic Sagittal Plane Analysis in Spondylolisthesis Insrumented to the Sacrum with New Techniques. *Orthop Trans* 1995–1996;19:593.

+ 18. Jonsson B, Shromqvist B. Lumbar Spine Surgery in the

Elderly: Complications and Surgical Results. *Spine* 1994; 19:1431.

+ 19. Kostuik J, Hall B. Spinal Fusions to the Sacrum in Adults with Scoliosis. *Spine* 1983;8:489.

+ 20. Kuslich S, Ulstrom C, Griffith S, et al. The Bagby and Kuslich Method of Lumbar Interbody Fusion. *Spine* 1998;23:1267.

+ 21. Mandelbaum BR, Tolo VT, McAfee PC, Burest P. Nutritional Deficiencies after Staged Anterior and Posterior Spinal Reconstructive Surgery. *Clin Orthop* 1988;234: 5.

\# 22. Nuber G, Schafer M. Surgical Management of Adult Scoliosis. *Clin Orthop* 1986;208:228.

! 23. Pashman RS, Hu S, Schendel MJ, Bradford DS. Sacral Screw Loads in Lumbosacral Fixation for Spinal Deformity. *Spine* 1993;18:2465.

+ 24. Powell ET, Krengel WF, King HA, Lagrone MO. Comparison of Same-day Sequential Anterior and Posterior Spinal Fusion with Delayed Two-staged Anterior and Posterior Spinal Fusion. *Spine* 1994;19:1256.

+ 25. Pritchett J, Bortel D. Degenerative Symptomatic Lumbar scoliosis. *Spine* 1993;18:700.

+ 26. Regan J, Ben-Yishay A, Mack M. Video-assisted Thoracoscopic Excision of Herniated Thoracic Disc: Description of Technique and Preliminary Experience in the First 29 Cases. *J Spinal Disord* 1998;11:183.

+ 27. Velis KP, Healey JH, Schneider R. Osteoporosis in Unstable Adult Scoliosis. *Clin Orthop* 1988;237:132.

CHAPTER 161
SURGERY FOR KYPHOSIS DEFORMITY

Jack K. Mayfield

PRINCIPLES OF TREATMENT

Kyphosis is a posteriorly directed convex curvature of the spine in the sagittal plane. In the thoracic spine, the normal kyphosis ranges from 20° to 40° as measured from the superior endplate of the second thoracic vertebra to the inferior endplate of the twelfth thoracic vertebra. In the adult cervical and lumbar spine, both of which are normally lordotic, any posteriorly directed curvature of 5° or greater is considered abnormal kyphosis.

J. K. Mayfield: Phoenix Spine Center, St. Luke's Hospital Medical Center, Phoenix, Arizona, 85006; and Department of Materials, Chemical and Bioengineering, Arizona State University.

A distinction should be made between *sagittal kyphosis* and *rotational kyphosis*. In sagittal kyphosis, the vertebral bodies remain in the sagittal plane and the spine angulates in that plane (Fig. 161.1). In rotational kyphosis, however, the vertebral bodies are rotated out of the sagittal plane, as is commonly seen in paralytic curvatures and kyphosis secondary to neurofibromatosis (Fig. 161.2). In either situation, once the anterior vertebral column is no longer in the sagittal plane, there is reduced resistance to kyphotic bending moments and thus an increased propensity for a kyphosis to progress. Most kyphotic deformities seem to fall within the sagittal kyphosis category.

A distinction should also be made between a short-radius and a long-radius kyphotic deformity. A short-radius curve is one that is more angular over a few verte-

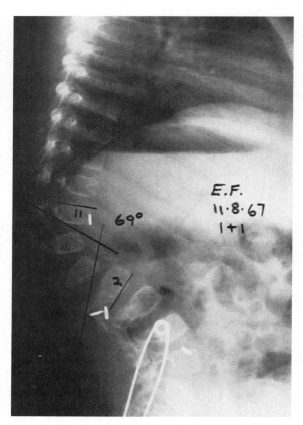

Figure 161.1. This 1-year-old child has a short-radius sagittal kyphosis secondary to radiation and laminectomy for neuroblastoma.

bral segments, and a long-radius kyphosis is a smooth curve of less acute angulation over many vertebral segments (Figs. 161.1, 161.3).

All kyphotic spinal deformities have variable degrees of rigidity and flexibility. Frequently there is an element of apical rigidity with variable degrees of flexibility at the ends of the curvature. The goal in correcting the kyphosis is to mobilize the rigid apex or to correct the flexible ends of the curve to bring the apex closer to the center of gravity, thereby placing the bone graft in the area of fusion under maximum compression (Fig. 161.4).

The degree of flexibility can be determined before surgery by a supine hyperextension lateral radiograph of the spine taken with a bolster placed under the apex of the kyphosis (Fig. 161.3) in short-radius kyphosis, and by a lateral radiograph of the spine with the patient in traction in long-radius paralytic curves.

Although traction as a means of correction has been gradually replaced by more aggressive anterior and posterior fusion and segmental instrumentation, in some situations traction can be helpful. Three traction techniques can be beneficial in the treatment of kyphosis: halo-wheelchair

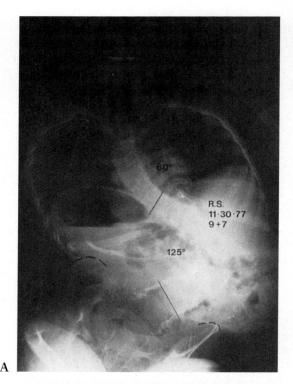

A

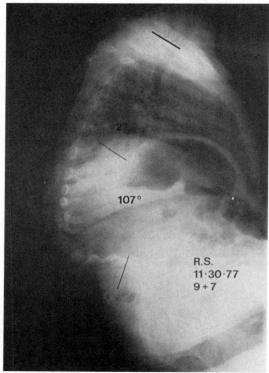

B

Figure 161.2. **A:** A 9-year-old child has a paralytic right thoracolumbar scoliosis of 125°. **B:** In addition to the paralytic scoliosis, a rotational thoracolumbar kyphosis of 107° is present. *(continued)*

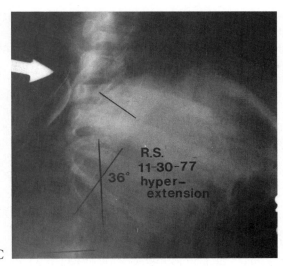

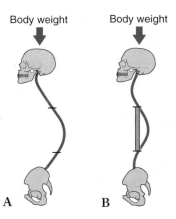

Figure 161.4. **A:** Diagram of kyphosis. **B:** The apex has been corrected somewhat and the flexible ends of the kyphosis are corrected so that the anterior strut graft is now in line with the body weight (*BW*).

Figure 161.2. *(continued)* **C:** The rotational kyphosis corrects to 36° on supine hyperextension (a flexible kyphosis).

traction, halo-femoral traction, and halo-hyperextension traction. Halo-wheelchair traction provides longitudinal traction against gravity and allows the patient mobility. Halo-femoral traction provides stronger, steady axial forces if continuous traction is essential.

A word of caution, however, is necessary about the use of heavy axial traction. If there is apical rigidity of the curve as determined by hyperextension lateral radiographs, paraplegia can be a complication because of the spinal cord's stretching over the rigid acute kyphotic apex. Mobilizing the apex of a kyphotic deformity is essential before heavy traction is used. In large kyphotic deformities

that have a short radius (neurofibromatosis), axial traction is more beneficial than three-point bending. In comparison, large kyphotic deformities with a long radius (such as Scheuermann's kyphosis) respond more effectively to three-point bending. In short-radius kyphotic deformities (such as spondylolisthesis), a combination of axial traction and three-point bending is needed (Fig. 161.5) (13).

Many disorders manifest kyphotic spine deformities that may need treatment. Any kyphosis that is increasing in magnitude may need surgical stabilization. It is helpful to classify the disorders by the degree of rigidity and flexibility as well as the magnitude of curve radius (Table 161.1).

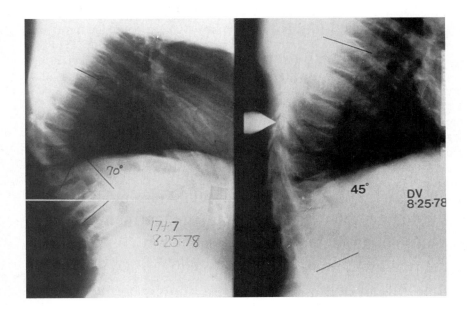

Figure 161.3. At age 17 years, this patient developed a long-radius thoracolumbar kyphosis of 70° as a result of radiation. This kyphosis corrects to 45° on a supine hyperextension lateral radiograph.

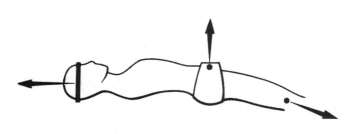

Figure 161.5.   Halo-femoral longitudinal and pelvic hyperextension traction for lumbosacral kyphosis from spondylolisthesis.

Table 161.1. *Classification of Kyphoses*	
Sagittal	*Rotational*
Short-radius rigid	Short-radius rigid
Long-radius rigid	Long-radius rigid
Short-radius flexible	Short-radius flexible
Long-radius flexible	Long-radius flexible

INDICATIONS FOR SURGERY

Indications for surgical treatment of kyphosis depend on the diagnosis, the etiology of the kyphosis, the curve progression, the location of the kyphosis, and the age of the patient. In general, the kyphotic spine deformity that is increasing in magnitude in an adult needs surgical stabilization. In the child, however, a brace may be helpful, depending on the age of the child, the etiology of the kyphosis, and the magnitude of the curve.

CONGENITAL TYPE I KYPHOSIS

The congenital type I kyphotic spinal deformity, in which there is incomplete vertebral formation, is usually diagnosed in childhood and has an average progression of 5° yearly (26,27,29). It usually involves only two to three vertebrae, and surgical stabilization is usually recommended when progression has been documented. There is a high incidence of spinal cord compression with large degrees of kyphosis, and early stabilization in a young child when the curve is small is ideal. An *in situ* posterior fusion before the age of 3 years will prevent late deformity. *In situ* posterior fusion must include the normal vertebrae above and below the congenital kyphosis. The posterior fusion will tether the posterior growth of these normal vertebrae so that their anterior growth will correct the deformity (these normal vertebrae will become trapezoidal in shape with growth) (Fig. 161.6).

Augment the posterior fusion at 6 months to achieve a thick posterior mass, thick enough to withstand the anterior growth forces. When an angulation of 50° or more is present, an anterior fusion is also needed. If the spinal cord is compressed anteriorly, perform an anterior decompression concomitantly with the anterior strut graft fusion. In the adult, I recommend a second-stage posterior fusion with instrumentation after the anterior correction. Osteotomies for deformity correction are not commonly used as in type II congenital kyphosis.

CONGENITAL TYPE II KYPHOSIS

In the congenital type II kyphotic disorder, in which failure of segmentation of the spine occurs anteriorly, progression of the kyphosis usually averages 5° yearly (15). The segmentation failure can involve only two vertebrae but also may involve many contiguous vertebrae. For young patients, I recommend an *in situ* posterior fusion to include one normal vertebral segment at each end of the curve. In the young child, an augmentation posterior spinal fusion may be necessary 6 months later to generate a thick fusion (Fig. 161.6). In the adolescent patient with an unacceptable kyphosis greater than 50°, a staged correction is indicated, with anterior osteotomy and anterior fusion using an intervertebral cage structural graft, followed by posterior fusion and instrumentation (15,26,27, 29). Spinal cord compression is usually not seen in type II congenital kyphosis.

POSTTRAUMATIC KYPHOSIS

Acute kyphosis associated with spinal instability due to fracture or dislocation usually requires reduction of the kyphosis, with spinal fusion (14,19). When the kyphosis occurs late and is increasing in magnitude, surgical stabilization and fusion are indicated. Particularly if the kyphosis spans multiple vertebral segments, a two-stage anterior and posterior fusion and stabilization are frequently necessary. In late posttraumatic kyphosis, the use of intervertebral structural cages with anterior fusion maintains lumbar lordosis below the fracture more effectively than an interbody fusion alone.

SPONDYLOLISTHESIS GRADES IV AND V

Anatomically, the grade IV and V spondylolistheses are usually lumbosacral kyphotic deformities and require reduction, stabilization, and fusion (4).

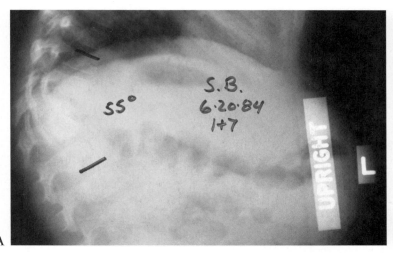
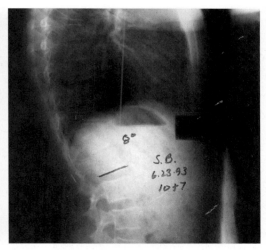

Figure 161.6. **A:** This 1½-year-old girl has type II congenital kyphosis at T-12–L-1 of 55°. **B:** At age 10, after *in situ* posterior fusion that included the normal vertebra above and below the congenital kyphosis. The kyphosis has corrected to 8°.

POSTLAMINECTOMY KYPHOSIS

Any progressive postlaminectomy kyphotic deformity (usually in a child) requires stabilization and fusion (11). Posterior segmental instrumentation and fusion will be necessary along with anterior fusion. Frequently, strut graft stabilization will be needed in larger kyphotic deformities. The entire kyphotic deformity must be instrumented and fused (11).

SCHEUERMANN'S KYPHOSIS

Scheuermann's kyphosis is seen in older adolescents and adults (19). In older adolescents with little vertebral growth remaining, a kyphosis of 70° or more usually requires surgical correction and fusion, especially if associated with back pain. In the adult, back pain associated with thoracic kyphosis greater than 75° to 80° is an indication for surgical treatment. If the kyphosis is located in the thoracolumbar spine, surgical treatment is indicated when the curve magnitude is much less than 70° because of the acute lumbar hyperlordosis below the kyphosis and associated problems with low back pain in an adult. A staged anterior interbody fusion followed by a posterior fusion with segmental instrumentation will effectively correct and stabilize this kyphosis; intervertebral cages could be used to maintain correction of the kyphosis and maintain lumbar lordosis (Fig. 161.7).

POSTRADIATION KYPHOSIS

Surgery in children is indicated when postradiation kyphosis (12) is documented to be progressive despite ade-

quate orthotic treatment. It is also indicated when the kyphosis is too large for orthotic control, or the deformity is cosmetically unacceptable. These curves are usually rigid and the potential for correction is limited.

PARALYTIC KYPHOSIS

Paralytic kyphoses are usually collapsing deformities that are seen in children (14,19). Surgical treatment of the kyphosis is usually planned when the child has a skeletal age of 10–12 years, when most of the axial skeletal growth has occurred. Until that age, orthotic treatment is recommended.

NEUROFIBROMATOSIS

Kyphosis in neurofibromatosis does not respond to orthotic treatment, and surgery is indicated when the kyphosis is 50° or more in a child or is documented to be increasing in magnitude (1,28). Anterior and posterior arthrodesis and instrumentation are usually necessary. Complications are common.

DIASTROPHIC DWARFISM

Progressive cervical kyphosis in diastrophic dwarfism should be stabilized early to prevent neurologic complications (2). Thoracic and thoracolumbar kyphoses usually appears in the juvenile years, is associated with scoliosis, and should receive early orthotic treatment. If progression occurs despite orthotic treatment, surgical treatment of the kyphosis is indicated.

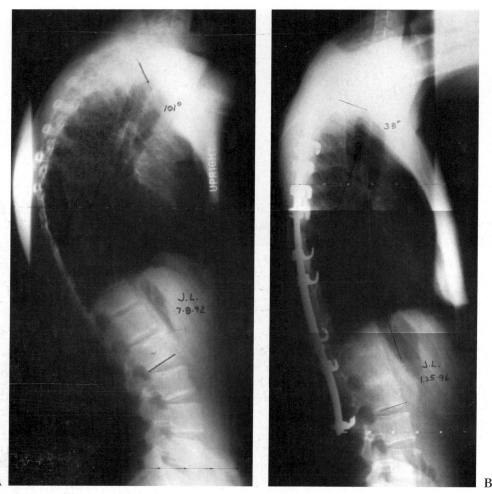

Figure 161.7. A: An 18-year-old man with 101° thoracic kyphosis from Scheuermann's disease. **B:** Four years after staged anterior interbody fusion and posterior fusion and segmental instrumentation. The kyphosis is corrected to 38°.

ACHONDROPLASIA

Kyphosis usually occurs in the thoracolumbar spine and may occur at an early age, but most kyphoses resolve. When apical vertebral hypoplasia is present (achondroplasia) (25), progression may occur and orthotic treatment is recommended. Surgical treatment of the kyphosis is indicated if progression occurs despite orthotic treatment or if anterior spinal cord compression occurs.

ADULT IDIOPATHIC KYPHOSCOLIOSIS

Rotational kyphosis in the adult is usually treated surgically when the kyphoscoliosis is progressing and if the scoliosis is greater than 60° to 70° (19). Frequently, the lumbar curve in kyphoscoliosis has rotational vertebral subluxation and is relatively kyphotic. Adult scoliosis fre-

quently requires anterior and posterior arthrodesis and instrumentation. Structural intervertebral cage grafts anteriorly are useful in creating and maintaining lumbar lordosis.

FLATBACK SYNDROME

Flatback syndrome results from the loss of lumbar lordosis and normal sacral slope. For patients with flatback syndrome to stand, their trunks must remain bent forward. To maintain this position, they are required to flex their knees, and they complain of pain and fatigue (6,8, 10). This syndrome is frequently seen after posterior distraction instrumentation in the lumbar spine, especially if the instrumentation approaches L-5 or the sacrum without supplemental anterior support (Fig. 161.8).

In young children with osteopenic bone, posterior

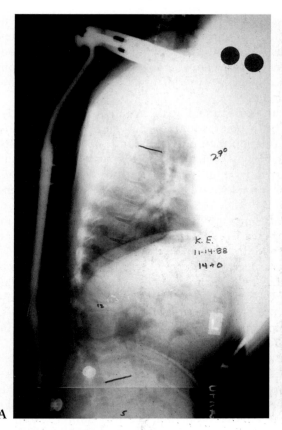

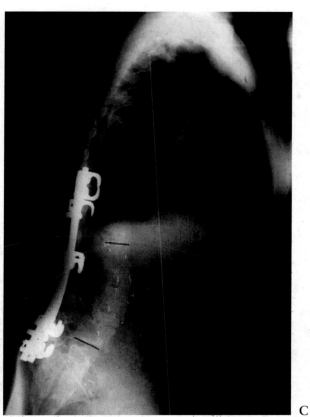

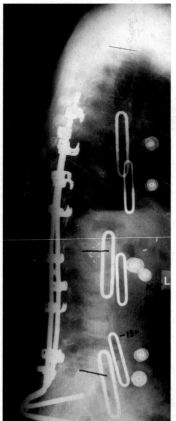

Figure 161.8. **A:** This 14-year-old boy has Gauché's disease with collapse of T-12, L-2, and L-5, with kyphosis and back pain. He has been treated for several years with an orthosis. **B:** Six months after posterior fusion and instrumentation to the sacrum, the lumbar lordosis was minus 13°. He had difficulty maintaining an upright posture (flatback syndrome). **C:** After anterior/posterior osteotomies, fusion, and instrumentation, the sagittal alignment is much improved.

compression instrumentation cannot maintain correct sagittal alignment. In this situation, intervertebral structural cage arthrodesis may be helpful to correct and maintain lumbar lordosis, in conjunction with posterior segmental instrumentation and arthrodesis. A flatback from a previous fusion needs posterior osteotomies along with anterior and posterior stabilization and arthrodesis.

RHEUMATOID SPONDYLITIS

Progressive kyphosis in rheumatoid spondylitis (Marie-Strümpel Kyphosis) is common and requires surgical treatment to maintain an upright head position. Usually, anterior and posterior osteotomies with segmental instrumentation are necessary. Single-level or multiple-level osteotomies may be utilized (5,7,9,21,22,24) (see Chapters 153, 154).

PREOPERATIVE PLANNING

In preoperative planning, distinguish between a short-radius and a long-radius kyphosis, and determine whether the curve is flexible or rigid. In short-radius curves, obtain a hyperextension cross-table lateral radiograph with a bolster under the apex of the kyphosis. Two interpretations should be made: the correctability of the apex of the kyphosis and the correctability of the ends of the kyphosis (Fig. 161.4) (13).

In Figure 161.4, the correction occurs in the more flexible ends of the kyphotic curve. When the ends of the kyphosis are flexible, a long-radius, unstable kyphosis can be converted to a short-radius stable curve. In this situation, use an anterior strut and interbody fusion as a first stage to stabilize the apical rigid component. Follow with a posterior approach to correct the flexible ends of the kyphosis, usually with segmental instrumentation. The goal at completion is to have the body weight in line with the apical strut graft, a curve configuration that is biomechanically stable (Fig. 161.4) (13).

In long-radius curves, a cross-table lateral radiograph, with the patient in longitudinal traction, is more helpful, particularly in paralytic curves. In general, rigid kyphotic deformities require strut grafting and interbody fusion of the rigid apical component in addition to posterior fusion and stabilization. Some mobilization of the rigid apex can be accomplished with disc excision and osteotomy, placing a strong strut graft in the corrected position.

Traction

Preoperative traction in rigid kyphotic curves (e.g., congenital kyphosis) is generally contraindicated because of the risk of precipitating anterior spinal cord compression. Preoperative traction for relatively inflexible long-radius curves is usually not beneficial, but it can be beneficial after an anterior disc excision, interbody fusion, and anterior release. In this situation, halo-hyperextension traction for 2 weeks between an anterior spinal release and fusion and a second-stage posterior fusion and instrumentation can be useful.

In neurofibromatosis with kyphoscoliosis and early spinal cord compression, careful and judicious halo-femoral traction may provide enough correction to improve neurologic function before surgical stabilization. Preoperative traction is useful in this situation, because the apex of the kyphosis is frequently rotated and inherently more flexible (28). A preoperative myelogram and computed tomography (CT) scan are recommended in neurofibromatosis because of the high incidence of dural ectasia and intradural and extradural tumors.

In cervical kyphosis resulting from diastrophic dwarfism and in thoracolumbar kyphosis in achondroplasia, obtain a CT scan to verify the spinal-canal size and bony architecture before surgery. Preoperative somatosensory, evoked potentials are useful for baseline measurements in preparation for intraoperative spinal cord monitoring.

In preoperative planning, determine the levels of posterior instrumentation. To be mechanically sound, the posterior instrumented end vertebrae should be close to the weight-bearing line. Include the entire length of the kyphotic curve in the fusion and instrumentation.

 ## SURGICAL TECHNIQUES

The anterior surgical techniques used in the surgical treatment of kyphosis are as follows:

- Strut graft (fibula or rib)
- Inlay rib graft
- Interbody fusion
- Vascularized rib or fibular graft
- Anterior vertebral osteotomy
- Interbody screw and rod instrumentation for rotational kyphosis
- Intervertebral structural cages

The posterior techniques for the surgical treatment of kyphosis are the following:

- Posterior spinal fusion with Moe facet fusion
- Posterior segmental instrumentation
- Posterior vertebral osteotomy
- Eggshell technique

ANTERIOR STRUT GRAFT

In all nonrotational kyphosis surgery, a subperiosteal exposure of the spine is recommended for maximal bone exposure for arthrodesis.

- Note the end vertebrae of the kyphosis and perform complete discectomies at each disc space between the end vertebrae. Incise the annulus fibrosus with a knife and excise the annulus with a narrow Luxsell rongeur.
- Incise the periphery of the cartilaginous endplate down to bone with a knife and peel it off the bony vertebral endplate with a narrow Cobb elevator.
- Remove the endplates with rongeurs, and remove the remaining disc with straight and angled curets.
- Pack the disc space with thrombin-soaked Gelfoam.

  Once all disc spaces are cleaned back to the posterior annulus, curet the endplates and interior of the bodies of the end vertebrae to create a seating hole for the strut.

- Correct the kyphosis by pushing on the apex of the curve and measure the length of strut required in the corrected position.
- Cut the graft (rib or fibula) longer than measured and round the ends with bone cutters.
- Insert one end of the strut in the end vertebra. Cut a trough in the lateral aspect in the other end vertebra. Correct the kyphosis by pushing on its apex, and impact the strut through the side trough and into the undercut end vertebra (Fig. 161.9). The intervening vertebra may have to be fashioned to allow the strut graft to fit.

- Pack the intervertebral disc spaces solidly with morselized rib graft.
- If the kyphosis is larger and angular, several parallel struts may have to be used. Use Pinto distractors to correct the kyphosis while the struts are inserted. These distractors are nonimplantable and come in three sizes. Each distractor is a turnbuckle with pronged feet at each end that anchor in the vertebral bodies. When maximum correction of the apical kyphosis is achieved, insert the struts and remove the Pinto distractors (Fig. 161.10).

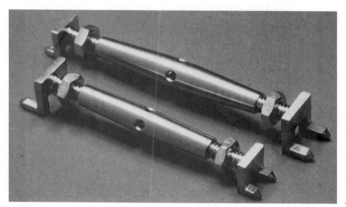

A

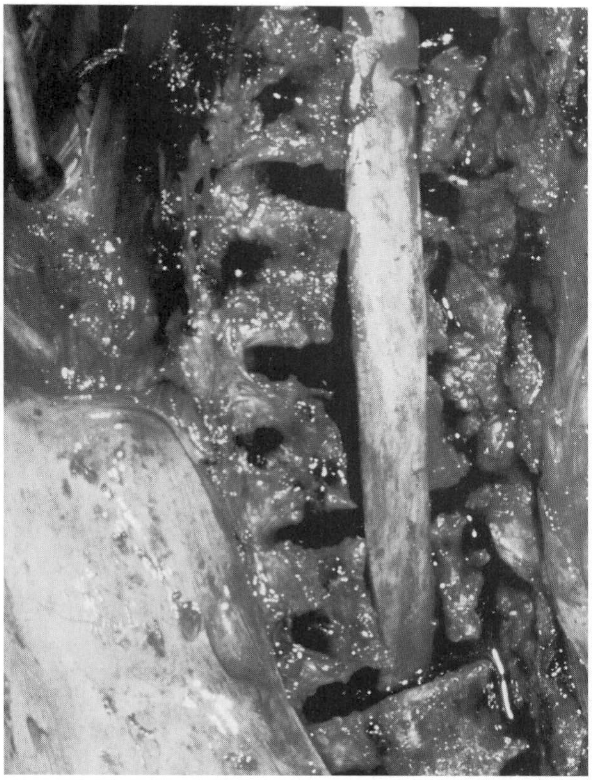

Figure 161.9. Intraoperative picture of an anterior strut graft.

B

Figure 161.10. **A:** Pinto distractors (nonimplantable). **B:** Acute angular kyphosis with two Pinto distractors holding the deformity in a corrected position. *(continued)*

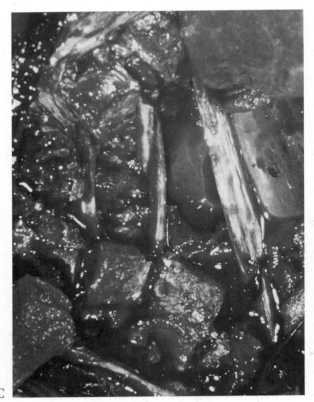

C

Figure 161.10. *(continued)* C: The Pinto distractors are removed and the three strut grafts are anchored in the vertebrae.

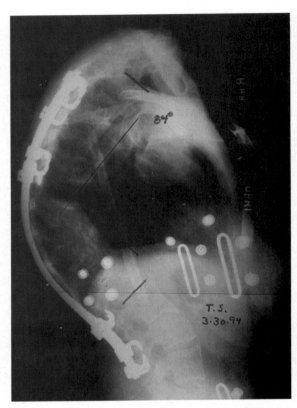

Figure 161.11. Radiograph shows an anterior fibular graft with bone graft positioned back to the vertebral bodies.

■ In large kyphotic deformities it is important to fill the dead space between the vertebral bodies and the strut graft with bone graft (Fig. 161.11) (19).

In rotational kyphosis, an additional and very useful strut graft technique, originally pioneered by P. Stagnara, consists of creating an osteoperiosteal flap from the vertebral bodies that are in the kyphotic area (23).

■ Use a wide osteotome to reflect the anterior portion of the vertebrae for the length of the kyphotic curve. This technique creates a good vascular bed.
■ Countersink the fibular or rib strut graft, with the bony flap adjacent to the graft, usually on the concavity of the scoliotic curve.
■ Pack the intervertebral disc spaces with bone graft (Fig. 161.12).

INTERBODY ARTHRODESIS

Perform an intervertebral disc excision as previously described. Break the bony endplates with an angled Lambotte osteotome or curet, and pack the entire disc space with rib graft (see Chapters 146, 155).

INLAY GRAFT

The inlay graft technique is useful when the kyphosis is not acutely angulated.

■ Clean all the intervening disc spaces and prepare each end vertebra of the curve as described in the strut graft technique.
■ Cut a trough in the interposed vertebral bodies with large Luxsell and Adson rongeurs and curved curets. The trough should be deep enough to bury the rib or fibular graft.
■ The trough may also be filled with morcelized bone graft if anterior flexibility is needed during the posterior instrumentation.
■ Correct the kyphosis by pushing on the apex of the curve, countersink the premeasured graft in the trough, and lock it in the end vertebrae.

VASCULARIZED RIB GRAFT

A vascularized rib graft has a distinct advantage in circumstances when early stabilization, earlier arthodesis, and shorter immobilization are needed.

■ When the thoracotomy is performed, make the entrance to the chest cavity through the intercostal muscle of the

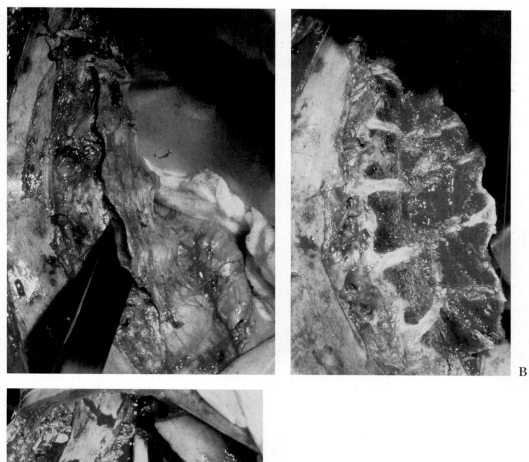

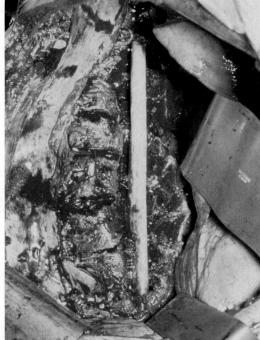

Figure 161.12. **A:** A Lambotte osteotome is used to create a vertebral flap. **B:** The vertebral flap is mobilized. **C:** The fibular strut graft is placed with the intervertebral disc spaces filled with bone graft. Bone graft is then placed from the flap to the vertebral bodies.

rib that articulates with the superior end vertebra of the kyphosis.

■ Determine the length of the vascular pedicle needed. Measure the length of the strut graft that is needed on the anterior portion of the rib and cut it free with a rib cutter, leaving all soft tissue attached.

■ Sharply dissect the neurovascular pedicle back to the rib base to allow mobilization of the strut. Expose each end of the strut subperiosteally for approximately 2 cm and impact and countersink these graft ends in the prepared end vertebra of the kyphosis, being careful not to kink the vascular pedicle (Fig. 161.13) (3).

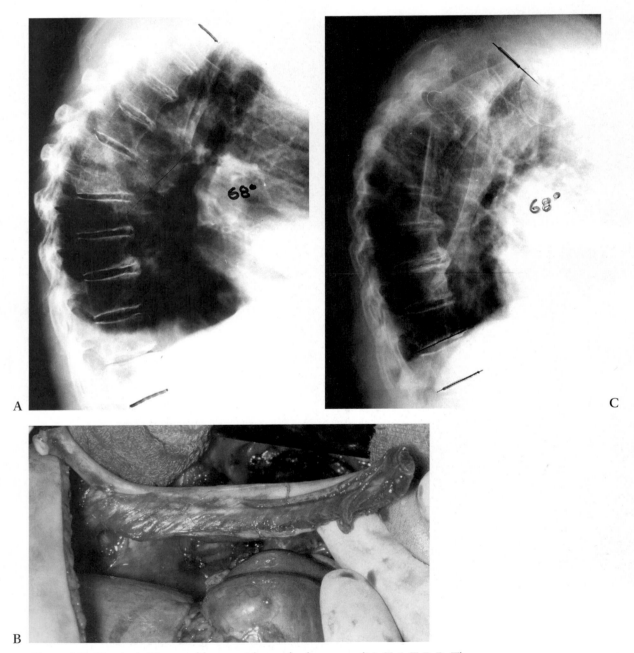

Figure 161.13. **A:** A 72-year-old man with vertebral osteomyelitis T-6–T-7. **B:** The vascularized rib graft with the neurovascular pedicle is at the left. **C:** This postoperative radiograph shows the anchored vascularized rib graft. Note the supplemental inlay and interbody grafts in the area of the osteomyelitis.

ANTERIOR VERTEBRAL OSTEOTOMY

After performing a subperiosteal exposure of the vertebra in a type II congenital kyphosis, the remnant of the posterior disc can be visualized. If the disc remnant cannot be visualized, perform the osteotomy at the level of the vertebral foramina to allow sagittal correction after the osteotomy.

- Perform multiple vertebral osteotomies at the levels of the posterior disc remnants or foramina using gouges, osteotomes, and curets. A power burr can be helpful for a portion of the osteotomy.
- Clean the disc spaces of all soft tissue back to the posterior annulus using curets and rongeurs.
- Use angled curets to complete the osteotomy on the opposite side, back to the posterior annulus.
- Check mobility of each intervertebral space with a Blount spreader, and pack each space with rib graft cut into small pieces (Fig. 161.14) (19).
- Use intervertebral structural cages to correct sagittal alignment and prevent vertebral collapse at the site of the osteotomies. The longer kyphotic curves will also need strut graft support.

ANTERIOR INSTRUMENTATION TO CORRECT ROTATIONAL KYPHOSIS

- Expose the anterior spine extraperiosteally on the convex side.

- Using rongeurs and curets, clean the disc space of its annulus fibrosus and nucleus pulposus, along with the cartilage endplates at each vertebral level to be instrumented (the same technique as an interbody fusion).
- Measure the vertebral body size with a caliper to determine the appropriate length of screw to be used.
- Prepare a hole with a trocar in each vertebral body to be instrumented at the midlateral aspect of the rotated vertebra.
- Insert a vertebral screw and washer, aiming each screw toward the opposite pedicle or anterior to the pedicle.
- Take great care to identify the anterior longitudinal ligament at each level so that the degree of vertebral rotation is appreciated before the screw is inserted.
- Prepare the disc spaces for grafting by breaking the bony endplates with an osteotome and curets to ensure good cancellous bony exposure.
- Distract the disc spaces with a Blount spreader, and hold them open with whole-rib grafts.
- After assembling the rod-and-screw construct, correct the sagittal deformity.
- With the Zielke system, attach the derotation bar and derotate the spine as the nuts are sequentially tightened. As the spine is derotated, the scoliosis and rotational kyphosis are corrected.
- With segmental rod-and-screw systems, sequentially distract the intervertebral segments as the rod is introduced into one screw at a time.

The whole-rib intervertebral grafts prevent interverte-

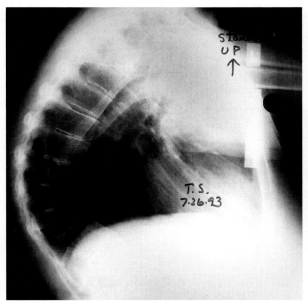
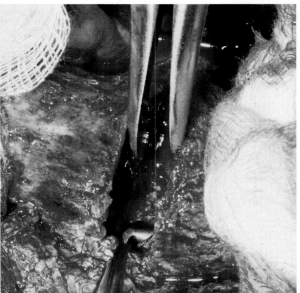

A   B

Figure 161.14. **A:** Type II congenital kyphosis. Note the posterior disc remnants in the area of the anterior bar. **B:** After osteotomy is completed with angled curets, gouges, and rongeurs. Mobility is then checked with a Blount spreader. See Figure 161.11 for the postoperative radiograph.

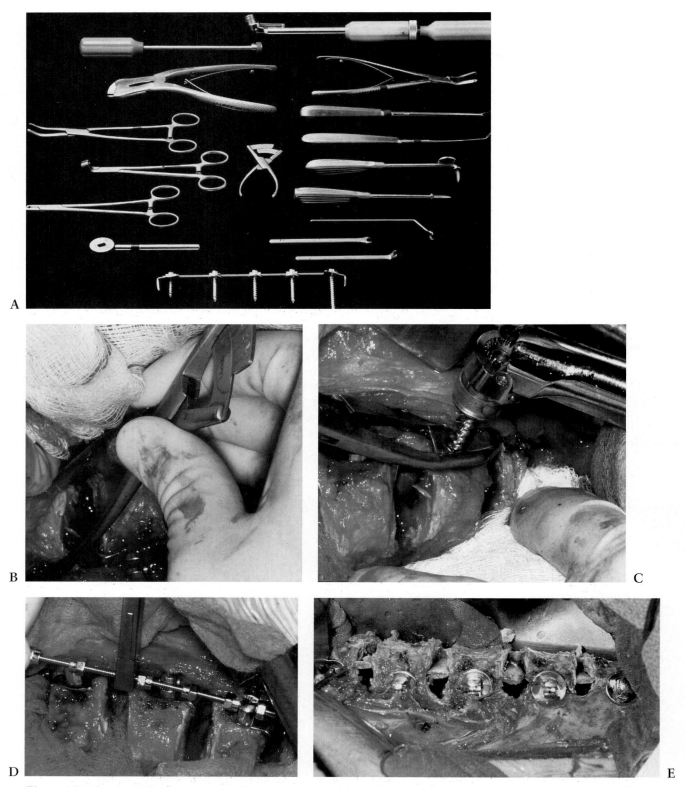

Figure 161.15.   **A:** Zielke instrumentation. **B:** Measuring the vertebral size with a caliper. **C:** Inserting a vertebral screw with a plate (a washer may be used instead). **D:** Rod insertion. Double nuts are used at the end of the construct and single nuts are used at other levels compressing toward the apex of the curve. **E:** Whole-rib grafts may be used to prevent collapse and sagittal kyphosis. Intervertebral cages may be useful in this situation. *(continued)*

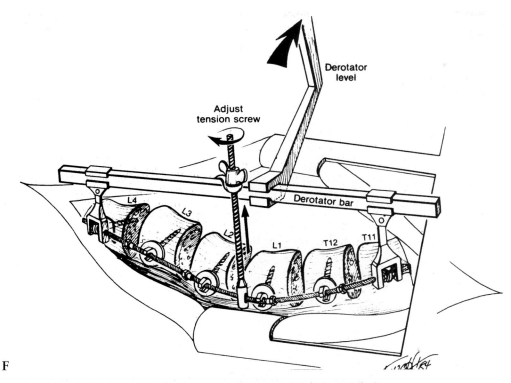

F

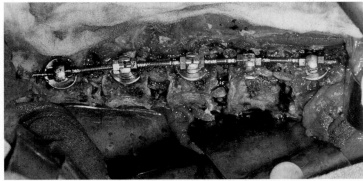

G

Figure 161.15. *(continued)* **F:** The derotator bar is used to pull the vertebral bodies back toward the sagittal plane, derotating the spine and correcting rotational kyphotic collapse. **G:** After derotation, the system is locked and the nuts are tightened.

bral collapse and the development of sagittal kyphosis after derotation has occurred. A supplementary posterior fusion and segmental instrumentation is usually done as a second-stage procedure (Fig. 161.15).

INTERVERTEBRAL CAGES AND FEMORAL ALLOGRAFT DOWELS OR RINGS

The use of metallic intervertebral cages and femoral allograft dowels or rings as structural grafts has been useful in correcting and maintaining correction of kyphosis. They unload the posterior segmental instrumentation by participating in load sharing. This combination creates a more rigid construct for arthrodesis. They are especially useful in maintaining lumbar lordosis.

- Expose the spine extraperiosteally and create a flap of the annulus. Tag the flap with suture, then clean the disc spaces of all soft tissue as previously described.
- The most useful cages are those that allow abundant bony ingrowth through a mesh design and add sufficient structural support. The allografts are hollow in the center for autografts, for early bony ingrowth.
- Insert a wedge into the disc space and impact it. Measure the height of the disc space and select the size of the cage. Fill the cage or allograft with bone graft and insert and impact it into place.
- Remove the wedge and insert the second cage or allograft.
- Decorticate the remaining vertebral endplates and fill the remaining space with autogenous graft (20).

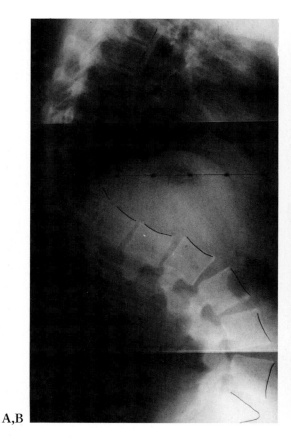

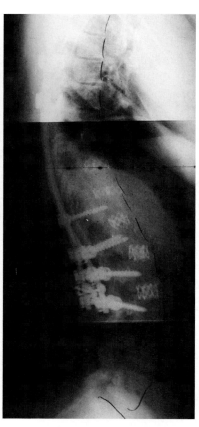

A,B

Figure 161.16. **A:** Postlaminectomy sagittal thoracolumbar kyphosis from resection of an arteriovenous malformation. **B:** Postoperative radiograph with intervertebral Harm's cages used as structural intervertebral grafts and posterior segmental instrumentation [three-stage (posterior–anterior–posterior), same-day surgery]. (Images courtesy of Dr. Harry Schufflebarger, Miami, FL.)

■ Reapproximate the annular flap and suture the margins together to act as a barrier for the bone graft.

Two small cages side by side or one large cage may be used, depending on the circumstances; usually a single allograft is sufficient. Follow the anterior procedure by a posterior arthrodesis and segmental instrumentation (Fig. 161.16).

SEGMENTAL SPINAL INSTRUMENTATION

The posterior surgical techniques used in correcting kyphosis are (a) segmental spinal instrumentation and Moe facet fusion and posterior arthrodesis, (b) posterior spinal osteotomy, and (c) the eggshell procedure.

Multiple segmental spinal instrumentation systems are now available, and most are strong enough to be acceptable. Which system to use is based on the experience of the surgeon. It is important to note, however, that some systems have a lower design profile than others. It is important to minimize the prominence of the instrumentation beneath the skin (see Chapter 156).

POSTERIOR SPINAL OSTEOTOMY

In previously fused patients, especially those with flatback syndrome, posterior osteotomies will be necessary for cor-

rection. When the spine is also fused anteriorly, combined anterior and posterior osteotomies will be necessary. The osteotomy site is selected by locating the vertebral foramina across which the osteotomy will be performed. The cranial–caudal width of the osteotomy is determined by the degree of closure that is necessary. Multiple osteotomies will spread the degree of correction across multiple levels and reduce the risk of neurologic compromise as compared with a single-level osteotomy. Single-level osteotomies can be useful, however, in ankylosing spondylitis and in patients with paralysis.

■ Perform the osteotomy with osteotomes, gouges, curets, and Kerrison rongeurs (see Chapter 163). Remove the bone in sizable pieces and save them for later use as an autograft.

■ A power burr can be used, although bone that can be used as an autograft is often lost. By attaching a Luken's trap to the suction system, much of the fine bone removed by the burr can be recaptured.

■ Carry the osteotomy down to the inner cortical table, which is then osteotomized with Kerrison rougeurs.

■ It is important to adequately decompress the spinal canal and undercut the osteotomy at the edges of the canal to prevent nerve root entrapment or central canal stenosis upon closure of the osteotomy (10,17).

■ Provide adequate fixation to maintain correction and prevent displacement of the osteotomy.

In patients who have not had a previous fusion, the osteotomy should include removal of lamina, spinous processes, facets, and bilateral pars interarticularis. The amount of bone removal is determined by the degree of correction that is desired and that is judged to be safe (7, 16,17,21,22,24).

EGGSHELL PROCEDURE

The eggshell procedure (9) is an operative technique that allows the spine surgeon to operate on the anterior thoracic or lumbar vertebral column through a posterior approach. It is most useful caudal to T-6 because of the more rigid conduit to the anterior spine (transpedicular vertebrectomy) (18). This approach can be used for a vertebral biopsy or decompression of a vertebral body abscess, but most eggshell procedures are done for chronic or acute deformity. In deformity surgery, the eggshell procedure is performed in addition to other procedures done for correction, arthrodesis, and stabilization.

■ Position the patient prone on a spinal frame.
■ Prepare the spine for segmental posterior instrumentation by inserting all hooks and screws in preparation for stabilization at the time of deformity correction.
■ Locate the pedicle by plain radiographs or image intensification. The location of the pedicle is identified by the bifurcation of a line transecting the transverse process and a line along the lateral margin of the pars interarticularis (Fig. 161.17).
■ Enter the pedicle with either a power burr or osteotomes and curets. Introduce a small curet into the pedicle and into the vertebral body.
■ Enlarge the pedicle hole by progressively increasing the size of the curets.
■ Leave the posterior elements intact and do not disturb the medial wall of the pedicles at this time. An extension moment promotes kyphosis correction and posterior bone removal may not be necessary.

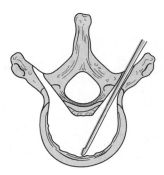

Figure 161.18. The curet is in the vertebral body to perform decancellation. The vertebral body is entered from both pedicles. An eggshell is created.

■ Use a sweeping motion to remove progressively more of the cancellous bone of the vertebral body.
■ The surgeon can operate at an angle of approximately 45° from lateral to medial and decancellate an area directly anterior to the spinal canal.
■ Perform the same procedure through the opposite pedicle (Fig. 161.18) and continue until the desired amount of material (e.g., bone, tumor) is removed.
■ To remove additional bone from just anterior to the spinal canal, remove the lateral wall of the pedicle to allow a more oblique angle for the curet to approach this area. Once this is accomplished, an eggshell is created (Fig. 161.18).
■ If correction of localized kyphosis is planned, fracture the lateral wall of the pedicles and extend the fracture into the shell of the vertebral body. An extension moment applied to the spine may assist in this technique. If additional correction is necessary, perform a sequential posterior decompression by removing the spinous process, lamina, pars interarticularis, and pedicles (Posterior Subtraction Osteotomy) (Fig. 161.19).
■ In the thoracic spine, it is often necessary to remove the

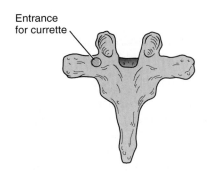

Entrance for currette

Figure 161.17. Entrance to the pedicle posteriorly.

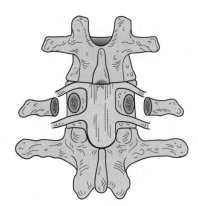

Figure 161.19. Complete posterior decompression is done.

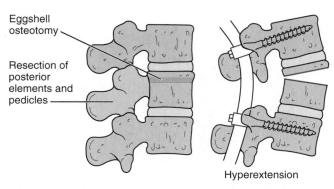

Eggshell osteotomy

Resection of posterior elements and pedicles

Hyperextension

Figure 161.20. Extension of the eggshell osteotomy and posterior segmental fixation.

proximal ribs and rib heads for adequate correction and closure of the osteotomy.

- Pack morcelized bone graft anteriorly before closing the osteotomy for anterior arthrodesis.
- Complete this wedge osteotomy and use segmental posterior instrumentation to correct the kyphosis and stabilize the spine. When the posterior elements are removed, a slow correction of the deformity is recommended to be sure that there is no encroachment of bone on the spinal canal or malalignment of the vertebra causing dural compression. Be careful of nerve root impingement.
- The inferior and superior laminae need to be undercut to avoid impingement on the dura during closure of the osteotomy.
- The axis of the closure of the osteotomy is anterior to the spinal canal, thus shortening the neural tube.
- Stable posterior fixation is required to maintain osteotomy stability, kyphotic correction, and arthrodesis (Fig. 161.20).
- The ultimate stability of the spinal construct depends on whether or not facet-to-facet or bone-to-bone apposition is obtained.

POSTOPERATIVE CARE AND REHABILITATION

Between the stages of operative correction, maintain patients on egg-crate or air mattresses, and log-roll them frequently to prevent decubiti and atelectasis. Prescribe daily bedside physical therapy for muscle strengthening, and joint range-of-motion exercises. Remove any chest tube and posterior drains on the second postoperative day or when the drainage is minimal.

At 5–7 days after the last staged procedure, place the patient in a bivalved polypropylene body jacket. If the patient is a teenager or young adult with good fixation and good-quality bone, bracing may not be needed. If there is any question about the stability of the instrumentation, bone weakness, or situations in which instrumentation cannot be used in the cervicothoracic spine (e.g., achondroplasia, diastrophic dwarfism), use a halo brace. In cervical kyphosis, apply a halo brace intraoperatively. Then allow patients to ambulate in the brace.

In patients with shorter kyphotic curves, do the anterior and posterior procedures at the same surgical setting to minimize anesthesia and recovery times. Sometimes a staged procedure may be indicated in patients who have had previously failed attempts at correction with resultant pseudarthroses and progressive curves, depending on the individual circumstances (19).

PITFALLS AND COMPLICATIONS

Many potential pitfalls are recognized:

- Failing to fuse the entire kyphotic curve (fusion too short) may allow progression of the kyphosis. This is especially true in children due to the adding-on phenomenon, in which vertebrae cranially and caudally tilt into the curve and are added to the curve.
- Placing the strut graft too far anteriorly with no bony contact with the apex of the kyphosis will lead to graft fracture.
- Placing the anterior strut graft too far posterior to the weight-bearing axis may lead to failure and progressive deformity.
- Failure to supplement an anterior procedure with a posterior fusion and instrumentation may lead to inadequate correction or late failure.
- Inadequately countersinking the strut graft may result in graft dislodgement after surgery.
- Failure to make osteotomies wide enough and the vertebral canal edges round enough may lead to nerve root entrapment at osteotomy closure.
- Dural, spinal cord, and nerve root injuries from too aggressive disc removal can occur.
- Inadequate disc removal will lead to failed fusion or to late progression of the deformity.
- Focusing on spinal instrumentation and inattention to fusion technique may lead to pseudoarthrosis and failure.
- Inadequate placement of posterior instrumentation may result in incomplete correction or an unbalanced torso, and failure to maintain lumbar lordosis below the kyphosis will lead to unbalanced sagittal alignment.
- Too-vigorous correction of the kyphotic deformity with posterior instrumentation in osteopenic bone can lead to bony failure, with loss of fixation and correction.

- Too-vigorous derotation with the Zielke instrumentation can cause spinal root injuries.
- With any anterior instrumentation, take care to prevent flatback syndrome.
- When there is severe vertebral rotation, anterior screw placement is critical so that spinal canal penetration does not occur.
- Finally, a well-applied brace is extremely important in some patients and should not be delegated to the inexperienced surgeon, or a less-than-ideal result may occur in an otherwise masterfully performed surgical procedure.

REFERENCES

Each reference is categorized according to the following scheme: *, classic article; #, review article; !, basic research article; and +, clinical results/outcome study.

\# 1. Akbarnia B. Spine Deformity in Neurofibromatosis. In: Bradford DS, Hensinger RM, eds. *The Pediatric Spine*. New York: Thieme, 1985;356.

+ 2. Betham D, Winter RB, Luther L. Disorders of the Spine in Diastrophic Dwarfism. *J Bone Joint Surg Am* 1980; 62:529.

* 3. Bradford DS. Anterior Vascular Pedicle Bone Grafting for the Treatment of Kyphosis. *Spine* 1980;5:318.

\# 4. Bradford DS. Spondylolysis and Spondylolisthesis in Children and Adolescents: Current Concepts in Management. In: Bradford DS, Hensinger RM, eds. *The Pediatric Spine*. New York: Thieme, 1985;416.

+ 5. Bradford DS, Schumacher WL, Lonstein JE, Winter RB. Ankylosing Spondylitis: Experience in Surgical Management of 21 Patients. *Spine* 1987;12:238.

+ 6. Bradford DS, Tribus CB. Current Concepts and Management of Patients with Fixed Decompensated Spinal Deformity. *Clin Orthop* 1994;306:64.

* 7. Briggs H, Keats S, Schlesinger PT. Wedge Osteotomy of the Spine with Bilateral Intervertebral Foraminotomy. *J Bone Joint Surg* 1947;29:1075.

\# 8. Canale ST, Beaty JH. *Operative Pediatric Orthopaedics*. St. Louis, MO: Mosby Year Book, 1991.

\# 9. Chewning SJ, Heinig CF. Eggshell Procedure. In: Bradford DS, ed. *Master Techniques in Orthopaedic Surgery*. Philadelphia: Lippincott-Raven, 1997;199.

* 10. Lagrone MO, Bradford DS, Moe JH, et al. Treatment of Symptomatic Flatback after Spinal Fusion. *J Bone Joint Surg Am* 1988;70:569.

+ 11. Lonstein JE. Postlaminectomy Kyphosis. In: Chou SN, Seljesky ED, eds. *Spinal Deformities and Neurological Dysfunction*. New York: Raven Press, 1978;53.

\# 12. Mayfield JK. Post-Radiation Spinal Deformity. *Orthop Clin North Am* 1979;10:829.

\# 13. Mayfield JK. Biomechanics of Spinal Deformities in Management of Spinal Deformity. In: Dickson R, Bradford D, eds. *Butterworths Int. Med. Rev. Orthop*, vol. 2, 1984;38.

+ 14. Mayfield JK, Erkkila J, Winter RB. Spine Deformity Subsequent to Acquired Childhood Spinal Cord Injury. *J Bone Joint Surg Am* 1981;63:1401.

* 15. Mayfield JK, Winter RB, Bradford DS, Moe JH. Congenital Kyphosis Due to Defects of Anterior Segmentation. *J Bone Joint Surg Am* 1980;62:1291.

* 16. McMaster MJ, Coventry MB. Spinal Osteotomy in Ankylosing Spondylitis. *Mayo Clin Proc* 1977;128:65.

* 17. McMaster PE. Osteotomy of the Spine for Fixed Flexion Deformity. *J Bone Joint Surg Am* 1962;44:1207.

* 18. Michelle A, Krudger FJ. A Surgical Approach to the Vertebral Body. *J Bone Joint Surg Am* 1949;31:873.

\# 19. Moe JH, Bradford DS, Lonstein JE, Winter RB. *Scoliosis and Other Spinal Deformities*. Philadelphia: WB Saunders, 1987.

+ 20. Shufflebarger H. Complex Revision Spinal Surgery: Posterior-Anterior-Posterior Sequence. In: *Proceedings of the Scoliosis Research Society*, St. Louis, 1997.

* 21. Simmons EH. Kyphotic Deformity of the Spine in Ankylosing Spondylitis. *Clin Orthop* 1977;128:65.

* 22. Smith-Peterson MN, Larson CB, Aufranc OE. Osteotomy of the Spine for Correction of Flexion Deformity in Rheumatoid Arthritis. *J Bone Joint Surg* 1945;27:1.

* 23. Stagnara P. *Spinal Deformity*. London: Butterworths, 1988.

* 24. Thomasen E. Vertebral Osteotomy for Correction of Kyphosis in Ankylosing Spondylitis. *Clin Orthop* 1985; 194:142.

\# 25. Tolo V. Spinal Deformity in Dwarfs. In: Bradford DS, Hensinger RM, eds. *The Pediatric Spine*. New York: Thieme, 1985.

\# 26. Winter RB, Lonstein JE, Boachie-Adjei O. Congenital Spinal Deformity. *Instr Course Lect* 1996;45:117.

\# 27. Winter RB, Lonstein JE, Leonard AS. *Congenital Deformities of the Spine*. New York: Thieme-Stratton, 1983.

* 28. Winter RB, Moe JH, Bradford DS, et al. Spine Deformity in Neurofibromatosis. *J Bone Joint Surg Am* 1979;61: 1677.

* 29. Winter RB, Moe JH, Wang JF. Congenital Kyphosis. *J Bone Joint Surg Am* 1973;55:223.

CHAPTER 162
SPONDYLOLISTHESIS

John D. Miles and Robert W. Gaines, Jr.

The concepts of spondylolysis, spondylolisthesis, and spondyloptosis have caused considerable confusion for students of orthopaedics. This chapter conveys the essentials of what is understood about these lesions to provide a foundation for rational treatment.

Spondylolisthesis is derived from the Greek *spondylos* (vertebra) and *olisthanein* (to slip or fall). This most commonly describes the forward slippage of a cephalad vertebra on a caudal vertebra (Fig. 162.1*A*). The term *spondylolysis* is also derived from the Greek word *lysis* (loosening). Spondylolysis is now specifically used to describe a bony defect in the pars interarticularis, the portion of the neural arch just caudal to the confluence of the pedicle and the superior articular process and at the most cephalad part of the lamina and inferior articular process (Fig. 162.1*B*). Spondylolisthesis can be present with or without spondylolysis (Fig. 162.1*C*). *Spondyloptosis* has similar origins, with the same root appended to the Greek word *ptosis* (falling). In modern usage, this refers to the most severe form of spondylolisthesis, when the body of L-5 has slipped into the pelvis and is positioned directly anterior to the sacrum (Fig. 162.1*D*).

PATHOPHYSIOLOGY

Two processes—dysplastic and traumatic—can give rise to spondylolisthesis. These can occur simultaneously, but generally one predominates.

The first, so-called dysplastic pathway is initiated by a congenital defect in the bony hook or its catch. The hook is composed of the pedicle, pars interarticularis, and inferior articular process of the cephalad vertebra, and the catch is the superior articular process of the caudal level. Dysplasia of any of these structures sets the stage for olisthesis when the weight of the trunk is transferred through the area at the initiation of upright stance and ambulation. The olisthesis is only potential at birth. Subluxation occurs when the soft-tissue restraints (intervertebral disc, anterior and posterior longitudinal ligaments,

J. D. Miles and R. W. Gaines, Jr.: Columbia Spine Center, Columbia Orthopaedic Group.

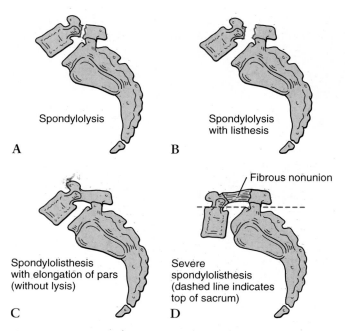

A Spondylolysis

B Spondylolysis with listhesis

C Spondylolisthesis with elongation of pars (without lysis)

D Severe spondylolisthesis (dashed line indicates top of sacrum)

Fibrous nonunion

Figure 162.1. **A:** Spondylolysis. **B:** Spondylolysis with listhesis. **C:** Spondylolisthesis and elongation of the pars interarticularis (without lysis). **D:** Severe spondylolisthesis (*dashed line* indicates top of sacrum).

ligamentum flavum, and posterior ligamentous complex) undergo plastic deformation due to repetitive loading unopposed by bony constraints. If pronounced subluxation occurs while significant growth still remains, the slippage will be accompanied by abnormal growth in the involved vertebral bodies or sacrum. These dysplastic changes form the basis for various classification schemes. Such changes include a trapezoidal shape of L-5, rounding of the superoanterior aspect of the sacrum, vertical orientation of the sacrum, junctional kyphosis at the involved segments, and a compensatory hyperlordosis at adjacent levels. There is evidence to support a genetic predisposition to this process, although no pattern of inheritance has been identified.

The second, so-called traumatic pathway is initiated by repetitive cyclic loading that ultimately results in a stress fracture. Impingement between the inferior articular process of the cephalad vertebra and the superior articular process of the caudal vertebra creates a bending moment that must be resisted by the pars (Fig. 162.2). Repetitive impingement causing loads in excess of the fatigue limit results in a fatigue (stress) fracture of an otherwise normal pars interarticularis. This repetitive loading is the same process that causes stress fractures in other anatomic locations, such as the femoral neck or the fifth metatarsal. The hard cortical bone of the pars predisposes it to fatigue fracture, as well as nonunion, decreasing the likelihood of spontaneous healing. If healing occurs, the pars often heals in an elongated position. Either outcome (nonunion or healing with elongation) permits vertebral subluxation.

This fundamental change in bony anatomy exposes the disc to increased shear load, even though the axial load remains unchanged. The increased shear load on the disc causes premature disc degeneration. Activities involving repetitive maximal flexion and extension (e.g., interior line play in football, pole vaulting, or gymnastics) are notoriously associated with fatigue fractures of the pars.

Spondylolisthesis may also be caused by other processes, although these are sufficiently different as to be considered distinct entities. They are included here for completeness.

Degenerative spondylolisthesis represents segmental instability and subluxation caused solely by degenerative change in the intervertebral disc and facet joints. The degree of subluxation is necessarily mild because the intact neural arch provides a bony limit to forward translation. Relatively more sagittal orientation of the facet joints is associated with degenerative spondylolisthesis (2,22).

A local or systemic pathologic process may cause a defect in the neural arch that can then permit subluxation. This is a pathologic fracture with resultant translational deformity.

High-energy trauma can cause translational deformity. In this setting, the spine will have sustained multiple bony and soft-tissue injuries, which may include a fracture in the pars. Other skeletal and visceral injuries will typically be present. This traumatic type of spondylolisthesis is a fracture–dislocation from high-energy trauma, not from repeated low-energy injuries.

Finally, a laminectomy that removes an entire articular process or more than half of each articular process can functionally destabilize the spine and permit translational deformity. This is iatrogenic postsurgical instability. Segments adjacent to previously fused segments are also at risk for development of degenerative spondylolisthesis (45). This subluxation is likely due to resection of the capsular, interspinous, or supraspinous ligaments at the adjacent level, but the loss of motion of the fused segment may contribute by increasing the motion demands at the next open level.

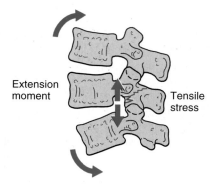

Extension moment

Tensile stress

Figure 162.2. Extension of the lumbar spine causes a tension load in the pars interarticularis.

Table 162.1.   Wiltse–Newman–Mcnab Classification of Spondylolisthesis

Type	Name	Description
I	Congenital	Dyplastic abnormalities in the posterior elements or the upper sacrum cause olisthesis
II	Isthmic	Three types are recognized: A: lytic, presumed to be a stress fracture of the pars B: a healed version of the lytic type, resulting in an elongated but intact pars C: an acute fracture of the pars interarticularis from a high-energy injury
III	Degenerative (pseudospondylolisthesis)	Neural arch (including the pars) is intact and the olisthesis results from longstanding segmental instability.
IV	Traumatic	Fracture of the bony hook other than the pars interarticularis (i.e., articular processes)
V	Pathologic	Generalized or localized bone disease that predisposes to olisthesis
VI	Postsurgical	Iatrogenic slippage as a result of loss of the posterior elements secondary to surgery

CLASSIFICATIONS

The classification scheme of Wiltse et al. (58) has gained wide acceptance (Table 162.1). It combines both anatomic and etiologic elements; however, this combination is one criticism of this system.

Table 162.2.   Marchetti and Bartolozzi Classification of Spondylolisthesis

I. Developmental
   A. High dysplastic
      With lysis
      With elongation
   B. Low dysplastic
      With lysis
      With elongation

II. Acquired
   A. Traumatic
      Acute fracture
      Stress fracture
   B. Postsurgery
      Direct (from excessive removal of facet articulation)
      Indirect (usually immediately above an arthrodesis)
   C. Pathologic
      Local pathology
      Systemic pathology
   D. Degenerative
      Primary (intact bony arch with degeneration in disc and facet joints)
      Secondary (adjacent to nonsurgically fused segments)

Marchetti and Bartolozzi (34) proposed a classification scheme based on etiologic criteria that has also gained wide acceptance (Table 162.2). The principal distinction in their system is between developmental and acquired forms, which correspond respectively to the dysplastic and traumatic pathways discussed previously.

CLINICAL ASSESSMENT

The symptoms associated with spondylolisthesis are caused by chronic muscle contraction (spasm) as the body attempts to limit motion around a painful pseudarthrosis of the pars interarticularis, by tears in the annulus fibrosus of the degenerating discs, or by compression of nerve roots. Pain may also derive directly from impingement at the fibrous pars nonunion, as nerve endings have been identified there (47). Children and younger adults who have symptomatic high-grade spondylolisthesis commonly complain of back fatigue and back pain on movement, particularly with hyperextension, as well as hamstring fatigue and pain. On examination, the paraspinal muscles are in chronic reactive contraction (spasm) to splint the painful underlying motion segment, and the hamstring muscles are in reactive contraction to stabilize the pelvis under the painful spinal motion segments. After months of continuous contraction in a growing child, fixed contractures of the hamstrings and paraspinal muscles may occur, limiting forward bending and hip flexion. These may be evident on clinical examination (Fig. 162.3*A*). Palpation elicits tenderness over the pars defect when the patient is lying prone with the spinal muscles relaxed, similar to the tenderness that exists over any other skeletal nonunion.

As aging proceeds and disc degeneration occurs (either

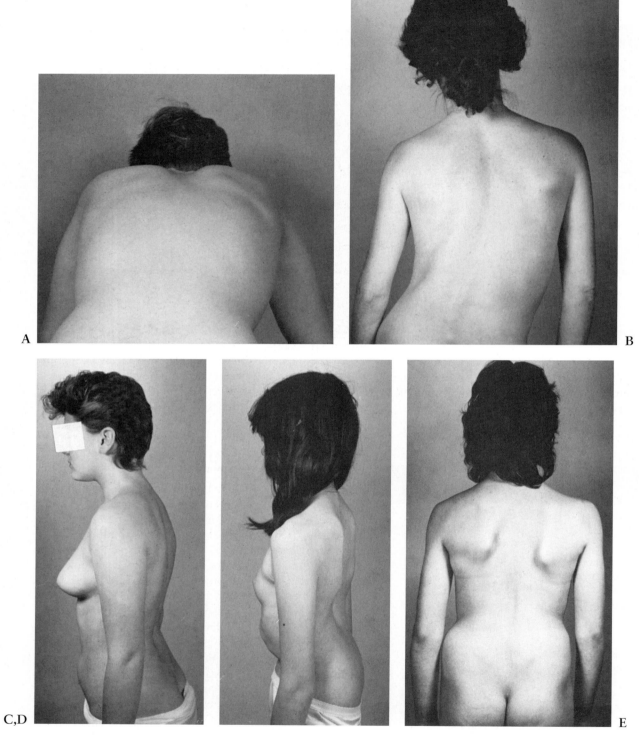

Figure 162.3. Physical findings in spondylolisthesis. **A:** Severely limited forward bending in a patient with moderate slippage and paravertebral muscle and hamstring spasm. **B:** Sciatic scoliosis in a patient with a disc rupture at the level above a pars defect. This patient's chief complaint was sciatica with mild back pain. **C:** Accentuated lordosis in a patient with mild slippage and a low slippage angle. **D:** Severe posterior tilting of the pelvis and secondary thoracolumbar lordosis are evident in this patient with a high-grade spondylolisthesis and high slippage angle. **E:** Heart-shaped buttocks and trunk foreshortening are visible in this patient with a high-grade slip. *(continued)*

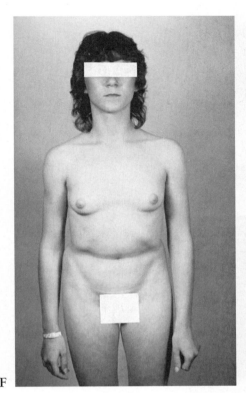
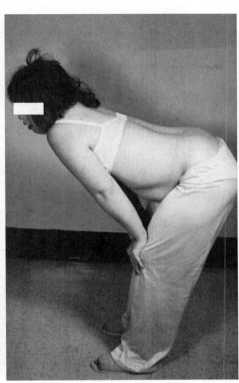

F   G

Figure 162.3. *(continued)* **F:** The same patient demonstrates an abdominal crease. **G:** Standing posture of a patient during olisthetic crisis with severe deformity, canal occlusion, and multiple root compression.

at the level of the slippage or at the level above it), episodes of the back "giving out" may occur. These episodes may or may not involve sciatica and vary in severity. As disc degeneration or subluxation increases, both the spinal canal and the lateral root foramina narrow, often causing symptoms related to nerve root compression (Fig. 162.3B). Such compression is manifested by sciatic pain radiating from the buttock into the posterior thigh and into the calf and foot. It is associated with numbness in a similar dermatomal distribution and with positive nerve stretch signs, such as straight-leg raising. Symptoms of spinal claudication indicate high-level stenosis. Compression of the central canal is confirmed by one or more of the following:

- Bowel or bladder symptoms or dysfunction
- Bilateral leg symptoms
- Positive straight-leg-raising test bilaterally
- Positive crossed straight-leg-raising test

Patients with spondylolysis or minor slips have no spinal deformity. As the amount of subluxation increases, spinal deformity becomes increasingly visible on inspection of the patient's torso. As the spine slides forward, the pelvis rotates posteriorly so that the top of S-1 becomes progressively more horizontal. This produces lumbosacral kyphosis and a relative posterior prominence of the posterior parts of the iliac crests (Fig. 162.3C,D). The gluteal muscles become less prominent. Patients with high-grade spondylolisthesis are often described as having heart-shaped buttocks (Fig. 162.3E). As the amount of telescoping approaches total dislocation (spondyloptosis), foreshortening of the lumbar spine becomes obvious on physical examination, and a crease appears across the abdomen (Fig. 162.3F). Patients in olisthetic crisis with total canal occlusion (the most severe type of spinal stenosis) relieve disc pressure and reduce nerve root tension by supporting trunk weight with hands on knees (Fig. 162.3G).

RADIOGRAPHIC ASSESSMENT

Plain anteroposterior and lateral radiographs document the amount of vertebral subluxation; often, they also reveal a pars interarticularis defect if one is present (Fig. 162.4). Oblique views have also been used to highlight the Scotty-dog sign (Fig. 162.5). In young patients, flex-

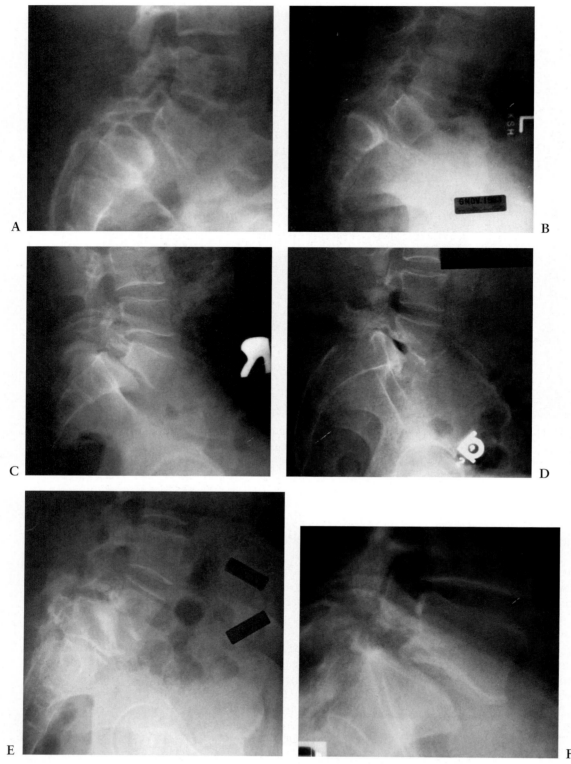

Figure 162.4. Spondylolisthesis in five patients with varied combinations of slippage, slippage angle, sacral inclination, sacral rounding, and disc degeneration. **A:** Moderate dysplastic spondylolisthesis. No pars defect is seen, and the slippage angle is low. **B:** Moderate isthmic spondylolisthesis. A pars defect is seen, and the slippage angle is higher than in the previous image. **C:** Moderate isthmic slip with moderate disc degeneration. The slippage angle is low, but striking retrolisthesis is present at the level above (L4-5). **D:** Moderate isthmic slippage with severe disc degeneration and a vacuum disc. **E:** High-grade slip with a higher slippage angle, vertical sacrum, high lumbar index, and severe disc degeneration. **F:** Low-grade slip with low slippage angle and minimal disc degeneration. A pars defect is present.

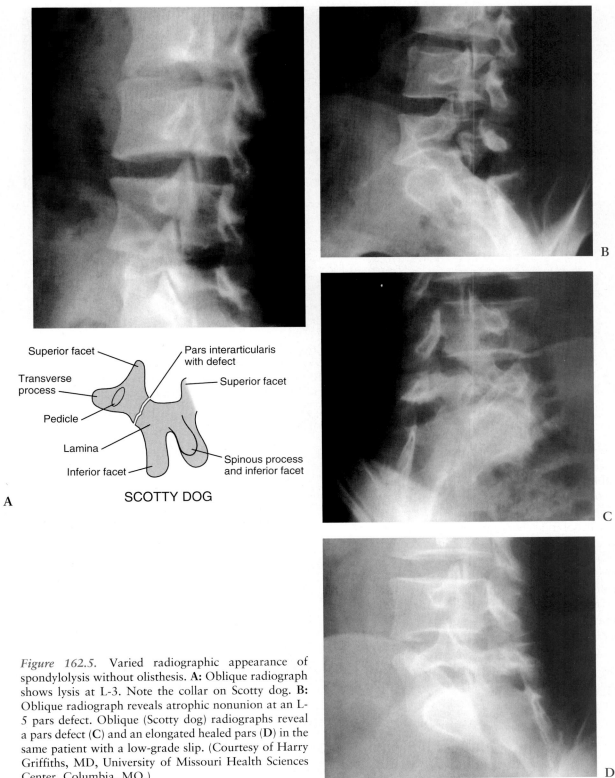

Figure 162.5. Varied radiographic appearance of spondylolysis without olisthesis. **A:** Oblique radiograph shows lysis at L-3. Note the collar on Scotty dog. **B:** Oblique radiograph reveals atrophic nonunion at an L-5 pars defect. Oblique (Scotty dog) radiographs reveal a pars defect (**C**) and an elongated healed pars (**D**) in the same patient with a low-grade slip. (Courtesy of Harry Griffiths, MD, University of Missouri Health Sciences Center, Columbia, MO.)

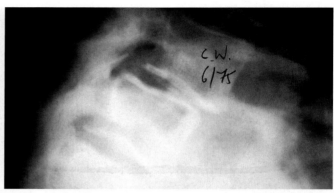

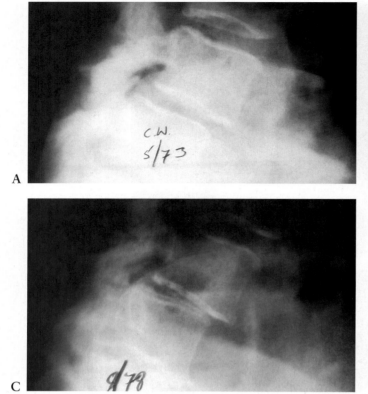

Figure 162.6. Progression of degenerative spondylolisthesis at L4-5 over a 5-year period as seen on lateral radiographs. **A:** 1973. **B:** 1975. **C:** 1978. (Courtesy of Harry Griffiths, MD, University of Missouri Health Sciences Center, Columbia, MO.)

ion–extension views can be used to show excessive movement across the site of pseudarthrosis in the pars interarticularis and subluxation of the vertebral body as the patient moves from extension into flexion. This motion may be more evident if the films are taken with the patient lying in the lateral decubitus position rather than standing (60). Plain standing radiographs are also quite useful for documenting progression of deformity (Fig. 162.6).

Older references grade the degree of vertebral subluxation by the Meyerding classification, which is based only on the amount of anterior (forward) subluxation of the cephalad vertebra in reference to the caudal vertebra (Fig. 162.7A). Slippage is graded as a percentage relative to the sagittal diameter of the inferior body:

Grade I	0% to 25%
Grade II	25% to 50%
Grade III	50% to 75%
Grade IV	75% to 100%
Grade V	Greater than 100%

This classification is particularly useful for low-grade (grade I or II) slips.

Boxall et al. (5) described the many adaptive changes in vertebral and disc anatomy that occur in response to chronic vertebral subluxation (Fig. 162.7B–D). In particular, they emphasized the importance of the kyphotic

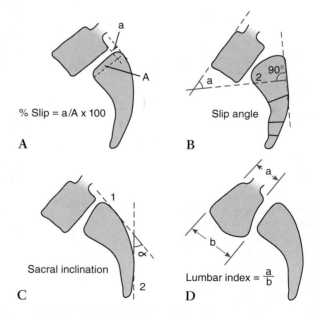

Figure 162.7. **A:** Calculation of the slippage percentage for spondylolisthesis. **B:** For a domed sacrum, the slippage angle is calculated from the posterior sacral body cortex and the superior endplate of L-5. **C:** The sacral inclination is the angle between the posterior sacral body cortex at S-1 and a vertical line (standing radiograph). **D:** Calculation of the lumbar index.

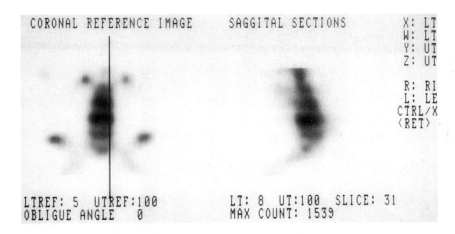

Figure 162.8. Bone scan shows increased activity in a patient with bilateral pars defects. (Courtesy of Harry Griffiths, MD, University of Missouri Health Sciences Center, Columbia, MO.)

component of the deformity in producing canal narrowing and sagittal-plane malalignment. Correction of kyphosis is very important in treating the condition, especially with regard to achieving a solid fusion (13). The radiographic measurement techniques described by Boxall et al. (5) emphasize the importance of the slippage angle as the best way to quantify the degree of kyphosis in a patient with spondylolisthesis.

Bone scintigraphy or single-photon emission computed tomography may occasionally be useful in symptomatic patients without radiographic evidence of spondylolis-

thesis (Fig. 162.8) (33). These studies document increased bone metabolic activity in an acutely injured pars interarticularis; however, they may revert to normal in a chronic unhealed defect or after a stress fracture heals (33).

Plain radiographs are sufficient for evaluating patients with solely mechanical complaints. If root symptoms, bowel or bladder complaints, or physical evidence of cord or root compression are present, then evaluate the soft tissues of the back with magnetic resonance imaging (MRI) (Fig. 162.9), myelography (Fig. 162.10), computed tomography, or a combination of these studies. MRI find-

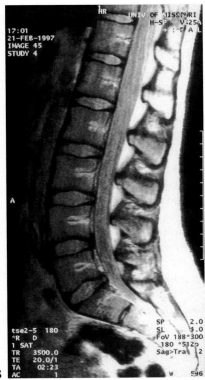

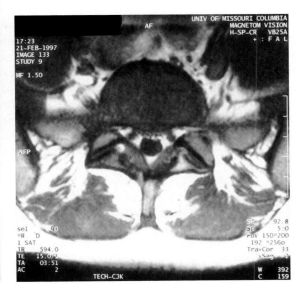

A,B

Figure 162.9. Sagittal (**A**) and axial (**B**) MR images reveal a herniated nucleus pulposus in a patient with spondylolysis and complaints of sciatica.

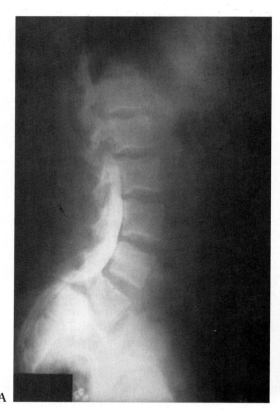

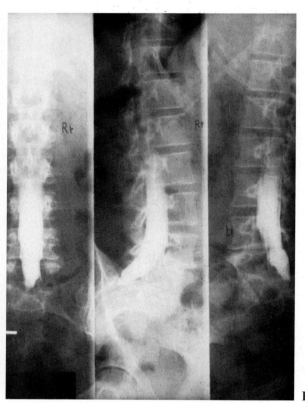

Figure 162.10. **A:** Myelogram reveals a block as the dural sac is tethered over S-1 in a high-grade slip. **B:** Lateral disc herniation is evident at L4-5 in a patient with an L-5 pars defect.

ings have been well correlated with clinical evidence of radiculopathy (28). Cystometric studies are helpful in patients with bladder dysfunction, although they are often confirmatory rather than diagnostic. Somatosensory-evoked cortical or spinal potentials may be of diagnostic value but are usually only confirmatory.

NATURAL HISTORY AND RISK FACTORS FOR PROGRESSION

Dysplastic spondylolisthesis most commonly occurs at the lumbosacral junction, with decreasing frequency at more cephalad levels in the lumbar spine. It is seldom seen in the cervical spine and rarely in the thoracic spine. Pars defects (spondylolysis) have not been reported at birth. However, the prevalence by early childhood is between 4% and 5% (17). By adulthood, the prevalence has increased to 6% or 7% (57,31). The great majority of patients with spondylolysis (radiographic evidence of a pars defect) are asymptomatic, and substantial slippage (spondylolisthesis) never develops (11,18,49). In a long-term study of adolescents with isthmic spondylolisthesis, 90% of slips occurred at the time of the initial presentation,

and the only factor predictive of progression was the magnitude of the initial slippage (50). Pronounced vertebral subluxation (>75%), if it occurs, generally arises during late childhood, at the time of the adolescent growth spurt, or during pregnancy (1,44). In patients who manifest a major deformity during adulthood, it is generally thought that the deformity developed before 20 years of age. The prevalence of spondylolisthesis is no higher in groups with chronic debilitating low back pain than in the general population (20). The association between low-back pain and spondylolisthesis is weak but is significant in women (56). The degree of dysplasia, including spina bifida occulta and small transverse processes, has been associated with progression but has not proven to be predictive. Rounding of the sacral promontory, trapezoidal wedging of L-5, vertical position of the sacrum, and segmental kyphosis all contribute to the mechanics of progression but are believed to be secondary changes. Similar to Harrington's stable zone in scoliosis, there may be a point of no return, beyond which progression is a certainty; however, documentation of this has not yet occurred.

Conversely, slippages that develop after 20 years of age (acquired) tend to be more stable, less symptomatic, and less likely to progress (38). Spondylolisthesis due to a fatigue fracture of the pars interarticularis will frequently occur in a high-level athlete. However, participation in athletics has little effect on progression of symptoms (35).

Degenerative spondylolisthesis usually occurs after 60 years of age, and progression is limited by the intact neural arch. Symptoms are generally due to stenosis, and progression to surgery is variable. A more sagittal orientation of the facet joints at L4-5 is strongly associated with the development of degenerative and postlaminectomy spondylolisthesis (22,43). Oophorectomy has also been identified as a risk factor for degenerative spondylolisthesis (26).

Both postsurgical and pathologic spondylolisthesis are relatively uncommon. Each patient must be evaluated and treated individually. Nerve root decompression and instrumented spinal fusion are the fundamentals of treatment.

Traumatic spondylolisthesis is a fracture–dislocation, and hence it is extremely unstable (24). Surgical stabilization is usually required.

NONOPERATIVE MANAGEMENT

Most patients who have a greater proportion of back pain than leg pain can be managed nonsurgically. In the pediatric population, symptoms may be controlled by a period of bed rest, bracing, or cessation of aggravating activities. For adults with any type of spondylolisthesis, initial nonoperative treatment is the rule.

- A corset and activity modifications are usually beneficial.
- For exacerbations, prescribe periods of bed rest.
- Palliate symptoms with hot or cold therapy, and use massage to treat the muscle fatigue or spasm resulting from disproportionate effort to limit movement across a painful motion segment.
- Initiate a program of aerobic conditioning; specific back exercises have variable effectiveness.
- Obese patients should lose weight to return to their healthy physiologic range.
- Nonsteroidal antiinflammatory medications and epidural steroid injections may be of some value.

These conservative measures are usually effective because fewer than 10% of symptomatic patients eventually require operative treatment. Surgery should be contemplated only after a trial of nonoperative care. In adult patients with predominantly sciatic complaints, nonoperative treatment may be less effective.

INDICATIONS AND SURGICAL TECHNIQUES

The surgical indications are different for children and adolescents than for adults. For children and adolescents, the indications for surgery are as follows:

- Documented progression of a slip beyond 25%
- Presentation with a high-grade slip (>50%)
- Intractable pain or neurologic symptoms
- Progressive postural deformity or gait abnormality

For adults, the usual surgical indication is persistent back pain and neurologic or radicular symptoms unresponsive to nonoperative management. As with other spine surgery, sciatica is more responsive than back pain to surgery (9). Patients with more severe symptoms will generally experience greater benefit from surgery than those with milder symptoms. Poor outcomes following surgery have been strongly associated with active workers' compensation claims and smoking (46,55).

TREATMENT OF SPONDYLOLYSIS AND LOW-GRADE (<50%) SPONDYLOLISTHESIS

PRIMARY REPAIR OF PARS DEFECT

In 1970, Buck (7) described a technique for direct repair of a pars defect with a screw placed through the lamina across the defect. There have since been other direct-repair techniques involving wires, hooks, and pedicle screws (30). The appropriate patient has spondylolysis but no olisthesis and a normal disc. Good results have been reported with these techniques, but because of the simplicity and predictability of fusion *in situ*, repair is not performed as often as fusion (3).

INSTRUMENTED POSTEROLATERAL FUSION *IN SITU*

The majority of symptomatic patients with mild to moderate (<50%) slips can be successfully treated with posterolateral fusion *in situ* (typically from L-5 to S-1) (8,19,27). Even patients with radicular symptoms may get good relief with fusion *in situ* (12). Wiltse et al. (58) advocated a muscle-splitting approach with two paramedian incisions; we favor a midline approach.

Internal fixation is rarely needed for children, although it is commonly used for adolescents and adults. The most popular systems today use pedicle screws. The biomechanical superiority of these systems for stabilizing spondylolisthesis has been demonstrated. Their effect on fusion rates and clinical outcomes is less clear, although generally beneficial (16,42,53,54,61).

- Position the patient prone on a Jackson table or blanket rolls without changing the patient's kyphosis or lordosis.
- Make a midline incision of sufficient length, and expose the posterior elements laterally to the tips of the transverse processes and sacral ala and thoroughly decorticate.

- For most adult-sized patients, we then place pedicle screws across the defect.
- We now routinely perform a laminectomy of the loose arch to provide local graft, instead of iliac crest, to reduce postoperative morbidity.
- Place morcelized autologous bone graft from the laminectomy in the prepared gutter under the plates (between the screws).
- Place rods or plates.
- Perform routine closure over a suction drain and epidural catheter.

Postoperatively, allow patients to be ambulatory, as tolerated, in a corset. Prohibit driving and sitting, except on a raised toilet seat, for 2 months.

The healing rate for a one-level fusion is approximately 95%. Most children have good or excellent results, with eventual return to full activity. As in other spine surgery, children do better than adults. The most common long-term problem is degenerative change at the level above the fusion (59).

DECOMPRESSION

Neural decompression is seldom required for children unless there is a cauda equina syndrome. Although foraminal stenosis with associated root pain is common in adults with isthmic spondylolisthesis, the indications for decompression are unclear because the addition of decompression may increase the rate of postoperative pseudarthrosis (10). Some authors have reported excellent fusion rates and relief of sciatica with fusion *in situ* (39), whereas others advocate formal decompression (6).

Adults with degenerative spondylolisthesis and secondary stenosis commonly present with claudication. Pedicle-to-pedicle posterior decompression is generally accepted, although the addition of intertransverse fusion has been shown to produce significantly better results than decompression alone for the treatment of degenerative spondylolisthesis (23).

The Gill procedure (excision of the loose laminar arch), long considered adequate decompression, actually fails to decompress the root in the neural foramen. A thorough decompression must include a foraminotomy, especially in the patient with radicular complaints. The best use of the loose laminar arch is as bone graft. We routinely perform Gill's procedure to obtain bone graft, not for the purpose of neural decompression.

ANTERIOR INTERBODY FUSION

Anterior interbody fusion is rarely indicated as a primary treatment for low-grade spondylolisthesis. It can be useful for failed posterior spinal fusion, however. Complications are potentially severe and include injury of the great ves-

sels, sexual dysfunction, and retrograde ejaculation (see Chapter 146).

TREATMENT OF HIGH-GRADE SPONDYLOLISTHESIS (>50%)

High-grade spondylolisthesis is rare but is a clinical challenge. Opinions vary widely as to optimal management.

ARTHRODESIS

Essentially, all authors would incorporate a bilateral posterolateral fusion in the treatment plan, but the agreement would stop there. Some authors have reported good results with isolated posterior fusion *in situ* (14,27,29). However, the pseudarthrosis rates are high, and progression is common, even with a radiographically solid fusion. In addition, fusion *in situ* fails to correct the clinical deformity and sagittal imbalance that generally accompany these severe deformities (51).

INSTRUMENTATION AND REDUCTION

The indications for instrumentation and reduction remain controversial (41). The relative indications for instrumented reduction include olisthetic crisis, cauda equina syndrome, a slip greater than 50% with a slippage angle greater than 30°, and major clinical deformity with global sagittal imbalance. Most intraoperative reduction techniques involve insertion of pedicle screws into L-4, L-5, and the sacrum. Often, a second point of pelvic fixation is added (iliac screws, intrasacral rods, or S-2 screws) to gain mechanical advantage. The forces applied are distraction, posterior translation of L-5, and sacral flexion. The terminal portion of the reduction maneuver has been shown to produce a disproportionate amount of nerve root tension, suggesting that postural reduction is a reasonable intermediate alternative (40). Many authors stress the importance of sacral flexion for restoring sagittal-plane balance (40). All series of instrumented reductions have reported nerve root injury, typically L-5, which manifests as foot drop. For the majority of affected patients, there is complete or partial recovery. These procedures are technically demanding and should be attempted only by experienced surgeons for patients who understand the potential risks. At long-term follow-up, most series have reported durable correction and clinical improvement with acceptable complication rates (15,25,37).

ANTERIOR INTERBODY FUSION

The addition of anterior interbody fusion is controversial (36). Some series report good results with isolated posterior spinal fusion, whereas others report higher fusion rates, less progression, and fewer implant failures with circumferential fusion (4,6). The relative indications are incomplete reduction, residual kyphotic slippage angle, and revision for previous pseudarthrosis. We favor the addition of anterior interbody fusion because of the relative difficulty of obtaining arthrodesis on the tension side of the lumbosacral kyphosis. The anterior interbody fusion generally heals readily on the compression side, but the lower pseudarthrosis rate must be weighed against the increased morbidity.

DECOMPRESSION

The need for decompression is also controversial. Decompression is commonly used in conjunction with fusion for patients with radicular or neurologic symptoms (52). However, relief of radicular symptoms has been reported with isolated posterior fusion (39). We use the presence of a positive seated straight-leg-raising test as an indication for nerve root exploration.

TREATMENT OF SPONDYLOPTOSIS

A patient with spondyloptosis presents a difficult, and fortunately rare, clinical challenge. In spondyloptosis, the entire body of L-5 is caudal to the sacrum. Although the slippage angle varies widely, the inferior endplate of L-4 is always closer than the inferior endplate of L-5 to the S-1 endplate. This observation provides the anatomic rationale for our technique, which is the resection of L-5 and reduction of L-4 onto the sacrum. The relative paucity of cases and the variable clinical presentation have led to a plethora of suggested techniques (4,6,13,27,36,37,39, 41,48,52). Treatment options include observation, reduction and casting, fusion *in situ*, reduction of L-5 onto the sacrum, and resection of L-5 with reduction of L-4 onto the sacrum. All options, including nonoperative management, have been associated with similar complications, including motor and sensory deficits or a cauda equina syndrome (48). The two-stage technique described in the following section is designed to eliminate lumbosacral kyphosis, restore sagittal-plane balance, and realign the spinal and nerve root canals while avoiding distraction and potentially devastating iatrogenic cauda equina injury.

AUTHORS' PREFERRED TECHNIQUE FOR SPONDYLOPTOSIS

Our preferred technique for spondyloptosis involves resection, instrumentation, and reduction of L-4 onto S-1.

As in other forms of spondylolisthesis, the severity of clinical symptoms in patients with spondyloptosis does not necessarily correlate with the degree of subluxation. Thus, L-5 vertebrectomy and reduction are advised only for severely disabled patients (Fig. 162.11).

The procedure consists of two parts performed 1 week apart (21).

■ Perform the first part through an anterior retroperitoneal approach (see Chapter 146).
■ Resect the L4-5 disc, the body of L-5, and the L5–S1 disc.
■ Take the resection back to the base of each pedicle, and take care to avoid injury to the L-5 root.
■ Remove the inferior cartilage endplate of L-4. Retain the bony endplate.

Postoperatively, place the patient in an intensive care unit for 1 week to await the second stage. Nursing care includes use of a rotokinetic bed.

■ Perform the second stage through a midline posterior approach.
■ Place Harrington outriggers from L-2 onto the sacral ala to provide very gentle (1–2 cm) distraction. (This step may be omitted after the surgeon gains more experience.)
■ Remove the loose posterior elements, transverse processes, and pedicles of L-5. Take special care to avoid injury to the L-5 root.
■ Remove the cartilage endplate of S-1 before reduction. Preserve the bony endplate.
■ Place pedicle screws into L-4 and S-1. Cortical purchase is essential.
■ Accomplish reduction of L-4 onto the sacrum by removing the outriggers or by gentle distraction and translation applied to the screws in L-4. Constantly assess the L-4 and L-5 nerve roots during reduction both visually and with a nerve hook.
■ Decorticate the transverse processes of L-4 and the sacral ala.
■ Place autograft retained from the vertebrectomy and from the posterior elements of L-5 in the lateral gutter.
■ Apply rods or plates to the screws. Two nerve roots (L-4 and L-5) will pass through the reconstructed neural foramen at L4–S1. Check to ensure that there is no impingement on the nerve roots before and after application of the rods or plates.

Postoperatively, keep patients at bed rest in a thoracolumbar spinal orthosis for 6 weeks, at which time begin mobilizing patients.

With this technique, 18 of 27 patients have experienced weakness in dorsiflexion postoperatively. This has been transient for all but two. All patients with preoperative cauda equina syndrome recovered postoperatively; no patient has had iatrogenic cauda equina injury (because the

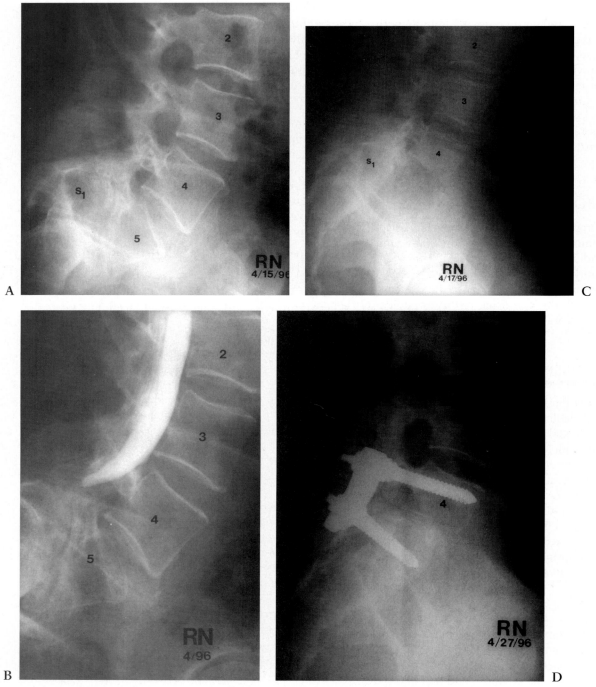

Figure 162.11.   **A:** Preoperative lateral radiograph of a 42-year-old man with spondyloptosis and debilitating back and leg pain. **B:** Preoperative myelogram shows total blockage. **C:** Lateral radiograph after first-stage L-5 anterior vertebrectomy. **D:** Lateral radiograph after second-stage reduction of L-4 onto the sacrum and pedicle-screw fixation. Alignment and lordosis have been restored.

spine is not lengthened). When reviewed by an independent observer, patients reported very high satisfaction, with significant improvements in pain, function, and appearance (32).

PITFALLS AND COMPLICATIONS

The resection described is one of the most difficult operations in spinal reconstruction. It should be only performed by surgical teams that are accustomed by experience to performing spinal osteotomies on a routine basis and are very experienced in handling the dural tube and nerve roots.

The anterior exposure requires extensive mobilization of the aorta, vena cava, and both internal and external iliac arteries and veins. Two to four assistants are regularly required to retract major vessels, roots, or vertebrae during various portions of the procedure.

Incomplete removal of the L4-5 or L5-S discs or the L-5 vertebra creates the potential for iatrogenic single- or multiple-root injury or incomplete reduction. Slow rehabilitation of patients is essential. One month of bed rest is routine before ambulation in a brace. No work or physical rehabilitation is started until convincing evidence of union is obvious.

REFERENCES

Each reference is categorized according to the following scheme: *, classic article; #, review article; !, basic research article; and +, clinical results/outcome study.

\# 1. Blackburne JS, Velikas EP. Spondylolisthesis in Children and Adolescents. *J Bone Joint Surg Br* 1977;59:490.

\+ 2. Boden SD, Riew KD, Yamaguchi K, et al. Orientation of the Lumbar Facet Joints: Association with Degenerative Disc Disease. *J Bone Joint Surg Am* 1996;78:403.

\+ 3. Bonnici AV, Koka SR, Richards DJ. Results of Buck Screw Fixation in Grade I Spondylolisthesis. *J R Soc Med* 1991;84:270.

\+ 4. Boos N, Marchesi D, Zuber K, Aebi M. Treatment of Severe Spondylolisthesis by Reduction and Pedicular Fixation: A 4–6 Year Follow-up Study. *Spine* 1993;18:1655.

* 5. Boxall D, Bradford DS, Winter RB, Moe JH. Management of Severe Spondylolisthesis in Children and Adolescents. *J Bone Joint Surg Am* 1979;61:479.

\+ 6. Bradford DS, Boachie-Adjei O. Treatment of Severe Spondylolisthesis by Anterior and Posterior Reduction and Stabilization: A Long-term Follow-up Study. *J Bone Joint Surg Am* 1990;72:1060.

* 7. Buck JE. Direct Repair of the Defect on Spondylolisthesis. *J Bone Joint Surg Br* 1970;52:432.

\+ 8. Burkus JK, Lonstein JE, Winter RB, Denis F. Long-term Evaluation of Adolescents Treated Operatively for Spondylolisthesis: A Comparison of *in Situ* Arthrodesis Only with *in Situ* Arthrodesis and Reduction Followed by Immobilization in a Cast. *J Bone Joint Surg Am* 1992;74:693.

\+ 9. Butterman GR, Garvey TA, Hunt AF, et al. Lumbar Fusion Results Related to Diagnosis *Spine* 1998;23:116.

\+ 10. Carragee EJ. Single Level Posterolateral Arthrodesis, with or without Posterior Decompression, for the Treatment of Isthmic Spondylolisthesis in Adults: A Prospective, Randomized Study. *J Bone Joint Surg Am* 1997;79:1175.

\+ 11. Danielson BI, Frennered AK, Irstam LK. Radiologic Progression of Isthmic Lumbar Spondylisthesis in Young Patients. *Spine* 1991;16:422.

\+ 12. de Loubresse CG, Bon T, Deburge A, et al. Posterolateral Fusion for Radicular Pain in Isthmic Spondylolisthesis. *Clin Orthop* 1996;323:194.

\# 13. Dubousset J. Treatment of Spondylolysis and Spondylolisthesis in Children and Adolescents. *Clin Orthop* 1997;337:77.

\+ 14. Esses SI, Natout N, Kip P. Posterior Interbody Arthrodesis with a Fibular Strut Graft in Spondylolisthesis. *J Bone Joint Surg Am* 1995;77:172.

\+ 15. Fabris DA, Constantini S, Nena U. Surgical Treatment of Severe L5-S1 Spondylolisthesis in Children and Adolescents: Results of Intraoperative Reduction, Posterior Interbody Fusion, and Segmental Pedicle Fixation. *Spine* 1996;21:728.

\+ 16. Fischgrund JS, Mackay M, Herkowitz HN, et al. Degenerative Lumbar Spondylolisthesis with Spinal Stenosis: A Prospective, Randomized Study Comparing Decompressive Laminectomy and Arthordesis with and without Spinal Instrumentation. *Spine* 1997;22:2807.

* 17. Frederickson BE, Baker D, McHolick WJ, et al. The Natural History of Spondylolysis and Spondylolisthesis. *J Bone Joint Surg Am* 1984;66:699.

\+ 18. Frennered AK, Danielson BI, Nachemson AL. Natural History of Symptomatic Isthmic Low-grade Spondylolisthesis in Children and Adolescents: A Seven-year Follow-up Study. *J Pediatr Orthop* 1991;11:209.

\+ 19. Frennered AK, Danielson BI, Nachemson AL, Nordwall AB. Midterm Follow-up of Young Patients Fused *in Situ* for Spondylolisthesis. *Spine* 1991;16:409.

\+ 20. Frennered K. Isthmic Spondylolisthesis among Patients Receiving Disability Pension under the Diagnosis of Chronic Low Back Pain Syndromes. *Spine* 1994;19:2766.

\+ 21. Gaines RW, Nichols WK. Treatment of Spondyloptosis by Two Stage L5 Vertebrectomy and Reduction of L4 onto S1. *Spine* 1985;10:680.

\! 22. Grobler LJ, Robertson PA, Novotney JE, Pope MH. Etiology of Spondylolisthesis: Assessment of the Role Played by Lumbar Facet Joint Morphology. *Spine* 1993;18:80.

\+ 23. Herkowitz HN, Kurz LT. Degenerative Lumbar Spondylolisthesis with Spinal Stenosis: A Prospective Study

Comparing Decompression with Decompression and Intertransverse Process Arthrodesis. *J Bone Joint Surg Am* 1991;73:802.

+ 24. Hilibrand AS, Urquhart AG, Graziano GP, Hensinger RN. Acute Spondylolytic Spondylolisthesis: Risk of Progression and Neurologic Complications. *J Bone Joint Surg Am* 1995;77:190.

+ 25. Hu SS, Bradford DS, Transfeldt EE, Cohen M. Reduction of High-grade Spondylolisthesis Using Edwards Instrumentation. *Spine* 1996;21:367.

+ 26. Imada K, Matsui H, Tsuji H. Oophorectomy Predisposes to Degenerative Spondylolisthesis. *J Bone Joint Surg Br* 1995;77:126.

+ 27. Ishikawa S, Kumar SJ, Torres BC. Surgical Treatment of Dysplastic Spondylolisthesis: Results after *in Situ* Fusion. *Spine* 1994;19:1691.

! 28. Jinkins JR, Rauch A. Magnetic Resonance Imaging of Entrapment of Lumbar Nerve Roots in Spondylolytic Spondylolisthesis. *J Bone Joint Surg Am* 1994;76:1643.

+ 29. Johnson JR, Kirwan EO. The Long-term Results of Fusion *in Situ* for Severe Spondylolisthesis. *J Bone Joint Surg Br* 1983;65:43.

+ 30. Kakiuchi M. Repair of the Defect in Spondylolysis: Durable Fixation with Pedicle Screws and Laminar Hooks. *J Bone Joint Surg Am* 1997;79:818.

+ 31. Leboeuf C, Kimber D, White K. Prevalence of Spondylolisthesis, Transitional Anomalies and Low Intercrestal Line in a Chiropractic Patient Population. *J Manipulative Physiol Ther* 1989;12:200.

+ 32. Lehmer SM, Steffee AD, Gaines RW Jr. Treatment of L5-S1 Spondyloptosis by Staged L5 Resection with Reduction and Fusion of L4 onto S1 (Gaines Procedure). *Spine* 1994;19:1916.

! 33. Lusins JO, Elting JJ, Cicoria AD, Goldsmith SJ. SPECT Evaluation of Lumbar Spondylolysis and Spondylolisthesis. *Spine* 1994;19:608.

* 34. Marchetti PG, Bartolozzi P. Classification of Spondylolisthesis as a Guideline for Treatment. In: Bridwell KH, DeWald RL, eds. *The Textbook of Spinal Surgery*, 2nd ed. Philadelphia: Lippincott–Raven Publishers, 1997: 1211.

+ 35. Muschik M, Hahnel H, Robinson PN, et al. Competitive Sports and the Progression of Spondylolisthesis. *J Pediatr Orthop* 1996;16:364.

+ 36. Muschik M, Zippel H, Perka C. Surgical Management of Severe Spondylolisthesis in Children and Adolescents: Anterior Fusion *in Situ* versus Anterior Spondylodesis with Posterior Transpedicular Instrumentation and Reduction. *Spine* 1997;22:2036.

+ 37. O'Brien JP, Mehdian H, Jaffray D. Reduction of Severe Lumbosacral Spondylolisthesis: A Report of 22 Cases with a Ten-year Follow-up Period. *Clin Orthop* 1994; 300:64.

+ 38. Ohmori K, Ishida Y, Takatsu T, et al. Vertebral Slip in Lumbar Spondylolysis and Spondylolisthesis: Long-term Follow-up of 22 Adult Patients. *J Bone Joint Surg Br* 1995;77:771.

+ 39. Peek RD, Wiltse LL, Reynolds JB, et al. *In Situ* Arthrodesis without Decompression for Grade III or IV Isthmic

Spondylolisthesis in Adults Who Have Severe Sciatica. *J Bone Joint Surg Am* 1989;71:62.

! 40. Petraco DM, Spivak JM, Cappadona JG, et al. An Anatomic Evaluation of L-5 Nerve Stretch in Spondylolisthesis Reduction. *Spine* 1996;21:1133.

+ 41. Poussa M, Schlenzka D, Seitsalo S, et al. Surgical Treatment of Severe Isthmic Spondylolisthesis in Adolescents. *Spine* 1993;18:894.

+ 42. Ricciardi JE, Pflueger PC, Isaza JE, Whitecloud TS 3rd. Transpedicular Fixation for the Treatment of Isthmic Spondylolisthesis in Adults. *Spine* 1995;20:1917.

! 43. Robertson PA, Grobler LJ, Novotney JE, Katz JN. Postoperative Spondylolisthesis at L4-5: The Role of Facet Joint Morphology. *Spine* 1993;18:1483.

+ 44. Sanderson PL, Fraser RD. The Influence of Pregnancy on the Development of Degenerative Spondylolisthesis. *J Bone Joint Surg Br* 1996;78:951.

+ 45. Schlegel JD, Smith JA, Schleusener RL. Lumbar Motion Segment Pathology Adjacent to Thoracolumbar, Lumbar, and Lumbosacral Fusions. *Spine* 1996;21:970.

+ 46. Schnee CL, Freese A, Ansell LV. Outcome Analysis for Adults with Spondylolisthesis Treated with Posterolateral Fusion and Transpedicular Screw Fixation. *J Neurosurg* 1997;86:56.

! 47. Schneiderman GA, McLain RF, Hambly MF, Nielson SL. The Pars Defect as a Pain Source: A Histologic Study. *Spine* 1995;20:1761.

+ 48. Schoenecker PL, Dole HO, Herring HA, et al. Cauda Equina Syndrome after *in Situ* Arthrodesis for Severe Spondylolisthesis at the Lumbosacral Junction. *J Bone Joint Surg Am* 1990;72:369.

+ 49. Seitsalo S. Operative and Conservative Treatment of Moderate Spondylolisthesis in Young Patients. *J Bone Joint Surg Br* 1990;72:908.

+ 50. Seitsalo S, Osterman K, Hyvarinen H, et al. Progression of Spondylolisthesis in Children and Adolescents: A Long-term Follow-up of 272 Patients. *Spine* 1991;16: 417.

+ 51. Shelokov A, Haideri N, Roach J. Residual Gait Abnormalities in Surgically Treated Spondylolisthesis. *Spine* 1993;18:2201.

+ 52. Smith MD, Bohlman HH. Spondylolisthesis Treated by a Single-stage Operation Combining Decompression with *in Situ* Posterolateral and Anterior Fusion: An Analysis of Eleven Patients Who Had Long-term Follow-up. *J Bone Joint Surg Am* 1990;72:415.

+ 53. Soini J, Laine T, Pohjolainen T, et al. Spondylodesis Augmented by Transpedicular Fixation in the Treatment of Olisthetic and Degenerative Conditions of the Lumbar Spine. *Clin Orthop* 1993;297:111.

+ 54. Thomsen K, Christensen FB, Eiskjaer SP, et al. The Effect of Pedicle Screw Instrumentation on Functional Outcome and Fusion Rates in Posterolateral Lumbar Fusion: A Prospective, Randomized Clinical Study. *Spine* 1997; 22:2813.

+ 55. Vaccaro AR, Ring D, Scuderi G, et al. Predictors of Outcome in Patients with Chronic Back Pain and Low-grade Spondylolisthesis. *Spine* 1997;22:2030.

+ 56. Virta L, Ronnemaa T. The Association of Mild–Moderate Isthmic Spondylolisthesis and Low Back Pain in Middle-aged Patients is Weak and It Only Occurs in Women. *Spine* 1993;18:1496.

+ 57. Virta L, Ronnemaa T, Osterman K, et al. Prevalence of Isthmic Lumbar Spondylolisthesis in Middle-aged Subjects from Eastern and Western Finland. *J Clin Epidemiol* 1992;45:917.

* 58. Wiltse LL, Newman PH, MacNab I. Classification of Spondylolysis and Spondylolisthesis. *Clin Orthop* 1976; 117:23.

+ 59. Wimmer C, Gluch H, Krismer M, et al. AP-translation in the Proximal Disc Adjacent to Lumbar Spine Fusion: A Retrospective Comparison of Mono- and Polysegmental Fusion in 120 Patients. *Acta Orthop Scand* 1997;68:269.

! 60. Wood KB, Popp CA, Transfeldt EE, Geissele AE. Radiographic Evaluation of Instability in Spondylolisthesis. *Spine* 1994;19:1697.

+ 61. Zdeblick TA. A Prospective, Randomized Study of Lumbar Fusion: Preliminary Results. *Spine* 1993;18:983.

Chapman's Orthopaedic Surgery, third edition. Edited by Michael W. Chapman. Lippincott Williams & Wilkins, Philadelphia © 2001.

CHAPTER 163

REVISION AND SALVAGE AFTER SURGERY FOR SPINAL DEFORMITY

Robert F. McLain

Surgical therapy for scoliosis has evolved considerably over the years, from *in situ* fusions and fusion with casting, to fusion using Harrington and Luque instrumentation, to the current generation of segmental systems that attempt to correct spinal deformity in three planes. Regardless of the treatment method, there have always been some patients who lose correction—either because of a pseudarthrosis or by progression of the curve—or who have poor results because of pain. Although acute failures can be treated by immediately reinstrumenting and augmenting the fusion, patients who have lost correction over time typically require a more aggressive approach to reconstruction. To successfully manage these patients, the surgeon must understand why the loss of correction occurred, develop a sound preoperative plan, and choose a surgical approach designed to provide a painless arthrodesis, good correction of deformity, and a well-balanced trunk.

CAUSES OF FAILURE

The therapeutic failures of the past have led to changes in the way fusions are performed, the way fusion levels are selected, and the types of instrumentation used to stabilize the spine (2,7,9,21). Despite technical advances, the following remain the most common causes of failure:

- Pseudarthrosis
- Fixation failure
- Inadequate fusion length

R. F. McLain: Department of Orthopaedics, The Cleveland Clinic Foundation, Cleveland, Ohio, 44195.

- Progression of deformity due to the "crankshaft" phenomenon
- Addition of new segments to the old curve
- Progression of an untreated, secondary curve

PSEUDARTHROSIS

In 1964, Moe and Gustilo (21) reported the results of 196 patients treated by cast correction and posterior fusion. They noted that 46 patients (23%) required reoperation for pseudarthrosis repair or a combination of pseudarthrosis repair and osteotomy. McMaster and James (20) reviewed the experience of a number of authors and concluded that pseudarthrosis rates ranged from 3.3% to 68.3% (average, 22.5%) in patients treated without internal fixation. When internal fixation was used, this rate was significantly lower (2% to 17%; average, 6.4%). With current instrumentation techniques, a pseudarthrosis rate of between 2% and 5% is typical in adolescent idiopathic scoliosis (1,5,7,10). However, other deformity groups remain at much greater risk. Adults treated for idiopathic and paralytic scoliosis have a 10% to 15% incidence of pseudarthrosis (12,23,25,26,28). Patients with myelodysplasia and paralytic scoliosis have a 20% to 45% incidence of pseudarthrosis (18,22).

Three factors have contributed to improved fusion rates. First, the fusion technique itself has improved over the years. Decortication of transverse processes, removal of facet joints, and meticulous exposure of the lumbar transverse processes have all resulted in improvements in fusion rates. Second, the use of autograft bone to augment the fusion mass has greatly improved success rates. Finally, the use of spinal instrumentation and the subsequent improvement in instrumentation constructs have further reduced pseudarthrosis rates. Still, some failures are inevitable. The surgeon has no control over the patient's age at the time of surgery, the nature of the deformity (paralytic, congenital, or those associated with neurofibromatosis or Marfan's syndrome), or the location and severity of the curve at presentation. All of these factors have an impact on fusion rates. Regardless of technique or instrumentation, pseudarthroses will continue to occur in patients with severe and recalcitrant curves.

FIXATION FAILURE

Despite a variety of hook types, construct patterns, and the addition of pedicle screws, instrumentation failures are inevitable. Excessive distraction and rotational forces applied to large, rigid curves can result in hardware displacement if the hook fractures through the lamina. Poor purchase of the hook over a deformed or rotated lamina may result in hook displacement at either end of the curve. Transverse process fractures may compromise the transversopedicular claw even in a well-designed scoliosis construct. Patients with poor bone quality or osteomalacia are also at increased risk for hardware displacement. Rod breakage, seen in 7% to 10% of Harrington constructs, is less common with current segmental systems but can still occur as either an acute or a late complication (7). Whether fixation is lost because of failure through the bone or failure of the hardware itself, the patient is exposed to a great risk of pseudarthrosis, pain, and loss of any correction gained at the initial surgery.

INADEQUATE FUSION LENGTH

In 1973, Kostuik et al. (12) reported that, among adult patients requiring revision surgery, the initial spinal fusion had been too short in a significant number. Cummine et al. (4) found that 40 of 59 patients requiring reconstruction for failed scoliosis fusion had curve progression due to incorrect selection of fusion levels at the initial operation. Inadequate fusion length may result in the following situations:

- The initial surgery stopped short of the appropriate end vertebra, leaving part of the primary curve unfused.
- The surgeon inadvertently selected a fusion level that did not address all the involved segments, particularly when there were a number of parallel end-vertebrae in the primary curve.
- Sagittal malalignment was not corrected, leaving an unfused kyphosis that tended to increase over time (17).
- In children fused at a young age, progression can be seen even when the initial fusion correctly addressed the entire primary curve. Over time, additional vertebrae not part of the original scoliotic curve may become involved.

CRANKSHAFT PHENOMENON

Bending of the fusion mass may occur in children fused at an early age. These patients, through growth and remodeling, experience an increase in curve magnitude without an increase in curve length. One of the earliest descriptions of what is now considered the "crankshaft" phenomenon was provided in Ponseti and Friedman's 1950 paper on progressive deformity after fusion (24). Letts and Bobechko (16) reviewed the outcome of children undergoing spine fusion before the age of 8 years and found that 26% had significant curve progression despite successful arthrodesis. They found that progression was an even bigger problem in children fused at less than 4 years of age. Curve progression was greatest during the rapid growth phase, and the patients who had the greatest problem with this type of curve progression were those with a congenital scoliosis requiring fusion at a very early age. The progressive bending of an apparently solid fusion mass has been explained as the continued growth of the anterior vertebral elements within a spinal segment that has been fused (tethered) posteriorly (6,14). As the anterior elements elongate, the vertebral bodies are forced farther out from the midline, increasing both the sagittal and scoliotic deformities. Anterior fusion at the time of the initial posterior surgery prevents this phenomenon.

PROGRESSION OF THE SECONDARY CURVE

A small number of patients present with progressive imbalance and deformity despite appropriate initial treatment and a successful primary fusion. In these patients, the progression occurs in the secondary curve either above or below the primary curve, resulting in significant trunk imbalance and an increase in apparent deformity. Whether this happens because of relentless progression of the secondary curve or the patient's progressive inability to compensate for the fused primary curve, the problem generally begins with a mild to moderate compensatory curve that, with age, becomes more severe and structural.

Progressive lumbar curves are a particular problem in the adult population. Curve progression in the lumbar segments results in low back pain, degenerative disc disease, translational deformities, and, in some cases, nerve root compression in the concavity of the curve. Once these curves become structural, correction may not be possible without simultaneously addressing the previously fused primary curve.

INDICATIONS FOR SURGERY

PAIN

Pain is the most common symptom in patients requiring reconstructive surgery of the spine (2,17). Generalized pain may involve either the convexity or the concavity of the curve. In the thoracic region, pain over the convexity of the curve usually involves paraspinous muscles overlying the ribs and bony prominence. Patients may also complain of subscapular or interscapular pain in the region of the rhomboid and levator muscle attachments. Pain on the concavity may be localized to the paraspinous muscles or may be radicular in nature. In thoracolumbar and lumbar curves, pain in the concavity is frequently associated with degenerative disease and facet arthrosis. Translational shifts, commonly seen in degenerative curves of the lumbar spine, may cause severe and debilitating pain related to both segmental instability and muscle spasm, as well as nerve root impingement and stenosis.

Conservative therapy is as appropriate for these patients as for any patient with chronic low back pain. Patients complaining primarily of pain without evidence of curve progression warrant a full course of nonoperative treatment, including physical therapy, anti-inflammatory medications, pain behavior modification, and a trial of bracing, before entertaining surgical options. All reasonable conservative measures should be explored prior to scheduling surgery.

When pain is severe and well localized to a region of previous fusion, suspect a pseudarthrosis. Pain from pseudarthrosis usually increases with activity and improves with rest. The area may be tender; however, if spinal instrumentation is in place, palpation may not produce symptoms. The patient may complain of a popping or grating sensation with movement, fatigue at the end of the day, or a sense that the deformity is progressing. Fixation failure, broken hardware, and progressive deformity strongly suggest the presence of a pseudarthrosis. Standard tomography is the most reliable method of demonstrating the defect.

Patients with pain at the end of a spinal fusion usually suffer at the levels immediately caudal to the fusion mass. This may be related either to discogenic pain or to facet arthrosis. Cochran et al. (3) demonstrated a proportionally greater incidence of degenerative disc disease as fusions are carried more distally. Their study showed that patients with fusions to L-2 had a 20% incidence of symptomatic disc degeneration; those with fusions to L-3, a 40% incidence; those with fusions to L-4, a 60% incidence; and those with fusions to L-5, an 80% incidence. Changes in spinal mechanics result in degeneration of the intervertebral disc and facet joints at the junction of the fused and mobile segments. Disc prolapse, facet hypertrophy, and translational deformities may produce spinal or foraminal stenosis. Patients with these disorders typically have radicular symptoms as well as back pain. Discography, done correctly, is frequently helpful in confirming the diagnosis of a painful disc below a previous fusion (2, 11).

DEFORMITY

A perception of increased deformity is the second most common symptom among patients presenting for revision surgery. Patients frequently sense that the curve has changed in magnitude or contour, and they complain of changes in shoulder alignment, height, or comfort when sitting or standing. They may also complain of alteration in waistline contour or discomfort in the flank caused by impingement of their ribs on the iliac crest. Patients may develop progressive deformity in either the sagittal or coronal plane, or both.

IMBALANCE

Although progressive trunk imbalance is related directly to progression of the deformity, it is a more particular concern in patients with a previous fusion; increasing curvature below a solid fusion, which allows no compensation, can generate a disproportionate imbalance relative to the change in curvature. With age, a previously compensatory curve may become structural, compromising the patient's ability to compensate for the original, static curve. As trunk imbalance increases, the patient's function is progressively impaired, and the pain may increase dramatically.

DYSPNEA

While only 15% of patients with idiopathic curves complain of dyspnea, pulmonary dysfunction is much more common in neuromuscular and postpoliomyelitic patients (4,17). Winter et al. (31) and Weinstein et al. (29) noted that patients with idiopathic scoliosis develop pulmonary insufficiency only when their curves become severe. However, advanced age may significantly aggravate this problem in patients undergoing revision surgery. Scoliosis surgery is more often done to *prevent* pulmonary complications in high-risk patients than to treat existing or progressive dysfunction.

PREOPERATIVE PLANNING

Obtain upright anteroposterior (AP) and lateral scoliosis radiographs to carefully document the magnitude of deformity and establish the correct end-vertebrae. The lateral view is particularly important because sagittal imbalance is common and debilitating in these patients. Loss of normal lordosis, or marked lateral decompensation, may cause the patient to stand with one or both knees flexed; it is important that upright radiographs be taken with the knees extended to adequately represent the deformity. Other studies include supine, oblique radiographs to evaluate the fusion mass, and tomograms to confirm the presence of pseudarthrosis. Assess spinal rigidity through side-bending views in scoliotic patients, and use hyperextension views, supine over a bolster, for kyphotic deformities. Side-bending films should visualize the full extent of both upper and lower curves, assessing the cervicothoracic junction in thoracic curves and the lumbosacral junction in thoracolumbar or lumbar curves. Use magnetic resonance imaging (MRI) or myelography to evaluate any neurologic abnormality in a patient with progressive scoliosis. Diastematomyelia, tethered cord, syrinx, and cord or root compression may be ruled out by using these studies.

Careful evaluation of pulmonary reserve is always important in adults, where pulmonary complications are common and potentially life-threatening. Pulmonary function testing is indicated in any patient complaining of dyspnea and in all those with neuromuscular or chronic pulmonary disease. Patients with a severe thoracic lordosis, with a reduced AP chest diameter, may also need pulmonary function testing even if asymptomatic. A medicine consultation is often appropriate for middle-aged patients preparing to undergo a major spine reconstruction, and it is particularly important in those with underlying cardiovascular, pulmonary, or renal disease.

Autologous blood donation is beneficial and should be initiated 3–4 weeks prior to the operation. Prescribe supplemental iron for any patient donating her own blood.

TREATMENT

The key to treating most failures of scoliosis fusion is early identification of the problem. If a pseudarthrosis or failure of fixation is identified in the early postoperative phase, reinstrumentation can be carried out easily without osteotomies or major reconstruction. Likewise, if progression of an adjacent compensatory curve is identified early, it may be corrected by simply extending the fusion while the curve is still supple. If these problems are neglected for long, however, compensatory curves may become structural and pseudarthroses may lead to progressive deformity and decompensation. In these patients, reconstruction and hardware revision can be challenging.

PSEUDARTHROSIS

Pseudarthrosis may be present with or without progressive deformity. In cases with no loss of correction, the surgeon may address the pseudarthrosis directly, retaining or replacing hardware as necessary.

- After exposing the fusion mass over its full length, strip the thickened periosteum laterally with Cobb elevators. Carefully expose the cortical bone of the fusion mass throughout its length and from transverse process to transverse process.
- At the pseudarthrosis, the periosteum will be bound down to the fibrous tissue insinuated into the bony defect. At this point, it becomes difficult to strip the periosteum away, and the persistent fibrous tissue left behind reveals the defect.
- The fusion defect is usually located at the level of unfused facets. Using curets and rongeurs, remove this fibrous tissue completely from the pseudarthrosis.
- Expose the facet joints, remove any residual fibrous tissue or articular cartilage, and pack the joints with cancellous autograft bone. If the transverse processes

were not previously exposed, strip away the soft tissue and decorticate the bone prior to applying the bone graft.

If pseudarthrosis is associated with progressive deformity, correct the deformity at the time of the pseudarthrosis repair. Better curve correction at the time of revision surgery correlates with a significantly better fusion rate (15). Increased age, lower lumbar pseudarthrosis, and nonsegmental instrumentation are associated with a significantly higher rate of salvage failure.

■ If segmental instrumentation is in place and in good alignment, do not remove it to treat the pseudarthrosis. Revise hardware that has failed or is loose, however.
■ Remove and replace nonsegmental instrumentation with segmental fixation: Pseudarthrosis repair using Harrington rods is successful in fewer than 60% of patients, while repair using segmental instrumentation has provided 100% success in some series (15,30).
■ Substitute a shorter compression construct at the site of the pseudarthrosis, if possible, to avoid reinstrumenting the entire spine.
■ In a mature fusion, insert compression hooks through the dorsal cortex of the fusion mass without entering the neural canal.
■ Place pedicle screws in the thoracolumbar region to restore fixation where hooks have failed. Position pedicle screws under fluoroscopic or stereotactic control.
■ Once the pseudarthrosis has been debrided of all soft tissue, decorticate the facets and pack the defect with cancellous bone. Then reapply the instrumentation, decorticate the fusion mass extensively with a gouge, and reapply local and autograft bone to obtain fusion.

In patients with failed pseudarthrosis repairs, and in adult patients with risk factors for delayed healing or recurrent pseudarthrosis, perform anterior interbody fusion in conjunction with the posterior repair. Particularly in pseudarthroses of the lower lumbar spine or where fusion crosses the lumbosacral junction, anterior interbody fusion increases the chances of a successful arthrodesis. Likewise, in patients with pseudarthrosis and progressive deformity, anterior release and fusion may be necessary to obtain sagittal correction and maximize the chance of a solid fusion. The debilitating sagittal imbalance associated with the lumbar flatback syndrome is most successfully corrected through a combined approach, coupling anterior osteotomy and interbody fusion with posterior osteotomy or pseudarthrosis repair and instrumentation (13).

FIXATION FAILURE

Failure of fixation in the early postoperative period is usually heralded by the sudden onset of severe pain. Pain is usually well localized to the region of failure, and the displaced hook or rod is sometimes palpable through the skin. There is sometimes an associated episode of trauma, and symptoms may begin several days before the instrumentation actually displaces. If the patient's curve was particularly rigid, or if poor bone quality or severe rotation made fixation particularly difficult, have a higher index of suspicion for hardware displacement.

There are three options for treatment:

1. First, if correction has not been lost and the patient's pain is tolerable, postpone surgical revision and treat the patient in a rigid orthosis until fusion occurs. Solid fusion of the operated segments will eliminate the problem of the displaced hardware, and any prominent hardware can be removed at a later date if necessary.

2. A second option is to reoperate, and either reinsert the dislodged hook or remove it, shortening the construct. This may reduce the patient's pain and eliminate the prominent hardware, but it could lead to a loss of correction.

• If the dislodged hook is surgically replaced, take care to see that other fixation hooks are not displaced during the revision.
• Carefully inspect the lamina under which the hook was seated to ensure that it is not fractured and that the bone is sound enough to allow rigid fixation; reinstrumenting a damaged or disrupted lamina is unwise.
• If you choose to remove the displaced hook and shorten the instrumentation construct, you may significantly compromise construct stiffness. Only when fusion is established and curve progression is unlikely does removal of an end-hook make good sense.

3. The third option is to revise the hardware with a modified construct. This is most often necessary in patients with end-hook displacement, particularly those with rigid curves. In these cases, revising the terminal segment fixation may salvage the overall construct.

• Where a single hook has pulled out or dislodged, a claw configuration may provide rigid fixation and salvage the construct.
• Salvage a transverse process fracture by applying a sublaminar hook in place of the transverse process hook.
• Use one or two pedicle screws on the convex side to salvage hook failure in lower lumbar curves (Fig. 163.1).

When the vertebral lamina has been so disrupted by hook pullout that it is unsalvageable, you must make a critical judgment. If shortening the construct to the next intact lamina will compromise fixation of the appropriate segments of the curve, then the instrumentation must be extended over a longer segment. This may necessitate removal of the previous instrumentation.

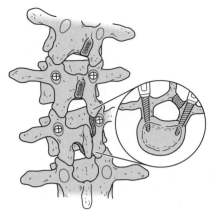

Figure 163.1. Pedicle screws can be used to salvage sites where hooks have loosened or pulled through the lamina. Orientation of the pedicles is determined on preoperative computed tomography. Pedicle screw fixation allows the surgeon to reinstrument the spine without extending the fusion to adjacent segments.

- In some cases it may be possible to salvage and lengthen an instrumentation construct by using "domino" rod connectors, extending the construct to the next stable level. This provides a bulky construct, however, which is more acceptable in the lumbar region than in the upper thoracic segments. This technique is particularly useful if fusion must be extended to the sacrum. Short segmental rods may be fixed to the sacrum either directly, using pedicle screws, or using a Galveston technique to instrument the iliac wings. These rods are then joined to the original construct using the "domino" connectors.

If the fixation rod has broken, then the whole construct must be replaced. All hook and screw attachments should be checked in the process. Reactive bone often reinforces the hook or screw insertion site, and these implants may be left in place. If the hook or screw site has been eroded by excessive motion or has fractured, a new fixation point must be chosen, or a different implant used—exchanging a pedicle screw for a hook, for example.

PROGRESSIVE DEFORMITY

In patients who have progressive deformity because of multiple pseudarthroses, adding unfused segments or bending the fusion mass may require multiple osteotomies, reinstrumentation, and extensive fusion before the spine is adequately corrected, stable, and balanced over the sacrum.

- When a progressive curve develops below a previous thoracic fusion, correct the upper curve when you cor-rect the lumbar curve to avoid causing significant coronal imbalance (19) (Fig. 163.2).
- Use preoperative radiographic studies to determine the stiffness of the previously fused curve, as well as the potential to correct the progressive compensatory curve.
- If pseudarthrosis is contributing to curve progression, obtain tomograms to document the extent and location of the defect.
- Obtain a bone scan to confirm the level of pseudarthrosis in difficult cases. Oblique radiographs can often identify the suspicious level.

OPERATIVE TECHNIQUE

In cases where the deformity is severe and rigid, it is necessary to perform anterior release and interbody fusion prior to posterior reconstruction. Both procedures may be performed under one anesthetic, but the two procedures in combination are time-consuming and demanding on both surgeon and patient. If excessive blood loss occurs or the patient experiences problems, perform a two-staged procedure.

- *For the anterior procedure*, place the patient in a lateral decubitus position. Establish appropriate monitoring lines prior to positioning the patient: Arterial and central venous lines are usually indicated, and some patients may require Swan-Ganz catheterization to more carefully monitor pulmonary pressures and cardiac output.
- Position the patient with the convexity of the most rigid and severe curve upward.
- Use a transthoracic or thoracolumbar surgical approach, taking one rib, or in some cases two, to expose the anterior spinal column.
- Expose as many interspaces as can be reached and excise the discs.
- Isolate and ligate segmental vessels on one side only, and spare particularly prominent vessels.
- If the patient has a severe kyphosis, peripheral vascular disease, or any other risk factor for cord ischemia, place a "bull-dog" vascular clip across the segmental vessels to temporarily occlude segmental flow. Spinal cord monitoring may then determine whether the vessel is crucial to cord perfusion.
- Once the interspaces are exposed, remove the discs with a scalpel and rongeurs, and remove the endplates with a sharp osteotome directed away from the spinal canal. In very rigid deformities, it may be necessary to release the entire posterior longitudinal ligament and lateral annulus before correction can be obtained. This is not necessary in more supple curves.
- When the endplates have been removed, morcelize iliac

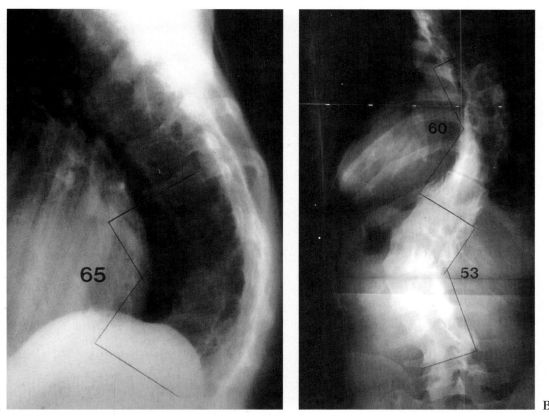

Figure 163.2. AP (**A**) and lateral (**B**) views of a 36-year-old woman with Marfan syndrome who presented 20 years after an *in situ* thoracic fusion for scoliosis (T-6 to T-12). She had low-back pain, progressive shoulder asymmetry, and progressive thoracic and lumbar deformities. The lateral view shows a significant thoracolumbar kyphosis, centered at T-9, which resulted in sagittal imbalance. The thoracic fusion was substantial and solid. (From McLain RF. Revision and Salvage in Deformity Surgery. *Semin Spine Surg* 1993;5:214, with permission.)

crest or rib graft and gently pack it into the interspace. Do not entirely fill the interspace with bone, as this may interfere with correction during the posterior procedure.

- Correct kyphotic segments by distracting the disc space anteriorly with a large vertebral body spreader and inserting a tricortical graft or titanium cage to restore sagittal lordosis.
- At the end of the anterior procedure, pull the pleura, or the paraspinous muscles in the thoracolumbar region, gently over the spinal column to prevent graft extrusion.
- Place a chest tube and close the wound.
- *For the posterior part of the procedure,* turn the patient or dress the wound and return the patient to the intensive care unit in anticipation of a staged posterior fusion.
- Perform the posterior reconstruction through the old

surgical wound. Expose the old fusion mass and the spinous processes and lamina of the secondary curve.
- Obtain a radiograph after the rigid and compensatory curves are fully exposed, to verify levels.
- Perform thoracic osteotomies at levels previously chosen in the preoperative plan (Fig. 163.3). Center the initial osteotomy over the apex of the curve, and subsequent osteotomies at every second level above and below the apex for the length of the previous fusion (8).
- Take care to complete the osteotomy across the full width of the fusion, and to take a wide enough wedge to allow correction of the scoliosis.
- Remove the outer cortex with either a burr or rongeurs, creating a defect that spans the fusion mass just below the transverse processes (Fig. 163.4*A*).
- Remove the cancellous bone down to the anterior, or volar, cortex of the fusion mass. To avoid plunging

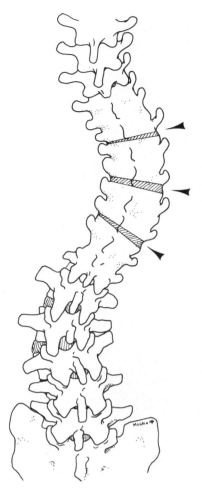

Figure 163.3.   The preoperative plan for the patient in Figure 163.2. To correct the progressive lumbar curvature without precipitating a marked thoracic imbalance, multiple osteotomies were planned as indicated. The initial osteotomy was centered over the curve apex; subsequent ones were located at every second level above and below the apex. (From McLain RF. Revision and Salvage in Deformity Surgery. *Semin Spine Surg* 1993;5: 214, with permission.)

through the inner cortex, direct the forces away from the midline and in an axial direction (Fig. 163.4*B*).

▪ After exposing the anterior cortex, penetrate it on the convexity with a burr or curet, creating a window large enough to admit the Kerrison rongeur. Use the Kerrison punch to complete the osteotomy across the full width of the fusion mass (Fig. 163.4*C*).

▪ After completing the osteotomy, use the Kerrison punch to undercut the margins of the osteotomy defect. This will reduce the chances that the cut edge of the fusion mass might impinge on the thecal sac when the osteotomy is closed, a particular risk when a kyphotic defor-

mity is being corrected. Cut the osteotomies so that they are wider posteriorly than anteriorly (again, particularly if a kyphotic deformity is being corrected) (Fig. 163.4*D*).

▪ Once the osteotomy is complete, the spinal segments above and below the cut should be independently mobile. Position hooks or pedicle screws proximally and distally for correction of both scoliotic curves.

Segmental instrumentation allows simultaneous correction of the scoliotic deformity with compression of the osteotomy sites.

▪ If the fusion mass is sufficient, place sublaminar wires or hooks through the dorsal cortex of the fusion without entering the canal.

▪ Carefully prepare and decorticate the area of the spine that was not previously fused, and pack the facet joints with cancellous bone graft prior to instrumentation.

▪ Once the segmental wires or hooks have been placed, apply the rods and correct the deformity either by tightening the segmental wires to bring the spine to the contoured rod or by gently rotating the rod, and sequentially distracting and compressing the hook combinations (Fig. 163.5).

▪ Pack local bone and iliac crest autograft around the osteotomy sites and over the previously unfused segment of spine.

At the end of the procedure, evaluate the patient for pneumothorax. If he has not undergone an anterior procedure and a chest tube was not previously placed, it is important to obtain a radiograph in the operating or recovery room to look for a pneumothorax and to place a chest tube if necessary.

POSTOPERATIVE CARE

In the first few postoperative days, the patient is carefully mobilized:

• Encourage the patient to sit up in bed or on a bedside chair on the first postoperative day.

• Independent ambulation is not possible until a molded thoracolumbosacral orthosis (TLSO) is available.

• The TLSO is usually molded by postoperative day 3 or 4, when the chest tube is removed.

• Begin transfers and ambulation when the brace arrives, and discharge the patient when he is independent.

The TLSO is worn full-time for 3–6 months, but it may not be needed at night after the third month. Wean the patient from the TLSO by 5–6 months, and begin physical rehabilitation for lifting and trunk strengthening at 6–8 months. Take oblique radiographs to evaluate the maturing fusion and thus ensure that the timing of brace removal and rehabilitation is appropriate.

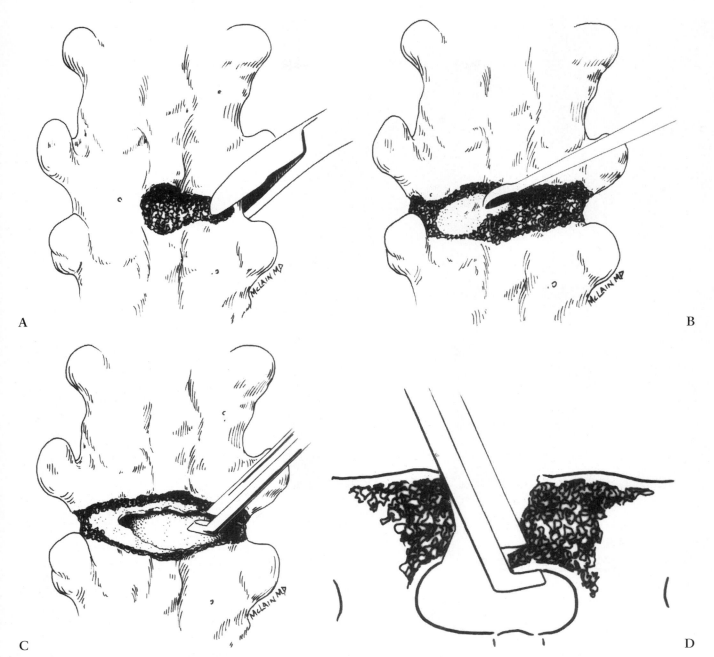

A

B

C

D

Figure 163.4. Osteotomy technique. See text for details. (From McLain RF. Revision and Salvage in Deformity Surgery. *Semin Spine Surg* 1993;5:214, with permission.)

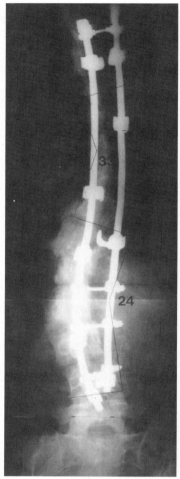
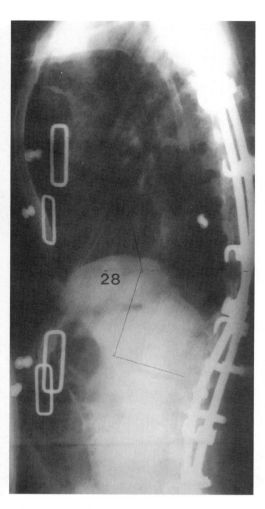

A,B

Figure 163.5. Postoperative radiographs of patient in Figure 163.2. After multiple osteotomies from T-6 to T-10, segmental instrumentation was used to correct the double curve to less than 50% of the preoperative deformity. Both sagittal and coronal deformities were improved, and shoulder asymmetry was corrected. (From McLain RF. Revision and Salvage in Deformity Surgery. *Semin Spine Surg* 1993;5:214, with permission.)

PITFALLS AND COMPLICATIONS

Complications are common in adults undergoing scoliosis surgery, and even more frequent when it is revision surgery. Complications in revision scoliosis surgery include the following:

- Pneumothorax, pneumonia, and/or respiratory insufficiency
- Infection
- Persistent or adjacent-level pseudarthrosis
- Instrumentation failure
- Neurologic injury
- Sagittal or coronal imbalance
- Thromboembolic disease and pulmonary embolism
- Death (a 1% to 2% mortality rate)

Swank et al. (26) demonstrated that the risks associated with scoliosis surgery appear to go up with each decade of life. The overall complication rate for primary surgery ranges from 53% to 62%, with a mortality rate of roughly 1.5% (23,25,26). The complication rates in patients undergoing revision surgery are even more daunting. Floman et al. (8) reported that 52% of revision patients had a serious complication; 10% developed pseudarthrosis, 14.5% had a significant neurologic complication, 11% had significant pulmonary complications, and 1.6% died (other complications made up the remaining 12.9%). Considering the young age of this group of patients (average, approximately 21 years), this is a high rate of complications. Kostuik (11) discussed outcomes in 31 patients undergoing revision surgery for scoliosis. The overall incidence of pseudarthrosis in this group was 23%, as opposed to a 6.5% incidence in adults undergoing primary fusion. He noted a 10% incidence of pulmonary complications, including nine pneumothoraces.

Cummine et al. (4) reviewed 59 patients undergoing reconstructive surgery for failed scoliosis fusion. The overall complication rate was 71%, with two postoperative deaths (3.4%) in the group. They noted a 17% incidence of pseudarthrosis, a 5% incidence of pulmonary complica-

HINTS AND TRICKS

- Monitor patients postoperatively to maintain an adequate blood pressure. Postoperative hypotension can lead to cord ischemia, particularly after extensive anterior dissection or multiple procedures that may have compromised collateral blood flow. Case reports have documented transient and permanent neurologic injuries associated with episodes of postoperative hypotension (27,30).

tions, and an 8% incidence of deep wound infections. There was one fatal and one nonfatal pulmonary embolism in this study group.

Current protocols for deep venous thrombosis prophylaxis and the routine use of prophylactic antibiotics have significantly reduced the incidence of pulmonary embolism and deep wound infections over those seen in previous studies. Likewise, the use of autograft bone and improved techniques in instrumentation and surgical fusion should reduce pseudarthrosis rates. Nonetheless, complications in revision scoliosis surgery are likely to remain high, particularly in older patients and those with neuromuscular or paralytic disorders.

Improvements in preoperative planning, patient management, surgical technique, and instrumentation technology will not eliminate the common complications associated with reconstructive surgery of the scoliotic spine. Early recognition of curve progression or pseudarthrosis remains the most reliable way to limit the complexity of these challenging reconstructions. In those patients who do develop rigid curvatures with marked loss of correction, careful preoperative planning is the key to a good surgical result.

REFERENCES

+ 1. Aurori BF, Weierman RJ, Lowell HA, et al. Pseudarthrosis after Spinal Fusion for Scoliosis. *Clin Orthop* 1985;199:153.

2. Bradford DS. Adult Scoliosis. *Clin Orthop* 1988;229:70.

+ 3. Cochran T, Irstram L, Nachemson A. Long-term Anatomic and Functional Changes in Patients with Adolescent Scoliosis Treated by Harrington Rod Fusions. *Spine* 1983;8:576.

+ 4. Cummine JL, Lonstein JE, Moe JH, et al. Reconstructive Surgery in the Adult for Failed Scoliosis Fusion. *J Bone Joint Surg Am* 1979;61:1151.

+ 5. Dodd CAF, Fergusson CM, Freedman L, et al. Allograft

versus Autograft Bone in Scoliosis Fusion. *J Bone Joint Surg Br* 1988;70:431.

* 6. Dubousset J, Herring JA, Shufflebarger H. The Crankshaft Phenomenon. *J Pediatr Orthop* 1989;9:541.

* 7. Erwin WD, Dickson JH, Harrington PR. Clinical Review of Patients with Broken Harrington Rods. *J Bone Joint Surg Am* 1980;62:1302.

+ 8. Floman Y, Penny N, Micheli L, Riseborough EJ. Osteotomy of the Fusion Mass in Scoliosis. *J Bone Joint Surg Am* 1982;64:1307.

* 9. King HA, Joe JH, Bradford DS, Winter RB. The Selection of Fusion Levels in Thoracic Idiopathic Scoliosis. *J Bone Joint Surg Am* 1983;65:1302.

+ 10. Knapp DR, Jones ET. Use of Cortical Cancellous Allograft for Posterior Spinal Fusion. *Clin Orthop* 1988;229:99.

+ 11. Kostuik JP. Recent Advances in the Treatment of Painful Adult Scoliosis. *Clin Orthop* 1980;147:238.

+ 12. Kostuik JP, Israel J, Hall JE. Scoliosis Surgery in Adults. *Clin Orthop* 1973;93:225.

+ 13. Lagrone MO, Bradford DS, Moe JH, et al. Treatment of Symptomatic Flatback after Spinal Fusion. *J Bone Joint Surg* 1988;70:569.

+ 14. Lapinksy AS, Richards BS. Preventing the Crankshaft Phenomenon by Combining Anterior Fusion with Posterior Instrumentation. Does It Work? *Spine* 1995;20:1392.

+ 15. Lauerman WC, Bradford DS, Transfeldt EE, Ogilvie JW. Management of Pseudarthrosis after Arthrodesis of the Spine for Idiopathic Scoliosis. *J Bone Joint Surg* 1991;73:222.

+ 16. Letts RM, Bobechko WP. Fusion of the Scoliotic Spine in Young Children. *Clin Orthop* 1974;101:136.

17. Lonstein JE. Salvage and Reconstructive Surgery. In: Bradford DS, Moe JH, Lonstein JE, et al., eds. *Moe's Textbook of Scoliosis and Other Spinal Deformities.* Philadelphia: WB Saunders, 1987.

+ 18. Mayfield JK. Severe Spine Deformity in Myelodysplasia and Sacral Agenesis. *Spine* 1981;65:498.

+ 19. McLain RF. Revision and Salvage in Deformity Surgery. *Semin Spine Surg* 1993;5:214.

+ 20. McMaster MJ, James JIP. Pseudarthrosis after Fusion for Scoliosis. *J Bone Joint Surg Br* 1976;58:305.

* 21. Moe JH, Gustilo RB. Treatment of Scoliosis. Results in 196 Patients Treated by Cast Correction and Fusion. *J Bone Joint Surg Am* 1964;46:293.

+ 22. Osebold WR, Mayfield JK, Winter RB, et al. Surgical Treatment of Paralytic Scoliosis Associated with Myelomeningocele. *J Bone Joint Surg Am* 1982;64:841.

+ 23. Ponder C, Dickson J, Harrington P, et al. Results of Harrington Instrumentation and Fusion in the Adult Idiopathic Scoliosis Patient. *J Bone Joint Surg Am* 1975;57:797.

* 24. Ponseti IV, Friedman B. Changes in the Scoliotic Spine after Fusion. *J Bone Joint Surg Am* 1950;32:751.

* 25. Sponseller PD, Cohen MS, Nachemson AL, et al. Results of Surgical Treatment of Adults with Idiopathic Scoliosis. *J Bone Joint Surg Am* 1987;69:667.

* 26. Swank S, Lonstein JE, Moe JH, et al. Surgical Treatment

of Adult Scoliosis. *J Bone Joint Surg Am* 1981;63: 268.

+ 27. Taylor BA, Webb PJ, Hetreed M, et al. Delayed Postoperative Paraplegia with Hypotension in Adult Revision Scoliosis Surgery. *Spine* 1994;19:470.

+ 28. Van Dam BE, Bradford DS, Lonstein JE, et al. Adult Idiopathic Scoliosis Treated by Posterior Spinal Fusion and Harrington Instrumentation. *Spine* 1987;12:32.

* 29. Weinstein SL, Zavala DC, Ponseti IV. Idiopathic Scoliosis: Long-term Follow-up in Untreated Patients. *J Bone Joint Surg Am* 1981;63:702.

+ 30. Winter RB, Denis F, Lonstein JE, Dezen E. Salvage and Reconstructive Surgery for Spinal Deformity using Cotrel-Dubousset Instrumentation. *Spine* 1991;16:S412.

+ 31. Winter RB, Lovell WW, Moe JH. Excessive Thoracic Lordosis and Loss of Pulmonary Function in Patients with Idiopathic Scoliosis. *J Bone Joint Surg Am* 1975; 57:972.

SECTION IX
PEDIATRIC DISORDERS

SECTION EDITOR

George T. Rab

CHAPTER 164

OPERATIVE TREATMENT OF CHILDREN'S FRACTURES AND INJURIES OF THE PHYSES

George T. Rab and Brian E. Grottkau

GENERAL APPROACH TO SURGERY

Fracture treatment in children is often simpler than in adults because of the rapid healing and remodeling of bone that occurs in children. A perceptive surgeon realizes that children differ a great deal from adults and care of

 G. T. Rab: Department of Orthopaedics, University of California, Davis, Sacramento, California, 95817.
 B. E. Grottkau: Department of Orthopedics, Tufts University School of Medicine Floating Hospital for Children, Boston, Massachusetts 02111.

their fractures can be affected by a child's preinjury status, the specific fracture mechanics of childhood injuries, the response to injury, and the unique treatment problems and complications that occur in the pediatric age group.

 Although fracture management in children is usually nonoperative, there are certain instances when surgical management is required, desirable, or optional. Open surgical treatment is indicated in certain physeal fractures where there is joint incongruence and closed reduction has not led to satisfactory position, and where exact reduction improves the chances of normal physeal growth. Open reduction should be performed when anatomic reduction is required for normal function, as in a displaced, both-bone forearm fracture in an older adolescent. Surgical treatment should be considered in children with multiple trauma if stabilization of major long-bone fractures will enhance nursing care and pulmonary management. It should also be considered in children with major long-bone fractures (especially femoral shaft) in the presence of a severe head injury.

An additional relative indication for open reduction and internal fixation is to alleviate the psychological stress of either children or parents associated with prolonged hospitalization. An example is a 13-year-old boy with a closed midshaft femoral fracture that would eventually heal with skeletal traction and spica-cast treatment—a treatment that might take 8 weeks or more. A closed intramedullary nail would allow rapid mobilization, discharge from the hospital in a few days, and return to home and school within 1 week.

PHYSEAL INJURIES

The Salter–Harris classification of injuries to the growing physis is widely accepted in North America (Fig. 164.1):

Type I	Separation of the epiphysis
Type II	Separation of the epiphysis with fracture through the metaphysis
Type III	Intra-articular fracture of part of the epiphysis that extends through the physis, causing it to separate from the metaphysis
Type IV	Intra-articular fracture of part of the epiphysis that extends through the physis and the metaphysis (malreduction of the physis results in bony union across the growth plate at the fracture site).
Type V	Crush injury to the physis resulting in premature closure of the growth plate
Type VI	Avulsion or crushing of the peripheral physis

Specific injuries are covered elsewhere in this chapter, but some general principles will be reviewed here. Nondisplaced fractures through the growth plate tend to be stable and require immobilization without internal fixation. Minimally displaced growth-plate injuries do not require reduction, and the chance of growth arrest is not increased by leaving them displaced. Displaced fractures requiring reduction should be treated early (within 48 hours) because growth arrest is common after attempts at late reduction. Atraumatic fracture reduction and suitable fixation (casting or surgical) are mandatory.

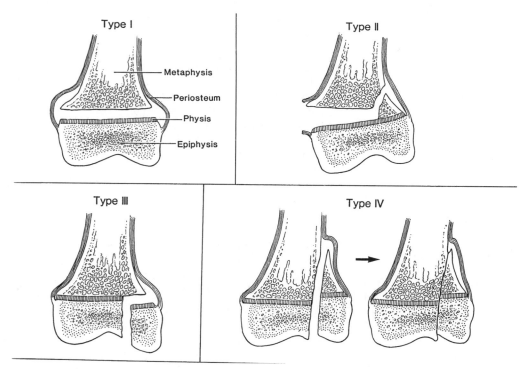

Figure 164.1. Salter–Harris classification of physeal fractures. See text for description of types. (Redrawn from Salter RB, Harris WR. Injuries Involving the Epiphyseal Plate. *J Bone Joint Surg Am* 1963;45:587, with permission.) *(continued)*

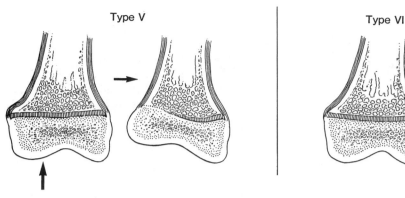

Figure 164.1.   (continued)

The younger the patient, the more remodeling potential exists and greater degrees of displacement are acceptable. However, younger patients in whom physeal arrest develops have a greater potential for deformity. Likewise, a growth plate that requires higher energy to cause failure because of its geometry tends to have a higher rate of problems with growth arrest. For instance, the distal femoral and proximal tibial growth plates are only rarely injured but are responsible for the majority of longitudinal and angular growth abnormalities following growth-plate fracture. Salter–Harris types III and IV fractures require anatomic reduction of both the growth plate and the articular surface; thus they frequently require open reduction with internal fixation.

An extensive discussion of operative fracture management of children's fractures is beyond the scope of this chapter. Following are descriptions of techniques that we have found useful for the surgical treatment of common pediatric injuries, as well as uncommon injuries requiring surgery. This chapter includes some generalizations and personal preferences in both indications and treatment options; readers should consult fracture textbooks and the scientific literature for more extensive descriptions.

UPPER EXTREMITY

PROXIMAL HUMERAL EPIPHYSEAL FRACTURES

Fractures of the proximal humerus (6,16,40,49) are most frequently seen in neonates and adolescents. Neonatal fractures are typically Salter–Harris type I injuries caused by an abduction–external rotation force imparted during the process of delivery. Orthopaedic consultation is obtained in these cases because a neonate will not actively move the involved extremity. Fracture of the clavicle, Erb's palsy, and infection are the main differential diagnoses. Radiographs may not be helpful, although ultraso-

nography yields a clear representation of this cartilaginous injury. Simple immobilization of the arm to the trunk with a loose elastic bandage for 1–2 weeks allows complete healing.

Adolescents are more prone to Salter–Harris type II and metaphyseal fractures of the humerus. Most of these can be managed by splinting because remodeling is rapid in this region and anatomic reduction is not required for excellent function. Fortunately, physeal growth arrest is rare and neurovascular injury uncommon. Closed reduction is generally necessary only in patients near skeletal maturity whose fracture has greater than 50° to 70° of angulation in either the sagittal or the coronal plane. After initial muscle spasms abate after treatment in a sling for 5–7 days, however, fracture alignment frequently improves enough to eliminate the need for closed reduction. If closed reduction does not yield an acceptable position, reduction under anesthesia with shoulder spica-cast immobilization usually suffices. On occasions when a spica cast may not be appropriate (e.g., when there is a chest injury), surgical fixation may be accomplished by introducing a large, smooth Steinmann pin into the reduced humeral head through a 1 cm incision over the deltoid tubercle. Bend the pin end to decrease the chance of proximal migration, and immobilize the arm with a sling and swath. Image intensification is necessary, and it is surprisingly difficult to place the pin in the head with enough purchase to fix the fracture. Remove the pin at 3–4 weeks.

SUPRACONDYLAR FRACTURES OF THE HUMERUS

Supracondylar humeral fractures (2,24,41,54,64,68,73) have the highest rates of complications of any pediatric fracture. Volkmann's ischemic contracture due to compartment syndrome, neurologic or vascular compromise, and cubitus varus have historically complicated the treatment of these fractures. Supracondylar fracture of the humerus is often a surgical emergency, and prompt reduction and stabilization will reduce the incidence of complications. Although closed methods of immobilization may be used, percutaneous pin fixation has emerged in the last decade as the preferred method for unstable, displaced fractures. Pin fixation, properly done, is a low-risk procedure that provides excellent control of fracture fragments, nearly eliminating the risk of cubitus varus that accompanies cast immobilization. In addition, percutaneous pinning allows partial extension of the elbow without loss of reduction, which is much safer when there is swelling and vascular compromise.

Before attempting reduction, carefully evaluate the extremity for neurovascular compromise or compartment syndrome (usually in the flexor compartment of the forearm), and document the findings in the chart. An absent radial pulse is an indication for prompt reduction but is not in itself an indication for surgical exploration if the capillary refill is intact and the hand well perfused after reduction is accomplished. Neurologic deficits are common in supracondylar fractures but generally disappear spontaneously within 3 months after treatment. Exploration of the nerve is probably indicated only when closed reduction is impossible in the face of a preexisting nerve deficit (implying interposed nerve tissue in the fracture), or when nerve deficit occurs coincident with reduction.

Approximately 2% of supracondylar fractures are anteriorly displaced as a result of a flexion force applied to the elbow. The remaining supracondylar fractures are caused by hyperextension injuries of the elbow. They have been classified by Wilkins (74) as follows:

Type I   Nondisplaced
Type II   Displaced with an intact posterior cortex
Type III   Completely displaced

Posteromedial displacement is more common than posterolateral displacement. Regardless of the direction of displacement of the distal fragment in an extension-type supracondylar fracture, the posterior periosteum is generally intact and may be used to assist reduction. Most supracondylar fractures occur with the forearm in pronation; therefore, the distal fragment is internally rotated relative to the proximal fragment. Thus, most are more unstable after reduction with the arm internally rotated, a fact that has implications when radiographs are obtained (see later discussion).

Closed Reduction and Percutaneous Pinning

- Place the patient in the supine position, and administer a general anesthetic. Use an image intensifier in a vertical position next to the table. The receiver can be used as a minitable to set the arm on.
- Perform closed reduction by manually distracting the fracture with the elbow slightly hyperextended and the forearm in supination. Correct the medial or lateral displacement, and then align the varus–valgus position of the arm to match the opposite normal elbow. While

still distracting, flex the supinated arm while pushing posteriorly on the distal portion of the humeral shaft (proximal fragment). Flex the elbow acutely, and temporarily hold it flexed by wrapping a gauze or tape between the wrist and shoulder (Fig. 164.2A); pronation of the forearm to "lock" the fracture is unnecessary if percutaneous fixation is to be used. The pulse may not be palpable at this time.

- Check an anteroposterior (AP) image, using the image intensifier. Obtain a lateral view by externally rotating the flexed arm on the image intensifier (Fig. 164.2B); internal rotation can destabilize the fracture at this point and cause loss of reduction. Exact anatomic reduction is unnecessary, but the carrying angle should be restored. Some translation or angulation on the lateral x-ray film is acceptable because it should correct with remodeling.
- Percutaneous pinning requires two pins, usually 0.045 Kirschner wires (K-wires), both of which may be inserted from lateral and parallel or from medial, lateral, and crossed. If crossed, they should not cross at the fracture site. Although crossed pins have been shown to be biomechanically advantageous, two parallel lateral pins are safer. An ulnar nerve palsy may result from injury to the nerve at the time of insertion of a medial pin or from chronic contact with the pin throughout the course of treatment. These neurotmeses usually resolve in 3–4 months. When a medial pin is used, massage the medial epicondyle for a few minutes to "milk out" edema to be sure that the ulnar nerve is avoided, or insert the pin through a 1 cm incision under direct visualization. If the medial epicondyle cannot be palpated, two lateral pins must be used. In either event, the pins must pass through the distal fragment and engage the opposite cortex of the proximal (shaft) fragment by passing just through the entire cortex. We always use two lateral pins, if possible.
- To make pinning easier, insert a 14-gauge needle into the periosteum of the distal fragment laterally at the desired angle of the pin (Fig. 164.2C). Obtain AP and lateral views (by external rotation), using the image intensifier. After adjustment of the direction of the needle, insert an 0.045 K-wire through the needle, and drill it through the opposite cortex of the proximal fragment. Place a second pin in a similar manner. Withdraw the needles, bend the pins outside the skin to avoid migration, and apply pin caps (Fig. 164.3).
- Extend the arm fully, and check the carrying angle of the elbow; if it is not correct, repeat the preceding procedure after a second reduction. Anatomic reduction on x-ray images is not necessary, but cubitus varus will not remodel and must be avoided. Flex the elbow to 90° (or less if the pulse disappears with flexion), and immobilize with a posterior splint, sling, and swath.

Obtain radiographs 1 week postoperatively to check

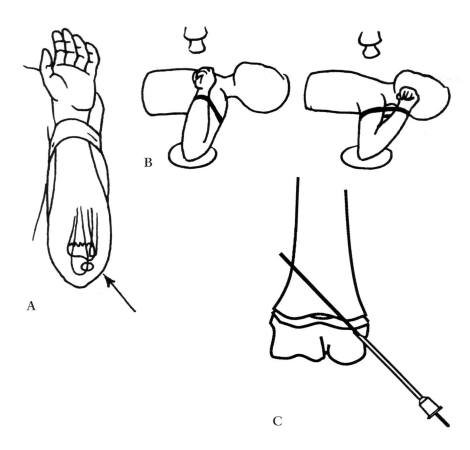

Figure 164.2. Surgical technique for percutaneous pinning of supracondylar fracture of the humerus. **A:** The hand and wrist are secured to the upper arm. **B:** AP and lateral image intensifier views are obtained by rotating the arm. **C:** A 14-ga needle is useful as a pin guide. See text for explanation.

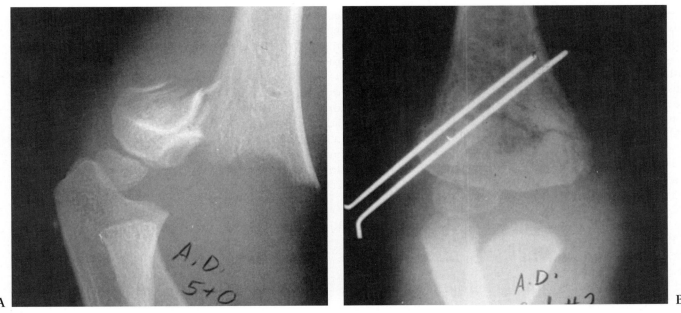

Figure 164.3. Displaced supracondylar fracture of the humerus fixed by closed reduction and percutaneous pinning with two parallel lateral pins. Note the engagement of the cortex of the medial proximal fragment.

position. Remove the pins and splint at 4 weeks after the fracture, and begin motion as tolerated. Immobilization beyond 4 weeks is unnecessary, and physical therapy is not appropriate.

The most serious complication following supracondylar fracture is compartment syndrome (Volkman's ischemic contracture). It is more common when there has been vascular compromise or massive swelling has occurred, but it can appear in less dramatic clinical situations. The hallmark feature of compartment syndrome is pain with passive finger extension, but it is easy to misinterpret the examination in a frightened or sedated child. Measure compartment pressures if necessary; this is facilitated by the stability achieved with percutaneous pinning.

Loss of position rarely occurs if pinning is adequate and both fragments are engaged by the pins. If loss of position is detected at 1 week, it may be possible to salvage a satisfactory carrying angle by extending the arm fully, adjusting the carrying angle back into valgus, and applying a long-arm cast with the forearm in supination and the elbow extended. Do not remove the pins. Continue immobilization for a total of 4 weeks.

Complete loss of position requires re-reduction and pinning in the operating room. This is not advisable or possible after approximately 10 days, as healing is too far advanced.

Supracondylar Fractures with Vascular Injury

Displaced (Salter–Harris type III) supracondylar humeral fractures may be associated with injury to the brachial artery. The brachial artery and the median nerve are juxtaposed to the fracture site and thus are subject to direct and stretch injury at the time of fracture and reduction. A well-documented neurovascular examination before closed reduction is mandatory to avoid unnecessary exploration afterward. Brachial artery compromise may be due to acute thrombi, intimal tears, laceration, transection, or entrapment within the fracture site. Absence of a radial pulse or the presence of a mottled arm and hand is an indication to proceed urgently to surgery for closed reduction. Do not delay treatment because circulation returns with fracture reduction. Because the site of vascular compromise is known, angiography is usually not necessary.

If an absent pulse does not return after reduction and extension, make a decision based on clinical examination of the hand. If the fingers are pink and well perfused, it is safe to observe, even if pulses are present. If the fingers are dusky, exploration of the artery is indicated.

If the pulse was present before reduction but absent afterward, obtain a vascular surgery consultation. The vascular surgeon may choose to obtain an angiogram with the image intensifier on the operating-room table or proceed directly to exploration. If revascularization is needed, closely monitor the patient for compartment syndrome, and give serious consideration to performing prophylactic forearm compartment releases.

Open Reduction

If an adequate closed reduction cannot be attained, consider an open reduction. Remember that anterior-to-posterior translation and angulation are generally acceptable, and even the AP radiograph does not need to be anatomic as long as the carrying angle is satisfactory with the elbow extended. Open reduction usually proves to be more difficult than anticipated. Use a surgical approach on the side of the largest fracture gap. Periosteum and the brachial muscle, nerve, and artery can all block reduction and should be looked for and extricated. Open reduction has not been associated with increased stiffness in children with this complication.

LATERAL CONDYLAR FRACTURES OF THE HUMERUS

Lateral condylar fractures (4,22,23,30,37,47,65,74) usually occur as the result of a fall on an outstretched hand and consequently are Salter–Harris type IV intra-articular fractures, with the initial failure beginning at the capitellar or trochlear surface. Errors in interpretation of the radiograph can lead to a missed diagnosis. Such fractures may be mistaken for type II fractures because of their metaphyseal component (Fig. 164.4A), but they are usually highly unstable injuries that require surgical treatment. Lateral condylar fractures that are truly nondisplaced may be treated nonoperatively, but they must be radiographed weekly because they have a propensity to displace late.

True type II fractures (transcondylar fractures) may be seen in children approximately 2 years of age. They are usually hyperextension injuries and are analogous to supracondylar fractures. They can be distinguished from lateral condylar fractures by their longer, more posterior metaphyseal fragment. Closed reduction (occasionally together with percutaneous pinning) is appropriate for these injuries.

The indication for surgical management of lateral condylar fractures is displacement, either acute or progressive, of the visible fragments by more than 2 mm. Some have advocated closed reduction and pinning for selected minimally displaced lateral condylar injuries (47) as determined by intraoperative arthrography. We generally perform open reduction because the joint surface is often remarkably displaced.

Open Reduction

- Under tourniquet control, make a curved longitudinal incision over the lateral humeral condyle. There is usually a longitudinal rent in the brachioradialis muscle; develop this interval and carefully expose the lateral margin of the condyle. Take great care at this point to keep all subsequent dissection anterior to the condyle because the blood supply of the capitellum lies posteriorly and a major complication of this procedure is osteonecrosis of this fragment.

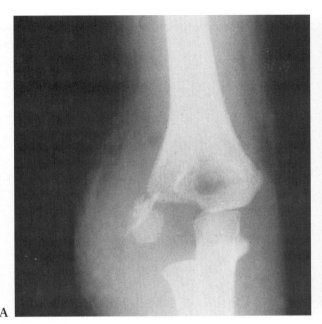
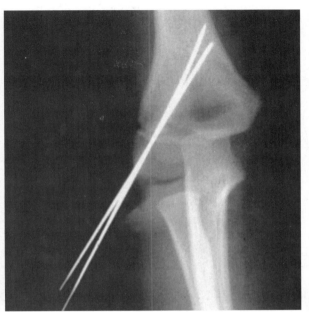

A   B

Figure 164.4.   Lateral condylar fracture of the humerus treated by open reduction and pinning. **A:** AP radiograph of acute fracture. **B:** Fracture is anatomical after fixation with two K-wires.

- Open the elbow joint, and retract the synovium anteriorly, using the long end of an army–navy retractor. The distal fragment is frequently rotated up to 90° and may be much larger than expected, including a sizable portion of the cartilaginous trochlea.
- Gently clean the fracture ends of hematoma and fibrous tissue, and reduce the fracture. Reduction may be unstable. Sometimes, stability is facilitated by inserting a K-wire in the fragment and using it as a "joystick" to control the fragment; however, be careful to plan its insertion point so that it may be used later to fix the fracture.
- Fix the fracture with two K-wires (Fig. 164.4B). If the metaphyseal fracture is large, they may pass through it, but often they must begin in the distal cartilaginous portion of the condylar fragment. Leave a space of at least 3 mm between the wires, and pass them just through the medial cortex of the proximal shaft to ensure stability. Bring the wires out through small stab wounds in the skin in the appropriate site. Bend the ends to prevent migration and place pin caps.
- Close the wound with fine, absorbable suture. Apply a splint at 90° of elbow flexion.

Remove the pins and splint at 4 weeks postoperatively, and begin motion as tolerated. Immobilization beyond 4 weeks is unnecessary.

The most common complications of lateral condylar fractures in children are missed diagnosis, nonunion, malunion, lateral growth arrest, and cubitus valgus. Tardy ulnar nerve palsy is possible late but fortunately is rare. Fractures treated by cast immobilization only that do not heal by 8 weeks after the injury should be treated with pin fixation and *in situ* bone grafting of the metaphyseal portion. If an arthrogram shows contrast agent between the capitellum and the trochlea, then do an open reduction with pin fixation. This can be done as late as 8 weeks after the injury. If contrast does not penetrate the fracture, then we pin the fracture percutaneously to add stability and facilitate healing. Leave wires in for 6 weeks, and then remove them.

Nonunions that are older than 12 weeks are difficult to treat. If the fracture is pain-free and there is no joint instability, treatment is not required. This avoids the possibility of stiffness secondary to bone grafting.

RADIAL NECK FRACTURES

Radial neck fractures (27,38,50,57,67,72) generally occur as a consequence of a fall on an outstretched hand that cause buckling and impaction of the radial neck. They are uncommon injuries. Their treatment is highly controversial because they often have good potential for remodeling and the results of open reduction are often poor. Despite the relatively minor appearance of some of these fractures, they are significant injuries, and compartment syndrome may occur.

Unless there are other considerations, we do not reduce fractures with angulations of 45° or less, particularly in

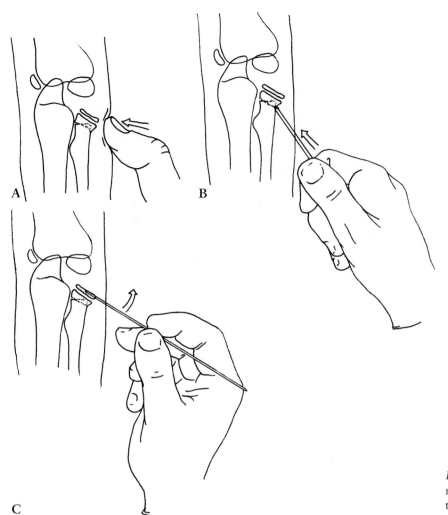

A

B

C

Figure 164.5. Three options for management of a severely angulated radial neck fracture that may allow avoidance of open reduction. See text for description.

children younger than 10 years. With greater angulation, closed manipulative reduction or percutaneous reduction techniques are indicated (Fig. 164.5). Remember that open reduction can be complicated by elbow stiffness, heterotopic ossification, growth arrest, and synostosis. A percutaneous technique described by Metaizeau uses a curved K-wire inserted retrograde into the canal from the distal radius (27). We have no experience with this technique, but it has been reported to be simple and effective.

Closed or Percutaneous Reduction

■ Under general anesthesia, attempt a closed reduction first; an assistant is helpful. Supinate the forearm, apply traction and varus stress to the elbow, and place the thumb over the radial head. By pronation and supination of the forearm, the deformity may be palpable. When the radial head feels most prominent, reduce the fracture by forceful pressure with the thumb (Fig.

164.5*A*). An image intensifier may be helpful for localizing the deformity. If reduction to 45° or less is obtained, accept the reduction, and immobilize the elbow in a splint for 3 weeks.

■ If reduction fails, rotate the forearm so that the tilt of the radial head is maximal, and pass a Steinmann pin percutaneously just below (distal to) the physis of the radial head, using the image intensifier. Use the Steinmann pin to push the head fragment back to an acceptable position (Fig. 164.5*B*). If this succeeds, immobilize the elbow for 3 weeks.

■ If this fails in an older child with an ossified radial head, a third option is to carefully pass an 0.035 K-wire transversely into the ossified radial head (be sure not to damage the physis). Use this wire to manipulate the head fragment into an improved position (Fig. 164.5*C*).

■ In both of these percutaneous techniques, if the fracture is unstable, it may be held for 2–3 weeks with a small

K-wire inserted percutaneously obliquely, usually from proximal to distal, from the radial head to the shaft fragment. Be careful when using pins for manipulation or fixation near the radial head not to pass through the radius into the ulna; even one pass may cause synostosis.

MEDIAL EPICONDYLAR FRACTURES OF THE HUMERUS

There has been much debate in the literature regarding the proper treatment of medial epicondylar fractures of the humerus (24,76), with particular concern about how much displacement of the fragment is acceptable. The true significance of this fracture, however, is that avulsion of the epicondyle is due to a subluxation or dislocation of the elbow joint. Consequently, the fracture should be thought of as similar to a medial collateral ligament injury, and the proper treatment is dictated by the instability of the elbow and not by some arbitrary degree of fracture displacement seen on radiographs.

The prognosis after medial epicondylar fractures is guarded. Periarticular injury may accompany an elbow dislocation, whether recognized or not, and can lead to permanent loss of elbow motion of a magnitude unexpected in a child. Warn parents about this early in the course of treatment. The medial epicondyle has a tendency to enlarge because of hyperemia after surgery; thus, the cosmetic result may be compromised after treatment.

Indications for operative reduction and fixation of medial epicondylar fractures include the following:

Incarceration of the medial epicondylar fragment in a dislocated, unreducible elbow
Gross valgus instability of the elbow
Displacement of 1.5–2 cm if accompanied by rotation of the fragment and marked weakness of the forearm flexors
Displacement of 1–2 cm in the dominant elbow of a child heavily involved in throwing sports

However, these indications, which we use, are arbitrary, and each child must be individually evaluated. The surgical technique is straightforward, but take care to avoid injury to the ulnar nerve during the dissection. Fixation may involve either K-wires or small-fragment screws because the amount of growth remaining in the usual patient is so small that cubitus varus will not develop.

FOREARM FRACTURES

In children younger than 10–12 years, closed management of forearm fractures (3,17,51,56,62,77) is usually successful. Growing children exhibit excellent remodeling potential, and angular and rotational deformities up to 15° are well tolerated. In older children, treatment can be closed, as long as reduction achieves satisfactory alignment, because union is rapid and stiffness unlikely. Adolescents with both-bone forearm fractures, however, represent a transitional situation between that of young children (who tolerate imperfect reduction) and that of adults (who generally require open reduction). We treat both-bone forearm fractures in older adolescents with open distal radial or ulnar physes, regardless of age, by performing closed reduction first; if the reduction is anatomic or nearly so, we accept it and follow the child with weekly radiographs until union occurs. If the reduction is not acceptable, we proceed with open reduction, using either one-third tubular plates or 3.5 mm compression plates and the same technique employed in adults (see Chapter 16). In most cases, it is wise to use the larger, 3.5 mm plate because nonunion is not unusual in this age group. After open reduction, immobilize the forearm in a long-arm cast until union occurs.

Occasionally, in younger children, diaphyseal both-bone forearm fractures either cannot be reduced by closed means or, once reduced, are too unstable to maintain the reduction in a cast (usually when the fractures are at the same level in the bone). Unreducible fractures may require a small incision to remove soft tissues blocking the reduction. An intramedullary K-wire or flexible nail can then be introduced either proximally through the olecranon in the ulna or distally in the radial metaphysis. Flynn (22) showed that intramedullary fixation of a single bone in both-bone forearm fractures in conjunction with long-arm casting results in excellent fracture fixation. The pins are left outside the skin and the ends bent over. They can be removed in the office 4–6 weeks after insertion.

Noonan and Price (51) outlined the acceptable limits of reduction for pediatric forearm fractures. In children younger than 9 years, 15° of angulation, 45° of malrotation, and complete displacement can be accepted. In children age 9 years or older, bayonet apposition, 30° of angulation, and 10° of malrotation are acceptable. The closer the fracture is to the growth plate and the younger the child, the greater is the remodeling potential in all planes, except for rotational malalignment.

A special situation requiring open reduction arises in younger children (approximately 10 years) with distal both-bone fractures in which the ulnar fracture is a greenstick fracture and the radial fracture is displaced and translated dorsally with shortening of approximately 1 cm. The radial fragment is often buttonholed through a rent in the periosteum and cannot be reduced back to length. In such cases, make a small dorsal incision, and pry the fragment back with an elevator. Usually, no internal fixation is required after reduction is achieved.

LOWER EXTREMITY

PELVIS

Relevant literature on pediatric pelvic fractures spans four decades (9,26,28,33,46,55,59). Unlike adults, most children with massive pelvis injuries do not exhibit gross instability of the fragments. Pubic symphysis widening is well tolerated and tends to decrease after the child begins to walk. Proximal displacement of the iliac bone is rare, but patients with fracture patterns susceptible to displacement must be followed with serial radiographs. In rare instances, they require external or internal fixation, as in adults. For most children, bed rest followed by mobilization to a chair and progression to weight bearing as tolerated, along with pain control, is all that is required.

Acetabular fractures in children are likewise rare and can usually be treated nonoperatively. When fragment displacement is wide, assessment with computed tomography (CT) or, especially, magnetic resonance imaging (MRI) will determine whether there is involvement of the triradiate cartilage. The surgical principles for the management of acetabular fractures in adults are outlined in Chapter 18. They must be applied sparingly in children because triradiate cartilage closure can be a serious complication in younger children, and nonoperative treatment may be safer. Sometimes, cartilage joint surfaces may remain intact, even though the underlying bone is displaced, and these fractures need not be surgically treated (Fig. 164.6).

Avulsion fractures of an iliac or ischial apophysis, seen in adolescent athletes, are known as transitional fractures because they occur when the muscle forces approximate those in adults but the bone is still immature. Surgical reattachment of the avulsed fragment usually results in redisplacement; therefore, symptomatic treatment is best for these injuries.

PROXIMAL FEMORAL FRACTURES

Femoral neck and intertrochanteric fractures in children (12,18,33,35,42,48,58) are dangerous injuries and do not behave similarly to their adult counterparts. Because they are so rare, few orthopaedic surgeons have extensive experience with them, and there is a natural tendency to treat them as one would in adults, which can lead to significant complications. Most proximal femoral fractures in children require operative management (Fig. 164.7). General principles and guidelines for surgical management include the following:

- Do not cross the proximal femoral physis with internal fixation devices. The exception to this occurs in older children with a very proximal femoral neck fracture (e.g., Salter–Harris type I fracture of the hip) in whom fixation into the head is necessary and leg-length discrepancy may be addressed later. Depending on the patient's age and the fracture configuration, devices may

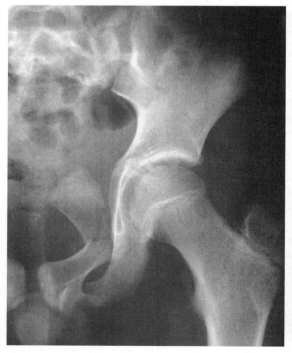
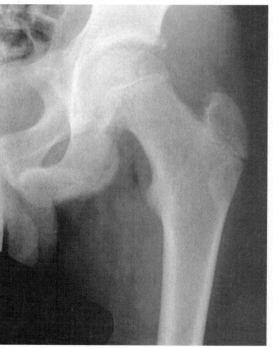

A   B

Figure 164.6. An 11-year-old boy with a fracture of the pubic ramus apparently involving the acetabulum. In reality, the triradiate cartilage and acetabular articular cartilage were intact, and the acetabulum was normal 1 year later without reduction.

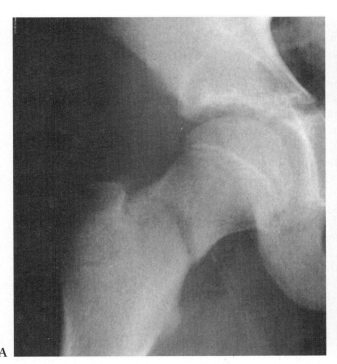
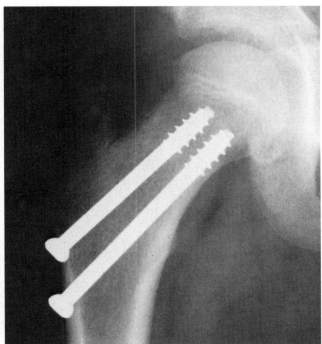

A   B

Figure 164.7. Operative fixation used for pediatric femoral neck fracture. The patient was immobilized in a spica cast.

include pins, cancellous screws, cannulated screws, or specialized pediatric blade-plate or screw-plate devices.

- Use a spica cast as supplemental fixation for all proximal femoral fractures, whether or not they are surgically stabilized. For most children, we prefer a full double-spica cast because it provides more effective mobilization.
- Treat most nondisplaced fractures of the femoral neck in a spica cast. Internal fixation with a Steinmann pin or cancellous bone screw, combined with a cast, is used by some surgeons for additional protection against displacement.
- Gently reduce and internally fix displaced fractures of the femoral neck, and supplement this with a spica cast until union.
- Intertrochanteric fractures of the femur in children have a tendency to drift late into varus. If they are nondisplaced, treat in a double-spica cast. Follow with serial radiographs, and continue cast immobilization for 8–10 weeks. If they are displaced, treat with closed reduction and fixation, using a pediatric hip screw-plate device supplemented by spica-cast immobilization.
- Most subtrochanteric fractures of the femur are treated in 90°/90° traction with the use of a distal femoral traction pin. A below-knee cast with a suspension loop to support the leg makes this form of traction easy to adjust and comfortable for children. Once callus is present,

bring the leg into extension, and apply a spica cast. An alternative to traction is operative reduction and fixation with a screw and plate device, but this must be supplemented with a spica cast during healing.

Avascular necrosis may follow hip fracture in children. The involvement may be epiphyseal (partial or complete), physeal (limiting growth potential or causing angulation of the femoral neck with growth), or metaphyseal. Long-term follow-up of pediatric hip fractures is therefore essential to allow prompt detection of complications and timely intervention if required.

FEMORAL-SHAFT FRACTURES

Treatment of fractures of the femoral shaft (1,5,13,32,33, 34,36,44,52,60,69,71,78,79) differs for young children and older children. Simple skin traction and early spica-cast application generally work well for younger children with fractures of the femoral shaft. Although such treatment leads to shortening, the predictable overgrowth of 1–2 cm that occurs in children 2–10 years of age allows excellent functional results. Angulation of up to 15° in the frontal plane and up to 30° in the sagittal plane will quickly remodel.

However, in children age 10 years or older, traction treatment is more difficult. Because overgrowth does not occur, prolonged traction (up to 4 weeks) may be required to ensure maintenance of length before cast application. The callus that forms in such patients may be flexible, and early angulation is common after casting; often, the angulated femur then heals rapidly with resulting malunion. The expense (both emotional and financial) of prolonged traction may be considerable, and school education can be severely disrupted. For these reasons, we often favor operative treatment of femoral-shaft fractures in children older than 10 years.

Surgical fixation may involve plate and screws (generally with a cast for additional protection) or external fixation; however, we usually favor intramedullary fixation. There are two general approaches to intramedullary fixation in children.

In highly unstable fractures, especially in older adolescents, standard intramedullary fixation with interlocking may be used. Use nails as small as 9 mm in diameter, and take great care to avoid penetrating the distal femoral physis with either the guidewire or the nail. Keep the proximal entry site as lateral as possible; using an entry guide pin is safer than using an awl to avoid inadvertently slipping posteriorly. Standard interlocking techniques, when required, can be safely applied to children (Fig. 164.8). It is wise to leave the proximal rod a little "proud" to facili-

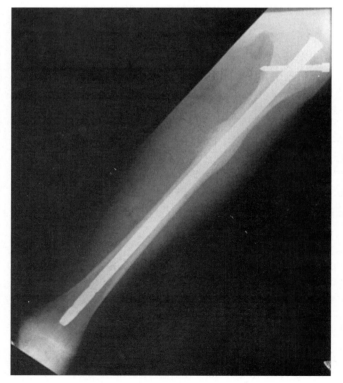

Figure 164.8. Interlocked intramedullary nail used to fix femoral-shaft fractures in children with open physes.

tate later removal. Heterotopic bone often forms at the insertion site and may be symptomatic, but the pain resolves when the rod and heterotopic bone are removed 1 year postinjury. There have been reports of avascular necrosis of the proximal femoral epiphysis with intramedullary nailing, especially with larger nails or posterior and medial insertion sites. For this reason, we prefer flexible nails, such as the Ender nail (See Chapters 19 and 20). In stable fractures, flexible intramedullary nails can be inserted antegrade or retrograde without risk to the blood supply to the femoral head.

The second option is external fixation of closed pediatric femoral fractures. Use a stable unilateral fixator along the lateral aspect. Once callus appears, apply compression across the fracture because early callus is soft and flexible and reducing distraction may help the callus mature. Do not remove the fixator too early, as malunion will occur. A main disadvantage of external fixation is the high rate of refracture; it is difficult to tell when the fracture is healed enough to discontinue the fixator. Dynamize the fixator, if possible, to minimize the risk.

Indications for operative treatment of pediatric femoral fractures include open femoral fractures and fractures in patients with multiple injuries or a serious head injury. Grade I open femoral fractures can be treated as outlined above after thorough irrigation and debridement. Fractures with more extensive wounds may require external fixation, although skeletal traction is often a viable option. If a head injury is likely to lead to spasticity and posturing, fixation of femoral fractures by one of the methods outlined previously is helpful. Even in younger head-injured children, intramedullary nailing with antegrade Ender nails, Rush rods inserted antegrade distal to the greater trochanter, flexible Nancy nails, or external fixation is usually necessary. It has been our experience that children with head injuries recover neurologic function more completely than adults; therefore, pay careful attention to the management of long-bone fractures to avoid malunion (see Chapters 14 and 20).

Flexible Intramedullary Nail Fixation of Femoral-shaft Fractures

- Place the child supine on a fracture table. Skin or foot traction usually suffices for children younger than 11–12 years with recent fractures, but the fracture should be reducible under fluoroscopy before the skin incision is made. If necessary, use skeletal traction while avoiding injury to the physes (see Chapter 20).
- For antegrade nailing, size the Ender nail by holding it over the leg, with the eye at the greater trochanter. The nail should end short of the distal femoral physis. Make a longitudinal incision from the lateral prominence of the trochanter proximally for about 5–7 cm. Incise the fascia lata to expose the trochanter. The entry point is the flat lateral surface of the trochanter (Fig. 164.9A).

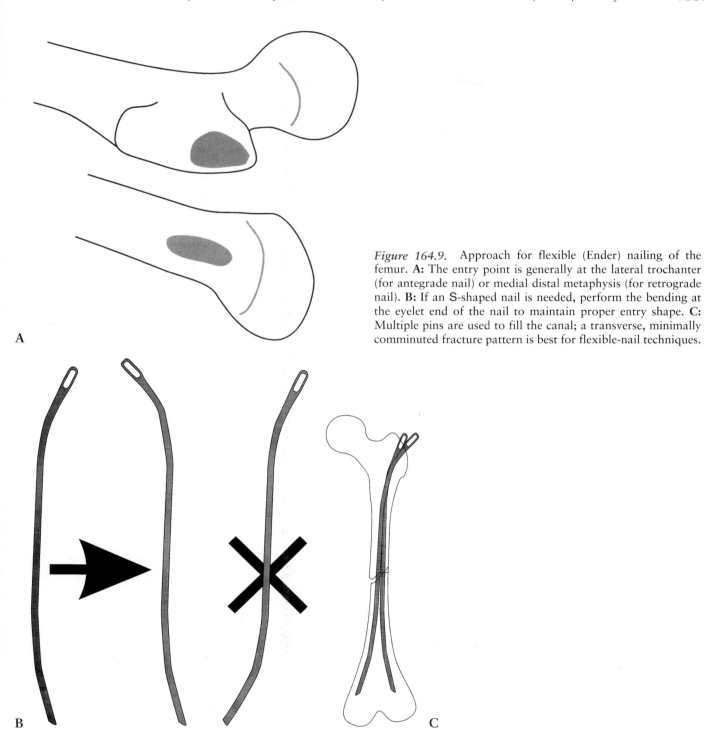

Figure 164.9. Approach for flexible (Ender) nailing of the femur. **A:** The entry point is generally at the lateral trochanter (for antegrade nail) or medial distal metaphysis (for retrograde nail). **B:** If an S-shaped nail is needed, perform the bending at the eyelet end of the nail to maintain proper entry shape. **C:** Multiple pins are used to fill the canal; a transverse, minimally comminuted fracture pattern is best for flexible-nail techniques.

■ Make an entry hole with a 6.5 mm drill, and introduce a curved Ender nail. Keep it aligned with the longitudinal axis of the femur. Gently tap it down the shaft, allowing the oblique blunt end to "bounce" off the medial cortex and pass down the canal. Verify its position on the image intensifier in two planes. At the fracture site, use the curve of the nail to hook the distal fragment, or make a small incision to openly reduce the fracture so that the nail can be passed. Once it is past the fracture, trap the nail distally so that it ends up in the lateral condyle, short of the physis. Leave the eye of the nail outside the cortex proximally for later removal.

- If the canal is large enough, insert a second nail. Many surgeons bend the nail into an S shape so that it will anchor in the medial condyle distally. Place the S curve at the proximal end of the nail to maintain the proper orientation of the oblique blunt entry tip (Fig. 164.9B). For most pediatric patients, two nails across the fracture give sufficient longitudinal stability. Adding a third (or occasionally a fourth) nail is optional. These extra nails may be shorter, just long enough to pass the fracture site and fill the canal. This helps align transverse fractures (Fig. 164.9C).
- For retrograde nailing (usually for subtrochanteric or intertrochanteric fractures), place the patient on the fracture table with the legs abducted. Approach the distal medial femur from the medial side, using a longitudinal incision just proximal to the physis. Elevate the vastus medialis, and cauterize the leash of geniculate vessels that sits against the bone.
- Make a 6.5 mm drill hole proximal to this leash, and carefully insert the first Ender nail from below. There is slightly more risk of penetrating the weaker cortex as the rod passes up the canal, and adding a slight curve to the end of the nail helps pass into the canal, as well as into the femoral neck. Reduce the fracture as for antegrade nailing, and carefully rotate the nail as it is inserted up into the neck. Stop short of the proximal physis. Two-plane fluoroscopy is essential to accomplish this maneuver. Use two or more nails as described for antegrade nailing.

PHYSEAL INJURIES OF THE DISTAL FEMUR

Most physeal injuries of the distal femur are Salter–Harris type I or II fractures. Unlike similar fractures in other anatomic locations, these have a likelihood of growth arrest as high as a 50%. This is both because high energy is required to fracture the distal femur and because the physeal mamilary processes are frequently sheared off during injury. Leg-length inequality can ensue from altered growth of this rapidly growing physis.

Distal femoral physeal fractures are occasionally accompanied by neurovascular injuries but not as frequently as are knee dislocations in adults. They are often unstable and may require internal fixation.

Closed Reduction and Fixation of Distal Femoral Physeal Fractures

- Use general anesthesia and muscle relaxation for the reduction. Closed reduction may require surprising force. Occasionally, the bone end will buttonhole through the periosteum, making closed reduction impossible and necessitating open reduction. Once the fracture is reduced, test the stability of the reduction, as internal fixation is usually required. If there is a large

metaphyseal component, it may be possible to stabilize the fracture by inserting a screw percutaneously across the metaphyseal fracture parallel to the physis. Otherwise, stabilize the fracture with two medium-sized, smooth Steinmann pins inserted from the medial and lateral femoral condyles at a 45° angle. Be sure that the pins pass into and just through the opposite cortex of the proximal fragment; otherwise, the fracture may remain unstable. Drive the pins slowly so as not to cause thermal damage.

- Bury the pin ends because they are intra-articular and the risk of infection is great if they are left protruding. After fixation, check the stability of the fixation. If it is stable, apply an above-knee cast; if there is any question, use a one-half hip spica cast with the knee in extension.
- Postoperatively, remove the pins under general anesthesia after 3–4 weeks. Immobilization for 4–6 weeks is sufficient for healing. Obtain follow-up radiographs every 3 months to look for evidence of growth arrest; if it occurs, it can be managed by methods outlined in Chapter 170 on leg-length discrepancy. In older children, however, an early epiphysiodesis of the contralateral distal femur may be a simple solution.

TIBIAL TUBERCLE AVULSION

Avulsion of the tibial tubercle (15,29,33) is characteristically a jumper's injury and occurs most commonly in boys 14 years of age. It usually happens when the patient lands, and the quadriceps muscles contract to support the falling weight. The avulsion may involve only the tubercle or may extend through the condyles and the tibial articular surface of the knee. Use CT to delineate the exact fracture pattern.

Anatomically reduce and rigidly fix displaced fractures of the tibial tubercle. Because the fracture usually occurs in a physis that is in the process of closing, it is unnecessary to avoid crossing the growth plate because growth arrest that can cause hyperextension will not be significant. For this reason, use fixation that provides the optimal strength and stability.

OPEN FRACTURES OF THE TIBIAL SHAFT

Treatment of open fractures of the tibial shaft is easier in children than in adults because children possess excellent healing potential (10,33,61,63,70). Initially, administer antibiotics, and irrigate and debride all open tibial-shaft fractures under a general anesthetic as described in Chapter 12. In younger children with Gustilo type I injuries and little periosteal injury, it is usually possible to treat the fracture with a long-leg cast. Some children may exhibit overgrowth, but this is unpredictable. In older children or children with severe soft-tissue wounds, external fixation is usually required to manage the soft-tissue injury.

Although plate fixation is possible, we prefer external fixation for the vast majority of open tibial-shaft fractures with a Gustilo type II or III wound. This allows excellent fracture control for repeated wound debridements as required. Usually, a single unilateral half-pin anterior frame is sufficient if supplemented by a posterior splint or cast. In most cases, we have achieved excellent immobilization and pain control, using a supplementary below-knee cast. This can be placed directly over the fixator if fluff gauze is packed in the recesses of the device, and the whole construct is then covered with cast padding. It can be removed and replaced by splitting the cast and opening it like a clamshell. Leave the fixator in place until callus is present, which usually requires 8 weeks or more, or until pin loosening occurs. Remove the fixator under a general anesthetic, and apply a long-leg cast with the knee straight until the fracture has united.

DISTAL TIBIAL EPIPHYSEAL FRACTURES

The anatomy of physeal closure as maturity approaches and the susceptibility of the distal tibial physis to fracture produce a group of fractures that may require operative management (20,21,39,45,66). The physis begins to close centrally, and then over 18 months to 2 years closure progresses medially, posteriorly, and laterally, sweeping like the hand of a clock. The last portion of the physis to close is the anterolateral corner (Fig. 164.10).

Depending on the portions of physis that are closed, stresses may be directed to open physeal regions, leading to a specific group of fracture patterns (Fig. 164.11). Before physeal closure (age 11 years and younger), Salter–Harris type II fractures are common and can usually be managed by nonoperative means. When inversion is included in the mechanism, Salter–Harris type III or IV injuries can be seen, and joint incongruence and physeal alignment may necessitate open reduction if closed reduction is not anatomic. It has been our experience that Salter–Harris type III fractures are quite rare; if radiographs are taken in various degrees of rotation, a metaphyseal fragment is usually detectable (type IV). Plan surgical fixation to avoid the physis, if at all possible, because growth remains in the distal tibia and a varus deformity may be a complication of treatment.

When the central or centromedial physis closes (age 12–14 years), a triplane fracture, originally described by Marmor (45), becomes common. This complex fracture may consist of two, three, or occasionally more parts, and the fibula may be fractured (Fig. 164.11). Open reduction may be required for joint incongruence. Interpret standard radiographs cautiously because the fragments can be spread posteriorly while reduced anteriorly, giving a false sense of security on the AP view, or there may be out-of-plane fractures. A transverse plane CT cut is often most helpful for exact delineation of the fracture pattern and displacement. We generally recommend open reduction if displacement after closed reduction is greater than 2 mm or if there is an articular surface step-off visible on the AP view, which is rare. Because the physis is in the process

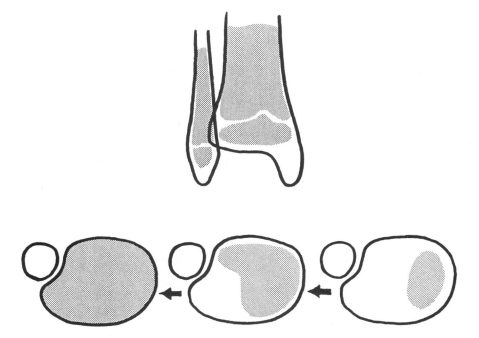

Figure 164.10. The sweep of closure of the distal tibial physis is a process that takes 18 months to 2 years to complete. Fracture patterns often parallel this pattern.

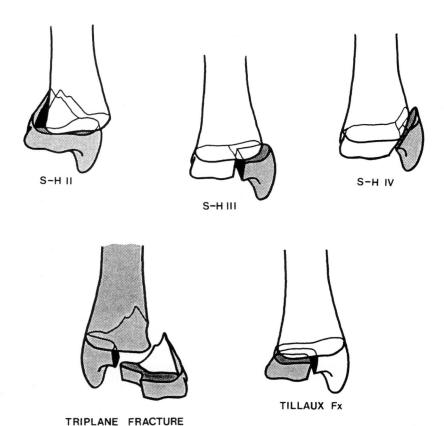

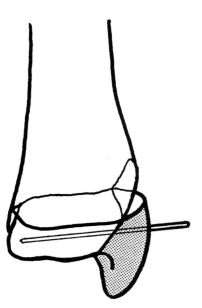

Figure 164.11. Common fracture patterns seen in the region of the distal tibial physis (*S-H*, Salter–Harris; *Fx*, fracture).

of closing, angular deformity does not occur if fixation devices cross it; fixation may therefore be planned for maximum fixation effectiveness.

When the medial and posterior portions of the physis close, which occurs age 15 years or older, the remaining anterolateral component may be avulsed by the ligaments of the anterior syndesmosis during forced external rotation. This is known as a juvenile Tillaux fracture, and surgical treatment is indicated if closed reduction does not close the gap to 2–3 mm or less. Like the triplane fracture, this fracture does not lead to late angular deformity because the physis is nearly closed.

Open Reduction of Salter–Harris Type III or IV Fractures of the Distal Tibial Physis

■ Make a medial or anteromedial incision over the malleolus. Take care not to strip more periosteum than is required, and do not further injure the physis. Carefully reduce the fracture; a fluoroscopic image intensifier may be helpful. If a Salter–Harris type IV fracture has a small metaphyseal component, carefully remove it with a rongeur to allow better visualization and alignment of the physeal plate (Fig. 164.12).

■ Fix the fracture with a transverse screw directed entirely within the epiphysis (a small cannulated screw works

Figure 164.12. A metaphyseal fragment may be removed for better physeal visualization when open reduction of a Salter–Harris type IV fracture of the distal tibial epiphysis is performed.

well if available). Try not to cross the physis, even with a smooth K-wire, because of the risk of physeal closure.

Postoperatively, immobilize the limb in a below-knee cast for 6 weeks. Weight bearing may then be increased as tolerated.

Open Reduction of Triplane Fractures

- Two incisions may be required. Reduce the medial epiphyseal fragment first through a medial or anteromedial incision, and fix it by stabilizing the posterior metaphyseal fragment with small-fragment screws or K-wires. Reduce the lateral (Salter–Harris type III) component through a lateral incision, and fix it with a cancellous small-fragment screw. It is unnecessary to avoid the physis because so little growth remains in the distal tibia.
- A Tillaux fracture is treated surgically in the same fashion as the Salter–Harris type III component of a triplane fracture.

Postoperatively, immobilize the limb in a below-knee cast for 6 weeks. Weight bearing may then be increased as tolerated.

MANAGEMENT OF GROWTH-PLATE INJURIES AND PHYSEAL BARS

The majority of growth-plate injuries heal uneventfully and proceed with no alteration in growth of the extremity. Occasionally, complete growth arrest will result in limb-length inequality, or partial growth arrest through formation of a bony bar will result in longitudinal and angular bone deformity. These complications are less significant the closer a patient is to skeletal maturity. In the lower extremity, if the limb-length difference is projected to be greater than 2–3 cm at skeletal maturity, consider treatment.

Base the treatment of significant posttraumatic growth arrest on a patient's (and parent's) height, projected degree of longitudinal or angular deformity, extent of physeal injury (size of the bony bar), and the patient's tolerance for the proposed treatment. Partial arrests of more than 30% to 50% of the cross-sectional area of the growth plate are not amenable to treatment designed to restore growth; they can be treated by early contralateral epiphysiodesis (see Chapter 170) or bone lengthening (Chapter 171). Children who are projected to be tall may be more easily treated by epiphysiodesis of the noninjured side than very short children. Partial arrest of less than 30% of the area of the growth plate in a patient with at least 2 years of growth remaining may be considered for excision of the bony bar if it is surgically accessible. The most common sites requiring surgery are the distal femur, prox-

imal tibia, or distal radius, where significant loss of length will have functional consequences.

When there is angular deformity, it is preferable in some instances to treat by acute opening-wedge osteotomy. This gains length and avoids complex, prolonged treatment. Such osteotomies, utilizing a tricortical wedge of iliac bone and appropriate internal fixation, heal rapidly in adolescents. If osteotomy is carried out before skeletal maturity, remember to complete the growth arrest by total epiphysiodesis to avoid recurrent deformity, with epiphysiodesis of the opposite extremity if indicated.

The feasibility of bar excision depends on its size and location within the physis. Plain x-ray films, scanogram, and bone-age determinations are important initially in determining which patients should be considered for bar excision (7,8,11,14,19,31,43,75). Standard tomography, trispiral tomography, CT, and MRI have each been advocated for physeal mapping. Plain tomography has long been utilized for characterizing physeal bars, but resolution is frequently inadequate. Images must be taken in two projections, and radiation exposure is quite high. Spiral and hypocycloidal tomography improve the resolution, but radiation exposure and scanning time remain high.

Axial CT of physeal bars requires precise placement of the extremity within the scanner and multiple thin cuts. The transverse section of these studies is inadequate, so sagittal and coronal reconstructions must be used and detail is poor. Direct and specific communication with the radiologist is frequently required to obtain clinically useful images. Helical CT has been reported to offer many advantages over other methods of growth-plate mapping. These include excellent bony detail, diminished radiation exposure, ability to manipulate the images into multiple perspectives, and significantly decreased scanning times that obviate sedation or anesthesia (Fig. 164.13). Advocates of MRI mapping cite the lack of ionizing-radiation exposure and excellent detail afforded. Scanning times are prolonged, and children frequently require sedation or general anesthesia. MRI data can be processed by either three-dimensional (3D) rendering or 3D projection to provide excellent detail to assist preoperative planning.

When significant angular deformity accompanies partial physeal arrest, the surgeon must decide whether to correct the angulation and complete the epiphysiodesis, correct the angulation and resect the physeal bar, or resect the physeal bar alone and allow remodeling with growth. Even though there are no simple answers to this dilemma, the basic guidelines used for management of postfracture angular deformities may be applied. For example, a 25° flexion deformity of the distal femur in an 8-year-old child might be expected to remodel after resection of a peripheral posterior bar, but a similar degree of varus deformity with a medial bar would not remodel, necessitating concurrent osteotomy. Central bars that are readily approached from a metaphyseal osteotomy site may lead to

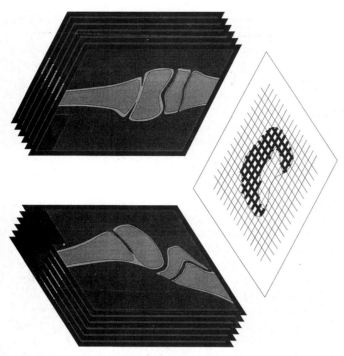

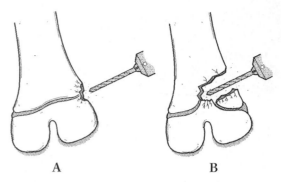

Figure 164.14. Approach to a physeal bar depends on its location. **A:** Peripheral bars are approached directly. **B:** Central bars may be approached through a metaphyseal window or osteotomy. Use a burr for this procedure.

Figure 164.13. Reconstruction of the position of a physeal bar by AP and lateral tomograms. Scaled graph paper is used to plot the presence of physeal bar on all radiographs in two planes; the resulting graph gives a good indication of the extent and location of the area of growth arrest.

region of the bar, using an image intensifier as necessary to confirm the location. With a #15 blade, sharply incise the perichondrial ring and a small cuff of proximal periosteum at the resection site, and completely remove both structures to a point where the edge of the resection contains the visualized physis; this helps prevent peripheral recurrence.

■ Use a small, high-speed burr to carefully remove the bar in layers; it will have a dense, slightly yellow appearance that will change into the normal cancellous-bone appearance as the edge of the bar is reached. Use irrigation to avoid overheating. Do not stray too far distally; if deeper visualization is required, burr more proximally. Eventually, the blue-gray cartilage of the physis will be visible, and with patience the physeal line will be exposed completely around the cavity of the resected bar (Fig. 164.15). Carefully sweep the burr up and down to smooth the edge of the physis and the contiguous bone.

■ When resecting a central bar, remove a large cortical window in the metaphysis through a periosteal win-

a decision to perform full early correction of an angular deformity. In the upper extremity, completion of epiphysiodesis and closure of the physis of the other forearm bone (usually the ulna) may be technically easier and appropriate, given the functional unimportance of equal upper-limb length.

Excision of a Physeal Bar

Assess the extent of the bar and its anatomic location with tomography or CT or MRI reconstructions. If a bar is 30% or less of the total physeal area, resection has a fairly high likelihood of success; with bars greater than 50% of the physeal area, failure is almost certain.

Plan the best approach to the bar (Fig. 164.14). If the bar is peripheral, it can be directly approached from the surface. Approach central bars through a large metaphyseal window proximal to the physis. If osteotomy is required, it is usually easiest to perform a transverse osteotomy and position the limb to avoid neurovascular damage; the bar is then approached from above through the distal face of the osteotomy.

■ Complete exsanguination and tourniquet control are essential for a dry field.
■ When resecting a peripheral bar, directly expose the

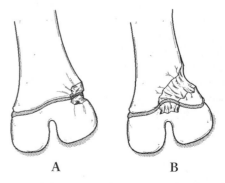

Figure 164.15. A burr is used to remove the dense, yellowish bar material until the physis is visualized throughout the cavity.

dow, taking care not to damage the actual physis or perichondrial ring. Alternatively, perform a transverse osteotomy with a saw, and displace it by bending to allow visualization from above.

- Using the burr and generous irrigation, slowly advance until the dense, yellow bony bridge is identified, and carefully burr in layers to follow the yellowish structure down through the physeal plane. An image intensifier will help avoid burring too far. Use a dental mirror to view difficult corners, and enlarge the cortical window proximally as necessary for exposure. Eventually, identify the length of the blue-gray cartilage physis completely as it surrounds the cavity, and smooth it and the attached bone with an up-and-down motion of the burr.
- At this point, place radiographic markers such as vascular clips or small K-wire fragments in the epiphyseal and metaphyseal portions of the bone to allow later measurement of longitudinal growth (Fig. 164.16).
- Before deflating the tourniquet, fill the cavity to prevent blood and eventual fibrous tissue from filling the space. We prefer Cranioplast, a slow-polymerizing polymethyl methacrylate (PMMA) that gives off very little heat as it cures. This material, familiar to orthopaedic surgeons, fully fills the cavity and leaves very little space for accumulation of organizing fibrous tissue. Alternatively, autogenous fat may be used, harvested locally or from the buttock. Fat tends to float out of the wound, and

provides no structural compressive strength, so we no longer recommend it. Medical-grade Silastic has also been used; however, it is not available to surgeons for this use and offers no distinct advantages. The object of the filling is to completely obliterate the cavity without interlocking with cancellous bone above and below the physis.

- Allow the PMMA to become doughy before inserting it, and gently push (do not "pressurize") it while it cures, irrigating with cool saline to minimize thermal damage. Once the PMMA is cured, replace the cortical window or fix the osteotomy if one has been made (see discussion above). Use iliac bone graft as needed for stability in opening-wedge osteotomies.
- Close the wound, and immobilize the limb, even if internal fixation has been used for an osteotomy.

Postoperatively, protect the patient until the bone is well healed, usually 6 weeks, and gradually begin increasing protected weight bearing. PMMA is load-sharing and allows safe weight bearing once muscle strength has recovered.

Physes that have been injured and partially closed will often exhibit premature closure after several years of normal growth after successful bar resection. Patients must be carefully monitored with periodic clinical, radiographic, and limb-length examinations until skeletal maturity. Be prepared to reassess late physeal closure and to carry out prompt treatment by epiphysiodesis, osteotomy, or other indicated procedure.

REFERENCES

Each reference is categorized according to the following scheme: *, classic article; #, review article; !, basic research article; and +, clinical results/outcome study.

+ 1. Allen BJ Jr, Kant AP, Emery FE. Displaced Fractures of the Femoral Diaphysis in Children: Definitive Treatment in a Double Spica Cast. *J Trauma* 1977;17:8.
+ 2. Aronson DD, Prager BI. Supracondylar Fractures of the Humerus in Children: A Modified Technique for Closed Pinning. *Clin Orthop* 1987;219:174.
* 3. Bado J. The Monteggia Lesion. *Clin Orthop* 1967;50:71.
+ 4. Bast SC, Hoffer MM, Aval S. Nonoperative Treatment for Minimally and Nondisplaced Lateral Humeral Condyle Fractures in Children. *J Pediatr Orthop* 1998;18:448.
+ 5. Beaty JH, Austin SM, Warner WC, et al. Interlocking Intramedullary Nailing of Femoral-shaft Fractures in Adolescents: Preliminary Results and Complications. *J Pediatr Orthop* 1994;14:178.
+ 6. Beringer DC, Weiner DS, Noble JS, Bell RH. Severely Displaced Proximal Humeral Epiphyseal Fractures: A Follow-up Study. *J Pediatr Orthop* 1998;18:31.

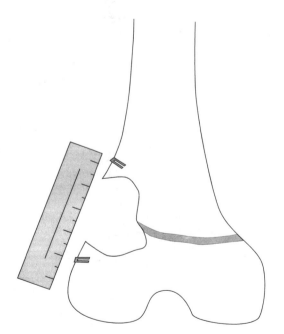

Figure 164.16. Small radiolucent markers (wires, staples, or vascular clips) help in the assessment of longitudinal growth after surgery for partial physeal growth arrest.

+ 7. Birch JG. Surgical Technique of Physeal Bar Resection. *Instr Course Lect* 1992;41:445.

+ 8. Broughton NS, Dickens DR, Cole WG, Menelaus MB. Epiphyseolysis for Partial Growth Plate Arrest: Results after Four Years or at Maturity. *J Bone Joint Surg Br* 1989;71:13.

+ 9. Bryan WJ, Tullos HS. Pediatric Pelvic Fractures: Review of 52 Patients. *Trauma* 1979;19:799.

+ 10. Buckley SL, Smith G, Sponseller PD, et al. Open Fractures of the Tibia in Children. *J Bone Joint Surg* 1990; 72-A:1462.

+ 11. Burke SW. Principles of physeal bridge resection. *Instr Course Lect* 1989;38:337.

+ 12. Canale ST, Bourland WL. Fracture of the Neck and Intertrochanteric Region of the Femur in Children. *J Bone Joint Surg Am* 1977;59:431.

+ 13. Carey TP, Galpin RD. Flexible Intramedullary Nail Fixation of Pediatric Femoral Fractures. *Clin Orthop* 1996; 332:110.

+ 14. Carlson WO, Wenger DR. A Mapping Method to Prepare for Surgical Excision of a Partial Physeal Arrest. *J Pediatr Orthop* 1984;4:232.

+ 15. Christie MJ, Dvonch VM. Tibial Tuberosity Avulsion Fracture in Adolescents. *J Pediatr Orthop* 1981;1:391.

+ 16. Dameron TB Jr, Reibel DB. Fractures Involving the Proximal Humeral Epiphyseal Plate. *J Bone Joint Surg Am* 1969;51:289.

+ 17. Davis DR, Green DP. Forearm Fractures in Children: Pitfalls and Complications. *Clin Orthop* 1976;120:172.

+ 18. Davison BL, Weinstein SL. Hip Fractures in Children: A Long-term Follow-up Study. *J Pediatr Orthop* 1992;12: 355.

+ 19. DeCampo JF, Boldt DW. Computed Tomography of Partial Growth Plate Arrest: Initial Experience. *Skeletal Radiol* 1986;15:526.

+ 20. Dias LS, Giegerich CR. Fractures of the Distal Tibial Epiphysis in Adolescence. *J Bone Joint Surg Am* 1983; 65:438.

+ 21. Ertl JP, Barrack RL, Alexander AH, Van Buecken K. Triplane Fracture of the Distal Tibial Epiphysis: Long-term Follow-up. *J Bone Joint Surg Am* 1988;70:967.

+ 22. Flynn JC. Nonunion of Slightly Displaced Fractures of the Lateral Humeral Condyle in Children: An Update. *J Pediatr Orthop* 1989;9:691.

+ 23. Foster DE, Sullivan JA, Gross RH. Lateral Humeral Condylar Fractures in Children. *J Pediatr Orthop* 1985;5: 16.

+ 24. Fowles JV, Kassab MT. Displaced Supracondylar Fractures of the Elbow in Children: A Report on the Fixation of Extension and Flexion Fractures by Two Lateral Percutaneous Pins. *J Bone Joint Surg Br* 1974;56:490.

+ 25. Fowles JV, Slimane N, Kassab MT. Elbow Dislocation with Avulsion of the Medial Humeral Epicondyle. *J Bone Joint Surg Br* 1990;72:102.

+ 26. Garvin KL, McCarthy RE, Barnes CL, Dodge BM. Pediatric Pelvic Ring Fractures. *J Pediatr Orthop* 1990;10: 577.

+ 27. Gonzalez-Herranz P, Alvarez-Romera A, Burgos J, et al. Displaced Radial Neck Fractures in Children Treated by Closed Intramedullary Pinning (Metaizeau Technique). *J Pediatr Orthop* 1997;17:325.

+ 28. Hamsa WR. Epiphyseal Injuries about the Hip Joint. *Clin Orthop* 1957;10:119.

+ 29. Hand WL, Hand CR, Dunn AW. Avulsion Fractures of the Tibial Tubercle. *J Bone Joint Surg Am* 1971;53:1579.

+ 30. Hardacre JA, Nahigian SH, Froimson AI, Brown JE. Fractures of the Lateral Condyle of the Humerus in Children. *J Bone Joint Surg Am* 1971;53:1083.

+ 31. Havranek P, Lizler J. Magnetic Resonance Imaging in the Evaluation of Partial Growth Plate Arrest after Physeal Injuries in Children. *J Bone Joint Surg Am* 1991;73: 1234.

+ 32. Heinrich SD, Drvaric D, Darr K, MacEwen GD. Stabilization of Pediatric Diaphyseal Femur Fractures with Flexible Intramedullary Nails (a Technique Paper). *J Orthop Trauma* 1992;6:452.

33. Hensinger RN, ed. *Operative Management of Lower Extremity Fractures in Children.* Park Ridge, IL: American Academy of Orthopaedic Surgeons, 1992:11.

+ 34. Herndon WA, Mahnken RF, Yngve DA, Sullivan JA. Management of Femoral Shaft Fractures in the Adolescent. *J Pediatr Orthop* 1989;9:29.

+ 35. Ingram AJ, Bachynski B. Fractures of the Hip in Children. *J Bone Joint Surg Am* 1953;35:867.

+ 36. Irani RN, Nicholson JT, Chung SM. Long-term Results in the Treatment of Femoral Shaft Fractures in Young Children by Immediate Spica Immobilization. *J Bone Joint Surg Am* 1976;58:945.

+ 37. Jakob R, Fowles JV, Rang M, Kassab MT. Observations Concerning Fractures of the Lateral Condyle in Children. *J Bone Joint Surg Br* 1975;57:430.

+ 38. Jones ERL, Esah M. Displaced Fractures of the Radial Neck in Children. *J Bone Joint Surg Br* 1971;53:429.

+ 39. Klieger B, Mankin HJ. Fracture of the Lateral Portion of the Distal Tibial Epiphysis. *J Bone Joint Surg Am* 1964;46:25.

+ 40. Kohler R, Trillaud JM. Fracture and Fracture Separation of the Proximal Humerus in Children: Report of 136 Cases. *J Pediatr Orthop* 1983;3:326.

+ 41. Labelle H, Bunnell WP, Duhaime M, Poitras B. Cubitus Varus Deformity Following Supracondylar Fracture of the Humerus in Children. *J Pediatr Orthop* 1982;2:539.

+ 42. Lam SF. Fractures of the Neck of the Femur in Children. *J Bone Joint Surg Am* 1971;53:1165.

+ 43. Loder RT, Swinford AE, Kuhns LR. The Use of Helical Computed Tomographic Scan to Assess Bony Physeal Bridges. *J Pediatr Orthop* 1997;17:356.

+ 44. Lombardo SJ, Harvey JP Jr. Fractures of the Distal Femoral Epiphysis: Factors Influencing Prognosis. *J Bone Joint Surg Am* 1977;59:742.

+ 45. Marmor L. An Unusual Fracture of the Tibial Epiphysis. *Clin Orthop* 1970;73:132.

+ 46. McDonald GA. Pelvic Disruptions in Children. *Clin Orthop* 1980;151:130.

+ 47. Mintzer CM, Waters PM, Brown DJ, Kasser JR. Percutaneous Pinning in the Treatment of Displaced Lateral Condyle Fractures. *J Pediatr Orthop* 1994;14:462.

48. Morrissey R. Hip Fractures in Children. *Clin Orthop* 1980;152:202.

+ 49. Neer CS II, Horwitz BS. Fractures of the Proximal Humeral Epiphyseal Plate. *Clin Orthop* 1965;41:24.

+ 50. Newman JH. Displaced Fractures of the Neck of the Radius in Children. *Injury* 1977;9:114.

51. Noonan KJ, Price CT. Forearm and Distal Radius Fractures in Children. *J Am Acad Orthop Surg* 1998;6:146.

+ 52. O'Malley DE, Mazur JM, Cummings RJ. Femoral Head Avascular Necrosis Associated with Intramedullary Nailing in an Adolescent. *J Pediatr Orthop* 1995;15:21.

+ 53. Peters CL, Scott SM. Compartment Syndrome in the Forearm Following Fractures of the Radial Head or Neck in Children. *J Bone Joint Surg Am* 1995;77:1070.

+ 54. Pirone AM, Graham HK, Krajbich JI. Management of Displaced Extension-type Supracondylar Fractures of the Humerus in Children. *J Bone Joint Surg Am* 1988; 70:641.

* 55. Ponseti IV. Growth and Development of the Acetabulum in the Normal Child: Anatomical, Histological, and Roentgenographic Studies. *J Bone Joint Surg Am* 1978; 60:575.

+ 56. Price CT, Scott DS, Kurzner ME, Flynn JC. Malunited Forearm Fractures in Children. *J Pediatr Orthop* 1990; 10:705.

+ 57. Radomisli TE, Rosen AL. Controversies regarding Radial Neck Fractures in Children. *Clin Orthop* 1998;353: 30.

58. Ratliff AHC. Fractures of the Neck of the Femur in Children. In: Salvati EA, ed. *The Hip: Proceedings of the Ninth Open Scientific Meeting of the Hip Society, 1981.* St. Louis, MO: Mosby, 1981:188.

+ 59. Reichard SA, Helikson MA, Shorter N, et al. Pelvic Fractures in Children: Review of 120 Patients with a New Look at General Management. *J Pediatr Surg* 1980;15: 727.

+ 60. Riseborough EJ, Barrett IR, Shapiro F. Growth Disturbances Following Distal Femoral Physeal Fracture-separations. *J Bone Joint Surg Am* 1983;65:885.

+ 61. Robertson P, Karol LA, Rab GT. Open Fractures of the Tibia and Femur in Children. *J Pediatr Orthop* 1996; 16:621.

+ 62. Sanders WE, Heckman JD. Traumatic Plastic Deformation of the Radius and Ulna: A Closed Method of Correction of Deformity. *Clin Orthop* 1984;188:58.

+ 63. Shannak AO. Tibial Fractures in Children: Follow-up Study. *J Pediatr Orthop* 1988;8:306.

+ 64. Shifrin PG, Gehring HW, Iglesias LJ. Open Reduction and Internal Fixation of Displaced Supracondylar Fractures of the Humerus in Children. *Orthop Clin North Am* 1976;7:573.

+ 65. Shimada K, Masada K, Tada K, Yamamoto T. Osteosynthesis for the Treatment of Non-union of the Lateral Humeral Condyle in Children. *J Bone Joint Surg Am* 1997;79:234.

+ 66. Spiegel PG, Mast JW, Cooperman DR, Laros GS. Triplane Fractures of the Distal Tibial Epiphysis. *Clin Orthop* 1984;188:74.

+ 67. Steinberg EL, Golomb D, Salama R, Weintraub S. Radial Head and Neck Fractures in Children. *J Pediatr Orthop* 1988;8:35.

+ 68. Thometz JG. Techniques for Direct Radiographic Visualization during Closed Pinning of Supracondylar Humerus Fractures in Children. *J Pediatr Orthop* 1990;10: 555.

+ 69. Thompson JD, Stricker SJ, Williams MM. Fractures of the Distal Femoral Epiphyseal Plate. *J Pediatr Orthop* 1995;15:474.

+ 70. Tolo VT. External Skeletal Fixation in Children's Fractures. *J Pediatr Orthop* 1983;3:435.

+ 71. Viljanto J, Kiviluoto H, Paananen M. Remodeling after Femoral Shaft Fracture in Children. *Acta Chir Scand* 1975;141:360.

+ 72. Vocke AK, Von Laer L. Displaced Fractures of the Radial Neck in Children: Long-term Results and Prognosis of Conservative Treatment. *J Pediatr Orthop B* 1998;7: 217.

+ 73. Weiland A, Meyer S, Tolo VT, et al. Surgical Treatment of Displaced Supracondylar Fractures of the Humerus in Children: Analysis of Fifty-two Cases Followed for Five to Fifteen Years. *J Bone Joint Surg Am* 1978;60: 657.

74. Wilkins KE. Fractures and Dislocations of the Elbow Region. In: Rockwood CA Jr, Wilkins KE, King RE, eds. *Fractures in Children.* Philadelphia: JB Lippincott Co, 1984:432.

+ 75. Williamson RV, Staheli LT. Partial Physeal Growth Arrest: Treatment by Bridge Resection and Fat Interposition. *J Pediatr Orthop* 1990;10:769.

+ 76. Wilson JN. The Treatment of Fractures of the Medial Epicondyle of the Humerus. *J Bone Joint Surg Br* 1960; 42:778.

+ 77. Yung SH, Lam CY, Choi KY, et al. Percutaneous Intramedullary Kirschner Wiring for Displaced Diaphyseal Forearm Fractures in Children. *J Bone Joint Surg Br* 1998;80:91.

+ 78. Ziv I, Blackburn N, Rang M. Femoral Intramedullary Nailing in the Growing Child. *J Trauma* 1984;4:432.

+ 79. Ziv I, Rang M. Treatment of Femoral Fracture in the Child with Head Injury. *J Bone Joint Surg Br* 1983;5: 276.

CHAPTER 165

CONGENITAL SHOULDER AND ELBOW MALFORMATIONS AND DEFORMITIES

Michelle A. James and Karen D. Heiden

Congenital malformations of the shoulder and elbow are frequently accompanied by hand malformations or absence; in these cases, treatment of the shoulder and elbow must be integrated with treatment of the hand. Surgical reconstruction of the shoulder or elbow, or both, is not indicated if the hand is absent or nonfunctional, unless the goal of surgery is to reduce pain. See Chapter 69, Congenital Hand Malformations, for a discussion of pathophysiology and principles of treatment of congenital malformations of the upper extremity.

ARTHROGRYPOSIS

PATHOPHYSIOLOGY AND PRINCIPLES OF TREATMENT

Arthrogryposis multiplex congenita (sometimes termed amyoplasia) is characterized by multiple, symmetric, non-progressive, congenital joint contractures (45) (Fig. 165.1A). Many etiologic factors have been associated with arthrogryposis (including fetal exposure to mutagens, toxins, hyperthermia, neuromuscular blocking agents, and mechanical immobilization) (158). The final common pathway for these etiologies is probably lack of fetal movement. Because fetal movement is necessary for joint development, immobile joints fail to develop normally and become contracted (43,108,182).

Although myopathic arthrogryposis has been reported,

M. A. James: Associate Clinical Professor, Department of Orthopaedic Surgery, University of California–Davis, Shriners Hospital for Children, Northern California Sacramento, California, 95817.
K. D. Heiden: Department of Orthopaedic Surgery, University of California, Davis Medical Center, Sacramento, California, 95817.

most cases studied show evidence of a neuropathic condition, possibly a disorder of the anterior horn cells, which partially paralyzes the fetus. Even though many different fetal exposures to drugs, chemicals, and mutagens have been associated with arthrogryposis in humans, in most cases, the cause remains unknown (50,72). Arthrogryposis is not an inherited condition (121), but many other syndromes that feature multiple joint contractures are inherited (72), and most children with this condition should be seen by a geneticist. The incidence of arthrogryposis is unknown, although congenital joint contractures are seen in about 1 in 3,000 live births (72).

Treatment of arthrogryposis focuses on enhancing the child's ability to perform activities of daily living, especially eating, toileting, and dressing (30).

ASSESSMENT, INDICATIONS, AND RELATIVE RESULTS

Arthrogryposis is a clinical diagnosis, usually made at birth. Mothers of children with this condition frequently report that fetal movement was diminished compared with their other pregnancies. Oligohydramnios is a frequent finding.

Joint contractures associated with arthrogryposis are usually more severe distally than proximally, and most patients have upper extremity involvement (58). The shoulder lacks abduction and external rotation (178), and the elbow (one of the most frequently involved joints) (108) may lack flexion or extension (161,167). The wrist is usually flexed and deviated ulnarward (176), the fingers flexed, and the thumb flexed in the palm (184) (see The Fingers: Camptodactyly and The Thumb: Clasped Thumb in Chapter 69, Congenital Hand Malformations). Severe clubfoot, knee flexion contracture, dislocated hip, and

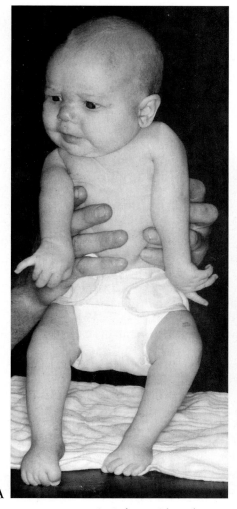

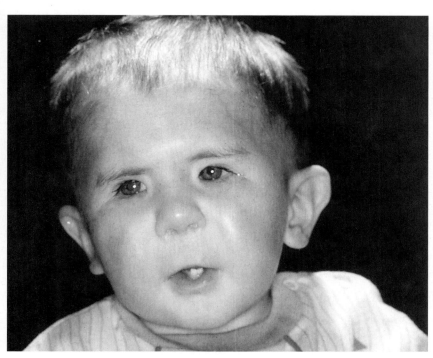

Figure 165.1. **A:** Infant with arthrogryposis. **B:** Facial features of child with Freeman–Sheldon syndrome (craniocarpal-tarsal dysplasia).

scoliosis are frequently associated with arthrogryposis (45,161). Joint contractures similar to those seen in arthrogryposis are associated with syndromes such as cranio-carpo-tarsal dysplasia (Freeman–Sheldon syndrome) (Fig. 165.1*B*) (53,161).

Shoulder contractures do not usually limit performance of activities of daily living (20) and are not usually amenable to range-of-motion exercises, splinting, or surgery. The most limiting deficit, lack of active elbow flexion, prevents the child from reaching the mouth and head, especially when accompanied by an elbow extension contracture. Children with only passive elbow flexion frequently discover "tricks" to help get their hand to their face, such as leaning the forearm on the edge of a table or on their leg. Serial casting, splinting, and range-of-motion exercises may improve elbow range of motion. If less than 90° of passive elbow flexion is gained after 6 months of super-

vised elbow stretching, posterior capsulotomy with triceps lengthening is indicated (167). In one study of this operation, postoperative improvement in passive elbow flexion was maintained for at least 2 years, although range of motion was occasionally limited by intra-articular incongruity (167).

Many different tendon transfers have been used to provide active elbow flexion, including pectoralis major, latissimus dorsi, triceps-to-biceps transfers, or proximal reattachment of the wrist and finger flexor muscles (Steindler flexorplasty) (12,44,167,178). Tendon transfer is indicated in children older than 4 years of age who lack active elbow flexion and have at least 90° of passive elbow motion, reasonable ipsilateral hand function, absent contralateral active elbow flexion, and an available donor muscle. Bilateral tendon transfer is not usually indicated; asymmetric function is usually desirable, especially when the triceps is the best donor available, and elbow extension is sacrificed for elbow flexion. Potential donor muscles must be carefully assessed preoperatively because they may be weak and therefore unsuitable for transfer. Triceps-to-biceps transfer gives the most reliable results (167), although this operation creates an elbow flexion contracture (31) and is contraindicated in children who need active elbow extension to ambulate or transfer because of lower extremity contractures. The pectoralis major is the best donor when the triceps is unavailable, but the scar left by this operation is large (extending from sternum to antecubital fossa) and crosses the breast, and transfer of the pectoralis may cause breast asymmetry. Latissimus dorsi and finger and wrist flexors are frequently weak in arthrogryposis, so latissimus dorsi-to-biceps transfer and Steindler flexorplasty are rarely indicated.

CLASSIFICATIONS

Many different terms have been used to describe arthrogryposis, including arthrogryposis multiplex congenita, multiple congenital articular rigidities, amyoplasia congenita, myodystrophia foetalis deformans, and congenital arthromyodysplasia (162). No classification scheme useful to orthopaedists has been described for this disorder.

PREOPERATIVE MANAGEMENT

Stretching, splinting, and serial casting of contracted elbows and wrists may increase passive range of motion, particularly for infants younger than 1 year of age. A creative occupational therapist may help the child improve function with the use of mechanical aids.

OPERATIVE TECHNIQUES

Posterior Elbow Capsulotomy with Triceps Lengthening

- Use loupe magnification (for the ulnar nerve dissection) and perform the operation under general anesthesia and a tourniquet. A sterile tourniquet may be necessary.
- Through a longitudinal incision on the posterior elbow, find the ulnar nerve. Open the cubital tunnel and retract the nerve with a Penrose drain, taking care not to damage branches to the flexor carpi ulnaris.
- Perform a V-Y lengthening of the triceps tendon. First, make a V incision through the tendon, with the point of the V proximal. Expose the humeroulnar joint, leaving the triangular tail of tendon attached to the olecranon.
- Using scissors, transect the posterior elbow joint capsule. If necessary to obtain flexion, transect the lateral and medial capsule, including collateral ligaments.

- Repair the triceps tendon with nonabsorbable suture while holding the elbow in maximum flexion.
- The ulnar nerve does not usually require transposition.
- Close the skin with an absorbable, running subcuticular suture. Apply a long-arm cast with the elbow in maximum flexion.

Remove the cast after 2 weeks and begin a program of frequent gentle passive elbow flexion exercises, supervised by an occupational therapist. Supplement with night splinting in maximum flexion, to be continued indefinitely.

Triceps-to-Biceps Transfer

Figure 165.2 shows a typical triceps-to-biceps transfer (31).

- Perform the operation under general anesthesia and a tourniquet. A sterile tourniquet may be required.
- Through a posterolateral longitudinal elbow incision, expose the triceps tendon and divide it at its insertion. Dissect it from the posterior aspect of the distal fourth of the humerus, and transfer it around the lateral aspect, superficial to the radial nerve.
- Through a separate anterior zigzag elbow incision, expose the biceps tendon.
- Pass the triceps tendon through a longitudinal slit in the biceps tendon, and suture it under tension with the elbow in flexion.
- Close the skin with an absorbable, running subcuticular suture. Apply a long-arm cast with the elbow in maximum flexion and neutral rotation.

Immobilize the elbow for 6 weeks, then begin a program of active elbow flexion exercises. Supplement with

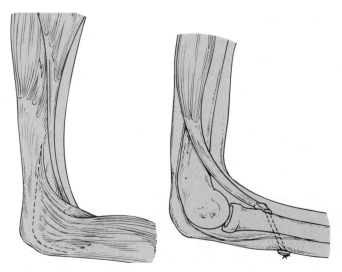

Figure 165.2. Triceps-to-biceps transfer (Reprinted from ref. 44, with permission).

night splinting until active flexion strength is at least anti-gravity.

Pectoralis Major-to-Biceps Transfer

For the surgical technique for a pectoralis major-to-biceps transfer, see the article by Schottstaedt et al. (147).

COMPLICATIONS

Inadequate lengthening of the triceps tendon will restrict elbow flexion following posterior elbow capsulotomy. The outcome of elbow flexion tendon transfer is frequently unsatisfactory, even when the donor muscle is normal; in arthrogryposis, donor muscles are likely to be weak and have poor excursion.

CONCLUSIONS

Children with arthrogryposis frequently function much better than their strength and range-of-motion measurements would predict. Surgery should be directed at functional goals shared by the surgeon, child, and family.

Although triceps-to-biceps transfer provides the best elbow flexion, patients may not like the mandatory elbow flexion contracture that accompanies this operation.

BRACHIAL PLEXUS BIRTH PALSY

PATHOPHYSIOLOGY AND PRINCIPLES OF TREATMENT

Brachial plexus birth palsy (BPBP), also known as obstetric palsy, occurs when the brachial plexus is injured by traction during birth. The mechanism of injury is forceful separation of the head from the shoulder by lateral flexion of the cervical spine and depression of the shoulder (Fig. 165.3). This most commonly occurs during a cephalic vag-

inal birth, owing to shoulder dystocia. The primary cause of shoulder dystocia is fetal macrosomia, which may be associated with maternal diabetes or a multiparous mother. The brachial plexus may also be injured during a breech delivery; injury during caesarian section is very rare (7,55). Obstetrics literature indicates that injury may occur prenatally (56,130,133), although this finding is controversial (38,60).

BPBP occurs in 0.5 to 2.6 per 1,000 live births, with the incidence unchanged or possibly increasing in the past 30 years, in spite of an increasing rate of caesarian sections (64,75,76,88,103,117,118,134,170). Although BPBP may often be attributable to poor prenatal care or obstetrician error, some cases cannot be reliably predicted or prevented. Macrosomia (fetal weight greater than 4,500 g) is difficult or impossible to detect with current prenatal diagnostic techniques (62), and shoulder dystocia, which occurs in up to 2% of deliveries, may be difficult to recognize and treat (63,74,80,118). In addition, shoulder dystocia and BPBP frequently occur in normal birth-weight fetuses (64,128). Other variables, including prolonged gestation, prolonged labor, use of oxytocin, use of forceps or vacuum suction, and previous maternal obstetric history of macrosomia are all associated with birth injuries, but even when combined, these problems fail to predict most birth injuries (134). BPBP in an older sibling is the only factor that may reliably predict BPBP (4) (Fig. 165.4).

The disability caused by BPBP varies from mild, partial, and transient upper extremity weakness [approximately 80% of newborns have full or near-full recovery of function (66,76,88,122)] to complete permanent upper extremity paralysis. Most of the improvement gained from nerve recovery is seen in the first 12 months of life, and the remainder by 2 years of age (5); recovery of sensation is more complete than recovery of motor function. Residual disability depends on the severity and location of the plexus injury (78) (Fig. 165.5). Injury to the upper trunk, where the C5 and C6 nerve roots join and the suprascapu-

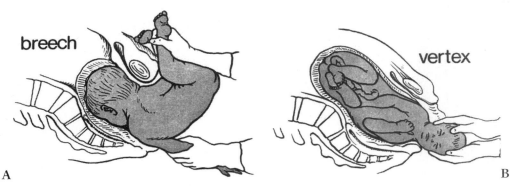

Figure 165.3. Breech (**A**) and Vertex births (**B**), showing wide separation of the head from the downside shoulder.

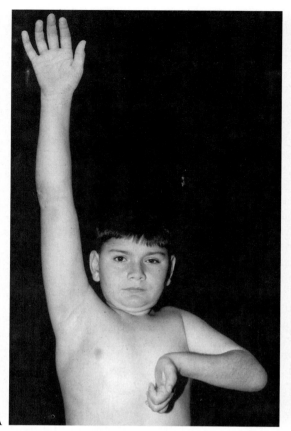

A

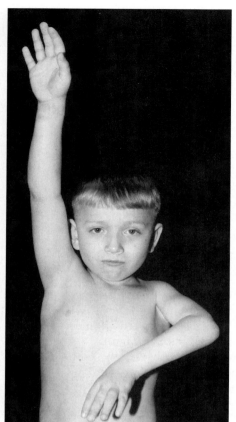

B

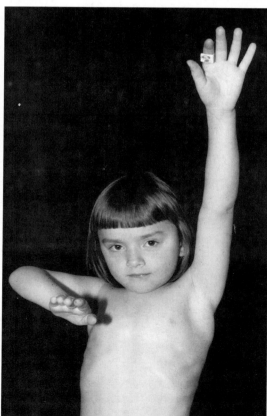

C

Figure 165.4. **A to C:** Three siblings with brachial plexus birth palsy. Both boys (A, B) have Horner's syndrome.

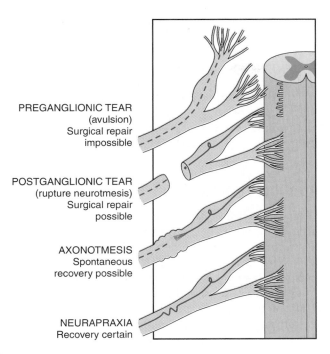

Figure 165.5. Different types of brachial plexus injury (78).

PREGANGLIONIC TEAR
(avulsion)
Surgical repair
impossible

POSTGANGLIONIC TEAR
(rupture neurotmesis)
Surgical repair
possible

AXONOTMESIS
Spontaneous
recovery possible

NEURAPRAXIA
Recovery certain

lar nerve leaves the plexus, is called Erb's palsy (49). This the most common type of plexus injury; the child with this type of BPBP has weakness or paralysis of shoulder external rotation and possibly abduction. The next most common type is global plexus palsy. Isolated injury to the lower trunk (C-8 and T-1 nerve roots), called Klumpke's palsy, is the least common type (6,90) and may actually represent partial recovery from global plexus palsy rather than injury to the lower trunk alone (172) (Fig. 165.6).

The muscle imbalance resulting from BPBP may cause multiple deformities at the shoulder, including internal rotation contracture and posterior subluxation or dislocation, as well as at the elbow, including flexion, supination, or pronation contracture, radial head dislocation, or complete elbow dislocation (3,13,41,83,104,110,174). The affected arm is smaller than the opposite side, in proportion to the severity of the BPBP (Fig. 165.7).

The goals of treatment are to prevent the formation of contractures while recovery is occurring, to restore neurologic function, to augment weak muscles, and to improve the appearance of deformities that occur as a result of muscle imbalance. Treatment depends on age and extent of weakness, and may include passive range-of-motion exercises (PROM), goal-directed occupational therapy, brachial plexus exploration and grafting, tendon transfers,

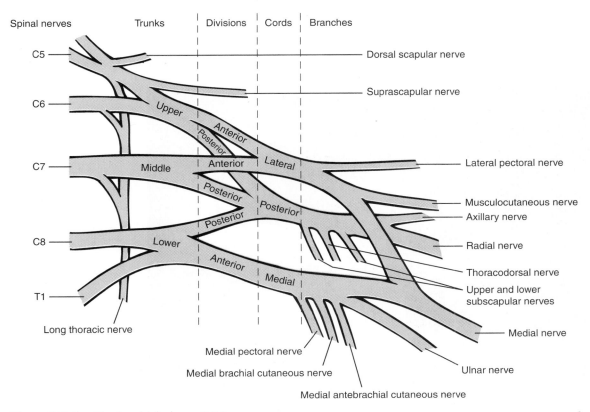

Figure 165.6. The brachial plexus (172).

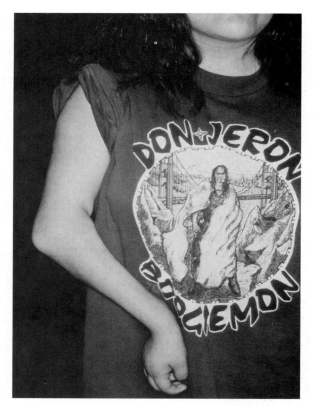

Figure 165.7. Severe brachial plexus birth palsy in a teenager.

osteotomies, and arthrodeses. Because of the complexity of their care, children with BPBP benefit from a multidisciplinary team approach (36). The BPBP team may include an orthopaedic surgeon, a surgeon with microneurosurgery expertise, a physiatrist, a pediatric neurologist, occupational and physical therapists, a social worker, and a therapeutic recreation specialist. Parents and older children appreciate team-sponsored activities, such as play groups and peer contacts (Fig. 165.8).

ASSESSMENT, INDICATIONS, AND RELATIVE RESULTS

The infant with BPBP presents with asymmetric upper extremity motion. The affected side is typically held in internal rotation at the shoulder, with the elbow extended and the wrist flexed (Fig. 165.9). The differential diagnosis includes hemiparesis, a septic glenohumeral joint, and congenital elevation of the scapula (Sprengel's deformity). Clavicle fracture and proximal humeral epiphyseal separation may be either differential diagnoses or associated lesions (5,59,103). Although most infants with BPBP recover useful function, those with an ipsilateral Horner's syndrome (due to injury to the sympathetic ganglia, associated with avulsion of the C-8 and T-1 nerve roots off the spinal cord) or hemidiaphragm paralysis (injury to the phrenic nerve) have a poor prognosis for recovery (122).

Teach parents to begin PROM exercises of the shoulder when the infant is 3 to 4 weeks of age. Examine the infant every 1 to 2 months for signs of recovery. The Infant Ac-

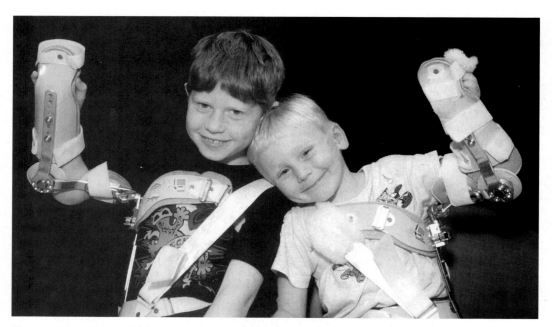

Figure 165.8. Two children who met through a peer contact program, wearing shoulder abduction splints following shoulder external rotation tendon transfers.

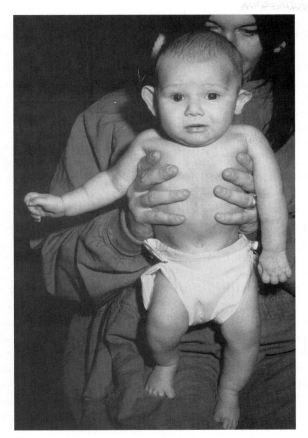

Figure 165.9. Infant with left brachial plexus birth palsy.

Table 165.1. *Infant Active Movement Scale*

Observation	Muscle grade
Gravity eliminated	
No contraction	0
Contraction, no motion	1
Motion ≤1/2 range	2
Motion >1/2 range	3
Full motion	4
Against gravity	
Motion ≤1/2 range	5
Motion >1/2 range	6
Full motion	7

From Clarke HM, Curtis CG. An Approach to Obstetrical Brachial Plexus Injuries. *Hand Clin* 1995;11:563, with permission.

tive Movement Scale (36) (Table 165.1) helps the examiner measure muscle recovery more accurately than do scales devised for adults because it does not require cooperation for testing muscles against resistance. Brachial plexus exploration with nerve grafting and transfer may be indicated if the infant does not recover elbow flexion strength.

Recovery of active elbow flexion is closely monitored for three reasons: It is easy to observe; the timing of natural recovery of elbow flexion may be a prognostic sign for plexus recovery; and early nerve grafting to the lateral cord of the plexus (Fig. 165.6) may be the best way to restore elbow flexion, which is difficult to replace with tendon transfers (112). In one often-quoted but unpublished study, children with full recovery from BPBP at 5 years of age showed antigravity elbow flexion and shoulder abduction by age 3 months (59,160). Later recovery of elbow flexion (between 3 and 6 months of age) has been associated with residual shoulder weakness (160,171). In contrast, however, other investigators have reported that most children with biceps recovery after 3 months of age are likely to have a good ultimate outcome, but lack of sensation and wrist extension at 3 months are poor prognostic signs (21).

Electromyography (EMG), nerve conduction studies (NCS), contrast computerized tomography (CT) myelography, magnetic resonance imaging (MRI), and intraoperative somatosensory-evoked potentials have all been used to measure and provide images of damage to the neonatal brachial plexus, with the goal of differentiating nonrepairable preganglionic rupture from postganglionic injury, which may be repairable or may recover without surgical treatment (52,77,78,123,153). EMG and NCS may help differentiate neuropraxia from axonal degeneration. CT myelography and MRI can identify preganglionic nerve root injuries (avulsions) if they are associated with traumatic pseudomeningoceles, as they are in many avulsions; however, root avulsions may occur without creating a pseudomeningocele, and pseudomeningoceles may be visualized at the level of a root that has not been avulsed. All tests require sedation, and CT myelography is invasive. Testing should be reserved for infants who are candidates for nerve surgery, to help the surgeon plan the operation.

Thus, the indications for brachial plexus exploration with nerve grafting and transfer are unclear. Some surgeons recommend this procedure for all children without full recovery of active elbow flexion and shoulder abduction by 3 months of age (59); others prefer to allow more time for recovery (35,79,102,137). Most surgeons agree that complete avulsion of the plexus is rare, so at least one root has a repairable injury in most cases, and the results are poor for surgical plexus reconstruction for BPBP performed after 12 months of age. Most surgeons resect the scarred plexus and graft nonavulsed roots to the lateral cord, suprascapular nerve, and posterior cord (79) (see Chapter 60). Nerve transfer (neurotization) of the accessory nerve may be helpful (94), but neurolysis of

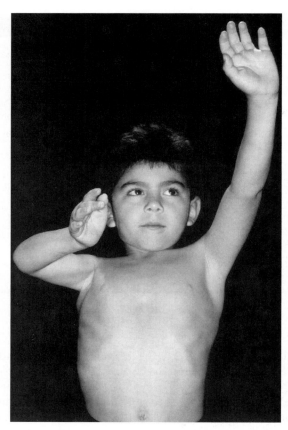

Figure 165.10. Decreased shoulder abduction and external rotation due to right brachial plexus birth palsy.

a neuroma-in-continuity probably is not (35). The results of plexus surgery vary, and few patients have had long-term follow-up, but nerve grafting and transfer in infants with poor prognostic signs probably result in better function than if no surgery was performed, and complications are unusual in the hands of experienced surgeons (59,79).

Children with upper-trunk BPBP frequently have residual weakness of shoulder external rotation and abduction (Fig. 165.10). Such a child may have difficulty positioning his or her hand in space, particularly to reach the head and face, or to throw, climb, turn a jump rope, or play a musical instrument. Eventually, the child may develop a shoulder internal rotation contracture, with glenohumeral joint changes and eventual posterior dislocation of the humeral head (70,81,174). Shoulder function may be classified using Mallet's scale (109,172) (Fig. 165.11). To diminish unopposed internal rotation, Sever (150), in 1925, recommended releasing the pectoralis major and subscapularis. In 1934, L'Episcopo (101) described the results of combining Sever's anterior release with transferring the teres major to the proximal humerus in order to provide active shoulder external rotation. This operation was later

modified by Hoffer and colleagues (19,84,136), who described latissimus dorsi and teres major transfer to the supraspinatus, with release of the pectoralis major only (because release of the subscapularis can cause glenohumeral instability); and Covey et al. (39), who described latissimus dorsi and teres major rerouting around the proximal humerus.

Shoulder external rotation tendon transfer and rerouting both reliably increase abduction, as well as external rotation in abduction by an average of 20° to 40° each. Abduction is increased because the transfer helps stabilize the glenohumeral joint, allowing the deltoid to function more efficiently. The rerouting procedure is more technically demanding and requires more excursion of the teres and latissimus muscles but may provide more external rotation than the transfer procedure (92). Other patient requirements for these operations include sufficient maturity to work with a therapist postoperatively to strengthen the transfer (4 years of age or older), minimal changes in the glenohumeral joint from unopposed internal rotation (usually 12 years of age or younger), and enough deltoid strength to abduct to at least 60° against gravity. However, Hoffer and Phipps (83) have reported that when posterior shoulder dislocation occurs early (before 4 years of age) latissimus and teres transfer and pectoralis release can be combined with closed shoulder reduction with good results and maintenance of reduction (83).

Tendon transfers do not reliably restore elbow flexion (112,127) but they may restore wrist extension, finger extension and flexion, and thumb opposition if adequate donors are available (26). For forearm supination deformity, biceps rerouting and forearm osteoclasis improve forearm position (23,106,110,185). Elbow flexion contractures can be treated with serial elbow drop-out casts (long-arm casts applied in maximum elbow extension, with the posterior above-elbow aspect cut out so that the elbow can extend farther but cannot flex). Surgical release of elbow flexion contractures is not usually indicated.

For the untreated older child or teenager, glenohumeral deformity and contracture may make shoulder tendon transfers less effective. External rotation osteotomy of the humerus improves the appearance and function of a limb with a shoulder internal rotation contracture in the older child (61,174).

If the deltoid is completely paralyzed, shoulder arthrodesis may improve function by conferring stability (139) (see Chapter 101). Wrist arthrodesis can improve hand position when wrist motors are paralyzed and no muscles are available for transfer (see Chapter 72). Arm-lengthening procedures are not indicated for treating the global extremity hypoplasia associated with severe BPBP.

Throughout childhood, the child with BPBP may benefit from goal-directed occupational and physical therapy.

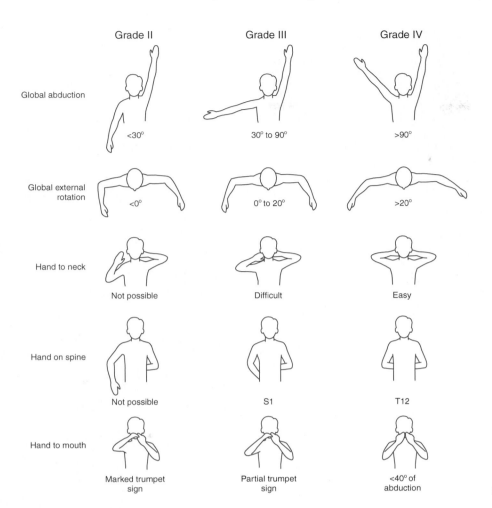

Figure 165.11. Modified Mallet's classification (172). Grade I has no function.

CLASSIFICATIONS

There is no standard classification system for BPBP, aside from classification by level of plexus involvement, as described previously. Shoulder limitation has been classified by Mallet (60,109,172) (Fig. 165.11).

PREOPERATIVE MANAGEMENT

PROM exercises help prevent or diminish contractures due to BPBP. PROM is especially important in the infant, because the shoulder can become fixed in internal rotation and subluxate or dislocate before the child is old enough to undergo shoulder external rotation tendon transfer or rerouting (83,164). Weekly manipulation by a therapist is not adequate; the child's shoulder should undergo PROM several times each day, so the child's caregivers must be trained to do shoulder PROM exercises.

PREOPERATIVE PLANNING

CT myelography or MRI may be helpful for planning brachial plexus exploration and nerve grafting, although the decision to proceed with this operation is based on lack of clinical recovery, and the most helpful planning information is gained from somatosensory-evoked potentials performed intraoperatively.

Before shoulder external rotation tendon transfer or rerouting, the waist portion of the shoulder spica cast can be applied with the child standing, to improve fit, then removed and reapplied at the end of the operation. Postoperative therapy is especially important following these procedures, so arrangements for this should be made prior to surgery.

OPERATIVE TECHNIQUES

Brachial Plexus Exploration and Nerve Grafting

See Chapter 60 and Figure 165.12 for details on surgical techniques for brachial plexus exploration. Repair of BPBP differs slightly from repair of traumatic brachial plexus palsy in adults. The differences stem from the following aspects of BPBP:

• Nerve transfer (neurotization) is not usually necessary;

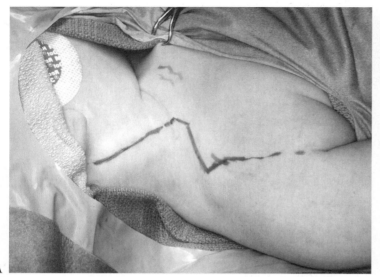

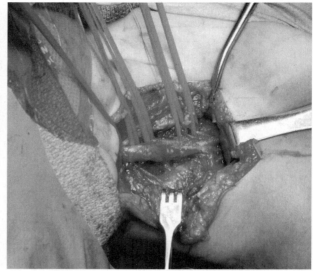

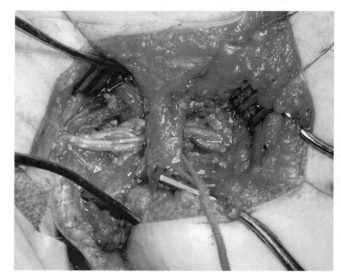

Figure 165.12. **A:** Marks indicate planned incision for brachial plexus exploration (child is supine, with head to the left). **B:** Intraoperative view of scarred plexus (same child as in *A*). The head is to the left, vessel loops surround the roots; the central horizontal structure is the plexus. **C:** Intraoperative view of clavicle and sural nerve cable grafts (same child as *A* and *B;* head is to the left, central vertical structure is clavicle).

at least one root is usually available as a proximal source of intact neurons.

- The entire plexus is often shifted distally, so landmarks such as the clavicle crossing the plexus at the level of the divisions are not reliable.
- Clavicular osteotomy is not usually necessary.

If sural nerve grafts are obtained and the child is ambulatory, apply short-leg walking casts. Apply a custom-fabricated chest and neck splint at the end of the operation (Fig. 165.13). The ipsilateral arm can be placed in a sling or attached to the chest splint with a Velpeau wrap. Remove the chest and neck splint, sling, and short-leg walking casts and resume shoulder PROM exercises 3 weeks after surgery. Return of function may take 6 months to 2 years.

Shoulder External Rotation Tendon Transfer

Tendon transfers (84,136) (Figs. 165.14 and 165.15) are methods used to improve shoulder motion in children with BPBP. The surgical technique is as follows:

- Perform the operation under general anesthesia.
- Place the patient in a lateral decubitus position and hold with a beanbag. Isolate the affected axilla and arm with a U drape. Range the shoulder under anesthesia; if there is less than 80° passive external rotation when the arm is abducted to 90°, perform the pectoralis major lengthening as described later. If there is more than 80° rotation, pectoralis lengthening is not necessary.
- Make a transverse axillary incision after infiltrating the area with bupivacaine with epinephrine. Extend the incision posteriorly to the deltoid-triceps interval.

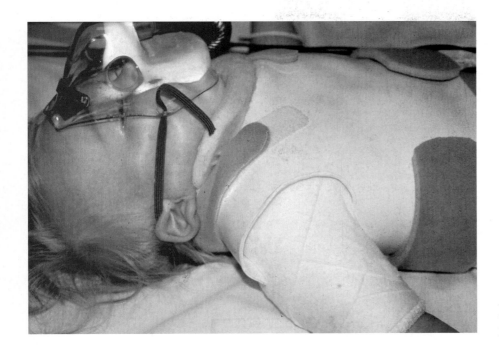

Figure 165.13. Infant in custom-fabricated neck brace following brachial plexus exploration and grafting.

- In the anterior end of the incision, locate the pectoralis major muscle. The tendon is short and most prominent on the deep side of the muscle. Using Bovie cautery, transect the tendinous and fascial portions of the muscle near its insertion on the humerus. Do not transect the entire muscle. Subscapularis lengthening is rarely necessary and may destabilize the shoulder.
- In the posterior part of the incision, locate the teres major and latissimus dorsi muscles. Trace them to their humeral insertions, using blunt dissection; these tendons are frequently conjoined (19). The axillary nerve

and posterior humeral circumflex artery cross from anterior to posterior deep to the latissimus and teres major tendons, just proximal to their insertions. They are easier to visualize after detaching the tendons.
- Detach the teres major and latissimus tendons from their humeral insertions. Bluntly free the muscle bellies from surrounding attachments, avoiding the circumflex scapular and thoracodorsal vessels. Tag the tendons with 0 nonabsorbable suture.
- Through the deltoid-triceps interval, locate the rotator cuff tendon. Stay proximal to avoid the axillary nerve.

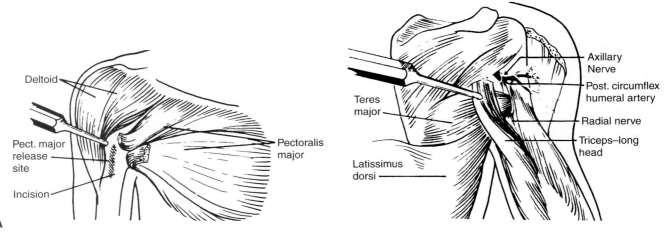

A

B

Figure 165.14. Tendon transfer procedure (84). **A:** Pectoralis major release. **B:** Teres major and latissimus dorsi, before attachment from humerus. *(continued)*

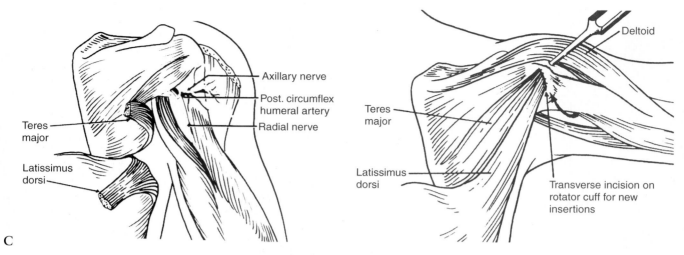

C

D

Figure 165.14. *(continued)* **C:** Teres major and latissimus dorsi, after detachment from humerus. **D:** Teres major and latissimus dorsi transferred to rotator cuff.

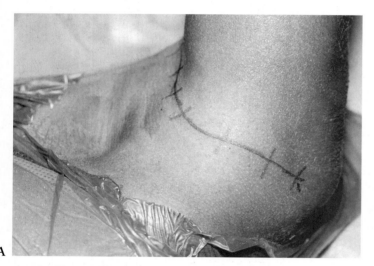

A

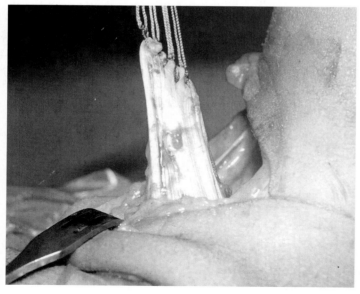

B

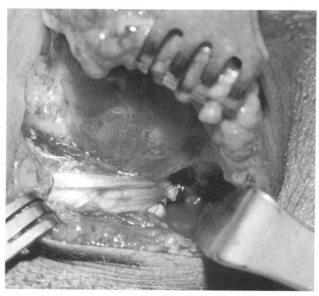

C

Figure 165.15. Shoulder external rotation tendon transfer. **A:** Transverse axillary incision. The patient is in right lateral decubitus position, with left arm abducted to 90°. **B:** Latissimus dorsi and teres major tendons after detachment from humerus. **C:** Latissimus dorsi and teres major tendons have been sutured to supraspinatus tendon (at tip of Army-Navy retractor).

teres major muscle belly; avoid excess tension, or mobilization of the teres will be difficult. Tag the latissimus tendon, which is still attached to the humerus at its insertion, with 0 nonabsorbable suture.

- Detach the teres major from its humeral insertion. Tag it with 0 nonabsorbable suture.
- Make a 3 cm incision starting at the acromion, at the posterior one third or anterior two thirds junction of the deltoid, after infiltrating with bupivacaine and epinephrine. Split the deltoid fibers bluntly down to the humerus. Stay proximal to the axillary nerve insertion.
- Bluntly make tunnels around the proximal humerus, starting at the humeral insertion site of the teres major. Each tunnel should reach the deltoid incision superiorly. The posterior tunnel must be large enough to ac-

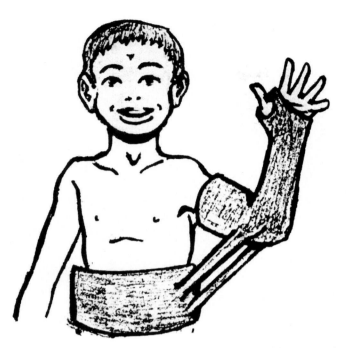

Figure 165.16. Shoulder spica cast used after shoulder external rotation tendon transfer or rerouting. (Drawing by Anthony Marotta, with permission).

- Position the arm in 90° of abduction and 60° to 80° of external rotation, bring the latissimus and teres major tendons posterior to the triceps muscle, and suture them into the rotator cuff tendon as high as possible.
- Close the skin incision in two layers. Apply the prefabricated waist portion of the spica cast, and attach a long-arm cast to the waist portion (Fig. 165.16).

Remove the shoulder spica cast 6 weeks after surgery. Apply an adjustable removable shoulder abduction splint (Fig. 165.8). Prescribe twice-daily occupational therapy (OT) for 2 weeks. The OT program is designed to strengthen the tendon transfer. Have the child wear the splint for the first week whenever he or she is not in therapy; in the second week, the splint can be discontinued during the day. The child should continue to wear the splint at night for 6 months. Continue OT at less frequent intervals for 6 to 12 months.

Shoulder External Rotation Tendon Rerouting

The surgical technique for tendon rerouting (39) (Figs. 165.17 and 165.18) follows the same first five steps as those used for tendon transfer (preceding technique). If the teres major and latissimus tendons are conjoined, this operation cannot be performed; the tendons must be transferred instead of rerouted. The surgical technique continues as follows:

- Transect the latissimus at the muscle–tendon junction. Attach the latissimus muscle belly side to side to the

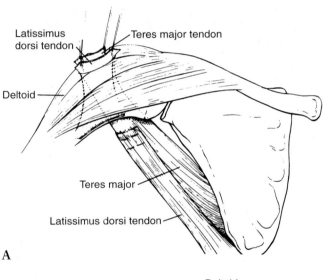

A

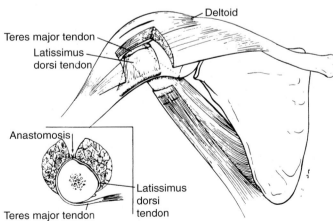

B

Figure 165.17. Tendon rerouting procedure. **A:** Latissimus dorsi tendon and teres major tendon pulled through a split in the deltoid. **B:** Latissimus dorsi tendon and teres major tendon after anastomosis. Reprinted from ref. 39, with permission.

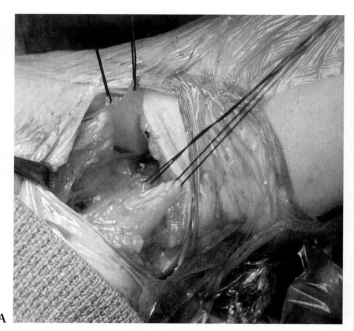
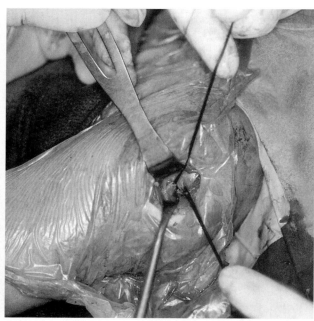

Figure 165.18.   Tendon rerouting procedure. **A:** Left axilla, upper sutures are in the latissimus dorsi tendon, lower sutures are in the teres major tendon. **B:** Left shoulder, head is to the right. Latissimus dorsi and teres major tendons pulled through a split in the deltoid muscle.

commodate the teres major muscle; the latissimus tendon will pass through the anterior tunnel.

■ Pass the latissimus tendon anteriorly, and the teres major muscle posteriorly. Both should be visible through the deltoid incision.

■ Attach the latissimus tendon to the teres major muscle by tying their tag sutures together through the deltoid incision, with the shoulder in 90° of abduction and 45° to 90° of external rotation.

■ Close the skin incision in two layers. Apply the prefabricated waist portion of the spica cast, and attach a long-arm cast to the waist portion (Fig. 165.16).

External Rotation Osteotomy of Humerus

Goddard and Fixsen (61) address the rotational osteotomy of the humerus for birth injuries of the brachial plexus. The surgical technique for osteotomy is as follows:

■ Perform the operation under general anesthesia.

■ Place the patient in supine position with a small bean-bag under the scapula. Examine the arm carefully, estimating the amount of external rotation necessary for the patient to reach the face and head. Prepare and drape the affected arm using a U drape.

■ Make a longitudinal anterolateral shoulder incision after infiltrating with bupivacaine and epinephrine. Approach the humerus through the deltopectoral and anterior deltoid–biceps intervals (between the radial and musculocutaneous nerves, neither of which are usually

visualized). The radial nerve will be more anterior than usual because of the internal rotation contracture.

■ Select the osteotomy site at the deltoid insertion, with enough exposure proximally and distally to apply a small six-hole AO plate. Predrill, measure, and tap two holes proximal to the osteotomy site before making the osteotomy.

■ Make the osteotomy after making a longitudinal mark across the osteotomy site.

■ Rotate the distal fragment the amount previously estimated to allow the patient to reach the face and head. Insert two screws proximally and one distal to the osteotomy, and carefully range the shoulder to make sure the new position is optimal. Remove the distal screw and adjust the rotation if necessary. Insert the remaining screws, check the position of the fixation on a radiograph, if necessary, and close the wound in layers.

■ Apply a shoulder immobilizer with an abduction pillow.

Remove the shoulder immobilizer 6 weeks after surgery and check radiographs for bridging callus. If callus is present, discontinue immobilization. Postoperative rehabilitation is not usually necessary.

Biceps Rerouting and Forearm Osteoclasis for Supination Deformity

Manske and McCarroll (110) discuss biceps rerouting (Fig. 165.19) and osteoclasis (Fig. 165.20) in treating supi-

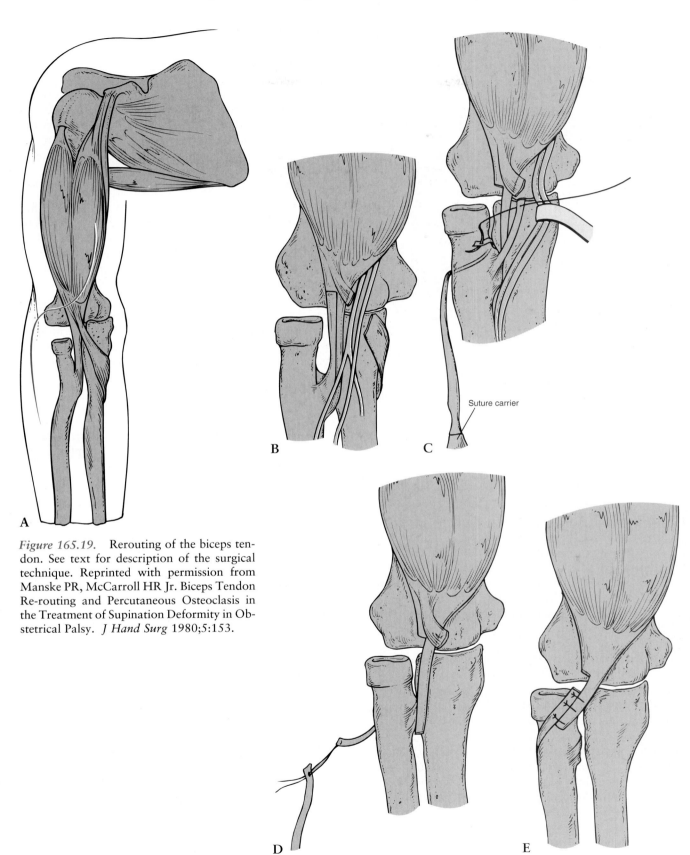

Figure 165.19. Rerouting of the biceps tendon. See text for description of the surgical technique. Reprinted with permission from Manske PR, McCarroll HR Jr. Biceps Tendon Re-routing and Percutaneous Osteoclasis in the Treatment of Supination Deformity in Obstetrical Palsy. *J Hand Surg* 1980;5:153.

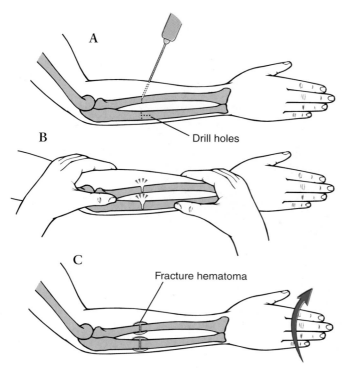

Figure 165.20.   Osteoclasis of the forearm. See text for a description of technique (110).

nation deformity in obstetric palsy. The general surgical technique is as follows:

■ Perform the operation under general anesthesia, and use a tourniquet. A sterile tourniquet may be necessary.
■ Approach the biceps tendon through an anterior zigzag incision, placing the transverse limb of the zigzag along the elbow flexion crease (Fig. 165.19A).
■ Incise the lacertus fibrosis, and retract the median nerve and brachial artery ulnarward (Fig. 165.19B).
■ Expose the biceps tendon to its insertion on the bicipital tuberosity of the radius. Divide the biceps tendon by a Z lengthening (the Z should be as long as possible). Protect the radial artery, which crosses the palmar surface of the tendon near its insertion.
■ Pass a folded wire suture or a curved suture carrier around the neck of the radius. Reroute the distal tendon segment so that it has a pronating torque by attaching it to the suture carrier (Fig. 165.19C).
■ Reattach the distal tendon to the proximal tendon in a side-to-side fashion using nonabsorbable suture. The biceps tendon usually requires 1.5 cm of lengthening to be repaired after rerouting (110). Close the wound in layers and apply a long-arm cast in neutral forearm rotation, with the elbow flexed 90° (Fig. 165.19D,E).
■ If biceps rerouting does not achieve adequate correction of the supination deformity, perform two-stage forearm

osteoclasis any time after the rerouting has healed (Fig. 165.20).
■ Perform the operation under general anesthesia, and use a tourniquet.
■ Through small incisions, use a one-eighth-inch drill to make three bicortical drill holes in the middle third of the radius and ulna (Fig. 165.20A). Fracture the bones by manipulating the forearm (Fig. 165.20B). Do not rotate the distal fragment at this time, or the fragments will displace. Close the wounds.
■ Place the arm in a long-arm cast, with the elbow at 90°.

After 10 to 14 days, under sedation or general anesthesia, remove the cast and manipulate the distal forearm to the desired position (0° to 40° of pronation) (Fig. 165.20C). Enough callus will have formed by this time that the fragments will not displace. Reapply the long-arm cast, with the elbow at 90° and the forearm in the desired position of rotation. Immobilize for 6 weeks after biceps rerouting. Focus the postoperative rehabilitation on active elbow flexion and extension, and forearm rotation. Then immobilize for 3 to 4 weeks after the second stage of forearm osteoclasis. Postoperative rehabilitation is not usually necessary.

Other Surgical Techniques

See Chapter 55 for the surgical technique for the wrist extension transfer, Chapter 56 for the opponensplasty, Chapter 101 for shoulder arthrodesis, and Chapter 72 for wrist arthrodesis.

COMPLICATIONS

Most pitfalls related to brachial plexus exploration and nerve grafting occur in patient selection. If the surgeon underestimates the infant's potential for recovery, resection and grafting of the plexus may do more harm than good. If the surgeon waits too long to operate (after 1 year of age), the limited improvement achieved before surgery will be lost and may not be recovered.

Just as in nerve exploration and grafting, most pitfalls related to shoulder external rotation tendon transfer and rerouting occur in patient selection. If the deltoid is too weak, the tendon transfer will not improve range of motion. If the patient is unable to cooperate with postoperative therapy, the tendon transfer will probably not function as well. If the shoulder contracture is due to extensive glenohumeral changes, or if long-standing posterior shoulder dislocation is present, the tendon transfer will not improve range. The transverse axillary scar in this procedure is nearly invisible.

In a external rotation osteotomy of the humerus, if the elbow flexion contracture is severe (more than 45°), the patient will probably be unhappy with the position of the forearm after the humerus is rotated externally. With the shoulder internally rotated, the forearm can lie across the front of the body, but after an external rotation osteotomy, the forearm and hand will "stick out." Also, the anterolateral arm scar widens and is quite noticeable.

Likewise, the anterior elbow scar from biceps rerouting and forearm osteoclasis often widens and is quite noticeable.

CONCLUSIONS

BPBP is very distressing to parents, perhaps because of the etiology, that is, because it is an injury rather than a congenital malformation. BPBP is a common cause of malpractice claims against obstetricians. The well-documented increased risk of recurrent BPBP with subsequent pregnancies has not been featured in the obstetrics literature; we advise parents of this risk so they can pass this information along to their obstetrician.

Although most series show high rates of full recovery, these data are based on relatively short follow-up. We frequently see 3- to 4-year-old children with functional limitations from BPBP who were declared fully recovered at 3 to 6 months of age, before they could cooperate with a thorough active motion and strength examination. However, many children with slightly limited shoulder range of motion and strength can function almost normally, and even when function is limited, older children and parents may be bothered more by the decreased size of the extremity and length discrepancy than the decreased function.

CONGENITAL TRANSVERSE FAILURE OF FORMATION OF THE UPPER EXTREMITY

PATHOPHYSIOLOGY AND PRINCIPLES OF TREATMENT

Transverse failure of formation, often inaccurately termed "congenital amputation," occurs when the upper limb fails to form below a certain level. Finger nubbins usually form at the distal end of the limb, regardless of level (Fig. 165.21); their presence helps differentiate this condition from congenital constriction ring syndrome, in which nubbins do not form (see Chapter 69).

Transverse failure of formation is not inherited. The leading hypothesis for the etiology of transverse failure of formation is the subclavian artery supply disruption sequence theory: disruption of the embryonic subclavian blood supply causes transverse failure of formation, Poland anomaly, symbrachydactyly, Mobius syndrome, or other conditions, depending on the location of the blockage and the timing and duration of disruption (16,154, 175). One study (86) showed evidence of fetal vascular occlusive disease in the placentas of infants with transverse failure of formation, and hypothesized that emboli-

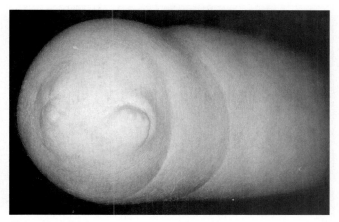

Figure 165.21.   Nubbins at end of below elbow transverse failure of formation.

zation from placental vascular thrombi caused this condition. Others (85,115) have found an increased incidence of transverse failure of formation and other limb defects in infants whose mothers underwent chorionic villus sampling before 10 weeks' gestation.

The most common level of transverse failure of formation is proximal forearm (below elbow), followed by transcarpal, distal forearm, and through humerus (above elbow) (181) (Fig. 165.22). This condition is almost always unilateral (148), and the left side is more commonly affected (91). Children with this condition have remarkably few functional deficits, and surgery has not been proven to improve their abilities (18). A prosthesis enhances prehension and possibly appearance but blocks sensory feedback. When indicated, goal-directed occupational therapy may help the school-aged child learn to perform activities of daily living with and without a prosthesis.

ASSESSMENT, INDICATIONS, AND RELATIVE RESULTS

Transverse failure of formation is usually an isolated anomaly, but children with amelia (failure of formation at the shoulder level) have a high incidence of scoliosis (138) (Fig. 165.23). Cognition and developmental milestones are usually normal, except that the child with a very short arm may not crawl.

The child with above-elbow or below-elbow failure of formation should be assessed by a prosthetic team (which includes a physician, a prosthetist, and an occupational therapist, and may include a recreation therapist and social worker) at around 6 months of age, and fitted with a prosthesis with a passive hand or mitt when able to sit independently (91) (Fig. 165.24). Parents are encouraged to gradually increase wearing time until the child tolerates

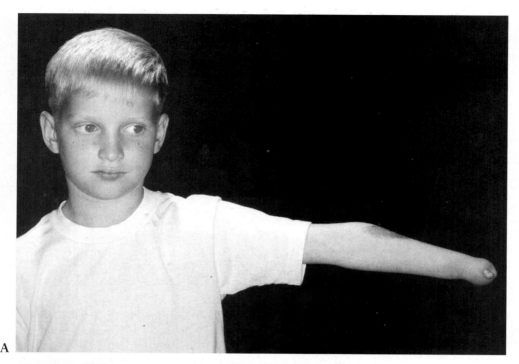

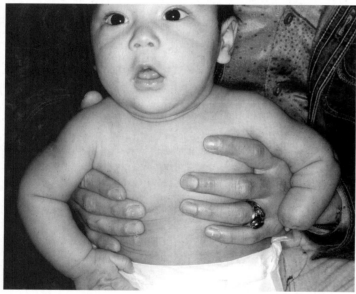

Figure 165.22.   **A:** Transcarpal transverse failure of formation with thumb nubbin. **B:** Long below-elbow transverse failure of formation. *(continued)*

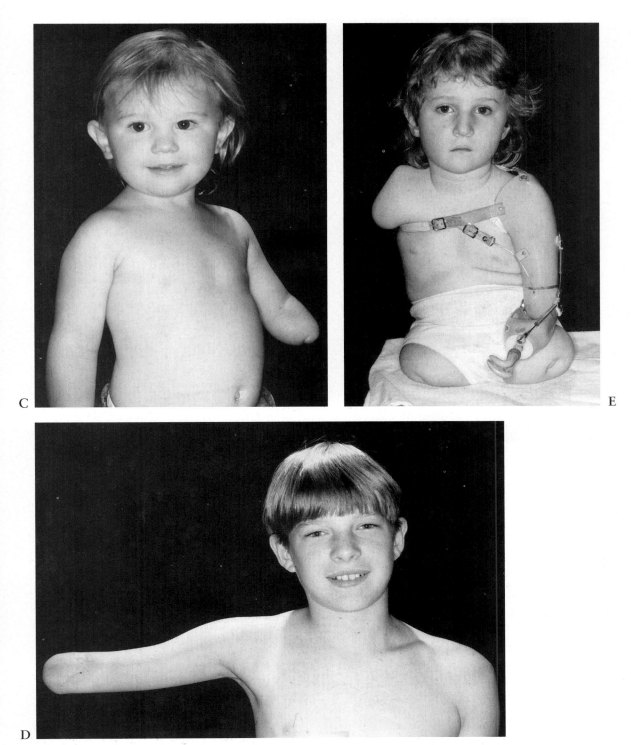

Figure 165.22. (continued) C: Short below-elbow transverse failure of formation. D: Through elbow amputation. E: Above-elbow transverse failure of formation.

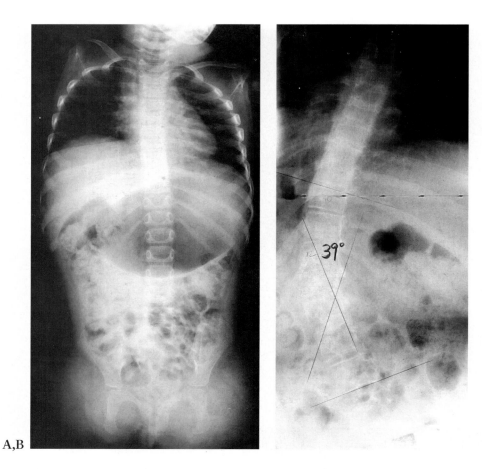

A,B

Figure 165.23. Girl with transverse failure of formation of upper (and lower) extremities. **A:** Radiograph of the spine (the child was 2 years of age). **B:** Radiograph of the spine (12 years of age) with 39° scoliosis.

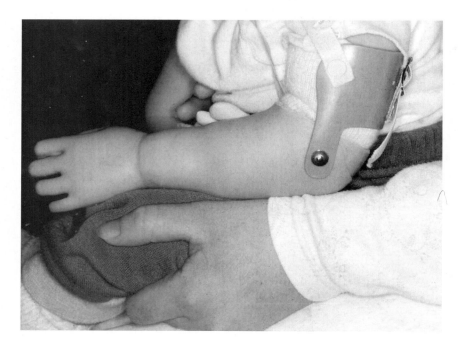

Figure 165.24. Passive below-elbow upper-extremity prosthesis.

the prosthesis for the majority of the waking hours. Children with more proximal or distal failure of formation are not usually fitted with a prosthesis in infancy. If the deficiency is at shoulder level, the prosthesis is too heavy for comfortable wear; if the deficiency is at the distal forearm or through the carpus, the child functions better without a prosthesis (148).

Follow the child's condition closely (three to four times each year) to check prosthesis fit and reinforce the importance of regular wear. Children who are fitted with a prosthesis before 2 years of age are more likely to continue to use the prosthesis throughout childhood (148). To enhance acceptance and use of the prosthesis by the family and child, the prosthetic team may organize supervised play groups for children who use prostheses, and the prosthetist can fabricate dolls with prostheses (Fig. 165.25). At 2 to 3 years of age, evaluate the child for readiness for an active terminal device (TD). If the child readily bears weight on the passive prosthesis when crawling and uses it for pulling up, balance, and two-handed activities, such as throwing and catching, he or she is probably ready to learn to use an active TD.

At this point, the physician and parents choose between a body-powered (cable-operated) prosthesis, which works best with a hook or similar type TD, and a prosthesis powered by electrical signals from proximal forearm muscle contractions (myoelectric prosthesis), which usually has a TD that looks like a hand and uses a chuck pinch (Fig. 165.26 and Table 165.2). Each of these prostheses has advantages and disadvantages; fortunately, because the growing child needs a new prosthesis every 1 to 2 years, no choice is permanent. The body-powered hook prosthesis is more difficult to learn to use, but children who learn to use this type of prosthesis first can usually learn to use a myoelectric prosthesis easily. Children who learn to use a myoelectric prosthesis first have more difficulty learning to use a body-powered hook prosthesis. Most studies comparing performance of body-powered and myoelectric prostheses use a hand TD on both prostheses. The cosmetic glove used with this TD increases resistance to opening, which is easily overcome by the myoelectric motor but makes the body-powered prosthesis very difficult to use. In spite of this handicap, however, these studies show that children perform most tasks faster with the body-powered prosthesis (47), and consistent users of a body-powered prostheses are more likely to be pleased with prosthetic function (100). However, parents and older children are often influenced by the

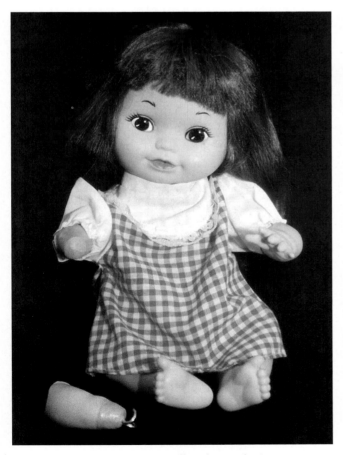

Figure 165.25. Doll with prosthesis.

Table 165.2. Comparison of Upper-Extremity Prostheses: Body vs. Myoelectric Power

	Body powered	Myoelectric
Weight	Lighter	Heavier
Speed	Faster	Slower
Strength	Weaker	Stronger
Noise	Quiet	Audible motor
Suspension	Figure 8 or 9 shoulder harness	No harness
Terminal device	Hook works best	Hand or hook
Maintenance	Infrequent, simple	Frequent, complex
Accommodation for growth	Growth liner can be removed when prosthesis becomes too small, extending prosthetic life	Can't use growth liners
Cost	$7000	$15000

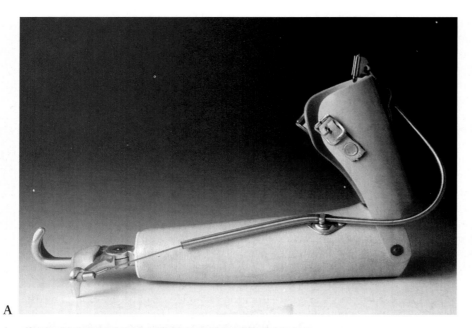

A

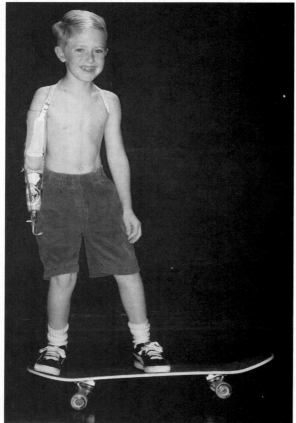

B

Figure 165.26.   **A and B:** Body-powered hook prosthesis. *(continued)*

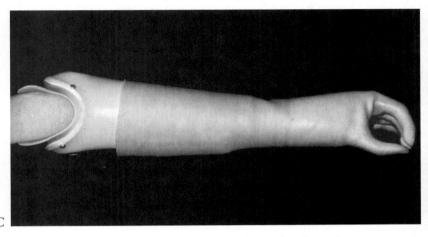

C

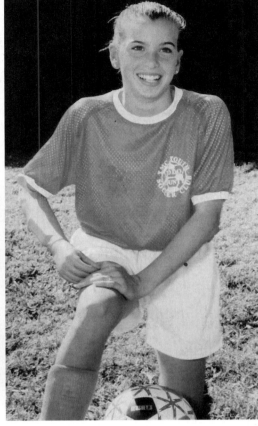

D

Figure 165.26. (continued) **C** and **D**: Myoelectric hand prosthesis.

"high-tech" image of the myoelectric prosthesis and the fact that the TD most commonly used with this prosthesis looks like a hand.

Forearm lengthening has been described for the very short below-elbow stump to improve prosthetic fitting (149); this is very rarely indicated. The Krukenberg procedure, in which the radius and ulna are separated and muscles reattached so that the radius pinches against the ulna, is most useful for blind bilateral distal forearm amputees, because it provides unilateral prehension with sensory feedback. This operation may occasionally be indicated for a sighted child with above-wrist failure of formation who does not have access to prosthetic facilities (34,69, 157). However, because children with unilateral above-wrist failure of formation have very few functional deficits and the appearance of the Krukenberg forearm is strikingly abnormal, this operation is rarely indicated for the child with a unilateral deficiency.

CLASSIFICATIONS

There is no classification system for transverse failure of formation other than level, which has been previously described.

CONCLUSIONS

The biggest challenge in the treatment of children with transverse failure of formation is helping parents adjust their often unrealistically high expectations of prosthetic technology. The importance of good communication with the child and family cannot be overstressed. We focus on

- The remarkable abilities of the child with or without the prosthesis (most children with below-elbow failure of formation tell us that the only activity they cannot perform is traveling hand over hand on the monkey bars)
- The opportunity to try a different type of prosthesis when the child outgrows the current one.
- The need for improved prosthetic technology [well documented in a recent nationwide survey of upper-extremity prosthesis users (11)].
- The importance of maintaining the prosthesis so that the child can use it, and the responsibilities of the child, family, prosthetist, and physician in accomplishing this task.

We prefer to prescribe a body-powered hook TD prosthesis, but will prescribe a myoelectric prosthesis if the family strongly prefers it and has demonstrated that they can keep their clinic appointments and return promptly if the prosthesis breaks or if the child outgrows it. Older children who use a body-powered prosthesis may appreciate interchangeable TDs: a hook for function and a prosthetic hand when appearance is more important than function.

CONGENITAL DISLOCATION OF THE RADIAL HEAD

PATHOPHYSIOLOGY AND PRINCIPLES OF TREATMENT

Congenital dislocation of the radial head (CDRH) is the most common congenital anomaly of the elbow (1,9,125). Although the etiology of CDRH is unknown, it is known to be associated with dysplasia of the capitellum and proximal radius, as well as shortening of the ulna (95,125). In CDRH, the radial head may be dislocated in an anterior, posterior, or lateral direction; in one series, 47% were anterior, 43% posterior, and 10% lateral (9).

CDRH is usually bilateral (1,9,97,111,125). It may be isolated and either sporadic or familial, or it may be associated with congenital radioulnar synostosis (124), or with a syndrome, such as Klinefelter's, Cornelia de Lange, Ehlers–Danlos, and nail-patella syndrome (1,9,46,71,97, 111,125,140,156). Not all cases are congenital; progressive subluxation of the radial head progressing to dislocation has also been reported (97).

ASSESSMENT, INDICATIONS, AND RELATIVE RESULTS

CDRH may be noted in infancy but often escapes detection until the child is of school age (97). The presenting complaint is usually posterolateral elbow prominence, restricted elbow extension and forearm rotation, elbow "popping," or pain with activity (1,95), although pain is uncommon before adolescence. Often, the limitations due to CDRH are first perceived after an unrelated elbow injury and may be erroneously attributed to that injury. When the condition is unilateral, CDRH may be difficult to distinguish from chronic traumatic dislocation (29) (Table 165.3).

The dislocated radial head is palpable just distal to the cubital fossa in anterior CDRH, and palpable and visible laterally in posterior CDRH (see Figs. 165.27 and 165.28). Elbow motion deficits are often minimal, usually nonprogressive, and worse in anterior than posterior CDRH. Loss of supination is the most prominent limitation in both anterior and posterior CDRH. Anterior CDRH blocks full flexion, and posterior CDRH blocks full extension, causing a flexion contracture (usually 30° or less). Wrist range of motion may also be limited (1,9, 97,111). In the infant, the unossified dislocated radial head may be visualized with diagnostic ultrasound (14), but the diagnosis is most commonly made by plain radiography (Figs. 165.27 and 165.28).

Surgical intervention is seldom necessary in childhood because most children are asymptomatic and have mini-

Table 165.3.   Congenital vs Traumatic Radial Head Dislocation

	Congenital	Traumatic
Anterior dislocation, radial head		
Radial head	Head is dome shaped with no central depression	Head has normal shape with central depression
Ulna	Palmar bow	Normal
Posterior dislocation, radial head		
Radial head	Head is elongated & narrow	Head has normal shape with central depression
Ulna	Accentuated dorsal bow	Normal
Capitellum	Hypoplastic or absent	Normal
Bilateral	Common	Rare
Other anomalies	Common	Rare
Trauma	Possible	Necessary

Data from Mardam-Bey, Ger E. Congenital Radial Head Dislocation. *J Hand Surg* 1979;4:316–320; and Kelly DW. Congenital Dislocation at the Radial Head: Spectrum and Natural History. *J Pediatr Orthop* 1981;1:295–298, with permission.

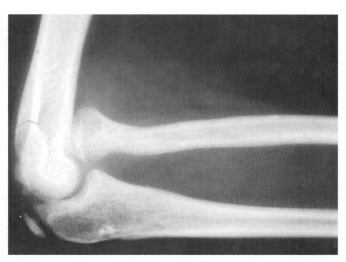

Figure 165.27. Anterior congenital dislocation of the radial head.

mal functional limitations (46,125). Radial head resection before skeletal maturity has been associated with several different complications (see Complications, later). Surgical reduction of the radial head and reconstruction of the annular ligament or rotational radial and ulnar osteotomies have not been consistently successful (9,124,125). In adolescence or adulthood, the laterally or posteriorly dislocated radial head may become painful owing to degenerative changes at the contact point between the radial head and the distal humerus; radial head excision relieves pain, improves appearance, and may improve range of motion (29,97).

CLASSIFICATIONS

CDRH is classified by the direction of the dislocation, as previously described.

PREOPERATIVE PLANNING

Examine the wrist for distal radioulnar joint (DRUJ) instability, and obtain bilateral wrist radiographs before radial head resection. If the DRUJ is unstable and the symptomatic side is ulna positive, resection of the radial head may cause wrist pain.

OPERATIVE TECHNIQUE

Resection of the Radial Head (Posterior or Lateral Dislocation)

- Perform the operation under general anesthesia, and use a tourniquet.
- Make a longitudinal incision using a Kocher approach over the dislocated radial head. Develop the interval between the extensor carpi ulnaris and anconeus muscles.
- Incise the capsule with the forearm in maximal pronation, and do not extend the capsular incision distal to the radial neck, to avoid injuring the posterior interosseous nerve. Preserve the annular ligament to enhance proximal radius stability and protect the posterior interosseous nerve. Avoid violating the periosteum of the proximal ulna to prevent radioulnar synostosis.
- Excise the radial head with an oscillating saw, osteotome, or rongeur perpendicular to the radial neck. Check elbow flexion and extension and forearm pronation and supination to make sure that the proximal radius does not contact the distal humerus; if it does, resect more until it moves freely. Remove any loose intraarticular osteochondral fragments.
- Close the capsule with nonabsorbable suture. Close the subcutaneous tissue with interrupted absorbable suture, and close the skin with running subcuticular suture.

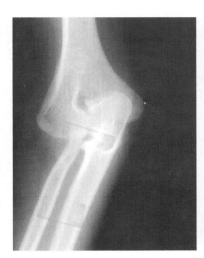

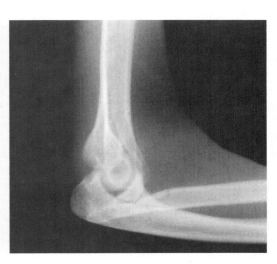

Figure 165.28. AP and lateral views of a posterior dislocation of the radial head.

■ Immobilize the elbow at 90° of flexion in a long-arm splint.

Remove the splint after 7 to 10 days, and begin early range-of-motion exercises.

COMPLICATIONS

If radial head resection is performed before skeletal maturity, several complications can occur, including regrowth of the proximal radius, postoperative radioulnar synostosis (29), and cubitus valgus deformity. However, radial head resection for a variety of indications, including CDRH, did not cause cubitus valgus in 27 elbows of 25 children with an average age of 14 years (range 5 to 18 years) (87). Other potential complications include injury to the posterior interosseous nerve, radioulnar synostosis, proximal migration of the radius, valgus elbow instability, cubitus valgus, and wrist pain (9,29,97,111).

CONCLUSIONS

If the dislocated radial head rubs against the distal humerus, painful degenerative changes can occur. Radial head resection reliably relieves pain and is sometimes necessary, even when the DRUJ is unstable. When wrist pain occurs following radial head resection for CDRH, it is usually mild and activity related.

CONGENITAL ELEVATION OF THE SCAPULA (SPRENGEL'S DEFORMITY)

PATHOPHYSIOLOGY AND PRINCIPLES OF TREATMENT

Congenital elevation of the scapula results from a failure of the normal caudal migration of the scapula during the fetal period of development (32,48). The scapula with this malformation is usually hypoplastic with decreased vertical length and increased horizontal width-to-height ratio (27), which is 2 to 10 cm more cephalad than normal (Fig. 165.29). The inferior pole is rotated medially with the glenoid displaced inferiorly. The periscapular muscles may be hypoplastic or absent, causing scapular winging (32,33). In 20% to 30% of cases, the superomedial scapula is connected to the spinous processes, laminae, or transverse processes by a fibrous tissue, cartilage, or bone called the omovertebral connection; this connection is diagnostic of congenital elevation of the scapula (27,32,33). Right and left sides are affected with equal frequency, and bilateral involvement occurs in 10% to 30% of the cases (168).

The majority of patients with congenital elevation of

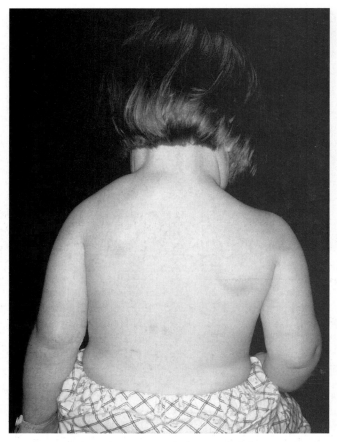

Figure 165.29.   Congenital elevation of the scapula.

the scapula have associated anomalies, most commonly congenital scoliosis, Klippel-Feil syndrome, fused or absent ribs, spina bifida, and VATER association (17,27,32, 33).

This condition is usually treated nonoperatively, except for resection of the omovertebral connection. Surgical mobilization and caudal repositioning of the scapula have been recommended, but most children with congenital elevation of the scapula do not need surgical treatment (168).

ASSESSMENT, INDICATIONS, AND RELATIVE RESULTS

Children usually present with evaluation of scapular asymmetry, diminished shoulder motion, and fullness at the base of the neck. The affected scapula appears to be elevated and hypoplastic. Shoulder abduction is significantly limited in 40% of patients, and elevation is often limited (33,73). Basilar neck fullness is due to the prominence of the superomedial angle of the scapula (32). Congenital elevation of the scapula is usually not painful.

Differential diagnosis includes brachial plexus birth

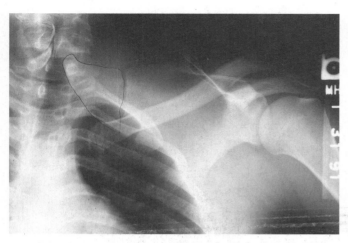

Figure 165.30. Bony omovertebral connection.

palsy and isolated scoliosis or Klippel-Feil syndrome (33). An anteroposterior (AP) radiograph of the shoulder demonstrates scapular elevation, especially when compared with the contralateral normal side. A bony omovertebral connection may be seen on the AP view (Fig. 165.30) or on lateral oblique views and CT scan. Examine the child for scoliosis and other associated anomalies.

Function may be limited by decreased shoulder abduction, but many children with this condition have excellent shoulder function. Passive stretching and abduction early in infancy may improve shoulder range of motion, and removal of an omovertebral connection may also improve range of motion.

The cosmetic deformity and degree of disability are proportional to the severity of deformity; children with mild grade 1 to grade 2 elevation (see next section, on classifications and terminology) have little functional impairment.

For more severe malformations with functional impairment, surgical repositioning of the scapula may be indicated in addition to resection of the omovertebral connection, with the goal of improving appearance and range of motion. Various methods of scapular mobilization have been described. Woodward (180) recommended moving the trapezius and rhomboid muscle origins to a more caudal position along the spine. Borges et al. (27) modified Woodward's procedure to include excision of the superomedial scapular prominence, to improve appearance. Clavicular osteotomy is recommended to allow further scapular descent and prevent damage to the brachial plexus (27, 33,67).

One long-term study (67) of 23 patients who underwent four different operations for congenital elevation of the scapula found that the average reduction of elevation was 2.7 cm, and average improvement in abduction was 19 degrees for repositioning procedures, with the best re-

sults in patients who underwent Woodward's procedure. Optimal age for surgery is probably between 3 and 8 years of age (32,68). Good results of scapular mobilization have been reported in older patients, but with less functional improvement (27). Normal appearance and function should not be expected at any age (33).

CLASSIFICATIONS AND TERMINOLOGY

Although congenital elevation of the scapula is commonly called Sprengel's deformity, it is actually a malformation instead of a deformity (see Chapter 69). The condition has been classified by severity (Table 165.4). This classification helps the surgeon determine treatment and prognosis and evaluate the postoperative result (33).

OPERATIVE TECHNIQUES

Resection of Omovertebral Connection
Figure 165-31 is an intraoperative photo of a resection of an omovertebral connection for the same patient whose radiograph is shown in Figure 165-30. The surgical procedure is as follows:

- Place the patient in the prone or lateral decubitus position with the affected side up.
- Place the incision directly over the omovertebral connection, in a transverse direction, if possible. Inject skin and subcutaneous tissue with bupivacaine and epinephrine; this provides pre-emptive analgesia and improves hemostasis.
- Expose and transect the connection at its scapular and spinous connections, and remove it.
- Close the incision in layers, and immobilize the arm in a sling or shoulder immobilizer.

Table 165.4.   Classification of Congenital Elevation of the Scapula

Grade	Description
1	Very mild; shoulders are level; deformity is not visible when patient is dressed
2	Mild; shoulder joints are almost level; deformity visible as lump in web of neck
3	Moderate; affected shoulder elevated 2–5 cm; deformity is easily visible
4	Severe; superior angle of scapula near occiput

From Cavendish ME. Congenital Elevation of the Scapula. *J Bone Joint Surg BR* 1972;54:395, with permission.

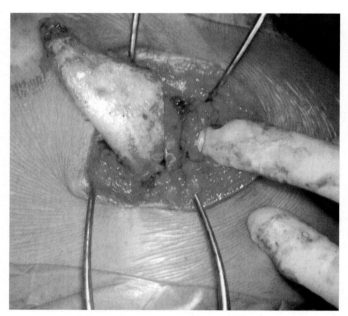

Figure 165.31. Intraoperative view of resection of omovertebral connection (same patient as in Fig. 165.30).

Allow normal use of the shoulder as soon as postoperative pain has diminished.

Surgical Repositioning of the Scapula
This operation is rarely indicated, and its description is beyond the scope if this text. For details, please see Woodward (180), Wilkinson and Campbell (177), Klisic et al. (99), and Borges et al. (27).

COMPLICATIONS

Complications of omovertebral resection are uncommon. Complications of surgical repositioning of the scapula include scar widening and residual scapular elevation (27, 32,33,177,180). Brachial plexus and vascular injury can occur (27); clavicular osteotomy (or morcellation) may prevent neurovascular injury with scapular repositioning (142). In addition, the suprascapular nerve may be injured with resection of the superior scapula.

CONCLUSIONS

Resection of the omovertebral connection is simple and usually improves appearance and range of motion. Scapular repositioning, a major operation with considerable risk of neurovascular injury and a good possibility of inadequate correction, is rarely indicated.

CONGENITAL PSEUDARTHROSIS OF THE CLAVICLE

PATHOPHYSIOLOGY AND PRINCIPLES OF TREATMENT

Congenital pseudarthrosis of the clavicle is a rare anomaly that results from failure of normal clavicular ossification (8,82,131). The etiology is unknown; one hypothesis suggests that the subclavian artery may compress the developing right clavicle, which might explain the predominance of right-sided lesions and the occurrence of left-sided lesions in association with dextrocardia. Bilateral involvement is rare (57,107,163). Another hypothesis is that the pseudarthrosis is caused by the failure of two ossification centers to fuse (82), but the normal clavicle in the developing embryo has only one ossifcation center (146). Unlike congenital pseudarthrosis of the tibia and ulna, this condition is not associated with neurofibromatosis, although it may be inherited in an autosomal recessive fashion (8,57, 146).

This condition does not usually require surgical treatment, and historically surgery for clavicular pseudarthrosis has had a high rate of serious complications (8, 68,131,163). Surgical resection of the pseudarthrosis and internal fixation may be indicated if the pseudarthrosis is very prominent or painful.

ASSESSMENT, INDICATIONS, AND RELATIVE RESULTS

Children with this rare condition are often noted to have a prominent middle third of the right clavicle at birth or soon thereafter; the prominence may increase with age (146). The pseudarthrosis is usually not painful, and shoulder range of motion is normal. Radiographs of the pseudarthrosis reveal an osseous separation with enlarged, rounded bone ends, and a distinctive absence of fracture callus (Fig. 165.32). Although case reports indicate that the natural history of pseudarthrosis of the clavicle is benign (151), no large series of cases has been reported.

Differential diagnosis includes traumatic clavicle fracture (a common birth injury, which is accompanied by pseudoparalysis of the involved limb, painful range of motion, and radiographic callus) and cleidocraniodysostosis (a bilateral inherited disorder of fetal membranous bone ossification, with clavicle, cranial, and pelvic dysplasia) (2,8,68,131,146,168).

Occasionally the pseudarthrosis is so prominent that surgical removal and repair with internal fixation is indicated (Fig. 165.32). Multiple complications of surgery have been reported, including sepsis, nonunion, and brachial plexus injury (8,163). Simple excision of the clavicular prominence without internal fixation or any attempt

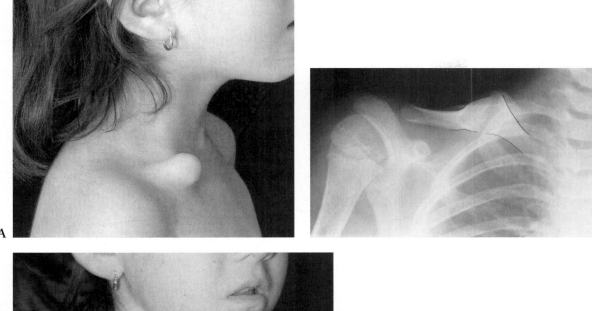

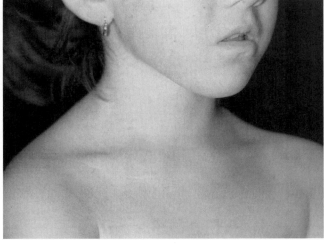

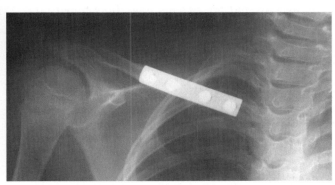

Figure 165.32.   Congenital pseudarthrosis of the clavicle. **A:** Preoperative photo. **B:** Preoperative radiograph (pseudarthrosis outlined). **C:** Postoperative photo. **D:** Postoperative radiograph.

to obtain union is generally recommended in the postpubertal patient who wishes to improve appearance. In prepubertal children, most authors who advocate surgical treatment recommend excision of the pseudarthrosis, bone grafting, and plating (8,57,68,82,131,146).

CLASSIFICATIONS

There are no classification systems for congenital pseudarthrosis of the clavicle.

OPERATIVE TECHNIQUE

Pseudarthrosis Resection and Bone Grafting

- Position the patient supine, with a pad under the affected scapula.

- Incise the skin longitudinally along the inferior clavicular border, and expose the pseudarthrosis.
- Incise the periosteum longitudinally. Resect the pseudarthrosis subperiosteally. Measure the defect.
- Obtain autologous corticocancellous iliac crest bone graft to span the clavicular defect created by resection of the pseudarthrosis, if necessary.
- Internally fix the clavicle with a semitubular or small low-profile dynamic compression plate. Avoid inferior placement of the plate or graft, which could cause subclavian vessel or brachial plexus injury (the subclavian artery passes between the clavicle and first rib immediately deep to the clavicular defect) (146).
- Close the incision in layers, and immobilize the arm in a sling.

    Remove the sling 6 weeks after pseudarthrosis and

grafting. The osteotomy sites are difficult to see on radiographs. If the plate or screws are prominent, they should be removed after osteosynthesis has occurred.

COMPLICATIONS

Many complications of pseudarthrosis resection, grafting, and plating have been described, including hypertrophic scar formation, infection, nonunion, neurovascular injury, and bone graft donor site morbidity (8,131). Steinmann pin fixation should never be used because it provides inadequate fixation and pins have been reported to migrate or cause neurologic injury (163). Simple excision of the pseudarthrosis without bone graft or internal fixation causes the affected shoulder to droop (68,131).

CONCLUSIONS

Surgical treatment of this condition is indicated only when the malformation is conspicuous and bothersome to the patient or the patient's parents. As with any elective operation, the patient and the parents must fully understand the potential risks. Resection, grafting, and plating can improve the patient's appearance considerably in this condition.

CONGENITAL PSEUDARTHOSIS OF THE ULNA

PATHOPHYSIOLOGY AND PRINCIPLES OF TREATMENT

Congenital pseudarthrosis of the ulna is a very rare condition that is usually associated with neurofibromatosis (114). Pseudarthrosis may be present at birth, or it may develop spontaneously after a fracture or after osteotomy; it has been reported to occur in the tibia, ulna, femur, clavicle, radius, and humerus (40). The etiology of congenital pseudarthrosis is unknown; in the majority of cases, the pseudarthrosis contains fibrous tissue, not neurofibroma (40) (see Chapter 169).

Congenital pseudarthrosis of the ulna causes a progressive forearm deformity. The forearm is short and bowed, and eventually the radial head dislocates (114) (Fig. 165.33). The goal of treatment is to obtain union without sacrificing motion.

ASSESSMENT, INDICATIONS, AND RELATIVE RESULTS

Pseudarthrosis of the ulna causes deformity, instability, weakness, and sometimes pain, although motion is usually not limited. Like the same condition in the tibia, union can be achieved with bone grafting and immobilization, but pseudarthrosis usually recurs. Historically, creation

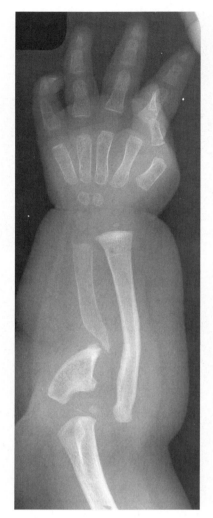

Figure 165.33.   Congenital pseudarthrosis of the ulna.

of a one-bone forearm was the only option available. This operation successfully restores forearm stability (169) but eliminates forearm rotation. Although the Ilizarov technique may successfully restore union in tibial pseudarthrosis (132), the use of prolonged immobilization and differential lengthening of the forearm bones is also likely to result in loss of forearm rotation.

Several authors (54,114,116,183) have reported treating ulnar pseudarthrosis with free vascularized fibular graft; in most cases, union was achieved, length was maintained, and forearm rotation was diminished but not completely lost. The indications for vascularized fibular graft, including the optimal age of the patient, have not yet been established, but this technique is promising.

CLASSIFICATIONS

There is no classification system for congenital pseudarthrosis of the ulna.

PREOPERATIVE PLANNING

When a free vascularized fibular graft is planned, preoperative arteriograms of the donor and recipient sites help identify possible vascular abnormalities (54).

OPERATIVE TECHNIQUE

Free Vascularized Fibular Graft to the Ulnar Pseudarthrosis

Gerwin and Weiland (54) discuss this technique. See Chapter 36 for the surgical technique of harvesting a free fibular graft.

■ Resect the pseudarthrosis and fix the graft in place using short plates at the proximal and distal ends, before performing vascular anastomoses. Avoid using intramedullary fixation or a long plate that spans both ends of the graft because these fixation methods interfere with graft vascularity.
■ Use an end-to-side anastomosis in the forearm, if possible, to minimize reduction of hand perfusion.
■ Use a supplemental cancellous bone graft at each end of the fibular graft to enhance union.

   Allow ambulation 3 to 5 days after surgery in a short-leg walking cast, which can be removed after 3 to 4 weeks. Immobilize the arm with a long-arm cast and check radiographs out of plaster every 6 weeks. Continue immobilization until graft incorporation is seen on radiographs; the average time to graft incorporation is 3 to 6 months.

COMPLICATIONS

Union may be difficult to achieve, and subsequent regrafting with cancellous allograft may be necessary. Even after union is achieved, pseudarthrosis may recur. If painful pseudarthrosis recurs and regrafting fails, creation of a one-bone forearm is the only remaining surgical option.

CONCLUSIONS

Because this condition is so rare, the indications for vascularized fibula grafting are not well established, and follow-up to skeletal maturity is lacking. The best indications probably are pain and progressive deformity.

CONGENITAL PROXIMAL RADIOULNAR SYNOSTOSIS

PATHOPHYSIOLOGY AND PRINCIPLES OF TREATMENT

Congenital proximal radioulnar synostosis (PRUS) is a malformation caused by failure of normal prenatal separa-

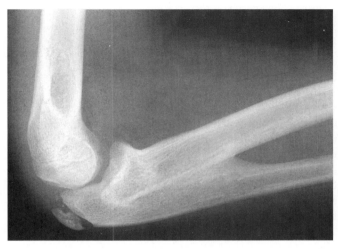

Figure 165.34.   Proximal radioulnar synostosis.

tion of the radius and ulna. The persistent connection between the two bones is nearly always proximal; distal radioulnar synostosis is extremely rare (15,96,144,152, 173). The connection is initially cartilaginous, but it usually eventually ossifies, forming a bony synostosis (Fig. 165.34). The forearm is usually fixed in pronation, probably because this is the normal fetal position (96,173).

   PRUS is usually an isolated malformation, but it may be associated with other malformations or syndromes in up to one third of affected children (152). Other malformations associated with PRUS include thumb hypoplasia, carpal coalition, symphalangism, and clubfoot (124); syndromes associated with PRUS include Apert's syndrome, arthrogryposis, fetal alcohol syndrome, and Klinefelter's syndrome (98,152,165,166). Familial occurrence (37,71) with autosomal dominant inheritance (141) has also been reported.

ASSESSMENT, INDICATIONS, AND RELATIVE RESULTS

Children with PRUS usually present between 2.5 and 6 years of age with painless limitation of forearm rotation and a slight flexion contracture (37,152), although occasionally PRUS is not noted until adolescence (71). Typically, a parent or teacher notices that the child has difficulty positioning the hand to catch a ball, drink from a cup, or accept small objects in an open palm and tends to hold objects in a backhanded, or hyperpronated, position. Bilateral involvement (60% to 80%) (129,152) and fixation in more than 60° of pronation (up to 40%) (152) are usually noted earlier because they cause more significant impairment.

   On examination, children with PRUS have an elbow flexion contracture, altered carrying angle, and short forearm in addition to a fixed forearm pronation deformity (129,144,152). Children with PRUS partially compensate for lack of forearm rotation by developing rotational hypermobility at the wrist and positioning the shoulder in internal rotation, flexion, and abduction (37,65,129).

PRUS usually does not cause significant functional impairment (15). In one study of the natural history of untreated PRUS (37), 96% of patients had mild or no limitations in daily activities regardless of forearm position, and the authors concluded that treatment of PRUS is rarely indicated. Other authors (157) consider fixed pronation between 15° and 60° a relative indication, and forearm fixation in greater that 60° pronation a definite indication for surgery, if functional limitations are significant.

Surgery to regain forearm rotation has nearly always been unsuccessful (126), although recently a free vascularized fascial flap placed between the separated forearm bones has been reported to successfully block postoperative recurrence of the synostosis (93). At present, however, the generally accepted surgical treatment is derotation osteotomy through the fusion mass, using K-wires or small Steinmann pins to fix the osteotomy (65,126,129,152). Others have described gradual correction to neutral following osteotomy, using the Ilizarov method (25), and two-stage osteoclasis without internal fixation (105).

The optimal position of the forearm is controversial because the best position of rotation varies with the task. Some surgeons recommend placement of the dominant forearm in 10° to 20° of pronation, and the nondominant forearm in neutral rotation, if necessary; and for unilateral PRUS, placement in 0° to 15° of pronation (152). Others (65,126) advocate placing the nondominant forearm in 20° to 35° of supination first, and the dominant forearm in 30° to 45° only, if necessary; and for unilateral involvement, 0° to 20° supination.

CLASSIFICATION

Radiographic classification based on radial head position and the presence of a radioulnar synostosis does not predict function (37). PRUS is part of a spectrum of malformations ranging from radial head abnormalities to complete synostosis with marked forearm shortening and absence of the radial head (124,152), although these have not been formally divided into types.

PREOPERATIVE PLANNING

Preoperative evaluation by an occupational therapist helps determine the child's functional deficits and optimal forearm position. If possible, surgery should be performed before school age (152), but this timing precludes considering the child's future intended occupation to determine the optimal forearm position, as recommended by some surgeons (37).

OPERATIVE TECHNIQUE

Rotational Osteotomy

Green and Mital (65) discuss surgical treatment of congenital radioulnar syntosis. The general surgical technique follows:

- Perform the operation under general anesthesia and a tourniquet.
- Make a dorsal longitudinal incision just radial to the subcutaneous border of the ulna. Incise the fascia in the interval between the anconeus and extensor carpi ulnaris muscles (Kocher approach). Expose the fusion mass subperiosteally.
- Pass a smooth K-wire from the olecranon apophysis into the intramedullary canal of the ulna under fluoroscopic guidance. This wire helps maintain longitudinal position while allowing adjustment of rotation.
- Make a mark across the osteotomy site to determine rotation. Perform the osteotomy around the wire, using multiple drill holes and an osteotome or oscillating saw. The osteotomy should be distal to the coronoid and radial head (if present).
- Rotate the forearm to the desired position and transfix the osteotomy site with a K-wire, passing obliquely from proximal ulna to distal radius. Leave the end of this wire through the skin to facilitate urgent removal for postoperative derotation if vascular compromise occurs.
- If a large change in forearm rotation is necessary, consider resecting 5 mm of bone at the osteotomy site (129), prophylactic forearm fasciotomy (152), or two-stage derotation to decrease the risk of postoperative neurovascular traction or compartment syndrome.
- Close the subcutaneous tissues and skin, and place the arm in a splint or long-arm cast with the elbow flexed to 90°.

Keep the forearm elevated and monitor the patient's neurovascular status closely for at least 48 hours postoperatively. If a long-arm splint was applied, change to a long-arm cast after 1 to 2 weeks. Remove the cast 6 weeks postoperatively to check forearm radiographs. Remove pins when the forearm bones show signs of healing. Therapy is not usually necessary.

COMPLICATIONS

The complication rate for forearm rotational osteotomy was 36% in one series (152), and the reoperation rate was 23% in another (65). The most serious complications are vascular compromise and compartment syndrome, which occur more frequently with rotational position change of greater than 85°. If this much correction is needed, obtain it in two stages. If either of these complications occur, remove the transfixion pin and return the forearm to its original position; if forearm compartment pressures are elevated, perform fasciotomies (see Chapter 13). Rotational correction can be reachieved 5 to 10 days later (152). Other complications include nerve palsy (due to either intraoperative damage to the posterior interosseous nerve or traction from rotational change), wound infection, loss of correction, and nonunion (37,105,129,152).

CONCLUSIONS

In our experience, children with PRUS associated with fetal alcohol syndrome have more severe pronation contractures than most other children with PRUS. Children with fetal alcohol syndrome are often mentally retarded, and they may be unable to describe symptoms of nerve traction following rotational osteotomy.

ELBOW AND FOREARM DEFORMITY DUE TO MULTIPLE HEREDITARY EXOSTOSES

PATHOPHYSIOLOGY AND PRINCIPLES OF TREATMENT

Multiple hereditary exostoses (MHE) is a disorder of enchondral bone growth in which cartilaginous exostoses (also called osteochondromas) grow from the physes of long bones and from the pelvis, ribs, scapula, and vertebrae (10,135). The exostoses may be sessile or pedunculated (Fig. 165.35). They grow until the patient is skeletally mature and eventually ossify. The forearm is affected in 30% to 67% of patients with this condition (22,89, 145), and the proximal humerus is also commonly involved (Fig. 165.36).

The prevalence of MHE is approximately 1 in 50,000 (145). MHE is inherited in an autosomal dominant pattern with high penetrance (145) and variable expressivity.

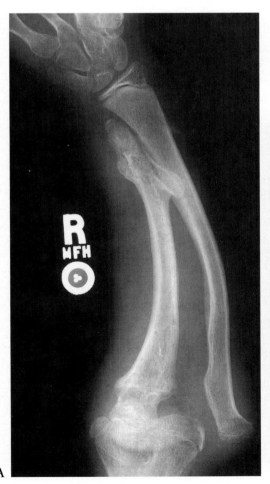
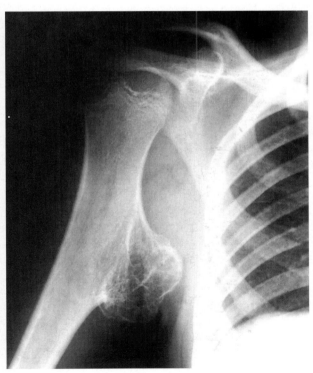

A   B

Figure 165.35. Multiple hereditary exostoses. **A:** Forearm, with distal ulna growth arrest and radial head dislocation. **B:** Proximal humeral exostosis.

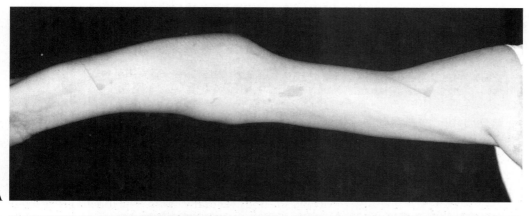

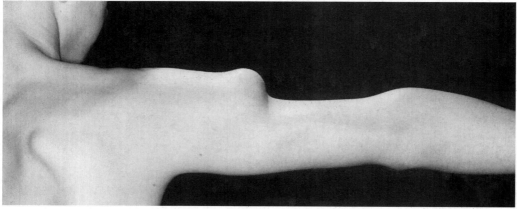

Figure 165.36.   Multiple hereditary exostoses. Forearm deformity associated with radial head dislocation (same patient as in Fig. 165.35A).

Although MHE has an equal prevalence in both sexes, boys tend to have more severe involvement (120). Genetic studies of families with this condition have mapped the chromosomal abnormality to at least three different loci (119,120), indicating that the MHE phenotype can be subdivided into at least three different genotypes. Multiple exostoses also occur in other conditions, such as meta-chondromatosis and the Langer–Giedion syndrome (120).

Estimates of the risk of malignant degeneration of os-teochondromas (secondary chondrosarcoma) in MHE vary from 0.5% to 50% of patients; the lower incidence is most likely correct. Malignant degeneration is quite rare in the upper extremity; the pelvis and proximal femur are the most common locations of secondary chondrosar-coma (159). Malignant degeneration in children is also very rare (120,135).

Most exostoses are asymptomatic and do not need to be surgically removed; exostoses removed before skeletal maturity may recur. However, exostoses can cause local discomfort, nerve or tendon impingement, decreased range of motion, and longitudinal and angulatory growth abnormalities (135). Growth abnormalities may also occur in MHE in the absence of radiologically visible exos-toses (24).

ASSESSMENT, INDICATIONS, AND RELATIVE RESULTS

The patient's history of local pain, crepitance, or de-creased range of motion, combined with a clinical exami-nation for bony bumps of the upper extremity, helps the physician determine which areas to radiograph. Most ex-ostoses have a cartilage cap and, therefore, are larger than their radiograph appearance suggests.

Local pain, often due to nerve, tendon, or vessel im-pingement, is a frequent indication for exostosis removal. Subscapular exostoses are common but do not usually cause pain or require removal. Proximal humeral exosto-ses may impinge on muscle tissue, the brachial plexus, or the axillary nerve, causing pain, paresthesias, or paresis; exostoses of the distal radius and ulna may impinge on the dorsal radial sensory, median, or ulnar nerves or the radial or ulnar arteries. These are indications for surgical removal, which effectively relieves symptoms of impingement (135). An exostosis in the interosseous space that is blocking forearm rotation should also be removed. Recurrence is unlikely if the patient is near skeletal maturity.

The forearm deformities caused by growth arrest due to MHE are complex, and their interrelationships are not well understood. Distal ulnar growth arrest is a common sequelae of MHE, even when osteochondromas of the distal ulna are not visible on radiographs. The radial articular angle may increase, and the carpus may "slip" ulnarward, but neither of these findings appears to be associated with negative ulnar variance (28). Radius bowing, radial head dislocation (179) (Fig. 165.35), and forearm shortening also occur, causing loss of forearm rotation.

Early osteochondroma removal may (113,135) or may not (51) retard these progressive growth disturbances. Hemiepiphyseal stapling of the radial side of the distal radius retards the growth of that side while allowing the ulnar side to continue to grow, which corrects the increased radial articular angle (179) (Fig. 165.37). This procedure may be performed in conjunction with ulnar lengthening (51,135). Resection of a dislocated radial

head relieves pain and removes the associated prominence (10,113) but probably does not improve forearm rotation significantly. This procedure should be reserved for skeletally mature patients because removal of the radial head in the growing child may cause cubitus valgus or proximal radial overgrowth (95,97). Single-stage ulnar lengthening with or without radial osteotomy can be performed (179), or using the Ilizarov technique, the ulna and radius can be differentially lengthened, radial bowing corrected, and the dislocated radial head reduced (42) (Fig. 165.38). Differential lengthening requires several months of external fixation and may diminish forearm rotation. Finally, radioulnar fusion may be performed as a salvage procedure (143).

Two recent studies show that skeletally mature people with untreated forearm deformities due to MHE maintain function are comfortable with their appearance (10,155). The authors of these studies recommend a less aggressive approach to surgical treatment of the forearm in MHE. They point out that relatively simple procedures, such as removal of symptomatic osteochondromas and dislocated radial heads, can improve appearance and relieve pain,

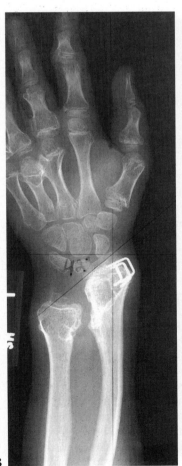
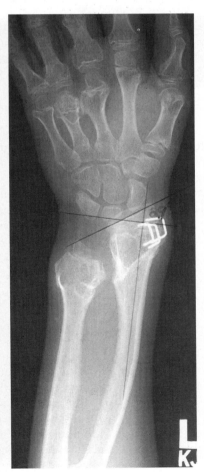

A,B

Figure 165.37. Correction of increased radial articulation angle (radial tilt) in multiple hereditary exostoses by hemiepiphyseal stapling. **A:** Forty-two degree radial tilt, immediately following distal radial stapling. **B:** Twenty-nine degree tilt, 2 years following distal radial stapling.

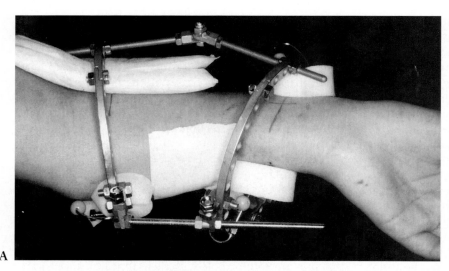

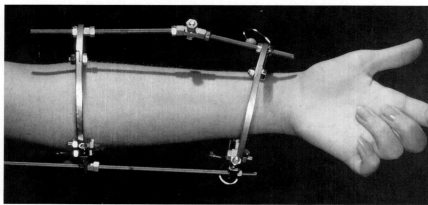

Figure 165.38. Differential radius and ulna lengthening for multiple hereditary exostoses. **A:** After application of Ilizarov fixator, before initiation of lengthening. **B:** After lengthening.

but no surgical treatment has been shown to improve forearm function in MHE.

One final indication for surgery in MHE is an enlarging osteochondroma in a skeletally mature person because this condition may be a sign of malignant degeneration.

CLASSIFICATIONS AND TERMINOLOGY

Many different names have been used to describe MHE, including multiple cartilaginous exostoses, diaphyseal aclasis, dyschondroplasia, hereditary deforming chondrodysplasia (89,179), and osteochondromatosis. The individual tumors may be called exostoses or osteochondromas. MHE is frequently confused with multiple enchondromatosis (Ollier's disease), an entirely different condition (89).

Two different classification systems have been described for forearm deformity caused by MHE. In the first, type I forearms are the most common type (24,113) (Table 165.5).

In the second classification system (159), forearm involvement is used as an index of overall disease severity (Table 165.6). Group III, with forearm shortening, had earlier initial symptoms, more frequent lower extremity deformity, a higher number of osteochondromas, and a shorter height; the authors hypothesize, but do not prove, that group III patients may be at higher risk of malignant degeneration.

OPERATIVE TECHNIQUES

Removal of Osteochondroma (Proximal Humerus or Distal Forearm)

- Perform the operation under a tourniquet, if possible.
- Approach the osteochondroma through a longitudinal incision, centered over the tumor.
- Use the most readily available anatomic interval. Usually the osteochondroma splits the surrounding structures, and approach is not difficult. Watch for nerves or vessels wrapped around the pedicle of the tumor, or a nerve flattened over its surface.

Table 165.5.   Classification of the Forearm with Multiple Hereditary Exostoses

Type	Ulna	Radius
I	Short, with distal osteochondromas	Bowed
IIa	Short, with distal osteochondromas	Radial head dislocated, with proximal osteochondromas
IIb	Short, with distal osteochondromas	Radial head dislocation
III	Relatively unaffected	Short, with distal osteochondromas

From Bock GW, Reed MH. Forearm Deformities in Multiple Cartilaginous Exostoses. *Skeletal Radiol* 1991;20: 483–486, and Masada K, Tsuyuguchi Y, Kawai H, et al. Operation for Forearm Deformity Caused by Multiple Osteochondromas. *J Bone Joint Surg* 1989;71B:24–29, with permission.

■ Remove the entire tumor, leaving a smooth contour.

Postoperatively, a soft dressing and wrist splint for 2 to 3 weeks is adequate immobilization.

Distal Radius Hemiepiphyseal Stapling
■ Perform the operation under a tourniquet, with fluoroscopic guidance.
■ Approach the radial aspect of the distal radial physis through a longitudinal incision. Find and protect the dorsal radial sensory nerve.
■ Under fluoroscopic guidance, place three extraperiosteal epiphyseal staples across the distal radial physis: one directly radial, one slightly palmar, and one slightly dorsal, all outside of the first dorsal compartment.

A soft dressing and wrist splint for 2 to 3 weeks postoperatively is adequate immobilization. Obtain radiographs of the distal radius twice a year, and remove the staples when the desired amount of radial tilt (usually 20°) is attained.

Radial Head Excision (Posterolateral Dislocation)
This technique is discussed in Chapter 16.

Differential Forearm Lengthening
This complex operation is rarely indicated and beyond the scope of this text. See Dahl (42) for a detailed description of planning osteotomies, designing fixation, ulnar lengthening and angular correction, and radial head reduction.

COMPLICATIONS

If the periosteum and physis are disrupted during insertion of hemiepiphyseal staples, permanent physeal arrest and overcorrection could occur. Hemiepiphyseal staples usually require removal at the end of growth, if not sooner, because of adequate correction or local irritation.

CONCLUSIONS

Hemiepiphyseal stapling and removal of osteochondromas and the radial head are simple operations with good results. We measure forearm rotation twice a year for children with MHE with forearm involvement, and consider progressive loss of forearm rotation an indication for osteochondroma removal.

Table 165.6.   Classification of Forearm Involvement as an Index of Overall Disease Severity in Multiple Hereditary Exostoses

Group	Distal forearm	Forearm shortening
I	Not involved	No
II	Radius or ulna involved	No
III	Radius or ulna involved	Yes

From Taniguchi K. A Practical Classification System for multiple Cartilaginous Exostoses in Children. *J Pediatr Orthop* 1995;15:585, with permission.

ACKNOWLEDGMENTS

The authors thank Deanna Simonis, medical librarian, Shriners Hospital Northern California, for her assistance with references, and Julia Serat, photographer, Shriners Hospital Northern California, for her assistance with clinical photographs and radiographic studies.

REFERENCES

Each reference is categorized according to the following scheme: *, classic article; #, review article; !, basic research article; and +, clinical results/outcome study.

+ 1. Agnew DK, Davis RJ. Congenital Unilateral Dislocation of the Radial Head. *J Pediatr Orthop* 1993;13:526.

* 2. Ahmadi B. Steel HH. Congenital Pseudarthrosis of the Clavicle. *Clin Orthop* 1977;126:129.

* 3. Aitken J. Deformity of the Elbow Joint as a Sequel to Erb's Obstetrical Paralysis. *J Bone Joint Surg* 1952;34B:352.

+ 4. Al-Qattan MM, Al-Kharfy TM. Obstetric Brachial Plexus Injury in Subsequent Deliveries. *Ann Plast Surg* 1996;37:545.

+ 5. Al-Qattan MM, Clarke HM, Curtis CG. The Prognostic Value of Concurrent Clavicular Fractures in Newborns with Obstetrical Brachial Plexus Palsy. *J Hand Surg* 1994;19B:729.

+ 6. Al-Qattan MM, Clarke HM, Curtis CG. Klumpke's Birth Palsy: Does in Really Exist? *J Hand Surg* 1995;20B:19.

+ 7. Al-Qattan MM, el-Sayed AA, Al-Kharfy TM, al-Jurayyan NA. Obstetrical Brachial Plexus Injury in Newborn Babies Delivered by Caesarean Section. *J Hand Surg* 1996;21B:263.

* 8. Alldred AJ. Congenital Pseudarthrosis of the Clavicle. *J Bone Joint Surg* 1963;45B:312.

* 9. Almquist EE, Gorden LH, Blue AL. Congenital Dislocation of the Head of the Radius. *J Bone Joint Surg* 1969;51A:1118.

+ 10. Arms DM, Strecker WB, Manske PR, Schoenecker PL. Management of Forearm Deformity in Multiple Hereditary Osteochondromatosis. *J Pediatr Orthop* 1997;17:450.

+ 11. Atkins DJ, Heard DCY, Donovan WH. Epidemiologic Overview of Individuals with Upper-limb Loss and Their Reported Research Priorities. *Journal of Prosthetics and Orthotics* 1996;8:2.

+ 12. Atkins RM, Bell MJ, Sharrard WJ. Pectoralis Major Transfer for Paralysis of Elbow Flexion in Children. *J Bone Joint Surg* 1985;67B:640.

+ 13. Ballinger SG, Hoffer MM. Elbow Flexion Contracture in Erb's Palsy. *J Child Neurol* 1994;9:209.

+ 14. Bar-On E, Howard CB, Porat S. The Use of Ultrasound in the Diagnosis of Atypical Pathology in the Unossified Skeleton. *J Pediatr Orthop* 1995;15:817.

+ 15. Bauer M, Jonsson K. Congenital Radioulnar Synostosis. Radiological Characteristics and Hand Function: Case Reports. *Scand J Plast Reconstr Surg Hand Surg* 1988;22:251.

+ 16. Bavinck JN, Weaver DD. Subclavian Artery Supply Disruption Sequence: Hypothesis of a Vascular Etiology for Poland, Klippel-Feil, and Mobius anomalies. *Am J Med Genet* 1986;23:903.

17. Beals RK, Rolfe B. VATER Association: A Unifying Concept of Multiple Anomalies. *J Bone Joint Surg* 1989;71A:948.

18. Beasley RW. Hand and Finger Prostheses. *J Hand Surg* 1987;12A:144.

+ 19. Beck PA, Hoffer MM. Latissimus Dorsi and Teres Major Tendons: Separate or Conjoint Tendons? *J Pediatr Orthop* 1989;9:308.

20. Bennett JB, Hansen PE, Granberry WM, Cain TE. Surgical Management of Arthrogryposis in the Upper Extremity. *J Pediatr Orthop* 1985;5:281.

+ 21. Benson L, Ezaki M, Carter PR, Knetzer D. Brachial Plexus Birth Palsy: A Prospective Natural History Study. *Orthopaedic Transactions* 1996;20:311.

+ 22. Black B, Dooley J, Pyper A, Reed M. Multiple Hereditary Exostoses. An Epidemiologic Study of an Isolated Community in Manitoba. *Clin Orthop* 1993;287:212.

* 23. Blount WP. Osteoclasis for Supination Deformities in Children. *J Bone Joint Surg* 1940;22:300.

+ 24. Bock GW, Reed MH. Forearm Deformities in Multiple Cartilaginous Exostoses. *Skeletal Radiol* 1991;20:483.

+ 25. Bolano LE. Congenital Proximal Radioulnar Synostosis: Treatment with the Ilizarov Method. *J Hand Surg* 1994;19A:977.

+ 26. Bonnard C, Narakas AO. Restoration of Hand Function after Brachial Plexus Injury. *Hand Clin* 1995;11:647.

+ 27. Borges JL, Shah A, Torres BC, Bowen JR. Modified Woodward Procedure for Sprengel Deformity of the Shoulder: Long-term Results. *J Pediatr Orthop* 1996;16:508.

+ 28. Burgess RC, Cates H. Deformities of the Forearm in Patients Who Have Multiple Cartilaginous Exostosis. *J Bone Joint Surg* 1993;75A:13.

+ 29. Campbell CC, Waters PM, Emans JB. Excision of the Radial Head for Congenital Dislocation. *J Bone Joint Surg* 1992;74A:726.

+ 30. Carlson WO, Speck GJ, Vicari V, Wenger DR. Arthrogryposis Multiplex Congenita. A Long-term Follow-up Study. *Clin Orthop* 1985;194:115.

* 31. Carroll RE, Hill NA. Triceps Transfer to Restore Elbow Function. *J Bone Joint Surg* 1970;52A:239.

+ 32. Carson WG, Lovell WW, Whitesides TE. Congenital Elevation of the Scapula. *J Bone Joint Surg* 1981;63A:1199.

* 33. Cavendish ME. Congenital Elevation of the Scapula. *J Bone Joint Surg* 1972;67A:539.

+ 34. Chan KM, Ma GFY, Cheng JCY, Leung PC. The Krukenberg Procedure: A Method of Treatment for Unilateral Anomalies of the Upper Limb in Chinese Children. *J Hand Surg* 1984;9A:548.

+ 35. Clarke HM, Al-Qattan MM, Curtis CG, Zuker RM. Obstetrical Brachial Plexus Palsy: Results Following Neurolysis of Conducting Neuromas-in-Continuity. *Plast Reconstr Surg* 1996;97:974.

+ 36. Clarke HM, Curtis CG. An Approach to Obstetrical Brachial Plexus Injuries. *Hand Clin* 1995;11:563.

+ 37. Cleary JE, Omer GE Jr. Congenital Proximal Radioulnar Synostosis. *J Bone Joint Surg* 1985;67A:539.

+ 38. Coene LN. Mechanisms of Brachial Plexus Lesions. *Clin Neurol Neurosurg* 1993;95(Suppl):S24.

+ 39. Covey DC, Riordan D, Milstead ME, Albright JA. Modification of the L'Episcopo Procedure for Brachial Plexus Palsies. *J Bone Joint Surg* 1992;74B:897.

40. Crawford AH. Neurofibromatosis. In: Lovell WW, Winter RB, ed. *Pediatric Orthopaedics*. Philadelphia: J.B. Lippincott Company, 1986:1121.

+ 41. Cummings RJ, Jones ET, Reed FE, Mazur JM. Infantile Dislocation of the Elbow Complicating Obstetric Palsy. *J Pediatr Orthop* 1996;16:589.

+ 42. Dahl MT. The Gradual Correction of Forearm Deformities in Multiple Hereditary Exostoses. *Hand Clin* 1993;9:707.

+ 43. Del Torto U, Bianchi O, Pone G, Sante G. Experimental Study on the Etiology of Congenital Multiple Arthrogryposis. *Ital J Orthop Traumatol* 1983;9:91.

+ 44. Doyle JR, James PM, Larsen LJ, Ashley RK. Restoration of Elbow Flexion in Arthrogryposis Multiplex Congenita. *J Hand Surg* 1980;5A:149.

45. Drennan JC. Neuromuscular Disorders. In: Lovell WW, Winter RB, ed. *Pediatric Orthopaedics*. Philadelphia: J.B. Lippincott Company, 1986:259.

+ 46. Echtler B, Burckhardt A. Isolated Congenital Dislocation of the Radial Head. Good Function in 4 Untreated Patients after 14–45 Years. *Acta Orthop Scand* 1997; 68:598.

+ 47. Edelstein JE, Berger N. Performance Comparison Among Children Fitted with Myoelectric and Body-powered Hands. *Arch Phys Med Rehabil* 1993;74:376.

* 48. Engel D. The Etiology of the Undescended Scapula and Related Syndromes. *J Bone Joint Surg* 1943;25A:613.

* 49. Erb W. Veber Eine Eigen Thumliche Localisation von Lahmungen in Plexus Brachialis. *Verh Dtsch* 1874;2: 130.

+ 50. Fahy MJ, Hall JG. A Retrospective Study of Pregnancy Complications Among 828 Cases of Arthrogryposis. *Genet Couns* 1990;1:3.

+ 51. Fogel GR, McElfresh EC, Peterson HA, Wicklund PT. Management of Deformities of the Forearm in Multiple Hereditary Osteochondromas. *J Bone Joint Surg* 1984; 66A:670.

+ 52. Francel PC, Koby M, Park TS, et al. Fast Spin-echo Magnetic Resonance Imaging for Radiological Assessment of Neonatal Brachial Plexus Injury. *J Neurosurg* 1995;83:461.

* 53. Freeman EA, Sheldon JH. Cranio-carpal-tarsal Dystrophy: An Undescribed Congenital Malformation. *Arch Dis Child* 1938;13:277.

+ 54. Gerwin M, Weiland AJ. Vascularized Bone Grafts to the Upper Extremity. Indications and Technique. *Hand Clin* 1992;8:509.

+ 55. Geutjens G, Gilbert A, Helsen K. Obstetric Brachial Plexus Palsy Associated with Breech Delivery. *J Bone Joint Surg* 1996;78B:303.

+ 56. Gherman RB, Goodwin TM, Ouzounian JG, et al. Brachial Plexus Palsy Associated with Cesarean Section: An In Utero Injury? *Am J Obstet Gynecol* 1997;177: 1162.

+ 57. Gibson DA, Carroll N. Congenital Pseudarthrosis of the Clavicle. *J Bone Joint Surg* 1970;52B:629.

+ 58. Gibson DA, Urs NDK. Arthrogryposis Multiplex Congenita. *J Bone Joint Surg* 1970;52B:483.

+ 59. Gilbert A, Brockman R, Carlioz H. Surgical Treatment of Brachial Plexus Birth Palsy. *Clin Orthop* 1991;264: 39.

+ 60. Gilbert A, Razaboni R, Amar-Khodja S. Indications and Results of Brachial Plexus Surgery in Obstetrical Palsy. *Orthop Clin North Am* 1988;19:91.

+ 61. Goddard NJ, Fixsen JA. Rotation Osteotomy of the Humerus for Birth Injuries of the Brachial Plexus. *J Bone Joint Surg* 1984;66B:257.

+ 62. Gonen R, Spiegel D, Abend M. Is Macrosomia Predictable, and Are Shoulder Dystocia and Birth Trauma Preventable? *Obstet Gynecol* 1996;88:526.

+ 63. Gonik B, Hollyer VL, Allen R. Shoulder Dystocia Recognition: Differences in Neonatal Risks for Injury. *Am J Perinatol* 1991;8:31.

+ 64. Graham EM, Forouzan I, Morgan MA. A Retrospective Analysis of Erb's Palsy Cases and Their Relation to Birth Weight and Trauma at Delivery. *Journal of Maternal-Fetal Medicine* 1997;6:1.

+ 65. Green WT, Mital MA. Congenital Radioulnar Synostosis: Surgical Treatment. *J Bone Joint Surg* 1979;61:738.

+ 66. Greenwald AG, Schute PC, Shiveley JL. Brachial Plexus Birth Palsy: A 10-year Report on the Incidence and Prognosis. *J Pediatr Orthop* 1984;4:689.

+ 67. Greitemann B, Rondhuis JJ, Karbowski A. Treatment of Congenital Elevation of the Scapula. 10 (2–18) Year Follow-up of 37 Cases of Sprengel's Deformity. *Acta Orthop Scand* 1993;64:365.

+ 68. Grogan DP, Love SM, Guidera KJ, Ogden JA. Operative Treatment of Congenital Pseudarthrosis of the Clavicle. *J Pediatr Orthop* 1991;11:176.

+ 69. Gu Y, Zhang L, Zheng Y. Introduction of a Modified Krukenberg Operation. *Plast Reconstr Surg* 1996;97: 222.

+ 70. Gudinchet F, Maeder P, Oberson JC, Schnyder P. Magnetic Resonance Imaging of the Shoulder in Children with Brachial Plexus Birth Palsy. *Pediatr Radiol* 1995; 25:S125.

+ 71. Guma M, Teitel AD. Adolescent Presentation of Congenital Radioulnar Synostosis. *Clin Pediatr* 1996;35: 215.

+ 72. Hall JG. Genetic Aspects of Arthrogryposis. *Clin Orthop* 1985;44.

+ 73. Hamner DL, Hall JE. Sprengel's Deformity Associated with Multidirectional Shoulder Instability. *J Pediatr Orthop* 1995;15:641.

+ 74. Hankins GD, Clark SL. Brachial Plexus Palsy Involving the Posterior Shoulder at Spontaneous Vaginal Delivery. *Am J Perinatol* 1995;12:44.

+ 75. Hansen OH, Andersen NO. Congenital Radio-ulnar Synostosis: Report of 37 Cases. *Acta Orthop Scand* 1970;41:225.

+ 76. Hardy AE. Birth Injuries of the Brachial Plexus: Incidence and Prognosis. *J Bone Joint Surg* 1981;63B:98.

+ 77. Hashimoto T, Mitomo M, Hirabuki N, et al. Nerve Root Avulsion of Birth Palsy: Comparison of Myelography with CT Myelography and Somatosensory Evoked Potential. *Radiology* 1991;178:841.

\# 78. Hentz VR. Brachial Plexus Injuries. In: Manske PR, ed. *Hand Surgery Update*. Rosemont, IL: American Academy of Orthopaedic Surgeons, 1996:243.

\# 79. Hentz VR, Meyer RD. Brachial Plexus Microsurgery in Children. *Microsurgery* 1991;12:175.

+ 80. Hernandez C, Wendel GD. Shoulder Dystocia. *Clin Obstet Gynecol* 1990;33:526.

+ 81. Hernandez RJ, Dias L. CT Evaluation of the Shoulder in Children with Erb's Palsy. *Pediatr Radiol* 1988;18:333.

+ 82. Hirata S, Miya H, Mizuno K. Congenital Pseudarthrosis of the Clavicle. Histologic Examination for the Etiology of the Disease. *Clin Orthop* 1995;242.

+ 83. Hoffer MM, Phipps GJ. Closed Reduction and Tendon Transfer for Treatment of Dislocation of the Glenohumeral Joint Secondary to Brachial Plexus Birth Palsy. *J Bone Joint Surg* 1998;80A:997.

+ 84. Hoffer MM, Wickenden R, Roper B. Brachial Plexus Birth Palsies. Results of Tendon Transfers to the Rotator Cuff. *J Bone Joint Surg* 1978;60A:691.

+ 85. Holmes LB. Report of National Institute of Child Health and Human Development Workshop on Chorionic Villus Sampling and Limb and Other Defects. *Teratology* 1992;48:7.

+ 86. Hoyme HE, Jones KL, Van Allen MI, et al. Vascular Pathogenesis of Transverse Limb Reduction Defects. *J Pediatr* 1982;101:839.

+ 87. Hresko MT, Rosenberg BN, Pappas AM. Excision of the Radial Head in Patients Younger than 18 Years. *J Pediatr Orthop* 1999;19:106.

+ 88. Jackson ST, Hoffer MM, Parrish N. Brachial-plexus Palsy in the Newborn. *J Bone Joint Surg* 1988;70A:1217.

* 89. Jaffe HL. Hereditary Multiple Exostoses. *Arch Pathol* 1943;36:335.

+ 90. Jahnke AH Jr, Bovill DF, McCarroll HR Jr, et al. Persistent Brachial Plexus Birth Palsies. *J Pediatr Orthop* 1991;11:533.

+ 91. Jain S. Rehabilitation in Limb Deficiency: The Pediatric Amputee. *Arch Phys Med Rehabil* 1996;77:S-9.

+ 92. James MA, McCarroll HR Jr. Shoulder External Rotation Tendon Transfers in Brachial Plexus Birth Palsy: Results of Two Techniques. *Orthopaedic Transactions* 1996;20;311.

+ 93. Kanaya F, Ibaraki K. Mobilization of a Congenital Proximal Radioulnar Synostosis with Use of a Free Vascularized Fascio-fat Graft. *J Bone Joint Surg* 1998;80A:1186.

+ 94. Kawabata H, Kawai H, Masatomi T, Yasui N. Accessory Nerve Neurotization in Infants with Brachial Plexus Birth Palsy. *Microsurgery* 1994;15:768.

+ 95. Kelikian H. Dislocation of the Radial Head. In: Kelikian H, ed. *Congenital Deformities of the Hand and Forearm*. Philadelphia: W.B. Saunders Company, 1974:902.

+ 96. Kelikian H. Radioulnar Synostosis. In: Kelikian H, ed. *Congenital Deformities of the Hand and Forearm*. Philadelphia: W.B. Saunders Company, 1974:939.

+ 97. Kelly DW. Congenital Dislocation of the Radial Head: Spectrum and Natural History. *J Pediatr Orthop* 1981;1:295.

+ 98. Kitoh H, Nogami H, Oki T, et al. Antley-Bixler Syndrome: A Disorder Characterized by Congenital Synostosis of the Elbow Joint and the Cranial Suture. *J Pediatr Orthop* 1996;16:243.

+ 99. Klisic P, Filipovic M, Uzelac O. Relocation of Congenitally Elevated Scapula. *J Pediatr Orthop* 1981;1:43.

+ 100. Kruger LM, Fishman S. Myoelectric and Body-powered Prostheses. *J Pediatr Orthop* 1993;13:68.

* 101. L'Episcopo JB. Tendon Transplantation in Obstetrical Paralysis. *Am J Surg* 1934;25:122.

+ 102. Laurent JP, Lee RT. Birth-related Upper Brachial Plexus Injuries in Infants: Operative and Nonoperative Approaches. *J Child Neurol* 1994;9:111.

+ 103. Levine MG, Holroyde J, Woods JRJ, et al. Birth Trauma: Incidence and Predisposing Factors. *Obstet Gynecol* 1984;63:792.

+ 104. Liggio FJ, Tham S, Price A, et al. Outcome of Surgical Treatment for Forearm Pronation Deformities in Children with Obstetric Brachial Plexus Injuries. *J Hand Surg* 1999;24B:43.

+ 105. Lin HH, Strecker WB, Manske PR, et al. A Surgical Technique of Radioulnar Osteoclasis to Correct Severe Forearm Rotation Deformities. *J Pediatr Orthop* 1995;15:53.

+ 106. Lipskeir E, Weizenbluth M. Derotation Osteotomy of the Forearm in Management of Paralytic Supination Deformity. *J Hand Surg* 1993;18A:1069.

* 107. Lloyd-Roberts GC, Apley AG, Owen R. Reflections Upon the Aetology of Congenital Pseudarthrosis of the Clavicle. *J Bone Joint Surg* 1975;57B:24.

* 108. Lloyd-Roberts GC, Lettin AWF. Arthrogryposis Multiplex Congenita. *J Bone Joint Surg* 1970;52B:494.

* 109. Mallet J. Paralysie Obstetricale du Plexus Brachial Symposium: Traitement des Sepuelles: Primaute du Traitement de l'Epaule—Methode d'Expression des Resultats. *Rev Chir Orthop* 1972;58:166.

+ 110. Manske PR, McCarroll HR Jr. Biceps Tendon Rerouting and Percutaneous Osteoclasis in the Treatment of Supination Deformity in Obstetrical Palsy. *J Hand Surg* 1980;5:153.

+ 111. Mardam-Bey T, Ger E. Congenital Radial Head Dislocation. *J Hand Surg* 1979;4:316.

+ 112. Marshall RW, Williams DH, Birch R, Bonney G. Operations to Restore Elbow Flexion after Brachial Plexus Injuries. *J Bone Joint Surg* 1988;70B:577.

+ 113. Masada K, Tsuyuguchi Y, Kawai H, et al. Operations for Forearm Deformity Caused by Multiple Osteochondromas. *J Bone Joint Surg* 1989;71B:24.

+ 114. Masterson E, Earley MJ, Stephens MM. Congenital Pseudarthrosis of the Ulna Treated by Free Vascularized Fibular Graft: A Case Report and Review of Methods of Treatment. *J Hand Surg* 1993;18B:285.

+ 115. Mastroiacovo P, Tozzi AE, Agosti S, et al. Transverse Limb Reduction Defects after Chorion Villus Sampling: A Retrospective Cohort Study. GIDEF: Gruppo Italiano Diagnosi Embrio-Fetali. *Prenat Diagn* 1993;13:1051.

+ 116. Mathoulin C, Gilbert A, Azze RG. Congenital Pseudarthrosis of the Forearm: Treatment of Six Cases with Vascularized Fibular Graft and a Review of the Literature. *Microsurgery* 1993;14:252.

+ 117. McFarland LV, Raskin M, Daling JR, Benedetti TJ. Erb/Duchenne's Palsy: A Consequence of Fetal Macrosomia and Method of Delivery. *Obstet Gynecol* 1986;68:784.

+ 118. McFarland MB, Langer O, Piper JM, Berkus MD. Perinatal Outcome and the Type and Number of Maneuvers in Shoulder Dystocia. *Int J Gynaecol Obstet* 1996; 55:219.

+ 119. McKusick VA. *Exostoses, Multiple, Type II;EXT2.* Online Mendelian Inheritance in Man, OMIM (TM) MIM Number:133701.1998. Baltimore, MD: Johns Hopkins University, 1998.

+ 120. McKusick VA. *Exostoses, Multiple, Type I;EXT1.* Online Mendelian Inheritance in Man, OMIM (TM) MIM Number:133700.1998. Baltimore, MD: Johns Hopkins University, 1998.

+ 121. Mennen U, Williams E. Arthrogryposis Multiplex Congenita in a Monozygotic Twin. *J Hand Surg* 1996;21B: 647.

+ 122. Michelow BJ, Clarke HM, Curtis CG. The natural history of obstetrical brachial plexus palsy. *Plast Reconstr Surg* 1994;93:675.

+ 123. Miller SF, Glasier CM, Griebel ML, et al. Brachial Plexopathy in Infants after Traumatic Delivery: Evaluation with MR Imaging. *Radiology* 1993;189:481.

+ 124. Mital MA. Congenital Radioulnar Synostosis and Congenital Dislocation of the Radial Head. *Orthop Clin North Am* 1976;7:375.

+ 125. Miura T. Congenital Dislocation of the Radial Head. *J Hand Surg* 1990;15B:477.

+ 126. Miura T, Nakamura R, Suzuki M, Kanie J. Congenital Radio-ulnar Synostosis. *J Hand Surg* 1984;9B:153.

+ 127. Moneim MS, Omer GE Jr. Latissimus Dorsi Muscle Transfer for Restoration of Elbow Flexion after Brachial Plexus Disruption. *J Hand Surg* 1986;11:135.

+ 128. Morrison JC, Sanders JR, Magann EF, Wiser WL. The Diagnosis and Management of Dystocia of the Shoulder. *Surg Gynecol Obstet* 1992;175:515.

+ 129. Ogino T, Hikino K. Congenital Radioulnar Synostosis: Compensatory Rotation Around the Wrist and Rotation Osteotomy. *J Hand Surg* 1987;12B:173.

+ 130. Ouzounian JG, Korst LM, Phelan JP. Permanent Erb Palsy: A Traction-related Injury? *Obstet Gynecol* 1997; 89:139.

+ 131. Owen R. Congenital Pseudarthrosis of the Clavicle. *J Bone Joint Surg* 1970;52B:644.

+ 132. Paley D, Catagni M, Argnani F, et al. Treatment of Congenital Pseudoarthrosis of the Tibia Using the Ilizarov Technique. *Clin Orthop* 1992;81.

+ 133. Paradiso G, Granana N, Maza E. Prenatal Brachial Plexus Paralysis. *Neurology* 1997;49:261.

+ 134. Perlow JH, Wigton T, Hart J, et al. Birth Trauma. A Five-year Review of Incidence and Associated Perinatal Factors. *J Reprod Med* 1996;41:754.

+ 135. Peterson HA. Multiple Hereditary Osteochondromata. *Clin Orthop* 1989;222.

+ 136. Phipps GJ, Hoffer MM. Latissimus Dorsi and Teres Major Transfer to Rotator Cuff for Erb's Palsy. *J Shoulder Elbow Surg* 1995;4:124.

+ 137. Piatt JH Jr, Hudson AR, Hoffman HJ. Preliminary Experiences with Brachial Plexus Exploration in Children: Birth Injury and Vehicular Trauma. *Neurosurgery* 1988;22:715.

+ 138. Powers TA, Haher TR, Devlin VJ, et al. Abnormalities of the Spine in Relation to Congenital Upper Limb Deficiencies. *J Pediatr Orthop* 1983;3:471.

+ 139. Pruitt DL, Hulsey RE, Fink B, Manske PR. Shoulder Arthrodesis in Pediatric Patients. *J Pediatr Orthop* 1992;12:640.

+ 140. Reichenbach H, Hormann D, Theile H. Hereditary Congenital Posterior Dislocation of Radial Heads. *Am J Med Genet* 1995;55:101.

+ 141. Rizzo R, Pavone V, Corsello G, et al. Autosomal Dominant and Sporadic Radio-ulnar Synostosis. *Am J Med Genet* 1997;68:127.

+ 142. Robinson RA, Braun RM, Mack P, Zadek R. The Surgical Importance of the Clavicular Component of Sprengel's Deformity. *J Bone Joint Surg* 1967;49A: 1481.

+ 143. Rodgers WB, Hall JE. One-bone Forearm as a Salvage Procedure for Recalcitrant Forearm Deformity in Hereditary Multiple Exostoses. *J Pediatr Orthop* 1993; 13:587.

+ 144. Sachar K, Akelman E, Ehrlich MG. Radioulnar Synostosis. *Hand Clin* 1994;10:399.

+ 145. Schmale GA, Conrad EU, Raskind WH. The Natural History of Hereditary Multiple Exostoses. *J Bone Joint Surg Am* 1994;76:986.

+ 146. Schnall SB, King JD, Marrero G. Congenital Pseudarthrosis of the Clavicle: A Review of the Literature and Surgical Results of Six Cases. *J Pediatr Orthop* 1988;8:316.

* 147. Schottstaedt ER, Larsen LJ, Bost FC. Complete Muscle Transposition. *J Bone Joint Surg* 1955;37A:897.

+ 148. Scotland TR, Galway HR. A Long-term Review of Children with Congenital and Acquired Upper Limb Deficiency. *J Bone Joint Surg* 1983;65B:346.

+ 149. Seitz WH. Distraction Osteogenesis of a Congenital Amputation at the Elbow. *J Hand Surg* 1989;14A:945.

* 150. Sever JW. Obstetric Paralysis: Report of Eleven Hundred Cases. *JAMA* 1925;85:1862.

+ 151. Shalom A, Khermosh O, Wientroub S. The Natural History of Congenital Pseudarthrosis of the Clavicle. *J Bone Joint Surg* 1994;76B:846.

+ 152. Simmons BP, Southmayd WW, Riseborough EJ. Congenital Radioulnar Synostosis. *J Hand Surg Am* 1983; 8:829.

+ 153. Smith SJM. The Role of Neurophysiological Investigation in Traumatic Brachial Plexus Lesions in Adults and Children. *J Hand Surg* 1996;21B:145.

+ 154. St. Charles S, DiMario FJJ, Grunnet MS. Mobius Sequence: Further In Vivo Support for the Subclavian Artery Supply Disruption Sequence. *Am J Med Genet* 1993;47:289.

+ 155. Stanton RP, Hansen MO. Function of the Upper Extremities in Hereditary Multiple Exostoses. *J Bone Joint Surg* 1996;78A:568.

+ 156. Steel HH, Piston RW, Clancy M, Betz RR. A Syndrome of Dislocated Hips and Radial Heads, Carpal Coalition, and Short Stature in Puerto Rican Children. *J Bone Joint Surg* 1993;75A:259.

+ 157. Swanson AB, Swanson GC. The Krukenberg Procedure in the Juvenile Amputee. *Clin Orthop* 1980;148:55.

+ 158. Swinyard CA, Bleck EE. The Etiology of Arthrogryposis (Multiple Congenital Contracture). *Clin Orthop* 1985;194:15.

+ 159. Taniguchi K. A Practical Classification System for Multiple Cartilaginous Exostosis in Children. *J Pediatr Orthop* 1995;15:585.

+ 160. Tassin JL. Paralysies Obstetricales du Plexus Brachial. Evolution Spontanee, Resultats des Interventions Reparatrices Precoces (Thesis). Universite Paris VII 1983.

161. Temtamy SA, McKusick VA. Contracture Deformities of Digits. In: Bergsma D, Mudge JR, Paul NW, Greene SC, eds. *The Genetics of Hand Malformations.* New York: Alan R. Liss, Inc., 1978:441.

+ 162. Thompson GH, Bilenker RM. Comprehensive Management of Arthrogryposis Multiplex Congenita. *Clin Orthop* 1985;194:6.

+ 163. Toledo LC, MacEwen GD. Severe Complication of Surgical Treatment of Congenital Pseudarthrosis of the Clavicle. *Clin Orthop* 1979;139:64.

+ 164. Troum S, Floyd WEI, Waters PM. Posterior Dislocation of the Humeral Head in Infancy Associated with Obstetrical Paralysis. *J Bone Joint Surg* 1993;75A:1370.

+ 165. Tsukahara M, Matsuo K, Furukawa S. Radio-ulnar Synostosis, Short Stature, Microcephaly, Scoliosis, and Mental Retardation. *Am J Med Genet* 1995;58:159.

+ 166. Uthoff K, Bosch U. [Proximal Radioulnar Synostosis within the Scope of Fetal Alcohol Syndrome]. *Unfallchirurg* 1997;100:678.

+ 167. Van Heest A, Waters PM, Simmons BP. Surgical Treatment of Arthrogryposis of the Elbow. *J Hand Surg* 1998;23A:1063.

+ 168. Van Heest AE. Congenital Disorders of the Hand and Upper Extremity. *Pediatr Clin North Am* 1996;43:1113.

+ 169. Vitale CC. Reconstructive Surgery for Defects in the Shaft of the Ulna in Children. *J Bone Joint Surg* 1952;34A:804.

+ 170. Walle T, Hartikainen-Sorri AL. Obstetric Shoulder Injury. Associated Risk Factors, Prediction and Prognosis. *Acta Obstet Gynecol Scand* 1993;72:450.

+ 171. Waters PM. *When Is the Timing of Biceps Return of Function Reliable in Patients with Obstetrical Brachial Plexopathy?* San Francisco: American Society for Surgery of the Hand, 1995.

172. Waters PM. Obstetric Brachial Plexus Injuries: Evaluation and Management. *Journal of the American Academy of Orthopaedic Surgeons* 1997;5:205.

173. Waters PM, Simmons BP. Congenital Anomalies: Elbow Region. In: Peimer CA, ed. *Surgery of the Hand and Upper Extremity.* New York: McGraw-Hill, 1996:2049.

+ 174. Waters PM, Smith GR, Jaramillo D. Glenohumeral Deformity Secondary to Brachial Plexus Birth Palsy. *J Bone Joint Surg* 1998;80A:668.

175. Weaver DD. Vascular Etiology of Limb Defects: The Subclavian Artery Supply Disruption Sequence. In: Herring JA, Birch JG, ed. *The Child With a Limb Deficiency.* Rosemont, Ill: American Academy of Orthopaedic Surgeons, 1998;25.

+ 176. Wenner SM, Saperia BS. Proximal Row Carpectomy in Arthrogrypotic Wrist Deformity. *J Hand Surg* 1987;12A:523.

+ 177. Wilkinson JA, Campbell D. Scapular Osteotomy for Sprengel's Shoulder. *J Bone Joint Surg* 1980;62B:486.

+ 178. Williams PF. Management of Upper Limb Problems in Arthrogryposis. *Clin Orthop* 1985;194:60.

+ 179. Wood VE, Sauser D, Mudge D. The Treatment of Hereditary Multiple Exostosis of the Upper Extremity. *J Hand Surg* 1985;10A:505.

* 180. Woodward JW. Congenital Elevation of the Scapula. Correction by Release and Transplantation of Muscle Origins: A Preliminary Report. *J Bone Joint Surg* 1961;43A:219.

+ 181. Wynne-Davies R, Lamb DW. Congenital Upper Limb Anomalies: An Etiologic Grouping of Clinical, Genetic, and Epidemiologic Data from 387 Patients with "Absence" Defects, Constriction Bands, Polydactylies, and Syndactylies. *J Hand Surg* 1985;10A:958.

+ 182. Wynne-Davies R, Williams PF, O'Connor JC. The 1960s Epidemic of Arthrogryposis Multiplex Congenita: A Survey from the United Kingdom, Australia and the United States of America. *J Bone Joint Surg Br* 1981;63-B:76.

+ 183. Yajima H, Tamai S, Ono H, Kizaki K. Vascularized Bone Grafts to the Upper Extremities. *Plast Reconstr Surg* 1998;101:727.

+ 184. Yonenobu K, Tada K, Swanson AB. Arthrogryposis of the Hand. *J Pediatr Orthop* 1984;4:599.

* 185. Zancolli EA. Paralytic Supination Contracture of the Forearm. *J Bone Joint Surg* 1967;49A:1275.

## CHAPTER 166

SURGERY FOR DEVELOPMENTAL DYSPLASIA OF THE HIP

George T. Rab

Abnormalities in newborns or in children consisting of dysplasia of the acetabulum and subluxation or dislocation of the femoral head from the acetabulum, if present at birth, have been known in the past as dysplasia or dislocation of the hip. Westin et al. (30) reported on late dislocation of the hip in children with apparently normal neonatal clinical and radiographic examinations, which they termed *developmental dysplasia of the hip* (DDH). Since then, the term *DDH* has come to be used to describe all dysplasias of the hip, reflecting the uncertainty about the exact time of onset and detection of the condition. Many mechanisms for DDH have been proposed, including the following:

Mechanical factors including breech delivery and postnatal positioning of the hips in extension and adduction
Hormone-induced joint laxity
Genetic inheritance
Primary acetabular dysplasia

Dysplasia of the hip occurs in approximately 1 in 1,000 live births. Involvement of the left hip alone or bilateral involvement is more common than involvement of the right hip alone.

Risk factors increasing the incidence of DDH have been identified; examiners should be alert to the following:

Female sex (5:1 female-to-male ratio)
Breech delivery
First-born child
Positive family history
White or Navajo Indian race
Associated disorders such as metatarsus abductus, talipes calcaneovalgus, and congenital torticollis

G. T. Rab: Department of Orthopaedics, University of California, Davis, Sacramento, California, 95817.

Early detection of DDH in newborns with early initiation of treatment is important to avoid the severe disability that results in late diagnosis, particularly after 5 years of age. Physicians and other paraprofessionals involved in delivering children must be competent in routine clinical screening with Ortolani's test and Barlow's provocative maneuver.

Use of ultrasound screening of newborns has proven useful in the hands of experienced ultrasonographers (9, 15). False-positive sonography is common in the first 10 weeks of life; practitioners should take this into account when making treatment decisions.

In children between 6 and 18 months of age in whom a dislocated hip was missed at birth or who subsequently dislocate a dysplastic hip, reduction of the hip or dislocation of the hip by Ortolani's test and Barlow's maneuver becomes impossible. Important clinical findings in this age group include asymmetry in abduction of the hip because of adductor muscle contractures, asymmetric skin folds with gathering on the dislocated side, and Galeazzi's sign showing apparent shortening of the femur on the side of the dislocation. Bilateral dislocations are more difficult to detect because they are symmetrically abnormal. If affected children reach walking age, they will usually demonstrate a waddling (Trendelenburg) gait.

Radiographic findings are not reliable in newborns because the lack of ossification of the proximal femur makes detection difficult. Indications of DDH in newborns include the following:

Acetabular index of more than 30°
Decreased center–edge angle of Wiberg
Disruption of Shenton's line
Location of the metaphyseal beak of the proximal femur outside the inner lower quadrant of the grid formed by the vertical line of Perkins and the horizontal line of Hilgenreiner (Fig. 166.1)

NONOPERATIVE TREATMENT

Most patients with DDH or dislocation can be treated by nonoperative methods if the condition is detected in the first 6 months of life. Pavlik harness treatment in this age group has a high rate of success, and I have been able to achieve reduction of hips in some children up to 9 months of age with this harness.

Pavlik-harness adjustment is critical to success. The shoulder harness portion should be tight enough to cover the chest at the nipple line. The anterior (medial) foot straps are tensioned enough so that the hips are flexed greater than 90°. The posterior (lateral) straps are tensioned enough so that the knees cannot touch in the midline; they must not be too tight.

The Pavlik harness should be worn full-time. I reexamine a child in 1–2 weeks and readjust the device, which is often necessary because it is confusing to parents. After it is accepted by the family and properly adjusted, the harness will rapidly produce a reduction of the hip if Pavlik treatment is going to be successful. If the hip reduces, the device should be worn for 3 or more months until stable reduction is accompanied by resolution of acetabular dysplasia (e.g., normal acetabular index, appearance of proximal femoral ossific nucleus).

If the Pavlik harness fails to effect a reduction in 2 weeks of wear after the initial readjustment, it should be discontinued, as it will not be effective if utilized longer. When Pavlik-harness treatment fails to achieve congruent reduction, closed reduction and casting must be considered. Prereduction traction, long considered to reduce the incidence of avascular necrosis, is now controversial; I personally do not use it.

When closed reduction fails, open reduction is indicated. Open reduction is a delicate, specialized operation with complications that can affect a patient for a lifetime, and it should not be undertaken by an inexperienced surgeon. Surgery for the residual dysplasia that can follow closed or open treatment of DDH also requires adequate follow-up and experienced judgment in its applications and execution. The techniques described in this chapter are those that I have found most effective in surgical management of this condition, but they are not exclusive and

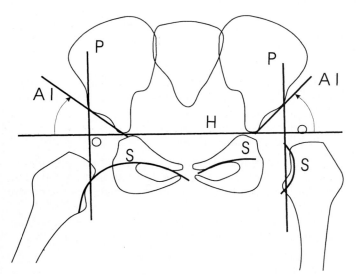

Figure 166.1. Radiographic signs of subluxation and dysplasia on an AP view. The proximal femoral ossification center has been drawn but may be absent before age 6 months (*H,* Hilgenreiner's line; *P,* Perkins' line; *S,* Shenton's line (broken on left); *AI,* acetabular index). Note the subluxation in the left hip.

many alternatives can be found in the literature (3,4,7,8, 13,16,18).

OPEN REDUCTION OF THE HIP

INDICATIONS

Open reduction of a dislocated hip is indicated when closed reduction fails or when closed reduction would result in such extremes of position that avascular necrosis would be a likely consequence. It is also indicated in children older than 12–18 months, when it is frequently combined with femoral shortening to decrease the overall time of immobilization required to achieve remodeling of the hip. Open reduction is indicated in a subluxated hip when abduction fails to reposition the femoral head deeply into the true acetabulum; in this instance, osteotomy of the pelvis or proximal femur is usually performed simultaneously.

Failures of closed reduction under anesthesia that obviously do not allow the femoral head to be centered in the acetabulum or that result in extremes of position are easy to detect and should be followed with prompt open reduction, preferably as a continuation under the same anesthetic. In children younger than 12 months, closed reduction that results in a reduction that is stable but not deep and concentric may be accepted initially. Follow these reductions by arthrography in 8–12 weeks; if soft-tissue remodeling has not occurred and the reduction is not congruent and deep, proceed with open reduction.

The use of prereduction traction and femoral shortening in 1–3-year-old children is somewhat controversial (8, 13,20,22,23,25). Standard open reduction can be performed with relative safety in some children, but many surgeons (including myself) elect femoral shortening in a walking child because it allows prompt open reduction without preoperative traction and with an extremely low incidence of avascular necrosis. It also permits derotation of the anteverted femur, thus stabilizing the reduction. This allows early ambulation and may speed hip remodeling; both of these goals are admirable in a child who has never had a reduced hip joint before surgery. Open reduction is occasionally useful in diseases other than congenital hip dysplasia, such as cerebral palsy or reconstruction following trauma or infection.

PREOPERATIVE CONSIDERATIONS

The use of preoperative traction, once so universally accepted, has been widely questioned in recent years (2,10, 20); I personally no longer use it. In general, open reduction and its variants should be done without the use of blood transfusions. This requires great care on the surgeon's part. The use of X or 3X loupes is valuable in the dissection, and electrocautery greatly facilitates dissection without excessive bleeding. All tissues must be handled extremely gently, and the surgeon should have a thorough knowledge of hip anatomy. For children younger than 2–3 years, attempt a closed reduction immediately before proceeding with an open procedure because occasionally a stable reduction can be achieved with good long-term prognosis for resolution of the dysplasia.

I prefer open reduction from an anterior approach because capsulorrhaphy and other reconstructive procedures can easily be accomplished. Open reduction from a medial (adductor) approach does not give sufficient exposure for these essential parts of the operation and is indicated only in very young children who will undergo prolonged casting to maintain reduction while the capsulotomy heals and remodels. The medial approach is not described here; see Chapter 3 and Ferguson's (7) description for details.

Although the standard exposure is a classic Smith–Petersen approach, I prefer a skin incision that falls in, or is parallel and superior to, the inguinal crease. Inguinal incisions can be extended medially and laterally, and they allow excellent deep longitudinal exposure with a nearly undetectable scar that is hidden beneath standard clothing. If open reduction and femoral shortening are combined, the use of an inguinal incision for the open reduction and a lateral incision for the femoral shortening yields a more cosmetic appearance and permits simple removal of internal fixation devices later through the lateral incision.

CLOSED REDUCTION

With the patient under a deep general anesthetic, gently flex, lift, and abduct the femur with the knee flexed until reduction is felt. In older children, the reduction is usually either definite or unobtainable, but younger children may not have distinct stability. Arthrography and fluoroscopy greatly improve assessment of the reduction (Fig. 166.2). Occasionally, percutaneous adductor-longus tenotomy enhances stability. If the hip is unstable in less than 55° of abduction, strongly consider open reduction. Full double-spica casting is safest in 90° to 100° of flexion, neutral rotation, and less than 55° of abduction, which is Salter's (18,19) "human" position.

Change the cast every 6–8 weeks until fluoroscopy demonstrates stability in the weight-bearing position. Usually, 12–18 weeks in a spica cast is required. Abduction bracing may be used long-term, although there is no scientific evidence of its value in this circumstance.

OPEN REDUCTION

■ Drape the affected limb and hip free with the pelvis elevated on a small towel.

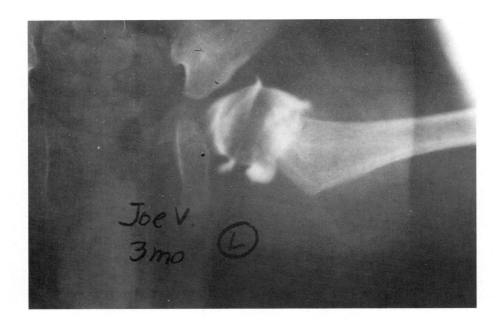

Figure 166.2. Arthrography during closed reduction can delineate anatomic features and aid in assessment of stability.

- Make a transverse inguinal incision directly in the most prominent flexion crease of the hip (Fig. 166.3A). After incising the skin, use electrocautery to expose the fascial layer.
- Dissect subcutaneously both proximally to the iliac crest and sufficiently distally to mobilize the skin and subcutaneous tissue and allow a longitudinal incision of the deeper layers of the wound.
- Identify the lateral femoral cutaneous nerve as it emerges from the sartorius. Isolate and protect it with Silastic tape (Fig. 166.3B).
- If an innominate osteotomy is to be done, now split the apophysis, but for standard open reduction, it is unnecessary to dissect the proximal iliac apophysis.
- Carefully develop the interval between the sartorius and the tensor fasciae latae. Retract the sartorius medially and the tensor laterally to expose the rectus femoris.
- Using a Kidner dissector, identify, tag, and transversely section the tendinous attachment of the rectus femoris to expose the reflected head of the rectus femoris, which is the key to the anterior capsule (Fig. 166.3C).
- Expose the capsule, using gentle blunt dissection with a periosteal elevator and a Kidner dissector. Use electrocautery for any bleeders. The capsule will be found to be large, redundant, and extending superiorly and posteriorly.
- Carry the capsular exposure medially under the adherent iliopsoas muscle and distally until the lesser trochanter can be palpated with a fingertip.
- At the medial border of the capsule, identify the iliopsoas muscle, hook its tendon with a right-angle clamp,

and bring it into the wound, where it is sectioned (Fig. 166.3D).
- Next, divide the capsule in a T fashion, taking care to avoid damage to the underlying femoral head (Fig. 166.3E). The vertical limb of the T lies parallel to the femoral neck, with the cross of the T lying parallel and 0.5 cm distal to the labrum of the hip joint. Scissors may be used to extend the superior border of the cross part of the T around to the upper and posterior portions of the hip capsule. At this point, place suture tags in the two corners of the capsulotomy for later use in repairing the capsule.
- Now inspect the hip joint (Fig. 166.3F). Unless the patient is older, the ligamentum teres will be seen as a large, hypertrophic, flattened structure. Carefully excise it sharply from its attachment on the femoral head. Leave its acetabular attachment intact, and follow the ligament into the acetabular fovea to locate the true acetabulum (Fig. 166.3G). With external rotation or flexion and adduction, the femoral head can be pulled out of the way to allow full exposure of the acetabulum.
- After the fovea has been clearly identified, cut the remaining stump of the ligamentum teres. Clean any fibro-fatty tissue from the acetabulum, using rongeurs and Kidner dissectors, being careful to avoid damage to the articular surface. Sometimes, the anterior capsule is adherent to the acetabulum and must be painstakingly dissected free to expose the entire "horseshoe" of the acetabular surface. In nearly every case, the transverse acetabular ligament (a capsular thickening that lies across the base of the horseshoe of the acetabular surface) will need to be sectioned. This ligament is hy-

pertrophic and prevents the descent of the femoral head into the depths of the true acetabulum.

Management of the labrum is controversial. Occasionally, the labrum may actually be inverted, but more often it is rolled and hypertrophic. If an actual inversion can be demonstrated and it cannot be adequately dissected to allow placement of the femoral head, use axial (radial) incisions to allow part of the labrum to be teased out of the acetabulum. This is rarely necessary. Do not excise the labrum because it contributes to future growth of the acetabular rim.

■ Now reduce the hip by traction, abduction, and internal rotation. The femoral head is often flattened on its medial border and somewhat bullet-shaped; this is usually not a problem if the hip is abducted and the apex of the femoral head can be brought inside the acetabular labrum. If any force is required to bring the femoral head into the acetabulum, perform a femoral shortening osteotomy. If the hip reduces but is stable only when the hip is flexed and abducted, consider performing an innominate osteotomy (usually Salter osteotomy), especially if the child is near 3 years of age. In addition, if severe internal rotation is required in an older child, consider a derotation osteotomy through a lateral incision.
■ With the hip held in internal rotation, close the capsulotomy (Fig. 166.3*H*). Bring the superior flap corner (tagged A in Fig. 166.3*H*) into the inferomedial portion of the capsule, at the lower end of the T. The redundant lower flap can then be either excised or sewn over the superior flap (tagged B in Fig. 166.3*H*). After additional capsular repair, the hip joint should be stable.
■ Close the wound by reattaching the tendons of the rectus femoris and by subcutaneous and subcuticular skin closure with absorbable 5-0 synthetic suture. Drainage is usually unnecessary.

Immobilize the child in a double-hip spica cast with the legs in 30° of abduction, 20° of flexion, and gentle internal rotation (Fig. 166.3*I*). The position is safe if the femur has been shortened and the iliopsoas lengthened. After open reduction in older children, this extended internally rotated position is more appropriate than the flexed "human" position used after closed reduction.

Postoperative radiographs must show a reduced femoral head, although the small ossific nucleus is often seen to be somewhat inferior to its expected position. This results from the misshapen femoral head and the hypertrophic labrum, and will remodel (Fig. 166.3*J*). Casting for 6 weeks is usually sufficient to allow healing of any osteotomy and development of satisfactory joint stability after open reduction. Ambulation with or without abduction bracing, as the clinical situation dictates, may begin immediately.

COMBINED OPEN REDUCTION AND FEMORAL SHORTENING

Femoral shortening is done during open reduction of the hip to minimize the compressive force across the joint (thus decreasing the risk of avascular necrosis) and to avoid preoperative traction in older children. It is also done in combination with derotation osteotomy to stabilize the reduction in the weight-bearing position (5,20, 22).

I prefer a second longitudinal lateral incision for the femoral-osteotomy portion of the combined procedure (Fig. 166.4*A*). This lateral approach is more cosmetic and facilitates plate removal, if desired. However, the proximal femoral shaft can, with more difficulty, also be reached anterolaterally through the lower arm of an extended standard Smith–Petersen incision.

■ Carry the lateral approach longitudinally through the fascia lata distal to the trochanteric apophysis.
■ Free the proximal origin of the vastus lateralis from the trochanter, and dissect the muscle from its posterior attachment longitudinally along the shaft of the femur. This avoids denervation of the vastus lateralis, but take care to cauterize perforating vessels that enter the muscle posteriorly. Then reflect the entire muscle subperiosteally anteriorly to expose the proximal femoral shaft.
■ Select a small plate for internal fixation; I use a four-hole $\frac{1}{3}$-tubular small-fragment plate. Place the plate along the lateral shaft of the femur just below the trochanteric flare.
■ Drill, measure, and tap the two proximal screw holes (because the shaft is so small, this is more easily done before the osteotomy).
■ Between the second and third holes of the plate, make a transverse osteotomy with a small, sharp oscillating saw.
■ After completion of the osteotomy, the proximal femur can easily be reduced into the hip joint through the anterior incision. Gently pull the thigh, and observe the bayonet overlap of the femoral fragments; this determines the amount of shortening to be done (usually 2 cm). Remove the selected length of shaft by a second transverse osteotomy of the distal fragment (Fig. 166.4*B*).
■ Secure the plate to the proximal femoral fragment, and temporarily fix the plate to the distal fragment with a small bone clamp. Adjust anteversion by putting the hip through the full range of motion while observing the joint through the anterior incision. Derotation should not be excessive; usually there should be 15° to 20° of residual anteversion after the osteotomy is fixed. I do not routinely increase varus; however, varus derotation osteotomy with shortening is an alternative at this point.
■ Once the three-dimensional position of the fragments

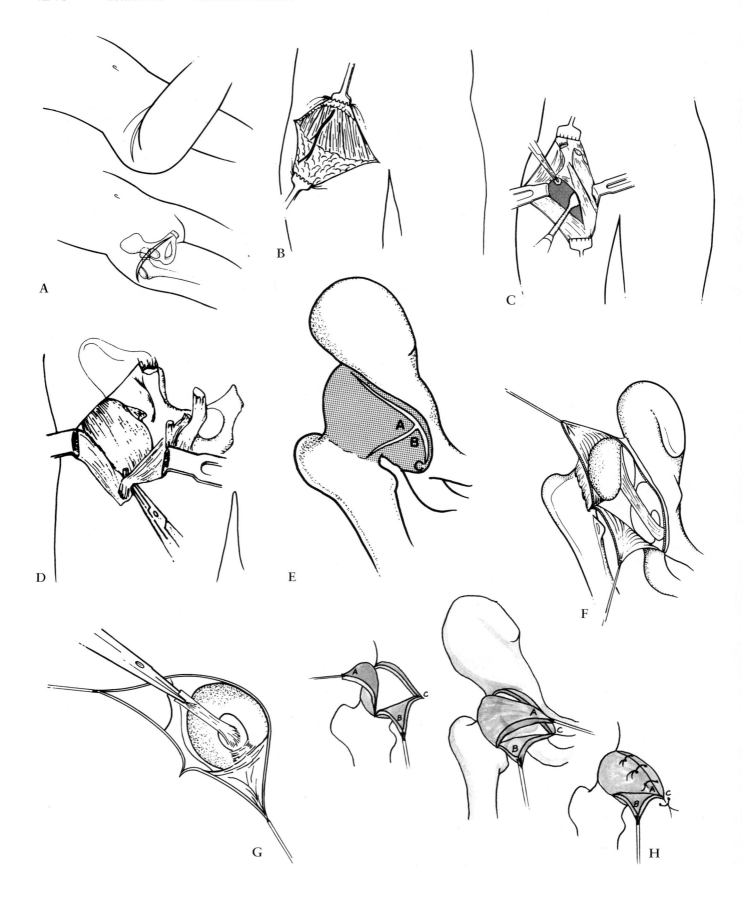

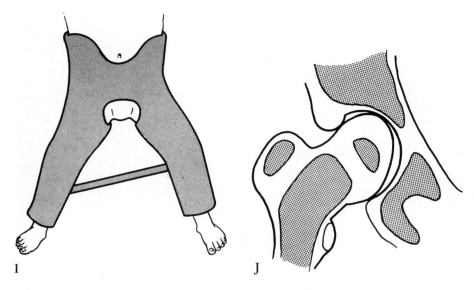

Figure 166.3. Surgical technique for open reduction of the hip through an anterior approach. See the text for a full description. **A:** Skin incision. **B:** Subcutaneous dissection and lateral femoral cutaneous nerve. **C:** Deep dissection exposes the hip joint capsule. **D:** Isolation and section of the iliopsoas tendon. **E:** Capsular incisions. **F:** Intra-articular pathology. **G:** Use of the sectioned ligamentum teres to locate the true acetabulum. **H:** Repair and reefing of the joint capsule. **I:** Double-hip spica cast. **J:** The hip and its ossific nuclei as seen on an AP radiographic view after reduction.

is satisfactory, fix the distal two holes of the plate to the distal shaft with screws (Fig. 166.5).

■ After a final check of hip coverage by the acetabulum during motion, close the lateral wound with fine, absorbable synthetic suture.

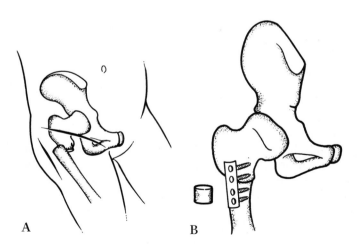

Figure 166.4. Surgical technique for femoral shortening derotation osteotomy combined with open reduction of the hip. **A:** Surgical incisions and osteotomy. **B:** Resection of a femoral segment and plate fixation.

COMPLICATIONS

Infection

Infection is rare, but if it occurs, open all wounds, including a second lateral incision (if done), down to the skeletal structures. Leave the plate in place if a femoral shortening osteotomy was done. Thoroughly irrigate and debride the wound. The hip capsule may be opened if necessary to irrigate the joint, but it must be repaired in the same fashion as the original capsulorrhaphy. The wounds may be packed open or closed over suction drains, depending on the severity of infection and the surgeon's preference. Cast immobilization is mandatory. Administer appropriate antibiotic therapy.

Redislocation

Early redislocation is evidence that the capsulorrhaphy has failed. If it is detected early, simple manipulation under general anesthesia and application of a spica cast should suffice to restore reduction. Late redislocation is often associated with residual stiffness. It may occur because of insufficient immobilization, capsulorrhaphy failure, or excessive derotation. Rarely, it can be secondary to severe ligamentous laxity, even when appropriate surgery has been done, usually in an older child with a markedly dysplastic acetabulum. Management of late redislocation must be based on careful radiographic studies to

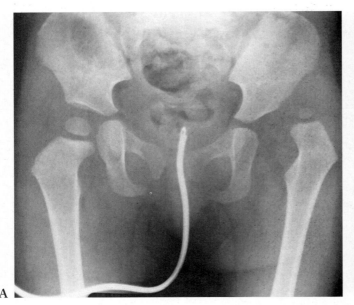 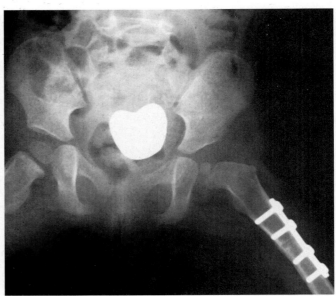

Figure 166.5. **A:** Radiographic appearance of complete congenital dislocation of the hip treated with primary open reduction and femoral shortening using plate fixation of the osteotomy (**B**).

determine the cause. Sometimes, fluoroscopy or arthrography is helpful. A proper diagnosis will suggest the most appropriate treatment.

Subluxation

Late subluxation of the hip following open reduction can occur, particularly in older children. Assessment is almost always radiographic. If subluxation is subtle and mild, I postpone additional surgical treatment for 6 months to allow complete rehabilitation of the hip girdle musculature and joint remodeling; abduction bracing during this period may be appropriate.

If a previous femoral shortening or derotation osteotomy was performed, subluxation is usually best treated by an innominate osteotomy. Repeat open reduction may be required. Unless the surgeon is extremely experienced in all aspects of congenital hip surgery, it is safer to perform such acetabular procedures as secondary treatment, even if it is initially thought that both femoral and acetabular surgery will be necessary. If previous femoral surgery was not done, the surgeon may elect either pelvic or femoral osteotomy, especially if the child is younger than 5 years.

Stiffness

A hip that has been properly reduced should not be stiff, even if open reduction was required. Stiffness is almost always a sign of subluxation or avascular necrosis. Make every attempt to accurately diagnose the problem; fluoroscopy and arthrography can be helpful.

Avascular Necrosis

Avascular necrosis may be mild and subtle (e.g., delayed or irregular ossification in a clinically normal joint) and require observation only. More extensive avascular necrosis may lead to temporary subluxation, which should be managed by casting, ambulatory abduction bracing, or surgical treatment. Severe subluxation associated with avascular necrosis may require reorientation of the acetabulum by innominate osteotomy (1), although it is safe to wait and observe if the hip is reduced in an abduction brace. Arthrography to visualize cartilaginous structures is recommended before surgical treatment for avascular necrosis. Avascular necrosis is a potential complication of all additional treatment options for patients and reduces the success of reconstructive surgery. It can also lead to early osteoarthrosis of the hip.

Extensive avascular necrosis involving the growth plate will be followed by leg-length discrepancy and deformity of the proximal femur. These deformities (head deformity, coxa breva, coxa valga) may appear late. Initiate a regular program of leg-length evaluation and x-ray observation to detect these complications and plan long-term management (11,27).

Proximal Femoral Growth Arrest and Leg-length Discrepancy

A leg-length discrepancy after congenital hip dysplasia usually occurs as a result of vascular damage to the proximal femoral physis (14). In most children (except very short ones), the appropriate management is properly timed epiphysiodesis of the contralateral limb, based on routine yearly leg-length measurements through childhood. Occasionally, femoral lengthening may be necessary (see Chapter 171). The slight temporary discrepancy that accompanies femoral shortening osteotomy is usually followed by slight femoral overgrowth, so treatment is unnecessary.

Surgery for Residual Dysplasia

After reduction has been achieved in DDH, treatment must be continued until remodeling has eliminated the secondary dysplastic features of the acetabulum and the proximal femur. Monitor dysplasia and residual subluxation both radiographically (acetabular index, center–edge angle) (21) and clinically (subtle loss of abduction, Trendelenburg gait). The use of casts, abduction braces, and surgery for residual dysplasia is somewhat arbitrary and should be based on the patient's age, the parents' wishes, and the surgeon's experience. However, failure of significant remodeling of dysplasia by 5 years of age makes additional surgery worth considering because there is good evidence that excellent remodeling can occur if correction is achieved by that age. Obvious subluxation warrants a more aggressive surgical approach because prompt treatment improves the dysplasia and the prognosis. Both femoral and pelvic osteotomies can be done for residual dysplasia.

FEMORAL OSTEOTOMY

INDICATIONS

Proximal femoral derotation or varus osteotomy is indicated in subluxation or dysplasia of the hip when reorientation can stabilize a reduction, resolve mild subluxation, or stimulate remodeling of the joint (4,5,12,22,25). Often, it is used to achieve a congruent joint in the weight-bearing position after closed or open reduction to allow a child of walking age to ambulate with less risk of subluxation. When acetabular dysplasia persists after reduction, femoral osteotomy can stimulate remodeling of the acetabulum, if done by 5 years of age (12). The choice of femoral or pelvic osteotomy in this situation is often a matter of the surgeon's personal preference; I prefer the pelvic procedure.

The usual deformity of the femur in congenital hip dysplasia is excessive anteversion. This contributes to anterolateral subluxation in the weight-bearing position and encourages superolateral subluxation in the sitting position. Femoral derotation alone is generally sufficient to correct the deformity. This becomes obvious when radiographs are taken with the legs internally rotated and a normal neck–shaft angle (135°) is seen. If abduction is also neces-

sary to produce a congruent reduction, then varus can be added, as well. Take great care not to overcorrect the femoral deformity. Avoid retroversion; increased varus of greater than 20° is rarely indicated. If a varus osteotomy is done, the hip must have an adequate range of abduction to allow functional motion after surgery. In my opinion, the prerequisites for femoral osteotomy in hip dysplasia are critical and should be the same as those for innominate osteotomy: congruent reduction of the hip and a full range of motion.

Internal fixation is necessary for femoral osteotomy. Some have advocated single-screw fixation or multiple smooth pins, but I strongly prefer rigid fixation with a small plate (for derotation alone) or a pediatric blade plate (for a varus osteotomy in an older child). This allows more accurate control of position during healing.

INTERTROCHANTERIC VARUS DEROTATION OSTEOTOMY

- Perform the operation with the hip and leg draped free, the patient on a radiolucent table, and an image intensifier available positioned anteroposteriorly. This allows testing of range of motion and reduces the chance of overcorrection, compared to the more conventional fracture table.
- Make a longitudinal lateral incision from the greater trochanter to a point distant enough to accommodate the fixation device selected. Incise the fascia lata and reflect the vastus lateralis anteriorly from its posterior femoral insertion, taking care to cauterize perforating vessels. Expose the proximal femoral shaft subperiosteally to the apophysis of the greater trochanter.
- The osteotomy site is critical. It must be intertrochanteric because internal rotation of the proximal fragment would otherwise increase iliopsoas tension (Fig. 166.6). If a subtrochanteric osteotomy is preferred, expose and release the tendinous portion of the iliopsoas insertion.
- Position the guide pins for a blade plate, using anteroposterior (AP) and frog-lateral image intensification. Use appropriate reamers or blade chisels according to the manufacturer's directions, depending on the specific fixation system being used. Drill and tap any proximal fixation holes before cutting the femur.
- Perform the osteotomy with a saw, taking an appropriate wedge out medially if varus positioning is desired. Fix the plate to the proximal fragment, externally rotate the distal fragment, and temporarily clamp the plate to the shaft. Now put the hip through a full range of motion while studying the joint with fluoroscopy, making special note of anteversion (which should not be less than 15°). Readjust the position until you are satisfied that subluxation has been adequately treated, and fix the plate to the distal fragment.
- Close the wound with fine, absorbable suture, including

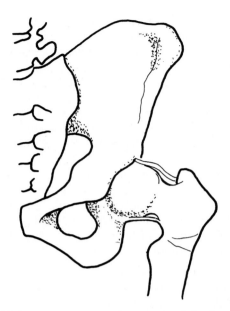

Figure 166.6.   Proper intertrochanteric level for femoral derotation osteotomy. This allows relaxation rather than tightening of the iliopsoas muscle.

the skin; I prefer 5-0 undyed polyglycolic acid subcuticular suture. Apply a double-spica cast.

Remove the cast at 8 weeks postoperatively or after radiographic union. Allow ambulation as tolerated. Physical therapy is unnecessary. Warn the family that the perineum will appear wide until the child grows and that a limp may persist for 2–3 months but will eventually disappear.

PELVIC OSTEOTOMY

INDICATIONS

Pelvic osteotomy is indicated when there is primary acetabular dysplasia, residual subluxation of the hip, or failure of gradual improvement of radiographic dysplasia following reduction of a dislocated hip. In general, pelvic osteotomy should be done when severe dysplasia is accompanied by significant radiographic changes (high acetabular index, failure of lateral acetabular ossification) on the acetabular side of the hip joint, as opposed to changes on the femoral side (e.g., marked anteversion), which are best treated by femoral osteotomy (5). Surgical treatment of definite hip subluxation by either pelvic or femoral osteotomy before age 4 years will be accompanied by at least partial remodeling and resolution of anatomic abnormalities on the opposite surface of the joint (12).

Pelvic osteotomy is ideal for treatment of dysplasia when expected remodeling has ceased (as assessed by serial radiographs) and dysplasia or subluxation persists (5). Often, after the hip is reduced, pelvic osteotomy can be postponed until 4 years of age to allow adequate time for remodeling.

Pelvic osteotomy is also indicated when necessary to stabilize reduction during or after open reduction of the hip.

PREREQUISITES AND SELECTION OF OSTEOTOMY SITE

The many osteotomies described for acetabular dysplasia may be categorized as indicated either for primary treatment of dysplasia (Salter innominate osteotomy, Pemberton osteotomy, triple innominate osteotomy) or for salvage of a poor result in the later stages of dysplasia when complete remodeling is not expected (Chiari osteotomy). The primary osteotomies are generally reorientation procedures for the acetabulum, although the Pemberton procedure allows actual diminution of acetabular volume at the expense of some acetabular congruity. The Salter and Pemberton osteotomies are the most common osteotomies performed in North America.

To be successful as a primary treatment of dysplasia, an osteotomy must be done only in the presence of a congruent reduction, satisfactory range of motion, and reasonable femoral sphericity. These prerequisites have been popularized primarily by Salter (18,19) for his innominate osteotomy, and they are appropriate preoperative goals for any primary osteotomy about the hip (acetabular or femoral).

The Salter and Pemberton osteotomies differ somewhat in concept, although both are designed to limit anterolateral subluxation by improving coverage in this area. The Salter osteotomy, because it goes completely through the pelvis, allows anterior and lateral rotation of the acetabulum through an axis formed by the sciatic notch and the pubic symphysis. There is a limit to the degree of correction that can be obtained, and the procedure does not change acetabular shape (17). Conversely, the Pemberton osteotomy is an incomplete osteotomy that hinges the anterolateral acetabular roof on the flexible triradiate cartilage for correction (16). This actually changes the configuration of the acetabulum and introduces joint incongruence that must be corrected by remodeling during growth. For these reasons, the Pemberton procedure may be indicated when there is an elongated, dysplastic acetabulum, but it is most effectively done in children younger than 8 years, as there is still flexibility in the triradiate cartilage and growth remains for remodeling of the joint surfaces (29).

In older children with deficient, dysplastic acetabulae but a relatively congruent reduction, the Salter osteotomy does not provide sufficient angular correction to improve stability. When the triradiate cartilage is closed, the Ganz periacetabular osteotomy (see Chapter 104) can achieve the extremes of reorientation required. When the triradiate cartilage is open, the same freedom to reorient the acetabulum in space can be achieved by cutting the ischium and pubis in addition to the ilium (triple innominate osteotomy). Variations of this technique have been described by Steel (24), Tönnis et al. (28), and Tachdjian (25). All are complex operations that should not be attempted by an inexperienced surgeon.

In older children, salvage of a hip that is too deformed to remodel for the growth time remaining requires a different type of procedure. The Chiari (3) osteotomy is probably the most commonly used operation. It is a displacement osteotomy that essentially provides a shelf or buttress to limit further proximal subluxation of the femoral head. The superior hip capsule provides an interpositional surface between the cancellous bone of the shelf and the femoral head, and the capsular tissue may undergo metaplasia into fibrocartilage. Thus, the functional size of the acetabulum can be increased by the operation. If done properly, the Chiari osteotomy also moves the hip joint center medially and improves the mechanical advantage of the abductor muscles, both of which tend to decrease the intra-articular resultant force across the hip joint. The Chiari osteotomy does not require a concentric reduction; it may be done above a subluxated hip. The chief indication for Chiari osteotomy is pain associated with a subluxated, dysplastic hip in an older child. It should not be performed if degenerative changes are present or the hip is stiff. Do not do a capsulotomy at the same time as a Chiari osteotomy.

The exact indications for salvage surgery in congenital hip dysplasia are controversial. The goal of surgery most often stated is to treat chronic hip pain in an adolescent who has significant dysplasia as seen on radiographs. For many surgeons, another appropriate indication is radiographically demonstrated progressive subluxation, often associated with increasing degenerative changes of the hip. Although it may be unwise to consider surgery in an adolescent who has no pain, regardless of the radiographic appearance of the hip, there are surgeons who are exploring the use of late reconstructive procedures (e.g., the Ganz osteotomy) in asymptomatic patients who have severe radiographic dysplasia (see Chapter 104).

SALTER INNOMINATE OSTEOTOMY

■ Prepare and drape the affected hip and leg free. Use a transverse inguinal skin incision as described earlier in this chapter (Salter describes a slightly more oblique incision), and identify the lateral femoral cutaneous nerve where it exits at the upper border of the sartorius; protect it with Silastic tape. Develop the proximal interval between the sartorius and the tensor fasciae latae muscles and between the straight head of the rectus femoris and the tensor fasciae latae muscles.

■ Split the iliac apophysis with a single longitudinal scalpel cut from the anterosuperior spine to the mid crest (Fig. 166.7A), and carefully pull the cartilage away from the crest. Strip the inner and outer walls of the ilium subperiosteally. Strip the anteroinferior spine medially with its attached rectus femoris. Carry the subperiosteal dissection to the sciatic notch. The notch is best exposed by gently teasing the periosteum away from it both medially and laterally with right-angle clamps; the tips of the two clamps should touch when stripping is complete. Stay subperiosteal to avoid sciatic nerve injury.

■ In the inferior wound, identify the hip capsule and the iliopsoas muscle anterior to it. Pull the tendinous portion of the muscle into the wound with a right-angle clamp and sever it.

■ Pass a Gigli saw through the notch with right-angle clamps. Saw a straight osteotomy from the notch to the anteroinferior iliac spine (Fig. 166.7B), keeping the hands as far apart as possible to avoid binding; protect the skin with ribbon retractors. Incline the osteotomy slightly in the frontal plane so that the lateral edge is superior to the medial edge.

■ Open the osteotomy by externally rotating, abducting, and extending the hip to place the extremity into a figure-four position while holding the posterior osteotomy site closed and slightly anteriorly with a tenaculum. Do not pull the proximal ilium upward; this tends to displace the proximal ileum rather than the distal fragment containing the acetabulum. Do not use a lamina spreader because damage to the fragile ilium may result.

■ With an oscillating saw (my preference) or a large rib cutter, fashion a triangular graft with one angle of 30° from the anterior portion of the proximal fragment. Place the graft into the osteotomy site, keeping the posterior osteotomy closed, and fix it with two threaded pins inserted from the proximal fragment, through the graft, and into the distal ischium posterior to the hip joint (Fig. 166.7C). Check the pin length carefully, and move the hip joint to feel for any crepitus, which might indicate pin protrusion into the joint. Temporarily leave the pin ends long.

■ Irrigate the wound and reapproximate the apophysis over the pins with simple absorbable sutures passed directly around the cartilaginous apophysis. Cut the pins so they will be palpable beneath the skin, and close the subcutaneous tissue and skin with fine, absorbable suture.

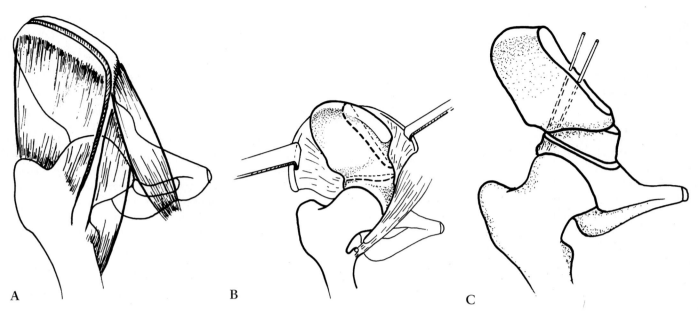

Figure 166.7. Surgical technique for Salter innominate osteotomy. **A:** Split of the iliac apophysis and fascial incision. **B:** Exposure of the ilium and sites of the osteotomy. **C:** Completed osteotomy.

■ Apply a well-molded one-and-one-half spica cast with the hip in 25° of flexion, 25° of abduction, and slight internal rotation.

Remove the cast and pins 8 weeks after surgery, when radiographic union has occurred, under a brief general anesthetic. The patient can then begin weight bearing as tolerated. Physical therapy is usually unnecessary.

PEMBERTON PERICAPSULAR OSTEOTOMY

■ Perform the operation on a radiolucent table with image-intensifier control.
■ Make a transverse skin incision in the inguinal crease, but use subcutaneous dissection to mobilize the proximal and distal flaps. Then use a standard Smith–Petersen exposure of the hip (see Chapter 3). Protect the lateral femoral cutaneous nerve.
■ Develop the interval between the sartorius and tensor fasciae latae muscles, and incise the iliac apophysis longitudinally with a sharp scalpel.
■ Expose the anterior two thirds of the inner and outer tables of the pelvis with a periosteal elevator. The subperiosteal stripping does not need to go behind the sciatic notch (as in the Salter osteotomy) but must proceed distally to the triradiate cartilage. This can be felt as a line of resistance to further stripping; facilitate a safe

approach to the area by teasing subperiosteally with a right-angle clamp.
■ Beginning on the outer wall of the pelvis, use a small, curved osteotome to make a cortical pericapsular osteotomy, starting at the anteroinferior iliac spine and continuing parallel to the joint. This osteotomy curves down to, but not into, the triradiate cartilage and must end anterior to the sciatic notch (Fig. 166.8A).
■ Make a similar cortical osteotomy in the inner wall of the pelvis, again ending at the triradiate cartilage but avoiding both the sciatic notch and the joint itself (Fig. 166.8B).
■ Join the two osteotomies, using a curved or spherical osteotome and taking care to avoid penetration of the sciatic notch or the joint. Use the image intensifier at this point to confirm the safe position of the osteotome.
■ Carefully pry the anterolateral acetabular fragment distally with the osteotome and a smooth, broad lamina spreader, without too much force. When this is properly done, the triradiate cartilage should be visible in the depths of the osteotomy.
■ Cut a triangular graft from the proximal ilium; a saw helps to make this cut without crushing the bone (Fig. 166.8C). Flatten a notch in the faces of the pelvic osteotomy, as needed, to receive the graft and lock it in place. Carefully wedge the triangular graft into the osteotomy site, and remove the lamina spreader; the graft should be secure and require no fixation (Fig 166.8D).

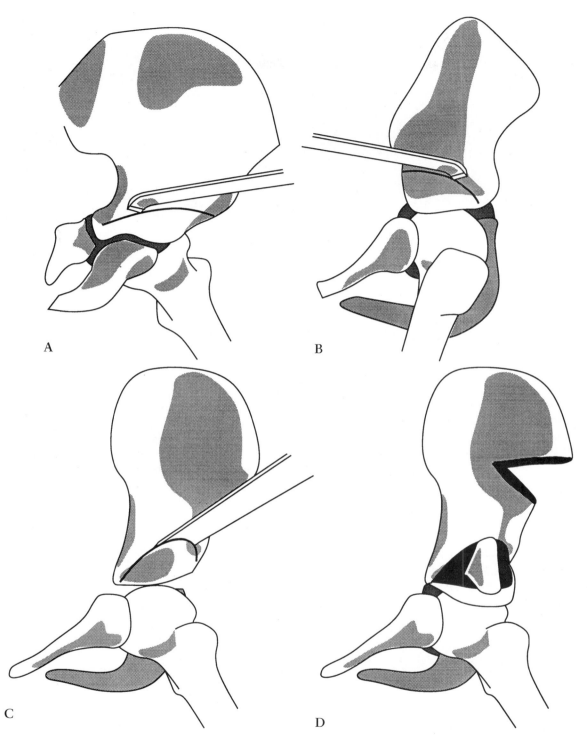

Figure 166.8. Pemberton osteotomy. **A:** Make a cortical pericapsular osteotomy cut. **B,C:** Make a similar cortical osteotomy in the inner wall of the pelvis. **D:** Cut a triangular graft from the proximal ilium, and carefully wedge the graft into the osteotomy site.

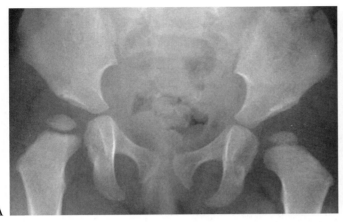
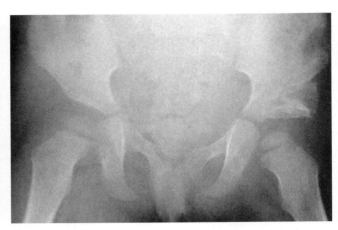

Figure 166.9.   Radiographs of a Pemberton osteotomy of a dysplastic left hip. **A:** Preoperative radiograph. **B:** Radiograph taken 6 weeks postoperatively.

■ Close the wound with absorbable sutures, and apply a spica cast as described in the technique of Salter osteotomy.

Remove the cast 8 weeks after surgery (Fig. 166.9). Allow weight bearing as tolerated. Physical therapy is unnecessary. Older children may exhibit transient stiffness of the hip joint because of changes in the acetabular surface configuration caused by the Pemberton osteotomy.

TRIPLE INNOMINATE OSTEOTOMY

General approaches to the variations in triple innominate osteotomy are presented here (24,26,28). These are highly specialized operations, and their powerful ability to reorient the acetabulum can lead to overcorrection (6). There is also significant potential risk of neural and vascular injury; these are not operations for the inexperienced. Of the operative approaches, I prefer Tachdjian's (26), but each has its proponents. For fully detailed descriptions, readers are referred to the originators of each approach (24,26,28).

■ Drape the patient on a radiolucent table with the leg free. The iliac portion of the osteotomy (usually performed last) is performed exactly as in the Salter osteotomy.

Steel Variation

Steel (24) makes the pubic cut through an inguinal incision and the ischial cut through the buttock (Fig. 166.10*A*).

■ Flex the hip 90° to expose the buttock and ischial tuber-osity. Make the ischial cut first through a transverse incision positioned 1 cm proximal to the gluteal crease. Retract the gluteus maximus laterally, and sharply dissect the origin of the biceps femoris from the ischium. Identify the sciatic nerve, using a nerve stimulator if necessary, and protect it throughout the procedure.

■ Separate the origins of the semimembranosus and semitendinosus muscles, and pass a very curved hemostat subperiosteally around the ischium, starting from the obturator foramen and emerging posterior to the ischial ramus. Stay carefully on the bone to avoid vascular injury. Cut the ramus, using the clamp as protection, with an osteotome as wide as the ischial ramus directed 45° posteriorly and laterally. Then close the wound. Steel recommended changing gloves, gowns, and instruments at this stage because of the risk of contamination in this area of the perineum.

■ Expose the anterior pelvis as for a Salter osteotomy (see above), continuing the dissection medially to identify the pectineus muscle. Detach the pectineus from the pubic ramus, clearing the pubis to about 1 cm medial to the pectineal tubercle. Pass a significantly curved hemostat subperiosteally from above the pubis and around the bone to emerge in the obturator foramen. Again using the instrument for protection, cut the pubic ramus by directing an osteotome posteriorly and medially.

■ Then make the iliac cut as described for the Salter osteotomy, and under image-intensifier control reposition the entire acetabular unit to its desired position. A towel clip or Steinmann pin (inserted as a "joystick") can be helpful in controlling the fragment.

■ Position a triangular graft in the iliac osteotomy site, and fix the ilium with threaded pins directed either as

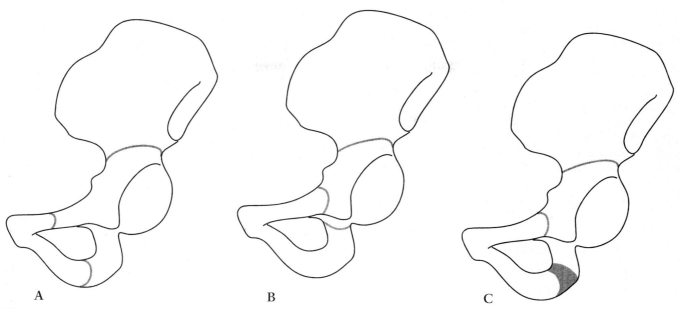

Figure 166.10. Site of iliac, pubic, and ischial osteotomies in the various triple innominate osteotomy procedures. **A:** Steel osteotomy. **B:** Tönnis osteotomy. **C:** Tachdjian triple osteotomy.

in the Salter osteotomy or from the distal fragment upward into the wing of the ilium.

- Close the wound, and immobilize the hip in a one-and-one-half hip spica cast for 8 weeks. Follow-up care is similar to that for Salter osteotomy.

Tönnis Variation

Tönnis (28) uses a posterior gluteal approach for the ischial cut (Fig. 166.10B). He felt that redirection should emphasize more lateral and less anterior coverage of the hip than advocated by Salter or Steel.

- With the patient lying prone, expose the ischial tuberosity through an oblique incision in the direction of the fibers of the gluteus maximus, which are split bluntly and separated. Cut the obturator internus and the inferior and superior gemellus muscles to expose the ischial ramus. Protect the sciatic nerve and the gluteal vessels with a blunt retractor in the sciatic notch, and place special retractors around the ischial ramus, preserving the sacrotuberous and sacrospinalis ligaments for stability. Make the ischial cut as frontal as possible, from lateral to medial, connecting the ischial and obturator foramina. The osteotomy must be complete, without spikes remaining on the cut surfaces of the bone.

- Close the wound and reposition the patient supine.

Rather than using an extended inguinal incision (see the Steel technique above), make a small incision over the pubis where it is palpable just medial to the psoas. Insert two retractors above the pubis and through the obturator foramen, and make the osteotomy cut parallel with the hip joint.

- The remaining procedure is performed similarly to the Steel osteotomy, except that in the frontal plane the iliac osteotomy is oriented from superolateral to inferomedial, which allows easier lateral rotation of the fragment.

Tachdjian Variation

Tachdjian (26) performs the ischial cut anteromedially through a subinguinal incision between the adductor magnus and obturator externus (Fig. 166.10C).

- With the extremity in the frog-leg position, make a transverse adductor incision over and posterior to the adductor longus. Although Tachdjian (26) released the adductors, I have found that the ischium can usually be exposed by bluntly developing the interval between adductor brevis and magnus and then carefully dissecting toward the ischial tuberosity on a line between the adductor magnus and obturator externus insertions. Expose the ischium subperiosteally, and protect the soft tissues with Chandler retractors. The ischial osteotomy is a laterally based about 1.5 cm wide wedge that allows moving the acetabulum medially.

■ Expose the pubis through the same incision by retracting the iliopsoas muscle (which may be fractionally lengthened) laterally and elevating the pectineus to expose the iliopectineal eminence. Protect the pubis subperiosteally with two Chandler retractors. Make the pubic osteotomy parallel to the joint, 1.5 cm medial to the acetabulum as seen on image intensification, with the osteotome directed 15° medially.

■ Using a second incision (or an extension of the medial one), perform the iliac osteotomy in a similar fashion to that in the Steel osteotomy.

CHIARI OSTEOTOMY

Perform a Chiari (3) osteotomy on a radiolucent table with AP image-intensifier control.

■ Drape the hip and leg free, with the affected side elevated on a small towel or sandbag.

■ Make an extended transverse inguinal incision as previously, carrying it well lateral to the mid-lateral line. Undermine the subcutaneous tissue to expose the proximal crest of the ilium, and isolate and protect the lateral femoral cutaneous nerve.

■ Detach and tag the straight head of the rectus femoris. Split the iliac apophysis longitudinally, and expose the inner and outer walls of the ilium by subperiosteal dissection down to the sciatic notch. Carefully cut the reflected head of the rectus femoris, and dissect it free to expose the edge of the capsule.

■ Under the reflected head of the rectus femoris, identify the edge of the capsule where it attaches to the pelvis. Use an instrument and the image intensifier to confirm the position of the capsular attachment on the ilium. The correct spot will be several millimeters above the superior edge of the acetabulum as seen on the fluoroscope because of the thickness of the capsule.

The original osteotomy described by Chiari (3) was straight from the front to the back of the pelvis. Most surgeons (including myself) prefer a curved cut, which limits anteroposterior sliding of the osteotomy. However, if the cut is made as a conical rather than cylindric curve three-dimensionally, the fragments will not displace; therefore, accurate three-dimensional control is mandatory.

■ Make the osteotomy just at the superior edge of the thickened hip capsule at a 15° upward angle as viewed in the AP plane with the image intensifier. Use two alternate ¾ in (1.5–2.0 cm) straight osteotomes and frequent radiographs to make a slightly curved osteotomy

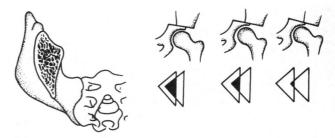

Figure 166.11.   The Chiari osteotomy is made through a triangular section of the ilium. Avoid excessive displacement of the distal fragment, which reduces the contact area and may result in delayed union.

from the front of the pelvis to near the notch. Both osteotomes must be kept absolutely parallel to each other (at 15° inclination); otherwise, the osteotomy will not slide properly. Although logic suggests that the entire osteotomy should follow the arc of the hip joint, there has never been any demonstrated advantage to such a cut, and it is unrealistic to expect perfect congruence with the hip capsule, except by the rapid remodeling that follows Chiari osteotomy.

■ Protect the inner wall of the pelvis with malleable retractors. The cut must be smooth so there are no spikes of bone to catch during displacement.

■ Complete the posterior part of the osteotomy with a Gigli saw passed behind the sciatic notch with right-angle clamps, as described above for Salter osteotomy.

■ Displace the osteotomy by abducting the leg widely. The displacement should be one-half of the width of the ilium at the site of the cut; too much displacement reduces the contact area of the osteotomy surface and may lead to delayed union (Fig. 166.11). Do not pull the proximal ilium laterally in an attempt to move the fragments; if the cut will not displace, it is because the osteotomy is not complete or is irregular or conical or because spikes of medial cortex remain.

■ If there is a large anterior defect over the capsule after displacement, it may be filled with corticocancellous graft from the proximal ilium.

■ I prefer internal fixation with a long, 4.5 mm cancellous bone screw introduced from the lateral proximal ilium into the distal fragment. Use the image intensifier to ensure that the hip joint is not penetrated. Alternatively, threaded Steinmann pins may be used. Internal fixation is not absolutely necessary, but if it is not used, the leg must be immobilized in abduction (with a spica cast or traction) to maintain displacement until the pelvis begins healing in 2–3 weeks (Fig. 166.12).

■ Close the wound over a suction drain. If internal fixation was used and is stable, allow early touch-down crutch walking.

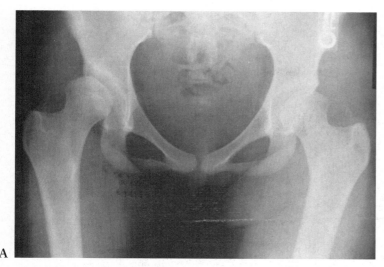

A

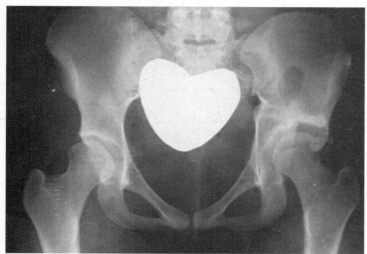

B

Figure 166.12. An adolescent girl with a painful dysplastic hip was treated by Chiari osteotomy. **A:** Preoperative radiograph. **B:** Postoperative radiograph. Note the upward inclination of the osteotomy. Postoperative hip function was excellent, with complete relief of pain.

REFERENCES

Each reference is categorized according to the following scheme: *, classic article; #, review article; !, basic research article; and +, clinical results/outcome study.

+ 1. Bar-On E, Huo MH, DeLuca PA. Early Innominate Osteotomy as a Treatment for Avascular Necrosis Complicating Developmental Hip Dysplasia. *J Pediatr Orthop B* 1997;6:138.

+ 2. Brougham DI, Broughton NS, Cole WG, Menelaus MB. Avascular Necrosis Following Closed Reduction of Congenital Dislocation of the Hip: Review of Influencing Factors and Long-term Follow-up. *J Bone Joint Surg Br* 1990;72:557.

* 3. Chiari K. Displacement Osteotomy of the Pelvis. *Clin Orthop* 1974;98:55.

* 4. Chuinard EG. Femoral Osteotomy in the Treatment of Congenital Dysplasia of the Hip. *Orthop Clin North Am* 1972;3:157.

5. Coleman SS. *Congenital Dysplasia and Dislocation of the Hip*. St. Louis, MO: Mosby, 1978.

+ 6. de Kleuver M, Kooijman MA, Pavlov PW, Veth RP. Triple Osteotomy of the Pelvis for Acetabular Dysplasia: Results at 8 to 15 Years. *J Bone Joint Surg Br* 1997;79:225.

* 7. Ferguson AB Jr. Primary Open Reduction of Congenital Dislocation of the Hip Using a Median Adductor Approach. *J Bone Joint Surg Am* 1973;55:871.

+ 8. Galpin RD, Roach JW, Wenger DR, et al. One-stage Treatment of Congenital Dislocation of the Hip in Older Children, Including Femoral Shortening. *J Bone Joint Surg Am* 1989;71:734.

+ 9. Gerscovich EO. A Radiologist's Guide to the Imaging in the Diagnosis and Treatment of Developmental Dysplasia of the Hip. II. *Skeletal Radiol* 1997;26:447.

+ 10. Kahle WK, Anderson MB, Alpert J, et al. The Value of Preliminary Traction in the Treatment of Congenital

Dislocation of the Hip. *J Bone Joint Surg Am* 1990;72:
1043.

+ 11. Kalamchi A, MacEwen GD. Avascular Necrosis Following Treatment of Congenital Dislocation of the Hip. *J
Bone Joint Surg Am* 1980;82:878.

+ 12. Kasser JR, Bowen JR, MacEwen GD. Varus Derotation
Osteotomy in the Treatment of Persistent Dysplasia in
Congenital Dislocation of the Hip. *J Bone Joint Surg Am*
1985;67:195.

+ 13. Klisic P, Jankovic L. Combined Procedure of Open Re-
duction and Shortening of the Femur in Treatment of
Congenital Dislocation of the Hips in Older Children.
Clin Orthop 1976;119:60.

+ 14. O'Brien T, Millis MB, Grifffin PP. The Early Identification and Classification of Growth Disturbances of the
Proximal End of the Femur. *J Bone Joint Surg Am* 1986;
68:970.

+ 15. Paton RW, Srinivasan MS, Shah B, Hollis S. Ultrasound
Screening for Hips at Risk in Developmental Dysplasia:
Is It Worth It? *J Bone Joint Surg Br* 1999;81:255.

* 16. Pemberton PA. Pericapsular Osteotomy for Congenital
Dislocation of the Hip: Indications and Techniques. *J
Bone Joint Surg Am* 1965;47:437.

+ 17. Rab GT. Preoperative Roentgenographic Evaluation for
Osteotomies about the Hip in Children. *J Bone Joint
Surg Am* 1981;63:306.

* 18. Salter RB. Innominate Osteotomy in the Treatment of
Congenital Dislocation and Subluxation of the Hip. *J
Bone Joint Surg Br* 1961;43:518.

* 19. Salter RB. The First 15 Years' Personal Experience with
Innominate Osteotomy in the Treatment of Congenital
Dislocation and Subluxation of the Hip. *Clin Orthop*
1974;98:55.

+ 20. Schoenecker PL, Strecker WB. Congenital Dislocation of
the Hip in Children: Comparison of the Effects of Femoral Shortening and of Skeletal Traction in Treatment. *J
Bone Joint Surg Am* 1984;66:21.

+ 21. Scoles PV, Boyd A, Jones PK. Roentgenographic Parameters of the Normal Infant Hip. *J Pediatr Orthop* 1987;
7:656.

+ 22. Simons GW. A Comparative Evaluation of the Current
Methods for Open Reduction of the Congenitally Displaced Hip. *Orthop Clin North Am* 1980;11:161.

23. Staheli LT, Coleman SS, Hensinger RN, et al. Congenital
Hip Dysplasia. *Instr Course Lect* 1984;33:350.

* 24. Steel HH. Triple Osteotomy of the Innominate Bone. *J
Bone Joint Surg Am* 1973;55:343.

25. Tachdjian MO, ed. *Congenital Dislocation of the Hip.*
New York: Churchill Livingstone, 1982.

26. Tachdjian MO, ed. *Pediatric Orthopedics,* 2nd ed. Phila-
delphia: WB Saunders, 1990:493.

+ 27. Thomas CL, Gage JR, Ogden JA. Treatment Concepts
for Proximal Femoral Ischemic Necrosis Complicating
Congenital Hip Disease. *J Bone Joint Surg Am* 1982;64:
817.

+ 28. Tönnis D, Behrens K, Tscharani F. A Modified Technique of the Triple Pelvic Osteotomy: Early Results. *J
Pediatr Orthop* 1981;1:241.

+ 29. Vedantam P, Capelli AM, Schoenecker PL. Pemberton
Osteotomy for the Treatment of Developmental Dysplasia of the Hip in Older Children. *J Pediatr Orthop* 1998;
18:254.

30. Westin GW, Ilfeld FW, Makin M, Paterson D. Develop-
mental Hip Dislocation. *Contemp Orthop* 1988;16:17.

## CHAPTER 167

CONGENITAL DEFORMITIES OF THE FOOT

George T. Rab and Peter B. Salamon

Foot deformities in children may be either congenital or acquired during childhood. Before starting a treatment program for congenital foot deformity, search for associated deformities that may also need treatment (e.g., congenital hip dysplasia, torticollis) and associated conditions that may require further evaluation and that might affect the prognosis of the foot deformity (e.g., arthrogryposis, spinal dysraphism, bone dysplasia). Deformities that develop during childhood are often manifestations of underlying neuromuscular disease that must be evaluated before intelligent treatment of the foot can be planned.

Primary treatment for congenital deformities often be-

gins the first day of life and generally should be concluded by the time the child begins walking. Secondary treatment and treatment of recurrence are often necessary, because mild muscular imbalance and incomplete correction of deformities are common. The foot may require long-term bracing or repeated surgery to maintain adequate function. For these reasons, experience and judgment are as important as surgical skill in the long-term management of foot deformities. The surgeon with only occasional exposure to these problems should not undertake treatment.

CONGENITAL CLUBFOOT

Congenital clubfoot (talipes equinovarus) is a hereditary foot deformity of unproven etiology. It affects males more

G. T. Rab and P. B. Salamon: Department of Orthopaedics, University of California Davis Medical Center, Sacramento, California, 95817.

often than females and may be unilateral or bilateral. It is often associated with other conditions, such as myelodysplasia, arthrogryposis, and congenital hip dysplasia. Pathologic changes seen in clubfoot include bony deformity, particularly of the talus (short neck, medial deviation of the neck, abnormal articular surface of the head) and soft-tissue contracture (muscle, tendon sheath, capsule, ligament, skin) (14). Externally, the clubfoot is smaller than the normal foot. There is equinus of the ankle, varus and internal rotation of the heel, accompanied by adduction, supination, and cavus of the midfoot. The calf is atrophic and smaller in circumference than the opposite calf. The leg lengths are generally equal. Internally, the deformity is most clearly defined as a rotational subluxation of the talocalcaneonavicular joint complex, with the talus in plantar flexion and the talocalcaneonavicular (subtalar) complex in medial rotation and inversion (20). There is controversy over whether the soft tissue or bony changes are the primary cause of the disorder, although nonoperative and surgical treatment both address the soft-tissue portion of the deformity with the expectation that at least some of the bony abnormalities will remodel. Regardless of the form of treatment, the resultant foot will be smaller and less mobile, and the calf relatively atrophic, when compared with a normal limb.

Management of the congenital clubfoot is initially nonoperative and, if possible, should begin on the first day of life. Serial manipulation of clubfoot and maintenance of correction with casting is a skill that all orthopaedic surgeons dealing with children should develop (15,26). It is essential to correct the midfoot adductus and hindfoot varus in the casts before you make any attempt to address the equinus. We have concern that overly aggressive attempts at dorsiflexion may damage the talus, and we often abandon casting once progression of the correction into dorsiflexion stops.

When casting fails, surgical release is indicated. The need for and the exact timing of the surgery depends on the severity of the clubfoot. We normally make a decision to treat surgically by 3–4 months of age. Surgery, however, can be timed so that the postoperative casting is completed at about the time the child begins to bear weight on the foot. Some surgeons prefer operative treatment at a much younger age, but there is also literature support for postponing surgery up to 1 year of age or beyond, if the surgeon feels technically more able to operate on a larger foot (33). In children with syndromes, delay of surgery until a year of age or beyond is often desirable or necessary.

Stress dorsiflexion lateral radiographs of an incompletely corrected clubfoot reveal inadequate dorsiflexion of the os calcis or parallelism of the talar and calcaneal axes. Anteroposterior (AP) views show medial deviation of the first metatarsal axis relative to the talar axis, a function of subluxation of the talonavicular joint (the navicu-

lar ossification center itself does not appear for several years, and its position must be inferred); the axes of the talus and calcaneus likewise become parallel because the external rotation of the subtalar joint is lost. Most of the angles described for evaluation of clubfoot are based on radiographs of older children, and they date from an era when treatment was nonoperative and involved prolonged casting. We have not found radiographs to be helpful in determining which children should have early surgery; the decision is made more easily on clinical grounds.

The aim of surgical treatment is to release soft-tissue restraints on proper positioning of the tarsal bones. The exact surgical procedure can be tailored to the residual deformity of the foot at the completion of casting. The usual surgical release always includes posterior structures (tendo Achillis, posterior tibial tendon, calcaneofibular ligament, posterior ankle, subtalar capsulotomy, and, sometimes, long toe flexors). If significant midfoot deformity remains (medial talonavicular subluxation), release the medial talonavicular joint and the tendon sheaths of posterior tibial, flexor digitorum longus (FDL), and flexor hallucis longus (FHL) muscles. Some clubfeet have significant medial subluxation of the calcaneocuboid joint, requiring capsular release (2,21). The medial subtalar capsule can be partially or completely released to correct hindfoot varus. These releases allow the talus to be dorsiflexed into neutral position, the navicular to be abducted and rotated onto the true axial head of the talus, and the os calcis to be brought out of varus and into lateral rotation under the talus to reduce the subtalar joint. Hold the reduction with pin fixation in a cast until the soft tissues heal.

Although surgeons have recognized for years that posterior and medial releases are necessary to correct clubfoot, recent attention to the posterolateral ankle structures (fibulocalcaneal ligament and peroneal sheaths) has emphasized the importance of correction of *internal rotation* of the subtalar joint if full correction of the clubfoot is to be achieved (20–22,28,29,32). The exact incision used may not be important, but it must provide adequate exposure of these structures or the correction is incomplete. We prefer the Cincinnati circumferential subtalar incision (or portions of it), because it gives the fullest visualization of the entire midfoot and hindfoot, including the posterolateral region; you can use portions of this incision for more limited releases (8). Because tarsal bones are largely cartilaginous in the small child, they are inevitably deformed at the time of reorientation, and the correction must be maintained for at least 3–4 months to allow remodeling. Many children require further bracing for a year or more to maintain position during walking.

Tailor the operative procedure to the deformity. If the releases performed are overly aggressive, the result may be an overcorrected clubfoot when the child becomes older. There are good methods that have been developed to later improve undercorrected feet or relapsed feet, but there are no good secondary procedures that adequately deal with the overcorrected clubfoot. Although our initial feeling was that complete correction of a clubfoot was necessary in most cases, the long-term follow-up of many of our earlier patients with clubfoot has led us to temper these beliefs. In the mild and moderate clubfoot, we now favor a more limited release of posterior structures, which generally leads to better foot function as the child matures.

CLUBFOOT RELEASE

- Perform clubfoot release with the patient prone or supine, using a pneumatic tourniquet.
- Make a full Cincinnati skin incision, extending it from the navicular tuberosity under the medial malleolus, arching slightly over the os calcis posteriorly, and extending obliquely around to the calcaneocuboid joint laterally (Fig. 167.1*A*). Portions of the incision may be used for less extensive releases.
- Keep the knife at a 90° angle to the skin, and carry the incision sharply through the subcutaneous tissue with minimal retraction. Use caution as the knife crosses the Achilles tendon, which is deep in the subcutaneous tissue of the posterior wound.
- Use a fine scissors for the remaining dissection.
- Identify and mobilize the neurovascular bundle in the posteromedial wound both proximally and distally (to the point where the nerve branches into the calcaneal branch and medial and lateral plantar nerves); retract it with a Silastic tape.
- Posterolaterally, identify the sural nerve running with the lesser saphenous vein; mobilize and protect these structures with a Silastic tape.

Posterior Release

Perform the posterior release portion of the procedure first.

- Protecting the neurovascular bundle and the sural nerve, perform a Z-lengthening of the Achilles tendon, making the distal transverse cut in the medial half of the tendon (the lateral half is left attached to the calcaneus). Tag each end with #0 absorbable suture (Fig. 167.1*C*).
- Just posterior and lateral to the neurovascular bundle lies the FHL tendon; incise its sheath, identify it, and protect it during the next stage with a Silastic tape, because it is easy to sever inadvertently.
- Excise the entire posterior capsule of the tibiotalar and subtalar joints and identify the joint lines; the subtalar joint will still be unyielding.
- If the midfoot deformity has been corrected by casting, the dissection just described may be enough to correct the deformity; in this case, the posterior tibial tendon

usually requires Z-lengthening, as may the FHL and FDL tendons.
- If you are satisfied with the correction obtained after posterior release alone, manipulate the forefoot into corrected position and blindly pin it from back (talus) to front, bringing the pin out the dorsum of the foot; bend the tip to prevent migration (Fig. 167.1*H*).
- Close the wound as will be described later.

Lateral Release

Frequently, additional release may be required.

- In the posterolateral portion of the wound, identify and transect the heavy fibulocalcaneal ligament (Fig. 167.1*D*); this allows external rotation of the os calcis as it is dorsiflexed (Fig. 167.1*E*). Use a pair of scissors to cut the sheaths of the peroneal tendons circumferentially, taking care not to injure the tendons. Slide the scissors along the posterolateral subtalar joint capsule to incise it.

Medial Release

- Incise the posterior tibial tendon sheath and perform a Z-lengthening of the tendon, grasping the distal tendon stump with a small Kocher clamp.
- Follow the tendon stump as it inserts into the navicular, and transversely incise the deep posterior tibial sheath and the medial, dorsal, and plantar talonavicular capsules.
- Blending with the inferior capsule are the spring ligament (connecting the navicular with the sustentaculum tali) and Henry's knot (where the flexor hallucis and flexor digitorum cross). While appearing in textbooks as discrete structures, these usually are difficult to separate and are released as the capsule is incised (Fig. 167.1*B*). One of us (GTR) separates the intact knot of Henry from the navicular, and one of us (PBS) incises it longitudinally, freeing the flexor tendons.
- Incise the anterior subtalar joint with scissors just above the sustentaculum. If the talus still does not mobilize, incise the remaining medial subtalar capsule. It is usually easiest to start from the posterior exposure of the subtalar joint at the site of the previous capsulectomy. Retract the FHL and the neurovascular bundle to cut the firm medial capsule, staying right at the joint level. It is very easy to inadvertently cut the FHL during this portion of the dissection.
- Incise the FDL tendon sheath transversely as you encounter it. Take care not to drift superiorly out of the subtalar joint, or injury to the deep deltoid ligament may occur.
- Once the subtalar capsule has been circumferentially incised to the anterior end of the os calcis, open the joint by everting the os calcis. This exposes the subtalar interosseous ligament, which can be seen through either

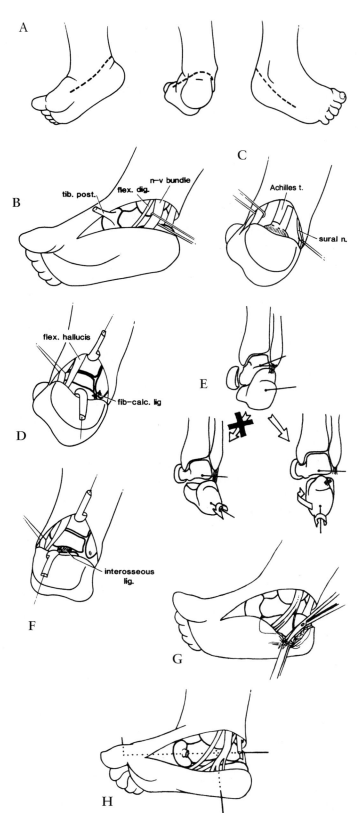

Figure 167.1. **A:** The Cincinnati incision used for standard clubfoot release. **B:** Isolation of the neurovascular bundle and posterior tibial tendon. The flexor digitorum longus (in its sheath) is visible medially. **C:** Preferred Z-plasty technique for the Achilles tendon. **D:** Incision of the fibulocalcaneal ligament and peroneal tendon sheaths. **E:** External rotation of the os calcis during dorsiflexion. **F:** The interosseous ligament, seen from the posterior incision. **G:** Release of the plantar fascia in the presence of cavus. **H:** Use of two pins to fix the talonavicular joint and subtalar joint. See text for details.

the medial or the posterior portions of the wound as a thick, ribbonlike band (Fig. 167.1*F*). You should not divide this ligament except in the most severe cases (usually arthrogryposis), because this can lead to significant overcorrection.

■ If the lateral border of the foot is still convex, or if preoperative radiographs demonstrate significant medial subluxation of the calcaneocuboid joint, release that joint. We prefer to dissect the medial wound distal to the anterior os calcis, which is now well exposed. Cut the long plantar ligament and identify the medial calcaneocuboid capsule; incise its entire medial surface and use a fine scissors to incise the superior and inferior capsule as well. If that does not free the joint sufficiently, expose the calcaneocuboid joint in the distal part of the lateral incision and release the capsule there.

■ If significant cavus is present, you may release the plantar fascia through the posteromedial wound. Identify the interval between the calcaneal sensory branch and the lateral plantar branch of the posterior tibial nerve, and gently retract the lateral branch anteriorly while dissecting down the medial and inferior side of the os calcis with scissors (Fig. 167.1*G*). Stay right on the bone, taking great care not to injure the neurovascular bundle, because after a Cincinnati incision it supplies the major vascularity to the heel pad. With a blunt scissors, cut the plantar fascia where it originates from the inferior os calcis; you will feel a palpable relaxation of the cavus.

■ Reduce the talonavicular joint, being careful not to overreduce it or allow it to subluxate dorsally (the most common malreduction), and hold it with an 0.035 Kirschner wire (K-wire), inserted from the posterior talus through the joint and out the skin of the dorsum of the foot (Fig. 167.1*H*). Pull the pin flush with the posterior talus, and cut and bend it superficial to the dorsal skin to prevent migration.

■ If you desire, insert a second pin through the heel pad longitudinally across the subtalar joint after it has been reduced into neutral varus–valgus and slight subtalar external rotation (Fig. 167.1*H*). Move the ankle to ensure that this pin stops before entering the ankle joint. Cut and bend the pin outside the heel skin.

■ Hold the ankle at 90° and use the two suture tags coming from the ends of the Achilles tendon to hold tension on the tendon so that the structure is snug at a neutral ankle position. Repair the tendon in this position. Be careful not to overlengthen the Achilles tendon, or calcaneus gait can result. Small gaps in the tendon fill in spontaneously in a child under 4–6 months of age.

■ Repair the Z-lengthened posterior tibial tendon, and perform sliding Z-lengthenings of the FDL (in the medial wound) and the FHL (in the posterior wound), if they are snug and prevent correction of the deformity.

■ Arrange the tendons properly in the wound, and close the skin with 4-0 absorbable sutures. We prefer deep, loose, through-and-through simple sutures, although subcutaneous and subcuticular suture may be used if there is minimal skin tension. If the wound seems too tight to close safely, allow the ankle to fall into slight plantar flexion and close the wound; the foot can easily be brought up in 3 weeks by changing the cast in the office, without risk to the skin.

■ Apply a well-padded, long-leg cast extending beyond the flexed toes, with the knee bent 90°; take care to gently externally rotate the heel. (If you used two subtalar pins, you can apply a short-leg cast at this point, because the hindfoot will not rotate.)

Postoperative Care   The cast is usually changed 6 weeks postoperatively, when the pins are removed. Apply a second cast for an additional 6 weeks. If the child is of walking age, the first 6–8 weeks of immobilization should be in a long-leg cast with a 90° bend to control subtalar rotation and prevent ambulation, but the last 6 weeks may be in a short-leg cast with a walking heel. Some surgeons use orthotic devices for the first 12–24 months following clubfoot release, but we have generally found them unnecessary. An exception may be made if a mild clubfoot has required only posterior release; in these cases, maintaining alignment with an ankle–foot orthosis (AFO) while postural muscles develop seems to lessen the flexible midfoot deformity.

MANAGEMENT OF RECURRENCE OR UNDERCORRECTION

Recurrence, relapse, or undercorrection occurs in up to 15% of operated clubfeet. The most common residual finding is adduction and supination of the forefoot so that the first metatarsal does not touch the ground during walking, and callosities develop on the lateral border of the foot. This can be associated with hindfoot varus and internal rotation. When noted early, it may be treated with an AFO, or a Perlstein brace (straight-last shoe, medial upright, lateral T-strap, and 90° plantarflexion stop). If the deformity persists, however, the treatment is surgical.

In a child younger than 2 years, you may manage recurrence by repeating the posterior medial release. In our experience, however, this is usually not enough, especially when adequate initial surgery was performed. Lateral column shortening is often extremely helpful to accomplish secondary correction (cuboid decancellation, Evans procedure, or Lichtblau osteotomy with a medial release). We use the Lichtblau procedure because it produces predictably good results.

After the age of 5 years, the joints of the foot are sufficiently formed that it is better to accept the malposition of the joints and perform secondary bony procedures to reorient the foot. Metatarsal or midfoot osteotomies (1) can be used to correct forefoot adduction, but they are of limited use since they do nothing for the main deformity in the hindfoot and midfoot. The soft-tissue alternative, mobilization of the tarsometatarsal joint by capsulotomies (Heyman-Herndon procedure), has been abandoned because it has been found to cause pain and midtarsal stiffness in an already stiff foot. The double tarsal osteotomy (opening wedge osteotomy of the medial cuneiform, accompanied by shortening of the lateral column of the foot) and a combination of a closing lateral column shortening procedure (cuboid osteotomy or Lichtblau procedure) and an opening wedge osteotomy of the medial cuneiform are excellent alternatives (19,23). Osteotomy of the os calcis can be used to correct the hindfoot inversion and varus (11).

Recurrence may be a manifestation of muscle imbalance in a growing foot (4). Regardless of the success of treatment, the clubfoot patient has an atrophic calf and a small foot on the affected side. Weakness of the peroneals or the peroneus tertius appears to contribute to the late tendency toward hindfoot varus, forefoot supination, and adductus. This can be improved with either lateral or split transfer of the anterior tibial tendon. The posterior tibial tendon transfer and FHL transfer have been described for residual anterior tibial muscle weakness in the clubfoot, but we have no personal experience with either procedure (22,34). Skeletal deformities should be corrected before the tendon transfers.

The last-resort salvage procedure, a triple arthrodesis, is best postponed until the age of 10–12, when the foot is fully grown.

LATERAL COLUMN SHORTENING PROCEDURES

- Perform lateral column shortening procedures (10,17) under pneumatic tourniquet control. Use the medial and lateral arms of the Cincinnati incision described for congenital clubfoot; leave the posterior portion of the skin intact.
- On the medial side, expose the posterior tibial tendon sheath and incise it, exposing the tendon.
- Perform a Z-lengthening of the tendon and tag both free ends.
- Use a fine curved scissors to dissect deep to the distal posterior tibial tendon stump, and identify the talonavicular joint; incise its capsule superiorly, medially, and inferiorly.
- In the lateral wound, expose the calcaneocuboid joint and incise its capsule sufficiently to mobilize it.
- If performing a *Lichtblau osteotomy* (Fig. 167.2A) (17), resect the distal portion of the os calcis to cancellous bone, using a small osteotome. This shortens the calcaneus at the same level as the talonavicular joint, allowing the midtarsal joint to translate easily to a corrected position.

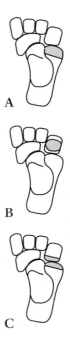

Figure 167.2. Lateral column shortening options for residual adduction deformity in clubfoot. **A:** Lichtblau osteotomy (resection distal os calcis). **B:** Cuboid decancellation. **C:** Evans procedure (calcaneocuboid fusion).

- Abduct the midfoot to check correction. If the medial release has been performed fully and enough os calcis has been resected, the foot should appear corrected. If it does not, resect more of the os calcis or release the medial foot more until the correction is adequate. Although the articular surface has been removed from the calcaneus, the cuboid articular cartilage remains, and a painless synchondrosis will develop.
- If performing a *cuboid decancellation* (Fig. 167.2B), incise only enough of the capsule to identify the joint surface plane (10). Use either a small osteotome or a curet to remove a wedge of bone from the middle portion of the cuboid. In younger children, it is usually easiest to simply curet out the ossific nucleus, leaving a shell of the cartilaginous anlage.
- Compress the cuboid closed as the released talonavicular joint is reduced. Check correction as for the Lichtblau osteotomy, and adjust the medial release and bone resection accordingly.
- If performing a *calcaneocuboid fusion* (Evans procedure) (Fig. 167.2C), curet or resect with an osteotome the articular surfaces of both joints. Excessive resection is unnecessary, since the fusion reduces lateral column growth potential and the midfoot will gradually abduct (10).
- Insert an 0.062 K-wire longitudinally across the corrected calcaneocuboid articulation. For the Evans and

Lichtblau procedures, this is done most easily by adducting the forefoot and placing the pin retrograde from the distal os calcis to the heel, correcting the lateral column, and advancing the pin antegrade into the forefoot, where it is withdrawn into the heel and left protruding on the dorsum of the foot.

- Carefully check forefoot pronation–supination, and reduce and pin the talonavicular joint with a second pin introduced from the dorsum of the foot. Bend the pins externally to prevent migration.
- Release the tourniquet, obtain hemostasis, and repair the posterior tibial tendon. Close the skin and subcutaneous layer loosely with a single layer of 4-0 interrupted absorbable sutures.
- Pad the pins and apply a long-leg cast with the foot in corrected position. Change the cast at 4–6 weeks, at which time you may remove the pins. Apply a second short-leg walking cast for an additional 4 weeks.

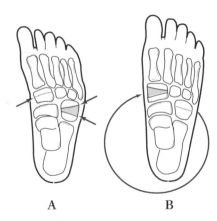

Figure 167.3. Double tarsal osteotomy for residual adductus deformity. Wedge resected from cuboid (**A**) is inserted into opening osteotomy of medial cuneiform (**B**).

DOUBLE TARSAL OSTEOTOMY

- Begin the double tarsal osteotomy (19,23) with an oblique or longitudinal incision over the cuboid.
- Identify the peroneal tendons, open the sheath, and retract these tendons in a plantar direction. Incise the periosteum of the cuboid bone.
- Using an oscillating saw, remove a laterally based trapezoidal fragment of bone from the cuboid. It is important to go through the medial cortex of the bone so that the osteotomy can be mobilized. Guide wires and image intensification facilitate these cuts and help prevent injury to the articular surfaces. Attempt to remove the trapezoid in a single piece.
- Make a second incision over the medial cuneiform. Protect the anterior tibial tendon and retract it dorsally and distally.
- Dissect the medial cuneiform subperiosteally and expose its plantar and dorsal aspects. Use an image intensifier at this point to identify the midportion of the bone.
- Make a single osteotomy cut transversely in the cuneiform (Fig. 167.3A). After you complete this osteotomy, place an instrument such as a small lamina spreader across the osteotomy and open it.
- Insert the bone graft that was taken from the cuboid into the osteotomy of the medial cuneiform (Fig. 167.3B). Usually the bone graft is quite stable, but a small K-wire can be used to secure the graft in place. Place it through the base of the first metatarsal and across the two fragments of the cuneiform, securing the bone graft.
- Close the cuboid osteotomy and hold it with K-wires. Close the wounds with 4-0 absorbable suture.
- Place the patient in a long-leg, bent-knee cast to prevent weight bearing. At 6 weeks, exchange the cast for a

weight-bearing short-leg cast, to be worn for an additional 4 weeks (19,23).

OS CALCIS OSTEOTOMY TO CORRECT HINDFOOT VARUS

- When performing an os calcis osteotomy to correct hindfoot varus, make a curved lateral incision just inferior and parallel to the peroneal tendon sheaths, and dissect down to the os calcis (Fig. 167.4A).
- Incise the periosteum parallel with the skin wound. Perform limited subperiosteal dissection to allow passage of a metatarsal (Hayes or Blount) retractor posteriorly between the Achilles tendon and bone, and inferiorly between the plantar structures and the calcaneus.
- After locating the site for the osteotomy, confirm the position with an image intensifier.
- With an osteotome or oscillating saw, cut an oblique osteotomy through the lateral cortex and medullary bone of the os calcis. Carefully complete the cut through the medial cortex with controlled use of an osteotome and varus manipulation of the heel (to crack the medial cortex). The neurovascular bundle lies on the medial side and must not be injured.
- Manipulate the heel to loosen the periosteum on the medial side, and slide the tuberosity of the os calcis laterally until the heel pad is positioned in the appropriate position.
- Hold the osteotomy with an oblique 0.065 K-wire or a small Steinmann pin inserted through the heel (Fig. 167.4B) and bent to prevent migration. Close the wound with subcuticular 4-0 synthetic absorbable suture.
- Apply a long-leg cast with the knee bent 90° to prevent weight bearing. Change the cast at 4 weeks and remove

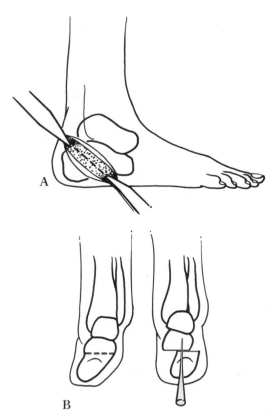

Figure 167.4. **A:** The lateral approach for osteotomy of the os calcis. **B:** Fixation with a small Steinmann pin inserted at a 45° upward angle from the tip of the os calcis.

the pin. Then use a weight-bearing short-leg cast until clinical and radiographic union is achieved, usually 6 weeks after surgery.

An alternative method is to do a closing wedge osteotomy in the same location. This is generally recommended in the older child.

METATARSAL OSTEOTOMIES

- The procedure for metatarsal osteotomies begins with three longitudinal incisions on the dorsum of the foot; the first is on the dorsomedial aspect of the proximal first metatarsal, and the remaining two are between the second and third metatarsals and the fourth and fifth metatarsals (Fig. 167.5). (An alternative is to use a curved transverse incision at the level of the tarsometatarsal joints.) Take care to protect the small dorsal veins, the superficial nerves, and the dorsalis pedis artery.
- Expose the proximal shaft of the first metatarsal by medial longitudinal subperiosteal dissection. The periosteum is adherent proximally, where the physis of the

first metatarsal is located. The physis must not be injured: Use a Keith needle or intraoperative radiograph, if necessary, to locate and protect it.

- Use a small oscillating saw to perform a transverse osteotomy 1 cm distal to the physis, starting from the medial side. If possible, do not quite complete the cut through the dorsolateral cortex, but instead create a greenstick-type fracture to act as a hinge, or leave an intact sleeve of periosteum laterally.
- Perform similar osteotomies of the remaining proximal four metatarsals using the saw; the physes of these bones are distal, so there is no risk of injury to them. Try not to injure the lateral periosteal sleeves.
- Manipulate the metatarsals into corrected position. Hold them in place with two K-wires inserted obliquely through the first and fifth metatarsal shafts into the midtarsus. Be sure to correct any forefoot supination (Fig. 167.5B) and cavus that are present. These must be evaluated clinically because axial deformity in particular will not be evident on radiographs. The foot should appear fully corrected externally when lying relaxed on the table, and the entire sole should be plantargrade from heel to metatarsals.
- Cut the wires outside the skin and bend them to prevent migration.
- Check the position of the wires on a radiograph. Minor displacement of the middle metatarsals remodels easily if the lateral periosteum has not been violated (Fig. 167.6). Gross displacement of lesser metatarsals can lead to nonunion, which, although not always painful, should be corrected. If the hindfoot is in rigid varus, perform an os calcis osteotomy, or perform any desired tendon transfers at this time.

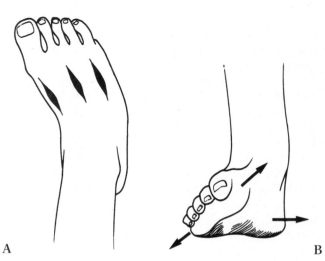

Figure 167.5. **A:** Preferred longitudinal incisions for metatarsal osteotomies. **B:** Supination of the forefoot relative to the heel must be corrected with the metatarsal osteotomies.

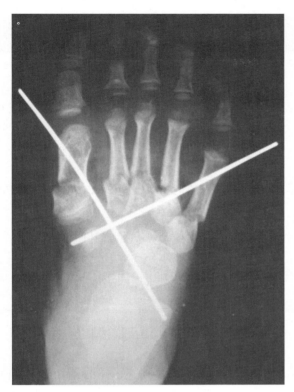

Figure 167.6. Radiograph of internal fixation used for metatarsal osteotomies.

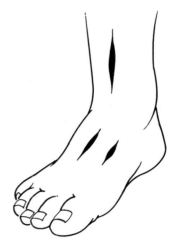

Figure 167.7. Preferred incisions for anterior tibial tendon transfer to the third cuneiform.

- Close the wounds with subcuticular 4-0 absorbable synthetic suture.
- Apply a well-padded short-leg cast. At 3–4 weeks, change the cast and remove the wires. Apply a new well-molded cast in the corrected position and allow weight bearing. Remove the cast 6–8 weeks after surgery.

ANTERIOR TIBIAL TENDON TRANSFER TO THE THIRD CUNEIFORM

Although Garceau (12) originally described anterior tibial tendon transfer to the cuboid, we have found that a less lateral position, to the third cuneiform, is more appropriate, especially when correction of fixed deformity is performed prior to the tendon transfer.

- Make a small dorsal medial incision (Fig. 167.7). Detach the insertion of the anterior tibial tendon close to bone through the wound, leaving the tendon as long as possible. Place a Bunnell suture of #1 or #0 synthetic absorbable suture in the tendon.
- Make a second, longitudinal incision over the anterior tibial muscle belly above the ankle, identify the muscle by pulling on the tendon, and pull the tendon into this incision.

- Make a third incision over the third cuneiform bone. Pull on the periosteum in line with the selected transfer insertion site to dorsiflex the foot, observing inversion–eversion. Modify the insertion site to obtain balanced dorsiflexion.
- Make a drill hole through the third cuneiform to the plantar surface. Pass the tendon through the subcutaneous tissue from the proximal wound to the third cuneiform (not beneath the ankle retinaculum). Thread the suture in the tendon into two Keith needles and pull it through the hole in the cuneiform. Bring the Keith needles out the plantar surface, tying the suture over a button or dental roll on the plantar aspect of the foot.
- Close the wounds with fine absorbable synthetic subcuticular suture.
- Apply a short-leg cast, which is worn for 6 weeks. Allow weight bearing after 4 weeks.

SPLIT ANTERIOR TIBIAL TENDON TRANSFER

- For a split anterior tibial tendon transfer (13), make a small medial incision (Fig. 167.8). Isolate the insertion of the anterior tibial tendon through the wound. There is usually a natural longitudinal division of the tendon. Split the tendon from proximal to distal. Do not attempt to split the tendon from below, because it is easy to rupture it. If rupture occurs, abandon the procedure and proceed with a standard anterior tibial transfer as described previously, using the remaining tendon stump. Free up the lateral half of the insertion into the navicular at this split, and place a suture of #1 or #0 synthetic absorbable suture in it using a crisscross Bunnell technique.

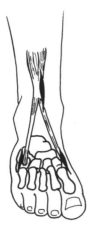

Figure 167.8.   The concept of split anterior tibial tendon transfer to cuboid. Incisions are shown.

- Make a second, longitudinal incision anteriorly above the ankle. Identify the anterior tibial muscle by pulling on the split tendon end, and pass a tendon passer from the proximal wound to distalward along the tendon, taking care to remain in the tendon sheath.
- Grasp the Bunnell stitch, pull it back into the second wound, and deliver the lateral half of the split tendon up into the proximal wound.
- Transfer the split portion of the tendon to the cuboid bone by the technique described previously for anterior tibial transfer. Adjust the tension so that the lateral arm of the transfer is just slightly tighter than the medial arm (observed through the superior wound). Anchor the transfer as described previously, or bring it through a hole in the cuboid and sew it back on itself.
- Closure and postoperative care are the same as for anterior tibial tendon transfer.

CAVUS FOOT

Rarely, cavus foot is idiopathic and seen in infancy. Cavus is a common component or residuum of clubfoot. However, isolated cavus or cavovarus deformity usually develops insidiously with growth and is a sign of occult neuromuscular disease. Some of the more common associated disorders are listed in Table 167.1.

Because the orthopaedic surgeon is often the first physician to recognize the deformity, it is important to do a careful neurologic examination and initiate necessary ancillary studies (e.g., electromyography, muscle enzyme studies, spine radiographs, and spine magnetic resonance imaging) and obtain appropriate consultation before attempting treatment.

Cavus is generally progressive until growth stops. Or-

Table 167.1. Common Conditions Associated with Cavus or Cavovarus Feet
Peripheral nervous system
Charcot-Marie-Tooth disease
Other hereditary peripheral neuropathies
Traumatic peripheral nerve lesions
Spinal cord
Spinal cord tumor
Tethered cord syndrome
Spina bifida
Poliomyelitis
Diastematomyelia
Central nervous system
Cerebral palsy
Friedreich's ataxia
Muscle disease
Duchenne's muscular dystrophy

thotic management is never successful; the deformity is either accepted or treated surgically. The mainstay of treatment is triple arthrodesis (see Chapter 115), but dorsal wedge osteotomy may be appropriate in selected cases. There is usually associated hindfoot varus. Determine whether hindfoot varus is fixed by the Coleman block test (Fig. 167.9). This test differentiates between rigid varus, which must be surgically treated by triple arthrodesis, and varus secondary to first metatarsal depression, which is flexible and corrects once the medial column cavus has been corrected using midfoot dorsal wedge osteotomy.

If cavus is severe and disabling in a young child, plantar release and metatarsal osteotomies can successfully temporize while the foot matures. However, bony procedures at maturity (after age 11 or 12 years) almost always are required, even after earlier soft-tissue release.

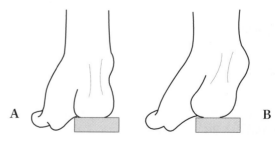

Figure 167.9.   Coleman block test. A block is placed beneath the heel and the fifth metatarsal head while the patient stands. **A:** The heel varus corrects, indicating hindfoot flexibility. **B:** Heel varus persists, indicating hindfoot rigidity.

DORSAL WEDGE OSTEOTOMY OF THE CUNEIFORMS

Dorsal wedge osteotomy of the cuneiforms is appropriate only if the hindfoot varus is flexible and fully correctable; otherwise, perform triple arthrodesis with appropriate wedge resection (see Chapter 115). Plan the osteotomy on a lateral radiographs of the foot so that the correction will bring the forefoot plantigrade when the hindfoot is in the weight-bearing position.

- Make a longitudinal midline dorsal incision from the mid talus to the base of the third metatarsal.
- Identify and protect the dorsal is pedis vessels, and incise the periosteum from the navicular to the cuneiform bones.
- Strip the periosteal and capsular structures medially and laterally to expose the cuneiforms dorsally, as far as the cuboid laterally and to the navicular medially.
- Under image intensification, insert two guide pins at the osteotomy edges, avoiding the talonavicular and cuneiform–metatarsal joints; converge the pins so that their tips meet at the plantar surface of the bones, producing a wedge large enough to correct the deformity (Fig. 167.10).
- Use an oscillating saw to cut the two faces of the wedge just inside the guide pins. Make the cut slowly, all in one pass, since the small bones shift and it is easy to lose the plane of the cut. Remove the wedge with an osteotome and a small rongeur.
- Close the wedge, correct for supination deformity, and carefully align the rotation of the forefoot with the

hindfoot. Fix the osteotomy with dorsal staples, or crossed smooth Steinmann pins or K-wires inserted from medially and laterally through the metatarsal bases.

- Close the wound with absorbable sutures.
- Apply a padded splint or a short-leg cast in neutral dorsiflexion. It is usually necessary to split the cast.

Aftercare
Change to a cast in neutral position when swelling in the foot resolves. Allow, but do not force, weight bearing as tolerated. Continue casting until union occurs, which is usually 6–8 weeks.

POLYDACTYLY

Polydactyly is a hereditary foot deformity inherited with an autosomal dominant pattern. The most common form is postaxial duplication of the fifth digit. Less common is preaxial duplication of the great toe. Rarest is middle toe duplication. Both preaxial and postaxial polydactyly may be associated with syndromes, which you should look for. The hand is often involved as well; when this is the case, the foot deformities are usually more severe than the hand deformities in that the duplications are more proximal. Generally, it is desirable to treat polydactyly of the toes because untreated patients experience difficulty with fitting shoes. In addition, extra digits, even though asymptomatic, can subject a child to ridicule from peers (9, 25,35).

POSTAXIAL POLYDACTYLY

In most postaxial (lesser toe) deformities, it is generally easiest and most effective to remove the peripheral (lateral) toes. The metatarsal is nearly always abnormal, ranging from a widened lateral metatarsal, through Y- or T-shaped distal metatarsals, to duplication of the entire bone. You must shave a widened or prominent metatarsal to reduce the width of the foot, or a bunionette will result. Preoperative radiographs are important for planning, because occasionally there is an obvious internal (central) duplication that requires more complex reconstruction. In such a case, it is desirable to preserve the toe that is more functional and has the best axial alignment. A risk of removing the intercalary digit may be the development of an angular deformity of the lateral toe. It may therefore be necessary to create a partial syndactyly between the remaining lateral toe and the fourth toe to prevent this from occurring. If the metatarsal is duplicated, you must remove this as well (Fig. 167.11).

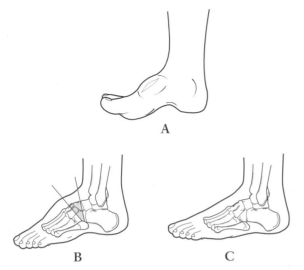

Figure 167.10. Dorsal wedge osteotomy for cavus foot. **A:** Dorsal skin incision. **B:** Bone resection is guided by K-wires. Talonavicular, calcaneocuboid, and tarsometatarsal joints are preserved. **C:** Closure of osteotomy corrects cavus. Residual pronation must be corrected as the osteotomy is closed.

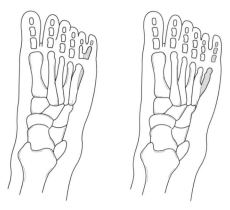

Figure 167.11. Examples of resection required (*shaded area*) for postaxial toe duplication correction. Trim the metatarsal so there is no lateral prominence.

RESECTION OF A SIXTH TOE

- To resect a sixth toe, make a dorsal curvilinear incision over the base of the toe (Fig.167.12). Make a longitudinal dorsal cut down the middle of the digit to be excised, and fillet it out.
- If the proximal phalanges of toes five and six are joined, cut the cartilaginous portion cleanly with a scalpel. Trim the metatarsal head to the size of a normal bone, using a sharp scalpel and osteotome; growth arrest will not occur. Wrap up the plantar flap dorsally, trim it, and stitch it with fine absorbable suture.
- Resect a fifth toe as a wedge, including the digit and any rudimentary metatarsal.
- Bring the fourth and sixth digits together, closing this wedge.

- Perform syndactylization if appropriate when drifting of the remaining toes is likely.
- A short-leg cast can be used for 3 or 4 weeks to allow the wounds to heal and the toes to stabilize.

HINTS AND TRICKS

If the postaxial digits are congenitally syndactylized, the principles of reconstruction remain the same. Preserve the most functional digits. A duplication of the nail frequently exists. It is important to carefully resect the nail and its matrix with the digit to be sacrificed to prevent recurrence of an abnormal nail. Plan skin flaps carefully.

PREAXIAL POLYDACTYLY

Preaxial duplications present a much more complex problem in reconstruction than postaxial duplications. Each of these reconstructions must be planned individually. The first metatarsal may be shortened and have a longitudinal epiphyseal bracket epiphysis that has an L or a C shape and acts as a medial tether to the growth of the toe (Fig. 167.13) (18,24). The hallux itself may be in varus. If a

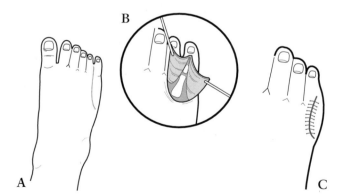

Figure 167.12. Excision of sixth digit. **A:** Curved dorsal incision and longitudinal sixth toe incision. **B:** Dorsal exposure of sixth toe allows complete excision and any necessary metatarsal trimming. **C:** Filleted skin flap is pulled dorsally, shaped, and closed. The resulting scar is dorsal and does not rub against shoewear.

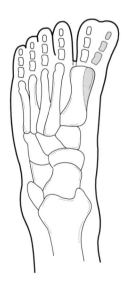

Figure 167.13. Duplicated first toe is frequently associated with a short, rounded first metatarsal with an epiphysis that surrounds both ends and the medial side of the bone—a longitudinal epiphyseal bracket. Excision (*shaded area*) at the time of toe removal may allow more normal longitudinal growth of the first metatarsal; failure to recognize this may lead to a very short first ray at maturity.

longitudinal epiphyseal bracket is present, central physeal lysis has been reported to be successful. The results of reconstruction of preaxial polydactyly can be disappointing. Residual or recurrent hallux varus occurs frequently and difficulties with shoe wear are common complications. Consider syndactylization of the first and second toes in the more difficult cases, especially if there is a recurrent deformity.

We recommend excising the toe that will allow the foot and remaining toes to assume the most normal contour. In most cases, this is the most medial or tibial toe in patients with duplication of the hallux. Sometimes it is appropriate to excise the tibial toe even if the second toe is more hypoplastic, since the risk of hallux varus is less. If a longitudinal epiphyseal bracket is present, excise the central portion of the bracket epiphysis. Because hallux varus has been the most common and most symptomatic long-term problem following surgery on duplicated great toes, make an effort to reinsert the adductor hallucis muscle into the proximal phalanx of the great toe. In addition, consider a partial syndactyly of the great and second toes. Syndactylization may be necessary at a separate procedure if extensive dissection would be necessary on both sides of the toe, resulting in an endangered blood supply. This combination of reconstructive procedures leads to an acceptable result for shoe wear. The cosmetic result is often less than satisfactory.

JUVENILE HALLUX VALGUS

Bunions, or hallux valgus deformities, are relatively common problems in children and adolescents (6,7,31). The incidence is unknown. It occurs much more commonly in girls than boys. Ill-fitting shoes have been implicated as a causative factor in adult hallux valgus, but the association of shoe wear with juvenile hallux valgus is unclear. There is often a positive family history. The deformity is usually bilateral. The age of onset may be as young as 10 years of age.

The general indications for surgical intervention are problems with shoe wear and dissatisfaction with the cosmetic appearance of the foot. Despite the fact that surgical intervention is noted to have a high failure rate, most reports on the correction of juvenile hallux valgus have presented the results of a single, specific technique of surgical reconstruction. We agree with Coughlin (6) that the operative procedure to correct juvenile hallux valgus must be customized to the specific deformities in the foot. Surgical correction prior to epiphyseal closure is controversial. Whereas there is rarely a rush to perform surgery to correct the deformities of juvenile hallux valgus, the notion that surgery performed on a patient with an open epiphysis is contraindicated has not been substantiated.

In assessing the patient with juvenile hallux valgus, obtain an AP weight-bearing radiograph of the foot. Measure the following: (a) the hallux valgus angle, (b) the first-to-second intermetatarsal angle, (c) the distal metatarsal articular angle, and (d) the first metatarsophalangeal joint congruency (the relationship of the articular surface of the base of the proximal phalanx to the articular surface of the 1st metatarsal) (Figs. 167.14, 167.15).

Operative procedures to correct juvenile hallux valgus can be grouped into four categories:

1. Distal soft-tissue procedures, such as the McBride operation. In most series, this has been associated with a high recurrence rate.
2. Distal metatarsal osteotomies, such as a chevron osteotomy or a Mitchell osteotomy. These procedures have a relatively high rate of patient satisfaction. They should be used for patients with less severe deformities

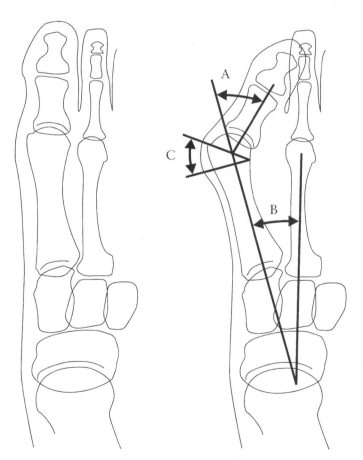

Figure 167.14. Lines used for assessing patient with juvenile hallux valgus. Normal values are in *parentheses.* **A:** Hallux valgus angle (<15°). **B:** First-to-second intermetatarsal angle (<9°). **C:** Distal metatarsal articular angle (useful for assessing subluxation and congruency).

and a relatively normal distal metatarsal articular angle. These procedures can be modified if the distal metatarsal articular angle is abnormal (see the fourth category).

3. A proximal metatarsal osteotomy with a distal soft-tissue procedure. These procedures can be used successfully in moderate hallux valgus deformities with fibular valgus subluxation of the metatarsophalangeal joint but are less successful in correcting a patient with a congruent joint and an increased distal metatarsal articular angle.

4. Double metatarsal osteotomies. We believe that this is the best method of correction in a patient with an increased first-to-second intermetatarsal angle and an increased distal metatarsal articular angle with a congruent joint. The proximal osteotomy corrects the first-to-second intermetatarsal angle (Fig. 167.16A), and the distal osteotomy corrects the hallux valgus and the increased distal metatarsal articular angle (Fig. 167.16B). The distal osteotomy can be a chevron or Mitchell type, with more bone resected on the tibial side of the osteotomy than on the fibular side.

These procedures are covered in more detail in Chapter 112. No one standard operation is suited for all juvenile patients with hallux valgus. Versatility is the surgeon's most important asset when treating the juvenile bunion. It is important not to stretch the indications for a particular technique to correct the deformity.

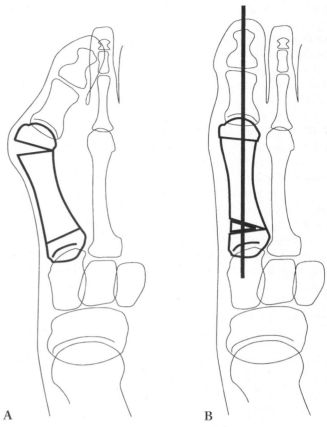

A   B

Figure 167.16. Double metatarsal osteotomy is used when a patient with hallux valgus has an increase of both the first-to-second intermetatarsal angle and the distal metatarsal angle. The proximal cut can be as shown or crescentic. The distal cut may also be a chevron type, with more resection on the tibial side of the osteotomy. **A:** The osteotomies. **B:** Completion of osteotomies and fixation with a longitudinal Kirschner wire.

TARSAL COALITION

Tarsal coalition (9,23) is a congenital fusion between two or more of the tarsal bones. The coalition can be a true bony fusion, or a cartilaginous or fibrous connection. The overall incidence of tarsal coalitions is unknown, but many are inherited with an autosomal dominant pattern. Many tarsal coalitions are not symptomatic and therefore go unrecognized. The most common symptomatic tarsal coalitions occur between the calcaneus and the talus, and between the calcaneus and the navicular. Complex coalitions also accompany fibular hemimelia and proximal femoral focal deficiency, but these rarely require treatment.

Pain is the principal presenting symptom, occurring when the coalition or bar begins to ossify. The usual age of onset is the second decade of life. The most common clinical finding is restriction of subtalar motion. The hind-

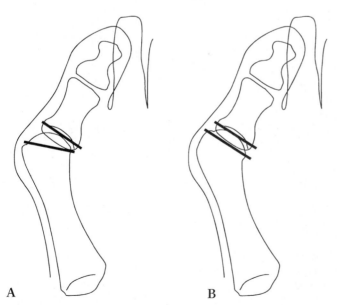

A   B

Figure 167.15. The first metatarsal phalangeal joint may be incongruent (**A**) with lateral subluxation of the joint, or congruent (**B**) with a tilted distal metatarsal articular surface.

foot is in valgus, and the patient may experience peroneal muscle spasm exhibiting in a rigid flatfoot. An attempt to invert the hindfoot, especially as a rapid maneuver, causes an increase in pain.

For radiographic evaluation, take AP, lateral, and oblique radiographs of the foot. The best radiographic view to detect a calcaneonavicular bar is the 45° oblique view (Fig. 167.17A). A lateral radiograph of the foot or of the ankle will usually demonstrate the so-called ant-eater nose sign, which is elongation of the anterosuperior aspect of the calcaneus as it is directed toward the navicular.

A talocalcaneal bar is much more difficult to demonstrate on plain radiographs. Oblique subtalar (Harris) views can be helpful, but often the best study to demonstrate a medial subtalar coalition is a computerized tomographic examination. When done in the coronal plane, this study usually successfully demonstrates talocalcaneal coalition.

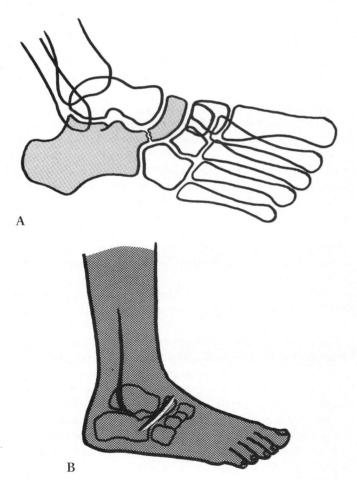

A

B

Figure 167.17. Tarsal coalition. **A:** Calcaneonavicular coalition is best visualized on a 45° oblique radiograph. **B:** Incision used to resect calcaneonavicular coalition.

The treatment of a symptomatic tarsal coalition is initially conservative. Start with 4–6 weeks of immobilization in a short-leg walking cast. If this and other conservative measures fail, consider resection of the tarsal coalition if the child is still young, particularly when some subtalar motion is present. Results are generally favorable with resection of calcaneonavicular tarsal coalitions. The results are less predictable with tarsal coalitions between the talus and calcaneus. The presence of symptoms for many years and advanced degenerative changes on midfoot radiographs are contraindications for resection of the coalition. In such cases, triple arthrodesis may be appropriate.

RESECTION OF CALCANEONAVICULAR TARSAL COALITION

- Using a thigh tourniquet, make an oblique incision across the sinus tarsi from near the heel to the head of the talus, or use a horizontal incision (Fig. 167.17B). Protect the branches of the sural nerve.
- Identify the fat of the sinus tarsi and the extensor digitorum brevis muscle, and reflect them distally from their origins on the calcaneus, exposing the sinus tarsi. Leave these tissues attached distally.
- Identify the calcaneonavicular coalition. Remove the coalition as a large rectangle of bone, using an osteotome and a rongeur. The removed bone is larger than one would expect when looking at the radiograph, and it must be rectangular in shape so that there is no bony impingement in the depths of the resection.
- Demonstrate motion between the calcaneus and the navicular, and between the talus and the calcaneus after the resection is complete. Apply bone wax to the cut bony surfaces.
- Place a Bunnell suture through the origin of the extensor digitorum brevis muscle. Pass the sutures through the coalition with Keith needles, and bring them out on the medial aspect of the midfoot.
- Pull the distally based pedicle flap of fat and the extensor digitorum brevis into the space created by resection of the coalition, and tie the sutures on the medial aspect of the foot over a dental roll.
- Close the wound with absorbable sutures.
- Place the patient in a non-weight-bearing cast for 3–4 weeks until soft tissues are healed. Generally, motion is regained over the following 6 weeks.

RESECTION OF MEDIAL SUBTALAR COALITIONS

Surgical resection of talocalcaneal tarsal coalitions is more controversial. In our opinion, it seems reasonable to attempt resection of the subtalar coalition when there are no associated degenerative changes in the joints of the foot. It has been observed that resection of even the more sizable subtalar tarsal coalitions can be successful. If the operation fails, a subtalar or triple arthrodesis can be a satisfactory salvage procedure. The technique involves a medial approach to the medial facet of the subtalar joint. Determine the exact location and size of the coalition preoperatively with coronal plane computerized tomography.

- Under pneumatic tourniquet, make a horizontal incision over the sustentaculum tali.
- Retract the muscle fibers of the abductor hallucis longus plantarward and divide the flexor retinaculum over the sustentaculum.
- Retract the FDL and neurovascular bundle plantarward.
- Identify the FHL (which is just beneath the sustentaculum tali) and retract it plantarward.
- Retract the posterior tibial tendon, above the sustentaculum, dorsally.
- Reflect the periosteum off the sustentaculum tali. Do this with care so that you can later approximate it to hold a fat graft in place.
- Identify the anterior and posterior boundaries of the coalition. We excise the coalition using a high-speed burr, gradually taking away bone until we identify the normal posterior facet of the subtalar joint. You must visualize the joint cartilage anteriorly, posteriorly, and laterally through the site of the excision. Once the excision is completed, subtalar motion should improve.
- The final step is to interpose fat between the two bony surfaces. You can obtain the fat locally, through a small incision at the ankle, or from a separate incision made in the suprapubic area, which gives a cosmetically invisible scar when the patient becomes more mature. Seal the resected bony surfaces with bone wax, and carefully push the fat graft into the defect created by the excision. Hold it in place by approximating the periosteum with sutures.
- Close the wound.
- Place the patient in a short-leg, non-weight-bearing cast for 4 weeks, and then allow progressive weight bearing as tolerated.

TRIPLE ARTHRODESIS

If resection of the tarsal coalition fails to relieve the patient's symptoms, triple arthrodesis is a successful salvage procedure. You can use it as a secondary procedure after a failed attempt at coalition resection, or as a primary procedure when the coalition is extremely large, symptoms have extended for years, or degenerative changes are present. This procedure is generally successful in relieving the pain associated with tarsal coalition. Techniques of triple arthrodesis are described in Chapter 115.

CONGENITAL VERTICAL TALUS

Congenital vertical talus (CVT), also know as congenital convex pes valgus, is a complex, rare, foot deformity that is resistant to conservative treatment. There is a continuum from a relatively mild, flexible form (oblique talus) to a rigid, severe deformity characterized by a plantarflexed talus, hindfoot equinus, and dorsal dislocations of the talonavicular and calcaneocuboid joints. The heel is always in rigid valgus. There are contractures of the Achilles tendon, peroneus tertius, long-toe extensors, and tibialis anterior muscle (Fig. 167.18). Lateral roentgenographs taken in full dorsi- and plantarflexion differentiate the more flexible oblique talus from the severe variety; oblique talus exhibits severe deformity in dorsiflexion but a relatively normal relation between the talus and calcaneus in full plantar flexion (16).

In more than 80% of cases, CVT is associated with other anomalies and syndromes (Marfan's syndrome, arthrogryposis, multiple pterygium syndrome), genetic abnormalities (trisomy 13–15, trisomy 18), or neuromuscular defects (myelomeningocele) (16). Unless the cause of the anomaly is clear, perform a thorough neuromuscular and genetic workup. Many children with CVT who would otherwise be candidates for surgery are wheelchair bound and can be treated by protecting the foot with a soft tennis shoe.

When indicated, treatment of rigid CVT is always surgical. Most experts recommend preliminary casting to mobilize the skin, but casting does not correct the bony deformity. Single-stage correction usually involves mobilization and reduction of all subluxed joints, internal fixation, and appropriate soft-tissue repair with transfer of the anterior tibial tendon to the neck of the talus to maintain dorsiflexion of the talus and minimize heel valgus (16,30).

The other commonly used approach is a two-stage method, with the procedures spaced 6–8 weeks apart (5). In this approach, first reduce the dorsally dislocated midfoot through an anterior incision, and lengthen contracted toe extensors and anterior tibialis muscles. Stabilize the subtalar joint in appropriate position with a subtalar bone block. Six weeks later, release the posterior ankle and subtalar joints, lengthen the heel cord, and reconstruct the anteriorly displaced posterior tibial muscle to support the talar head and neck. Whereas many surgeons attempt correction by soft-tissue means, this approach (using a subtalar fusion) can be highly effective in difficult cases.

Seimon (27) has described correction of deformities in CVT with a single dorsolateral longitudinal incision and a percutaneous posterior release. This procedure has been used with excellent success in patients under the age of 2 years.

Surgery is ideally done at 4–6 months of age, although accompanying anomalies and illnesses often require post-

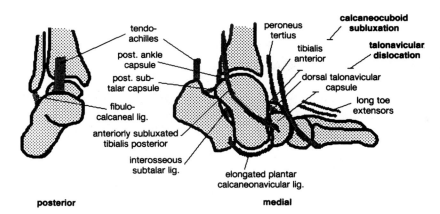

Figure 167.18. Contractures involved in severe congenital vertical talus.

ponement to age 1 year or later. After the age of 2 to 5 years, reduction is difficult unless the foot is decompressed by navicular excision (3). Partial talectomy and decancellation of the tarsal bones may be required. Triple arthrodesis may be necessary in neglected or severe cases, and it may be necessary in maturity even when surgery early in life has corrected the gross deformity. This is especially true when tarsal bones are excised, leading to late degenerative arthritis.

DORSOLATERAL APPROACH

- Approach the dorsolateral aspect of the foot with either an oblique incision or a longitudinal incision over the mid-dorsum of the foot (27).
- Lengthen the extensor digitorum longus and peroneus tertius tendons. Accomplish digital extensor lengthening by dividing a portion of the tendons proximally and a portion distally, and suturing the long proximal stumps to the long distal stumps in the elongated position.
- Identify the neurovascular bundle. Retract the tibialis anterior and extensor hallucis longus tendons medially.
- Generally, the peroneal tendons are contracted and lengthening is necessary.
- Divide the dorsal and lateral talonavicular joint capsule. This allows the navicular to be readily reduced onto the head of the talus. The dorsal and lateral calcaneocuboid capsule may require release as well. You can elongate the tibialis anterior and extensor hallucis longus tendons if they are obstacles to an easy reduction.
- Transfix the talonavicular joint with a smooth K-wire. If the calcaneocuboid joint is released (or subluxated), transfix it as well. Take care to correct midfoot supination when fixing these joints.
- Lengthen the Achilles tendon percutaneously.
- You may perform posterior capsulotomies of the ankle and subtalar joint to come to equinus, but usually this is not required.

- Once the hindfoot has been corrected, pass a second K-wire from the plantar aspect of the heel through the calcaneus and talus into the tibia.
- Apply an above-knee cast to be worn for 6 weeks. After 6 weeks, remove the two K-wires and apply a below-knee cast to be worn for a further 6 weeks.

SINGLE-STAGE REPAIR

- Make three incisions (Fig. 167.19): The first is concave downward over the medial talonavicular joint; the second is oblique over the sinus tarsi to expose the calca-

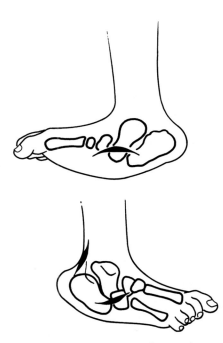

Figure 167.19. Preferred incisions for single-stage repair of congenital vertical talus (medial and lateral views).

neocuboid joint and peroneal and extensor tendons; the third is along the lateral border of the Achilles tendon to allow posterior release.

■ Begin laterally and make the dorsolateral approach already described. Inspect the calcaneocuboid joint, and release its capsule as necessary to correct lateral column alignment.

■ In the medial wound, divide the dorsal talonavicular (deltoid) ligament and open the capsule of the dorsolateral talonavicular joint.

■ Subluxate the posterior tibial tendon superiorly; divide it and tag it for later repair.

■ The navicular is riding on the anterior talar neck; continue mobilizing the joint capsules dorsally through both incisions until the midfoot can be brought into plantar flexion, with reduction of the talonavicular and calcaneocuboid joints.

■ Through the posterior incision, perform Z-lengthening of the Achilles tendon with the distal transverse cut directed laterally; tag the ends with #0 absorbable synthetic suture.

■ Incise or excise the posterior capsules of the ankle and subtalar joints, and release the contracted fibulocalcaneal ligament and tendon sheaths of the peroneals by cutting circumferentially with small scissors. In severe cases, the interosseous subtalar ligament may require full or partial release.

■ Reduce the talonavicular joint and pin it with a K-wire directed from the posterior tuberosity of the talus through the center of the joint. Bring the pin out anteriorly and bend it to prevent migration.

■ Check the ankle to be sure there is adequate dorsiflexion and slight heel varus. Obtain an intraoperative lateral radiograph. The first metatarsal axis should line up exactly with the long axis of the talus; if it does not, repeat the preceding steps until it is correct.

■ Repair the talonavicular joint capsule by reefing the elongated plantar calcaneonavicular ligament and remaining capsule, and repair the posterior tibial tendon, sewing it beneath the talar head and neck to assist in support.

■ Release the origin of the anterior tibial tendon and transfer it to the midtalar neck, using a drill hole and sewing it to itself, to prevent abnormal plantar flexion of the talus; in the young child, make a small gutter in the medial cartilage of the talar neck and sew the tendon over this and into the soft tissues below the neck (Fig. 167.20).

■ Repair the Achilles tendon with the heel in neutral position.

■ Close the skin with fine interrupted absorbable synthetic suture.

■ Apply a long-leg cast, molded in the arch. Change the cast at 3-week intervals; it is worn for 4 months. Often

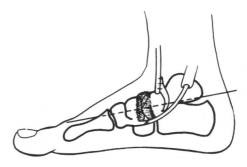

Figure 167.20. A completed repair of congenital vertical talus. See text for details.

a reverse Perlstein brace or AFO is necessary for 1–2 years.

Feet with CVT are invariably somewhat stiff after surgery; a normal foot never can be obtained. Persevere to obtain a plantigrade foot that fits easily into normal shoes and that has no pain or pressure sores. Late subtalar or triple arthrodesis may be required. The vertical talus associated with myelomeningocele or cerebral palsy may require modifications of the surgical treatment and individualized tendon transfer to achieve a balanced foot.

PITFALLS AND COMPLICATIONS

Do not miss associated anomalies and conditions. Misdiagnosis can lead to a poor outcome or, worse, a serious complication when there is serious associated systemic disease or other disorders.

Precise, careful surgical technique is necessary to avoid neuromas from inadvertently cutting superficial sensory nerves, more serious injury to the main neurovascular bundles and tendons, and skin sloughs. In small feet, magnifying loupes are quite helpful.

Avoid incomplete correction or overcorrection, particularly the latter as it is more difficult to correct, by careful preoperative planning.

REFERENCES

Each reference is categorized according to the following scheme: *, classic article; #, review article; !, basic research article; and +, clinical results/outcome study.

+ 1. Berman A, Gartland JJ. Metatarsal Osteotomy for the

Correction of Adduction of the Forepart of the Foot in Children. *J Bone Joint Surg Am* 1971;53:498.

\# 2. Carroll N. Pathoanatomy and Surgical Treatment of the Resistant Clubfoot. *Instr Course Lect* 1998;37:93.

\+ 3. Clark MW, D'Ambrosia RD, Ferguson AB Jr. Congential Vertical Talus: Treatment by Open Reduction and Navicular Excision. *J Bone Joint Surg Am* 1977;59:816.

\# 4. Coleman SS. *Complex Foot Deformities in Children.* Philadelphia: Lea & Febiger, 1983.

\+ 5. Coleman SS, Stelling FH, Jarrett J. Pathomechanics and Treatment of Congenital Vertical Talus. *Clin Orthop* 1970;70:62.

\+ 6. Coughlin MJ. Juvenile Hallux Valgus: Etiology and Treatment. *Foot Ankle Int* 1995;16:682.

\# 7. Coughlin MJ, Mann RA. The Pathophysiology of the Juvenile Bunion. *Instr Course Lect* 1987;36:123.

\+ 8. Crawford AH, Marxen JL, Osterfield DL. The Cincinnati Incision: A Comprehensive Approach for Surgical Procedures of the Foot and Ankle in Childhood. *J Bone Joint Surg Am* 1982;64:1355.

\# 9. Drennan JC. *The Child's Foot and Ankle.* New York: Raven Press, 1992.

\+ 10. Evans D. Relapsed Clubfoot. *J Bone Joint Surg Br* 1961;43:722.

\+ 11. Fisher RL, Shaffer SR. An Evaluation of the Calcaneal Osteotomy in Congenital Clubfoot and Other Disorders. *Clin Orthop* 1970;70:141.

* 12. Garceau GJ. Anterior Tibial Tendon Transfer for Recurrent Clubfoot. *Clin Orthop* 1972;84:61.

\+ 13. Hoffer MM, Reiswig JA, Garrett AM, Perry J. The Split Anterior Tibial Tendon Transfer in the Treatment of Spastic Varus Hindfoot of Childhood. *Orthop Clin North Am* 1974;5:31.

* 14. Irani RN, Sherman MS. The Pathological Anatomy of Clubfoot. *J Bone Joint Surg Am* 1972;45:45.

* 15. Kite HJ. Nonoperative Treatment of Congenital Clubfoot. *Clin Orthop* 1972;84:29.

\# 16. Kumar SJ, Cowell HR, Ramsey PL. Foot Problems in Children. Part I. Vertical and Oblique Talus. *Instr Course Lect* 1982;31:235.

\+ 17. Lichtblau S. A Medial and Lateral Release Operation for Clubfoot. A Preliminary Report. *J Bone Joint Surg Am* 1973;55:1377.

\+ 18. Light TR, Ogden JA. The Longitudinal Epiphyseal Bracket, Implications for Surgical Correction. *J Pediatr Orthop* 1981;1:299.

\+ 19. McHale KA, Lenhart MK. Treatment of Residual Clubfoot Deformity—The "Bean-Shaped" Foot—By Opening Wedge Medial Cuneiform Osteotomy and Closing Wedge Cuboid Osteotomy. *J Pediatr Orthop* 1991;11:374.

\+ 20. McKay DW. New Concept of and an Approach to Clubfoot Treatment. Section I. Principles and Morbid Anatomy. *J Pediatr Orthop* 1982;2:347.

\+ 21. McKay DW. New Concept of and an Approach to Clubfoot Treatment. Section II. Correction of the Clubfoot. *J Pediatr Orthop* 1983;3:10.

\+ 22. McKay DW. New Concept of and an Approach to Clubfoot Treatment. Section III. Evaluation and Results. *J Pediatr Orthop* 1983;3:141.

\# 23. Morrissy RT. *Atlas of Pediatric Orthopaedic Surgery.* Philadelphia: Lippincott-Raven, 1996.

\+ 24. Mubarak SJ, et al. Metatarsal Epiphyseal Bracket: Treatment by Central Physiolysis. *J Pediatr Orthop* 1993;13:124.

\+ 25. Phelps DA, Grogan DP. Polydactyly of the Foot. *J Pediatr Orthop* 1985;5:446.

* 26. Poseti IV, Smoley EM. Congenital Clubfoot: The Results of Treatment. *J Bone Joint Surg Am* 1963;45:261.

\+ 27. Seimon LP. Surgical Correction of Congenital Vertical Talus under the Age of Two Years. *J Pediatr Orthop* 1987;7:405.

\+ 28. Simons GW. Complete Subtalar Release in Clubfeet. Part I. *J Bone Joint Surg Am* 1985;67:1044.

\+ 29. Simons GW. Complete Subtalar Release in Clubfeet. Part II. *J Bone Joint Surg Am* 1985;67:1056.

\# 30. Tachdjian MO. Congenital Convex Pes Valgus. *Orthop Clin North Am* 1972;3:131.

\# 31. Thompson GH. Bunions and Deformities of the Toes in Children and Adolescents. *Instr Course Lect* 1996;45:355.

\+ 32. Turco VJ. Surgical Correction of the Resistant Clubfoot. *J Bone Joint Surg Am* 1971;53:477.

\# 33. Turco VJ. *Clubfoot.* New York: Churchill-Livingstone, 1981.

\+ 34. Turner JW, Cooper RR. Anterior Transfer of the Tibialis Posterior through the Interosseous Membrane. *Clin Orthop* 1972;83:241.

\# 35. Venn-Watson EA. Problems in Polydactyly of the Foot. *Orthop Clin North Am* 1976;7:909.

## CHAPTER 168

SURGICAL MANAGEMENT OF TORSIONAL DEFORMITIES OF THE LOWER EXTREMITIES

Vincent S. Mosca and Lynn T. Staheli

The most common reason for children to seek orthopaedic evaluation, except perhaps for trauma, is for suspected torsional or angular deformities of the lower extremities. Most of these children are normal. Studies have shown that measurements of torsion and angulation in children have wide ranges of normal values and that these values change spontaneously with age until they reach the narrower adult normal ranges (3,15,17,21,22).

Values within two standard deviations of the mean are termed *physiologic variations*. Those beyond two standard deviations are called *deformities*.

It is the role of the orthopaedist to identify the few true torsional or angular deformities, as well as to identify disease entities that mimic or resemble these deformities. Do this with a careful history and clinical assessment. Perform the torsional profile examination and document it for all children who are referred for evaluation of their

lower extremities or gait abnormalities (18). Clinical photographs are helpful for documentation, especially for serial evaluations. Accurate anatomic diagnosis can be made by routine radiographs for angular deformities and biplane radiographs or computed tomography (CT) scan for torsional deformities. These studies are reserved for severe deformities and for preoperative planning.

Having ruled out true deformities and other disease entities, convince the parents (and grandparents) that the apparent deformity is a normal finding, although it may not represent the average value. Point out that the apparent deformity will probably become "more normal" with time. There is no convincing evidence that orthotic management of torsional or angular variations or deformities has any beneficial effect over simple observation of the natural history alone (4,10). Therefore, the management decision is between observation with parent education, and surgery.

The parents' main concern is usually the child's appearance. Education about natural history, the uselessness and expense of orthotic devices, and the cost–benefit ratio of

---

V. S. Mosca and L. T. Staheli: Children's Hospital and Regional Medical Center, Seattle, Washington, 98105.

surgery establishes a rational basis for the observational approach. If the parents are not convinced, see their child yearly and review the torsional or angular profile with them. Clinical photographs are most helpful in this setting. Also stress that even if full spontaneous correction of torsional variations does not occur, the child may be able to volitionally change the foot-progression angle when self-appearance takes on increased meaning during adolescence.

Function is frequently the family's second concern. One study has shown that severe medial femoral torsion appears to adversely affect running, but a moderate amount of torsion does not (23). Marked genu valgum appears to adversely affect running performances as well, but this has not been documented.

Although secondary deformities have been attributed to some variations, only the concurrence of lateral tibial torsion with medial femoral torsion in late childhood has been documented (5). Likewise, genu valgum is often associated with foot pronation, but a cause-and-effect relationship has not been documented.

A final concern about torsional or angular variations or deformities is the development of arthritis (6,8,9,11,12,24,25). No documentation to date proves a cause-and-effect relationship between such variations or deformities and arthritis of the hip or patellofemoral joint.

It follows from the foregoing that indications for surgery for torsional or angular variations or deformities are extremely narrow. Because of the natural tendency for rotational deformities to remodel and improve with growth, surgical treatment is not indicated in children under 10–12 years of age. The decision hinges primarily on cosmetic concerns in the adolescent.

In most cases, variations or deformities are bilateral and often at more than one level; for example, medial femoral torsion often accompanies lateral tibial torsion. Surgical correction at one level frequently necessitates surgical correction at the other level. Staged unilateral surgery prolongs the period of temporary disability. Simultaneous bilateral surgery increases the extent of temporary disability.

The risk of complications from surgery is quite high. A 15% complication rate was found in a review of operative treatment for medial femoral torsion alone (20). In another study, a 13% incidence of peroneal nerve palsy was reported following proximal tibial rotational osteotomies if the fibula was not osteotomized (16).

Indications for surgery are subjective and must be individualized. The patient's general body habitus, the torsional and angular profile at all levels, the patient's emotional and psychologic makeup, and the torsional and angular variations of other family members must be considered. With these parameters carefully evaluated and in perspective, consider surgical correction when (a) femoral rotation values are more than three standard deviations

from the mean, (b) tibial rotation values are more than four standard deviations from the mean, or (c) there is more than 25° of genu valgum in a child older than 8 years. A busy, full-time pediatric orthopaedist may find one or two torsional or angular variations or deformities per year that require surgery. The operations to be described are used much more frequently to correct the anteversion and coxa valga in cerebral palsy, the lateral tibial torsion with ankle valgus in myelodysplasia, and the angular deformities from old infection, partial physeal arrest, metabolic disorders, ischemia, ionizing irradiation, or genetic conditions.

FEMORAL ROTATIONAL OSTEOTOMIES

Femoral rotational osteotomies can be carried out proximally, in the mid shaft, or distally. The intertrochanteric region of the femur is the preferred site for proximal osteotomies (19). Osteotomy at this level is safe, heals rapidly, and leaves an acceptable cosmetic scar. The intertrochanteric region is usually the site of the pathology and is easily accessible. The essence of the problem is torsional malalignment of the femoral neck and shaft, and it is in the intertrochanteric region that these two anatomic structures meet. If proximal femoral angulation is a problem in addition to torsion, simultaneous corrections can be made with osteotomy at this level. The technique and instrumentation for intertrochanteric osteotomy are simple and no special training or equipment is required. Early partial weight bearing is possible when rigid internal fixation is used.

Closed, mid-shaft, intramedullary rotational osteotomy of the femur is an alternative for the older adolescent in whom there is adequate intramedullary shaft diameter and little concern about iatrogenic arrest of the greater trochanter (26,27). The utility of this operation in the immature child, however, is limited both by its complexity and by the small but real risk of avascular necrosis of the femoral head related to the proximal insertion site for the nail. The scar is acceptable cosmetically and the patient may bear weight immediately. Special expertise and equipment are required, and after surgery the femur may tend to derotate around the rod unless a locked nail is used. Some angular deformities can be corrected simultaneously (see Chapter 30).

Distal femoral osteotomy in the supracondylar region gives the least acceptable scar, runs the highest risk of potential injury to growth plates, is more likely to leave residual angulation, and is farthest from the site of pathology, unless there is an associated marked patella-tracking problem (7).

OPERATIVE TECHNIQUES

Proximal Femoral Rotational Osteotomy

Use preoperative planning with radiographs and templates to determine which blade-plate angle will permit entrance of the blade just distal to the greater trochanteric apophysis, and to determine seating of the tip of the blade in the inferior proximal femoral neck.

- Place the patient supine on a radiolucent operating table extension to permit use of the image intensifier. Place folded towels under the buttocks in such a way as to allow the lateral soft tissues of the buttocks and thigh to overhang the edge of the towels. Isolate the perineum with an adherent plastic drape. Prepare both lower extremities from the iliac crests over most of the hemipelvis down to the toes.
- Make a straight lateral longitudinal incision extending distally from the greater trochanter. Incise the fascia lata longitudinally. Incise the vastus lateralis transversely just distal to the vastus ridge, and then longitudinally just anterior to the linea aspera. Bring the transverse cut in the vastus lateralis anteromedially, sufficient to see the base of the femoral neck. This creates an L-shaped flap of the muscle that can be easily reattached at the completion of the procedure.
- Expose the femur subperiosteally. Carefully incise the linea aspera with a scalpel at the proposed level of the osteotomy. Attempts at blunt elevation are difficult and may result in plunging into highly vascularized soft tissues. Using image intensification, internally rotate the extremity until the femoral neck is in the horizontal plane. Place a Steinmann pin along the anterior femoral neck in the proposed position of the blade and use the image intensifier to confirm the appropriateness of the chosen angle (Fig. 168.1).

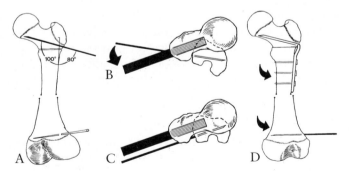

Figure 168.1. Proximal femoral rotational osteotomy with blade plate. **A:** Steinmann pin confirms appropriateness of 100° blade plate. Notice placement of distal femoral alignment pin. **B:** Initial position of distal pin and chisel. Angle represents degree of desired correction. **C:** Pin and chisel (which is actually the plate holder) aligned parallel after osteotomy. Note residual average amount of torsion. **D:** Final position with blade-plate fixation after intertrochanteric osteotomy.

- Introduce the seating chisel (13), mounted on the seating chisel guide, distal to the vastus ridge and in the anterior half of the greater trochanter when viewed laterally. Hold the chisel in the horizontal plane (which is the plane of the femoral neck as positioned earlier) and angled away from the femoral shaft by 180° minus the predetermined blade-plate angle. Most importantly, rotate the chisel until the flap of the seating chisel guide is exactly in line with the long axis of the femur. Incorrect alignment of this position will result in flexion or extension at the osteotomy site when fixing the plate to the shaft. The proximal femoral shaft must be well exposed to make this alignment possible. Insert the chisel to the desired depth under image intensifier control. Check the frog-leg lateral view as well as the anteroposterior view to guide your chisel correctly.
- Insert a smooth Steinmann pin in the distal femoral metaphysis perpendicular to the long axis of the femur and rotated away from the chisel (in the direction of the rotational deformity) by the desired degree of correction. Perform the osteotomy with an oscillating saw beginning 5–10 mm distal to the entrance point of the chisel and perpendicular to the long axis of the femur.
- Use a bone-holding clamp to stabilize the proximal fragment as the chisel is removed. Carefully insert the blade plate on the plate holder. It is vital to maintain your attention and orientation during this maneuver or the blade plate could easily find a new seat in the femoral neck. Confirm the position in two planes with the image intensifier.
- Rotate the femoral shaft until the Steinmann pin and plate holder are aligned parallel. Then clamp the plate firmly on the shaft and rotate the extremity with a finger on the osteotomy site to ensure that there is no false rotation at this level. If the arc of rotation of the extremity is as desired, the side plate can be attached to the shaft with cortical screws in the usual fashion. Make sure that the side plate sits squarely on the shaft prior to making drill holes. An oblique orientation will create undesired and uncalculated additional rotation as the screws are tightened. It is better to accept a few millimeters of translation than to accept an oblique plate. Once again, check rotation and confirm final position of instrumentation by image intensification.
- Reattach the vastus lateralis with 0 Vicryl sutures. Repair the fascia lata with the same suture material. Use an absorbable subcuticular suture for the skin.
- A soft sterile dressing is all that is required. Rigid external immobilization is not needed. The child may begin touch-down weight bearing with crutches when comfortable, usually within several days of surgery. If both femurs have been osteotomized, weight bearing is not permitted. Continue this for 6–8 weeks, at which time healing should be sufficient for full weight bearing. Re-

move the blade plate 1 year after surgery, with 6 weeks of protected weight bearing after plate removal.

Closed Intramedullary Femoral Rotational Osteotomy

Closed intramedullary femoral rotational osteotomy is described in detail in Chapter 30. A brief description follows:

- The patient can be either lateral or supine on a fracture table. Make a longitudinal incision just proximal to the greater trochanter. Incise the abductors in the direction of their fibers to expose the trochanteric recess just medial to the greater trochanter. Open the medullary canal and then pass a bulb-tipped guide down the canal. Ream the canal up to the desired diameter.
- Place a smooth Steinmann pin percutaneously in the lateral cortex of the proximal femur. Place a second pin through the lateral cortex of the distal femur rotated internally from the plane of the first pin by the desired amount of rotational correction.
- Introduce the intramedullary saw down to the mid diaphysis under image intensifier control and make the osteotomy (Fig. 168.2). Rotate the distal fragment until the two Steinmann pins are parallel; then drive the intramedullary nail. Statically lock the intramedullary nail with the osteotomy in compression. This guarantees that rotational correction will not be lost. Immediate weight bearing with assistive devices is usually possible.
- Begin crutch-assisted weight bearing when tolerated and continued for 6 weeks. Remove the nail approxi-

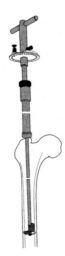

Figure 168.2. Closed femoral rotational osteotomy with an intramedullary saw. (From Winquist RA. Closed Shortening of the Femur: Utilizing a New Type of Intramedullary Saw. In: Hempel D, Fischer S, eds. *Intramedullary Nailing.* New York: Thieme-Stratton, 1982;214.)

mately 1 year after the operation or when healing is solid (see Chapter 30).

Distal Femoral Rotational Osteotomy

- Prep the entire leg and hip area free so the limb is free to move in space. Make a longitudinal incision over the posterolateral distal femur, but do not extend distally beyond the lateral epicondyle of the femur. Lift the vastus lateralis fibers from the posterior fascia lata, and incise the muscle along its femoral insertion. Take time to carefully identify and cauterize the two or three perforating vessels before dividing or tearing them.
- Strip the periosteum and retract it using a Bennett or Hohmann retractor. As the periosteum is gently stripped distally, a point of resistance will be felt; this is the region just above the physis, and dissection should not be carried more distally. An image intensifier may be used to confirm this position.
- Place a six-hole, 3.5 mm AO plate longitudinally along the femur with the distal portion just at the end of this subperiosteal dissection. Predrill, measure, record, and tap the distal three holes. Steinmann pins may be inserted proximally and distally to mark the desired rotational correction, as described before for proximal femoral osteotomy. Do not put the pins where they will interfere with the plate after derotation.
- Using an oscillating saw, make a transverse saw cut just above the proximal hole. Fix the plate to the distal three holes and rotate the femur into its corrected position, using a Lowman clamp to fix the proximal plate into place. Check clinical rotation, and, if correct, complete the fixation by attaching the proximal screws in compression. It is unnecessary to contour the plate to the minor bend of the lateral femur, since it will elastically conform, enhancing medial compression. Check rotation again, and close using absorbable sutures and subcuticular technique.
- Place the limb in a knee immobilizer and protect from weight-bearing until callus is seen medially (usually 4–6 weeks). At this time, allow weight bearing. Knee function spontaneously returns, and the plate may be electively removed at 1 year after the surgery.

COMPLICATIONS

There are few potential complications from proximal femoral rotational osteotomy other than those that accompany any surgical procedure—superficial and deep wound infections, anesthetic risk, and bleeding.

A potential complication with any form of fixation is malrotation. When using the blade plate, clamp the side plate on the femoral shaft and check rotation before inserting the screws. Also, recheck rotation after the screws have been inserted. The position may shift during screw insertion. Guide pins are not precisely accurate and final confirmation by intraoperative range of motion is required.

Rotational malunion should not occur if all the described steps are followed, and the final position is checked by image intensification and by range of motion on the table. Angular malunion can occur if the osteotomy is not precisely perpendicular to the femoral shaft. Should either occur, the same careful assessment used for the initial surgical decision should be made to determine if repeat osteotomy is indicated.

In adolescents, nonunion of femoral osteotomies in the intertrochanteric region is extremely rare. However, this could result from failure to achieve reasonable apposition of bone, or from distraction of the osteotomy by the hardware. In cases of delayed union, prolonged external immobilization or prolonged partial weight bearing is usually all that is necessary to achieve union.

The blade of the blade plate is extremely sharp and can easily miss the track left by the chisel. Maintain precise orientation during the switch and insert it by pushing manually. Check final position with the image intensifier.

Holes left in the bone after hardware removal are potential stress risers for fractures. If a blade plate has been used, there are multiple stress risers and temporary (6–8 weeks) partial weight bearing with crutches must be enforced after removal of the hardware.

If a fracture occurs, it should be treated as any intertrochanteric or subtrochanteric fracture—that is, by skin or skeletal traction followed by spica casting. Internal fixation may be used but is reserved for fractures that cannot be reduced or held well in a spica cast.

TIBIAL ROTATIONAL OSTEOTOMIES

Indications for tibial rotational osteotomies are even narrower than for femoral rotational osteotomies. They are perhaps most commonly performed in conjunction with femoral osteotomies in the case of medial femoral torsion with lateral tibial torsion. Cosmesis is the prime indication.

Preoperatively, the angle of the transmalleolar axis and the thigh–foot angle must be assessed to determine that the rotational problem is in the tibia and not in the foot. Tibial rotational osteotomy is reserved for tibial torsion problems. Transverse or coronal plane deformities of the foot should be managed by appropriate surgery on the foot.

Distal tibial rotational osteotomy is preferred for its accessibility, simplicity, safety, rapid healing, and cosmetically acceptable scar. It is also versatile in cases where rotational abnormalities are accompanied by distal angular abnormalities.

Proximal tibial osteotomy has the disadvantages of potential injury to the common peroneal nerve and the popliteal artery at its trifurcation, as well as damage to the tibial apophysis. There is a greater risk of compartment syndrome. Scars at the knee are perhaps less cosmetically acceptable than scars at the ankle.

Mid-shaft osteotomies have the disadvantages of potential for compartment syndrome and delayed union or nonunion.

For pure rotational deformity in the tibia, the advantages of distal osteotomy over proximal or mid-shaft osteotomy are overwhelming. We therefore feel there are no reasonable alternatives.

OPERATIVE TECHNIQUES

Distal Tibial Rotational Osteotomy

■ Position the patient supine on a radiolucent operating table extension. Prepare both limbs from the toes to the tourniquets on the proximal thighs (Fig. 168.3). The distal thigh and knee must be exposed in the surgical field. In the skeletally immature child, identify the distal tibial physis with the image intensifier and mark its level on the skin.

■ Make a 5 cm longitudinal incision 1–2 cm lateral and parallel to the tibial crest ending at the physeal line. Retract the anterior compartment tendons laterally and protect the anterior tibial neurovascular bundle. Incise the periosteum longitudinally down to, but not across, the physis, and expose the tibial metaphysis subperiosteally.

■ Through the same skin incision, make an extrafascial approach to the fibula between the lateral and anterior compartments. Expose the fibula subperiosteally at a level 1–2 cm proximal to the anticipated osteotomy of the tibia. Make a long oblique osteotomy with an osteotome.

■ Drill a smooth ³⁄₃₂-inch Steinmann pin into the anterior proximal tibia in the sagittal plane. Drill a second smooth pin into the distal metaphysis just proximal to the physis. This pin should be perpendicular to the long axis of the tibia and axially rotated away from the first pin (in the direction of the deformity) by the amount to be corrected. The goal is a transmalleolar axis of +20° and a corresponding thigh–foot angle of +10°.

■ Perform the osteotomy 1–1.5 cm proximal to and parallel with the physis using an oscillating saw. Then rotate the distal fragment until the two Steinmann pins are aligned parallel. Fix the osteotomy with crossed smooth ³⁄₃₂-inch Steinmann pins that enter each malleolus, cross the osteotomy, and engage the tibial cortex of the proximal fragment. Occasionally a third Steinmann pin will be needed for fixation across the osteotomy. Check fixation and bone apposition with the image intensifier. Check the angle of the transmalleolar axis and the

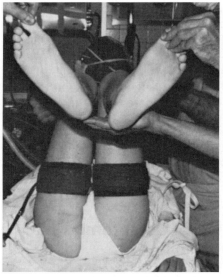
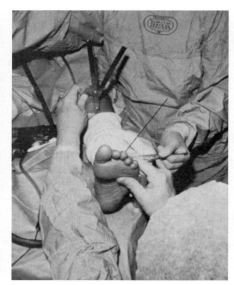
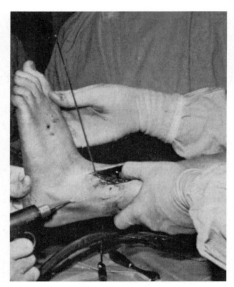

A,B

C

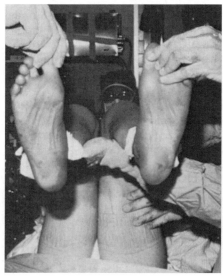

D,E

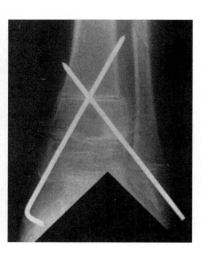

Figure 168.3. Distal tibial rotational osteotomy. **A:** Both limbs prepped and exposed up to tourniquets. **B:** Initial axial rotation between alignment pins checked with goniometer. **C:** Pins aligned parallel after osteotomy. Fixation pins enter malleoli and cross osteotomy. **D:** Final thigh–foot angle checked with hip and knee flexed 90° and also with joints in extension. **E:** Good early healing. Notice fibular osteotomy.

thigh–foot angle with the hip and knee flexed 90° and again with these joints in extension.

- Perform a blind, prophylactic, subcutaneous fasciotomy of the anterior and lateral compartments with Metzenbaum scissors. Be certain that the fascia is cut.
- Loosely reapproximate the tibial periosteal edges with 2-0 Vicryl sutures. Following irrigation and hemostasis, approximate the subcutaneous tissues with 3-0 Vicryl sutures, and approximate the skin with running subcuticular 4-0 Vicryl sutures. Bend the fixation Steinmann pins at the point they exit the skin and cut them long.
- Apply a well-padded, bent-knee, long-leg cast. A long-leg cast with 5° to 10° of knee flexion can be applied 3 weeks after surgery so partial weight bearing can begin. Remove the pins at approximately 6–8 weeks. Use ra-

diographs to determine the need for further immobilization in a short-leg cast.

COMPLICATIONS

Because you want to make the smallest incision possible, exposure of the fibula is necessarily limited. To avoid damage to the superficial peroneal nerve or the peroneal vascular structures, perform the fibular osteotomy with an osteotome.

Although the risk of compartment syndrome is lowest with distal tibial osteotomy, prophylactic subcutaneous anterior and lateral compartment fasciotomy is advised. Nevertheless, frequent careful postoperative assessment is mandatory to detect impending compartment syndrome early. Perform four-compartment fasciotomy if it occurs.

Malunion indicates failure to confirm correction intraoperatively, as described. The decision for repeat osteotomy should be made as carefully as the initial decision to operate.

Nonunion at this level is extremely unusual. Weight bearing in a cast with or without pins in place should effectively treat delayed union.

REFERENCES

Each reference is categorized according to the following scheme: *, classic article; #, review article; !, basic research article; and +, clinical results/outcome study.

 * 1. Blount WP. A Mature Look at Epiphyseal Stapling. *Clin Orthop* 1971;77:158.
 + 2. Bowen JR, Leahey JL, Zhang Z, MacEwen GD. Partial Epiphysiodesis at the Knee to Correct Angular Deformity. *Clin Orthop* 1985;198:184.
 # 3. Engel GM, Staheli LT. The Natural History of Torsion and Other Factors Influencing Gait in Childhood: A Study of the Angle of Gait, Tibial Torsion, Knee Angle, Hip Rotation, and Development of the Arch in Normal Children. *Clin Orthop* 1974;99:12.
 + 4. Fabry G. Torsion of the Femur. *Acta Orthop Belg* 1977;43:454.
 + 5. Fabry G, MacEwen GD, Shands AR Jr. Torsion of the Femur: A Follow-up in Normal and Abnormal Conditions. *J Bone Joint Surg Am* 1973;55:1726.
 + 6. Halpern AA, Tanner J, Rinsky L. Does Persistent Fetal Femoral Anteversion Contribute to Osteoarthritis? A Preliminary Report. *Clin Orthop* 1979;145:213.
 + 7. Hoffer MM, Prietto C, Koffman M. Supracondylar Derotational Osteotomy of the Femur for Internal Rotation of the Thigh in the Cerebral Palsied Child. *J Bone Joint Surg Am* 1981;63:389.
 + 8. Hubbard DD, Staheli LT, Chew DE, Mosca VS. Medial Femoral Torsion and Osteoarthritis. *J Pediatr Orthop* 1988;8:540.
 + 9. Insall J, Falvo KA, Wise DW. Chondromalacia Patellae: A Prospective Study. *J Bone Joint Surg Am* 1976;58:1.
 + 10. Knittel G, Staheli LT. The Effectiveness of Shoe Modifications for Intoeing. *Orthop Clin North Am* 1976;7:1019.
 # 11. MacEwen GD, Shands AR Jr. Rotation and Angulation Deformities of the Lower Extremity in Childhood. *Orthopedics* 1960;2:66.
 + 12. McSweeny A. A Study of Femoral Torsion in Children. *J Bone Joint Surg Br* 1971;53:90.
 # 13. Müller ME, Allgöwer M, Schneider R, Willenegger H. *Manual of Internal Fixation: Techniques Recommended by the AO Group*, 2nd ed. New York: Springer-Verlag, 1979.
 + 14. Pistevos G, Duckworth T. The Correction of Genu Valgum by Epiphysial Stapling. *J Bone Joint Surg Br* 1977;59:72.
 + 15. Salenius P, Vankka E. The Development of the Tibiofemoral Angle in Children. *J Bone Joint Surg Am* 1975;57:259.
 + 16. Schrock RD Jr. Peroneal Nerve Palsy Following Derotation Osteotomies for Tibial Torsion. *Clin Orthop* 1969;62:172.
 + 17. Shands AR Jr, Steele MK. Torsion of the Femur: A Follow-up Report on the Use of the Dunlap Method for Its Determination. *J Bone Joint Surg Am* 1958;40:803.
 # 18. Staheli LT. Torsional Deformity. *Pediatr Clin North Am* 1977;24:799.
 # 19. Staheli LT. Medial Femoral Torsion. *Orthop Clin North Am* 1980;11:39.
 + 20. Staheli LT, Clawson DK, Hubbard DD. Medial Femoral Torsion: Experience with Operative Treatment. *Clin Orthop* 1980;146:222.
 + 21. Staheli LT, Corbett M, Wyss C, King H. Lower-Extremity Rotational Problems in Children: Normal Values to Guide Management. *J Bone Joint Surg Am* 1985;67:39.
 + 22. Staheli LT, Engel GM. Tibial Torsion: A Method of Assessment and a Survey of Normal Children. *Clin Orthop* 1972;86:183.
 + 23. Staheli LT, Lippert F, Denotter P. Femoral Anteversion and Physical Performance in Adolescent and Adult Life. *Clin Orthop* 1977;129:213.
 + 24. Terjesen T, Benum P, Anda S, Svenningsen S. Increased Femoral Anteversion and Osteoarthritis of the Hip Joint. *Acta Orthop Scand* 1982;53:571.
 + 25. Turner MS, Smillie IS. The Effect of Tibial Torsion on the Pathology of the Knee. *J Bone Joint Surg Br* 1981;63:396.
 # 26. Winquist RA. Closed Shortening of the Femur: Utilizing a New Type of Intramedullary Saw. In: Hempel D, Fischer S, eds. *Intramedullary Nailing*. New York: Thieme-Stratton, 1982;214.
 + 27. Winquist RA, Hansen ST Jr, Pearson RE. Closed Intramedullary Shortening of the Femur. *Clin Orthop* 1978;136:54.

## CHAPTER 169

ANGULAR DEFORMITIES OF THE LOWER EXTREMITIES IN CHILDREN

George H. Thompson

Angular deformities of the lower extremities in children are common and are a frequent reason for orthopaedic referral. They predominantly occur in the tibia; the femur is much less frequently involved. Angulation may occur in the frontal plane (varus and valgus), the sagittal plane (anterior and posterior), or a combination of both (anterolateral or posteromedial). Torsion may also be involved. It is important to understand the various physiologic and pathologic causes of angular deformities, the methods of evaluation, and the natural histories of the abnormalities to determine appropriate treatment (50,115,287). The classification for the differential diagnoses of genu varum (bowleg), genu valgum (knock-knee), and congenital an-

gular deformities of the tibia and fibula are presented in Tables 169.1 to 169.3.

NORMAL DEVELOPMENTAL ALIGNMENT OF THE LOWER EXTREMITY

Mild to moderate bowing of the lower extremities is a common finding in infants and young children. It is the result of molding of the lower extremities *in utero*. The bowed appearance of the lower extremities is actually a combination of external or lateral rotation of the hip (tight posterior capsule) and internal or medial tibial torsion. This physiologic genu varum tends to persist during the first year of life with only minimal improvement. After a child begins to walk, the bowing corrects spontaneously.

G. H. Thompson: Division of Pediatric Orthopaedics, Case Western Reserve University, Cleveland, Ohio 44106.

Table 169.1. Classification of Genu Varum or Bowleg Deformities of the Lower Extremities in Children

Physiologic genu varum

Pathologic genu varum

Tibia vara (Blount's disease)
  Infantile
  Juvenile
  Adolescent

Focal fibrocartilaginous dysplasia

Physeal injury
  Trauma
  Infection
  Tumor

Metabolic disorders
  Vitamin D deficiency (nutritional rickets)
  Vitamin D–resistant rickets
  Hypophosphatasia

Renal osteodystrophy

Skeletal dysplasia
  Metaphyseal chondrodysplasia
  Achondroplasia
  Enchondromatosis

Osteogenesis imperfecta

Table 169.2. Classification of Genu Valgum or Knock-knee Deformities of the Lower Extremities in Children

Physiologic genu valgum

Pathologic genu valgum

Trauma
  Physeal injury
  Genu valgum following fracture of the proximal tibial metaphysis
  Malunion

Infection
  Physeal damage

Tumor
  Physeal involvement

Metabolic disorders
  Vitamin D deficiency (nutritional rickets)
  Vitamin D–resistant rickets
  Renal osteodystrophy

Skeletal dysplasia
  Multiple epiphyseal dysplasia
  Pseudoachondrodysplasia
  Kneist syndrome

Congenital abnormalities
  Congenital dislocation of the patella

Neuromuscular disorders
  Cerebral palsy
  Myelodysplasia

Table 169.3. Differential Diagnosis of Congenital Angular Deformities of the Tibia and Fibula

Posteromedial angulation

Anterolateral angulation

Congenital pseudarthrosis of the tibia

Congenital longitudinal deficiency of the tibia (paraxial tibial hemimelia)

Congenital longitudinal deficiency of the fibula (paraxial fibular hemimella)

Complete correction may require up to 36 months of ambulation.

Physiologic genu valgum may appear by 3–4 years of age. This is true genu valgum, not the result of a torsional combination from *in utero* positioning. This deformity also undergoes spontaneous correction with normal adult knee alignment of mild genu valgum obtained by 5–8 years of age. Cahuzac et al. (55) demonstrated that girls have a consistent genu valgum alignment by 10 years of age that remains constant as they finish musculoskeletal growth. Boys, however, tend to have a decreasing valgus alignment until approximately 16 years of age. Thus, men have less valgus at maturity than do women.

Salenius and Vankka (242) analyzed the femoro-tibial angles clinically and radiographically in 1,279 children between birth and 16 years of age (Fig. 169.1). They found a mean varus alignment of 15° in newborns. This decreased to approximately 10° of varus alignment by age 1 year. Neutral alignment occurred between 18 and 20

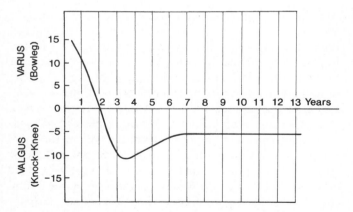

Figure 169.1. Normal development of knee alignment from infancy through childhood. (Adapted from Salenius P, Vankka E. The Development of the Tibio-femoral Angle in Children. *J Bone Joint Surg Am* 1975;57:259.)

months of age. The maximum valgus of approximately 12° was achieved by 3–4 years of age. The results were similar for boys and girls. By age 7 years, the children's valgus alignments had corrected to those of normal adults (8° in women, 7° in men). The researchers estimated that in approximately 95% of the children physiologic genu varum or valgum alignments resolved spontaneously with growth. In a follow-up study of 20 children between 1 and 4 years of age with pronounced physiologic varus (16° to 33°) or valgus (15° to 20°) deformities of the knees, Vankka and Salenius (279) found that even these pronounced deformities resolved during growth, although some did not completely correct until adolescence. They recommended that surgical correction be cautiously considered for children between 10 and 13 years of age, when corrective osteotomies are usually performed.

GENU VARUM

Genu varum, or bowleg, is a common childhood deformity and one of the most common causes of parental concern. In the majority of cases, it will be physiologic in origin and will correct with normal growth and development. However, there are pathologic genu varum disorders that may progress and produce functional impairment (Table 169.1).

The evaluation of a child with genu varum consists of a careful history and physical examination. The history will frequently distinguish physiologic from pathologic genu varum. Obtain a birth history, family history, the age at which developmental milestones occurred, a nutritional history, and the previous percentiles for height and weight. A family history of short stature or varus alignment or progression of the deformity may indicate a pathologic process.

On physical examination, measure height and weight, and determine the percentile for age. Shortening of the extremities relative to the trunk may indicate a skeletal dysplasia. In ambulatory children, the appearance to the lower extremities during standing and gait can provide important information. Determine the location of the deformity, as well as whether there is a lateral knee thrust while walking. Measure the range of motion of the hips, knees, and ankles. Assess the presence of ligamentous laxity. Measure the degree of genu varum in the standing and the supine positions. Measure and record the distance between the medial femoral condyles in centimeters. In addition, measure the torsional profile as described by Mosca and Staheli (see Chapter 168). This includes the foot progression angle, hip range of motion in extension, the thigh–foot angle, and the shape of the foot. Torsional changes in the femur and tibia are common in angular deformities of the lower extremities. Obtain serial photographs, if possible, and place them in the child's chart as an aid in documentation of improvement or worsening over time.

Radiographs are not routinely necessary in genu varum. However, if the child is short, the deformity is asymmetric, there is a history of progression, or the child is older than 3 years, obtain radiographs consisting of a standing anteroposterior (AP) projection of the lower extremities, including the hips, knees, and ankles. Position the patellae pointing forward. Measure the femoro-tibial angle, the mechanical axis, and the metaphyseal–diaphyseal angles. Assess the physes of the femur and tibia, especially those about the knee. Metaphyseal and physeal widening suggest an underlying metabolic disorder.

The history, physical examination, and radiographic evaluation then provide the basis for an accurate assessment of whether the child has a physiologic or pathologic genu varum deformity. The specifics of further evaluation and treatment are based on the diagnosis.

PHYSIOLOGIC GENU VARUM

Pathophysiology

Physiologic genu varum due to *in utero* positioning is a common finding in children between birth and 2 years of age. It is usually associated with a toe-in gait due to medial tibial torsion.

While the child is standing, the lower extremities appear bowed. However, physical examination demonstrates excessive lateral rotation of the extended hip and medial tibial torsion (Fig. 169.2). Contracture of the posterior capsule is a normal finding in children up to 1 year of age. It tends to improve during the first 3 years of life, and ultimately medial rotation slightly exceeds lateral rotation (222). Medial tibial torsion is the major component of physiologic genu varum. The knees are normal, except for possibly a slight residual knee-flexion contracture. A lateral knee thrust during gait is uncommon and indicates a pathologic genu varum deformity (161,163). The degree of varus can be measured by a goniometer (femoro-tibial angle) or the distance between the medial femoral condyles (55,65,126).

On radiographs, the typical features of physiologic genu varum include the following (268):

Transverse planes of the knees and the ankle joints are tilted medially.

Tibia is slightly bowed laterally at the junction of its proximal and middle thirds and the femur at its distal third.

Medial cortices of the tibia and femur are thickened and sclerotic.

Epiphyses, physes, and metaphyses have normal appearances, and there is no evidence of intrinsic bone disease.

Involvement is usually symmetric.

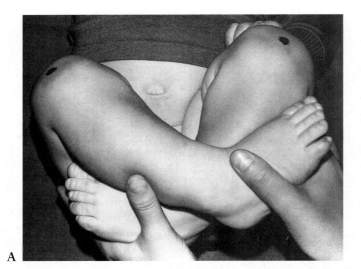

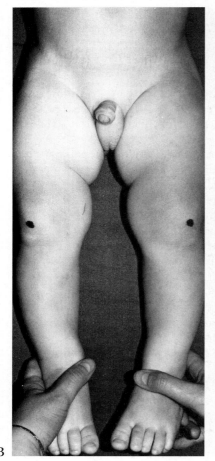

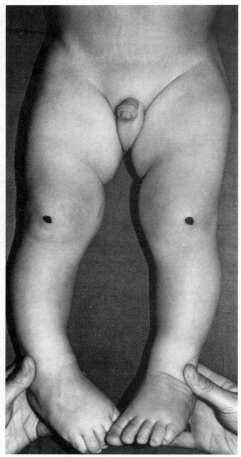

Figure 169.2. **A:** Physical examination of a 9-month-old boy with physiologic genu varum. The infant may still comfortably assume the *in utero* position with the hips flexed, abducted, and laterally rotated. The knees are flexed, with the lower legs and feet medially rotated. This position results in a hip flexion contracture, a contracture of the posterior aspect of the hip capsule, knee flexion contracture, and medial tibial torsion. **B:** When the lower extremities are extended, the posterior hip capsule contracture results in increased lateral rotation (80° to 90°) and limited medial rotation (0° to 10°). When the patellae point laterally, the medial tibial torsion is not readily apparent. **C:** When the hips are maximally rotated medially and the patellae are directed anteriorly, the medial tibial torsion is more apparent. The medial tibial torsion can be measured by the thigh–foot angle or the transmalleolar axis. The medial tibial torsion may also produce in-toeing during ambulation. This can be assessed by measuring the foot progression angle.

A

B

C

It can be difficult to differentiate radiographically between physiologic genu varum and tibia vara (Blount's disease) in children younger than 3 years of age. Levine and Drennan (176) developed the metaphyseal–diaphyseal angle to aid in differentiating these two disorders (Fig. 169.3). An angle of 11° or less indicates physiologic genu varum, and angles greater than 11° suggest that progressive tibia vara is likely (Fig. 169.4). However, a later study by Feldman and Schoenecker (101) indicated that angles greater than 16° are predictive of tibia vara, whereas angles of 9° or less suggest physiologic genu varum and angles between 10° and 15° are indeterminate. The metaphyseal–diaphyseal angle has been shown to have good interobserver and intraobserver reproducibility (104). However, it is important that standing radiographs be obtained with the knees in a neutral position, as rotational changes can alter measurements (265).

If a metabolic disorder is suspected, obtain serum calcium, phosphorus, and alkaline phosphatase levels. Ob-

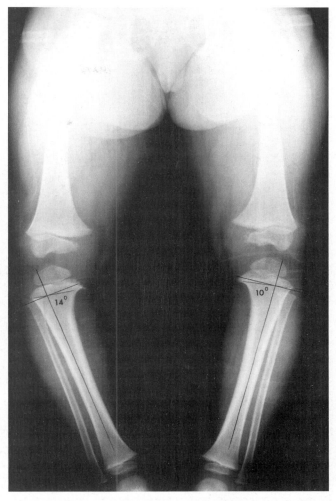

Figure 169.4. Standing AP radiograph of an 18-month-old girl with asymmetric bowing of the lower extremities. The metaphyseal–diaphyseal angle is 14° on the right, indicating infantile tibia vara; it is 10° on the left, representing physiologic genu varum. There is already medial metaphyseal irregularity and beaking, as well as mild medial epiphyseal flattening on the right.

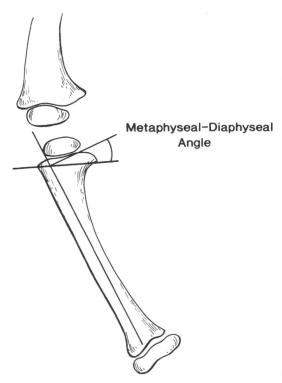

Metaphyseal–Diaphyseal Angle

Figure 169.3. Metaphyseal–diaphyseal angle. Draw a line between the radiographic corners of the medial and the lateral metaphyses of the proximal tibia, and another line parallel to the longitudinal axis of the tibial diaphysis. Then construct a line perpendicular to the diaphyseal line at the intersection of the metaphyseal and diaphyseal lines, and measure the angle between the right-angle line and the metaphyseal line. (Adapted from Levine AM, Drennan JC. Physiologic Bowing and Tibia Vara: The Metaphyseal–Diaphyseal Angle in the Measurement of Bowleg Deformities. *J Bone Joint Surg Am* 1982;64:1158.)

tain a pediatric endocrinology evaluation to assist in diagnosis and management.

Physiologic genu varum resolves spontaneously with normal growth and development (94,124,161,163,190, 242,252,268,279). Operative treatment is rarely indicated. Orthoses or corrective shoes are not recommended because there is no evidence that they improve alignment of the extremity. Follow infants and young children with physiologic genu varum at 6-month intervals (Fig. 169.5). Recording accurate clinical measurements is useful in reassuring anxious parents that improvement is occurring.

Operative Techniques

The techniques for correction of genu varum are listed in Table 169.4. The usual procedures for physiologic genu

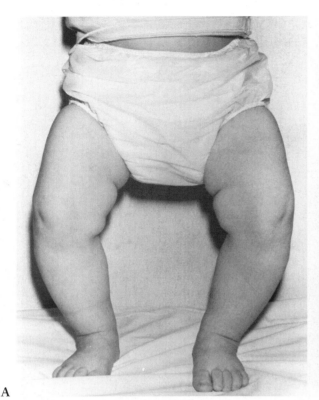
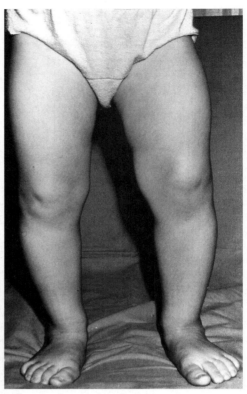

A   B

Figure 169.5. **A:** A 16-month-old girl with physiologic genu varum. Observe the lateral rotation of the thighs and knees and the medial tibial torsion. **B:** One year later, with no treatment, there has been complete resolution of the physiologic genu varum.

Table 169.4.   Surgical Options for Genu Varum Deformities

Distal femur

Valgus osteotomy
  Closing wedge
  Opening wedge
  Callotasis

Lateral hemiepiphyseal stapling

Lateral hemiepiphysiodesis

Proximal tibia

Valgus osteotomy (including derotation and diaphyseal fibular osteotomy)
  Closing wedge
  Opening wedge
  Dome
  Oblique
  Callotasis
  Other

Lateral hemiepiphyseal stapling

Lateral hemiepiphysiodesis

varum include a proximal tibial valgus derotation and diaphyseal fibular osteotomies, proximal tibial hemiepiphyseal stapling, or proximal tibial hemiepiphysiodesis. The latter two procedures are based on adequate remaining growth to achieve complete correction (39). The graph developed by Bowen et al. (38) can be helpful in determining proper timing.

Proximal Tibial Valgus Osteotomy and Diaphyseal Fibular Osteotomy   This is the most common procedure in persistent physiologic genu varum because it addresses both the varus and the medial tibial torsion. A variety of techniques can be used, including closing-wedge, opening-wedge, oblique, or dome osteotomies. These are essentially the same procedures as for tibia vara or Blount's disease. A diaphyseal fibular osteotomy is performed concomitantly because the fibula is usually too long and may be contributing to the deformity. The technique of a closing-wedge proximal tibial and diaphyseal fibular osteotomy is discussed in the section on tibia vara (see below). Internal or external fixation to maintain alignment is necessary and usually supplemented by a long-leg cast until complete healing has occurred.

Proximal Tibial Hemiepiphyseal Stapling   Temporary retardation of growth in the lateral aspect of the proximal tibial epiphysis with staples is an effective method for correction of persistent physiologic genu varum. If the deformity is severe or there is limited remaining growth, a combined lateral stapling of the distal femoral and the proximal tibial epiphyses may need to be performed. This procedure will not correct any coexistent medial tibial torsion.

Proximal Tibial Hemiepiphysiodesis Percutaneous closure of the lateral aspect of the proximal tibial epiphysis can be effective in correcting persistent physiologic genu varum in adolescents. The indications are essentially the same as for stapling. However, once complete correction has been achieved, a second procedure may be necessary on the medial side to prevent overcorrection. The proximal fibular epiphysis is usually closed concomitantly. This procedure will not correct any medial tibial torsion.

Rehabilitation and Postoperative Principles
In general, children treated with a proximal tibial valgus derotation and diaphyseal fibular osteotomies are managed similar to patients undergoing the same procedure for tibia vara. In children treated with a proximal tibial hemiepiphyseal stapling or hemiepiphysiodesis, apply a knee immobilizer postoperatively for approximately 2 weeks. This allows healing of the skin incision and minimizes discomfort. Then begin active range of motion exercises, and allow return to normal activities, typically at 4–6 weeks postoperatively.

Pitfalls and Complications
Complications of proximal tibial osteotomies have been well described in the orthopaedic literature (88,103,148, 187,202,204,263). There is a risk for injury to the peroneal nerve as it passes around the lateral aspect of the proximal fibula, and to the anterior tibial artery as it passes into the anterior compartment through the hiatus between the proximal tibia and fibula. Compartment syndromes have been described, and a child must be carefully evaluated for the first 24–48 hours postoperatively. Perform prophylactic anterior compartment fasciotomies at the time of surgery.

Complications of hemiepiphyseal stapling or epiphysiodesis occur much less frequently. Physeal damage with asymmetric closure and complete closure secondary to prolonged compression are the most common problems but are fortunately rare.

Conclusion
Physiologic genu varum rarely persists to such a degree that surgical intervention is necessary. There is a relationship between this disorder and tibia vara (Blount's disease). Persistent varus deformity may progress to the latter disorder. It has been my experience that the most common residual abnormality of physiologic genu varum is persistent medial tibial torsion. This is a more common indication for surgical treatment (see Chapter 168).

PATHOLOGIC GENU VARUM DEFORMITIES

Tibia Vara
Idiopathic tibia vara (Blount's disease) is the most common pathologic genu varum deformity. It is characterized by abnormal growth of the medial aspect of the proximal tibial epiphysis that results in progressive varus angulation beneath the knee. This disorder was first described by Erlacher (95) in 1922 and further analyzed by Blount (35) in 1937.

Classifications Tibia vara may occur at any age in a growing child. It was initially classified into two broad groups, depending on the age at clinical onset: infantile, with onset between 1 and 3 years of age; and adolescent, with onset inconsistently described as occurring after 6–8 years of age or just before puberty (33,35,97,110,111, 157,158,260). In 1984, Thompson et al. (275) proposed a three-group classification based on the age at onset: infantile (1–3 years), juvenile (4–10 years), and adolescent (11 years or older). The juvenile and adolescent forms are commonly combined as late-onset tibia vara. However, the incidence of recurrent deformity after a corrective valgus osteotomy of the proximal tibia is much higher in the juvenile group, justifying a three-group classification. All three groups share relatively common clinical characteristics, although the radiographic changes in the late-onset groups are less pronounced. Although the exact cause of tibia vara remains unknown, it appears to be secondary to growth suppression from increased compressive forces across the medial aspect of the knee (22,29,33,35,59,60, 69,111,157,168,171,172,274,275,286). Familial cases have been reported (23,111,173,250,253).

The natural history of tibia vara is one of progressive varus deformity. Infantile tibia vara can produce the greatest degree of deformity because of the greater amount of growth time remaining. In 1952, Langenskiöld (172) described six stages of progressive deformity in infantile tibia vara. Each grade advanced the degree of physeal growth inhibition (Fig. 169.6). It is possible to restore normal growth and development of the proximal tibial physes in grades I and II and probable grades III and IV. Grades V and VI represent severe damage to the medial proximal tibial physis and probable premature or asymmetric closure. The rate of deformity in grades V and VI is rapid, resulting in severe deformity and articular malformation. There is relatively good interobserver agreement with the use of this classification, especially for the early and late stages (264).

Assessment, Indications, Relative Results Comparison of the clinical characteristics of the infantile (22,23,33,

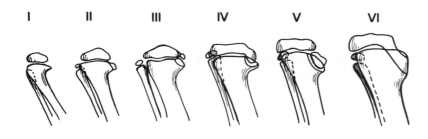

Figure 169.6.   Six grades of radiographic changes in infantile tibia vara as described by Langenskiöld (172). These represent a continuum of progressing deformity over time.

35,46,90,91,95,97,103,110,111,116,151,167,168,169, 172,173,180,181,223,248,260) and late-onset (juvenile and adolescent) (29,46,129,167,274,275,286) forms of tibia vara shows similarities as well as distinct differences (Table 169.5). The infantile form is the most common (Fig. 169.7). However, the late-onset forms also occur frequently (Fig. 169.8). Anterior cruciate ligament incompetence may occur in severe deformities (28).

Radiographically, fragmentation with a protuberant step deformity and beaking of the proximal medial tibial metaphysis are the major features of infantile tibia vara (Fig. 169.7*B*) (54,116,151,260). The changes in the proximal medial tibia are less conspicuous in the late-onset forms and are characterized by wedging of the medial portion of the epiphysis, a mild posteromedial articular depression, a serpiginous cephalad-curved physis, and mild or no fragmentation or beaking of the proximal medial metaphysis (Fig. 169.8*B*) (29,46,54,77,78,254–256, 274,275,286). The differences among the three tibia vara groups appear to be primarily due to the age at onset, the amount of remaining growth, and the magnitude of the medial compression forces on the involved side.

The major deformity that must be differentiated from tibia vara is physiologic genu varum deformity. It is difficult to differentiate these disorders in patients younger than 2 years. Children with tibia vara are typically African-American and obese and have a clinically apparent lateral thrust of the knee during the stance phase of gait. The deformities are progressive and may be asymmetric. Radiographic differentiation may be difficult. Standing radiographs of the lower extremities in children younger than 18 months of age with genu varum deformities are typically normal. However, normal knee radiographs do not eliminate infantile tibia vara from consideration. A metaphyseal–diaphyseal angle greater than 16° is an early prognosticator of infantile tibia vara (Fig. 169.3) (101). After 2–3 years of age, the radiographic characteristics become apparent, and the condition can be classified according to the six grades of Langenskiöld (172). The radiographic changes in late-onset forms of tibia vara are less dramatic but nevertheless diagnostic.

Pathophysiology   Histopathologic studies indicate a similar pathologic process for all three groups. Only a few biopsies of the proximal medial tibial condyle have been obtained from patients with infantile tibia vara (35,95, 111,171,173). Histopathologic abnormalities included islands of densely packed chondrocytes exhibiting a greater degree of hypertrophy than would be expected from their topographic position, areas of almost acellular cartilage, and abnormal groups of capillaries. Langenskiöld (171) and Golding and McNeil-Smith (111), in studies of nine

---

Table 169.5.   Comparison of the Clinical Characteristics of Tibia Vara

Infantile	Late-onset (juvenile and adolescent)
African-American race	African-American race
Female predominance	Male predominance
Marked obesity	Marked obesity
Bilateral involvement (80%)	Bilateral involvement (50%)
Medial metaphyseal beak	No medial metaphyseal beak
Medial tibial torsion	Minimal medial tibial torsion
Lower-extremity length inequality	Mild lower-extremity length inequality
	Pain rather than deformity
	Mild medial collateral ligament laxity
	Steadily progressive deformity

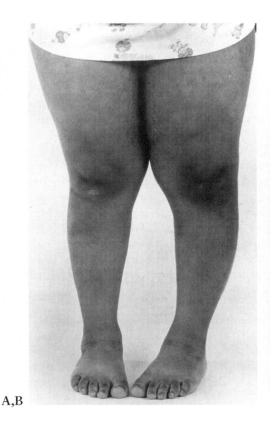

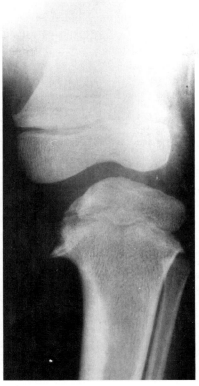

Figure 169.7. **A:** Clinical photograph of a 5-year-old African-American girl with left infantile tibia vara. Observe the obesity, the unilateral left genu varum deformity, and the associated medial tibial torsion. **B:** Standing radiograph of the left knee demonstrates Langenskiöld grade III changes in the medial aspect of the proximal tibial epiphysis and metaphysis. Notice the metaphyseal beaking.

A,B

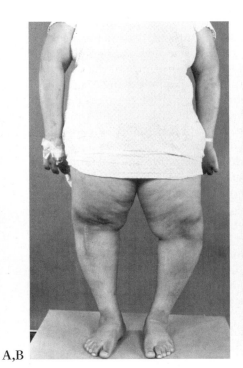

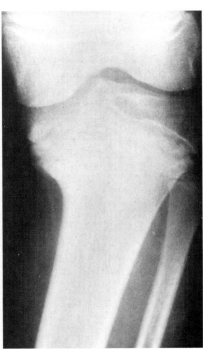

Figure 169.8. **A:** Standing preoperative photograph of a 13-year-old African-American boy with bilateral adolescent or late-onset tibia vara. A previous proximal tibial osteotomy was performed on the right, producing only partial correction. Observe the marked obesity and the untreated left genu varum deformity and its medial tibial torsion. The patient subsequently underwent a laterally based closing-wedge proximal tibial osteotomy, including the physis, and a diaphyseal fibular osteotomy for correction of this deformity. **B:** On a standing AP radiograph of the left knee, the radiographic changes in adolescent tibia vara are less striking than in the infantile form. There is narrowing of the medial aspect of the proximal tibial epiphysis, physeal irregularity, and increased height of the lateral aspect of the epiphysis.

A,B

and six biopsies, respectively, concluded that the abnormalities were localized principally to the physes and that there was no evidence of avascular necrosis.

More extensive histopathologic data are available for the late-onset forms of tibia vara (59,60,223,274,275, 286). The major histologic aberrations include the following:

Disorganization and misalignment of the physeal zones
Abnormal histochemical staining and excess of hypocellular matrix
Cystic degeneration and necrosis
Multidirectional clefts and fissures
Transphyseal canals of capillaries
Intraphyseal ossification centers
Increased necrotic chondrocytes throughout the proliferative and hypertrophic zones
Abnormal collagen fibers in the cartilage matrix
Chondrocytes at the apex of the vascular invasion front, which has increased width and length
Extension of noncalcified cartilaginous bars into the proximal and distal metaphyses

These changes are found uniformly throughout the medial and lateral aspects of the physes, although they are quantitatively greater on the medial side. They are remarkably similar to the changes observed in infantile tibia vara and in slipped capital femoral epiphysis, suggesting a common cause (1,2). Lovejoy and Lovell (182) described two patients with late-onset tibia vara associated with slipped capital femoral epiphysis.

The histopathologic abnormalities indicate that asymmetric compression and shear forces acting across the proximal tibial physis result in suppression and deviation of normal endochondral ossification, producing tibia vara. This concept, which reflects the Heuter–Volkmann law, has been confirmed experimentally by Arkin and Katz (13). Golding and McNeil-Smith (111) concluded that children who had significant physiologic varus deformity, walked early and stretched their knee ligaments. This resulted in asymmetric compression with subsequent suppression of posteromedial physeal growth and ultimate formation of an osseous bridge, producing a permanent and progressive varus deformity. This pathogenesis is consistent with Blount's (33,35) initial observations that infantile tibia vara is first recognized when there is an increase of physiologic bowing during the first 3 years of life. Langenskiöld (172,173) emphasized that necrosis of the physeal cartilage is the principal cause of growth disturbance, leading to varus deformity; he attributed the abnormal cartilage to abnormal pressure or shear in overweight children with physiologic bowleg. Others agreed that abnormal pressure is probably the primary etiologic factor in infantile tibia vara (22,35,46,111,157,162).

In predisposed older children or adolescents with minimal residual deformity after physiologic bowleg, rapid growth and weight gain repetitively injure the posteromedial portion of the proximal tibial physis, resulting in a cycle of varus-growth suppression similar to the cycle described by Golding and McNeil-Smith (111) for the infantile form (127,129,274,275,286). Progressive genu varum deformity is not due to an osseous bridge but is caused by suppression of normal endochondral growth after repetitive local injury (29,162,260,274,275,286). The concept of physeal growth suppression in tibia vara has been confirmed biomechanically by Cook et al. (69) in a finite element analysis. As varus increases, the forces in the proximal medial tibial physis increase. Obesity and mild varus (10°) in older children create enough force to suppress growth. However, Henderson and Green (127) reported a case of late-onset tibia vara in an adolescent with previously documented neutral mechanical alignment, suggesting that, at least in some cases, preexisting varus alignment is not a prerequisite.

Preoperative Management and Planning   If radiographic findings confirm the diagnosis of infantile tibia vara, begin treatment immediately. Orthotic management may be considered for children 3 years of age or younger with Langenskiöld's grade II and possibly grade III involvement. Approximately 50% to 65% of these in children can be corrected with an orthosis (151,180,232,248). Children with suspected infantile tibia vara with metaphyseal–diaphyseal angles of 10° to 15° are more likely to benefit from orthotic management (232). Use a knee–ankle–foot orthosis with a single medial upright without a knee hinge. Place pads, straps, or elastic webbing over the distal femur and proximal tibia to apply a valgus force. The orthosis should be worn for 22–23 hours each day. Tighten the straps at 1–2-month intervals to provide progressive correction. Obtain standing radiographs at 3-month intervals to document correction of the tibia vara deformity. The metaphyseal–diaphyseal angle should decrease (122). After obtaining an absolute valgus mechanical axis, begin weaning from the orthosis. Follow the child carefully thereafter to ensure maintenance of correction.

A maximum trial of 1 year of orthotic management is currently recommended. If correction is not obtained after 1 year of bracing, corrective osteotomy is indicated. Orthotic treatment is not indicated after 3 years of age or for severe deformities. Bracing children older than 3 years risks delaying performance of a corrective osteotomy. Loder and Johnston (180) showed that delay in performing corrective osteotomy, even by a few months, beyond 4 years of age risks failure to achieve lasting reversal of the physeal inhibition of the proximal tibia. This predisposes a child to repeated operative procedures to maintain a satisfactory result.

Conservative management in the late-onset forms of tibia vara is contraindicated. The children are too large and the remaining growth is too small to allow adequate correction. Compliance with an orthosis in this age group is difficult to achieve.

The indications for surgical treatment in infantile tibia vara include age 4 years or less, failure of orthotic management, and Langenskiöld grade III or higher. The possible procedures are presented in Table 169.4. Proximal tibial valgus osteotomy with fibular diaphyseal osteotomy is usually the procedure of choice. Perform an anterior compartment fasciotomy concomitantly. Tibial osteotomy techniques include closing-wedge, opening-wedge, dome, and oblique osteotomies. The procedure selected must correct the varus deformity and any associated medial tibial torsion. Tibial length is usually not a problem in infantile tibia vara. It is important that the selected osteotomy overcorrect the mechanical axis of the knee to 5° or more of valgus. This ensures that the supine correction obtained in the operating room is adequate. Overcorrection compensates for the tendency of the knee to fall back into varus after a patient resumes weight bearing because of the depression in the posteromedial articular surface and the ligamentous relaxation laterally. The goal is to transfer the line of weight bearing to the lateral compartment of the knee. Schoenecker et al. (248) reported that correction within 5° of neutral usually proves satisfactory. However, others recommend overcorrection (168,173,180,229). Considering the physeal inhibition phenomena as proposed by Cook et al. (69), overcorrection to absolute valgus alignment is necessary to relieve the excessive compressive forces medially.

Rab (229) described an oblique osteotomy of the proximal tibia for tibia vara. It is a single-plane osteotomy that allows simultaneous correction of the varus and medial tibial torsion deformities and permits postoperative cast wedging, if necessary, to improve position. This ability to adjust the osteotomy postoperatively is important because of the difficulty in achieving satisfactory alignment intraoperatively.

In older children with infantile tibia vara, especially those with Langenskiöld grade IV lesions or higher, a single osteotomy of the proximal tibia is usually insufficient to restore normal alignment and physeal growth. Langenskiöld grades IV and V act effectively as medial physeal arrests. Possible procedures for these children include the following (25,47,65,87,103,117,130,152,158, 159,166,177,195,217,229,245–248,255,261,274,275):

Multiple proximal tibial metaphyseal osteotomies and fibular diaphyseal osteotomies
Proximal tibial osteotomy with physeal resection
Intraepiphyseal osteotomy to elevate the medial tibial articular surface (elevation of the medial tibia plateau)
Physeal bridge resection and replacement with interposition material such as fat or Silastic
Hemiepiphysiodesis of the lateral aspect of the proximal tibial epiphysis

Oblique proximal tibial osteotomy
Ilizarov ring fixation system and callotasis technique

In the juvenile and adolescent forms of tibia vara, surgical correction is necessary to restore the mechanical axis of the knee. The same surgical options as those for older children with infantile tibia vara are applicable in these groups. Correction to physiologic genu valgum with careful preoperative biotrignometric planning for the tibial osteotomy is the goal (57). Kline et al. (160) demonstrated that distal femoral varus is a part of the deformity in late-onset tibia vara. Evaluate this possibility, and perhaps consider it in the treatment plan.

Obtain intraoperative radiographs with the knee in extension and with slight varus stress to ensure contact between the medial femoral condyle and the posteromedial articular depression of the proximal tibia. This technique can help minimize undercorrection of the deformity. Aim to achieve at least 5° of valgus at the time of osteotomy. The recurrence rate for the juvenile-onset group approaches 25% overall and is even higher in boys (274, 275). Evaluate all juvenile-onset patients with tomography or magnetic resonance imaging (MRI) before surgery for evidence of premature closure or impending closure of the proximal medial tibial physis. If premature closure is not present, a simple closing-wedge metaphyseal osteotomy or oblique proximal tibial osteotomy with correction to physiologic valgus may be performed (229). Correction using the Ilizarov ring fixation system and callotasis may be applicable, especially if there is a significant lower-extremity length discrepancy (227).

If the deformity recurs, indicating significant physeal inhibition, then additional surgery is necessary; techniques include physeal bridge resection and interposition graft, intraepiphyseal osteotomy, elevation of the medial tibial plateau, and physeal excision (117,152,174,177,185,245, 248,255,289). Internal or external fixation is usually necessary to maintain alignment until satisfactory healing occurs. Physeal distraction with an external fixator has also been used in Europe (86,88), but it is not widely used. The procedure selected depends on the patient's age, the amount of growth remaining, and the severity of the deformity. Proximal tibial physeal excision with proximal fibular epiphysiodesis is usually recommended for recurrent deformities with premature medial tibial physeal closure or for patients 12 years of age or older (274). Healing is rapid and the correction permanent. Measure any residual lower-extremity length discrepancy with scanograms, and manage by contralateral epiphysiodesis, when necessary.

Henderson et al. (128) reported results in nine children with late-onset tibia vara treated by hemiepiphysiodesis of the lateral aspect of the proximal tibial epiphysis. The average preoperative varus was 13° (range, 3° to 25°).

They found a correction rate of 7° per year. Three patients required a proximal tibial osteotomy because of incomplete correction. The authors thought that hemiepiphysiodesis was an effective procedure with less morbidity for managing varus deformities of the extremities of obese children. Similar results can probably be anticipated with staples, although they were not used in this study.

Operative Techniques
Proximal Tibial Valgus Osteotomy and Fibular Diaphyseal Osteotomy

- Make a 5 cm horizontal or transverse skin incision below the level of the tibial tubercle (Fig. 169.9).
- Expose the proximal tibia subperiosteally.
- Release the fascia of the anterior compartment. The fibers of the patellar tendon insertion are usually visible in the proximal portion of the incision.
- Perform a fibular diaphyseal osteotomy through a 3 cm vertical incision at the junction of the middle and proximal thirds of the fibula.
- Identify the muscles of the lateral compartment, and retract them anteriorly. Split the periosteum of the fibula longitudinally, and reflect it circumferentially.
- Make an oblique osteotomy with a small oscillating saw.
- With the fibular osteotomy completed, proceed with the proximal tibial osteotomy. This may be a closing-wedge, opening-wedge, or dome osteotomy. The procedure should allow correction of the medial tibial torsion and the varus deformity. I prefer a closing-wedge osteotomy. It is important to correct the medial tibial torsion first and then perform the laterally based, closing-wedge osteotomy. Excessive correction and unnecessary bone excision may occur if the torsion is not corrected first.
- Fix the osteotomy with crossed Steinmann pins, compression plate and screws, or an external fixation device. I prefer the latter because the pins can be removed in the outclinic without a separate operative procedure.
- Obtain intraoperative radiographs with the knee in extension to confirm that approximately 5° of valgus alignment have been obtained.
- After closure, immobilize the leg in a long-leg cast with the knee in extension and a slight valgus stress.

Oblique Tibial Osteotomy

- Make a transverse incision just beneath the tibial tubercle. Make a Y-shaped incision in the periosteum, and elevate it circumferentially
- Insert a small Steinmann pin at a cephalad angle of approximately 45° 1 cm distal to the tibial tubercle, and advance it under image-intensifier control until it passes through the posterior cortex distal to the proximal tibial physis. The angle of insertion determines the amount of correction for the varus and the medial tibial torsion. Have a nomogram available to assist in preoperatively determining the appropriate angle of guide-pin insertion.

- Carefully perform the osteotomy immediately beneath the Steinmann pin.
- After completion of the tibial osteotomy, perform a fibular diaphyseal osteotomy. This results in free mobility at the tibial osteotomy.
- Drill a hole in the anteroposterior direction across the osteotomy and lateral to the tibial tubercle.
- Insert a single 3.5 mm cortical or cancellous lag screw, align the osteotomy, and loosely tighten the screw to allow later adjustments, if necessary.
- After an anterior compartment fasciotomy, close the incisions. Insert a suction drain at the time of closure.
- Apply a long-leg cast. Rab (229) advised injection of contrast material into the knee to enhance the ability to check the radiographic alignment after the dressings are applied but before the long-leg cast is applied.

Excision of the Proximal Tibial Physis   If the deformity recurs in an older child with the adolescent form of tibia vara, excision of the proximal tibial physis may be advantageous.

- This procedure is similar to the proximal tibia osteotomy previously described. Make a similar incision, although more proximally.
- Mobilize the patellar tendon on its medial and lateral sides.
- Place a smooth Steinmann pin through the epiphysis just below the articular surface.
- Excise the entire physis in a closing-wedge osteotomy. Insert a second pin distally, and apply an external fixator.

Always perform a fibular diaphyseal osteotomy. The advantage of this procedure is that it is performed at the site of the deformity and therefore allows maximal correction and physiologic realignment of the tibia. Healing is usually rapid, and there is no risk of recurrent deformity. A contralateral proximal tibia epiphysiodesis may be performed at the same time. However, in most cases, the degree of lower-extremity length discrepancy is followed scanographically, and any residual leg-length discrepancy is corrected by a contralateral distal femoral epiphysiodesis at the appropriate time.

Other Techniques   In the late-onset form of the disease, a callotasis technique may be beneficial with either a cantilever or Ilizarov ring fixation system. The advantage of this procedure is that it allows slow, progressive correc-

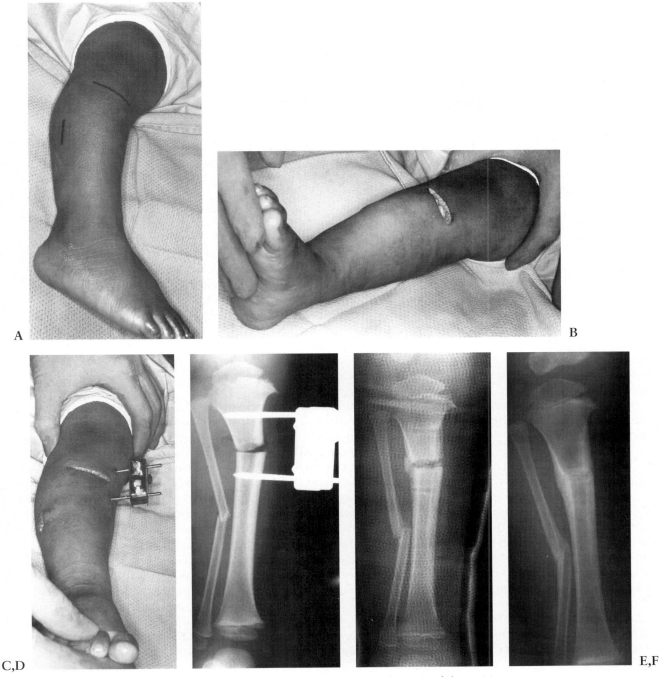

A

B

C,D

E,F

Figure 169.9.   **A:** Intraoperative photograph shows the location and extent of the incisions for a proximal tibial and diaphyseal fibular osteotomy. **B:** After a transverse osteotomy of the proximal tibia, derotate the leg to correct the associated medial tibial torsion. Remove an appropriate, laterally based wedge to correct the residual varus deformity. **C:** Insert a threaded Steinmann pin above and below the proximal tibial osteotomy. Take care to ensure that the proximal pin is inferior and posterior to the apophysis of the tibial tubercle. Secure the pins with an external fixation clamp. **D:** Postoperative radiograph after correction shows that there has been some distraction at the osteotomy site. This is usually not a problem. Ideally, the osteotomy should remain closed. The external fixation clamp is incorporated into the cast, providing secure fixation. **E:** AP radiograph in a long leg cast shows that there is partial healing and the external fixation system has been removed. **F:** AP radiograph obtained 3 months after surgery demonstrates satisfactory healing of the osteotomy and correction of the tibia vara deformity. The extremity is in approximately 5° to 7° of genu valgum.

tion. Because the patient is bearing weight, the precise degree of desired correction can be achieved. This procedure is being used more frequently today (see Chapter 171).

General Rehabilitation and Postoperative Principles   The postoperative management of children is similar after any corrective osteotomy of the proximal tibia. Continue immobilization until healing is complete; then place the children on a physical therapy program at home for approximately 2 weeks. After complete rehabilitation, allow them to return to normal activities. Because of associated obesity, these children frequently benefit from a dietary consultation.

Complications   Complications during and after a proximal tibial osteotomy are common. They include peroneal nerve palsy, injuries to the anterior tibial artery, and compartment syndromes (88,103,148,187,202,204,249,263). Occurrence of a compartment syndrome may be minimized by performing an anterior compartment fasciotomy at the time of surgery. If a compartment syndrome occurs, temporarily reduce the correction, and perform a four-compartment fasciotomy. Children with the infantile form of tibia vara require long-term follow-up to assess the results of surgery. The deformity may recur, especially in older children and those with advanced Langenskiöld grades. Deformity persisting after skeletal maturity predisposes to degenerative osteoarthritis (137,291).

Conclusion   I prefer a proximal tibial valgus derotation and fibular diaphyseal osteotomy to correct infantile tibia vara. This allows simultaneous correction of both components of the deformity. It is important that the deformity be slightly overcorrected so that the mechanical axis passes medial to the ankle joint. It can be difficult to assess the degree of correction intraoperatively because radiographs on a long cassette cannot be obtained. A helpful hint is to visualize the iliac crest on the involved side. The cord from the electrocoagulation knife can be used to measure the mechanical axis on the fluoroscope. This can be stretched between the anterosuperior iliac spine and the middle of the patella. Its distal extension can then be judged with respect to the ankle joint. Undercorrection is a common problem that prevents adequate alignment. Radiographic contrast material in the knee joint at the time of surgery may also be helpful. Manually manipulate the knee into varus after the osteotomy is internally stabilized, as this gives a more realistic feeling for the alignment of the extremity during weight bearing.

In older children with infantile or late-onset tibia vara, especially the juvenile type, a preoperative MRI may be helpful in assessing the integrity of the physis. However, even if the physis appears open, it may still be abnormal and not respond to normalization of the compressive forces postoperatively. Correction in these children can be accomplished using an Ilizarov frame and callotasis. This allows precise correction of the deformity. Weight-bearing radiographs may be obtained during treatment.

In children with recurrent deformities in whom a physeal bridge is suspected, I would suggest excision of the physis with concomitant correction of both the residual tibia vara deformity and any medial tibial torsion. Postoperatively, patients will need to be evaluated for residual lower-extremity length discrepancy. An appropriately timed contralateral epiphysiodesis will be necessary to achieve relatively equal leg lengths at skeletal maturity.

Tibia Vara Caused by Focal Fibrocartilaginous Dysplasia

Tibia vara secondary to focal fibrocartilaginous dysplasia involving the medial aspect of the proximal tibial metaphysis was first reported by Bell et al. (26) in 1985. Since then, additional cases have been reported (3,45,67,131, 145,208,290). Tibia vara may also involve other areas of the body. Lincoln and Birch (178) reported upper-extremity involvement. It is an uncommon cause of pathologic genu varum but one that must be differentiated from Blount's disease because the natural histories of the two disorders are distinctly different.

Pathophysiology   Biopsy of the lesion at the time of corrective osteotomy or for diagnostic purposes has shown consistent histopathologic features. Grossly, there is a white cartilaginous lesion with well defined margins deep to the insertion of the pes anserinus. Histopathologic findings include acellular or sparsely cellular collagenous tissue, inactive fibrocytes, plump cells resembling chondrocytes in lacunae, and dense, nondescript fibrous tissue (26, 45,155,192,208). No giant cells, osteoid, or bone are found within these lesions. The lesions suggest fibrocartilage centrally and tendinous tissues peripherally. They do not involve the physis or epiphysis. Bell et al. (26) observed that the tissue resembles that normally found at the site of the insertion of tendons into cortical bone, as described by Cooper and Misol (70) in 1970. They suggested that these children had abnormal development of fibrocartilage at the insertion of the pes anserinus. The exact mechanism of this abnormal growth is unknown. The defect may be congenital.

Assessment   All children with tibia vara caused by focal fibrocartilaginous dysplasia present with unilateral bowing. There is no apparent sex or side predilection. The onset is usually before age 1 year, and the deformity progresses until approximately age 2 years and then begins to resolve. During the time of progression, the deformity may become quite prominent, reaching 20° to 30° of varus. Medial tibial torsion and mild tibial length discrepancy (0.5–1.0 cm) are common associated findings (26,

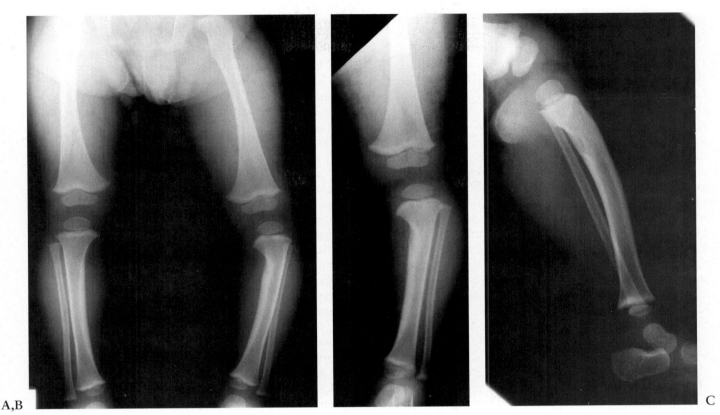

A,B   C

Figure 169.10. **A:** Standing AP radiograph of a 2-year-old Caucasian boy shows asymmetric genu varum involving the left lower extremity. **B:** Observe the typical radiographic features of focal fibrocartilaginous dysplasia of the proximal tibia. There is a cortical defect involving the medial aspect of the proximal tibial metaphysis. There is associated sclerosis, as well as the mild tibia vara deformity. **C:** The lateral radiograph is relatively normal.

45). The lesions are characteristically not tender to palpation, and there is no prominence of the proximal medial metaphysis, as seen in infantile tibia vara.

Radiographically, there is a cortical defect in the medial metaphyseal region of the proximal tibia with an area of surrounding sclerosis (Fig. 169.10). MRI will demonstrate dense fibroconnective tissue (192). Computed tomography shows similar findings, with an elliptical fibrous cortical defect but no soft-tissue mass (131,290). On the basis of reported cases, it appears that the metaphyseal lesion resolves spontaneously after age 2 years, followed by correction of the tibia vara deformity. Significant improvement is usually evident by 4 years of age (26,45). Use of an orthosis does not increase the rate of improvement.

Preoperative Planning Although data are limited, it appears that only children with no evidence of spontaneous correction by 4 years of age are candidates for corrective osteotomy (290). This typically involves a proximal tibial osteotomy distal to the apophysis of the tibial tubercle and a diaphyseal fibular osteotomy. Because of the associated

medial tibial torsion, the procedure of choice is a laterally based closing derotation osteotomy or an oblique proximal tibial osteotomy as described by Rab (229).

Operative Techniques The procedures for focal fibrocartilaginous dysplasia are the same as those for tibia vara. There is no intrinsic osseous pathology that interferes with bone healing. Immobilization in a long-leg cast or a one-and-one-half spica cast is necessary, depending on the child's age. A spica cast is usually advised for younger children. After healing, there is usually rapid rehabilitation and return to normal activities. Prolonged follow-up is necessary to assess resolution of the lesion and subsequent growth and development of the proximal tibia. Periodic scanograms are necessary to assess the length of the extremities.

Complications A peroneal nerve palsy and persistent valgus deformity into adolescence were reported by Bradish et al. (45) after corrective osteotomy. This appears to have been a technical problem. No other complications have been reported for operative treatment of this lesion.

Other Pathologic Genu Varum Deformities

Vitamin D–Resistant and Nutritional Rickets   Persistent or progressive genu varum deformities are common in children with metabolic disorders such as vitamin D–resistant rickets (hypophosphatemic rickets) or nutritional rickets. Vitamin D–resistant rickets is an X-linked dominant disorder due to vitamin D resistance that results in defective bone mineralization. Affected children typically have bilateral symmetric genu varum; they are relatively short, usually being in the tenth percentile. The varus deformity is due to a combination of bowing and involvement of the distal femur and the proximal tibia. Hematologic studies reveal normal serum calcium and decreased phosphate values. In nutritional rickets, the child has been receiving an unusual diet from the parents.

Radiographically, the features are widening of the metaphyses, widening of the physes, and a cup-shaped relationship between the physis and the metaphysis. The bowing is usually symmetric throughout the femur and the tibia. Marked osteopenia and thinning of the cortices are also common. Obtain serum calcium, phosphorus, and alkaline phosphatase levels, as well as a pediatric endocrinology consultation to confirm the diagnosis.

Medical treatment is important before any form of orthopaedic intervention is considered (96,239). This typically includes oral phosphate supplementation and high doses of vitamin D for vitamin D–resistant rickets, and dietary changes for nutritional rickets. Surgical measures to correct genu varum deformities are usually unsuccessful unless adequate medical control has been obtained preoperatively. If such control cannot be obtained, it is usually best to wait until skeletal maturity before attempting to realign the mechanical axes.

If metabolic control can be obtained and a child is young, observation is appropriate. Spontaneous improvement may occur in children younger than 5 years. However, in older children or those who are not improving spontaneously, surgical treatment is necessary (96,239). This may consist of osteotomies of the distal femur, proximal tibia, or both. If involvement is extensive, proximal femoral and distal tibial osteotomies may be necessary to adequately realign the lower extremities. Cast immobilization postoperatively may result in immobilization-induced hypercalcemia and may require modification of medical management. When osteotomies are done, healing time may be twice normal. It is often advantageous to postpone major alignment procedures until adolescence to minimize the recurrence that is common in younger children.

Renal Osteodystrophy   Children who have end-stage renal disease may manifest renal osteodystrophy. The physes in these children show the same pathologic changes found in tibia vara and slipped capital femoral epiphysis. These include disorganized endochondral ossification at the physeal–metaphyseal junctions. Because end-stage renal failure occurs more commonly in older children who have achieved physiologic valgus alignment, valgus deformities are much more common. Varus is more likely when renal failure occurs at 3 years of age or younger. Renal osteodystrophy has many of the same radiographic features as vitamin D–resistant and nutritional rickets. There is physeal cupping and widening at both the distal femoral and proximal tibial physes. Marked osteopenia and thinning of the cortical bone are also present.

Treatment of genu varum deformities secondary to renal osteodystrophy is similar to that for vitamin D–resistant and nutritional rickets. Surgical treatment is usually postponed until the renal status has stabilized in response to medical treatment, hemodialysis, or kidney transplantation. There will be a rapid recurrence of the deformity if the underlying metabolic bone disease is not corrected first.

Skeletal Dysplasias   Many skeletal dysplasias may result in a progressive genu varum deformity (Table 169.1). Metaphyseal chondrodysplasia (both Jansen and Schmid types), which results in abnormal chondroblast function and chondroid production, is a common cause. Occasionally, these may be difficult to distinguish from rickets. Although the physes are widened and cupped in the Schmid type, the epiphyses are normal, and the presence of short stature may be helpful in making the correct diagnosis.

Genu varum frequently occurs in achondroplasia. This rhizomelic dwarfing condition is due to abnormal endochondral bone formation. Affected children have short stature and characteristic craniofacial features. The genu varum deformity is due to asymmetric growth of the proximal tibial epiphysis and overgrowth of the fibula. These children rarely have knee pain.

For some surgeons, the treatment options for genu varum deformities secondary to achondroplasia must be surgical because orthotic management historically has not been effective. Their usual procedure is a proximal tibial valgus osteotomy and proximal fibular epiphysiodesis (Fig. 169.11). The latter must be done early in childhood to prevent recurrence and progression of the genu varum deformity. Others feel that genu varum in achondroplasia is not associated with functional difficulty or increased risk of osteoarthritis, and surgery may not be recommended (see Chapter 180).

Osteogenesis imperfecta results from a defect in type I collagen and produces varying degrees of skeletal fragility. Repeated fractures often lead to bowing and torsional malalignment of the lower extremities. The distal third of the femur is a common location for these fractures, which frequently result in anterolateral angulation. Residual de-

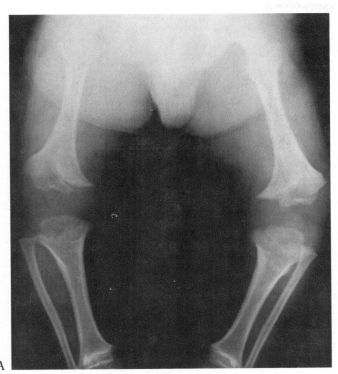

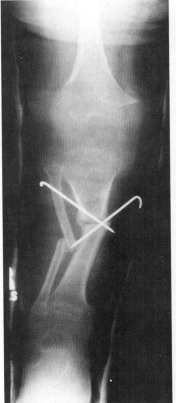
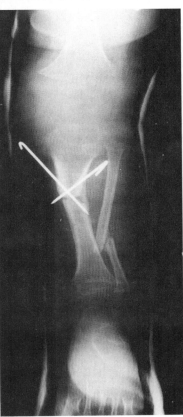
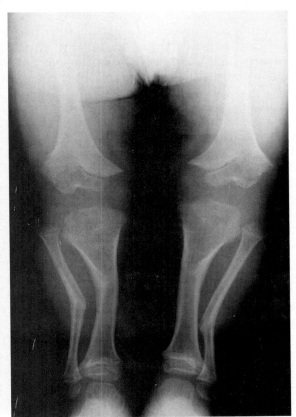

A

B,C

D

Figure 169.11. **A:** Standing preoperative radiographs of a 6-year-old Caucasian boy with achondroplasia genu varum demonstrating the typical epiphyseal and metaphyseal changes, as well as overgrowth of the fibulae. **B:** Postoperative radiograph after proximal tibial and fibular diaphyseal valgus derotation osteotomies of the right leg shows that internal fixation was achieved with percutaneous smooth Steinmann pins. **C:** Postoperative radiograph of the left lower leg. **D:** Standing radiographs 6 months postoperatively demonstrates satisfactory healing and excellent correction of the genu varum deformities.

formities after fractures are common, and the varus angulation often increases as a result of repeated fractures. Occasionally, in the more severe cases, osteotomies with intramedullary fixation may be beneficial (see Chapter 180).

Other Causes Any condition, such as infection or trauma, that damages the physis may result in asymmetric growth and deformity. The distal femur is the most common site of growth disturbance following a physeal fracture. Physeal fractures of the proximal tibia occur much less commonly. The management of genu varum deformities secondary to physeal growth disturbance is complex. If an asymmetric physeal bar is present, it may be resected and grafted with fat or Silastic. The deformity is corrected concomitantly by an osteotomy. If the physeal damage is extensive, complete physeal closure and management of the associated leg-length discrepancy may need to be considered (see Chapter 164).

GENU VALGUM

Genu valgum, or knock-knee, is a common condition affecting the lower limbs in children and adolescents. Physiologic genu valgum is the most common form, but pathologic genu valgum disorders occur and may require treatment (Table 169.2). The most common pathologic causes of genu valgum are posttraumatic and renal osteodystrophy.

Evaluation of a child with genu valgum is similar to that for genu varum and includes a careful history and physical examination. In the majority of children with genu valgum, the femoro-tibial angles are within the physiologic range of two standard deviations above or below the mean. Only those with an angle greater than two standard deviations from the mean are considered to have a deformity. Fat thighs, ligamentous laxity, and flat feet are often the results of associated out-toeing, and this can accentuate the appearance of the knock-knee, making physiologic genu valgum appear more severe. Measurements of the femoro-tibial angle (with a goniometer) and the intermalleolar distance are methods for assessing and following genu valgum (55,65,126). However, the intermalleolar distance may be misleading. The same intermalleolar distance in an individual of short stature may be more significant than the same distance in a taller individual. Torsional malalignment is less common in genu valgum, but the combination of femoral anteversion or torsion and compensatory external tibial torsion gives the appearance of a valgus knee.

The indications for radiographs for genu valgum are similar to those for genu varum. Short stature, asymmetry, history of injury, or history of progression are indications. Standing AP radiographs of the lower extremities, includ-

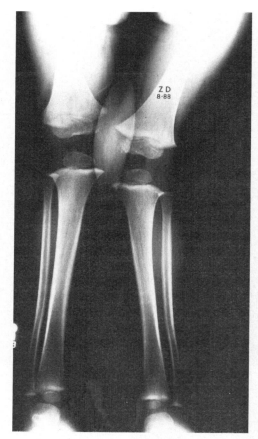

Figure 169.12.   Standing AP radiographs of the lower extremities of a 3-year-old boy with physiologic genu valgum show no radiographic abnormalities of the distal femoral or proximal tibial epiphyses or metaphyses.

ing the hip, knee, and ankle, are the best method (Fig. 169.12). The majority of children with genu valgum have physiologic genu valgum or its persistence into later childhood and early adolescence. However, there are other pathologic genu valgum disorders that may progress and cause functional impairment.

PHYSIOLOGIC GENU VALGUM

Pathophysiology
Physiologic genu valgum is a normal finding in children between 2 and 6 years of age (Fig. 169.13). The maximal deformity occurs between 3 and 4 years of age. It rarely causes symptoms or disability unless the deformity is severe. In these cases, the knees may rub, and the child walks and runs with a circumduction gait. With severe genu valgum deformities, the feet are pronated. In older children or adolescents, malalignment of the quadriceps mechanism may occur, resulting in patellar subluxation or dislocation. Severe genu valgum occurs more frequently in obese

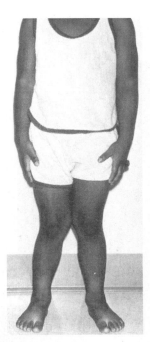

Figure 169.13. Typical appearance of physiologic genu valgum in a 4-year-old boy. With the knees approximated, there is a wide separation between the ankles. There is approximately 15° of genu valgum bilaterally.

Table 169.6. Surgical Options for Genu Valgum Deformities

Distal femur
Varus osteotomy
  Closing wedge
  Opening wedge
  Callotasis

Medial hemiepiphyseal stapling

Medial hemiepiphysiodesis

Proximal tibia
Varus osteotomy (may also include derotation and diaphyseal fibular osteotomy)
  Closing wedge
  Opening wedge
  Dome
  Oblique
  Callotasis
  Other

Medial hemiepiphyseal stapling

Medial hemiepiphysiodesis

children. The abnormal weight may produce a medial thrust that can result in laxity of the medial collateral ligament and possibly early degenerative osteoarthritis.

Preoperative Management and Planning

In 95% of cases, physiologic genu valgum resolves spontaneously with normal growth (94,161,163,190,197,207, 242,268,279). Use of an orthosis is controversial and is not recommended. Even significant deformities persisting into adolescence can be expected to improve or resolve if slow, steady improvement can be documented. Persistent deformities that are not improving may benefit from surgical treatment.

The major indication for surgical intervention in physiologic genu valgum is a persistent, severe deformity (>15°) in the immediate preadolescent years (ages 11 years in girls and 12 years in boys). After this age, significant spontaneous improvement is not likely to occur (141).

The methods for surgical correction of genu valgum are presented in Table 169.6. Three methods are usually employed for physiologic genu valgum:

Medial physeal stapling
Medial physeal hemiepiphysiodesis
Osteotomy

These procedures are applicable in the distal femur, proximal tibia, or both, depending on the patient's age and the severity and location of the deformity.

Operative Techniques

Medial Physeal Stapling of the Distal Femur or Proximal Tibia Retardation of growth about the medial aspect of the distal femur or proximal tibia by medial physeal stapling is a relatively easy, reliable method of correcting a genu valgum deformity if there is sufficient remaining growth to produce satisfactory alignment (Fig. 169.14) (36,105,141,193,221,282,294). If the deformity is pronounced or there is insufficient remaining skeletal growth, a combined stapling of the medial aspect of the distal femoral and the proximal tibial physes may be necessary (105, 221).

The medial aspect of the distal femoral epiphysis is palpable at the junction of the maximal metaphyseal flare and the medial femoral condyle. Stapling of the distal femoral epiphysis proceeds as follows.

■ Approach the physis through a 4–5 cm longitudinal incision between the anterior and posterior margins of the medial femoral condyle. Begin the incision approximately 1–1.5 cm distal to the physis, and extend it proximally.

■ Divide the subcutaneous tissues, deep fascia, and patellar retinaculum. If necessary, retract the medial margin of the vastus medialis anteriorly. Identify the physeal plate with a straight Keith needle or by fluoroscopy. Identification of the physis and insertion of the staples occur more quickly and more accurately with fluoroscopy. If the physeal plate is identified by probing with

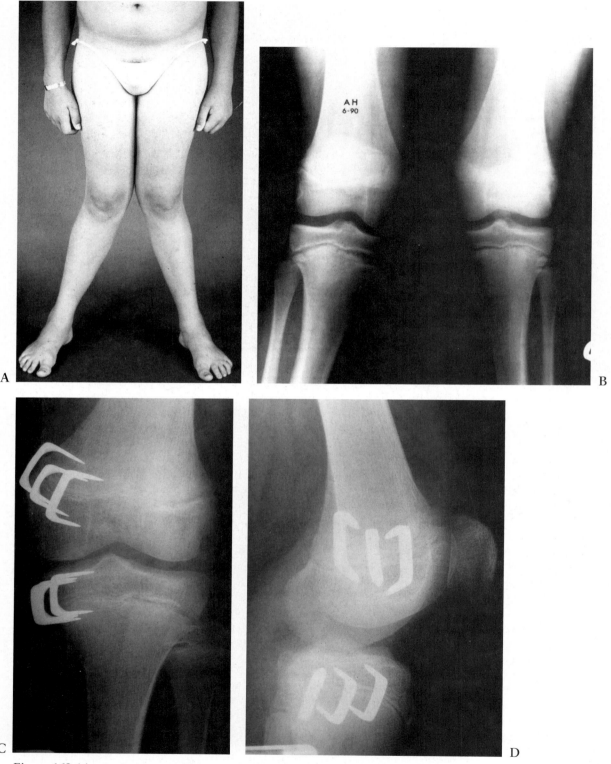

Figure 169.14.   **A:** A 14-year-old boy with persistent severe physiologic genu valgum. **B:** Standing AP radiograph of both lower extremities demonstrates a valgus deformity in the distal femora and proximal tibiae. Observe the physeal widening at the proximal tibial physes. A metabolic evaluation was normal. **C:** Postoperative radiograph of the left knee after stapling of the medial aspect of the distal femoral and proximal tibial epiphyses shows the three staples used to bracket each epiphysis. **D:** Lateral radiograph. *(continued)*

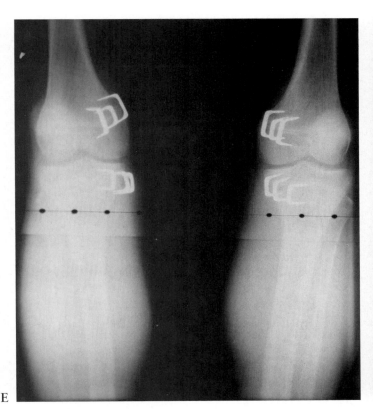

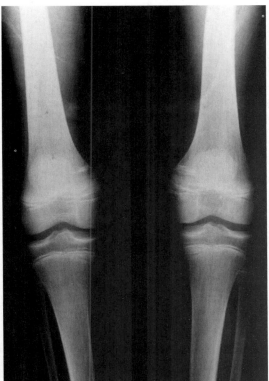

E
F

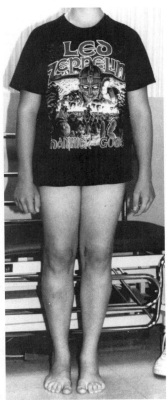

G

Figure 169.14. *(continued)* **E:** Standing radiograph of both knees 9 months postoperatively shows excellent correction of the genu valgum deformities. **F:** On a standing radiograph 6 months after staple removal, physiologic alignment is being maintained. **G:** Clinical photograph.

a Keith needle, the plate is softer than the adjacent cancellous bone.

- Select Blount staples that are rectangular or oblique, depending on the shape of the medial femoral condyle and metaphysis. Vitallium staples cause less reaction, are stronger, and are less likely to be extruded than stainless steel staples.
- Avoid subperiosteal stripping to protect the perichondrial ring and the physeal plate.
- With a staple holder, partially insert three staples. Insert one directly medially and one each in the anteromedial and the posteromedial aspects of the distal femur. Before completely setting the staples, confirm their location and orientation with radiographs or fluoroscopy. The physis should be in the mid portion of each staple. Insert the ends of the staple parallel to the physis to avoid physeal injury. If position and orientation are satisfactory, drive the staples flush with the periosteum. Do not bury the staples into the bone to avoid injury to the perichondrial ring.
- Close the patellar retinaculum and the deep fascia separately. It is important that the patellar retinaculum not be bound down by the staples because it can cause loss of knee motion, local swelling, and pain.
- Close the subcutaneous tissues and skin with absorbable sutures. A subcuticular closure of the skin gives the best cosmesis. Reinforce the incision with adhesive closure strips, and apply sterile dressings and a knee immobilizer.

If the proximal tibial physis is selected for stapling, the procedure is similar to that for the distal femur.

- Make a 4–5 cm longitudinal incision directly over the medial aspect of the knee. The incision usually begins just distal to the joint line and proceeds distally.
- Identify and retract anteriorly the medial border of the pes anserinus, if possible. Occasionally, the pes anserinus must be split. After the periosteum of the proximal tibia is visualized, identify the physeal plate with a Keith needle or by fluoroscopy.
- Insert one staple directly medially and one each in the anteromedial and the posteromedial aspects of the proximal tibia. The oblique or angulated Vitallium Blount staples are quite useful in this location because they conform to the flare of the medial aspect of the proximal tibia. Insert the staples parallel to the physis and the articular surface. Center the staples over the physeal plate. Before setting the staples, confirm the position radiographically.
- Close the wound in layers. If the pes anserinus is split, repair it with absorbable sutures. Close the subcutaneous tissues and skin in a similar manner, and apply sterile dressings.

Postoperatively, use a knee immobilizer for approxi-

mately 2 weeks. Follow up at 2–3-month intervals, and assess radiographically for correction. After the desired amount of correction has been achieved, remove the staples. However, there is frequently rebound overgrowth and slight recurrence of the deformity. Zuege et al. (294) recommended allowing 5° of rebound. Accomplish this by allowing the correction to proceed to slight overcorrection before staple removal. However, Fraser et al. (105) found that the amount of rebound overgrowth was minimal and unpredictable. They also advised against leaving the staples in place for longer than 1 year because of possible premature closure of the physis. The amount of correction can be calculated mathematically on the basis of the width of the physis and the amount of remaining growth (38).

Medial Hemiepiphysiodesis of the Distal Femur or Proximal Tibia   Partial or hemiepiphysiodesis of the medial aspect of the distal femur or proximal tibia has been proposed as a method for gradual correction of genu valgum deformity. The table devised by Bowen et al. (38) can be used to determine the appropriate time for epiphysiodesis. However, because of the variability in the data necessary to make these determinations, a second operative procedure is often required to close the remaining lateral portion of the epiphysis.

Rotational bone blocks, as described by Phemister (218), were once popular. However, the percutaneous techniques of epiphysiodesis using curet, drills, burrs, or a combination of these are now preferred (37,39,58,207, 276). These are as accurate and much more cosmetic than the open bone graft epiphysiodesis techniques. Although this technique is most commonly used for lower-extremity length discrepancies, it can also be used successfully in the correction of persistent angular deformities such as genu valgum and genu varum (39).

Percutaneous Epiphysiodesis
- Position the patient supine on a fluoroscopy table. Identify and mark the mid portion of the medial aspect of the distal femoral physis.
- Make a 2–3 mm incision directly over the physeal plate.
- Enter the medial aspect of the physis with a small curet or drill, and remove the medial portion of the physis. This allows the formation of a medial bone bridge. Do not extend the epiphysiodesis across the midline of the physis to avoid symmetric closure.
- Only a single subcutaneous suture is usually necessary to close the wound.

A similar procedure may be performed on the medial aspect of the proximal tibial epiphysis, if necessary.

After epiphysiodesis of the distal femur or proximal tibia, use a knee immobilizer for approximately 2 weeks. This allows skin and soft-tissue healing. The physis after epiphysiodesis is weak and must be protected for a short period to prevent complete physeal separation. At the end of 2 weeks, discontinue the knee immobilizer and allow the child active range-of-motion exercises and full weight bearing. Continue restriction of activities until 6 weeks postoperatively. Institute quadriceps and hamstring strengthening exercises at that time, with a gradual return to normal activities. After the desired correction has been achieved with medial epiphysiodesis, a lateral epiphysiodesis of the distal femur or proximal tibia is necessary to prevent overcorrection if the lateral physes remain open.

Osteotomy of the Distal Femur or Proximal Tibia Correction of a genu valgum deformity by distal femoral or proximal tibial and fibular diaphyseal osteotomies allows full correction of the deformity with a single operative procedure. However, both procedures are extensive and require internal or external fixation to maintain alignment until healing has occurred. In the correction of a valgus deformity, attention must be given to the peroneal nerve because neurapraxia or partial paralysis may occur if the nerve is stretched. The osteotomy may be performed in early adolescence or after skeletal maturity. Several techniques are available, including opening-wedge, closing-wedge, and dome osteotomies. The choice of technique is frequently based on the length of the lower extremity and the individual bones. An opening-wedge or dome-shaped osteotomy adds length to the extremity. DePablos et al. (87) described a progressive opening-wedge osteotomy using an external fixator; a fibular osteotomy is not required, and the osteotomy allows progressive and adjustable correction. Both lower extremities can be corrected simultaneously. Ordinarily, osteotomies are considered for boys age 14 years or older and girls age 12 years or older.

Varus osteotomy of the proximal tibia and diaphyseal osteotomy of the fibula are indicated if the valgus deformity is in the proximal tibia below the knee joint and there is no associated lateral tilt to the articular surface. The osteotomy is usually performed at the junction of the metaphysis and the diaphysis, just distal to the tibial tubercle. If there is associated lateral torsion of the tibia, derotation may also be accomplished. If a closing-wedge osteotomy is to be performed, perform the derotation initially because it frequently decreases the amount of bone requiring resection to correct the angular deformity. After satisfactory correction has been achieved, internal or external fixation is required. Compression plate and screws, crossed Steinmann wires, or an external fixator are suitable. In some cases, the Ilizarov ring fixator and the callotasis technique may be beneficial; this allows slow correction of the valgus and the derotation. Hemichondrodiastasis, or asymmetrical physeal lengthening, has been recommended by some, but it is not popular in the United States. This procedure allows simultaneous correction of limb-length inequality and correction of the genu valgum defor-

mity. Because the physeal plate closes after this procedure, it is best performed for patients in late adolescence.

Treat a genu valgum deformity associated with a valgus alignment of the distal femur with an osteotomy of the distal femur. Deformities in this area are associated with a lateral tilt to the joint line that cannot be corrected by a proximal tibial osteotomy. The osteotomy may be performed through a medial or a lateral approach to the distal femur. The medial approach is more complex because of the proximity of the femoral artery, but it allows easier visualization of the operative site. The lateral approach is simpler, and there is less risk to the femoral artery as it passes posteriorly at the upper margin of a medial incision. Opening- or closing-wedge osteotomies are commonly performed because it is difficult to perform a dome osteotomy of the distal femur. After the osteotomy is complete, internal or external fixation is performed with a compression plate and screws, crossed threaded Steinmann pins, or an external fixation device. See Chapters 30 and 31 for additional information on osteotomies of the femur and the tibia, respectively.

General Rehabilitation and Postoperative Principles

After an osteotomy has been performed, postoperative management depends on the type of internal or external fixation. If rigid internal fixation has been achieved with a compression plate and screws, immobilization is usually unnecessary, other than perhaps a knee immobilizer for 1–2 weeks for comfort. Allow only toe-touch weight bearing until early callus formation; then increase weight bearing, although not to full weight bearing, until the osteotomy site is completely healed. Remove the compression plate and screws 12–18 months postoperatively.

If simple external fixation is used, supplement it with a long-leg cast. Have the patient avoid weight bearing for 3–4 weeks, until there is early radiographic callus formation. Then allow toe-touch weight bearing. Usually, at 4–6 weeks after surgery, there is sufficient healing to allow removal of the external fixation device in the clinic. Apply a cylinder cast for an additional 2 weeks to allow solid union. After this has been accomplished, institute range-of-motion exercises. Failure to obtain a full range of motion at the end of 2 weeks is an indication for a referral to physical therapy. After full motion has been regained, begin strengthening exercises of the quadriceps and hamstring muscles. Return the patient to full activities after rehabilitation of the leg is complete.

Complications

The problems of asymmetric growth retardation associated with physeal stapling were outlined by Tachdjian (268): unpredictability of growth after the staples have been removed, possibility of asymmetric medial physeal closure, widening or loosening of the staples with eventual extrusion requiring revision, irregular patterns of initial growth retardation after stapling, the need for a second surgical procedure to remove the staples or to perform a lateral epiphysiodesis, and long and frequently wide operative scars due to stretching with knee motion. In 49 patients with genu valgum treated with stapling by Pistevos and Duckworth (221), there were no complications other than scarring, although six patients did not obtain complete correction. Staples may be painful; however, this resolves after removal.

Osteotomies of the distal femur or proximal tibia may result in peroneal nerve palsy, injury to the femoral or anterior tibial arteries, and anterior compartment syndrome (148,187,202,204,249,263,268). These severe complications are more common after proximal tibial osteotomies. Monitor patients closely postoperatively so that immediate intervention can be taken if a complication occurs. Postoperative wound infection, delayed union, nonunion, overcorrection, and undercorrection may occur after corrective osteotomies.

Conclusion

Because physiologic genu valgum does not usually have a rotational component, medial physeal stapling is my procedure of choice. This is usually performed on the proximal tibial epiphysis. In severe deformities, however, the distal femur may be included. I have not used the chart described by Bowen et al. (38). Once slight overcorrection is achieved, I remove the staples, and I have not encountered a case of premature physeal closure. This procedure is simple and effective and requires minimal postoperative immobilization.

PATHOLOGIC GENU VALGUM DEFORMITIES

Genu Valgum after Fractures of the Proximal Tibial Metaphysis

Fractures of the proximal tibial metaphysis are relatively common and tend to occur most frequently in children between 3 and 6 years of age (range, 1–12 years) (79,146, 150,205,237). Three times as many boys are affected as girls, which is typical for all tibial fractures (123). Skak et al. (258) reported an incidence of 5.6 fractures per 100,000 children per year. The fractures are usually the result of direct injury to the lateral aspect of the extended knee. The primary injury patterns are compression (i.e., torus fracture), incomplete tension–compression (i.e., greenstick fracture), or complete fractures (235). The fibula is typically intact but may be fractured or have a plastic deformation. The incomplete tension–compression or greenstick fracture is the most common pattern. The medial cortex on the tension side fractures, whereas the lateral cortex on the compression side remains intact or hinges slightly. The distal fragment may angulate into a

slight valgus deformity, but there is no displacement and the apposition remains normal. However, most fractures are nondisplaced and without angulation.

The most common sequelae of the fracture of the proximal tibial metaphysis are valgus deformity and overgrowth of the tibia. In 1953, Cozen (72) reported on four patients with valgus deformities after nondisplaced or minimally angulated fractures of the proximal tibial metaphysis. Many other reports of this complication have been published (16,18,21,27,30,44,51,66,71,76,79,109, 113,133,146,147,150,153,183,184,226,258,273,281, 283,292,293). Similar valgus deformities were observed after other insults to the immature proximal tibial metaphysis, such as osteomyelitis, bone-graft harvest, osteochondroma excision, and osteotomy (18,243,280).

The incidence of genu valgum deformity after proximal tibial metaphyseal fractures varies. It appears to occur in approximately 50% of cases. Salter and Best (244) reported on 21 patients with proximal tibial metaphyseal fractures, observing the development of a valgus deformity of 11° to 22° in 13 (62%) of them. Robert et al. (235) reported the development of a genu valgum deformity in 12 (48%) of 25 patients. However, Skak et al. (258) reviewed 40 consecutive patients and found the development of deformity in only 4 (10%). Boyer et al. (44) reported no valgus deformity in seven children 2–5 years of age who sustained fractures while jumping on a trampoline with a heavier child or adult. Valgus deformities occur predominantly in association with greenstick or complete fractures and are uncommon after a torus fracture (235,258).

Theories about the cause of valgus deformity include injury to the lateral aspect of the proximal tibial physis, inadequate reduction, premature weight bearing, hypertrophic callus formation, dynamic muscle action, soft-tissue interposition, tethering from the intact fibula, and asymmetric physeal growth stimulation (14,16,18,21,27, 30,34,51,61,66,71,72,76,80,113,133,139,140,146,147, 153,183,184,191,205,206,226,230,237,243,244,257, 273,281,283,292,293).

In 1990, Ogden et al. (206) measured the medial and the lateral metaphyseal–diaphyseal–metaphyseal tibial distances in 17 children with 19 proximal tibial metaphyseal fractures. They found four patients in whom the medial distance of the injured tibia was longer than the lateral distance, which was the same distance as the uninjured tibia. In 11 patients, there was overgrowth on both the medial and the lateral sides of the injured tibia. This indicates that a valgus deformity following a proximal tibial metaphyseal fracture is usually due to eccentric proximal medial overgrowth.

Assessment, Indications, and Relative Results Valgus deformity usually develops within 5 months of injury, reaches its maximum in 1–2 years, stabilizes, and then

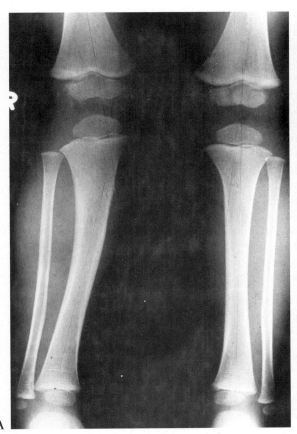
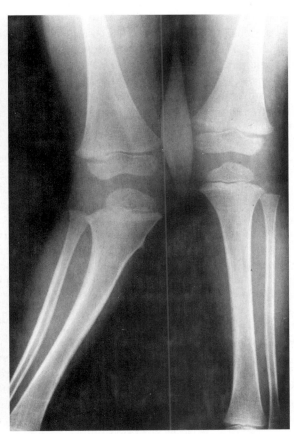

A

B

Figure 169.15. **A:** Standing AP radiograph of a 5-year-old boy after treatment for a greenstick fracture of the right proximal tibial metaphysis. At the time of cast removal, there was already 22° of genu valgum on the right but only 5° on the left. **B:** One year later, there was increased genu valgum deformity.

begins to improve by longitudinal growth through the proximal and distal physes (Fig. 169.15) (216). Unfortunately, there are no data indicating how much improvement can be anticipated. Salter and Best (244) found no improvement in 21 patients, and 13 later required proximal tibial varus osteotomies. Visser and Veldhuizen (281) reported no spontaneous improvement in the valgus deformity from the proximal tibial physis but observed some correction in alignment from the distal tibial epiphysis. Taylor (273) found improvement in some patients but not all. Of the 12 children with valgus deformity described by Jordan et al. (153), 11 had documented improvement, although four subsequently required corrective osteotomies. Two of these children had their deformities recur, and two had compartment syndromes. Six children had complete correction of their deformities.

Jackson and Cozen (147) and later Ippolito and Pentamalli (146) observed that deformities of 15° or less usually remodeled completely, especially in young children. The more severe deformities, however, did not completely

correct. Bahnson and Lovell (16) found some improvement in the valgus deformities in five children followed for a minimum of 3 years after injury. Balthazar and Pappas (18) reported that two of nine patients who were treated nonoperatively had resolution of their valgus deformity in 1–3 years. Skak et al. (258) found that valgus deformities tended to increase during the first year after injury and then remained constant for 1–2 years and finally improved. Only one of their six patients had residual deformity at final follow-up.

MacEwen and Zionts (183,293) followed seven children with posttraumatic tibial valgus deformities for a mean of 39 months after injury. These children were 11 months to 6 years of age. The valgus deformities progressed most rapidly during the first year after injury and then continued at a slower rate for as long as 17 months. Overgrowth of the tibia accompanied the valgus deformities. The mean overgrowth was 1 cm (range, 0.2–1.7 cm). Clinical correction with subsequent growth occurred in six of their seven patients. They recommended that the alignment of the lower extremities be measured by the mechanical femoro-tibial angle as described by Visser and Veldhuizen (281) rather than the metaphyseal–diaphyseal angle of Levine and Drennan (176). The latter measured only the alignment of the proximal tibia. Much of the late correction of the deformity is due to distal realignment (183,258,281). The distal epiphysis tends to realign itself perpendicular to the applied forces, resulting in asymmetric growth and an S-shaped appearance of the tibia radiographically (216).

Preoperative Management and Planning   The treatment of proximal tibial metaphyseal fractures must consist of correction of any associated valgus angulation by manipulative reduction and immobilization in a long-leg cast with the knee in extension for 4–6 weeks or until the fracture is well healed (238). If closed reduction is required, it is best performed under general anesthesia. Radiographic evaluation of fracture alignment may be difficult unless radiographs of both lower extremities with the knee in extension are obtained on a long cassette. Greenstick fractures with slight valgus angulation may require that the intact hinged lateral cortex be manually fractured. This usually allows correction of the deformity. Slight overcorrection is desirable (205).

Displaced fractures also require correction of any residual angulation. However, normal apposition is not always necessary. There are limited indications for open reduction of these fractures. Inability to correct a significant valgus deformity by manipulation under general anesthesia rather than failure to close the medial fracture gap is currently the major indication. Most angulated displaced fractures are amenable to reduction by nonoperative methods.

The final step in initial management is to advise the family that although anatomic alignment of the fracture has been obtained, the possibility of valgus angulation and tibial overgrowth exist as a natural consequence of this fracture. This information prepares the family for complications if they occur.

Assess fracture alignment radiographically at least weekly during the first 3 weeks after injury. Correct any loss of alignment. During this initial period, children should avoid bearing weight to minimize compression forces and the possibility of valgus angulation within the cast.

Treatment of valgus deformities after proximal tibial metaphyseal fractures is predominantly nonoperative with prolonged observation. The use of orthoses has been suggested, but there is no evidence to substantiate the efficacy of this method (89,133,146). MacEwen and Zionts (183) recommended observation until early adolescence. If spontaneous improvement fails to provide sufficient clinical correction, surgical intervention may be necessary. McCarthy et al. (188) reported no difference in the long-term results between 10 patients treated nonoperatively and five managed operatively.

The major indications for surgical intervention include severe valgus deformities (>25°) and failure to achieve satisfactory correction by the immediate preadolescent years. All children should be allowed 2–4 years of growth after injury to allow spontaneous correction to occur. Most deformities of 15° or less resolve, and those that are 25° or more may not. Deformities between 15° and 25° must be carefully followed. The development of a medial thrust during this observation period is an indication for surgical intervention to prevent laxity in the medial collateral ligament.

Operative Techniques   The operative procedures to correct genu valgum deformities after proximal tibial metaphyseal fractures are similar to those for other valgus deformities and include the following:

Medial physeal stapling
Medial physeal epiphysiodesis
Osteotomy with internal or external fixation

Because the deformity is usually restricted to the tibia, these procedures are most commonly applicable to the proximal tibia. They are described in the section on physiologic genu valgum. If surgical intervention is contemplated, it is important to assess the degree of tibial-length inequality. Surgery must address the valgus deformity and residual tibial overgrowth. In young children with severe genu valgum deformities that are not improving with spontaneous growth and development, a corrective osteotomy may be indicated. This should include shortening of the tibia by approximately 5 mm to allow recurrent overgrowth. Similar consideration is necessary in the early adolescent years when surgical intervention is planned.

Recurrence of Deformity   Recurrence has been attributed to the same overgrowth phenomenon that led to the initial valgus deformity. Balthazar and Pappas (18) reported that the valgus deformity recurred, although lesser in magnitude, in six children undergoing a proximal tibial varus osteotomy. Four of the six also had further longitudinal overgrowth of the tibia. DalMonte et al. (80) reported recurrent valgus deformities in 7 (44%) of 16 patients after proximal tibial osteotomies. The recurrence rate for children younger than 5 years was 60%, and for those between 5 and 10 years of age, it was 36%. The authors concluded that the osteotomy is essentially a second fracture and therefore has the same risks of deformity. If surgery is undertaken, families should be advised that the deformity can recur and that prolonged follow-up is required.

Conclusion   With the recent demonstration that the majority of children with genu valgum following a proximal tibial metaphyseal fracture will undergo spontaneous correction during growth, I now feel that these children should be observed for as long as possible. Only a severe disabling deformity should be considered for early surgical correction. Deformities persisting into adolescence can be corrected with a proximal tibial or distal femoral medial hemiepiphyseal stapling (or both). Typically, this allows for rapid correction of any residual deformity. I try to avoid corrective osteotomy because this may induce the same genu valgum deformity that followed the initial fracture.

Other Pathologic Genu Valgum Deformities

Metabolic Disorders Metabolic causes of pathologic genu valgum include vitamin D–resistant rickets, nutritional rickets, and renal osteodystrophy. These disorders are more likely to produce genu valgum rather than genu varum. This is due to their later onset, at which time the physiologic valgus alignment of the knee has already been achieved. Renal osteodystrophy is the most common metabolic disorder producing genu valgum (12,19,32,62,75, 81,132,143,210). Oppenheim et al. (210) described changes in the lateral proximal tibial epiphysis and me-

taphysis in children with renal osteodystrophy similar to those seen in the medial proximal tibia in Blount's disease.

Treatment is generally initiated after correction of the underlying metabolic disorder. Treatment before that time has a high incidence of recurrence. After the metabolic condition has been controlled, treatment may be by either osteotomy or physeal stapling of the distal femur or proximal tibia. The latter is a particularly effective method, provided there is sufficient remaining growth (Fig. 169.16).

Trauma Injuries to and about the distal femoral or proximal tibial epiphyses is a common cause of genu valgum (142,233). The deformities are progressive and require surgical treatment if there is an asymmetric physeal bar or bridge. The extent of the bar can be assessed by tomography or, preferably, MRI. Treatment options consist of physeal bar excision and grafting with fat or Silastic (Langenskiöld [169] procedure), together with a corrective osteotomy. If the bar is extensive, then complete physeal closure and corrective osteotomy may be performed, with delayed management of the leg-length discrepancy (see Chapter 164).

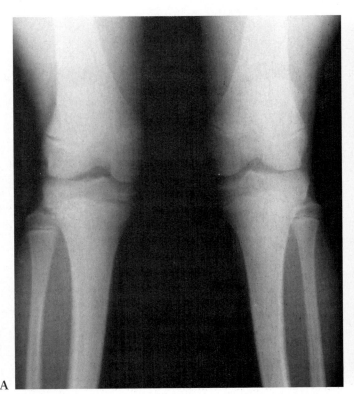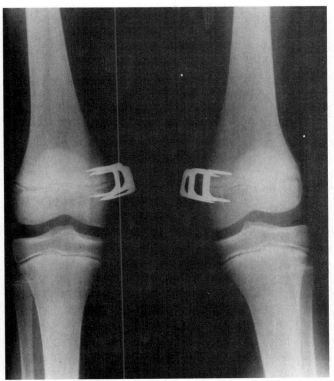

A   B

Figure 169.16. **A:** Preoperative standing radiograph of a 15-year-old boy 2 years after renal transplantation. His genu valgum has not been improving, although the physes now appear normal. **B:** Postoperative radiograph after insertion of staples about the medial aspect of the distal femoral epiphyses. *(continued)*

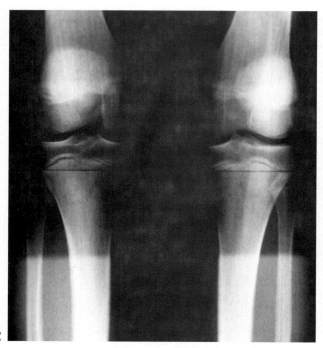

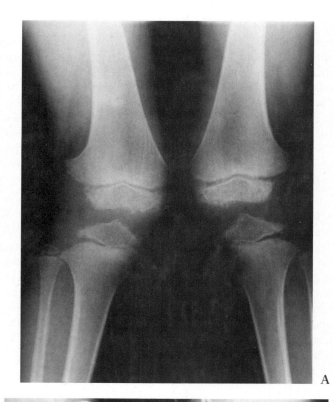

C

Figure 169.16. *(continued)* **C:** Standing radiograph at 18 months postoperatively and 9 months after staple removal demonstrates physiologic alignment and no evidence of growth disturbance.

Neuromuscular Ambulatory children with neuromuscular disorders, such as cerebral palsy, often have a pes valgus and excessive external tibial torsion that may produce a progressive genu valgum. This is more likely to be a torsional malalignment than a true genu valgum deformity. Treatment may involve soft-tissue releases to restore muscle balance and osteotomies to correct torsional and angular deformities (see Chapter 177).

Infection/Osteomyelitis Osteomyelitis may cause genu valgum directly by damaging the physis or producing a reactive hyperemia and asymmetric growth stimulation. Asymmetric physeal arrest is managed similarly to trauma (see Chapter 176).

Skeletal Dysplasia Genu valgum will occur in children with skeletal dysplasia, including multiple epiphyseal dysplasia, spondyloepiphyseal dysplasia, metaphyseal dysplasia, and pseudoachondroplasia. Treatment is based on the diagnosis. Orthotic management is usually ineffective in skeletal dysplasia. Surgery with either stapling or corrective osteotomies is usually necessary (Fig. 169.17) (see Chapter 180).

Inflammatory Disorders Juvenile rheumatoid arthritis may produce a progressive genu valgum deformity, but

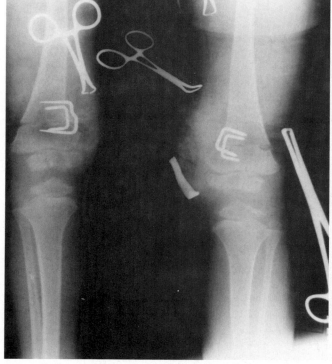

A

B

Figure 169.17. **A:** Preoperative standing radiograph of a 13-year-old boy with spondyloepiphyseal dysplasia and severe genu valgum. **B:** Intraoperative radiograph after closing-wedge distal femoral osteotomies. Staples were used to maintain alignment. *(continued)*

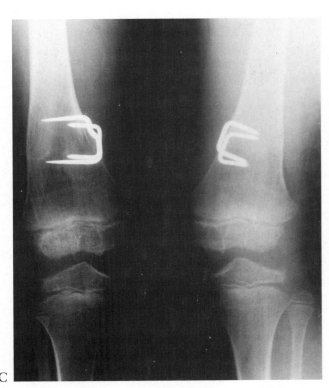

C

Figure 169.17. (continued) C: Standing radiograph 3 years postoperatively demonstrates that normal alignment is being maintained. Note the proximal migration of the staples with growth.

this is uncommon. Correction can be achieved by physeal stapling (240). In older children and adolescents, an osteotomy may be necessary.

CONGENITAL ANGULATION DEFORMITIES OF THE TIBIA AND FIBULA

Congenital angular deformities of the tibia and fibula are uncommon (Table 169.3). Anterior and anterolateral angulation or bowing is the most common form and is usually associated with other congenital anomalies, such as congenital pseudarthrosis (8,11,15,120,125,135,165, 200,212,231). Congenital posteromedial angulation is less common, resolves spontaneously, and is not associated with significant osseus pathology other than residual lower-extremity length inequality.

CONGENITAL ANTEROLATERAL BOWING OF THE TIBIA: CONGENITAL PSEUDARTHROSIS

Anterolateral bowing of the tibia is usually associated with significant pathologic disorders (Table 169.3). The

most common are congenital pseudarthrosis of the tibia, congenital longitudinal deficiency of the tibia (paraxial tibial hemimelia), and congenital longitudinal deficiency of the fibula (paraxial fibular hemimelia) (see Chapter 174).

Congenital pseudarthrosis of the tibia is a rare congenital malformation that includes all congenital fractures of the tibia and pseudarthrosis of the tibia arising after pathologic fracture in a tibia with congenital anterolateral angulation (4). Usually, anterior or anterolateral bowing of the tibia is recognized shortly after birth. Only occasionally are the fracture and pseudarthrosis present at birth, and the pseudarthrosis is therefore not truly congenital. Its incidence has been estimated to be 1 in 190,000 live births (149). The left side is affected slightly more often than the right (270); bilateral involvement is rare. Beals and Fraser (24,106) reported cases with bilateral and familial involvement. Congenital pseudarthrosis of the tibia is one of the most difficult and challenging deformities confronting orthopaedic surgeons (120,213, 270).

Pathophysiology
The exact cause of congenital pseudarthrosis of the tibia is unknown (43,49,52). Between 40% and 80% of children with this disorder are ultimately diagnosed with neurofibromatosis (5,49,52,56,74,186,203,213,214,262). Others have fibrous dysplasia or no associated disorders. Brown et al. (52), in a study of 17 children with a congenital pseudarthrosis, found that eight had neurofibromatosis, three had fibrous dysplasia, and six had no apparent disorder. Despite the clinical association with neurofibromatosis, the cause remains obscure.

Biopsy material removed from the tibia in the area of the pseudarthrosis shows a dense, cellular, fibrous connective tissue with variable areas of cartilage formation (43, 49,52,114). Electron microscopy reveals the lack of a basement membrane, and the cells resemble fibroblasts rather than Schwann cells or perineural cells, even in children with known neurofibromatosis (49). Only rarely is neurofibromatosis tissue observed in these specimens, and these samples are usually from intraosseous neurofibromas (114). In some cases, the tissue does resemble fibrous dysplasia (42). This dense, fibrous connective tissue with fibrocartilage and occasional bone trabeculae fills a poorly vascularized gap between the sclerotic bone ends to create the nonunion. This is not a true pseudarthrosis. The defective tissue occurs within the bone itself, the periosteum, the surrounding soft tissue, and possibly in the nerve and vascular supply to the involved area.

Assessment, Indications, and Relative Results
An infant predisposed to congenital pseudarthrosis of the tibia characteristically presents with anterior or anterolateral bowing of the tibia (Fig. 169.18). This rarely occurs

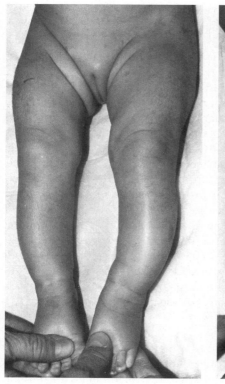
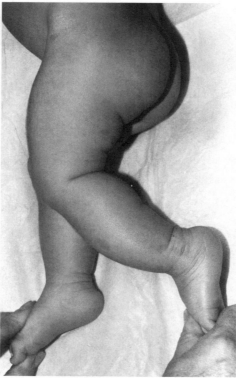
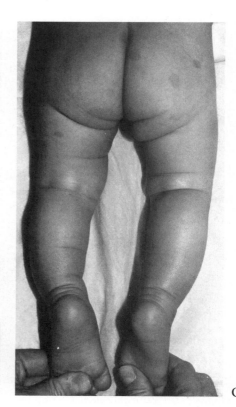

A,B   C

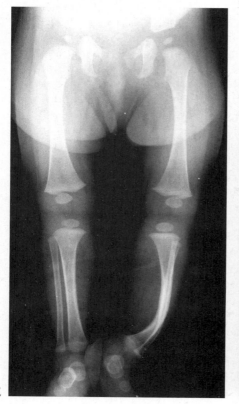
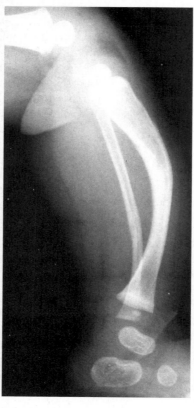

D,E

Figure 169.18. **A:** Photograph of a 3-month-old girl with anterolateral bowing of the left tibia shows numerous café-au-lait spots involving the left lower extremity. **B:** Lateral view shows anterior bowing of the tibia. **C:** On the posterior view, observe the café-au-lait spots. **D:** AP radiographs of the lower extremities demonstrate anterolateral bowing of the left tibia. The central portion of the tibia is sclerotic, and there is thinning of the fibula. This indicates a congenital pre-pseudarthrosis. **E:** Lateral radiograph demonstrates marked anterior bowing of the tibia. The apical sclerosis is more easily visualized in this view.

in conjunction with an acute fracture. The bowing is rarely anteromedial. The angular deformity of the tibia is congenital. Unless there is a fracture, the area is not tender, and a bony prominence is palpable. With an acute fracture, the area is unstable and is usually painful.

Because of the high incidence of neurofibromatosis in these patients, the hallmarks of this disease must be sought. The criteria used by Crawford (73) for diagnosis required at least two of the following:

Multiple café-au-lait spots
Positive family history
Definitive biopsy
Characteristic bony lesions, such as pseudarthrosis of the tibia, hemihypertrophy, or a short, sharply angulated spinal curvature

Café-au-lait spots are typically smooth-edged. The presence of at least five spots measuring more than 0.5 cm in diameter is considered diagnostic. The number of spots increases with the patient's age. Subcutaneous nodules (i.e., fibroma molluscum) are uncommon until adolescence and are typical of chronic disease. Although other bones may be involved in neurofibromatosis, involvement of more than one bone is extremely rare. Isolated cases of congenital pseudarthrosis of the fibula with an intact tibia have been reported (79,92,170). They were usually associated with anterior bowing of the tibia and ankle valgus. Curly and overlapping toes have been reported, as well as congenital constriction bands (201,271).

In children younger than 2 years presenting with anterior or anterolateral bowing of the tibia, there may be no clinical evidence of neurofibromatosis. The clinical features of neurofibromatosis usually become more apparent with growth and development. Radiographs of the tibia before the establishment of a pseudarthrosis may show an intact bowed tibia exhibiting sclerosis in the area of angulation without a medullary canal. After a fracture has occurred and a pseudarthrosis has been established, the proximal and the distal ends of the fracture site become tapered. Both tapered bone ends remain sclerotic.

Classification

Many classifications of pseudarthrosis have been based on the prognosis for various radiographic types (6,7,15, 20,40,73,125,186,270). The classification by Boyd (40) is one of the most commonly used methods of assessment (Table 169.7). Crawford (73) proposed a four-group functional classification:

Type I	Anterolateral bow with a normal medullary canal
Type II	Anterolateral bow with a narrow, sclerotic medullary canal (Fig. 169.19)
Type III	Anterior bow with a cystic lesion
Type IV	Anterolateral bow with a fracture, cyst, or frank pseudarthrosis (Fig. 169.20)

Table 169.7. Boyd Classification of Congenital Pseudarthrosis

Type I	Occurs in patients born with anterior bowing and a defect in the tibia (rare)
Type II	Occurs in patients born with anterior bowing and an hourglass constriction of the tibia Spontaneous fracture usually occurs before 2 years of age Is often associated with neurofibromatosis
Type III	Develops in a bone cyst, often at the junction of the upper and lower thirds of the tibia Anterior bowing may precede or follow a fracture
Type IV	Originates in a sclerotic segment of the tibia without any narrowing or fracture; the medullary canal is partially or completely obliterated Progresses to a stress-type fracture that fails to unite
Type V	Occurs in patients who also have a dysplastic fibula; pseudarthrosis develops later
Type VI	Occurs in patients with an intraosseous neurofibroma or schwannoma (very rare)

Adapted from Boyd HB. Pathology and Natural History of Congenital Pseudarthrosis of the Tibia. *Clin Orthop* 1982;166: 5, with permission.

The type of radiographic deformity is related to the recommended treatment. In Crawford's classification, a type I lesion has the best prognosis, and the remaining three types have progressively worse prognoses. However, the relation between the type of pseudarthrosis and the clinical result is not always predictable (4,73,183,198). The presence or absence of established neurofibromatosis makes no difference in the classification and is not a factor in determining treatment or prognosis. Cases in which bone-end resorption and sclerosis are evident radiographically and bone graft rapidly resorbs postoperatively have a poor prognosis. Those with a cystic lesion have a more favorable prognosis (198).

The natural history of anterior or anterolateral bowing of the tibia secondary to neurofibromatosis or fibrous dysplasia is a fracture with the establishment of a pseudarthrosis. The treatment of anterior and anterolateral bowing with an intact tibia is directed toward prevention

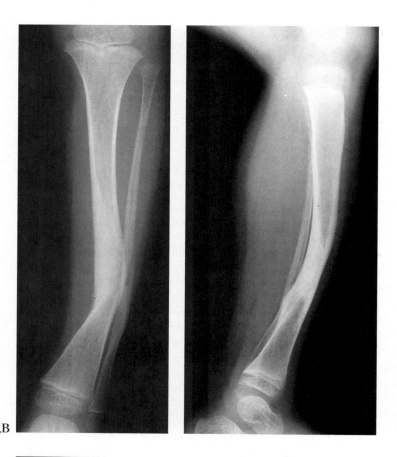

Figure 169.19.   A: AP radiograph of a 5-year-old boy with neurofibromatosis with a type II lesion of the left tibia. He has been managed in an ankle–foot orthosis since he began ambulation, and he has not had a fracture. B: Lateral radiograph demonstrates the apical sclerosis, which has been slowly improving.

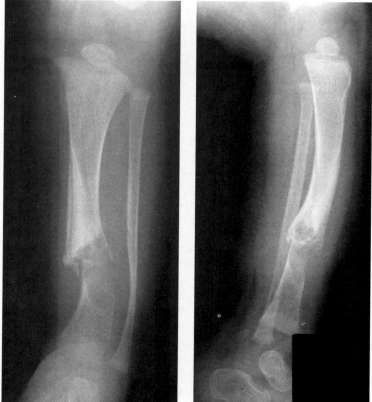

Figure 169.20.   A: AP radiograph of a 3-month-old child with a type IV congenital pseudarthrosis of the left tibia. Notice the cystic lesion and fracture. There is thinning of the distal aspect of the fibula. B: Lateral radiograph demonstrates anterior bowing.

of the fracture and pseudarthrosis. Congenital pseudarthrosis of the tibia is more than a mechanical problem (199); it represents a complex biologic problem because the established pseudarthrosis is extremely difficult to manage.

Preoperative Management and Planning

Patients with anterior or anterolateral bowing of the tibia without pseudarthrosis are best treated initially with a total-contact plastic orthosis. This is usually an ankle–foot orthosis. Prophylactic treatment may delay or prevent a fracture and subsequent pseudarthrosis. These orthoses are worn for years. With growth and in the absence of a fracture, the tibial bowing usually improves. There is typically some residual shortening within the bone. The medullary canal develops slowly over 5–10 years. It is possible, although unlikely, that a fracture and pseudarthrosis can be avoided with the use of an orthosis alone. If the tibia has straightened sufficiently, the medullary canal has reconstituted, and there is adequate cortical thickness, the orthosis may be discontinued as skeletal maturity is approached. Vigorous physical activities should be avoided. There are no long-term reports of successful orthotic management in adolescents or adults.

After a pathologic fracture and pseudarthrosis have occurred, the treatment is usually surgical. Casting alone rarely results in healing. However, Roach et al. (234) demonstrated that a late-onset fracture in a dysplastic tibia may heal with prolonged immobilization. Six of 11 fractures healed, but four of the six had a residual anterior bow susceptible to a stress fracture.

Operative Techniques

The indication for surgical management is an established pseudarthrosis. The goals of treatment include obtaining union at the pseudarthrosis site, maintaining union throughout growth and development, and obtaining an acceptable limb length at maturity (213,278). Previously, surgery was advised only for children age 4 years or older (6,125,203). Most physicians now recommend early surgical intervention and revision if the first procedure does not result in union of the pseudarthrosis (186,199,213, 214). Morrissey et al. (199) reported that a good result did not occur in any child whose tibia was not united by 6 years of age. Masserman et al. (186) reported that union was more related to the pathologic process than the age at surgery. Earlier union produces more normal growth of the distal tibial epiphysis and less lower-extremity length discrepancy.

The current methods of surgical treatment include bone grafting alone, bone grafting and internal fixation, electrical stimulation, microvascular bone grafting, Ilizarov external fixation methods, and amputation.

Bone Grafting Alone Prophylactic bone grafting has been used for the deformed tibia before a pathologic fracture occurs (179,191,266,270). This was thought to strengthen the deformed area and decrease the risk for pathologic fracture. The technique described by McFarland (191) is the most common procedure. A long corticocancellous graft from the opposite tibia is placed posteriorly, spanning the deformity in the normal biomechanical longitudinal axis of weight bearing. Lloyd-Roberts and Shaw (179), however, reported success in only three of their seven patients, while Tachdjian (270) reported success in all five children. Recently, Strong and Wong-Chung (266) prevented fracture in six of nine children with a prepseudarthrosis secondary to neurofibromatosis. Paterson (213), however, felt that the procedure was indicated primarily for cystic prepseudoarthrosis. Tachdjian (270) suggested concomitant curettage and bone grafting of any cystic lesions.

Many possible bone-grafting procedures have been used to treat an established congenital pseudarthrosis of the tibia (41–43,98,100,191,225,228). Morrissey et al. (199) reviewed 167 operations performed in 40 patients. The Farmer procedure, using a composite bone graft from the opposite tibia, demonstrated the best result, with a success rate of 53% (100). Other procedures had lower success rates, including onlay grafts (13%), bypass grafts (7%), Sofield procedure (25%), sliding grafts (33%), bone allograft (17%), and autogenous grafts (10%).

Bone Grafting and Internal Fixation Surgical excision of the pseudarthrosis, correction of the angular deformity of the tibia, and rigid internal fixation in addition to bone grafting have improved the rate of primary union. Stabilization has been achieved with compression plates and intramedullary rods. The former is rarely used because of difficulties involved in achieving adequate fixation (6, 213). The most common methods at this time are tibial or dual tibial and fibular intramedullary rods. These techniques usually transfix the ankle and subtalar joints to adequately stabilize the distal tibial segment (4,9,17,63, 108,278). These joints are progressively freed with growth of the tibia and proximal migration of the rod. This method does not result in significant stiffness of the joints. Postoperatively, immobilize with a unilateral hip spica cast followed by a long-leg cast and then a knee–ankle–foot orthosis. Anderson et al. (9) reported that 10 of 13 pseudarthroses healed with an intramedullary rod technique. However, their mean follow-up time was short (6.9 years).

Several researchers used extending intramedullary rods and bone grafting (e.g., double cortical onlay, cancellous) (31,102). These rods extended with growth, decreasing the need for revision surgery and protecting the union until skeletal maturity. They were not inserted across the ankle or subtalar joint. Bitan et al. (31) reported satisfactory extension of the rods in four of seven patients when these rods were used in revision surgery after primary union. Fern et al. (102) recommended that the outer sleeve of an extendable rod be inserted across the pseudarthrosis site to provide more strength and decrease the risk of refracture. They reported primary union in all five patients in whom extendable rods and bone grafting were used. All rods expanded with growth up to a maximum of 6.4 cm.

The use of intramedullary rods, especially those that stabilize the hind foot, and cancellous bone grafting increases the rate of primary union. The correction of anterior or anterolateral bowing undoubtedly enhances healing by allowing compression across the pseudarthrosis. These rods are not removed until after skeletal maturity because the tibia may undergo progressive bowing or refracture.

Electrical Stimulation   Electrical stimulation has been used in the treatment of congenital pseudarthrosis of the tibia for the past two decades (20,48,164,214,215,251, 267). The various techniques include implanted direct-current bone growth stimulators and external stimulation devices with pulsating electromagnetic fields. The addition of electrical stimulation has improved success rates after bone-grafting procedures (213,214). Most reports recommend that electrical stimulation be used in conjunction with internal fixation and bone grafting. In 1982, Kort et al. (164) observed that the most important variable in healing was the radiographic morphology of the nonunion. Patients with spindled bone ends, a large gap, and gross mobility had a poor prognosis, whereas those with a cystic or sclerotic transverse fracture and a gap of less than 5 mm had better responses.

Paterson and Simonis (214) described a technique of excision of the pseudarthrosis and abnormal tissue, fibular osteotomy, intramedullary rod fixation (i.e., large Steinmann pin or Kuntscher nail), cancellous bone grafting, and an implanted direct-current electrical bone growth stimulator. The leg was protected in a long-leg plaster cast until clinical and radiographic healing was achieved. Weight bearing was allowed and encouraged. They reported primary union in 20 (74%) of 27 patients. The average time for union was 7.2 months (range, 3–18 months). During a mean follow-up period of 3.8 years (range, 6 months to 10 years), no refractures were reported. The reasons for failure in seven patients included inadequate correction of the anterior tibial bowing, poor internal fixation, incorrect placement of the cathode, and extensively diseased bone. Brighton et al. (48) reported that only one of four patients with congenital pseudarthrosis of the tibia healed with direct-current stimulation from an implanted single cathode. However, they did not excise abnormal tissue, provide internal fixation, or use bone grafting. The extremities were immobilized in a plaster cast, and weight bearing was not allowed. They thought that the results did not prove the efficacy of this technique for congenital pseudarthrosis of the tibia.

In 1981, Bassett et al. (20) reported the results in 34 patients with congenital pseudarthrosis of the tibia treated with pulsed electromagnetic fields (PEMFs) by way of external coils. They reported that 17 of 34 patients achieved complete healing with reconstitution of the medullary canal. An additional seven (21%) patients achieved union with function but required continued protection with an orthosis. Healing of the pseudarthrosis occurred in 24 (71%) of 34 patients. Analysis of the failures demonstrated that most occurred in male patients with a history of early fracture (younger than 1 year) and with an atrophic, spindled, hypermobile pseudarthrosis. The researchers did not employ any additional surgical procedures in the initial treatment. However, after early healing was demonstrated radiographically, surgical realignment, immobilization, and bone grafting were combined with the PEMFs. This did not have an adverse affect on the ultimate outcome. In 1982, Sutcliffe and Goldberg (267) reported the results of 49 patients treated for congenital pseudarthrosis of the tibia with PEMFs. The definite end point of treatment was reached in 37 patients, and in 26 (70%) of them there was a successful outcome. Fifteen pseudarthroses healed with PEMFs alone. The remaining 11 patients required subsequent surgery, usually cancellous bone grafting, and a second course of PEMFs before healing was obtained.

It appears that electrical stimulation may help induce bone formation in the area of a pseudarthrosis and abnormal tissue. Electrical stimulation alone is effective in approximately 50% of the successful cases. In the remainder, additional procedures are necessary before primary union can be achieved, including excision of the pseudarthrosis and abnormal tissue, correction of existing deformity, intramedullary fixation, and cancellous bone grafting. However, in approximately 30% of cases, electrical stimulation with or without surgical intervention results in failure. The incidence of refracture appears to be low.

Microvascular Bone Graft   Free vascularized bone grafts represent another popular procedure for congenital pseudarthrosis of the tibia (64,68,84,85,93,108,112,121, 154,175,196,219,220,259,272,277,284,285,295). Vascularized rib, iliac crest, and fibula grafts have been used, and the latter appears to be superior in congenital pseudarthrosis of the tibia (64,68,84,85,92,108,121,154,175, 219,220,284,285). The graft can be ipsilateral if it is of sufficient size (68,196,259,295). The procedure consists of transferring the contralateral fibular diaphysis on its vascular pedicle with a cuff of muscle to maintain the periosteal blood supply into a defect created by resecting the pseudarthrosis and abnormal soft tissue on the involved side (Fig. 169.21). Supplemental cancellous bone

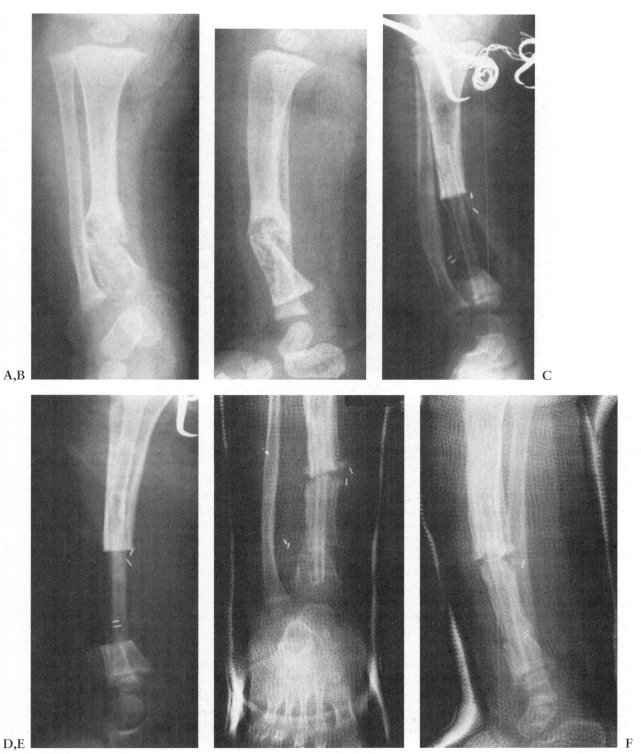

Figure 169.21. **A:** AP radiograph of the right lower leg of a 6-month-old boy with neurofibro-matosis and a congenital pseudarthrosis of the distal tibia. **B:** Lateral radiograph. **C:** A proce-dure using a vascularized fibula graft from the left leg was performed at 17 months of age. Internal fixation was not used, and the ends of the fibula graft were inserted into the medullary canal proximally and into the metaphysis distally. **D:** Lateral radiograph. **E:** Two months after vascularized-fibula grafting, there is extensive subperiosteal new bone formation and hypertrophy of the graft. **F:** Lateral radiograph. *(continued)*

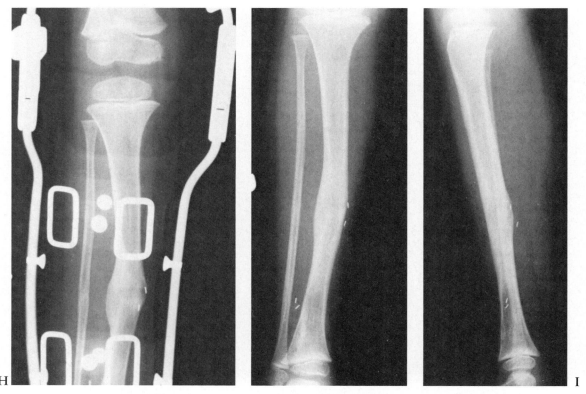

G,H   I

Figure 169.21. *(continued)* **G:** Twenty-two months later, the tibia is healed, but the leg is protected in a knee–ankle–foot orthosis. **H,I:** Thirty-three months postoperatively, the tibia has healed well, and the medullary canal is reforming in the area of the vascularized fibula.

grafting may be included to facilitate bone healing. The fibular graft is advantageous because it is straight, a long segment can be harvested, and it tends to hypertrophy after healing. Leung (175) reported three successful microvascularized iliac crest grafts in congenital pseudarthrosis of the tibia. He thought that it was easier to harvest the iliac crest and there was a more rapid healing because the graft was predominantly corticocancellous bone rather than cortical bone alone. Iliac crest grafts ranging from 3 to 10 cm may be obtained in children age 4 years or older. Rib grafts are less advantageous because of their curvature. Hagan and Buncke (121) reported that this curvature does not tend to correct with growth after satisfactory incorporation and the curvature may increase. Use of extensive corticocancellous grafting may prevent progressive bowing of the vascularized rib graft. Donor site problems after vascularized fibula transfers have been reported (209).

In 1990, Weiland et al. (285) reported on the long-term results in 19 consecutive children with congenital pseudarthrosis of the tibia treated with a vascularized fibula graft. The mean age at surgery was 5.1 years (range, 1.4–11.4 years). The mean follow-up was 6.3 years (range, 2–11 years). They reported that 18 (95%) of the

19 pseudarthroses healed. The lower-extremity length discrepancy at follow-up was a mean of 1.6 cm (range, 0–4 cm). Sixteen of the children had been treated with electrical stimulation techniques, which failed, for at least 1 year before surgery. However, the fibular graft hypertrophied rapidly, and no graft fractured during follow-up. Five patients required secondary procedures for nonunion and angulation. Only one child failed and subsequently required an amputation. Four patients ultimately achieved healing, although they required nine bone-grafting procedures. Two children had fractures through normal bone distal to the vascularized bone graft; they also required bone-grafting procedures to achieve union. Morbidity of the donor site was minimal, but one patient sustained a nondisplaced fracture of the tibia through a screw hole, and a 20° valgus deformity requiring osteotomy developed in another. Thirteen tibiae had residual deformity: valgus deformity (five patients); anterior angulation (two patients), or both (six patients). The mean valgus deformity was 25° (range, 5° to 45°), and the mean anterior angulation was 24° (range, 10° to 30°). Two patients with a valgus deformity required correction with an osteotomy. Four patients had anterior bowing of more than 20°, but none required additional surgery. All chil-

dren were treated with orthoses until skeletal maturity was achieved.

The five basic steps of free vascularized bone grafts are applicable whether iliac crest or fibula graft is used (220):

- Harvest of the vascularized bone with an intact vascular pedicle
- Excision of the tibial pseudarthrosis and abnormal tissue
- Fixation of the vascularized bone *in situ*
- Microvascular anastomosis
- Skin closure

The procedure is usually performed with two surgical teams. One team harvests the vascularized bone, and the second prepares the recipient site. Some form of internal fixation is usually necessary to maintain alignment of the extremity. One advantage of microvascularized bone grafts is the simultaneous correction of any residual deformity and possible tibial lengthening, depending on the mobility of the tibial segments. Prolonged immobilization is necessary until healing occurs, with protected weight bearing allowed thereafter. Weiland et al. (285) maintain their children in hip spica casts for 2–3 months to allow healing. After healing occurs, protected weight bearing with a knee–ankle–foot orthosis is allowed. The orthosis is worn until skeletal maturity (see Chapter 36).

Ilizarov Fixation System   The Ilizarov method has been shown to be effective in achieving union at the pseudarthrosis site and in simultaneously correcting any associated angular deformity and lengthening of the tibia to restore length (85,99,119,144,211,224). The apparatus can be used in four ways: compression of the pseudarthrosis, compression with metaphyseal tibial lengthening, compression followed by distraction for hypertrophic nonunion, and distraction alone for hypertrophic nonunion. Excellent short-term results for union were reported. Whether the union is maintained in the long term remains uncertain.

Amputation   In children with persistent congenital pseudarthrosis of the tibia after previous surgical procedures, an amputation may be advised. This should be a Boyd or Symes ankle-disarticulation amputation of the foot (82,134,149,189). See Chapter 175 on principles of pediatric amputation and Chapters 120 and 122 on lower-extremity amputations and prostheses. Amputation with appropriate prosthetic fitting allows rapid rehabilitation and return to normal function. McCarthy (189) recommended amputation for several criteria: failure to achieve bony union after three surgical attempts, a significant lower-extremity length inequality (usually 5 cm or greater), development of a deformed foot, undue functional loss from prolonged hospitalizations, and high medical costs.

The Boyd or Symes amputation is usually the procedure of choice. It preserves the heel pad and distal tibial epiphysis, which allows end bearing on the stump. The bone and skin are lengthened as a unit to avoid problems with overgrowth (82). A below-knee amputation through the pseudarthrosis produces a poor end-bearing stump for ambulation. The abnormal tissue and previous surgical scar provides poor skin coverage and predisposes to breakdown. There are also the problems of overgrowth and frequent revision. Amputation above the pseudarthrosis site provides better skin coverage, but there are problems with bony overgrowth.

Jacobsen et al. (149) reported the results of Symes amputation in eight children with pseudarthrosis of the tibia. The average age at amputation was 8.2 years, and the mean follow-up was 5.9 years. These children had a mean of 3.8 surgical procedures performed before amputation. None of the pseudarthroses healed, but with an appropriate Symes prosthesis, the children were able to engage in normal activities, including sports. The lower-extremity length inequality and some of the angular deformity were corrected within the prosthesis. Herring et al. (134) reported that 21 children (none with congenital pseudarthrosis) who had 23 Symes amputations had better psychological functioning than children undergoing multiple corrective surgical procedures. The better psychological function correlated with their better orthopaedic function. The level of family stress influenced the child's behavior, self-perception, and intelligence. The physicians thought that an early Symes amputation in a young patient was compatible with good athletic and psychological functioning, which closely approached that of a nonhandicapped child of the same age. Similar results were reported by Davidson and Bohne (82) for 23 children, including one with a congenital pseudarthrosis of the tibia that did not heal.

Because of the complexities associated with the treatment of pseudarthrosis of the tibia, it is recommended that Symes amputation be discussed as an alternative method of treatment with the parents and child from the outset. Discussion should not be delayed until later in the treatment. Tell the family of the difficulties that will be encountered in attempting to obtain primary tibial union and satisfactory function.

General Rehabilitation and Postoperative Principles

Each surgical procedure has its specific postoperative regimen, but all share long-term orthotic management. The extremity needs to be protected with a plastic ankle–foot orthosis. This helps prevent recurrent refracture. Protection is required at least until skeletal maturity and perhaps even longer. This decision is based on the radiographic appearance of the tibia, the degree of residual deformity, and the presence or absence of a reconstituted medullary canal.

Rehabilitation to restore maximum strength and function after healing of a congenital pseudoarthrosis of the tibia is very important. Karol et al. (156) recently performed gait analysis on 12 patients with healed lesions and four patients treated by amputation. Gait and muscle strength were markedly disturbed. Early onset of fracture, early surgery, and transankle fixation lead to an inefficient gait compared with that of amputees.

Complications

Congenital pseudarthrosis of the tibia is a difficult and challenging deformity. Refracture, tibial and lower-extremity length discrepancy, stiffness of the ankle and subtalar joints, progressive anterior angulation of the tibia, and ankle valgus are the major complications (270,285). Surgical complications are also common. Most children have had multiple surgical procedures and are at risk for infection and neurovascular injury. Because of these problems, the true outcome of a congenital pseudarthrosis cannot be fully assessed until skeletal maturity. Crossett et al. (74) found that the clinical results for their patients remained stable after skeletal maturity. Neurofibromatosis does not increase the incidence of complications or adversely affect the final clinical result (198).

Conclusion

Probably, the most important aspect of the management of children with congenital pseudarthrosis of the tibia is to minimize the number of operative procedures and to maintain as normal function as possible. Prevention of fractures in children with prepseudarthrosis lesions is critically important. This can sometimes be achieved with a clamshell ankle–foot orthosis. After a pseudarthrosis is established, the best results with respect to union are achieved with a vascularized fibula graft or intramedullary rod. I feel that the initial surgical procedure should be the latter. This allows straightening of the tibia, with weight bearing providing compression across the pseudarthrosis. The results of a vascularized fibula transfer are also good, but I am concerned about a major operative procedure on the uninvolved extremity. Once it is apparent that a pseudarthrosis cannot be satisfactorily healed, Symes amputation and prosthetic replacement permit restoration of relatively normal function.

CONGENITAL POSTEROMEDIAL ANGULATION OF THE TIBIA AND FIBULA

Pathophysiology

The cause of congenital posteromedial angulation of the tibia and fibula is unknown. There is some evidence to indicate a primary chondro-osseous defect in the embryo-

logic development of the distal tibial and fibular epiphyses (138,212). Pappas (212) demonstrated delayed development of the secondary center of ossification of the distal tibia and a relative reduction in the height of the distal epiphysis. Other possibilities include intrauterine fracture of the tibia and fibula with malunion, restriction of growth from soft-tissue contractures, or intrauterine malpositioning with the affected leg molded under the buttock (15,83,107,165).

Assessment, Indications, and Relative Results

Congenital posteromedial angulation of the tibia and fibula has three associated clinical problems (120,135,136, 194,212,231,236):

Angular deformity
Calcaneovalgus foot
Lower-extremity length inequality

The tibia and fibula are shortened and bowed posteriorly and medially at the junction of the middle and distal thirds of their shafts. The deformity, which is obvious at birth, is usually unilateral. The right and left sides are equally affected, and there is no sex predilection (138). Infants are typically normal, and there is no increased incidence of other congenital anomalies (288). Hofmann and Wenger (138) reported on a child who had a contralateral talipes equinovarus (clubfoot) deformity. Angulation can vary from 25° to 65°, with the magnitude of deformity in the posterior and medial directions being almost equal (241). The foot is hyperdorsiflexed and has a marked calcaneovalgus posture. It appears to fit into the anterior cavity of the lower leg. The anterior compartment muscles appear shortened and limit plantar flexion of the foot. The posterior bow of the shaft causes the distal portion of the tibia and fibula at the ankle to angulate anteriorly. This makes the limitation of plantar flexion seem even more severe. There is no true bone deformity of the ankle or foot. The calf musculature is usually slightly atrophic, and the foot is smaller than on the opposite, normal side (8,138). There may be a dimple at the apex of the posteromedial angulation (8,53,135,138,212). Occasionally, an extra skin crease is associated with the dimple (212).

Anteroposterior and lateral radiographs of the lower extremities of an affected child are necessary for complete assessment. The proximal aspects of the tibia and fibula, including their epiphyses, are normal. The degree of posteromedial angulation of the distal aspect of the tibia and fibula can be measured directly from the radiographs. The cortices in the concave aspect of the posterior and medial bows are thickened, and the distal aspects of the tibia and fibula are broader than the opposite, uninvolved side (212). The intramedullary cavities at the apex of the bowing are usually poorly developed or obliterated by sclerotic bone. The alignment of the tarsal and metatarsal bones is relatively normal, although occasionally there may be a slight valgus orientation. Radiographs of the femora and pelvis should be obtained for thorough assessment of the lower extremities. Special diagnostic studies, such as MRI, are rarely indicated.

The posteromedial angulation or bowing resolves with growth, especially during the first 3 years of life (Fig. 169.22). The posterior bowing resolves more quickly than the medial bowing, which may not resolve until 5 years of age (120,212). However, the associated shortening of the tibia and fibula, which is unrelated to the bowing, persists and progresses during growth (8,138,212,288). The fibula is frequently slightly shorter than the tibia; there is usually no shortening in the femur. The mean growth inhibition in the involved tibia and fibula averages 12% to 13% (range, 5% to 27%). This percentage of growth inhibition persists throughout growth and development. There appears to be a direct correlation between the degree of tibial shortening and the degree of posteromedial angulation: The greater the angulation, the more severe is the lower-extremity length discrepancy (135,136, 138,165). The mean tibial length difference is approximately 1.2 cm in the first 2 months of life, 2.4 cm by 5 years of age, 3.3 cm at 10 years, and 4.1 cm (range, 3.3–6.9 cm) at maturity (138,212). It is possible to determine the percentage of inhibition and the ultimate leg-length inequality by annual scanographic evaluation and bone-age determination after the posteromedial angulation has resolved. During the first 6 months of life, correction of the bowing is rapid, and by 2 years of age approximately 50% of the angulation has undergone spontaneous correction. After 3 years of age, improvement in the deformity occurs at a much slower rate.

The appearance of the foot gradually improves with growth and development. As the posterior bowing decreases, the degree of plantar flexion improves. A pes planovalgus appearance of the foot may persist. Hofmann and Wenger (138) found mild loss of ankle dorsiflexion in older children. They thought that this was due to mild equinus contracture from toe-walking to compensate for the length discrepancy. It may also be due to the slightly shorter fibula.

Preoperative Management
Because posteromedial angulation of the tibia and fibula in children undergoes spontaneous resolution, treatment is predominantly conservative. In newborn and young infants, passive stretching exercises of the hyperdorsiflexed foot may be performed to stretch the anterior compartment muscles and improve plantar flexion. It is important to assess maximal plantar flexion of the foot on a lateral radiograph because of the anterior angulation of the distal tibia, fibula, and ankle joint. What appears to be limited plantar flexion may only be secondary to the anterior tilt to the articular surface of the distal tibia. The talus may

be in full plantar flexion in the ankle mortise, but the foot still may not appear plantigrade.

In selected cases, use serial short-leg casts to hold the foot in maximal plantar flexion and inversion (83,194, 231,288). In 3–6 weeks, maximal stretching of the anterior compartment musculature and anterior ankle capsule is usually achieved. Yadav and Thomas (288) reported that six children with a unilateral posteromedial bow of the tibia did well with serial casting, although one patient underwent an anterior soft-tissue release before initiation of casting. After complete correction has been obtained, passive exercises may be continued to maintain alignment. In severe cases, Tachdjian (269) recommended the use of night splints to hold the foot in plantar flexion and inversion. After 2–3 years of age, a University of California Biomechanics Laboratory or similar foot orthosis may be worn to support the planovalgus foot deformity. However, in view of the natural history and management of posteromedial bowing, the use of casts and orthoses is probably not indicated. Heyman and Herndon (135) initially thought that an orthosis was necessary to reduce the posterior thrust at the apex of the deformity during weight bearing. However, in their later report, they stated that the use of an orthosis was unnecessary (136).

Follow children with posteromedial angulation of the tibia and fibula with annual scanograms and bone-age determinations (10,118,200) (see Chapter 170 on leg-length inequality).

Operative Techniques
Typically, there are only two operative procedures utilized in this disorder:

- Osteotomy to correct severe or persistent angulation
- Equalization of lower-extremity length inequality

Tibia and Fibula Osteotomy   Osteotomy to correct posteromedial bowing of the tibia is rarely indicated. If severe medial bowing persists after 3 or 4 years of age, corrective osteotomy may be considered. Bone healing is not a problem after a corrective osteotomy or a fracture because there is no underlying bone disorder affecting healing (8, 83,165,231). Hofmann and Wenger (138) suggested corrective osteotomy in cases of severe bowing with progressive shortening during the first 5 years of life. They thought that an osteotomy would add length by correcting the deformity and realigning the physes perpendicular to the axis of weight bearing, stimulating growth. These concepts were not confirmed clinically. Osteotomy can realign the tibia, but it has a minimal effect on the ultimate lower-extremity length inequality. Krida (165) reported that all three patients treated by corrective osteotomies had significant residual leg-length discrepancies.

Leg-length Equalization   Lower-extremity length discrepancy is the most common sequela of posteromedial

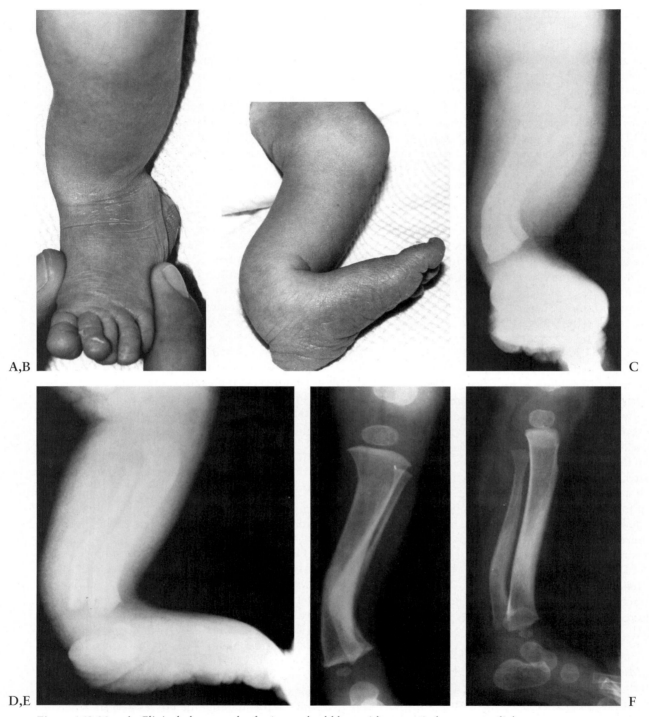

Figure 169.22.   **A:** Clinical photograph of a 1-month-old boy with congenital posteromedial bowing of the left tibia. Observe the medial bowing of the distal aspect of the tibia. **B:** The posterior bow of the distal tibia produces a calcaneovalgus appearance of the left foot. **C:** AP radiograph of the left leg confirms the severe medial bowing of the distal third of the tibia and fibula. **D:** Lateral radiograph demonstrates the posterior bowing and the calcaneovalgus appearance to the foot. The alignment of the foot is due to the dorsal angulation of the distal tibia and ankle. **E:** AP radiograph obtained at 1 year demonstrates decreased medial angulation of the distal tibia. **F:** Lateral radiograph shows a significant decrease in the posterior bow of the tibia and improved alignment of the ankle joint. *(continues)*

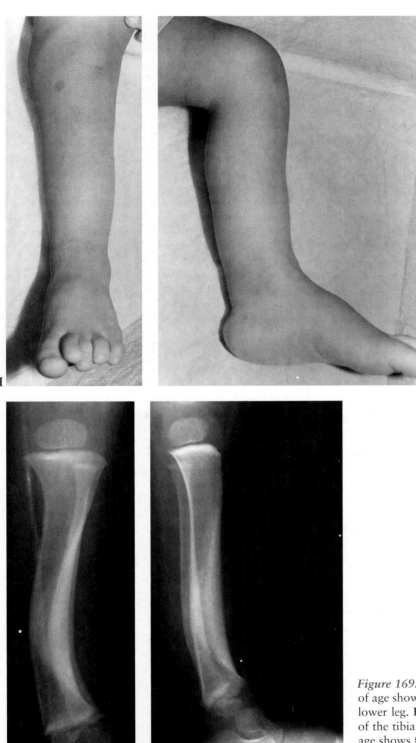

G,H

I,J

Figure 169.22. *(continued)* **G:** Clinical photograph at 2 years of age shows marked improvement in the appearance of the left lower leg. **H:** There is only slight residual posterior angulation of the tibia in the sagittal plane. **I:** AP radiograph at 2 years of age shows further improvement in the medial angulation of the distal tibia. **J:** Lateral radiograph confirms further improvement in posterior angulation.

angulation of the tibia and fibula. Most affected children have enough inequality (2 cm) to require equalization. The procedure performed to equalize the leg length depends on the estimated tibial length inequality at maturity and the predicted normal height of the child (see Chapter 170).

Conclusion

In patients with posteromedial angulation of the tibia, I prefer prolonged observation. Casting of the foot is rarely indicated, as the limitation of dorsiflexion is due primarily to the alignment of the ankle. This will correct with growth. The associated lower-extremity length inequality is followed by scanograms at 1- or 2-year intervals. An appropriately timed contralateral percutaneous proximal tibial and fibular epiphysiodesis is the procedure of choice for most patients. Leg-lengthening techniques are usually not necessary, unless the discrepancy is severe or the patient has short stature.

REFERENCES

Each reference is categorized according to the following scheme: *, classic article; #, review article; !, basic research article; and +, clinical results/outcome study.

+ 1. Agamanolis DP, Weiner DS, Lloyd JK. Slipped Capital Femoral Epiphysis: A Pathological Study. I. A Light Microscopy and Histochemical Study of 21 Cases. *J Pediatr Orthop* 1985;5:40.

+ 2. Agamanolis DP, Weiner DS, Lloyd JK. Slipped Capital Femoral Epiphysis: A Pathological Study. II. An Ultrastructural Study of 23 Cases. *J Pediatr Orthop* 1985;5:47.

+ 3. Albiñana J, Cuervo M, Certucha JA, et al. Five Additional Cases of Focal Fibrocartilaginous Dysplasia. *J Pediatr Orthop B* 1997;6:52.

+ 4. Andersen KS. Congenital Pseudarthrosis of the Leg: Late Results. *J Bone Joint Surg Am* 1976;58:657.

+ 5. Andersen KS. Congenital Pseudarthrosis of the Tibia and Neurofibromatosis. *Acta Orthop Scand* 1976;47:108.

+ 6. Andersen KS. Operative Treatment of Congenital Pseudarthrosis of the Tibia: Factors in Influencing the Primary Results. *Acta Orthop Scand* 1974;45:935.

+ 7. Andersen KS. Radiological Classification of Congenital Pseudarthrosis of the Tibia. *Acta Orthop Scand* 1973;44:719.

+ 8. Andersen KS, Bohr H, Sneppen O. Congenital Angulation of the Lower Leg: Crus Curvatum Congenitum. *Acta Orthop Scand* 1968;39:387.

+ 9. Anderson DJ, Schoenecker PL, Sheridan JJ, Rich MM. Use of an Intramedullary Rod for the Treatment of Congenital Pseudarthrosis of the Tibia. *J Bone Joint Surg Am* 1992;74:161.

! 10. Anderson M, Green WT, Messner MB. Growth and Prediction of Growth in the Lower Extremities. *J Bone Joint Surg Am* 1963;45:1.

+ 11. Angle CR. Congenital Bowing and Angulation of Long Bones. *Pediatrics* 1954;13:257.

+ 12. Apel DM, Millar EA, Moell DI. Skeletal Disorders in Pediatric Renal Transplant Population. *J Pediatr Orthop* 1989;9:505.

! 13. Arkin AM, Katz JF. The Effects of Pressure on Epiphyseal Growth: The Mechanism of Plasticity of Growing. *J Bone Joint Surg Am* 1956;38:1056.

! 14. Aronson DD, Stewart DC, Crissman JD. Experimental Tibial Fractures in Rabbits Simulating Proximal Tibial Fractures in Children. *Clin Orthop* 1990;255:61.

+ 15. Badgley CE, O'Connor SJ, Kudner DF. Congenital Kyphoscoliotic Tibia. *J Bone Joint Surg Am* 1952;34:349.

+ 16. Bahnson DH, Lovell WW. Genu Valgum Following Fractures of the Proximal Tibial Metaphysis in Children. *Orthop Trans* 1980;4:306.

+ 17. Baker JK, Cain TE, Tullos HS. Intramedullary Fixation for Congenital Pseudarthrosis of the Tibia. *J Bone Joint Surg Am* 1992;74:169.

+ 18. Balthazar DA, Pappas AM. Acquired Valgus Deformity of the Tibia in Children. *J Pediatr Orthop* 1984;4:538.

+ 19. Barrett IR, Papadimitriou DG. Skeletal Disorders in Children with Renal Failure. *J Pediatr Orthop* 1996;16:264.

+ 20. Bassett CAL, Caulo N, Kort J. Congenital "Pseudarthroses" of the Tibia: Treatment with Pulsing Electromagnetic Fields. *Clin Orthop* 1981;154:136.

+ 21. Bassey LO. Valgus Deformity Following Proximal Metaphyseal Fractures in Children: Experience in the African Tropics. *J Trauma* 1990;30:102.

+ 22. Bateson EM. The Relationship between Blount's Disease and Bow Legs. *Br J Radiol* 1968;41:107.

+ 23. Bathfield CA, Beighton PH. Blount Disease: A Review of Etiological Factors in 110 Patients. *Clin Orthop* 1978;135:29.

+ 24. Beals RK, Fraser W. Familial Congenital Bowing of the Tibia with Pseudarthrosis and Pectus Excavatum: Report of a Kindred. *J Bone Joint Surg Am* 1976;58:545.

+ 25. Beck CL, Burke SW, Roberts JM, Johnston CE II. Physeal Bridge Resection in Infantile Blount Disease. *J Pediatr Orthop* 1987;7:161.

* 26. Bell SN, Campbell PE, Cole WG, Menelaus MB. Tibia Vara Caused by Focal Fibrocartilaginous Dysplasia: Three Case Reports. *J Bone Joint Surg Br* 1985;67:780.

+ 27. Ben-Itzhak I, Erken EHW, Molkin C. Progressive Valgus Deformity after Juxta-epiphyseal Fractures of the Upper Tibia in Children. *Injury* 1987;18:169.

+ 28. Berg EE. Case Report: Anterior Cruciate Ligament Incompetence in Severe Blount's Disease. *J Pediatr Orthop* 1994;3:197.

+ 29. Beskin JL, Burke SW, Johnston CE II, Roberts JM. Clinical Basis for a Mechanical Etiology in Adolescent Blount's Disease. *Orthopaedics* 1986;9:365.

+ 30. Best TN. Valgus Deformity after Fracture of the Upper Tibia in Children. *J Bone Joint Surg Br* 1973;55:222.

+ 31. Bitan F, Rigault P, Padovani JP, Touzet P. Congenital Pseudarthrosis of the Tibia in Childhood: Results of

Treatment by Nailing and Bone Graft in 18 Cases. *Fr J Orthop Surg* 1987;1:331.

+ 32. Blockney NJ, Murphy AV, Mocan H. Management of Rachitic Deformities in Chldren with Chronic Renal Failure. *J Bone Joint Surg Br* 1986;68:791.

+ 33. Blount WP. Tibia Vara: Osteochondrosis Deformans Tibiae. *Curr Pract Orthop Surg* 1966;3:141.

34. Blount WP. *Fractures in Children*. Baltimore: Williams & Wilkins, 1955;171.

* 35. Blount WP. Tibia Vara: Osteochondrosis Deformans Tibiae. *J Bone Joint Surg* 1937;19:1.

* 36. Blount WP, Clarke GR. Control of Bone Growth by Epiphyseal Stapling: A Preliminary Report. *J Bone Joint Surg Am* 1949;31:464.

+ 37. Bowen JR, Johnson WJ. Percutaneous Epiphysiodesis. *Clin Orthop* 1984;190:170.

* 38. Bowen JR, Leahey JL, Zahang Z, MacEwen GD. Partial Epiphysiodesis at the Knee to Correct Angular Deformity. *Clin Orthop* 1985;198:184.

+ 39. Bowen JR, Torres RR, Forlin E. Partial Epiphysiodesis to Address Genu Varum or Genu Valgum. *J Pediatr Orthop* 1992;12:359.

! 40. Boyd HB. Pathology and Natural History of Congenital Pseudarthrosis of the Tibia. *Clin Orthop* 1982;166:5.

+ 41. Boyd HB. Congenital Pseudoarthrosis: Treatment by Dual Bone Grafts. *J Bone Joint Surg* 1941;23:497.

+ 42. Boyd HB, Fox KW. Congenital Pseudarthrosis: Follow-up Study after Massive Bone Grafting. *J Bone Joint Surg Am* 1948;30:274.

+ 43. Boyd HB, Sage FP. Congenital Pseudarthrosis of the Tibia. *J Bone Joint Surg Am* 1958;40:1245.

+ 44. Boyer RS, Jaffe RB, Nixon GW, Condon VR. Trampoline Fractures of the Proximal Tibia in Children. *AJR* 1986;146:83.

+ 45. Bradish CF, Davies SJM, Malone M. Tibia Vara Due to Focal Cartilaginous Dysplasia: The Natural History. *J Bone Joint Surg Br* 1988;70:106.

46. Bradway JK, Klassen RA, Peterson HA. Blount's Disease: A Review of the English Literature. *J Pediatr Orthop* 1987;7:472.

+ 47. Bright RW. Surgical Correction of Partial Growth Plate Closure: A Clinical Study of 24 Cases. *Orthop Trans* 1977;1:82.

+ 48. Brighton CT, Friedenberg ZB, Zemsky LM, Pollis PR. Direct-current Stimulation of Non-union and Congenital Pseudarthrosis. *J Bone Joint Surg Am* 1975;57:368.

! 49. Briner J, Yunis E. Ultrastructure of Congenital Pseudarthrosis of the Tibia. *Arch Pathol* 1973;95:97.

50. Brooks WC, Gross RH. Genu Varum in Children: Diagnosis and Treatment. *J Am Acad Orthop Surg* 1995;3:326.

+ 51. Brougham DI, Nicole RO. Valgus Deformity after Proximal Tibial Fractures in Children. *J Bone Joint Surg Br* 1987;69:482.

+ 52. Brown GA, Osebold WR, Ponseti IV. Congenital Pseudoarthrosis of Long Bones: A Clinical, Radiographic, Histologic and Ultrastructure Study. *Clin Orthop* 1977;128:228.

+ 53. Caffey J. Prenatal Bowing and Thickening of Tubular Bones with Multiple Cutaneous Dimples in the Arms and Legs. *Am J Dis Child* 1946;74:543.

+ 54. Caffey JP. *Pediatric X-ray Diagnosis*, 7th ed. Chicago: Year Book Medical Publishers, 1978.

+ 55. Cahuzac JPH, Vardon D, Sales de Gauzy J. Development of the Clinical Tibiofemoral Angle in Normal Adolescents: A Study of 427 Normal Subjects from 10 to 16 Years of Age. *J Bone Joint Surg Br* 1995;77:729.

+ 56. Campanacci M, Nicoll EA, Pagella P. Differential Diagnosis of Congenital Pseudarthrosis of the Tibia. *Int Orthop* 1981;4:283.

! 57. Canale ST, Harper MC. Biotrigonometric Analysis and Practical Applictions of Osteotomies of the Tibia in Children. *Instr Course Lect* 1981;30:85.

+ 58. Canale ST, Russell RA, Holcomb RL. Percutaneous Epiphysiodesis: Experimental Study and Preliminary Clinical Results. *J Pediatr Orthop* 1986;6:150.

+ 59. Carter JR, Leeson MC, Thompson GH, et al. Late-onset Tibia Vara: A Histopathologic Analysis: A Comparative Analysis with Infantile Tibia Vara and Slipped Capital Femoral Epiphysis. *J Pediatr Orthop* 1988;8:187.

+ 60. Carter JR, Thompson GH, Leeson MC, et al. Physeal Histopathology in Late-onset Tibia Vara. In: Uthoff HK, Wiley JJ, eds. *Behavior of the Growth Plate*. New York: Raven Press, 1988;285.

! 61. Carvell JE. The Relationship of the Periosteum to Angular Deformities of Long Bones: Experimental Operations in Rabbits. *Clin Orthop* 1983;173:262.

+ 62. Cattell HS, Levin S, Kopits S, Lyne ED. Reconstructive Surgery in Children with Azotemic Osteodystrophy. *J Bone Joint Surg Am* 1971;53:216.

+ 63. Charnely J. Congenital Pseudarthrosis of the Tibia Treated by the Intramedullary Nail. *J Bone Joint Surg Am* 1956;38:283.

+ 64. Chen CW, Yu ZJ, Wang Y. A New Method of Treatment of Congenital Pseudarthrosis Using Free Vascularized Fibular Graft: A Preliminary Report. *Ann Acad Med Singapore* 1979;8:465.

+ 65. Cheng JC, Chan PS, Chiang SC, Hui PW. Angular and Rotational Profile of the Lower Limb in 2630 Chinese Children. *J Pediatr Orthop* 1991;11:154.

+ 66. Coates R. Knock-knee Deformity Following Upper Tibial "Greenstick" Fractures. *J Bone Joint Surg Br* 1977;59:516.

+ 67. Cockshott WP, Martin R, Friedman L, Yuen M. Focal Fibrocartilaginous Dysplasia and Tibia Vara: A Case Report. *Skeletal Radiol* 1994;23:333.

+ 68. Coleman SS, Coleman DA. Congenital Pseudarthrosis of the Tibia: Treatment by Transfer of the Ipsilateral Fibula with Vascular Pedicle. *J Pediatr Orthop* 1994;14:156.

! 69. Cook SD, Lavernia CJ, Burke SW, et al. A Biomechanical Analysis of the Etiology of Tibia Vara. *J Pediatr Orthop* 1983;3:449.

! 70. Cooper RR, Misol S. Tendon and Ligament Insertion: A Light and Electron Microscopy Study. *J Bone Joint Surg Am* 1970;52:1.

+ 71. Cozen L. Knock-knee Deformity after Fracture of the Proximal Tibia in Children. *Orthopaedics* 1959;1:230.

* 72. Cozen L. Fracture of the Proximal Portion of the Tibia in Children Followed by Valgus Deformity. *Surg Gynecol Obstet* 1953;97:183.

73. Crawford AH. Neurofibromatosis in Childhood. *Instr Course Lect* 1981;30:56.

+ 74. Crossett LS, Beaty JH, Betz RR, et al. Congenital Pseudarthrosis of the Tibia: Long-term Follow-up Study. *Clin Orthop* 1989;245:16.

+ 75. Crutchow WP, David DS, Witsell J. Multiple Skeletal Complications in a Case of Chronic Renal Failure Treated by Kidney Homotransplantation. *Am J Med* 1971;50:390.

+ 76. Currarino G, Pickney LE. Genu Valgum after Proximal Tibial Fractures in Children. *AJR* 1981;136:915.

+ 77. Curriano G, Kirks DR. Lateral Widening of Epiphyseal Plates in Knees of Children with Bowed Legs. *AJR* 1977;129:309.

+ 78. Dalinka MD, Coren G, Hensinger RN, Irani RN. Arthrography in Blount's Disease. *Radiology* 1974;113:161.

+ 79. DalMonte A, Donzelli O, Sudanese A, Baldini N. Congenital Pseudarthrosis of the Fibula. *J Pediatr Orthop* 1987;7:14.

+ 80. DalMonte A, Manes E, Cammarota V. Post-traumatic Genu Valgum in Children. *Ital J Orthop Traumatol* 1985;11:5.

+ 81. Davids JR, Fisher R, Lumbar G, Von Glinski S. Angular Deformity of the Lower Extremity in Children with Renal Osteodystrophy. *J Pediatr Orthop* 1992;12:291.

+ 82. Davidson WH, Bohne WHO. The Syme Amputation in Children. *J Bone Joint Surg Am* 1975;57:905.

+ 83. Dawson GR. Intra-uterine Fracture of the Tibia and Fibula: Report of a Case with Correction by Osteotomy and Plating. *J Bone Joint Surg Am* 1949;31:406.

+ 84. DeBoer HH, Verbout AJ, Nielsen HK, van der Eijken JW. Free Vascularized Fibular Graft for Tibial Pseudarthrosis in Neurofibromatosis. *Acta Orthop Scand* 1988;59:425.

85. Delgado-Martinez AD, Rodriguez-Merchan EC, Olsen B. Current Concepts: Congenital Pseudarthrosis of the Tibia. *Int Orthop* 1996;20:192.

+ 86. DePablos J, Franzreb M. Treatment of Adolescent Tibia Vara by Asymmetrical Physeal Distraction. *J Bone Joint Surg Br* 1993;75:592.

+ 87. DePablos J, Azcaráte J, Barrios C. Progressive Opening-wedge Osteotomy for Angular Long-bone Deformities in Adolescents. *J Bone Joint Surg Br* 1995;77:387.

+ 88. deSanctis N, Della Corte S, Pempinello C, et al. Infantile Type of Blount's Disease: Complications concerning Etiopathogenesis and Treatment. *J Pediatr Orthop B* 1995;4:200.

89. Dias LS. Fractures of the Tibia and Fibula. In: Rockwood CH Jr, Wilkens KE, King RE, eds. *Fractures in Children*. Philadelphia: JB Lippincott Co, 1984:983.

+ 90. Dietz FR, Weinstein SL. Spike Osteotomy for Angular Deformities of the Long Bones in Children. *J Bone Joint Surg* 1988;70:848.

+ 91. Dietz WH Jr, Gross WL, Kirkpatrick JA Jr. Blount Disease (Tibia Vara): Another Skeletal Disorder Associated with Childhood Obesity. *J Pediatr* 1982;101:735.

+ 92. Dooley BJ, Menelaus MB, Paterson DC. Congenital Pseudarthrosis and Bowing of the Fibula. *J Bone Joint Surg Br* 1974;56:739.

+ 93. Dormans JP, Krajbich JL, Zucker R, Demuynk M. Congenital Pseudarthrosis of the Tibia: Treatment with Free Vascularized Fibular Grafts. *J Pediatr Orthop* 1990;10:623.

+ 94. Engel GM, Staheli LT. The Natural History of Torsion and Other Factors Influencing Gait in Childhood: A Study of the Angle of Gait, Tibial Torsion, Knee Angle, Hip Rotation and Development of the Arch in Normal Children. *Clin Orthop* 1974;99:12.

+ 95. Erlacher P. Deformierende Prozesse der Epiphysengegend bei Kindern. *Arch Orthop Unfallchir* 1922;20:81.

+ 96. Evans GA, Arulanantham K, Gage JR. Primary Hypophosphatemic Rickets: Effects of Oral Phosphate and Vitamin D on Growth and Surgical Treatment. *J Bone Joint Surg Am* 1980;62:1130.

+ 97. Evensen A, Steffenson J. Tibia Vara (Osteochondrosis Deformans Tibiae). *Acta Orthop Scand* 1957;16:200.

+ 98. Eyre-Brook HL, Bailey RAJ, Price CHG. Infantile Pseudarthrosis of the Tibia: Three Cases Treated Successfully by Delayed Autogenous Bypass Graft with Some Comments on the Causative Lesion. *J Bone Joint Surg Br* 1969;51:604.

+ 99. Fabry G, Lammens J, van Melkebeek J, Stuyck J. Treatment of Congenital Pseudarthrosis with the Ilizarov Technique. *J Pediatr Orthop* 1988;8:67.

+ 100. Farmer AW. The Use of a Composite Pedicle Graft for Pseudarthrosis of the Tibia. *J Bone Joint Surg Am* 1952;34:591.

+ 101. Feldman MD, Schoenecker PL. Use of the Metaphyseal–Diaphyseal Angle in the Evaluation of Bowed Legs. *J Bone Joint Surg Am* 1995;75:1602.

+ 102. Fern ED, Stockley I, Bell MJ. Extending Intramedullary Rods in Congenital Pseudarthrosis of the Tibia. *J Bone Joint Surg Br* 1990;72:1073.

+ 103. Ferriter P, Shapiro F. Infantile Tibia Vara: Factors Affecting Outcome Following Proximal Tibial Osteotomy. *J Pediatr Orthop* 1987,7:1.

+ 104. Foreman KA, Robertson WW Jr. Radiographic Measurement of Infantile Tibia Vara. *J Pediatr Orthop* 1985;5:452.

+ 105. Fraser RK, Dickens DRV, Cole WG. Medial Physeal Stapling for Primary and Secondary Genu Valgum in Late Childhood and Adolescence. *J Bone Joint Surg Br* 1995;77:733.

+ 106. Fraser W. Congenital Pseudarthrosis of the Tibia. *J Bone Joint Surg Br* 1964;46:167.

* 107. Freund E. Congenital Defect of Femur, Fibula, and Tibia. *Arch Surg* 1936;33:349.

+ 108. Gilbert A, Brockman R. Congenital Pseudarthrosis of the Tibia: Long-term Follow-up of 29 Cases Treated by Microvascular Bone Transfer. *Clin Orthop* 1995;314:37.

109. Goff CW. *Surgical Treatment of Unequal Extremities*. Springfield, IL: Charles C Thomas, 1960.

+ 110. Golding JSR, Bateson EM, McNeil-Smith JDG. Infantile Tibia Vara (Blount's Disease or Osteochondrosis Deformans Tibiae) In: Rang M, ed. *The Growth Plate and its Disorders.* Edinburgh: Churchill Livingstone, 1969:10.

+ 111. Golding JSR, McNeil-Smith JDG. Observations on the Etiology of Tibia Vara. *J Bone Joint Surg Br* 1963;45:320.

+ 112. Gordon L, Weulker N, Jergensen H. Vascularized Fibular Grafting for the Treatment of Congenital Pseudarthrosis of the Tibia. *Orthopaedics* 1986;9:825.

+ 113. Green NE. Tibia Valga Caused by Asymmetrical Overgrowth Following a Nondisplaced Fracture of the Proximal Tibial Metaphysis. *J Pediatr Orthop* 1983;3:235.

+ 114. Green WT, Rudo N. Pseudarthrosis and Neurofibromatosis. *Arch Surg* 1943;46:639.

115. Greene WB. Genu Varum and Genu Valgum in Children. *Instr Course Lect* 1994;43:151.

116. Greene WB. Instructional Course Lecture: Infantile Tibia Vara. *J Bone Jont Surg Am* 1993;75:130.

+ 117. Gregosiewicz A, Wosko I, Kandzierski G, Drabik Z. Double-elevating Osteotomy of Tibiae in the Treatment of Severe Cases of Blount's Disease. *J Pediatr Orthop* 1989;9:178.

! 118. Greulich WW, Pyle SI. *Radiographic Atlas of Skeletal Development of the Hand and Wrist.* Stanford, CA: Stanford University Press, 1959.

+ 119. Grill F. Treatment of Congenital Pseudarthrosis of the Tibia with the Circular Frame Technique. *J Pediatr Orthop B* 1996;5:6.

120. Grogan DP, Love SM, Ogden JA. Congenital Malformations of the Lower Extremities. *Orthop Clin North Am* 1987;18:537.

+ 121. Hagan KF, Buncke HJ. Treatment of Congenital Pseudarthrosis of the Tibia with Free Vascularized Bone Graft. *Clin Orthop* 1982;166:34.

+ 122. Hägglund G, Ingvarsson T, Ramgren B, Zayer M. Metaphyseal–Diaphyseal Angle in Blount's Disease: A 30-year Follow-up of 13 Unoperated Children. *Acta Orthop Scand* 1997;68:167.

+ 123. Hansen BA, Greiff J, Bergmann F. Fractures of the Tibia in Children. *Acta Orthop Scand* 1976;47:448.

+ 124. Hanson LI, Zayer M. Physiologic Genu Varum. *Acta Orthop Scand* 1975;46:221.

+ 125. Hardinge K. Congenital Anterior Bowing of the Tibia. *Ann R Coll Surg* 1972;51:17.

+ 126. Heath CH, Staheli LT. Normal Limits of Knee Angles in White Children: Genu Varum and Genu Valgum. *J Pediatr Orthop* 1993;13:259.

+ 127. Henderson RC, Green WB. Etiology of Late-onset Tibia Vara: Is Varus Alignment a Prerequisite? *J Pediatr Orthop* 1994;14:143.

+ 128. Henderson RC, Kemp GJ Jr, Greene WB. Adolescent Tibia Vara: Alternatives for Operative Treatment. *J Bone Joint Surg Am* 1992;74:342.

+ 129. Henderson RC, Kemp GJ Jr, Hayes PRL. Prevalence of Late-onset Tibia Vara. *J Pediatr Orthop* 1993;13:255.

+ 130. Henderson RC, Lechner CT, Demasi RA, Greene WB. Variability in Radiographic Measurement of Bowleg Deformity in Children. *J Pediatr Orthop* 1990;10:491.

+ 131. Herman TE, Siegel MJ, McAlister WH. Focal Fibrocartilaginous Dysplasia Associated with Tibia Vara. *Radiology* 1990;177:767.

+ 132. Herring JA. Instructional Case: Valgus Knee Deformity—Etiology and Treatment. *J Pediatr Orthop* 1983;3:527.

+ 133. Herring JA, Moseley C. Post-traumatic Valgus Deformity of the Tibia: Instructional Case. *J Pediatr Orthop* 1981;1:435.

+ 134. Herring JA, Barnhill B, Gaffney C. Syme Amputation: An Evaluation of the Physical and Psychological Function in Young Patients. *J Bone Joint Surg Am* 1986;68:573.

+ 135. Heyman CH, Herndon CH. Congenital Posterior Angulation of the Tibia. *J Bone Joint Surg Am* 1949;31:571.

+ 136. Heyman CH, Herndon CH, Heiple KG. Congenital Posterior Angulation of the Tibia with Talipes Calcaneus: A Long-term Report of Eleven Patients. *J Bone Joint Surg Am* 1959;41:476.

+ 137. Hofmann A, Jones RE, Herring JA. Blount's Disease after Skeletal Maturity. *J Bone Joint Surg Am* 1982;64:1004.

+ 138. Hofmann A, Wenger DR. Posteromedial Bowing of the Tibia: Progression of Discrepancy in Leg Lengths. *J Bone Joint Surg Am* 1981;63:384.

! 139. Houghton GR, Dekel S. The Periosteal Control of Long Bone Growth. *Acta Orthop Scand* 1979;50:635.

! 140. Houghton GR, Rooker GD. The Role of the Periosteum in the Growth of Long Bones: An Experimental Study in the Rabbit. *J Bone Joint Surg Br* 1979;61:218.

+ 141. Howorth B. Knock Knees: With Special Reference to the Stapling Operation. *Clin Orthop* 1971;77:233.

+ 142. Hresko MT, Kasser JR. Physeal Arrest about the Knee Associated with Non-physeal Fractures in the Lower Extremity. *J Bone Joint Surg Am* 1989;71:698.

+ 143. Hsu AC, Kooh SW, Fraser D, et al. Renal Osteodystrophy in Children with Chronic Renal Failure: An Unexpectedly Common and Incapacitating Complication. *Pediatrics* 1982;70:742.

+ 144. Huang SC, Yip KM. Treatment of Congenital Pseudarthrosis of the Tibia with Ilizarov Method. *J Formos Med Assoc* 1997;96:359.

+ 145. Husien AM, Kale VR. Tibia Vara Caused by Focal Fibrocartilaginous Dysplasia. *Clin Radiol* 1989;40:104.

+ 146. Ippolito E, Pentamalli S. Post-traumatic Valgus Deformity of the Knee in Proximal Metaphyseal Fractures in Children. *Ital J Orthop Traumatol* 1984;10:103.

+ 147. Jackson DW, Cozen L. Genu Valgum as a Complication of Proximal Tibial Metaphyseal Fractures in Children. *J Bone Joint Surg Am* 1971;53:1571.

+ 148. Jackson JP, Waugh W. The Technique and Complications of Upper Tibial Osteotomy: A Review of 226 Operations. *J Bone Joint Surg Br* 1974;56:236.

+ 149. Jacobsen ST, Crawford AH, Millar EA, Steel HH. The Syme Amputation in Patients with Congenital Pseudarthrosis of the Tibia. *J Bone Joint Surg Am* 1983;65:533.

+ 150. Johnson PH. Beware: Greenstick Fractures of the Proximal Tibial Metaphysis. *J Arkansas Med Soc* 1983;80:215.

+ 151. Johnston CE II. Infantile Tibia Vara. *Clin Orthop* 1990;225:13.

+ 152. Jones GB, Poiakoff SJ, Bright RW. Surgical Correction of Severe Blount's Disease by Physeal Bridge Resection and Silastic Interposition. *J Bone Joint Surg Br* 1988;70:680.

+ 153. Jordan SE, Alonso JE, Cook FF. The Etiology of Valgus Angulation after Metaphyseal Fractures of the Tibia in Children. *J Pediatr Orthop* 1987;7:450.

+ 154. Kanaya F, Tsai TM, Harkness J. Vascularized Bone Grafts for Congenital Pseudarthrosis of the Tibia. *Microsurgery* 1996;17:459.

+ 155. Kariya Y, Taniguchi K, Yagisawa H, Ooi Y. Focal Fibrocartilaginous Dysplasia: Consolidation of Healing Process. *J Pediatr Orthop* 1991;11:545.

+ 156. Karol LA, Haideri NF, Halliday SE, et al. Gait Analysis and Muscle Strength in Children with Congenital Pseudarthrosis of the Tibia: The Effect of Treatment. *J Pediatr Orthop* 1998;18:381.

+ 157. Kessel L. Annotations on the Etiology and Treatment of Tibia Vara. *J Bone Joint Surg Br* 1970;52:93.

+ 158. Khermosh O, Weintroub S. Serrated (W/M) Osteotomy: A New Technique for Simultaneous Correction of Angular and Torsional Deformity of the Lower Limb in Children. *J Pediatr Orthop B* 1995;4:204.

+ 159. Klassen RA, Peterson HA. Resection of Epiphyseal Bars. *Orthop Trans* 1982;6:134.

+ 160. Kline SC, Bostrum M, Griffin PP. Femoral Varus: An Important Component in Late-onset Blount's Disease. *J Pediatr Orthop* 1992;12:197.

161. Kling TF Jr. Angular Deformities of the Lower Limbs in Children. *Orthop Clin North Am* 1987;18:513.

+ 162. Kling TF Jr. Tibia Vara: A Mechanical Problem. *Orthop Trans* 1981;5:138.

163. Kling TF Jr, Hensinger RN. Angular and Torsional Deformities of the Lower Limbs in Children. *Clin Orthop* 1983;176:136.

+ 164. Kort JS, Schink MM, Mitchell SN, Bassett CAL. Congenital Pseudarthrosis of the Tibia: Treatment with Pulsating Electromagnetic Fields. The International Experience. *Clin Orthop* 1982;165:124.

+ 165. Krida A. Congenital Posterior Angulation of the Tibia: A Clinical Entity Unrelated to Congenital Pseudoarthrosis. *Am J Surg* 1951;82:98.

+ 166. Kruse RN, Bowen JR, Heithoff S. Oblique Tibial Osteotomy in the Correction of Tibial Deformity in Children. *J Pediatr Orthop* 1989;9:476.

+ 167. Langenskiöld A. Tibia Vara: A Critical Review. *Clin Orthop* 1989;246:195.

+ 168. Langenskiöld A. Tibia Vara: Osteochondrosis Deformans Tibiae—Blount's Disease. *Clin Orthop* 1981;158:77.

+ 169. Langenskiöld A. An Operation for Partial Closure of an Epiphyseal Plate in Children and its Experiential Basis. *J Bone Joint Surg Br* 1975;57:325.

+ 170. Langenskiöld A. Pseudarthrosis of the Fibula with Progressive Valgus Deformity of the Ankle in Children: Treatment by Fusion of the Distal Tibial and Fibular Metaphysis: Review of 3 Cases. *J Bone Joint Surg Am* 1967;49:463.

+ 171. Langenskiöld A. Aspects of the Pathology of Tibia Vara. *Ann Chir Gynaecol* 1955;44:58.

* 172. Langenskiöld A. Tibia Vara (Osteochondrosis Deformans Tibiae): A Survery of 23 Cases. *Acta Chir Scand* 1952;103:1.

+ 173. Langenskiöld A, Riska EB. Tibia Vara (Osteochondrosis Deformans Tibiae): A Survey of Seventy-one Cases. *J Bone Joint Surg Am* 1962;46:1405.

+ 174. Laurencin CT, Ferriter PJ, Millis MB. Oblique Proximal Tibial Osteoomty for the Correction of Tibia Vara in the Young. *Clin Orthop* 1996;327:218.

+ 175. Leung PC. Congenital Pseudarthrosis of the Tibia: Three Cases Treated by Free Vascularized Iliac Crest Graft. *Clin Orthop* 1983;175:45.

+ 176. Levine AM, Drennan JC. Physiologic Bowing and Tibia Vara: The Metaphyseal–Diaphyseal Angle in the Measurement of Bowleg Deformities. *J Bone Joint Surg Am* 1982;64:1158.

+ 177. Lichtblau PO, Waxman BA. Blount's Disease: Review of the Literature and Description of a New Surgical Procedure. *Contemp Orthop* 1981;3:526.

+ 178. Lincoln TL, Birch JG. Focal Fibrocartilaginous Dysplasia in the Upper Extremity. *J Pediatr Orthop* 1997;17:528.

+ 179. Lloyd-Roberts GC, Shaw NE. The Prevention of Pseudarthrosis in Congenital Kyphosis of the Tibia. *J Bone Joint Surg Br* 1969;51:100.

+ 180. Loder RT, Johnston CE II. Infantile Tibia Vara. *J Pediatr Orthop* 1987;7:639.

+ 181. Loder RT, Schaffer JJ, Bardenstein JA. Late-onset Tibia Vara. *J Pediatr Orthop* 1991;11:162.

+ 182. Lovejoy JF Jr, Lovell WW. Adolescent Tibia Vara Associated with Slipped Capital Femoral Epiphysis: Report of Two Cases. *J Bone Joint Surg Am* 1970;52:361.

183. MacEwen GD, Zionts LE. Proximal Tibial Fractures in Children. In: Uhthoff HK, Wiley JJ, eds. *Behavior of the Growth Plate.* New York: Raven Press, 1988:141.

+ 184. Mahnken RF, Yngve DA. Valgus Deformity Following Fracture of the Tibial Metaphysis. *Orthopaedics* 1988;11:1320.

+ 185. Martin SD, Moran MC, Martin TL, Burke SW. Proximal Tibial Osteotomy with Compression Plate Fixation for Tibia Vara. *J Pediatr Orthop* 1994;14:619.

+ 186. Masserman RL, Peterson HA, Bianco AJ Jr. Congenital Pseudarthrosis of the Tibia: A Review of the Literature and 52 Cases at the Mayo Clinic. *Clin Orthop* 1974;99:140.

+ 187. Matsen FA III, Steheli LT. Neurovascular Complications Following Tibial Osteotomy in Children. *Clin Orthop* 1975;110:210.

+ 188. McCarthy JJ, Kim DH, Eilert RE. Posttraumatic Genu Valgum: Operative versus Nonoperative Treatment. *J Pediatr Orthop* 1998;18:518.

+ 189. McCarthy RE. Amputation for Congenital Pseudarthrosis of the Tibia: Indications and Techniques. *Clin Orthop* 1982;166:58.

190. McDade W. Bow Legs and Knock Knees. *Pediatr Clin North Am* 1977;24:825.

+ 191. McFarland B. Pseudarthrosis of the Tibia in Childhood. *J Bone Joint Surg Br* 1951;33:36.

+ 192. Meyer JS, Davidson RS, Hubbard AM, Conrad KA.

MRI of Focal Fibrocartilaginous Dysplasia. *J Pediatr Orthop* 1995;15:304.

+ 193. Mielke CH, Stevens PM. Hemiepiphyseal Stapling for Knee Deformities in Children Younger than 10 Years: A Preliminary Report. *J Pediatr Orthop* 1996;16:423.

+ 194. Miller BF. Congential Posterior Bowing of the Tibia with Talipes Equinovarus. *J Bone Joint Surg Br* 1951; 33:50.

+ 195. Monticelli G, Spinelli R. A New Method of Treating the Advanced Stages of Tibia Vara (Blount's Disease). *Ital J Orthop Traumatol* 1984;10:295.

+ 196. Mooney JF III, Moore R, Sekiya J, Koman LA. Congenital Pseudarthrosis of the Tibia Treated with Free Vascularized Fibular Graft. *J South Orthop Assoc* 1997;6: 227.

197. Morley AJM. Knock Knees in Children. *Br Med J* 1957; 2:976.

+ 198. Morrissey RT. Congenital Pseudarthrosis of the Tibia: Factors that Affect Results. *Clin Orthop* 1982;166:21.

+ 199. Morrissey RT, Riseborough EJ, Hall JE. Congenital Pseudarthrosis of the Tibia. *J Bone Joint Surg Br* 1981; 63:367.

+ 200. Moseley CF. A Straight-line Graph for Leg-length Discrepancies. *J Bone Joint Surg Am* 1977;59:174.

+ 201. Moss MC, Davies MS, Simonis RB. Curly and Overlapping Toes in Congenital Pseudarthrosis of the Tibia. *J Bone Joint Surg Br* 1994;76:983.

+ 202. Mubarak SJ, Carroll NC. Volkmann's Contracture in Children: Aetiology and Prevention. *J Bone Joint Surg Br* 1979;61:285.

+ 203. Murray HH, Lovell WW. Congenital Pseudarthrosis of the Tibia: A Long-term Follow-up Study. *Clin Orthop* 1982;166:14.

+ 204. Mycoskie PJ. Complications of Osteotomies about the Knee in Children. *Orthopaedics* 1981;4:1005.

205. Ogden JA. Tibia and Fibula. In Ogden JA, ed. *Skeletal Injury in the Child*. Phildelphia: Lea & Febiger, 1990: 787.

+ 206. Ogden JA, Ogden DA, Pugh L, et al. Tibia Valga after Proximal Metaphyseal Fractures in Childhood: A Normal Biologic Response. *J Pediatr Orthop* 1995;15:489.

+ 207. Ogilvie JW, King K. Epiphysiodesis: Two-year Clinical Results Using a New Technique. *J Pediatr Orthop* 1990;10:809.

+ 208. Olney BW, Cole WG, Menelaus MB. Case Report: Three Additional Cases of Focal Fibrocartilaginous Dysplasia Causing Tibia Vara. *J Pediatr Orthop* 1990; 10:405.

+ 209. Omokawa S, Tamai S, Takakura Y, et al. A Long-term Study of the Donor-site Ankle after Vascularized Fibula Grafts in Children. *Microsurgery* 1996;17:162.

+ 210. Oppenheim WL, Shayestehfar BS, Salusky IB. Tibial Physeal Changes in Renal Osteodystrophy: Lateral Blount's Disease. *J Pediatr Orthop* 1992;12:774.

+ 211. Paley D, Catagni M, Argnani F, et al. Treatment of Congenital Pseudarthrosis of the Tibia Using the Ilizarov Technique. *Clin Orthop* 1992;280:81.

+ 212. Pappas AM. Congenital Posteromedial Bowing of the Tibia and Fibula. *J Pediatr Orthop* 1984;4:525.

+ 213. Paterson D. Congenital Pseudarthrosis of the Tibia: An Overview. *Clin Orthop* 1989;247:44.

+ 214. Paterson DC, Simonis RB. Electrical Stimulation in the Treatment of Congenital Pseudarthrosis of the Tibia. *J Bone Joint Surg Br* 1985;67:454.

+ 215. Paterson DC, Lewis GH, Cass CA. Treatment of Congenital Pseudarthrosis of the Tibia with Direct Current Stimulation. *Clin Orthop* 1980;148:129.

+ 216. Pauwels F. Grundriss einer Biomechanik der Fraktur Heilung. *Verh Dtsch Orthop Gesell* 1940;34:62.

+ 217. Peterson HA. Partial Growth Arrest and Its Treatment. *J Pediatr Orthop* 1984;4:246.

* 218. Phemister DB. Operative Arrestment of Longitudinal Growth of Long Bones in the Treatment of Deformities. *J Bone Joint Surg* 1933;15:1.

+ 219. Pho RWH, Levack B. Preliminary Observations of Epiphyseal Growth Rate in Congenital Pseudarthrosis of the Tibia after Free Vascularized Fibular Graft. *Clin Orthop* 1986;206:148.

+ 220. Pho RWH, Levack B, Satku K, Patradul A. Free Vascularised Fibula Graft in the Treatment of Congenital Pseudarthrosis of the Tibia. *J Bone Joint Surg Br* 1985; 67:64.

+ 221. Pistevos G, Duckworth T. The Correction of Genu Valgum by Epiphyseal Stapling. *J Bone Joint Surg Br* 1977; 59:72.

+ 222. Pitkow RB. External Rotation Contracture of the Extended Hip: A Common Phenomenon of Infancy Obscuring Femoral Neck Anteversion and the Most Frequent Cause of Out-toeing in Children. *Clin Orthop* 1975;110:139.

+ 223. Pitzen P, Marquardt WO. Beinbildung durch Umschriebene Epiphysen Wachstumsstörung (Tibia Vara Bilbung). *Z Orthop* 1939;69:174.

+ 224. Plawecki S, Carpentier E, Lascombes P, et al. Treatment of Congenital Pseudarthrosis of the Tibia by the Ilizarov Method. *J Pediatr Orthop* 1990;10:786.

+ 225. Pompe van Meedervort HF. Infantile Pseudarthrosis of the Tibia. *J Bone Joint Surg Br* 1978;60:296.

+ 226. Potthoff H. Ein Beitrag zur Behandlung der Proximalen Metaphysaren Tibia Fraktur in Kindesalter. *Aktuel Traumatol* 1982;12:127.

+ 227. Price CT, Scott DS, Greenberg DA. Dynamic Axial External Fixation in the Surgical Treatment of Tibia Vara. *J Pediatr Orthop* 1995;15:236.

+ 228. Purvis GD, Holder JE. Dual Bone Graft for Congenital Pseudoarthrosis of the Tibia: Variations of Technic. *South Med J* 1960;53:926.

+ 229. Rab GT. Oblique Tibial Osteotomy for Blount's Disease. *J Pediatr Orthop* 1988;8:715.

230. Rang M. *Children's Fractures*. Philadelphia: JB Lippincott Co, 1974;189.

+ 231. Rathgeb JM, Ramsey PL, Cowell HR. Congenital Kyphoscoliosis of the Tibia. *Clin Orthop* 1974;103:178.

+ 232. Richards BS, Katz DE, Sims JB. Effectiveness of Brace Treatment in Early Infantile Blount's Disease. *J Pediatr Orthop* 1998;18:374.

+ 233. Riseborough EJ, Barrett IR, Shapiro F. Growth Disturbance Following Distal Femoral Physeal Fracture-separations. *J Bone Joint Surg Am* 1983;65:885.

+ 234. Roach JW, Shindell R, Green NE. Late-onset Pseud-arthrosis of the Dysplastic Tibia. *J Bone Joint Surg Am* 1993;75:1593.

+ 235. Robert M, Khouri N, Carlioz H, Alain JL. Fractures of the Proximal Tibial Metaphysis in Children: Review of a Series of 25 Cases. *J Pediatr Orthop* 1987;7:444.

+ 236. Rabinowitz MS. Congenital Curvature of the Tibia with Talipes Calcaneo-valgus. *Bull Hosp Joint Dis* 1951;12:63.

237. Rooker GD, Coates RL. Deformity after Greenstick Fractures of the Upper Tibial Metaphysis. In: Houghton GR, Thompson GH, eds. *Problematic Musculo-skeletal Injuries in Children.* London: Butterworth 1983:1.

+ 238. Rooker GD, Salter R. Prevention of Valgus Deformity Following Fracture of the Proximal Metaphysis of the Tibia in Children. *J Bone Joint Surg Br* 1980;62:527.

+ 239. Rubinovitch M, Said SE, Glorieux FH, et al. Principles and Results of Corrected Lower Limb Osteotomies for Patients with Vitamin D–Resistant Hypophosphatemic Rickets. *Clin Orthop* 1988;237:264.

+ 240. Rydholm U, Brattstrom H, Bylander B, et al. Stapling of the Knee in Juvenile Chronic Arthritis. *J Pediatr Orthop* 1987;7:63.

+ 241. Sadiq SA, Varshney GK. Congenital Posterior Angula-tion of the Tibia. *Int Surg* 1977;62:48.

* 242. Salenius P, Vankka E. The Development of the Tibio-femoral Angle in Children. *J Bone Joint Surg Am* 1975; 57:259.

243. Salter RB, Best TN. Pathogenesis of Progressive Valgus Deformity Following Fractures of the Proximal Me-taphyseal Region of the Tibia in Young Children. *Instr Course Lect* 1992;45:409.

+ 244. Salter RB, Best T. The Pathogenesis and Prevention of Valgus Deformity Following Fractures of the Proximal Metaphyseal Region of the Tibia in Children. *J Bone Joint Surg Am* 1973;55:1324.

+ 245. Saski T, Yagi T, Monji J, et al. Transepiphyseal Plate Osteotomy for Severe Tibia Vara in Children: A Fol-low-up Study of Four Cases. *J Pediatr Orthop* 1986;6: 61.

+ 246. Scheffer MM, Peterson HA. Opening-wedge Osteot-omy for Angular Deformities of Long Bones in Chil-dren. *J Bone Joint Surg Am* 1994;76:325.

+ 247. Schoenecker PL, Johnston R, Rich MM, Capelli AM. Elevation of the Medial Plateau of the Tibia in the Treatment of Blount Disease. *J Bone Joint Surg Am* 1992;74:351.

+ 248. Schoenecker PL, Meade WC, Pierron RL, et al. Blount's Disease: A Retrospective Review and Recommenda-tions for Treatment. *J Pediatr Orthop* 1985;5:181.

+ 249. Schrock RD Jr. Peroneal Nerve Palsy Following Dero-tation Osteotomies for Tibial Torsion. *Clin Orthop* 1969;62:172.

+ 250. Sevastikoglou JA, Eriksson I. Familial Infantile Osteo-chondrosis Deformans Tibiae: Idiopathic Tibia Vara: A Case Report. *Acta Orthop Scand* 1967;38:81.

+ 251. Sharrard WJW. Treatment of Congenital and Infantile Pseudarthrosis of the Tibia with Pulsing Electromag-netic Fields. *Orthop Clin North Am* 1984;15:143.

+ 252. Sherman M. Physiologic Bowing of the Legs. *South Med J* 1960;53:830.

+ 253. Sibert JR, Bray PT. Probable Dominant Inheritance in Blount's Diseae. *Clin Genet* 1977;11:394.

+ 254. Siegling JA, Gillespie JB. Adolescent Tibia Vara. *Ra-diology* 1939;32:483.

+ 255. Siffert RS. Intraepiphyseal Osteotomy for Progressive Tibia: Case Report and Rationale for Management. *J Pediatr Orthop* 1982;2:81.

+ 256. Siffert RS, Katz JF. The Intra-articular Deformity in Osteochondrosis Deformans Tibiae. *J Bone Joint Surg Am* 1970;52:800.

+ 257. Skak SV. Valgus Deformity Following Proximal Me-taphyseal Fracture in Children. *Acta Orthop Scand* 1982;53:141.

+ 258. Skak SV, Toftgard T, Torben DP. Fractures of the Prox-imal Metaphysis of the Tibia in Children. *Injury* 1987; 18:149.

+ 259. Smit CS, Zeeman BJ, Wade WJ. Congenital Pseud-arthrosis of the Tibia: Treatment with Free Vasculari-sed Fibular Grafts. *S Afr Med J* 1993;83:750.

260. Smith CF. Current Concepts Review: Tibia Vara (Blount's Disease). *J Bone Joint Surg Am* 1982;64:630.

+ 261. Smith DN, Harrison MHM. The Correction of Angular Deformities of Long Bones by Osteotomy–Osteoclasis. *J Bone Joint Surg Br* 1979;61:410.

+ 262. Sofield HA. Congenital Pseudarthrosis of the Tibia. *Clin Orthop* 1971;76:33.

+ 263. Steel HH, Sandrow RE, Sullivan PD. Complications of Tibial Osteotomy in Children for Genu Varum and Valgum: Evidence That Neurologic Changes Are Due to Ischemia. *J Bone Joint Surg Am* 1971;53:1629.

+ 264. Stricker SJ, Edwards PM, Tidwell MA. Langenskiöld Classification of Tibia Vara: An Assessment of Interob-server Variability. *J Pediatr Orthop* 1994;14:152.

+ 265. Stricker SJ, Faustgen JP. Radiographic Management of Bow Leg Deformity: Variability Due to Method and Limb Rotation. *J Pediatr Orthop* 1994;14:147.

+ 266. Strong ML, Wong-Chung J. Prophylactic Bypass Graft-ing of the Prepseudarthrotic Tibia in Neurofibro-matoses. *J Pediatr Orthop* 1991;11:757.

+ 267. Sutcliffe ML, Goldberg AAJ. The Treatment of Con-genital Pseudarthrosis of the Tibia with Pulsating Elec-tromagnetic Fields: A Survey of 52 Cases. *Clin Orthop* 1982;166:45.

268. Tachdjian MO. Angular Deformities of the Long Bones of the Lower Limbs. In: Tachdjian MO, ed. *Pediatric Orthopaedics.* Philadelphia: WB Saunders, 1990:2820.

269. Tachdjian MO. Congenital Posteromedial Angulation of the Tibia and Fibula. In: Tachdjian MO, ed. *Pediatric Orthopaedics.* Philadelphia: WB Saunders, 1990:651.

270. Tachdjian MO. "Congenital" Pseudarthrosis of the Tibia. In: Tachdjian MO, ed. *Pediatric Orthopaedics.* Philadelphia: WB Saunders, 1990:656.

+ 271. Tanguy AF, Dalens BJ, Boisgard S. Congenital Con-stricting Band with Pseudarthrosis of the Tibia and Fi-bula: A Case Report. *J Bone Joint Surg Am* 1995;77: 1251.

+ 272. Taylor GI, Miller, GDH, Ham FJ. The Free Vascularized Bone Graft: A Clinical Extension of Microvascular Techniques. *Plast Reconstr Surg* 1975;55:533.

+ 273. Taylor SL. Tibial Overgrowth: A Cause of Genu Valgum. *J Bone Joint Surg Am* 1963;45:659.

+ 274. Thompson GH, Carter JR. Late-onset Tibia Vara (Blount's Disease): Current Concepts. *Clin Orthop* 1990;255:24.

* 275. Thompson GH, Carter JR, Smith CW. Late-onset Tibia Vara: A Comparative Analysis. *J Pediatr Orthop* 1984; 4:185.

+ 276. Timperlake RW, Bowen JR, Guille JT, Choi IH. Prospective Evaluation of Fifty-three Consecutive Percutaneous Epiphysiodeses of the Distal Femur and Proximal Tibia and Fibula. *J Pediatr Orthop* 1991;11:350.

+ 277. Townsend PL. Vascularized Fibular Graft Using Reverse Peroneal Flow in the Treatment of Congenital Pseudarthrosis of the Tibia. *Br J Plast Surg* 1990;43: 261.

+ 278. Umber JS, Moss SW, Coleman SS. Surgical Treatment of Congenital Pseudarthrosis of the Tibia. *Clin Orthop* 1982;166:28.

+ 279. Vankka E, Salenius P. Spontaneous Correction of Severe Tibiofemoral Deformity in Growing Children. *Acta Orthop Scand* 1982;53:567.

+ 280. Verhelst MP, Spaas FM, Fabry G. Progressive Valgus Deformity of the Knee after Resection of an Exostosis at the Proximal Medial Tibial Metaphysis: A Case Report. *Acta Orthop Belg* 1975;41:689.

+ 281. Visser JD, Veldhuizen AG. Valgus Deformity after Fracture of the Proximal Tibial Metaphysis in Childhood. *Acta Orthop Scand* 1982;53:663.

+ 282. Volpon JB. Idiopathic Genu Valgum Treated by Epiphysiodesis in Adolescence. *Int Orthop* 1997;21:228.

+ 283. Weber BG. Fibrous Interposition Causing Valgus Deformity after Fracture of the Upper Tibial Metaphysis in Children. *J Bone Joint Surg Br* 1977;59:290.

284. Weiland AJ. Vascularized Bone Transfers. *Instr Course Lect* 1984;33:446.

+ 285. Weiland AJ, Weis APC, Moore JR, Tolo VT. Vascularized Fibular Graft in the Treatment of Congenital Pseudarthrosis of the Tibia. *J Bone Joint Surg Am* 1990,72:654.

+ 286. Wenger DR, Mickelson M, Maynard JA. The Evolution and Histopathology of Adolescent Tibia Vara. *J Pediatr Orthop* 1984;4:78.

287. White GR, Mencio GA. Genu Valgum in Children: Diagnosis and Therapeutic Alternatives. *J Am Acad Orthop Surg* 1995;3:275.

+ 288. Yadav SS, Thomas S. Congenital Posteromedial Bowing of the Tibia. *Acta Orthop Scand* 1980;51:311.

+ 289. Zayer M. Hemicondylar Tibial Osteotomy in Blount's Disease: A Report of 2 Cases. *Acta Orthop Scand* 1992; 63:350.

+ 290. Zayer M. Tibia Vara in Focal Fibrocartilaginous Dysplasia: A Report of 2 Cases. *Acta Orthop Scand* 1992; 63:353.

+ 291. Zayer M. Osteoarthritis Following Blount's Disease. *Int Orthop* 1980;4:63.

+ 292. Zionts L, Harcke TH, Brooks KM, MacEwen GD. Post-traumatic Tibia Valga: A Case Demonstrating Asymmetric Activity of the Proximal Growth Plate on Technetium Bone Scan. *J Pediatr Orthop* 1987;7:458.

+ 293. Zionts LE, MacEwen GD. Spontaneous Improvement of Post-traumatic Tibia Valga. *J Bone Joint Surg Am* 1986;68:680.

+ 294. Zuege RC, Kempken TC, Blount WP. Epiphyseal Stapling for Angular Deformities of the Knee. *J Bone Joint Surg Am* 1979;61:320.

+ 295. Zumiotti A, Ferreira MC. Treatment of Congenital Pseudarthrosis of the Tibia by Microsurgical Fibula Transfer. *Microsurgery* 1994;15:37.

CHAPTER 170

LIMB-LENGTH DISCREPANCY IN CHILDREN

Kent A. Vincent and Colin I. Moseley

INTRODUCTION

Limb-length discrepancy problems are challenging because growth complicates the longitudinal evaluation of each patient. Therefore, the orthopaedic surgeon must have an understanding of growth and the methods by which to analyze and predict future changes; this is particularly important before considering any surgery to correct limb-length discrepancy.

Human height is the combined total of limbs, pelvis, torso, and head. The limbs constitute approximately half of this total height, and they are the most kinetic component of the body during gait. Length abnormalities of the limbs have the potential to affect both height and efficiency of gait.

INCIDENCE

The incidence of limb-length discrepancy is relatively common. Reports have suggested some level of discrepancy in up to 70% of adult males (72). In a review of more than 100 Swedish laborers, 30% had a limb-length discrepancy of 1.0 to 1.5 cm, 4% had 2.0 to 2.5 cm, and 0.7% had more than a 2.5 cm discrepancy (35). Estimates are especially difficult in the changing pediatric population, but for individual congenital conditions, the incidence could be predicted more reliably.

K. A. Vincent: Staff Surgeon, Shriners' Hospital for Children, Portland Department of Orthopaedics, Oregon Health Sciences University, Portland, Oregon, 97201.
C. I. Moseley: Shriners' Hospital for Children, Los Angeles, California, 90020.

NATURAL HISTORY

SPINE

Most important to the treating physician, as in many pediatric orthopaedic conditions, is the natural history of the condition. Parents are commonly concerned about the long-term effects of a limb-length discrepancy on the spine, but cause-and-effect relationships are unknown. Low back pain in the child is rare, even for a child with a limb-length discrepancy. Given the high rate of back pain in the normal adult population, we may assume that this rate of back pain must also exist for the same reasons in the population with limb-length discrepancies. Changes in adult spine radiographs, such as vertebral wedging and traction spurs, have been associated with limb-length differences of more than 9 mm, but these findings have not been correlated with symptoms (22,26,27,79). Reviews of adults with minor discrepancies have suggested a relatively low association with low back pain (62,77,92). Other studies confirm that adult patients presenting with low back pain associated with limb-length discrepancy appear to have symptomatic relief after equalization surgery (71,84).

An increased incidence of structural scoliosis over the general population is associated with limb-length discrepancies (66). However, the causative effects of one deformity on the other are unknown. Lumbar facet orientation does not correlate well with asymmetric changes in limb length (24). The direction of the curve is not always in the direction expected based on the limb-length difference (33). This makes it more difficult to postulate that the limb-length difference is the causative factor.

HIP

As limb-length discrepancy increases, so does the amount of uncoverage by the acetabulum of the high-side femoral head hip (59). Theoretically, this problem should result in force concentration on the lateral edge of the acetabulum, with resultant early arthritis. Gait lab studies, however, suggest the possibility that high-side hip forces may actually decrease during stance phase (13). Little long-term clinical information exists on the subject.

KNEE AND FOOT

Knee problems secondary to leg-length differences do not seem to be common in children. A report has been made of increased incidence of knee pain in athletes (47). The most common associated problem in the foot is equinus on the short side. When the problem is not followed closely, a contracture may result from years of compensation in this position.

GAIT

Children tend to be better able than adults to compensate for differences in limb length. Their increased joint flexibility and higher strength-to-weight ratio may result in adjustments that produce a smooth, even gait. With greater discrepancies between the two legs, compensation becomes more difficult. Coronal plane pelvic tilt may increase the energy consumption of gait.

Data from gait lab studies of children with length discrepancies have suggested a quite variable pattern of compensation among individuals (44,51,76). Those with less than 3% discrepancy do not require compensatory strategies. Compensation for greater discrepancies results in greater work and greater vertical displacement of the center of body mass. Each child applies compensatory mechanisms differently; the most common are walking with the short-side ankle in equinus or the long-side knee in flexion. Energy consumption studies have yet to be completed to confirm the meaning of these changes to gait efficiency.

GROWTH

LONGITUDINAL DATA

Growth of the limbs results from the combination of physeal new bone production and actual epiphyseal size increase. Epiphyseal size increase usually accounts for only about 5% of the total growth of the limb, but for calculation purposes, this increase is usually ignored (Fig. 170.1).

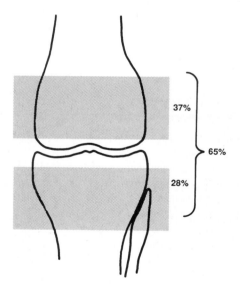

Figure 170.1. The distal femoral and proximal tibial physes contribute constant proportions to the growth of the leg. (From Moseley CF. Leg-Length Discrepancy. In: Morrissy RT, Weinstein SL, eds. *Lovell & Winter's Pediatric Orthopaedics.* Philadelphia: J.B. Lippincott, 1996:855, with permission.)

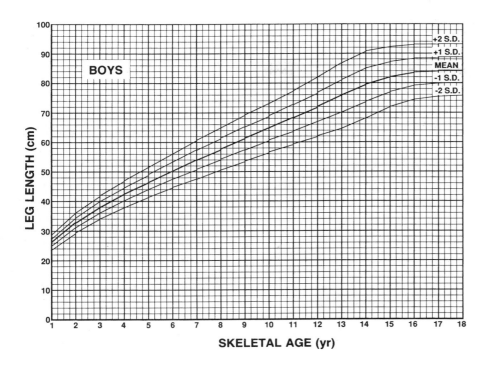

Figure 170.2. Graph of total limb length (femur plus tibia only) for boys. An individual boy may be plotted instantaneously and projected into the future based on his current situation. (From Anderson M, Messner MB, Green WT. Distribution of Lengths of the Normal Femur and Tibia in Children from One to Eighteen Years of Age. *J Bone Joint Surg* 1964;46A:1197, with permission.)

The growth plates at the knee contribute the most to total limb length, whereas the distal tibial and proximal femoral physes add lesser amounts.

Difficulty with measurement has prevented us from understanding patterns of growth in the short term. One study suggests that children have week-to-week variability in limb growth, with pulsatile patterns of miniature growth spurts every 30 to 55 days, alternating with periods of slower growth (32). In the longer term, however, the growth pattern evens out.

Data for growth calculation have come mainly from two studies by Anderson and colleagues (4,6). In one, data were collected instantaneously on children between 5 years of age and maturity. In the other, a group was followed longitudinally until maturity. Their data were reported in tabular and graphic forms as total limb length as a function of skeletal age (Fig. 170.2). These were converted into the growth-remaining charts for the distal femur and proximal tibia (Fig. 170.3).

SKELETAL AGE

The study of limb-length discrepancy problems involves the interaction of patient age, maturity, and limb length. Growth rate is maximal at the time of birth, both in percentage gain and in absolute terms. The absolute rate of growth relative to chronologic years drops slightly between 3 years of age and the adolescent growth spurt. During the adolescent growth spurt, the absolute rate of growth increases. Cessation of growth occurs in boys at

16 to 17 years of age, and in girls at 14 to 15 years of age. When we compare different people, it becomes quickly evident that their times of maturation, as measured in chronologic years, vary considerably. One child who may appear to be tall may just be going through the process of maturation at an earlier time. In fact, this "temporarily" tall child may then end up shorter than a second child who, although shorter initially, matures at a later time as measured by chronologic age.

The best method we have to measure level of maturity appears to be radiographs of the bones. The standard radiograph has become the anteroposterior view of the left wrist, although other x-ray techniques are available (81). The skeletal age of a patient is defined as the age at which the general population, on average, reaches the same level of bony development as that patient. This skeletal age correlates more closely than chronological age with other signs of maturation, including menarche, secondary sexual characteristics, height, and limb length. Measurement of skeletal age with the anteroposterior view of the wrist, however, remains the weak point in predicting limb-length discrepancy, both because of reliability of readings and because of more variability in children with limb-length discrepancy (15,18).

For any large group of normal children at the same chronologic age, the average skeletal age should equal chronologic age. However, time of maturation varies greatly between people; thus, for any given child, the skeletal age does not necessarily equal the chronologic age. A child who matures earlier than his peers appears to go

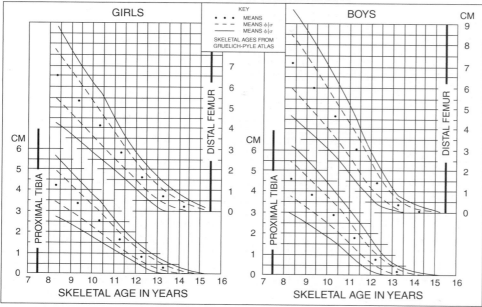

MEANS AND STANDARD DEVIATIONS DERIVED FROM
LONGITUDINAL SERIES 50 GIRLS AND 50 BOYS

THE CHILDREN'S MEDICAL CENTER, BOSTON, MASSACHUSETTES

Figure 170.3. Green-Anderson growth-remaining graph for girls and boys. This plots the amount of remaining growth from each of the distal femoral and proximal tibial epiphyses as functions of the skeletal age. The mean is in the center, whereas one and two standard deviations in each direction are represented by the other lines. This enables the calculation of results if an epiphysiodesis is done. (From Anderson M, Green WT, Messner MB. Growth and Predictions of Growth in the Lower Extremities. *J Bone Joint Surg* 45A: 1963, with permission.)

through a maturation spurt in which the skeletal age years are changing more quickly than the chronologic years. The other milestones of maturity (secondary sexual characteristics, menarche, and limb growth) are moving forward at a similar, early rate.

DIFFERENT GROWTH PATTERNS

Based on the change in discrepancy over time, Shapiro (74) has previously divided growth patterns in children with limb-length discrepancy into five types (Fig. 170.4). Three phases are used to describe the change over time: In the initial phase, the discrepancy develops; in the middle phase, a pattern of difference is established during further growth; and the final phase is the period of time before growth cessation. Patient age is plotted against the limb-length discrepancy on a graph. By definition, the initial phase results in an increase in discrepancy. During the middle phase, the discrepancies are variable; some continue to increase (e.g., a traumatic physeal closure), whereas others plateau (e.g., a patient being treated for juvenile rheumatoid arthritis). The final phase is also variable in that a discrepancy may increase, plateau, or decrease. Again, conditions that cause permanent physeal damage tend to cause a steady increase in discrepancy, whereas other conditions are associated with a plateau in differences (e.g., improvement in functional level in a paralytic limb, as with a brace). The most common scenario for an actual decrease in limb-length discrepancy is

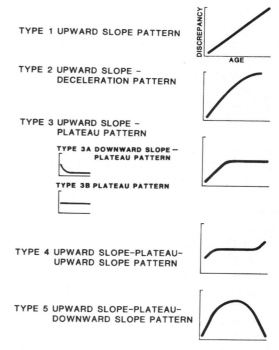

Figure 170.4. Various patterns of changes in limb-length discrepancy over time. The patterns shown are based on absolute magnitude of discrepancy, and thus the graphs do not take into account the natural slowing of growth near maturity. (Shapiro F. Developmental Patterns in Lower Extremity Length Discrepancies. *J Bone Joint Surg* 1982;64-A:639.)

that of a treated juvenile rheumatoid arthritis patient (75, 86).

A discussion of patterns of change in limb-length discrepancy by Shapiro's technique are useful for large groups of patients, but it may be less useful for the individual patient. This is because patterns are plotted to age 13 rather than maturity, and the differences are related to chronologic age rather than the skeletal age. This technique also does not compare the pattern of the limb-length difference curve with the normal growth curve or take into account lengthening of either leg with growth, whether it is normal or not.

ANATOMIC SITES OF LENGTH INEQUALITY

The femur and tibia are not the only components of the limbs that make up the leg's effective length. Variable heights of the two sides of the pelvis and pelvic obliquity to the floor result in a functional difference in limb lengths. Scoliosis and hip abduction and adduction contractures are common situations in which resultant changes in the orientation of the pelvis to the ground create apparent changes in the limb length. The other commonly overlooked source of difference between limb lengths is the foot. Some loss of height may be expected from either varus or valgus collapse of the foot, and the operated hindfoot may lose a portion of its vertical height.

CAUSES OF LIMB-LENGTH DISCREPANCY

Limb-length discrepancy may be due to factors that change length directly or from an alteration in growth. Fractures, dislocations, and surgery are the only mechanisms by which length is changed acutely.

INHIBITION OF GROWTH

A physis may be slowed by several mechanisms. The congenitally short limb is genetically programmed to be shorter via slower physeal growth. A growth plate injury may result in slowing or complete cessation of growth. External influences such as disuse, as may occur in polio or hemiplegia, may also cause slowing of growth. Experimental denervation of sciatic nerves in animal models suggest a slowed rate of maturation in denervated bone (20).

Congenital

Children with limbs of different lengths may be either hemihypertrophic or hemiatrophic, although distinguishing between the two may be difficult (7). Typically, the shortening involves all parts of the involved limb. It is probably best to consider each limb as being genetically programmed at a different rate of growth. Plotting sequential growth on the straight-line graph should confirm this.

Congenitally short bones may occur in conjunction with anomalies of other bones or independently. The congenital short femur is considered to be a variant of proximal focal femoral deficiency (43). The spectrum of the presentation includes anterior cruciate ligament deficiency, absence of the fibula, progressive ankle valgus deformity, absence of the lateral ray or rays of the foot, and tarsal coalitions. Congenitally short tibiae are commonly associated with both posterior and anterior bowing deformities.

Trauma

Fractures through the growth plate tend to occur through the zone of hypertrophy. Fortunately, this weak area of the physis is not responsible for the continued generation of growth cells, which occurs closer to the epiphysis. Thus in the Salter-Harris classification of epiphyseal fracture type I and II injuries (see Chapter 164) tend not to result in long-term growth disturbances, with a few exceptions. The type V crush injury, however, may permanently damage cells at all levels of the physis. Type III and IV fractures do cross the growth zone of the physis; thus, they are most prone to formation of a bridge of bone or physeal closure. Anatomic reduction of type III and IV fractures helps prevent physeal abnormalities. When physeal bars form or partial closure occurs, angular malalignment occurs because of asymmetric involvement of the growth plate. Physeal closure has also been recognized as a complication of diaphyseal fractures of the ipsilateral limb (8).

Infection

Disturbance of growth from infections tends to have more severe results because of the young age at which this occurs. Direct invasion of the physeal cells occurs in hematogenous osteomyelitis, sometimes in conjunction with a septic joint. The bridges that result tend to be broader and more central than those that result from fractures, and thus, they are more difficult to resect successfully. A so-called sick physis may develop when an infection has a global effect on a physis. The cellular effects of the infection on the physis then either slow the rate of growth or create a delayed complete or partial arrest. Meningococcemia is one of the more common infectious processes that create this delayed growth arrest.

Paralysis

The cause of limb-length differences in paralysis is not completely clear. Theories have included decreased blood flow, poor venous return, decreased neurogenic input to the physis, and disuse atrophy. Polio commonly results in significant differences in limb lengths. Hemiplegic cerebral palsy patients may have small differences in length, which seldom require surgical correction. Hemiplegic patients often appear to have more of a discrepancy because of asymmetric muscle tone and other joint contractures that result in pelvic obliquity.

Tumors

Tumors may directly invade the growth plate, having a destructive effect similar to infection. Abnormal cartilage emanating from the physeal cells may also disturb normal growth patterns. In enchondromatosis and Ollier's disease, abnormal physeal cells produce tumor cartilage rather than cartilage for longitudinal growth. Osteochondromata may have more of a mechanical effect on growth plates that may disturb growth, such as at the distal tibia. This is more commonly angular than longitudinal.

Avascular Necrosis

The proximal femur is the most common location for clinical problems arising secondary to avascular necrosis. Fortunately, the proximal femur is responsible for only about 15% of limb length. Clinical presentations include the treated developmental hip dislocation, traumatic hip dislocations and fractures, slipped capital femoral epiphysis, and Legg-Calvé-Perthes disease. A common situation with avascular necrosis of the proximal femur is a severe adduction contracture secondary to femoral head collapse. This results in a large apparent length discrepancy, which is actually due to a marked coronal plane pelvic obliquity.

STIMULATION OF GROWTH

A physis may be stimulated to increase growth by arteriovenous malformation, inflammation, fracture, and tumor. From a clinical standpoint, surgical creation of a situation that mimics these conditions has failed to provide reproducible increases in growth.

Tumor

Vascular malformations such as hemangiomas may result in growth stimulation, presumably via increased blood flow. Other nonvascular growths such as neurofibromatosis, fibrous dysplasia, and Wilms' tumor may result in overgrowth, usually of focal areas of bones.

Fracture

Overgrowth from fractures commonly occurs in the femur in children younger than 10 years of age (2,34). Studies of the factors most responsible for femoral overgrowth have been contradictory (45,52,54,67). The proximal tibia also has a tendency toward overgrowth following fracture (52,67). If the fibula is not also fractured, a relative increase in tibial length results in progressive valgus deformity at the knee.

Inflammation

Infection may damage the growth plate, but in some cases, chronic osteomyelitis may actually result in physeal stimulation. Another common example is pauciarticular juvenile rheumatoid arthritis, in which overgrowth of the involved limb is common, particularly before 3 years of age (75,86).

EVALUATION

CLINICAL EXAMINATION

The physical exam remains the central tool for clinical assessment in limb-length differences. Physicians may tend to focus on radiographic findings; however, radiographic methods can have inherent artifacts from patient movement or from poor conversion of an angular deformity to two-plane measurement. In addition, many other clinical factors not measured by radiographs are important in making treatment decisions. Once the complete historical and physical evidence has been obtained, radiographs may be used to fine-tune data and to follow the condition precisely.

The most useful clinical tool is to place blocks beneath the foot of the short side of the patient in the standing position. The height can be adjusted until the pelvis is level, as judged by the anterior superior iliac spines from the front or the posterior iliac crests from the back (Fig. 170.5) This technique is generally the most reliable and provides the most comprehensive information, because it allows the clinician to take into account pelvic obliquity, contractures, angular deformities, and differences in foot height. To use the technique even more effectively, shoe lifts of variable heights may be used; this allows evaluation of gait and dynamic events, with partial to complete correction of differences (Fig. 170.17).

A traditional method of determining the limb length has been to measure from the anterior superior iliac spine to the medial malleolus, in the supine or standing position, using a tape measure. (Fig. 170.6). This method has some value, but reproducibility may be poor because of poorly palpable landmarks, tenting of the tape, angular deformity at the knee, and differences in the height of the pelvis (49). In addition, this measurement does not take into account angular deformity (i.e., obliquity) about the pelvis.

RADIOGRAPHIC EVALUATION

Scanogram

Radiographic techniques may be inherently more accurate than clinical methods in measuring limb lengths, and thus,

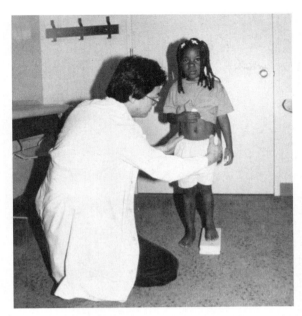

Figure 170.5. The standing technique of limb-length measurement is done with the patient standing on blocks on the short side until the anterior superior iliac spines are at the same level. It may also be visualized from behind the patient, using the top of the iliac crests as the measure of level.

they may be more valuable over the long term for evaluating growth trends. All of the radiographic techniques used have variability between readings because of differences in technician techniques, changes in patient position, and differences in techniques and landmarks of people reading the films. The orthopaedic surgeon must review all of the data derived from radiographs before considering surgery, check for consistency, and correlate the data with clinical findings.

Confusion exists over the terminology used for radiographic measurement techniques. The original scanogram was done with a collimated x-ray beam directed through a transverse slit that exposed a film beneath the patient as the x-ray tube was moved from one end of the limb to the other. The teleoradiograph is a single-exposure x-ray shot from a 2 m (6 ft) distance with a radiopaque ruler placed on the film cassette. It can reveal an angular deformity but has the disadvantage of increasing distortion through parallax of the x-ray beam (Fig. 170.7) The orthoradiograph avoids the parallax problem by taking three separate exposures on the same ruled cassette. Like the teleoradiograph, the large film size can be cumbersome (Fig. 170.8). The current scanogram technique uses three exposures, but the cassette is moved beneath the patient between each image. The ruler must be fixed to the x-ray table, which is not a necessity with the single exposure techniques (Fig. 170.9). The patient must be able to remain still between exposures with the teleoradiograph and the scanogram. For children younger than 5 or 6 years of age, the teleoradiograph is more appropriate.

The current standard of radiographic assessment for most situations is the scanogram. The images are captured

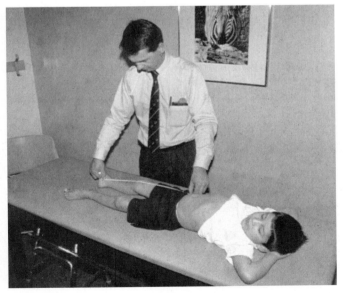

Figure 170.6. The supine technique of limb-length measurement is done with the tape measure from the anterior superior iliac spine to the medial malleolus with the knee straight. Because of difficulties in reproducing accurate measurements, the standing technique is generally preferred.

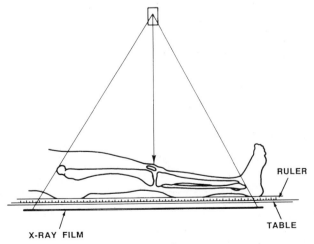

Figure 170.7. The supine teleoradiogram method. Parallax effect is greater with a single exposure. (From Moseley CF. Leg-Length Discrepancy. In: Morrissy RT, Weinstein SL, eds. *Lovell & Winter's Pediatric Orthopaedics*. Philadelphia: J.B. Lippincott, 1996:865, with permission.)

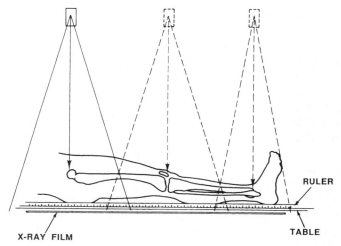

Figure 170.8. The orthoradiograph. When three separate exposures are used, parallax is minimized, but the patient must be able to hold still for three images to avoid inaccuracies. (From Moseley CF. Leg-Length Discrepancy. In: Morrissy RT, Weinstein SL, eds. *Lovell & Winter's Pediatric Orthopaedics*. Philadelphia: J.B. Lippincott, 1996:865, with permission.)

on one film of relatively convenient size. As long as the patient does not move between exposures and no joint contractures are present, this provides an accurate and relatively reproducible methodology (3,29). When knee contractures are present, the bones may be measured individually by placing the patient prone for a ruled radio-

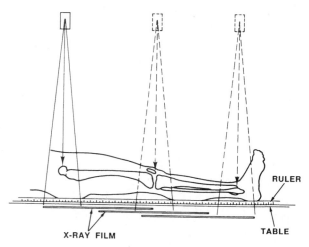

Figure 170.9. The scanogram: The three exposures are taken after positioning a portion of the 14-by-17-inch cassette behind each of the hip, knee, and ankle joints. (From Moseley CF. Leg-Length Discrepancy. In Morrissy RT, Weinstein SL, eds. *Lovell & Winter's Pediatric Orthopaedics*. Philadelphia: J.B. Lippincott, 1996:866.)

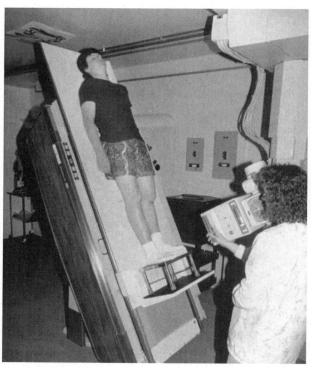

Figure 170.10. The semierect scanogram method. The tilt table allows for placement of lifts for leveling the pelvis, and will give more accurate information about joint and length changes with weight bearing. The three images of the hips, knees, and ankles are taken in the same way as with the supine technique shown in Figure 170.7.

graph of the femur, and in the lateral position for the film of the tibia.

The scanogram is most ideally taken with the patient semierect, with the short side blocked up beneath the foot to level the pelvis. Separate images are then taken of the hips, knees, and ankles, including the plantar portion of the foot (Fig. 170.10). The semierect position has the advantage of mimicking the upright weight-bearing position, leveling the pelvis for more accurate measurement, limiting patient motion between exposures, and allowing evaluation of the contribution of the foot to the discrepancy. The only disadvantage is that a tilting x-ray table is required.

The standard landmarks used from the orthoroentgenogram are the tops of the femoral head and the middle of the "saddle" formed by the subchondral bone of the distal tibial plafond. If separation into femoral and tibial components is required, use the medial femoral condyle. Then draw a horizontal line from the chosen points to the ruled area on the film. Each of these lines should be parallel to the edge of the film. (This assumes that the edge of the cassette is close to being perpendicular to the orientation of the leg.) By subtracting these numbers, the lengths

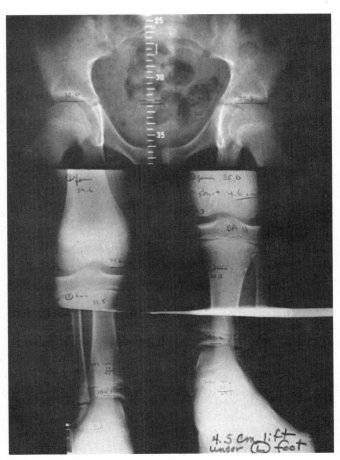

Figure 170.11. Sample orthoroentgenogram. Results may be analyzed on one film of convenient size, but this film does not allow accurate calculation of mechanical or anatomical axis.

of both legs and the femoral and tibial components may be calculated (Fig. 170.11.)

Other Methods

The computerized axial tomogram may be used in place of the orthoroentgenogram. It offers the advantage of being more accurate and delivering less radiation, but for many centers, the technique is more cumbersome and it is expensive to obtain (1,36). A decision should be made on the basis of cost and availability because the accuracy of the two techniques appears to be comparable.

Recently, real-time ultrasonography has been reported as an effective screening tool, although slightly less accurate than radiography, for limb-length determination (42, 82).

Skeletal Age

Determining skeletal age is done by comparing radiographic landmarks of maturity with standards. The Greulich-Pyle atlas is the most commonly used standard today

(30). The left hand and wrist are imaged in the anteroposterior plane; separate standards are used for boys and girls. The standard radiograph in the atlas represents the median level of bony maturity for the chronologic age. Given a random sampling of children at the same chronologic age, half of the left hand and wrist radiographs would appear more mature and half would appear less mature than the standard. For any given child, then, the skeletal age is that which corresponds with the best radiographic match from the atlas (Fig. 170.12).

Unfortunately, the skeletal age determination is the weakest link in the process of limb-length calculations. Differences between children in the order of bone maturation around the wrist, extrapolation between ages in the atlas, and congenital anomalies of wrist bones may result in different interpretations of the radiograph for skeletal age (15,18). Other methods have been used to determine skeletal age and are probably more exacting, but they are also more cumbersome. In addition, all of the predictive growth data derived by Green and Anderson are based on the Greulich-Pyle atlas. Other methods of skeletal age

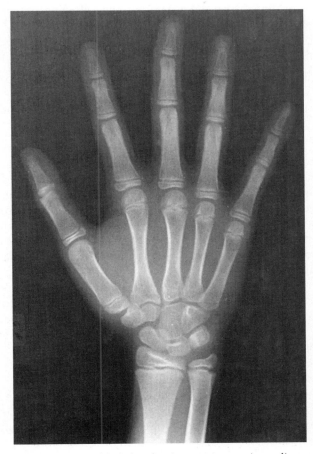

Figure 170.12. Left hand and wrist anteroposterior radiograph taken for bone age estimation.

determination do not necessarily correlate with the Greulich-Pyle skeletal age and, thus, should not be used with Green and Anderson's data for surgical calculations.

ANALYZING THE DATA

After skeletal maturity, limb-length differences do not change without surgical intervention. The growing child, on the other hand, is continuously changing. The goal of the orthopaedic surgeon must be to predict the situation at maturity. In most cases, this means analyzing the data from a young age to predict the limb-length difference at maturity. Treatment should be based on this prediction, so careful analysis of the data is crucial (10). At present, three general methods are used widely for data analysis—the arithmetic method, the growth-remaining method, and the straight-line graph method. They all use roughly the same steps of analysis but with different techniques. The first step is evaluation of past growth, the second step is prediction of future growth, and the third step is evaluation of what the results of surgical correction would be.

Arithmetic Method
The arithmetic method is based on the following assumptions of growth patterns (Fig. 170.13):

- Girls stop growing at chronologic age 14.
- Boys stop growing at chronologic age 16.
- The distal femur grows at a rate of ⅜ inch (10 mm) per year.
- The proximal tibia grows at a rate of ¼ inch (6 mm) per year.

This technique is convenient but has some inherent inaccuracies. The estimations of growth are most accurate during the last few years of growth, but are relatively inaccurate in younger children. In addition, the chronologic age is the basis for the measurements and determinations. As discussed earlier, the patient's chronologic age and bone age may vary considerably, but the bone age is a more reliable indicator of skeletal maturity for individual patients.

This technique should be used as a tool for estimation well before surgery is being considered. As the time for surgery nears, other, more precise methods should be used to minimize errors and make correction as exacting as possible.

Growth-Remaining Method
The growth-remaining method is based on the data and tables of Green and Anderson (4,5). The percentage of growth inhibition of the short leg is first calculated. Using these data, the lengths of long and short legs at maturity can be predicted. The graphs of the growth remaining from the distal femoral and proximal tibial physes are

used to determine appropriate times for epiphysiodesis (Fig. 170.14).

The growth-remaining method is based on skeletal age and uses growth percentile of the child to predict future growth. The technique does have some disadvantages: It requires two sets of graphs in making the calculations, and it relies heavily on the most recent skeletal age for predictions.

Straight-Line Graph Method
The straight-line graph method was conceived as a way of graphically representing the growth of the two limbs (61). It incorporates the data of Green and Anderson (5), and is used as a method of recording, analyzing, and predicting both growth and the results of treatment. The method is based on two principles: First, the growth of each leg can be graphically represented as a straight line, and second, a nomogram can be used to determine the growth percentile, based on skeletal age and limb length (Fig. 170.15).

Green and Anderson's graphs have a curved pattern at each end, representing the high rate of growth during infancy and the slowing rate before skeletal maturity. By manipulation of the scale of the x-axis at each end of the growth curve, the length of the limb can be graphically represented as a straight line. The long limb is thus assigned the graphic slope of 1.00, representing 100% of normal growth. If no variable disease process or treatment is changing the short limb, it will also follow a straight line on the graph over time. The discrepancy between the two limbs is thus represented by the vertical distance between the two growth lines, and the inhibition by the difference in the lines' slopes.

The nomogram for skeletal age has been set up on the graph to allow the long limb length to be compared with that of the Green-Anderson population. If a child grew such that the bone age and limb lengths progressed together exactly as the Green and Anderson data would suggest, the points on the nomogram would describe a perfect horizontal line. This rarely happens, both because of the inherent differences in the reading of bone ages and differences in growth of individual children. As an increasing number of estimates of bone age are obtained, these differences tend to diminish such that a more accurate best horizontal line estimate through the points can be obtained. Generally, heavier weighting is given to the most recent bone age readings when making a best horizontal line estimate.

Predictions of surgical results may be made with the graph as well. Changes in the growth rate of either leg result in a change in slope of the line representing that leg. Lengthening a limb results in simple upward vertical displacement of the line; shortening results in downward vertical displacement. When an epiphysiodesis is performed on a long limb, the slope of the line representing

Determining Leg Length Discrepancy: The Arithmetic Method

Leg length data
(for examples for all three methods):

Sex: Female

Age (yr)	Skeletal age (yr.)	Right leg length (cm)	Left leg length (cm)
7 + 10	8 + 10	60.0	58.2
8 + 4	9 + 4	64.4	61.9
9 + 3	10 + 3	70.0	66.2

Prerequisite growth information

Distal femoral plate grows 10 mm/yr.
Proximal tibial plate grows 6 mm/yr.

Girls stop growing at 14 years of age.
Boys stop growing at 16 years of age.

A Assessment of past growth

1. Longest time interval for data
   = age at last visit - age at first

2. Years of growth remaining
   = 14 (16 for boys) - age at last visit

3. Past growth of legs
   = present length - first measured length

4. Growth rate of long leg
   $= \dfrac{\text{past growth}}{\text{time interval}}$

5. Growth inhibition
   $= \dfrac{(\text{growth of long leg - growth of short leg})}{\text{growth of long leg}}$

1. Longest time interval for data
   = 9 yr 3 mo - 7 yr 10 mo = 1 yr 5 mo
   = 1.42 yr

2. Years of growth remaining
   = 14 yr - 9 yr 3 mo = 4 yr 9 mo = 4.75 yr

3. Past growth of:
   long leg = 70.0 - 60.0 = 10.0 cm
   short leg = 66.2 - 58.2 = 8.0 cm

4. Growth rate of long leg
   $= \dfrac{10.0}{1.42} = 7.04$ cm/yr

5. Inhibition
   $= \dfrac{(10.0 - 8.0)}{10.0} = 0.2$ cm

B Prediction of future growth

1. Future growth of long leg
   = years remaining X growth rate

2. Future increase in discrepancy
   = future growth of long leg X inhibition

3. Discrepancy at maturity
   = present discrepancy + future increase

1. Future growth of long leg
   = 4.75 X 7.04 = 33.4 cm

2. Future increase in discrepancy
   = 33.4 X 0.2 = 6.7 cm

3. Discrepancy at maturity
   = (70.0 - 66.2) + 6.7 = 10.5 cm

C Prediction of effect of surgery

Effect of epiphysiodesis
   = growth rate X years remaining

Effect of epiphysiodesis
   Femoral = 1.0 X 4.75 = 4.75 cm
   Tibial = 0.6 X 4.75 = 2.85 cm
   Both   = 1.6 X 4.75 = 7.6 cm

Figure 170.13. Arithmetic method of limb-length discrepancy determination. In the left column, a theoretical explanation, and on the right, a sample calculation. (From Moseley CF. Leg-Length Discrepancy. In: Morrissy RT, Weinstein SL, eds. *Lovell & Winter's Pediatric Orthopaedics.* Philadelphia: J.B. Lippincott, 1996:869.)

Determining Leg Length Discrepancy: The Growth-Remaining Method

A Assessment of past growth

1. Growth of both legs
= present length - first length

1. Growth of long leg
= 70.0 - 60.0 = 10.0 cm

1. Growth of short leg
= 66.2 - 58.2 = 8.0 cm

2. Present discrepancy
= length of long leg - length of short leg

2. Present discrepancy
= 70.0 - 66.2 = 3.8 cm

3. Growth inhibition

$$= \frac{(\text{growth of long leg} - \text{growth of short leg})}{\text{growth of long leg}}$$

3. Growth inhibition

$$= \frac{(10.0 - 8.0)}{10.0} = 0.2 \text{ cm}$$

B Prediction of future growth

1. Plot present length of long leg on Green-Anderson leg length graph for appropriate sex

1.

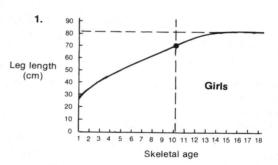

2. Project to right parallel to standard deviation lines until maturity to determine mature length of long leg

2. Length of long leg at maturity = 81.1 cm

3. Future growth of long leg
= mature length - present length

3. Future growth of long leg
= 81.1 - 70.0 = 11.1 cm

4. Future increase in discrepancy
= future growth long X inhibition

4. Future increase in discrepancy
= 11.1 X 0.2 = 2.2 cm

5. Predicted discrepancy at maturity
= present discrepancy + future increase

5. Discrepancy at maturity
= 3.8 + 2.2 = 6.0 cm

C Prediction of effect of surgery

1. The effect of epiphysiodesis of the distal femoral and proximal tibial plates for a given sex and skeletal age can be determined by the Green-Anderson growth = remaining graph.

1. Correction from proximal tibial arrest
= 2.7 cm

Correction from distal femoral arrest
= 4.1 cm

Correction from combined arrest
= 2.7 + 4.1 = 6.8 cm

2. The effect of lengthening is not affected by growth.

Figure 170.14.   Growth-remaining method of leg-length discrepancy determination. In the left column, a theoretical explanation, and on the right, a sample calculation. (From Moseley CF. Leg-Length Discrepancy. In: Morrissy RT, Weinstein SL, eds. *Lovell & Winter's Pediatric Orthopaedics.* Philadelphia: J.B. Lippincott, 1996:870.)

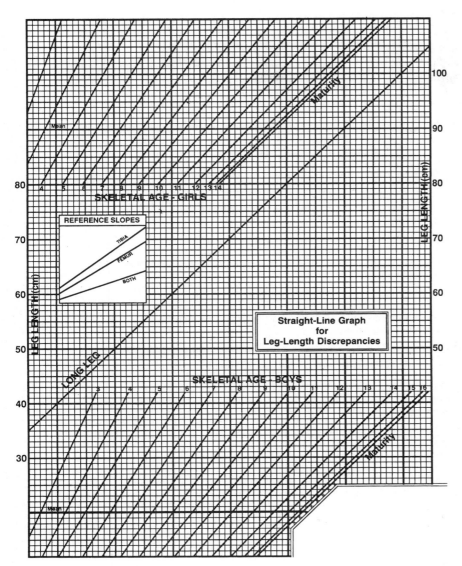

Figure 170.15. Straight-line graph, composed of three sections. The central line for plotting the length of the long leg in centimeters is predefined by the graph. The sloping lines are areas for plotting bone ages, with girls above and boys below. The reference slopes allow plotting of growth lines to predict changes after epiphysiodesis. (From Moseley CF. Leg-Length Discrepancy. In: Morrissy RT, Weinstein SL, eds. *Lovell & Winter's Pediatric Orthopaedics.* Philadelphia: J.B. Lippincott, 1996:871.)

that leg decreases by an exact amount. This is because each epiphysis contributes a known amount to the length of the leg. Reference slopes placed on the graph include slopes of lines representing a normal (long) limb after proximal tibial epiphysiodesis, after distal femoral epiphysiodesis, and after both epiphysiodeses done simultaneously. Figure 170.16 shows a sample calculation using the straight-line graph.

Note that with the straight-line graph, the left edge represents the time of birth, and the long limb begins at 35 cm, not zero. If calculations depend on inhibition from the time of conception (such as congenitally short limbs), the long-limb and the short-limb lines will converge off the graph to the left, where the limb length is zero. If the growth inhibition began at a later date after birth (such as early physeal closure from infection), then convergence of lines will occur at a later date on the graph.

This technique uses skeletal age for determination, takes into account growth percentile in prediction of future growth and results of surgery, decreases the inherent

Determining Leg Length Discrepancy: The Straight Line Graph Method

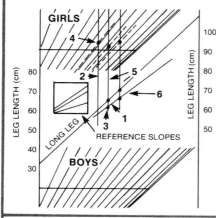

A Assessment of past growth

1. Plot the point for the long leg on the sloping line labeled "LONG LEG" at the appropriate length.

2. Draw a vertical line through that point representing the current assessment.

3. Plot the point for the short leg on the vertical line.

4. Plot the point for skeletal age with reference to the sloping lines in the nomogram.

5. Plot successive visits in the same fashion.

6. Draw a straight line through the short leg points to represent the growth of the short leg.

B Prediction of future growth

1. Draw the horizontal straight line that best fits the points previously plotted for skeletal age. The fit to later points is more important than to earlier points. This is the growth percentile line.

2. From the intersection of the growth percentile line with the maturity skeletal age line, draw a vertical line to intersect the growth lines of the two legs. This line represents the end of growth.

3. The points of intersection of the vertical line with the two growth lines indicate the predicted lengths of the legs at maturity.

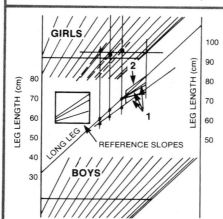

C Prediction of effect of surgery

1. To predict the outcome after epiphysiodesis, draw three lines to the right from the last point for the long leg parallel to the three reference slopes. The intersections of these lines with the vertical line representing the end of growth indicates the predicted lengths of the long leg after the three possible types of epiphysiodesis.

2. To predict the outcome after leg lengthening, draw a line parallel to the growth line of the short leg but elevated above it by the amount of length gained.

Figure 170.16.   Straight-line graph method of leg-length discrepancy determination. The step-by-step instructions for a sample patient are shown, using the same example as in Figure 170.13. (From Moseley CF. Leg-Length Discrepancy. In: Morrissy RT, Weinstein SL. *Lovell & Winter's Pediatric Orthopaedics.* Philadelphia: J.B. Lippincott, 1996:873.)

error of single skeletal age measurements, eliminates the need for cumbersome arithmetic, and spots values that appear to be out of line with others in longitudinal assessment. It also allows all data to be accumulated sequentially at a single place in the medical record.

Other Techniques

Recently, two additional graphic techniques have been described for limb-length inequality evaluation. One is based on data from Dutch children between 1979 and 1994. It suggests that children today have longer bones than the children in the study of Green and Anderson from the 1940s and 1950s (9). The technique uses principles similar to those of the straight-line graph. In the second technique, a graphic display is made based on plotting limb-length discrepancy versus chronologic age. This is a graphic variation of the arithmetic technique (21).

EVALUATION OF EFFICACY

In evaluating the various techniques used to assess limb-length discrepancy, studies vary with respect to interpretation of success. Theoretically, the Green and Anderson method and the straight-line graph methods should give the same prediction because they are derived from the same growth data. General success has been reported with both of these methods (19,48,61,69,78). Another recent review reported disappointing results with all three commonly used methods (50). Continued study and refinement are needed.

TREATMENT

GOALS

The goal in treatment of a patient with a limb-length discrepancy is based on a thorough assessment of the patient's problems, both clinically and radiographically. Each patient may have differing goals, reflecting a unique combination of associated problems. In general, it is best to consider correcting coexisting conditions before addressing the limb-length difference. Correcting a spinal deformity affects pelvic obliquity. Correcting angular deformity in the lower limb, whether it is at the level of a malunion or a contracture at a joint, usually has the effect of lengthening that limb.

Ideally, correction would result in limbs of exactly the same length, but this may not always be the best goal. In the patient with polio residuals, it is usually desirable to leave a weak extremity slightly short, which allows it to function better in the swing phase of gait. In the neuromuscularly normal child, it is best to plan for a limb-length difference of between 5 mm and 1 cm at maturity when considering epiphysiodesis. This allows for slight changes

in growth patterns after the epiphysiodesis and inaccuracies in the preoperative assessment while not compromising adult height any more than necessary.

Many factors will influence the decision on the exact level in the limb at which to correct a discrepancy. The ideal situation would be to lengthen the short bone or shorten the long bone to a normal length. A general goal is to keep the legs symmetric so that knee height is equal. However, in some cases, a well-timed epiphysiodesis at one level (for instance, the distal femur) will eliminate the need for a later procedure involving two growth plates (distal femur and proximal tibia), even though it may leave the knee heights at slightly different levels. During lengthening procedures, this may be of even more concern, because differences made up are often greater than with epiphysiodeses. If lengthening is proceeding well, it may be more desirable to continue lengthening the segment past the predicted length at maturity of that segment on the opposite side so as to avoid the necessity of another segment lengthening as well. Asymmetry of knee height is generally of little functional significance but is of some cosmetic concern.

Much of the prior discussion of the workup and assessment of limb-length discrepancy has focused on the magnitude of discrepancy at maturity. This is because the predicted amount of difference at maturity helps determine the exact amount to correct and the treatment group likely to be best for equalization. These treatment groups with their suggested approaches, given a normal height range, are as follows:

- Difference of 0 to 2 cm: no treatment
- Difference of 2 to 6 cm: shoe lift, epiphysiodesis, shortening
- Difference of 4 to 15 cm: lengthening procedure
- Difference of more than 15 cm: prosthetic fitting

Discrepancies of less than 2 cm, although quite common, do not have functional significance for the majority of adults of normal stature, and therefore do not need treatment (31,72). For those patients who feel unbalanced, a shoe lift can be tried.

In the 2 to 6 cm range, shortening procedures are generally the first choice for treatment. For greater levels of discrepancy, shortening procedures are usually not considered because of disproportionate appearance in the shortened segment and loss of stature. Also, if the limb is shortened acutely, the normal-sized muscle-tendon units also have difficulty adapting to the shortened bone, and consequently they become weaker. Correction of a difference of greater than 6 cm with epiphysiodesis may be considered when the long limb is clearly the abnormal side, because loss of stature and disproportionate appearance are not a concern.

For discrepancies of more than 4 cm, lengthening may be considered. In the 4 to 6 cm range, patient and family preference may be taken into consideration as the complications and long-term goals of lengthening versus shortening are weighed. For discrepancies greater than 6 cm, lengthening becomes the preferred treatment option. The total length possible from a lengthening procedure is variable. Generally the maximum length attainable at a single lengthening is 20% of the bone's length. Thus, if both the femur and tibia are lengthened (usually done in a staged manner), this may total more than 15 cm length gained. A complete assessment of patient needs and psychosocial situation are crucial before beginning any lengthening procedure, but the entire lengthening team must pay particularly close attention to these factors for the longer lengthenings. Consideration can be given to staged lengthenings of the same bones, spaced apart by several years for joint and soft-tissue recovery. An epiphysiodesis may also be used in combination with an opposite-side lengthening procedure as a method of limiting the amount of length required.

For discrepancies of more than 15 cm, or 20% of limb length, prosthetic fitting is the usual choice of treatment. Often, this is combined with an amputation, fusion of a joint, or rotationplasty for more functional prosthetic wear. Common clinical situations include the severe end of the spectrum of fibular hemimelia and proximal focal femoral deficiency. In many cases, discussion with the family centers on how quickly the child can return to normal function. The prosthetic option often allows a relatively fast return to a high functional level. If a lengthening device is used, much more time is required to attain the same functional level as that using a prosthetic device.

Shoe Lift

In a discrepancy of 2 to 5 cm, a shoe lift may be an acceptable method of treatment, particularly when the patient will not consider or is not an appropriate candidate for surgery. A lift becomes more unwieldy and thus a less viable alternative as more height is added. The weight of the lift and ankle instability are the chief problems with larger lifts. In addition, patients find them cosmetically unappealing. Lifts can be used as a trial in the preoperative period to determine the most comfortable or functional amount of lengthening or shortening (Fig. 170.17).

Limb Shortening

Epiphysiodesis Epiphysiodesis slows the rate of growth of the long limb to allow the short side to catch up. It is simple, effective, and predictable; is done in one stage; and has a low complication rate (25,28,55,78). It is the usual procedure of choice when predicted discrepancy at maturity is 2 to 6 cm (80). When the procedure is completed, the growth at that physis is assumed to be completely stopped. Loss of percentage contribution to limb length will be 38% for the distal femur, 27% for the proximal tibia, and 65% for the two combined. The distal tibia contributes 18% of leg length and occasionally is also considered for closure. The exact amount of shortening desired can be achieved only by completing the epiphysiodesis at exactly the correct time. Usually, this choice of timing comes down to three different options that correspond to the surgical site: femur only, tibia only, or both femur and tibia. Because proper timing is so important, close preoperative follow-up of patients is necessary for prediction of growth. In one review of 67 epiphysiodeses, more than half were deemed failures due solely to improper interpretation of growth data (10).

Many techniques of epiphysiodesis have been used. The goal of all of them is production of symmetric physeal closure to prevent future growth. The traditional Phemister technique uses removal of a rectangular block of bone medially and laterally at the level of the physis that is then replaced in a 18° rotated position (68) (Fig. 170.18). The rectangular window is also used to remove remaining bits of physis with a curet. White and Stubbins (90) described removal of a square block at the level of the lateral physis, which is then rotated 90° and replaced. Epiphysiodesis by stapling was originally thought to be a good technique to stop physeal growth temporarily, but problems developed

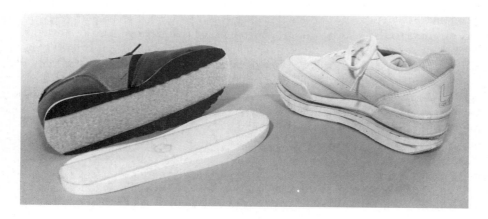

Figure 170.17. Variable sizes of lifts are attached to the bottom of the shoe with hook-and-pile strips. These allow trials of differing amounts, which are particularly helpful in deciding how much to shorten a limb.

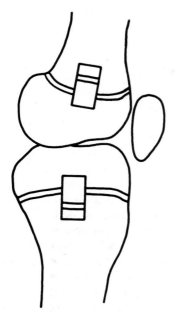

Figure 170.18. The Phemister technique of epiphysiodesis. An open exposure is done both medially and laterally. The rectangular blocks of bone are replaced in a reversed position to create a physeal bar and thus stop growth. (From Moseley CF. Leg-Length Discrepancy. In: Morrissy RT, Weinstein SL. *Lovell & Winter's Pediatric Orthopaedics.* Philadelphia: J.B. Lippincott, 1996:878.)

with asymmetric and complete physeal closure; thus it should be considered a permanent form of growth arrest (12). Stapling has fallen out of favor but may be appropriate in less developed areas of the world without routine access to fluoroscopy (73). Screw epiphysiodesis at the knee has also been described (56).

We recommend use of the percutaneous technique for most cases (63,83).

- Make longitudinal incisions medially and laterally. Use separate incisions for both the femur and tibia as necessary. If the tibia has been chosen, make an incision posterolaterally as well for the fibula. Incisions can be limited to approximately 1 cm in length or may be made longer if a rotated block is to be used.
- Under image control use a 2 mm wide curet to locate the medial and lateral borders of the physis. Then bore the curet into the physis both medially and laterally, using a turning motion with the curet. Sweeping from anteriorly to posteriorly with the curet scrambles the physeal cartilage.
- The lateral side of the femur and tibia can be completed through lateral incisions, and the medial side can be completed through the medial incisions. The curet tip can be crossed to the opposite side of the bone to allow more surface area to be reached. Close 50% to 75%

of the area of the growth plate using this method. The remaining amount ensures that strength remains for ambulation without immobilization.

- Complete the approach to the fibula in the same manner, but with a wide enough exposure to allow direct visualization of the edge of the physis. This extra exposure allows the common peroneal nerve to be protected.
- The technique can be modified slightly in the femur and tibia by using a power drill to complete the physeal closure. A drill bit or straight Steinmann pin with a slightly bent tip damages the growth plate enough to cause closure.

Follow-up care involves the use of a compressive bandage until the wound is healed. Allow the patient to have full range of motion about the knee postoperatively and to bear weight as tolerated with the aid of crutches initially. A knee immobilizer may be added for 2 to 3 weeks for pain relief. Full activities can usually be resumed in 6 to 8 weeks. Bony fusion across the physis occurs within 8 weeks.

Epiphysiodesis is a mainstay in the treatment of limb-length discrepancies. However, it is compensatory in that a normal leg is made abnormal and usually involves decreasing the patient's stature. For these reasons, other procedures are also considered.

Acute Shortening Procedures Shortening procedures are considered for patients with the same amounts of discrepancy as those for epiphysiodesis but who are too old for full correction with physeal closure. In the patient who has matured, it has a distinct advantage in that the exact amount of discrepancy is known and no future growth predictions are necessary.

In general, femoral shortening is preferred to tibial shortening. The amount of shortening tolerable in the femur is approximately 5 cm. Greater shortening results in ineffective recovery of muscle-tendon units. The tibia may also be shortened but to a lesser degree (14). Maximum shortening in the tibia should be 3 cm because of shorter muscle-tendon unit lengths. Also, tibial shortening by intramedullary technique is less feasible because the bone is subcutaneous. Thus, the femur is strongly preferred.

In the past, femoral shortening used step-cut osteotomies with interfragmentary screws for fixation, but better implants have made these procedures obsolete. Current techniques include open shortening with plate fixation or proximal femoral shortening with blade plate fixation. The plating technique offers the advantage of ease of fixation but requires hardware removal and may result in scarring and stiffness of the quadriceps mechanism. Blade plate fixation offers the advantage of being proximal to most of the quadriceps origins but has the disadvantage of a more involved operation.

More recently, closed femoral shortening has become popular (11,91). A standard closed intramedullary femoral nailing technique is used with the addition of a special eccentric cam saw. See Chapters 30 and 174 for more details. The intramedullary saw is used to make two transverse cuts in the femur. The segment of bone is then split vertically and displaced to the sides, and the femur is then shortened over an intramedullary femoral nail and locked proximally and distally. The technique is demanding technically and requires experience with closed intramedullary nailing techniques. Malrotation can be a problem; assess this before awakening the patient. In children, the nail is removed after complete healing has occurred. The procedure is cosmetic and allows secure intramedullary fixation with its inherent healing capabilities. Implant removal is less involved than plating techniques. However, this procedure causes temporary quadriceps weakness similar to that of femoral plating. Complications in the young patient have been reported, including intraoperative or postoperative fat embolus syndrome; one center reported that 4 out of 100 patients had this complication (53).

Growth Stimulation

Multiple techniques for stimulation of the short extremity have been tried, including electrical stimulation, sympathectomy, surgical construction of arteriovenous fistulae, placement of foreign bodies next to the physis, and packing bone beneath the periosteum near the physis. None of these techniques have produced reproducible or clinically significant results. At present, growth stimulation through the physis is not a realistic option.

Limb Lengthening

Lengthening the short limb initially appears to be the most desirable approach because it allows correction of the abnormal extremity to a normal length while not changing the normal limb. However, lengthening is generally reserved for those patients with the most severe deformities. This is because lengthening techniques are associated with multiple complications and a prolonged treatment time.

Usually, the patient who is considered for lengthening has a projected discrepancy of between 4 and 20 cm. Relatively stable joints above and below the level to be lengthened are a prerequisite. Rotational or angular malalignment usually decreases the total length attainable through lengthening procedures. The patient should be emotionally mature. The youngest child we generally consider for a lengthening is 8 to 9 years of age so that the patient can cooperate with physical therapy. Occasionally, a younger child is considered for lengthening when two different stages of lengthening are required. A decision is made preoperatively for a target goal of length.

Lengthening procedures have been widely used in the past with varying degrees of success, as described by Codivilla (17), Millis and Hall (57), Anderson and colleagues (4–6), Wagner (87,88), Ilizarov and colleagues (37–39), Wasserstein and colleagues (89), Monticelli and Spinelli (58), and Paley (64). Specific techniques are described in Chapters 32 and 171.

The use of the ring fixator with thin wires, as described by Ilizarov, has focused interest on the biology of lengthening. Lengthening success has been clearly related to the emphasis on the exact rate of small incremental lengthening of bone. Others have modified the technique of using only thin wires by adding thicker half pins for stability (16). In addition, lengthening with the uniplane frame over an intramedullary nail, which allows significantly reduced external fixator time, is gaining popularity (65). The uniplane frame alone also has a place in pure length correction when angular correction at the same time is not needed. In all of these techniques, the rate of lengthening should be the same whichever external frame is used because the recent successes have been based on a biology that is highly dependent on technique.

The biology of osteogenesis during distraction begins in the intramedullary area as multipotential cells differentiate into osteoblasts. Their bone formation resembles intramembranous growth because no cartilage matrix is laid down. Cells appear to lay down in a longitudinal direction of the retreating bone end (40). Patients are allowed to bear weight fully immediately postoperatively and participate vigorously in exercise to prevent joint contractures.

One of the most difficult decisions after bone is lengthened is when to remove the fixator. The actual length of time that the fixator is left on will vary because the amount of length gained and the bone quality laid down differs among patients.

There are several complications that result from lengthening techniques. Most series have reported more than one major complication per patient. Pin-track infection or inflammation is almost universally expected. Joint contractures are a persistent problem as well, particularly flexion or extension contracture of the knee and equinus position of the ankle. Joint subluxation or dislocation at the hip or knee are relatively common complications (41, 60). In addition, nonunion, malunion, and device failures have been reported.

Growth after lengthening is completed may be variable. One review suggested normal or even accelerated growth after moderate external fixator frame lengthening, whereas longer amounts of time and length may actually diminish later growth (70).

Prosthetic Fitting

Prosthetic fitting is generally the least desirable form of treatment, but it may be the best choice when a large discrepancy or severe deformity exists. When predicted discrepancy at maturity exceeds 15 to 20 cm, or 20% of the long side, this approach should be considered. A single operation can be performed during one hospitalization, so that multiple procedures and complications can be avoided.

A typical patient with fibular hemimelia, either with or without associated femoral shortening, has a large predicted discrepancy at maturity as well as progressive valgus in the foot. A Syme amputation followed by prosthetic fitting results in a functional below-knee amputation that results in a near-normal gait and activity level. This procedure is best performed when the child is younger than 1 year old. Waiting until a later age often results in a great emotional attachment of the family and the patient to saving the foot.

For the patient who has severe proximal focal femoral deficiency, Syme amputation with or without a knee fusion may be the best option. This is followed with fitting for an above-knee prosthesis. Another option is the Van Nes rotationplasty, which reverses the ankle joint to power a modified below-knee prosthesis (23,46,85). The Van Nes procedure can be performed on children at any age, but results are optimal when the procedure is completed at 3 or 4 years of age. It is particularly helpful to have parents of these patients see and talk with parents of older patients who have undergone these procedures.

REFERENCES

Each reference is categorized according to the following scheme: *, classic article; #, review article; !, basic research article; and +, clinical results/outcome study.

+ 1. Aaron A, Weinstein D, Thickman D, Eilert R. Comparison of Orthoroentgenography and Computed Tomography in the Measurement of Limb-Length Discrepancy. *J Bone Joint Surg* 1992;74-A:897.

+ 2. Aitken A, Blackett C, Ciacotti J. Overgrowth of the Femoral Shaft following Fractures in Childhood. *J Bone Joint Surg* 1939;21:334.

+ 3. Altongy JF, Harcke HT, Bowen JR. Measurement of Leg Length Inequalities by Micro-dose Digital Radiographs. *J Pediatr Orthop* 1987;7:311.

* 4. Anderson M, Green W. Lengths of the Femur and Tibia: Norms Derived from Orthoroentgenograms of Children from 5 Years of Age Until Epiphyseal Closure. *Am J Dis Child* 1948;75:279.

* 5. Anderson M, Green W, Messner M. Growth and Pedictions of Growth in the Lower Extremities. *J Bone Joint Surg* 1963;45A:1.

* 6. Anderson M, Messner M, Green W. Distribution of Lengths of the Normal Femur and Tibia in Children from One to Eighteen years of age. *J Bone Joint Surg* 1964; 46A:1197.

* 7. Beals RK. Hemihypertrophy and Hemiatrophy. *Clin Orthop* 1982;166:199.

+ 8. Beals RK. Premature Closure of the Physis following Diaphyseal Fractures. *J Pediatr Orthop* 1990;10:717.

+ 9. Beumer A, Lampe HI, Swierstra BA, et al. The Straight Line Graph in Limb Length Inequality. A New Design Based on 182 Dutch Childern. *Acta Orthop Scand* 1997; 68:366.

+ 10. Blair V, Walker S, Sheridan J, et al. Epiphyseodesis: A Problem of Timing. *J Pediatr Orthop* 1982;2:281.

+ 11. Blair VP, Schoenecker PL, Sheridan JJ, et al. Closed Shortening of the Femur. *J Bone Joint Surg* 1989;71A: 1440.

* 12. Blount W. Control of Bone Growth by Epiphyseal Stapling. A Preliminary Report. *J Bone Joint Surg* 1949;31: 464.

! 13. Brand RA, Yack HJ. Effects of Leg Length Discrepancies on the Forces at the Hip Joint. *Clin Orthop* 1996;333: 172.

+ 14. Broughton NS, Olney BW, Menelaus MB. Tibial Shortening for Leg Length Discrepancy. *J Bone Joint* Surg 1989;71-B:242.

+ 15. Carpenter CT, Lester EL. Skeletal Age Determination in Young Children: Analysis of Three Regions of the Hand/ Wrist Film. *J Pediatr Orthop* 1993;13:76.

16. Catagni MA. Current Trends in the Treatment of Simple and Complex Bone Deformities Using the Ilizarov Method. *Instr Course Lect* 1992;41:423.

* 17. Codivilla A. On the Means of Lengthening in the Lower Limbs, the Muscles and Tissues which Are Shortened through Deformity. *Am J Orthop Surg* 1905;2:353.

+ 18. Cundy P, Peterson D, Morris L, Foster B. Skeletal Age Estimation in Leg Length Discrepancy. *J Pediatr Orthop* 1988;8:513.

+ 19. Dewaele J, Fabry G. The Timing of Epiphysiodesis. A Comparative Study Between the Use of the Method of Anderson and Green and the Moseley Chart. *Acta Orthop Belg* 1992;58:43.

! 20. Dietz FR. Effect of Denervation on Limb Growth. *J Orthop Res* 1989;7:292.

+ 21. Eastwood DM, Cole WG. A Graphic Method for Timing the Correction of Leg-Length Discrepancy. *J Bone Joint Surg* 1995;77-B:743.

+ 22. Friberg O. Clinical Symptoms and Biomechanics of Lumbar Spine and Hip Joint in Leg Length Inequality. *Spine* 1983;8:643.

+ 23. Friscia DA, Moseley CF, Oppenheim WL. Rotational Osteotomy for Proximal Femoral Focal Deficiency. *J Bone Joint Surg* 1989;71A:1386.

+ 24. Froh R, Yong-Hing K, Cassidy JD, Houston CS. The Relationship between Leg Length Discrepancy and Lumbar Facet Orientation. *Spine* 1988;13:325.

+ 25. Gabriel KR, Crawford AH, Roy DR, et al. Percutaneous Epiphyseodesis. *J Pediatr Orthop* 1994;14:348.

+ 26. Gibson PH, Papaioannou T, Kenwright J. The Influence on the Spine of Leg-Length Discrepancy after Femoral Fracture. *J Bone Joint Surg* 1983;65B:584.

+ 27. Giles LG, Taylor JR. Lumbar Spine Structural Changes Associated with Leg Length Inequality. *Spine* 1982;7: 159.

* 28. Green WT, Wyatt GM, Anderson M. Orthoroentgenography as a Method of Measuring the Bones of the Lower Extremities. *J Bone Joint Surg* 1946;28:60.

* 29. Green W, Anderson M. Experiences with Epiphyseal Ar-

rest in Correcting Discrepancies in Length of the Lower Extremities in Infantile Paralysis. *J Bone Joint Surg* 1947; 29:659.

* 30. Greulich W, Pyle S. Radiographic Atlas of the Skeletal Development of the Hand and Wrist. Stanford, CA: Stanford University Press, 1959.

+ 31. Gross R. Leg Length Discrepancy: How Much is Too Much? *Orthopedics* 1978;1:307.

+ 32. Hermanussen M, Geiger-Benoit K, Burmeister J. Analysis of Differential Growth of the Right and the Left Leg. *Hum Biol* 1989;61:133.

+ 33. Hoikka V, Ylikoski M, Tallroth K. Leg-Length Inequality Has Poor Correlation with Lumbar Scoliosis. *Acta Orthop Trauma Surg* 1989;108:173.

+ 34. Holschneider A, Vogl D, Dietz H. Differences in Leg Length following Femoral Shaft Fractures in Childhood. *Z Kinderchir* 1985;40:341.

* 35. Hult L. The Munkfors Investigation. A Study of the Frequency and Causes of the Stiff Neck-Brachialgia and Lumbago-Sciatica Syndromes, as well as Observations on Certain Signs and Symptoms from the Dorsal Spine and the Joints of the Extremities in Industrial and Forest Workers. *Acta Orthop Scand* 1954:16(Suppl).

+ 36. Huurman WW, Jacobsen FS, Anderson JC, et al. Limb-length Discrepancy Measured with Computerized Axial Tomographic Equipment. *J Bone Joint Surg* 1987;69A: 699.

* 37. Ilizarov G, Deviatov A. Surgical Lengthening of the Shin with Simultaneous Correction of Deformities. *Ortop Travmatol Protez* 1969;30:32.

+ 38. Ilizarov G, Deviatov A. Surgical Elongation of the Leg. *Ortop Travmatol Protez* 1971;32:20.

+ 39. Ilizarov G, Deviatov A, Trokhova V. Surgical Lengthening of the Shortened Lower Extremities. *Vestn Khir I I Grek* 1972;107:100.

+ 40. Ilizarov G, Palienko L, Shreiner A. Bone Marrow Hematopoietic Function and Its Relationship to Osteogenesis Activity during Reparative Regeneration in Leg Lengthening in the Dog. *Ontogenez* 1984;15:146.

+ 41. Jones D, Moseley C. Subluxation of the Knee as a Complication of Femoral Lengthening by the Wagner Technique. *J Bone Joint Surg* 1985;67-B:33.

+ 42. Junk S, Terjesen T, Rossvoll I, Braten M. Leg Length Inequality Measured by Ultrasound and Clinical Methods. *Eur J Radiol* 1992;14:185.

+ 43. Kalamchi A, Cowell H, Kim K. Congenital Deficiency of the Femur. *J Pediatr Orthop* 1985;5:129.

! 44. Kaufman KR, Miller LS, Sutherland DH. Gait Asymmetry in Patients with Limb-Length Inequality. *J Pediatr Orthop* 1996;16:144.

+ 45. Kohan L, Cumming W. Femoral Shaft Fractures in Children: The Effect of Initial Shortening on Subsequent Limb Overgrowth. *Aust NZ J Surg* 1982;52:141.

+ 46. Kostuik JP, Gillespie R, Hall JE, Hubbard S. Van Nes Rotational Osteotomy for Treatment of Proximal Femoral Focal Deficiency and Congenital Short Femur. *J Bone Joint Surg* 1975;57-A:1039.

+ 47. Kujala U, Friberg O, Aalto T, et al. Lower Limb Asymmetry and Patellofemoral Joint Incongruence in the Eti-

ology of Knee Exertion Injuries in Athletes. *Int J Sports Med* 1987;8:214.

+ 48. Lampe HI, Swierstra BA, Diepstraten AF. Timing of Physiodesis in Limb Length Inequality. The Straight Line Graph Applied in 30 Patients. *Acta Orthop Scand* 1992; 63:672.

+ 49. Lampe HI, Swierstra BA, Diepstraten AF. Measurement of Limb Length Inequality. Comparison of Clinical Methods with Orthoradiography in 190 Children. *Acta Orthop Scand* 1996;67:242.

+ 50. Little DG, Nigo L, Aiona MD. Deficiencies of Current Methods for the Timing of Epiphysiodesis. *J Pediatr Orthop* 1996;16:173.

! 51. Liu XC, Fabry G, Molenaers G, et al. Kinematic and Kinetic Asymmetry in Patients with Leg-Length Discrepancy. *J Pediatr Orthop* 1998;18:187.

+ 52. Lorenzi G, Rossi P, Quaglia F, et al. Growth Disturbances following Fractures of the Femur and Tibia in Children. *Ital J Orthop Traumatol* 1985;11:133.

+ 53. Matson P, Johnson LO. *Fat Embolism following Closed Femoral Shortening for Limb Length Inequality.* Shriners Hospitals Orthopaedic Symposium, Los Angeles, 1987.

+ 54. Meals R. Overgrowth of the Femur following Fractures in Children: Influence of Handedness. *J Bone Joint Surg* 1979;61-A:381.

* 55. Menelaus M. Correction of Leg Length Discrepancy by Epiphyseal Arrest. *J Bone Joint Surg* 1966;48-B:336.

+ 56. Metaizeau JP, Wong-chung J, Bertrand H, Pasquier P. Percutaneous Epiphysiodesis Using Transphyseal Screws (PETS). *J Pediatr Orthop* 1998;18:363.

+ 57. Millis M, Hall J. Transiliac Lengthening of the Lower Extremity. A Modified Innominate Osteotomy for the Treatment of Postural Imbalance. *J Bone Joint Surg* 1979;61-A:1182.

+ 58. Monticelli G, Spinelli R. Leg Lengthening by Closed Metaphyseal Corticotomy. *Ital J Orthop Traumatol* 1983; 9:139.

+ 59. Morscher E. Etiology and Pathophysiology of Leg Length Discrepancies. *Prog Orthop Surg* 1977;1:9.

+ 60. Mosca V, Moseley CF. Results of Limb Lengthening Using the Wagner Device. *Orthop Trans* 1987;11:52.

* 61. Moseley CF. A Straight-Line Graph for Leg-Length Discrepancies. *J Bone Joint Surg* 1977;59-A:174.

+ 62. Nadler SF, Wu KD, Galski T, Feinberg JH. Low Back Pain in College Athletes. A Prospective Study Correlating Lower Extremity Overuse or Acquired Ligamentous Laxity with Low Back Pain. *Spine* 1998;23:828.

+ 63. Ogilvie JW. Epiphysiodesis: Evaluation of a New Technique. *J Pediatr Orthop* 1986;6:147.

64. Paley D. Current Techniques of Limb Lengthening. *J Pediatr Orthop* 1988;8:73.

+ 65. Paley D, Herzenberg JE, Paremain G, Bhave A. Femoral Lengthening Over an Intramedullary Nail. A Matched-Case Comparison with Ilizarov Femoral Lengthening. *J Bone Joint Surg* 1997;79-A:1464.

+ 66. Papaioannou T, Stokes I, Kenwright J. Scoliosis Associated with Limb-Length Inequality. *J Bone Joint Surg* 1982;64-A:59.

* 67. Parrini L, Paleari M, Biggi F. Growth Disturbances from

Fractures of the Femur and Tibia in Children. *Ital J Orthop Traumatol* 1985;11:139.

* 68. Phemister P. Operative Arrestment of Longitudinal Growth of Bodies in the Treatment of Deformities. *J Bone Joint Surg* 1933;15:1.

+ 69. Porat S, Peyser A, Robin GC. Equalization of Lower Limbs by Epiphysiodesis: Results of Treatment. *J Pediatr Orthop* 1991;11:442.

+ 70. Pouliquen JC, Etienne W. [Segmentary Growth of the Lower Limb after Surgical Lengthening in the Children]. In French. *Cir Pediatr* 1978;19:179.

+ 71. Rossvoll I, Junk S, Terjesen T. The Effect on Low Back Pain of Shortening Osteotomy for Leg Length Inequality. *Int Orthop* 1992;16:388.

* 72. Rush W, Steiner H. A Study of Lower Extremity Length Inequality. *Am J Roentgenol* 1946;56:616.

+ 73. Sengupta A, Gupta P. Epiphyseal Stapling for Leg Equalization in Developing Countries. *Int Orthop* 1993;17:37.

+ 74. Shapiro F. Developmental Patterns in Lower-Extremity Length Discrepancies. *J Bone Joint Surg* 1982;64-A:639.

+ 75. Simons S, Whiffen J, Shapiro F. Leg-Length Discrepancies in Monoarticular and Pauciarticular Juvenile Rheumatoid Arthritis. J Bone Joint Surg 1981;63-A:209.

! 76. Song KM, Halliday SE, Little DG. The Effect of Limb-Length Discrepancy on Gait. *J Bone Joint Surg* 1997;79-A:1690.

+ 77. Soukka A, Alaranta H, Tallroth K, Heliovaara M. Leg-Length Inequality in People of Working Age. The Association Between Mild Inequality and Low-Back Pain is Questionable. *Spine* 1991;16:429.

+ 78. Stephens DC, Herrick W, MacEwen GD. Epiphysiodesis for Limb Length Inequality: Results and Indications. *Clin Orthop* 1978;136:41.

+ 79. Stephens MM, Hsu LCS, Leong JCY. Leg Length Discrepancy after Femoral Shaft Fractures in Children: Review after Skeletal Maturity. *J Bone Joint Surg* 1989;71-B:615.

* 80. Straub L, Thompson T, Wilson P. The Results of Epiphyseodesis and Femoral Shortening in Relation to Equalization of Leg Length. *J Bone Joint Surg* 1945;27:254.

* 81. Tanner J, Whitehouse R, Marshall W, et al. *Assessment of Skeletal Maturity and Prediction of Adult Height (TW2 method)*. London: Academic Press, 1975.

+ 82. Terjesen T, Benum P, Rossvoll I, et al. Leg-Length Discrepancy Measured by Ultrasonography. *Acta Orthop Scand* 1991;62:121.

+ 83. Timperlake RW, Bowen JR, Guille JT, Choi IH. Prospective Evaluation of Fifty-three Consecutive Percutaneous Epiphysiodeses of the Distal Femur and Proximal Tibia and Fibula. *J Pediatr Orthop* 1997;11:350.

+ 84. Tjernstrom B, Rehnberg L. Back Pain and Arthralgia Before and After Lengthening. 75 Patients Questioned after 6(1–11) Years. *Acta Orthop Scand* 1994;65:328.

* 85. Van Nes CP. Rotationplasty for Congenital Defects of the Femur. *J Bone Joint Surg* 1950;32-B:12.

+ 86. Vostrejs M, Hollister J. Muscle Atrophy and Leg Length Discrepancies in Pauciarticular Juvenile Rheumatoid Arthritis. *Am J Dis Child* 1988;142:343.

* 87. Wagner H. Surgical Leg Prolongation. *Chirurg* 1971;42:260.

* 88. Wagner H. Operative Lengthening of the Femur. *Clin Orthop* 1978;136:125.

+ 89. Wasserstein I, Correll J, Niethard F. Closed Distraction Epiphyseolysis for Leg Lengthening and Axis Correction of the Leg in Children. *Z Orthop* 1986;124:743.

* 90. White J, Stubbins SJ. Growth Arrest for Equalizing Leg Lengths. *JAMA* 1944;126:1146.

* 91. Winquist RA. Closed Intramedullary Osteotomies of the Femur. *Clin Orthop* 1986;212:155.

+ 92. Yrjonen T, Hoikka V, Poussa M, Osterman K. Leg-Length Inequality and Low-Back Pain after Perthes' Disease: A 28–47-year Follow-up of 96 Patients. *J Spinal Disord* 1992;5:443.

## CHAPTER 171

PEDIATRIC APPLICATIONS OF CIRCULAR AND UNILATERAL EXTERNAL FIXATION

Deborah F. Stanitski

Over the past decade, external fixation has gained increasing acceptance as a surgical technique in children. The most common applications include incidences of trauma, correction of limb deformity, and limb-length equalization.

The numerous fixators available fall into two general categories: circular fixators and cantilever external fixators. Biomechanical studies have demonstrated that bone formation is enhanced by cyclic axial micromotion and, perhaps, by limited-bending micromotion (23). Torsion, on the other hand, is generally deleterious to bone formation. The Ilizarov-type of circular external fixator, which is less stable to axial loading than are most cantilever systems but relatively resistant to torsion, provides an excellent biomechanical environment for bone formation (42).

Another advantage of circular external fixation is that it is applicable to patients of virtually any size from toddler to large child, obese adolescent, or adult. The system provides three-dimensional adjustability, allowing angulation, translation, rotation, and lengthening when necessary. The Taylor Spatial Frame (5) now allows these parameters to be corrected simultaneously but currently has some ring-size limitations (Fig. 171.1). The traditional Ilizarov external fixator can be constructed with hinges to correct existing limb deformity (Fig. 171.2). Circular external fixation can be used to span adjacent limb segments, to protect potentially unstable joints, or to treat joint contractures (Fig. 171.3).

The disadvantages of the traditional circular external fixator are its bulk, the fact that it is difficult to apply and adjust, and that it requires multiple sites for transfixing wires. The traditional Ilizarov external fixator uses 1.5 or 1.8 mm transfixing tensioned wires for bone fixation, with half-pin fixation in the proximal femur. Over the last 5 to

D. F. Stanitski: Professor, Orthopaedic Surgery, Medical University of South Carolina, Charleston, SC, 29425.

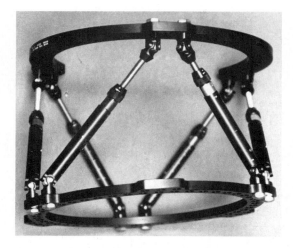

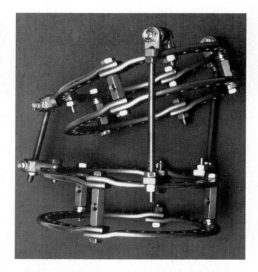

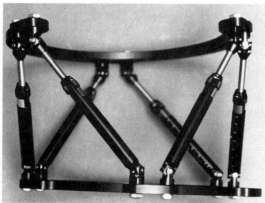

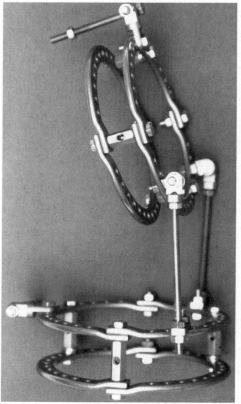

Figure 171.1. The Taylor Spatial frame allows simultaneous correction of angulation, rotation, length, and translation through the use of six struts and universal ball joints.

6 years, a number of surgeons have modified the originally described techniques, substituting half-pins for some of the wires. Specifically, in children, the traditional "medial face" tibial wire (parallel to the medial face of the tibia) has been eliminated in favor of an anteroposteriorly directed half-pin. Affixing half-pins to a circular fixator permits 360° adjustability at the same time it avoids some of the soft-tissue problems of transfixing wires.

Unilateral external fixators by contrast are easy to apply, require a limited number of pin sites, and are less bulky (33). They are applied to only one side of the limb and require usually no more than four to six half-pins per limb segment depending on the type of application. Cantilever systems have some disadvantages. They can be used only on limbs of a certain size, they have less stability to shear stress than circular fixators, they cannot span joints easily, and their ability to correct angulation, rotation, and translation gradually is limited. With many current systems, significant adjustments such as device and pin clamp exchange must be made under general anesthe-

Figure 171.2. Preconstructed Ilizarov tibial fixator mimics the deformity and allows gradual correction through hinges placed at the level of the deformity.

sia. Some systems, including the Heidelberg (5), Orthofix (5), and EBI (5) systems, have gradual but limited correction capabilities.

In this chapter, I provide specific application recommendations. I have had more than a decade of experience

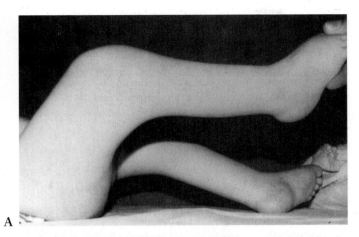

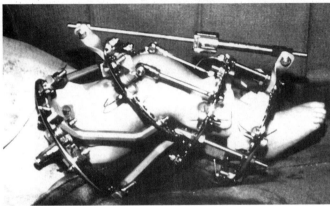

Figure 171.3. **A:** Preoperative photograph of a 3-year-old patient with arthrogryposis and a nearly 90° flexion deformity of the knee. **B:** Appearance of Ilizarov fixator affixed to the femur and tibia, spanning the knee joint with corrective hinges.

with both types of devices. The Ilizarov type of fixator remains the more versatile device, but patient acceptance and comfort clearly favor the monolateral fixator.

LARGE PIN AND CANTILEVER SYSTEMS

A number of cantilever devices are available in North America for trauma or limb reconstruction applications, including the Orthofix device (Orthofix, Winston-Salem, NC), EBI Dynafix (EBI Corp., Parsippany, NJ), Smith and Nephew Heidelberg fixator (Smith and Nephew, Memphis, TN), the Hex-Fix (Smith and Nephew, Memphis, TN), and the Synthes External Fixator (Synthes USA, Philadelphia, PA). In each case, application requires pin clamps or pin clamp templates through which half-pins are inserted. The choice of fixator is usually determined by the problem to be addressed and size of the patient.

The most commonly used limb reconstruction systems are the Orthofix and EBI, with the Heidelberg system having been recently introduced. These fixators are lightweight devices with the ability to telescope. The technique for insertion of the half-pins, and application of these types of fixators is discussed in detail in Chapter 11 and specifically for the tibia in Chapter 24.

ORTHOFIX UNIT

The Orthofix, available in pediatric and adult sizes, has variable body lengths (Fig. 171.4). The short or standard length devices are used most often on children. Orthofix has two articulating ball joints and uses tapered predrilled half-pin fixation. The telescoping body can be unlocked once fracture or osteotomy callus formation is evident radiographically. This capacity theoretically allows axial loading or dynamization of the bone facilitating callus formation and bone healing. The standard articulated device is used for fracture management and osteotomies (16, 35,40,50,53). Its ball-and-joint articulation permits approximately 30° to 35° of angulation; it can be freely rotated.

Use the straight slide-type device or LRS (5) (Limb Reconstruction System) for lengthening (Fig. 171.5). It allows placement of more than two pin clamps when necessary for situations such as bone transport. A swivel clamp

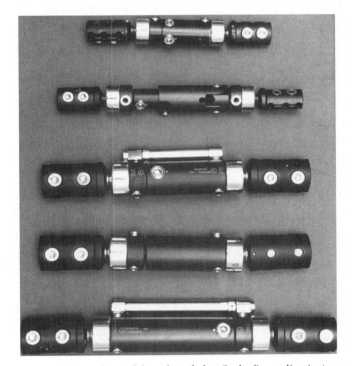

Figure 171.4. Several lengths of the Orthofix pediatric (top two) and adult (bottom 3) fixators are available.

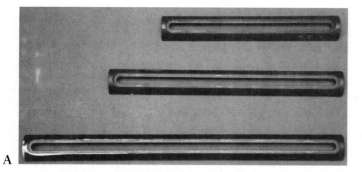
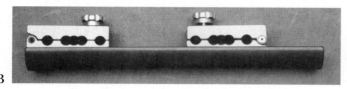
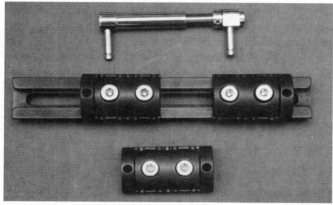
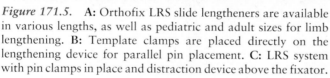

A

B

C

Figure 171.5. **A:** Orthofix LRS slide lengtheners are available in various lengths, as well as pediatric and adult sizes for limb lengthening. **B:** Template clamps are placed directly on the lengthening device for parallel pin placement. **C:** LRS system with pin clamps in place and distraction device above the fixator.

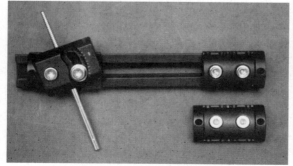

Figure 171.6. Swivel template clamps and swivel pin clamps are available for angular correction.

can be substituted for straight clamps at one or both ends of the bone (Fig. 171.6); this technique may be useful for bifocal osteotomies with acute deformity correction or to eliminate deformity that may develop during lengthening. A variety of angulation and rotation template clamps are now available for more accurate multiplanar corrections (Fig. 171.7). Do not use the standard swivel clamps for lengthening; they are less stable than the standard pin

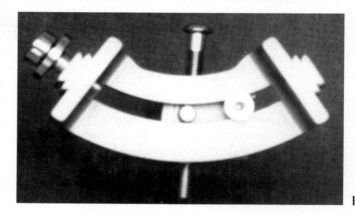

A

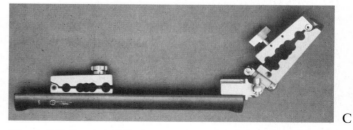

B

C

Figure 171.7. **A and B:** A new rotation template clamp is now available to allow accurate planning and pin insertion for acute rotational corrections. **C:** The new angulation template clamp can be affixed to the end of the slide for planned acute angular correction 90° orthogonal to the plane of the swivel clamp.

clamps. With either the standard articulated body fixator or LRS, insert tapered predrilled half-pins through the clamp templates. Then replace the template with the standard pin clamps and tighten them. For fractures and osteotomies, generally two half-pins above and below the fracture or osteotomy are adequate. The widest pin spread in the clamp provides the best stability. For limb lengthening, use three pins proximal to the lengthening site in the femur and tibia. Two or three are adequate distally, depending on the size of the patient and amount of anticipated lengthening (Fig. 171.8) (1,22,25,46,47,48).

The T-Garches device (Orthofix) is useful for gradual correction of frontal plane deformity in the tibia—for example, in adolescent Blount's disease (Fig. 171.9) (59). Small lengthenings can also be achieved with this device. A new template clamp allows correction of acute sagittal plane deformity before application of the device following osteotomy (Fig. 171.10). It is not recommended for large lengthenings; the hinge may not withstand large lengthening forces, and the device, for the most part, accommodates only two proximal tibial pins (Fig. 171.11).

In applying the LRS systems, standard ball-joint fixa-

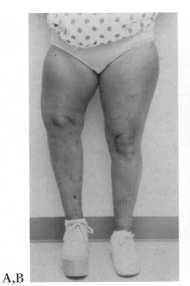
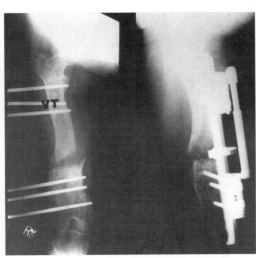

Figure 171.8. **A:** Clinical appearance of a patient with Ollier's disease after tibial lengthening with residual varus deformity of the femur and shortening. **B:** AP and lateral radiographs following application of LRS system and acute correction of femoral deformity. **C to E:** Clinical and radiographic appearance at the conclusion of lengthening and bone consolidation.

A,B

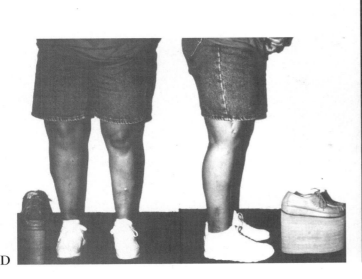
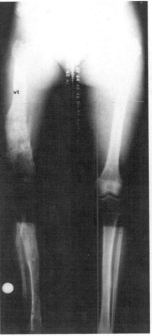
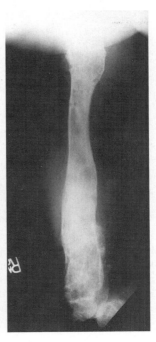

C,D   **E**

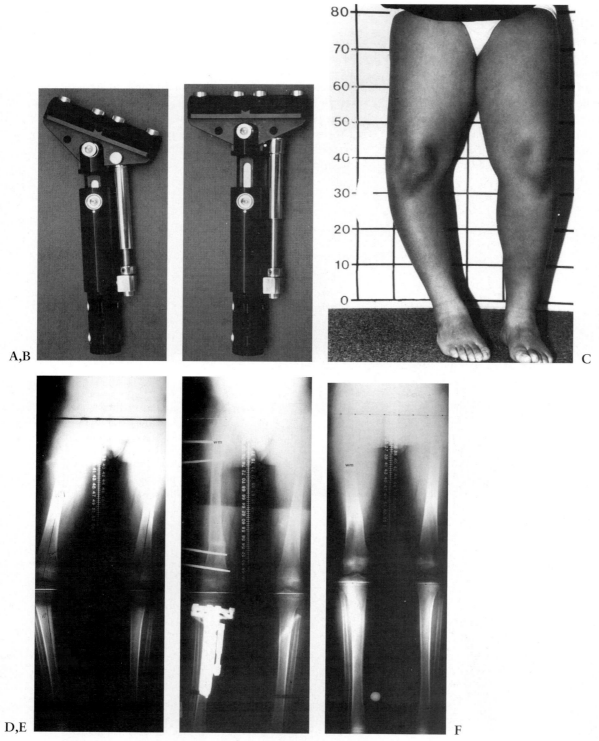

Figure 171.9.   **A and B:** The T-Garches external fixator is ideal for correction of proximal tibial frontal plane deformity. **C and D:** Clinical and radiographic appearance of a 12-year-old boy with adolescent Blount's disease and varus deformity of both the tibia and the femur. **E:** Radiographic appearance following osteotomy of the femur and tibia, and application of an Orthofix external fixator to the femur and T-Garches external fixator to the tibia. **F:** Radiograph following fixator removal with restoration of normal limb mechanical axis.

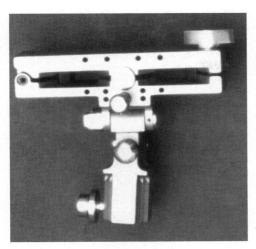

Figure 171.10. The new T-Garches template clamp allows accurate pin placement for simultaneous sagittal and frontal plane deformity correction.

tors, and the T-Garches, it is important to note the length of the device and the pin spread for the particular application. Be certain, for example, in a limb lengthening, that the device is long enough. At least 10% extra length is needed for the tibia and 20% for the femur. The bone-to-fixator distance is relatively large, particularly in the

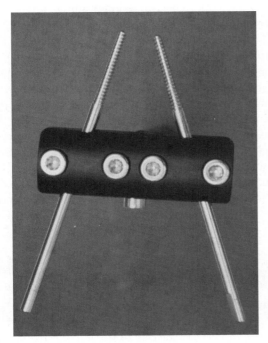

Figure 171.11. Only two pins can be placed in the proximal T-Garches fixator. This potentially limits its use, particularly for significant lengthenings.

femur. Thus, there is not always a 1:1 ratio between the amount of lengthening the device can achieve (ie, number of turns) and the actual distraction achieved in the limb. Start with some extra length in the device to avoid running out of space.

ORTHOFIX TECHNIQUE FOR FRACTURE AND OSTEOTOMIES

- In the case of fracture reduction or osteotomy, anticipate whether the device will need to be lengthened or shortened to achieve the correct bone position before determining pin placement. Add a supplemental pin to the fixator body if necessary for segmental fracture stabilization.
- Once pins are in place, remove the template. Obtain provisional reduction of a fracture or positioning of the bone ends following osteotomy before applying the fixator.
- Apply the fixator and tighten the pin clamps. Attach the reduction forceps to the clamps and fine-tune the bone position under image intensifier control.

Dynafix

The major generic difference between the Orthofix and the Dynafix (manufactured by EBI Medical Systems) is that the Dynafix itself is used as its own template. Tissue protectors and drill guides are placed directly through the pin clamps. The Dynafix articulated body fixator has mobile joints that allow angulation in the frontal and sagittal

---

HINTS AND TRICKS

- With the articulated body fixator, always secure the ball joints with methylmethacrylate to avoid slippage during weight bearing, which can lead to loss of position in fractures or after osteotomy.
- Small articulated fixators are available for specialized application in the pediatric forearm, humerus, and tibia (5).
- In general, an adult-size fixator is recommended for the femur of all except the smallest children (those weighing less than 50 to 60 lb); it can also be applied to the tibia in older children.
- Use the larger 6.0 to 5.0 mm tapered pins when possible except in the forearm or in bones smaller than 15 mm in diameter. Two pin sizes are available for small bones.

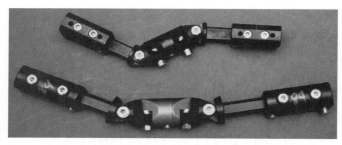

Figure 171.12. The EBI Dynafix external fixator allows angulation, translation, and rotation through its "snake-like" configuration.

plane and rotation through the center of the fixator (Fig. 171.12). The snakelike configuration of the device and the multiple fixator body joints permit translation and rotational corrections as well as approximately 30° of angulation at each joint. As with the standard Orthofix unit, these corrections need to be completed during surgery.

The lengthening system is similar in concept to the Orthofix LRS (Figs. 171.13 and 171.14). Both systems use pins with an external shaft diameter of 6.0 mm. The pin clamp spacing and configuration are different between the two devices; thus, it is impossible to exchange devices without changing pin locations.

A device similar to the Orthofix T-Garches is also available for correction of proximal tibial deformities (Fig.

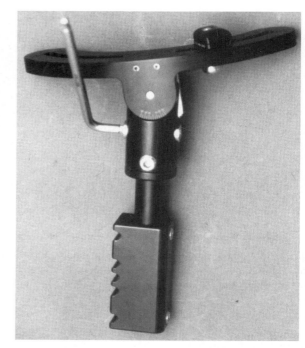

Figure 171.15. Like the T-Garches, the EBI T-fixator allows gradual angular correction in the proximal tibia and lengthening.

171.15). Because the pin clamps are applied to the T portion of the device, more than two pins can be inserted if desired. The pins may also be applied either proximal or distal to the T allowing some longitudinal spread of the proximal metaphyseal pins.

Heidelberg Fixator

Used in Europe for approximately 5 years, the Heidelberg fixator, designed by Dr. Joachin Pfeil, has recently been introduced to North America (Fig. 171.16). This device is yet another cantilever system. Its proposed benefit, however, is the ability to achieve gradual angular correction through a device called the angulator (Fig. 171.17). Pins are inserted through a drill guide template (Fig. 171-18), which can be applied to the fixator in any plane and allows correction of oblique plane deformity or correction of de-

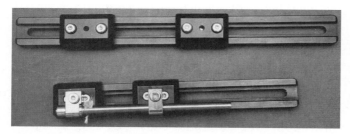

Figure 171.13. The EBI lengthening system is similar to the Orthofix LRS system.

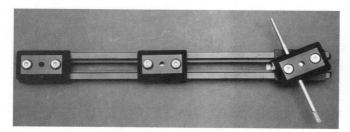

Figure 171.14. Swivel clamps are available for the Dynafix lengthening system.

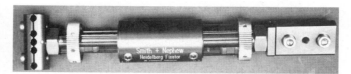

Figure 171.16. The Heidelberg fixator has been recently introduced to North America. Similar to other systems, it has several pin clamp types. Lengthening occurs through the body of the fixator itself.

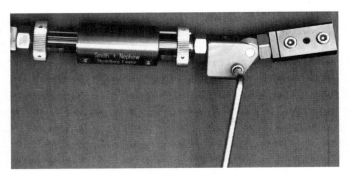

Figure 171.17. The Heidelberg "angulator" allows gradual deformity correction following lengthening.

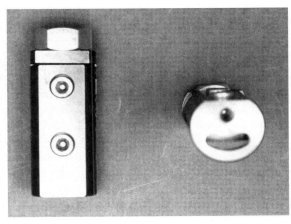

Figure 171.19. A special Heidelberg clamp allows fixator attachment to the Ilizarov ring system.

formity that may arise during limb lengthening such as procurvatum and valgus in the tibia. The surgeon can also apply supplemental bone screws when necessary to enhance stability. A special clamp is also available to allow fixation to the Ilizarov ring system (Fig. 171.19). Experience thus far in North America is limited, but the device has some potentially significant advantages, particularly when gradual deformity correction is desirable. Translational correction must nonetheless be obtained intraoperatively.

Hex-Fix

The Hex-Fix can be used to stabilize pediatric long-bone fractures definitively and in osteotomies in small children or children with particularly small bones, as in the skeletal dysplasias. I prefer to use it for proximal femoral fractures or fractures in very small children (those younger than 4 to 5 years of age) in whom stable fracture fixation is desired. The device can accommodate predrilled or self-drilling (eg, Schanz) half-pins of 4, 5, or 6 mm. There are

several types of pin clamps available that accommodate one or two bone pins (Fig. 171.20). The single pin clamps permit flexible pin spacing. The clamps also allow some angulation and rotation, enabling multiplanar half-pin fixation on a cantilever device.

Generally, insert two pins proximally and distally to the fracture or osteotomy; pin spacing is dependent on the individual situation. There is no limit to the number of pins that can be used other than the ability to put the pin clamps on the bar. The actual bar on which the pin clamps are assembled is available in several lengths, the shortest being 8 inches. Although a distractor unit is available for lengthening, I have no experience using this device for limb lengthening.

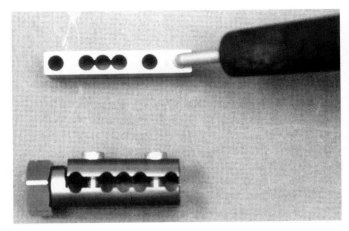

Figure 171.18. Pins are introduced through a hand-held template that matches the pin clamp.

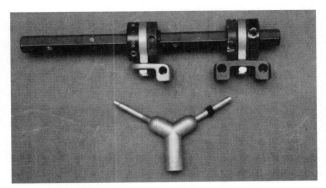

Figure 171.20. The Hex-Fix is particularly useful for fracture fixation in small children. Four, five, or six millimeter pins may be introduced through the pin clamps, which act as their own template. They are available as single or double clamps as shown. Pins and pin clamps are secured using the universal tool.

CIRCULAR EXTERNAL FIXATION

The most commonly used circular external fixator is the Ilizarov apparatus. This device is applicable to all limb segments in both the upper and the lower extremities and can be used for deformity correction of both bone and soft tissue, and for limb lengthening (3,5–12,15,17,19–21, 24,27,29–31,32,38–39,41–45,51,56–58,61–63). Acute trauma applications in the child are limited. It is used most commonly for segmental bone loss, in which it can be used for bone transport (11).

In children, the Ilizarov device is applied most com- monly to the femur or the tibia. The standard tibial fixator consists of one or two rings proximally and distally de- pending on the size of the patient. The standard tibial wire "formula" calls for the insertion of four wires proximally and distally (Fig. 171.21) (26). These wires are either 1.5 or 1.8 mm in diameter. Use 1.5 mm wires in the tibia of smaller children, and 1.8 mm wires in the femur and the tibia of heavier children. At each end of the bone, place two "olive" wires and two smooth wires. Generally, place the olive wires transversely in the frontal plane, one olive from the medial and one from the lateral aspect of the bone. Transfix the fibula and tibia with a smooth wire, both proximally and distally. Finally, place two wires

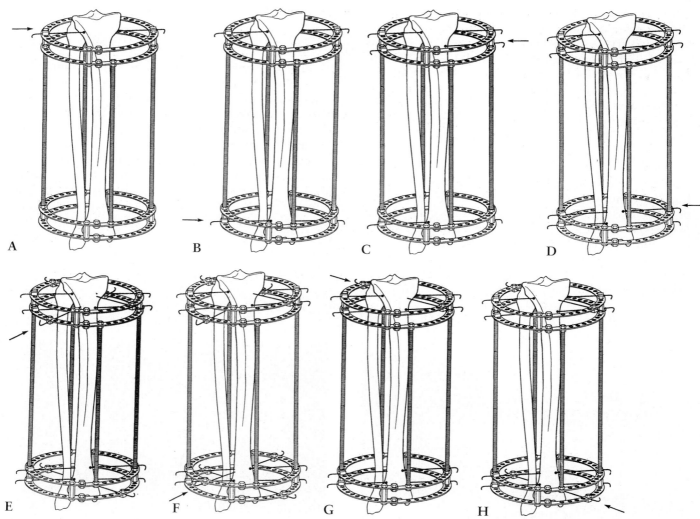

Figure 171.21.   **A and B:** Transverse "Olive" wires are first placed on the most proximal and distal rings. **C and D:** Two additional olive wires are placed from the opposite direction on the two middle rings. **E and F:** Smooth wires are placed from the lateral aspect of the leg, parallel to the medial face of the tibia both proximally and distally. **G and H:** Two smooth wires are placed through the proximal and distal fibula, transfixing the tibia.

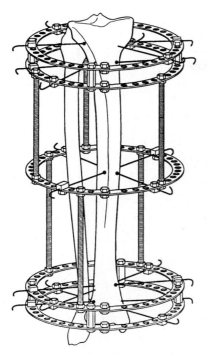

Figure 171.22. Bifocal treatment for deformity or lengthening requires an additional middle ring with two-wire or wire and half-pin fixation.

fixator. Because the standard medial face tibial wire can often interfere with the pes anserinus tendons, I substitute a half-pin for this wire, leaving the remaining wires as described earlier (Fig. 171.23). In the tibia, the addition of an extra ring in the diaphysis allows bifocal treatment. It is useful for patients with deformities at more than one level (Fig. 171.24), when extensive lengthening is necessary, and in bone transport (Fig. 171.25).

For femoral fixation I prefer an Italian modification using partial rings proximally, as compared with the original Russian technique, which uses full rings for both the proximal and distal thigh. My technique is as follows.

- Generally, I use four wires distally—two 1.8 mm olive wires and two plain wires fixed to one or two rings (Fig. 171.26).
- Connect these rings to an empty diaphyseal ring via lengthening rods or hinges depending on the application.
- Achieve proximal fixation by half-pin, rather than by wire fixation. Determine the diameter of the half-pin by the size of the child.
- Connect the distal rings to the proximal thigh fixation through oblique supports.
- Attach the proximal half-pins to one or two "arches," depending on the size of the patient.

from anterolateral to posterolateral (one proximal and one distal), parallel to the medial border of the tibia. When bifocal—proximal and distal tibial osteotomies—are planned, use another ring fixed to the mid-diaphysis by two wires (Fig. 171.22). These wires are often two olive wires, or an olive wire and plain wire, depending on the direction or nature of the deformity.

Many modifications have been made to this standard wire "formula" in recent years, generally the substitution of half-pins for wires (discussed in Chapter 32).

In children, I prefer a largely "wired-based" circular

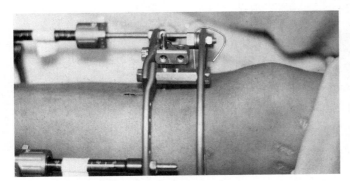

Figure 171.23. A half-pin is often substituted for the traditional Ilizarov medial face wire and affixed to a Rancho cube.

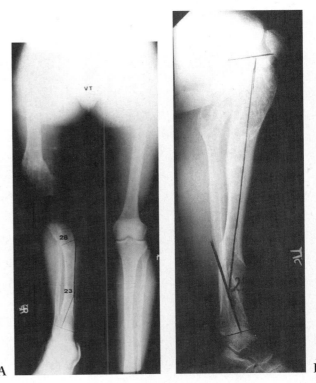

Figure 171.24. **A and B:** Standing and lateral teleoroentgenograms of a patient with Ollier's disease and a 13 cm limb-length inequality with bifocal tibial deformity. *(continued)*

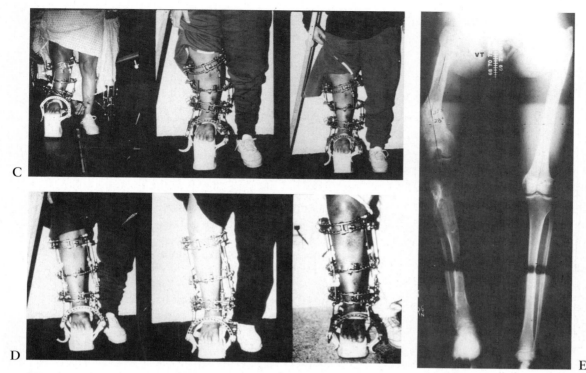

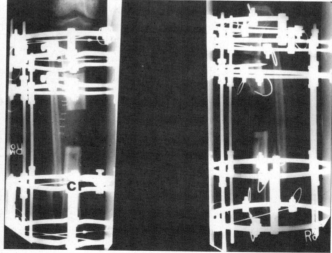

Figure 171.24. *(continued)* **C and D:** The Ilizarov external fixator with bifocal application was used for gradual correction of the proximal and distal deformities as well as 8 cm of lengthening. **E:** Radiographs at the conclusion of tibial consolidation.

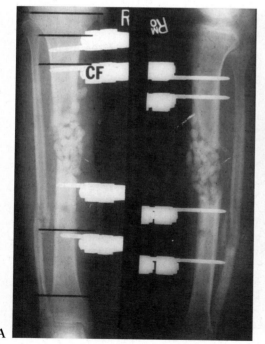

Figure 171.25. Tibial radiographs of a 16-year-old boy who presented following a pedestrian motor vehicle accident with 6 cm of missing bone. Antibiotic cement beads were used as a spacer, and external fixation was applied using a Synthes external fixator. **B:** The Ilizarov apparatus was applied over the Synthes fixator, which was then removed. A proximal osteotomy was performed and bone transport was initiated to restore the defect. *(continued)*

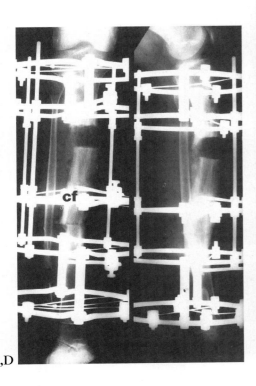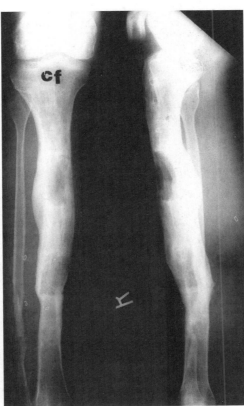

C,D

Figure 171.25. (continued) **C:** Radiographs at the conclusion of bone transport. **D:** Radiographs following fixator removal.

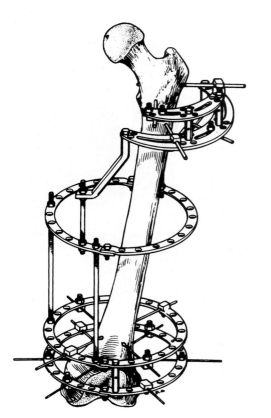

Figure 171.26. Schematic drawing of the Italian modification of standard Ilizarov fixation of the femur. Note that proximal fixation is achieved using half-pins. An empty middle ring is used to facilitate angular or rotation correction as well as lengthening. Distal fixation is traditional through four 1.8 mm transfixing wires.

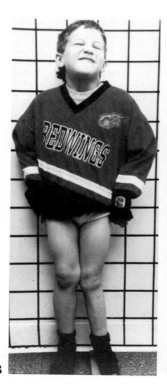
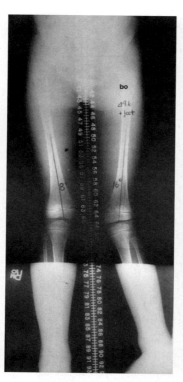
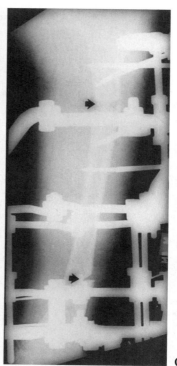

A,B

C

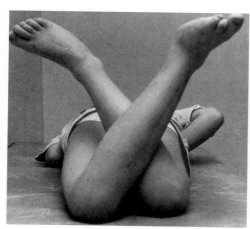

D,E

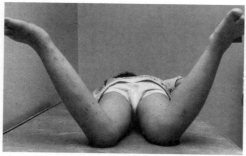

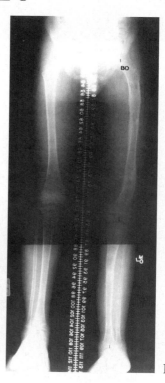

F

Figure 171.27.   **A and B:** Preoperative photographs and teleoroentgenogram of a 6-year-old boy with congenital shortening of the femur, fibular hemimelia, and a three-ray foot. **C:** The Ilizarov technique was used for bifocal application. Acute rotational correction was performed proximally. Elimination of distal femoral valgus and subsequent lengthening was done distally. **D and E:** The photographs demonstrate symmetric internal and external rotation at the conclusion of treatment. **F:** Radiographs demonstrate excellent healing of both femoral and tibial lengthening sites.

■ Introduce wires or half-pins on the diaphyseal ring for bifocal application to the femur. Although bifocal lengthening is not recommended, proximal angular or rotational osteotomy can be performed acutely (Fig. 171.27), combined with distal deformity correction and lengthening.

Circular fixation allows almost limitless modification of the fixator. During lengthening, adjacent joints are at risk for progressive contracture, subluxation, or dislocation. The risk of dislocation is particularly significant in the case of congenitally short limbs, such as the ankles associated with fibular hemimelia, knees or hips in the congenital short femur, and proximal femoral focal deficiency (PFFD). Pre-existing contracture due to trauma, burn, or infection may warrant use of circular fixation for gradual correction of deformity with combined femoral and tibial lengthening. Consider prophylactic incorporation of the foot or tibia in tibial or femoral lengthening, respectively, at the beginning or if there is any indication of subluxation or progressive contracture as lengthening proceeds. Consider extending the fixator to the pelvis when the hip is at risk for subluxation (Fig. 171.28). I recommend fixation of the foot at the initial surgery in any patient undergoing tibial lengthening who has fibular

hemimelia or a pre-existing equinus contracture. Comprehensive release of the foot can be maintained with foot fixation and combined with tibial lengthening (Fig. 171.29).

■ Try to use two metatarsal olive wires and two calcaneal olive wires.
■ In the forefoot, introduce the medially based olive wire through the first and second metatarsals and the lateral wire through the two lateral metatarsals. Fix them to an arch, tensioned no more than 50 to 80 kg. Place the wires in this fashion to avoid flattening the forefoot arch and preclude weight bearing on wires.
■ Introduce one calcaneal wire from the medial side and one from the lateral side, usually diverging no more than 45° (Fig. 171.30).
■ Fixation of both the hindfoot and forefoot avoids midfoot deformity and forefoot equinus, which can result from tension on the long toe flexors during lengthening.
■ Once the distraction phase has been completed, remove the foot fixation, allowing the ankle and foot to regain motion while the tibial lengthening site consolidates. If prophylactic circular fixation has been applied to the tibia during femoral lengthening, remove it once femo-

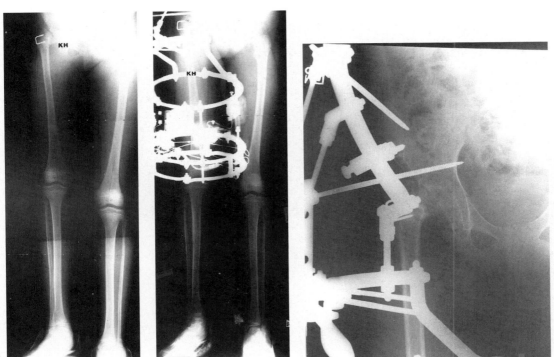

A,B   C

Figure 171.28. **A:** Radiographs of an 11-year-old girl with a painless fibrous pseudarthrosis of her right hip and a projected limb length inequality of 9 cm. **B and C:** Radiographs demonstrate Ilizarov fixation of the femur with extension of the fixation to the pelvis to protect the potentially unstable hip. *(continued)*

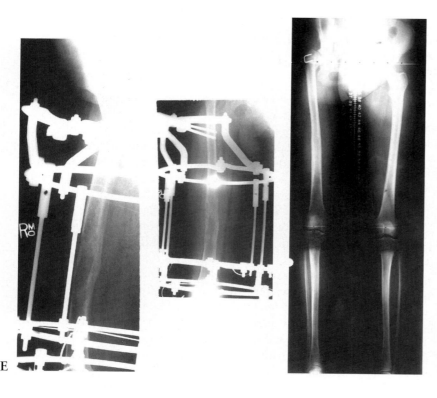

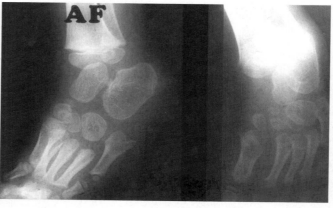

Figure 171.28. *(continued)* **D** and **E:** Radiographs at the conclusion of lengthening demonstrate excellent consolidation of the bone and no disruption of the hip joint.

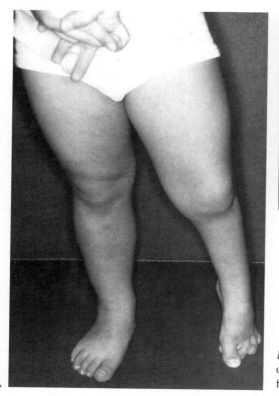

Figure 171.29. **A and B:** Clinical appearance and radiographs of a 2 1/2-year-old girl with hemisacral agenesis, recurrent club foot deformity, and a leg-length inequality. *(continued)*

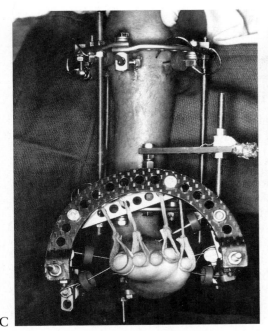

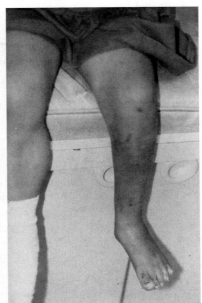

C

E

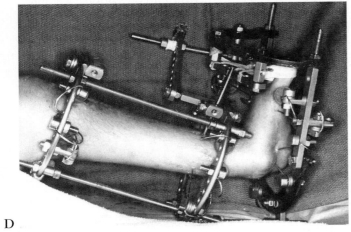

D

Figure 171.29. (continued) **C and D:** An open soft-tissue release of the foot was combined with gradual correction of residual foot deformity and tibial lengthening using the Ilizarov technique. **E:** Clinical appearance at the end of treatment.

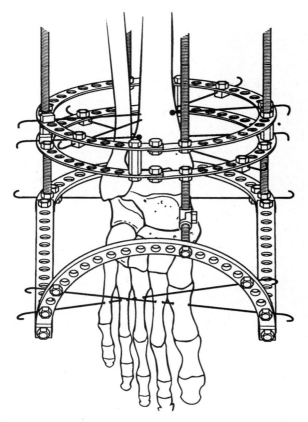

Figure 171.30. A variety of options are available for foot fixation using the Ilizarov technique. I prefer hindfoot fixation through the calcaneus using opposing olive wires and forefoot fixation, with the lateral olive wire transfixing the two lateral metatarsals and the medial Olive wire transfixing the two medial metatarsals.

ral distraction has been completed as long as there is no significant concurrent contracture of the hip.

OSTEOTOMY TECHNIQUE

■ Perform osteotomy of long bones for deformity correction or lengthening through a 1 to 1.5 cm incision, with minimal periosteal stripping generally using a sharp, thin ¼-inch osteotome.

■ Predrill the bone with a 2.7 mm or 3.2 mm drill to avoid crack propagation from the osteotomy into the adjacent half-pins, which could considerably weaken fixation.

■ Avoid large incisions with subperiosteal exposure of the bone and insertion of retractors to minimize scarring and promote bone healing.

■ There is no need to make a true "corticotomy" as described by Ilizarov, because the periosteal blood supply is more critical than the endosteal supply. Furthermore,

the endosteal blood supply usually re-establishes itself within a matter of days following osteotomy.

SPECIAL APPLICATIONS

THE FOOT

Circular external fixation is used to correct foot deformity (32) by one of three approaches: (1) correction by distraction alone; (2) soft-tissue release and tendon lengthening combined with distraction; and (3) osteotomy and distraction. The choice of method depends on the child's age and whether the deformity is bony alone or combined with soft-tissue contractures. Ilizarov originally described correction of all soft-tissue deformity through closed distraction or "bloodless" surgery (28,32). This situation may present itself in the child younger than 4 to 5 years old with a multiply operated club foot in poor position. In my experience, an attempt at correction by closed distraction alone may be unacceptably painful and, owing to the scar stiffness, may result in wire cut-out thorough osteopenic bone. In this situation, perform a conventional comprehensive release first, followed by fixation of the foot and tibia with appropriate hinge placement and subsequent gradual correction (Fig. 171.31). This surgery avoids the problem of wire migration.

Apply this technique only to stiff feet in poor position, the goal being to produce a plantigrade foot.

The distraction rate in soft-tissue corrections is limited by patient discomfort, skin tension, and the tolerance of neurovascular structures. Slight overcorrection is recommended due to soft-tissue elasticity which can cause rebound following apparatus removal. Once correction has been achieved, maintain the fixation an additional 6 to 8 weeks. Use orthotics after the removal of the fixator to maintain the correction.

Tibial fixation should span the leg with two rings. A total of four wires, or two wires and two half-pins, are adequate fixation in the tibia because there is no tibial osteotomy. The number of wires in the foot and complexity of the apparatus depends entirely on the nature of the deformity.

With bony deformity in the older child, osteotomy is usually necessary (Fig. 171.32). The nature of the deformity determines the location of the osteotomy. If the hindfoot is neutral and the problem is midfoot cavus or supination, use a midtarsal osteotomy. Hindfoot fixation can be neutral with respect to the tibial fixation. Place hinges between the hindfoot and forefoot, centered over the apex of the deformity. A hindfoot that is not in neutral may be addressed in one of two ways. If cavus exists with hindfoot deformity, use a V-shaped osteotomy to address the hindfoot and midfoot independently. Additional fulcrum wires are necessary, usually in the midfoot and talus to ensure that correction occurs through the osteotomy and not through joint distraction. If the midfoot and forefoot are relatively neutral with respect to one another and the hindfoot is the problem, use a crescent-shaped osteotomy. Perform the osteotomy from the lateral side through the calcaneus and neck of the talus. Place wires superior and

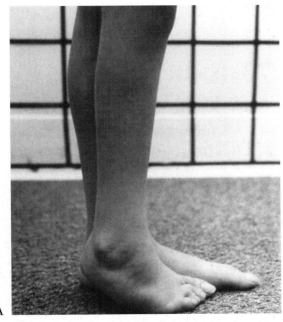

A

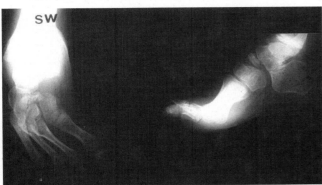

B

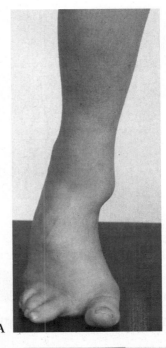

A

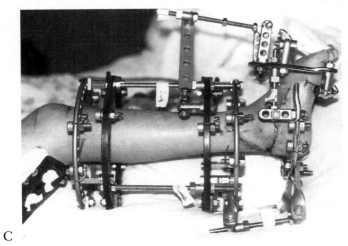

C

Figure 171.31. **A and B:** Clinical and radiographic appearance of a girl with fibular hemimelia and a four-ray equinovarus foot following two previous attempts to correct her foot deformity. **C:** Comprehensive foot release was combined with gradual independent correction of the forefoot and hindfoot deformities and tibial lengthening.

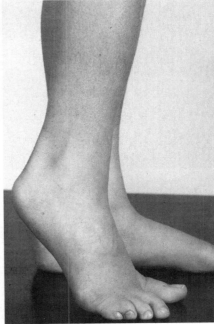

B

Figure 171.32. **A and B:** This nearly skeletally mature boy with fibular hemimelia has a fixed deformity of his foot and limb shortening. *(continued)*

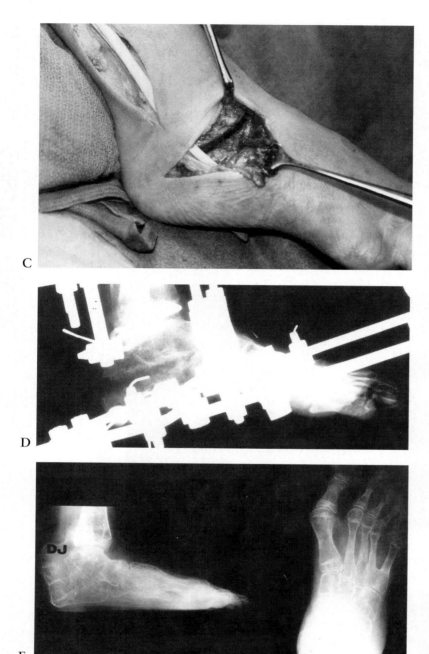

Figure 171.32. *(continued)* C: An open crescentic osteotomy was performed through the talus and calcaneus with resection of the deforming tight fibular anlage. D: Lateral foot radiograph at the conclusion of correction. E: Radiographs following fixator removal.

inferior to the osteotomy with appropriate hinge location to avoid translation of the foot during correction.

JOINT CONTRACTURES

Circular external fixation can be used to correct joint contractures in children due to trauma (Fig. 171.33), infection, and burns. Unfortunately, to date, most surgeons' long-term experience has been disappointing. As with conventional soft-tissue and capsular release, the recurrence rate is high despite prolonged periods of posttreatment bracing. Furthermore, as with conventional surgery, depending on the du   tion of the deformity and the nature of the articular cartilage, the surgeon's goal may be limited to reorienting rather than increasing the arc of motion. The joints most commonly involved in the pediatric patient are the knee and ankle. The usual deformities are knee flexion and ankle equinus contractures.

In the knee, the rate of correction is usually limited by the neurovascular bundles, in particular the sciatic nerve.

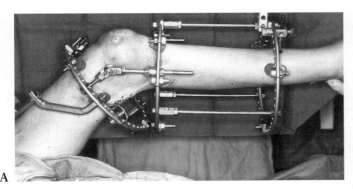

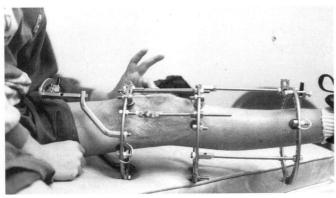

Figure 171.33. **A:** A lawnmower accident resulted in a severe flexion deformity of this knee. Open posterior release achieved no improvement in knee position, and the Ilizarov external fixator was applied to the femur and tibia with hinges at the approximate center of rotation of the knee. **B:** Appearance at the conclusion of correction.

Apply circular fixation to span the adjacent femur and tibia to provide an efficient lever arm. Hinges must be located as close to the center of rotation of the knee joint as possible to avoid joint compression or subluxation. After obtaining correction, depending on the preoperative range of motion, use the hinges to assist in moving the knee during physical therapy. At the ankle, center the hinge placement over the center of the talar dome to avoid anterior subluxation of the talus in the ankle mortise.

UPPER EXTREMITY

In general, it is easier to apply cantilever fixation than circular fixation to the upper extremity. At present, circular fixation is optimal for complex deformities that cannot be corrected acutely (Fig. 171.34). It is also useful if the wrist needs to be spanned, for example, in lengthening of radial or ulnar club hand (12,37). Metacarpal wires can be fixed to a half-ring and attached to the forearm fixation (10,12,37,49,64).

Cantilever fixation can be combined with circular fixa-

tion of the forearm, and the two methods can be used independently for deformities such as those associated with multiple hereditary exostosis (Fig. 171.35). In general, half-pin fixation is easier and safer to apply to the forearm than transfixing wires. The fact that the ulna is subcutaneous throughout its length makes half-pin fixa-

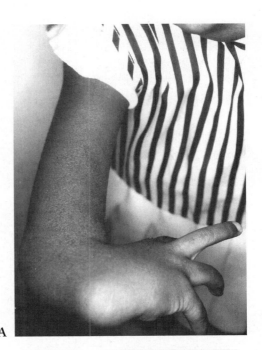

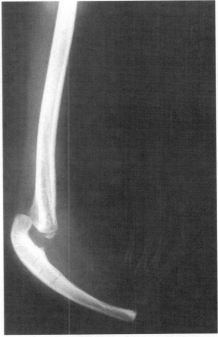

Figure 171.34. **A and B:** Clinical and radiographic appearance of 6-year-old girl with a right radial club hand and no history of prior intervention. *(continued)*

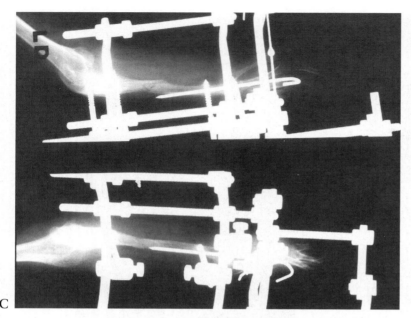

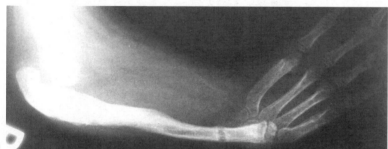

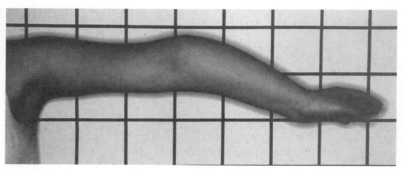

Figure 171.34. *(continued)* **C:** The ulna was centralized through an open procedure and the wrist stabilized with a transfixing Kirschner wire. Lengthening of forearm was then undertaken. **D:** The ulna was lengthened by more than 89%.

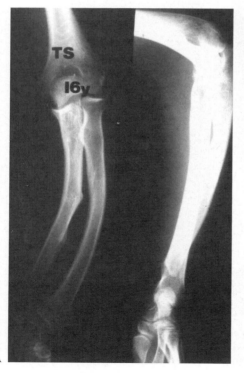

Figure 171.35. **A and B:** Radiographs and clinical appearance of a 16-year-old girl with multiple hereditary exostoses with forearm shortening and deformity. *(continued)*

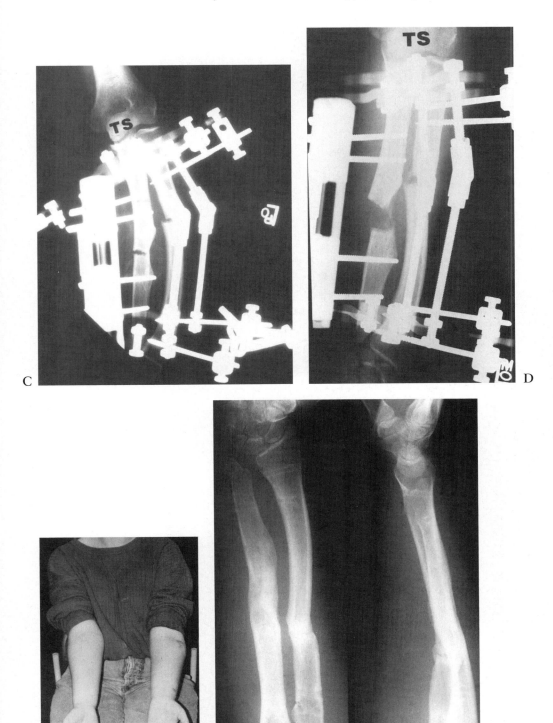

Figure 171.35. *(continued)* **C and D:** Circular fixation was applied to the radius around a small Orthofix LRS fixator for gradual correction of radial deformity and ulnar lengthening. **E and F:** Clinical and radiographic appearance of the forearm at the conclusion of treatment.

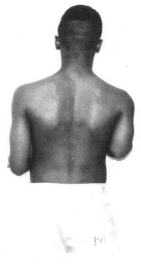

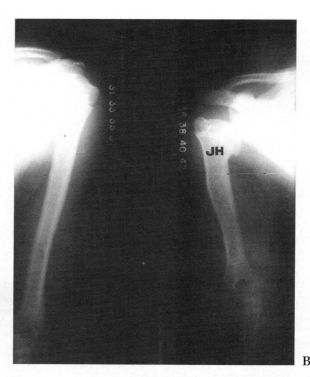

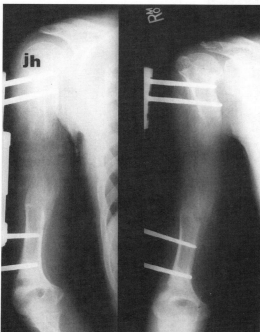

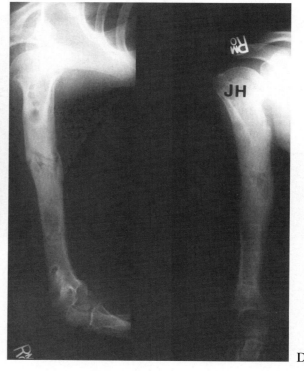

Figure 171.36.   **A and B:** Clinical appearance and radiographs of 13-year-old boy with 10 cm of right humeral shortening due to septic growth arrest of the proximal humerus at the age of 2 years. **C and D:** Radiographs at the conclusion of distraction and following consolidation.

tion attractive. Half-pins can be attached in a multidirectional fashion to rings if desired. Two half-pins proximal and distal to the osteotomy site are enough for deformity correction or lengthening.

The humerus is the most easily lengthened long bone (Fig. 171.36) (10). Perform osteotomy distal to the deltoid insertion. Two half-pins proximal and distal to the osteotomy or lengthening site are adequate in the arm. Insert the most distal pin just proximal to the olecranon fossa. The next most proximal pin must avoid the path of the radial nerve. Place it with open technique.

TRAUMA APPLICATIONS

OPEN FRACTURES

At present, open fracture is the most clear-cut indication for external fixation of pediatric long-bone fractures (4, 14,16,34,35,47,50,53,55,60). Depending on the size of the limb segment, apply a four-pin fixator (Hex-Fix, Orthofix, Dynafix) after irrigation and debridement of the open wound. Locate the fixator to minimize interference with subsequent wound management such as local or free flaps and skin grafts. In the case of segmental bone loss, circular fixation can be used to transport bone for definitive bone reconstruction of bone loss.

MULTIPLE TRAUMA

Multiple trauma, particularly if combined with a concurrent severe closed head injury, is a strong indication for fixation of major long bone fractures in the pediatric patient. Those patients who require frequent computed tomography (CT) scans, magnetic resonance imaging (MRI) studies, or the operations for treatment of their associated injuries are more easily managed with stable fracture fixation. Traction or spica casts make this difficult, and spica casts may interfere with management of abdominal or chest trauma. Patients who experience spasticity or who are uncooperative following head injury are best managed with rigid stabilization of their long-bone fractures. Even in the very young child, small cantilever unilateral external fixators, such as the Hex-Fix, can be adapted to long-bone fractures, particularly of the femur and tibia.

FEMORAL SHAFT FRACTURES

Operative management of isolated femoral diaphyseal fractures using external fixation has become accepted in patients older than 5 to 6 years of age (14,22,34,35,50,52, 55). Immediate spica treatment is still preferred in small children, and older adolescents may be treated with intramedullary rodding. Current literature supports operative treatment of this intermediate age group between age 5

and 11 to 12 years, reporting excellent results with external fixation decreasing hospitalization, promoting early patient mobilization and return to school, decreasing psychosocial family stress, with an acceptable complication rate (2,4,14,16,34,50,52,53,55). A recent report (18) also demonstrated a clear cost savings when compared with traditional skeletal traction followed by spica-cast immobilization. The major concern when using external fixation in these fractures is the risk of refracture. The incidence of refracture can be minimized by early weight bearing, early fixator dynamization, and mobilization of the knee. Anecdotal reference is made by some to suggest that the most common fracture pattern susceptible to refracture is a transverse diaphyseal fracture. In my experience, the most important factors in refracture are a stiff knee and lack of weight bearing during fracture healing.

FLOATING KNEE

Ipsilateral concomitant fracture of both the femur and the tibia produces a floating knee. Operative stabilization of both the tibia and the femur are indicated. Depending on the skeletal maturity of the patient, intramedullary fixation of the femur, using either reamed or flexible implants, can be combined with external fixation of the tibia. In the younger child, external fixation can be applied to both the femur and the tibia. It allows rapid mobilization of the patient, motion of the knee and ankle, and normal shoe wear. Weight bearing can be initiated as soon as patient can tolerate it in most cases.

PELVIC FRACTURES

Although they are relatively rare in children, unstable pelvic fractures, particularly open-book type fractures of the pelvis, can be treated with external fixation as in the adult (52). Posterior disruptions can be addressed by internal fixation and combined with an anterior fixator (see Chapter 17). For more details on the treatment of pediatric fractures, see Chapter 164.

REFERENCES

Each reference is categorized according to the following scheme. *, classic article; #, review article; !, basic research article; and +, clinical results/outcome study.

+ 1. Aldegheri R, Renzi-Brivio L, Agostini S. Callotasis Method of Limb Lengthening. *Clin Orthop Rel Res* 1989;241:137.
+ 2. Alonso JE, Horowitz M. Use of the AO/ASIF External Fixator in Children. *J Pediatr Orthop* 1987;7:594.
+ 3. Armstrong PF, Bell DF, Rajacich N. The Ilizarov Technique. In: Malcolm Menelaus, ed. *The Management of*

Limb Discrepancy. London: Churchill Livingstone, 1991:161.

+ 4. Aronson J, Tursky EA. External Fixation of Femur Fractures in Children. *Pediatr Orthop* 1992;12:157.

+ 5. Bell DF. Treatment of Adolescent Blount's Disease Using the Ilizarov Technique. In: Balderston RA, ed. *Operative Techniques in Orthopaedics*, Vol 3, No 2. Philadelphia: W.B. Saunders, 1993:149.

+ 6. Bell DF. Treatment of Post-traumatic Sequelae by the Ilizarov Technique. In. Letts M, ed: *Management of Pediatric Fractures*. London: Churchill Livingstone, 1993: 711.

+ 7. Bell DF, Armstrong P, Paley D. Extensive Two-level Limb Lengthening. Early Results Utilizing the Ilizarov Technique. *J Bone Joint Surg* 1990;72-B:538.

+ 8. Bell DF, Boyer MI, Armstrong PF. The Use of the Ilizarov Technique in the Correction of Limb Deformities Associated with Skeletal Dysplasia. *J Pediatr Orthop* 1992;12: 283.

+ 9. Cattaneo R, Catagni M, Johnson EE. The Treatment of Infected Nonunions and Segmental Defects of the Tibia by the Methods of Ilizarov. *Clin Orthop Rel Res* 1992; 280:143.

+ 10. Cattaneo R, Villa A, Catagni MA, Bell DF. Lengthening of the Humerus Using the Ilizarov Technique. Description of the Method and Report of 43 Cases. *Clin Orthop Rel Res* 1990;250:117.

+ 11. Cattaneo R, Villa A, Catagni MA, Tentori L. Limb Lengthening in Achondroplasia by Ilizarov's Method. *Int Orthop* 1988;12:173.

+ 12. Catagni MA, Szabo RM, Cattaneo R. Preliminary Experience with Ilizarov Method in Late Reconstruction of Radial Hemimelia. *J Hand Surg* 1993;18A:316.

! 13. Chao E, Hein T. Mechanical Performance of the Standard Orthofix External Fixator. *Orthopaedics* 1988;11: 1057.

+ 14. Clinkscales CM, Peterson HA. Isolated Closed Diaphyseal Fractures of the Femur in Children. Comparison of Effectiveness and Cost of Several Treatment Methods. *Orthopaedics* 1997;20:1131.

* 15. Dal Monte A, Donzelli O. Tibial Lengthening According to Ilizarov in Congenital Hypoplasia of the Leg. *J Pediatr Orthop* 1987;7:135.

* 16. DeBastiani G, Aldegheri R, Renzi-Brivio L. The Treatment of Fractures with a Dynamic Axial Fixator. *J Bone Joint Surg* 1984;66B:538.

* 17. DeBastiani G, Aldegheri R, Renzi-Brivio L, Trivella F. Limb Lengthening by Callus Distraction (Callotasis). *J Pediatr Orthop* 1987;7:129.

+ 18. Doane RM, Stanitski DF, Stanitski CL. Treatment Cost of Isolated Femoral Shaft Fractures in Children. External Fixation Versus Traction. Submitted to Journal Pediatric Orthopaedics.

+ 19. Eldridge JC, Bell DF. The Correction of Severe Growth Abnormalities Following Purpura Fulminant Using the Ilizarov Technique. *Orthop Trans* 1992–1993;16:861.

+ 20. Fabry G, Lammens J, Van Melkebeek J, Stuyck, J. Treatment of Congenital Pseudarthrosis with the Ilizarov Technique. *J Pediatr Orthop* 1988;8:67.

+ 21. Ghoneem HF, Wright JG, Cole WG, Rang M. The Ilizarov Method for Correction of Complex Deformities. *J Bone Joint Surg* 1996;78A:1480.

+ 22. Glorion C, Pouliquen JC, Langlais J, et al. Femoral Lengthening Using the Callotasis Method. Study of the Complications in a Series of 70 Cases in Children and Adolescents. *J Pediatr Orthop* 1996;16:161.

! 23. Goodship AE, Kenwright J. The influence of induced micro-movement on the healing of experimental tibia fractures. *J Bone Joint Surg* 1985;67B:650.

+ 24. Grill F. Correction of complicated extremity deformities by external fixation. *Clin Orthop Rel Res* 1989;241:166.

+ 25. Guidera KJ, Hess WF, Highhouse KP, Ogden JA. Extremity Lengthening. Results and Complications with the Orthofix System. *J Pediatr Orthop* 1991;11;90.

26. Hamdy RC, Stanitski DF. A Visual Presentation of Ilizarov Tibial Lengthening. *The Journal of Orthopaedic Techniques* 1995;3:55.

+ 27. Huang SC, Kuo KN. Differential Lengthening of the Radius and Ulna Using the Ilizarov Method. *J Pediatr Orthop* 1998;18;370.

28. Ilizarov GA. The Principles of the Ilizarov Method. *Bull Hosp Jt Dis* 1988;48:1.

28. Ilizarov GA. The Tension-Stress Effect on the Genesis and Growth of Tissues. Part I. *Clin Orthop* 1989;238: 249.

* 30. Ilizarov GA. The Tension-Stress Effect on the Genesis and Growth of Tissues. Part II. *Clin Orthop* 1989;239: 264.

* 31. Ilizarov GA. Clinical Application of Tension-Stress Effect for Limb Lengthening. *Clin Orthop* 1990;250:8.

+ 32. Ilizarov GA, Shevtsov VJ, Kuzmin NV. Method of Treating Talipes Equinocavus. *Ortop Travmatol Protez* 1983; 5:46.

+ 33. Kamegaya M, Shinohara Y, Shinada Y. Limb Lengthening and Correction of Angulation Deformity. Immediate Correction by Using a Unilateral Fixator. *J Pediatr Orthop* 1996;16;477.

+ 34. Kirschenbaum D, Albert MC, Robertson WW, Davidson RS. Complex Femur Fractures in Children. Treatment with External Fixation. *J Pediatr Orthop* 1990;10:588.

+ 35. Klein W, Pennig F, Brug E. *Dynamic Axial Fixation for Femoral Fractures in Children*. Presented at the International Congress. Evolution of External Fixation. June 1990, Montpellier, France.

+ 36. Knapp DR, Price CT. Correction of Distal Femoral Deformity. *Clin Orthop Rel Res* 1990;255:75.

+ 37. Lammens J, Mukherjee A, Van Eygen P, Fabry B. Forearm Realignment with Elbow Reconstruction Using the Ilizarov Fixator. A Case Report. *J Bone Joint Surg* 1991; 73B:412.

! 38. Lavini F, Renzi-Brivio L, deBastiani G. Psychologic, Vascular and Physiologic Aspects of Lower Limb Lengthening in Achondroplastics. *Clin Orthop Rel Res* 1990;250: 138.

+ 39. Miller LS, Bell DF. Management of Congenital Fibular Deficiency by Ilizarov Technique. *J Pediatr Orthop* 1992;12:651.

+ 40. Noonan KJ, Price CT. The Pearls and Pitfalls of Limb Lengthening and Deformity Correction via Unilateral External Fixation. *Iowa Orthop J* 1996;16:58.

41. Paley D. Current Techniques of Limb Lengthening. *J Pediatr Orthop* 1988;8:73.

+ 42. Paley D, Catagni M, Argnani F, et al. Treatment of Congenital Pseudarthrosis of the Tibia Using the Ilizarov Technique. *Clin Orthop Rel Res* 1992;280:81.

! 43. Paley D, Fleming D, Catagni M, et al. Mechanical Evaluation of External Fixators Used in Limb Lengthening. *Clin Orthop Rel Res* 1990;250:50.

+ 44. Plawecki S, Carpentier E, Lascombes P, et al. Treatment of Congenital Pseudarthrosis of the Tibia by the Ilizarov Method. *J Pediatr Orthop* 1990;10:786.

+ 45. Pouliquen JC, Coelin JD, Langlais J, Pauthier F. Upper Metaphyseal Lengthening of the Tibia by Callotasis. Forty-seven Cases in Children and Adolescents. *J Pediatr Orthop* 1993;2B:49.

+ 46. Pouliquen JC, Gorodischer S, Vernevet C, Richard L. Femoral Lengthening in Children and Adolescents. A Comparative Study of a Series of 82 Cases. *Fr J Orthop Surg* 1989;3:162.

+ 47. Price CT. Limb Lengthening for Achondroplasia. Early Experience. *J Pediatr Orthop* 1989;9:512.

48. Price CT. Metaphyseal and Physeal Lengthening. *Instr Course Lect* 1989;38:331.

+ 49. Price CT, Cole D. Limb Lengthening by Callotasis for Children and Adolescents. Early Experience. *Clin Orthop Rel Res* 1990;250:105.

+ 50. Price CT, Levengood G, Zink W. The Treatment of Pediatric Fractures with Dynamic External Fixation. *Techn Orthop* 1989;4:74.

+ 51. Rajacich R, Bell DF, Armstrong PF. Pediatric Application of the Ilizarov Method. *Clin Orthop Rel Res* 1992;280:72.

+ 52. Reff RB. The Use of External Fixation Devices in the Management of Severe Lower Extremity Trauma and Pelvic Injuries in Children. *Clin Orthop Rel Res* 1984;188:22.

+ 53. Scavenius M, Ebskov LB, Sloth C, Torholm C. External Fixation with the Orthofix System in Dislocated Fractures of the Lower Extremities in Children. *J Pediatr Orthop* 1993;2:161.

+ 54. Schlenzka D, Poussa M, Osterman K. Metaphyseal Distraction for Lower Limb Lengthening and Correction of Axial Deformities. *J Pediatr Orthop* 1990;10:202.

+ 55. Shih HN, Chen LM, Lee ZL, Shih CH. Treatment of Femoral Shaft Fractures with the Hoffman External Fixator in Prepuberty. *J Trauma* 1989;29:498.

+ 56. Stanitski DF. Treatment of Deformity Secondary to Metabolic Bone Disease with the Ilizarov Technique. *Clin Orthop Rel Res* 1994;301:38.

+ 57. Stanitski DF, Bullard M, Armstrong P, Stanitski CL. Results of Femoral Lengthening Using the Ilizarov Technique. *J Pediatr Orthop* 1995;15:224.

+ 58. Stanitski DF, Shahcheraghi H, Nicker DA, Armstrong PF. Results of Tibial Lengthening Using the Ilizarov Technique. *J Pediatr Orthop* 1996;16:168.

+ 59. Stanitski DF, Srivastava P, Stanitski CL. Correction of Proximal Tibial Deformities in Adolescents Using the T-Garches External Fixator. *J Pediatr Orthop* 1998;18:512.

+ 60. Tolo V. External Skeletal Fixation in Children's Fractures. *J Pediatr Orthop* 1983;3:435.

+ 61. Trivella GP, Brigadoi F, Aldegheri R. Leg Lengthening in Turner Dwarfism. *J Bone Joint Surg* 1996;78B:290.

+ 62. Velazquez RJ, Bell DF, Armstrong PF, et al. Complications Using the Ilizarov Technique in the Correction of Limb Deformities in Children. *J Bone Joint Surg* 1993;75A:1148.

* 63. Vilarrubias JM, Ginebreda I, Jimeno E. Lengthening of the Lower Limbs and Correction of Lumbar Hyperlordosis in Achondroplasia. *Clin Orthop Rel Res* 1990;250:143.

+ 64. Villa A, Paley D, Catagni MA, et al. Lengthening of the Forearm by the Ilizarov Technique. *Clin Orthop Rel Res* 1990;250:125.

! 65. Young NL, Bell DF, Anthony A. Paediatric Pain Patterns During the Ilizarov Treatment of Limb Length Discrepancy and Angular Deformity. *J Pediatr Orthop* 1994;14:352.

! 66. Young NL, Davis RJ, Bell DF, Redmond DM. Electromyographic and Nerve Conduction Changes after Tibial Lengthening by the Ilizarov Method. *J Pediatr Orthop* 1993;13:473.

CHAPTER 172
SLIPPED CAPITAL FEMORAL EPIPHYSIS

Randall T. Loder

PATHOPHYSIOLOGY

Slipped capital femoral epiphysis (SCFE) is the most common adolescent hip disorder (39). It is defined as a posterior and inferior slippage of the proximal femoral epiphysis relative to the metaphysis; it occurs through the hypertrophic physeal zone. In actuality, the relationship of the epiphysis and its articular surface relative to the acetabulum does not change, and the slippage is better defined as an anterior and superior slippage of the proximal femoral metaphysis (neck) relative to the epiphysis. Familiarity with this concept makes the surgical techniques much easier to visualize.

The cause of idiopathic SCFE is unknown, and it is probably multifactorial (90). Because it occurs during the adolescent growth spurt, a subtle endocrine influence is likely. Physeal shear strength decreases during that period (17), probably reflecting the increased physeal width in response to growth hormone. However, circulating hormone levels are usually normal when standard assays are used. The majority of children with SCFE are obese, typically above the 95th percentile for body weight for age (49). In an adolescent child who is above the 95th percentile for body weight, biomechanical studies have shown that the shear stress across the proximal femoral physis from simple running is enough to create an SCFE (17,68). This stress is further increased with femoral retroversion, an associated finding in obese children and in the contralateral "normal" hips of children with SCFE (28,29). In addition, children with SCFE demonstrate a more vertical physis, further increasing the susceptibility to slip (61).

PRINCIPLES OF TREATMENT

The goals of treatment are to (a) prevent further slipping until physeal closure; (b) avoid complications, primarily those of avascular necrosis (AVN) and chondrolysis; and (c) maintain adequate hip function. Four main treatments are described: (a) internal fixation, (b) epiphysiodesis, (c) proximal femoral osteotomy, and (d) spica cast immobilization.

ASSESSMENT, INDICATIONS, AND RELATIVE RESULTS

CLASSIFICATION AND ASSESSMENT

The traditional classifications of SCFE are acute, chronic, and acute-on-chronic (1,23). An acute SCFE is one with a symptom duration of less than 3 weeks; a chronic SCFE, greater than 3 weeks; and an acute-on-chronic SCFE is one with chronic symptoms for more than 3 weeks but with a sudden exacerbation of symptoms for less than 3 weeks. This classification scheme is unreliable because many children and parents cannot remember the exact duration of symptoms. It also gives no information regarding hip prognosis.

Newer classification systems account for SCFE stability, are easier to use, and impart prognostic information (37,52). A child with a stable SCFE is able to walk, with or without crutches; a child with an unstable SCFE is unable to walk, with or without crutches. The prognosis for a child with a stable SCFE is very good, with an incidence of AVN approaching zero. The prognosis for a child with an unstable SCFE is guarded because of the increased risk of AVN, which may be up to 50%. The vast majority (>95%) of SCFEs are stable.

A child with a stable SCFE has a history of intermittent limp for several weeks to months that may or may not be associated with thigh, knee, or groin pain. Hip pain is variably present, often resulting in diagnostic delay. Physical examination demonstrates loss of internal rotation and spontaneous external rotation with hip flexion. Abduction and flexion are usually decreased, especially in the more severe cases. In longstanding cases, shortening of the lower extremity with varying degrees of thigh atrophy is noted; the parents usually also describe a gradually increasing external rotation gait and limb-length discrepancy.

A child with an unstable SCFE presents with sudden, severe pain; there is often a history of a minor fall, such as tripping off a curb. The child lies perfectly still with the lower extremity in a position of flexion, abduction, and external rotation. The hip is extremely irritable, and any attempts toward active or passive hip motion are resisted. These SCFEs are analogous to an acute Salter Harris I fracture, which explains their painful nature and high AVN rate.

In a stable SCFE, the diagnosis is confirmed with anteroposterior (AP) and lateral pelvis radiographs; both views are needed because an early SCFE often is seen only on the lateral view. Always view both hips because the incidence of simultaneous bilaterally may approach 20%. Either frog-lateral or cross-table lateral radiographs may be used. Proponents of the cross-table lateral view argue that the variability with the frog positioning resulting from limitation of hip motion inaccurately represents the SCFE, and that the frog view can also theoretically convert a stable SCFE to an unstable SCFE. Proponents of the frog-lateral view argue that the lateral epiphyseal–shaft angle, a commonly used method to assess slip magnitude, is measured on the frog-lateral view. It is also the view many of the preoperative osteotomy plans depend on.

R. T. Loder: Chief of Staff, Shriner's Hospital for Children, Minneapolis, Minnesota, 55414.

Comparisons with the literature findings are also possible with this view because of its common use.

In an unstable SCFE, only an AP pelvis radiograph can be obtained, and the diagnosis is readily made. A cross-table lateral radiograph can be attempted, but clearly a frog-lateral radiograph should not be attempted, because of both the severe discomfort for the child and the risk of further slippage. A frog-lateral view of the opposite hip should be obtained; it is easy to forget this in the excitement of assessing the unstable side.

Slip magnitude is commonly measured using two methods. The first involves the amount of epiphyseal displacement relative to the metaphysis (16) (Fig. 172.1A). A mild SCFE is one with less than 33% displacement; moderate, 33% to 50%; and severe, greater than 50%. This can be measured on both the AP and the lateral radiographs. In the case of a stable SCFE of many months' duration, remodeling of the femoral neck makes this measurement less reliable, underestimating the true magnitude of slip.

Because of these concerns with the displacement method, the epiphyseal–shaft angle, which more accurately reflects the true slip magnitude, is used (78) (Fig. 172.1B). This angle is measured on the frog-lateral pelvis radiograph by the following method.

- Draw a line between the anterior and posterior tips of the epiphyseal at the physeal level.
- Then draw a line perpendicular to this epiphyseal line.
- Finally, draw a line along the mid axis of the femoral shaft.
- The epiphyseal–shaft angle is the angle formed by the intersection of the perpendicular line and the femoral shaft line.
- Measure this angle for both hips; the magnitude of slip displacement is the angle of the involved hip minus the angle of the contralateral normal hip.
- By using this angle, SCFEs can be classified as mild (<30°), moderate (30° to 50°), or severe (>50°).
- In the case of bilateral SCFEs, 10° to 12° is used as the normal hip angle.

Other imaging techniques are rarely needed. Computed tomography (CT) scans are useful when doubt exists regarding the status of physeal closure or when the postoperative screw position is not adequately determined with plain radiographs. Bone scans are helpful in the rare occasion when AVN or chondrolysis is suspected but not yet visualized on plain radiographs. Magnetic resonance imaging is unnecessary in either the diagnosis or treatment of SCFE.

INDICATIONS FOR TREATMENT

Any child with an SCFE and open physis needs treatment; without stabilization, progression is inevitable. Most authors advocate an *in situ* technique (either internal fixation or epiphysiodesis) for any mild or moderate SCFE. The treatment to use for severe SCFE is more controversial. Primary osteotomy has been advocated to improve joint mechanics, motion, and hip function. However, the incidence of complications is much higher with osteotomy than *in situ* fixation, and thus most surgeons recommend *in situ* fixation as the primary treatment of a severe SCFE. *In situ* fixation allows the synovitis to subside, which will in itself result in improved motion (77). After complete physeal closure (usually 1 or 2 years later), the child's functional limitations, gait pattern, and pain can be more leisurely assessed (36,44). A decision regarding the need for osteotomy can then be made after a thorough discussion of the risks and benefits with both child and parents.

In a patient with closed physes, the only surgical treatment in the absence of severe degenerative changes is proximal femoral osteotomy. Indications are functional limitations, unacceptable gait, or cosmetic deformity. Here again, a thorough discussion of the risks and benefits is needed before performing the procedure.

RESULTS OF TREATMENT

When selecting treatment, the results should be better than the natural history of the disease. The natural history of SCFE is one of gradual degenerative arthritis of the hip (16). The more severe the SCFE at diagnosis, the sooner the degenerative changes appear.

Stable SCFE

Proximal femoral osteotomy makes the most "orthopaedic sense" for stable SCFE (Tables 172.1, 172.2). Although some of the literature demonstrates low complication rates with osteotomy, the majority document a higher complication rate than with *in situ* stabilization. The complications, primarily AVN (13% with cuneiform osteotomy) and chondrolysis (23% with intertrochanteric osteotomy, 16% with cuneiform osteotomy, 7% with basilar neck osteotomy), result in poor long-term outcomes. No long-term study has demonstrated an improved outcome in severe SCFEs treated by osteotomy compared to *in situ* fixation (16,72).

Spica cast immobilization is difficult because of the typical body habitus of a child with SCFE, and it has an unacceptably high rate of chondrolysis (18%) and slip progression (8%) (9,59). Difficulties in mobility are encountered in these very large children in spica casts and with prolonged bed rest.

The best long-term results are with *in situ* treatment. The results of *in situ* fixation with a single central screw using today's intraoperative imaging technology are uniformly excellent (0% AVN and chondrolysis, 1% slip progression), as long as attention to technical details is maintained. The use of two screws does not double the biomechanical strength of the physeal–screw construct,

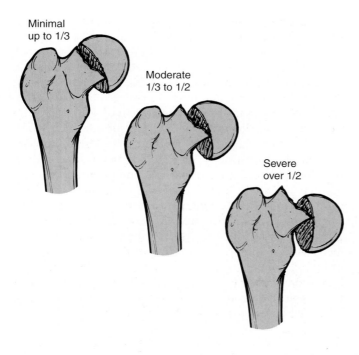

A

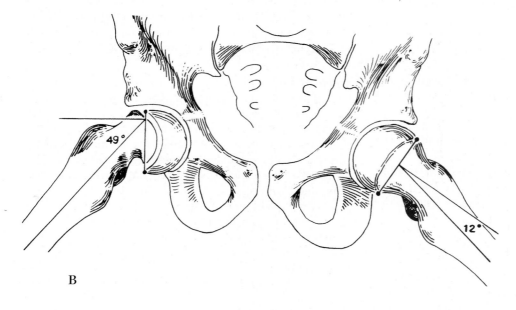

B

Figure 172.1.   Two common methods of magnitude measurement for slipped capital femoral epiphysis (SCFE). **A:** Measurement of the amount of displacement of the epiphysis relative to the metaphyseal width. The SCFE is considered mild if the measured tip is less than 33%, moderate if it is 33% to 50%, and severe if it is more than 50%. **B:** The head–shaft angle is measured on the frog-lateral pelvis radiograph of the pelvis to determine the degree of the slip, which is calculated by subtraction of the angle on the normal side from the angle of the affected hip: 49° − 12° = 37°. (From Aronson DD, Carlson WE. Slipped Capital Femoral Epiphysis: A Prospective Study of Fixation with a Single Screw. *J Bone Joint Surg Am* 1992;74:810, with permission.)

Table 172.1. Results of Various Treatment Methods for Stable Slipped Capital Femoral Epiphysis (SCFE)

Author	Year	Follow-up (yr, ave)	SCFEs (N)	AVN (N)	Chondrolysis (N)	SCFE Progression (N)	Nonunion[a] (N)
Cuneiform osteotomy							
Pearl et al. (66)	1961	5.8	17	4	—	—	—
Gage et al. (27)	1978	9.5	77	22	29	—	2
Kulick and Denton (46)	1980	4.7	9	3	—	—	—
Carlioz et al. (15)	1984	1 to 10	27	0	3	0	0
Szypryt et al. (83)	1987	5.3	22	4	0	0	0
Broughton et al. (13)	1988	12.92	70	3	6	—	—
Nishiyama et al. (65)	1989	10.3	18	1	1	—	—
Fish (25)	1994	13.3	50	0	1	0	0
DeRosa et al. (20)	1996	8.4	27	4	6	2	—
Total (%)			317	41 (13%)	46 (16%)	2 (3%)	2 (1%)
Basilar Neck Osteotomy							
Kramer et al. (45)	1976	2 to 11	56	0	1	—	0
Abraham et al. (2)	1993	9	36	0	5	0	0
Total (%)			92	0	6 (7%)	0	0
Intertrochanteric Osteotomy							
Southwick (78)	1967	>5	55	0	6	0	—
Southwick (79)	1973	—	24	0	8	0	1 DU
Frymoyer (26)	1974	—	9	0	5	—	—
Ireland and Newman (35)	1978	7.5	35	0	4	—	—
Salvati et al. (74)	1980	4.5	24	1	5	1	1 DU
Rao et al. (69)	1984	7.5	29	0	1	—	1 DU
Carlioz et al. (15)	1984	2.5 to 8.3	6	0	1	0	0
Total (%)			132	1 (0.8%)	30 (23%)	1 (1.7%)	3 DU (4%)
Epiphysiodesis							
Zahrawi et al. (95)	1983	6.6	28	0	0	1	2
Weiner et al. (92)	1984	≥1	169	1	0	4	0
Carlioz et al. (15)	1984	2.5 to 8.3	5	0	0	—	—
Irani et al. (34)	1985	—	48	1	0	—	—
Szypryt et al. (83)	1987	3.7	29	2	3	—	1
Ward and Wood (88)	1990	—	17	—	—	8	—
Schmidt et al. (76)	1996	3.5	40	0	0	3[b]	0
Rao et al. (70)	1996	2.3	46	3	2	1	0
Total (%)			382	7 (1.8%)	5 (1.3%)	14 (7%)	3 (1%)
In Situ fixation with a single central screw							
Koval et al. (43)	1989	2.9	67	0	0	0	—
Aronson and Carlson (3)	1992	3	50	0	0	1	—
Ward et al. (87)	1992	2.7	48	0	0	1	—
Total (%)			165	0	0	2 (1%)	—
Spica cast immobilization							
Betz et al. (9)	1990	4	37	0	5	1	—
Meier et al. (59)	1992	4.5	13	0	4	3	—
Total (%)			50	0	9 (18%)	4 (8%)	—

Note: In calculating the percentages, the denominator was the sum of only those series with available data.

AVN, avascular necrosis; DU, delayed union; —, data not available from study.

[a] Epiphysiodesis and osteotomy.

[b] Described as progressive coxa vara after physeal closure.

[c] Thirteen had both chondrolysis and AVN.

Table 172.2.   *Synopsis of Complication Rates with Different Treatments for Stable Slipped Capital Femoral Epiphysis (SCFE)*

Treatment method	Avascular Necrosis (%)	Chondrolysis (%)	SCFE progression (%)
Osteotomy			
Cuneiform	**13**[a]	16	3
Basilar neck	0	7	0
Intertrochanteric	1	**23**	2
Epiphysiodesis	2	1	7
Spica cast immobilization	0	18	**8**
In situ fixation with single central screw	0	0	1

[a] The treatment method with the highest complication rate for each complication is shown in bold type.

and it increases the risk of complications (e.g., joint penetration) (38,41). *In situ* epiphysiodesis does not give comparable results (2% AVN, 1% chondrolysis, 7% slip progression, 1% nonunion) and is also plagued with increased morbidity [e.g., blood loss, wound problems (hematoma/seroma, infection), longer operative time, larger incisions, failure of fixation, and further slippage]. For all these reasons, most surgeons presently recommend *in situ* fixation with a single central screw for all stable SCFEs (30).

Unstable SCFE

The results in the population of unstable SCFE are much worse, primarily because of the increased risk of AVN, up to 47% (52,82). If AVN does not occur, then the outcomes and results are similar to those of the stable SCFE.

PREOPERATIVE MANAGEMENT

STABLE SCFE

Once the diagnosis is made, do not allow the child to bear weight on the involved limb. The ideal treatment is immediate hospital admission, enforced bed rest, and next-day surgery. There is no need or role for preoperative traction. The goal is to obtain epiphyseal fixation before the SCFE can become unstable. However, it is often difficult to convince the family, and especially insurance companies, that this is a medical urgency. If such immediate procedures cannot be done, keep the child strictly nonweight-bearing; strongly counsel regarding the concerns

of walking, running, or falls that might create an unstable SCFE; and rapidly schedule stabilization in the next few days. Waiting several weeks for an opening on an elective surgical schedule is inappropriate management.

UNSTABLE SCFE

The controversies with unstable SCFEs concern the timing of surgical stabilization and the use of preoperative traction (5,82). If an unstable SCFE resembles a displaced femoral neck fracture in a young adult in terms of concerns about AVN, then an immediate anatomic reduction should be obtained (closed, or open if necessary), and the hip joint decompressed to relieve intracapsular pressure, all in the hopes of reducing the risk of AVN. However, the present data are inadequate to either support or refute this approach. My approach is to admit the child and schedule surgery within the next 24 hours. Some advocate keeping the child at bed rest for 1 or 2 weeks; this allows the joint to quiet down, early healing to occur, and a more stable situation to develop (5). Here again, the data are lacking to either support or refute this approach.

If surgery is scheduled within the next few days, the next question concerns preoperative traction (either skin or skeletal) (21). The proponents of gentle preoperative traction argue that it allows a gradual reduction in the hopes of reducing the risk of AVN. Again, the data are inadequate to answer the question. If traction is used, the hip should be flexed. Extension decreases intracapsular volume, makes the child more uncomfortable, and theoretically increases the risk of AVN. My approach is to keep the child comfortably positioned in bed with pillows and other supports until surgery.

PREOPERATIVE PLANNING

Take adequate AP and lateral radiographs of both hips to ensure that a contralateral SCFE is not missed. This is especially important when *in situ* fixation with a single screw is the selected treatment, because both hips should be treated under one anesthetic.

IN SITU FIXATION

No further special preoperative planning is needed for *in situ* fixation. The position and length of the cannulated screw is determined intraoperatively.

EPIPHYSIODESIS

Only adequate preoperative radiographs are needed.

PROXIMAL FEMORAL OSTEOTOMY

Proximal femoral osteotomy can be performed at several locations: (a) physis (Fish or Dunn cuneiform osteotomy); (b) basilar neck (e.g., Abraham); and (c) intertrochanteric/subtrochanteric level (Southwick, Müller osteotomy) (Fig. 172.2.). The physeal osteotomy is at the level of pathology and allows for maximal correction (20,25,65). Its serious disadvantage is a high rate of AVN. The few studies with low AVN rates indicate that its success depends on the individual surgeon (15,25). The object of the basilar neck osteotomy is to reduce the risk of AVN by operating immediately distal to the entry site of the epiphyseal blood supply, yet close enough to the deformity for adequate correction (2,45). The intertrochanteric/subtrochanteric osteotomies are compensatory and introduce a distal reverse deformity (69,78). Their advantage is a low risk of AVN. However, they do not allow as much correction and are complicated by chondrolysis and fixation problems. Later joint replacement arthroplasty is more difficult because of the distorted proximal femoral anatomy (19).

If proximal femoral osteotomy is selected as the treatment, accurate preoperative planning is mandatory. Use paper tracing cut-outs and implant templates to ensure that the osteotomy is properly performed and that the necessary internal fixation is available. In certain circumstances, the fixation device can be preoperatively bent and only fine adjustments need to be made intraoperatively.

The surgical technique for the intertrochanteric osteotomy (Southwick osteotomy) is as follows:

■ Use a standard technique to obtain AP and frog-lateral radiographs of the pelvis incorporating the proximal femurs. Maintain the pelvis flat on the x-ray table and center the beam midline between the hips. For the AP film, maintain the hips in as neutral a position as possible by keeping the patellae pointing as straight up as possible. For the frog-lateral film, place the hips in maximal abduction and external rotation, with the knees flexed, the plantar surface of the feet facing each other, and their lateral surfaces resting on the table. Determine the osteotomy angles by marking the angular relationships of the femoral head to the shaft on the radiographs; use the opposite normal side for comparison (78).

■ The AP measurement determines the amount of varus deformity, and the frog-lateral measurement determines the amount of posterior epiphyseal tilting (Fig. 172.3*A,B*). The difference in the epiphyseal–shaft angle on the AP view determines the anterior osteotomy. (If there is bilateral involvement, use 145° as the normal angle.) The difference in the epiphyseal–shaft angle on the frog-lateral view determines the lateral osteotomy. (If there is bilateral involvement, use 10° as the normal angle of retroversion.) Mark the wedges of bone to be removed on both radiographs, and fabricate templates for intraoperative use (Fig. 172.3*C,D*). Southwick initially used tin for the templates, but any malleable material that can be safely sterilized can be used; I have found metallic suture wrappers to be helpful (Fig. 172.3*E*). The template outlines the size and shape of the bone wedge to be removed. Typical angles are 20° to 30° anteriorly and 45° laterally. A wedge of 25° typically cuts through two thirds of the femoral shaft, and a wedge of 50° typically cuts through one half of the femoral shaft. Never exceed 45° anterior and 60° lateral.

■ Next, plan the internal fixation. After obtaining paper tracings of the proximal femurs in both AP and lateral projections, draw the intended osteotomy on paper. Use overlay templates of the selected internal fixation device(s) to plan their appropriate position and length (e.g., length and angle of side plate and lag screw if using a hip compression screw system, or the length and angle of the blade plate if using a blade-plate system). Take care to ensure that the tips of the lag screw or blade plate do not violate the posterior retinacular blood supply or penetrate the articular surface. The length of the lag screw or blade plate is often much shorter than expected; preoperative planning is imperative to ensure that the appropriate selection of devices is available at surgery. Note that some sizes of lag screws or blade plates may be special orders. After osteotomy, the femoral head should appear erect in the acetabulum in the AP view, and at a right angle to the long axis of the femoral shaft in the lateral view.

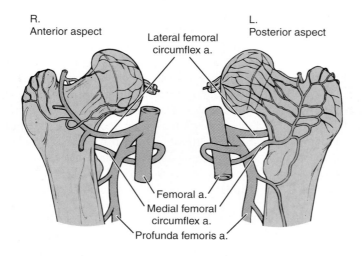

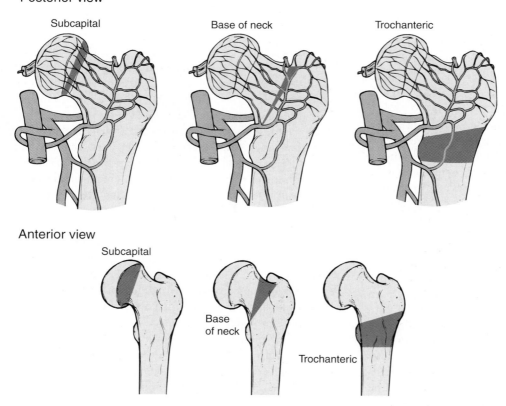

Figure 172.2. The three osteotomy locations for proximal femoral osteotomy for slipped capital femoral epiphysis as shown in both anterior and posterior views. These locations are subcapital, basilar neck, and trochanteric. The wedges of bone necessary for removal are different in shape anteriorly and posteriorly. On the posterior view it is noted that the vascular supply to the proximal femoral epiphysis enters the femur just proximal to the basilar neck osteotomy, whereas with the subcapital osteotomy the entry point of the vascularity is distal to the osteotomy which increases the risk of avascular necrosis with that osteotomy. The trochanteric osteotomy is safely distal to the entry point of the vessels into the femoral neck.

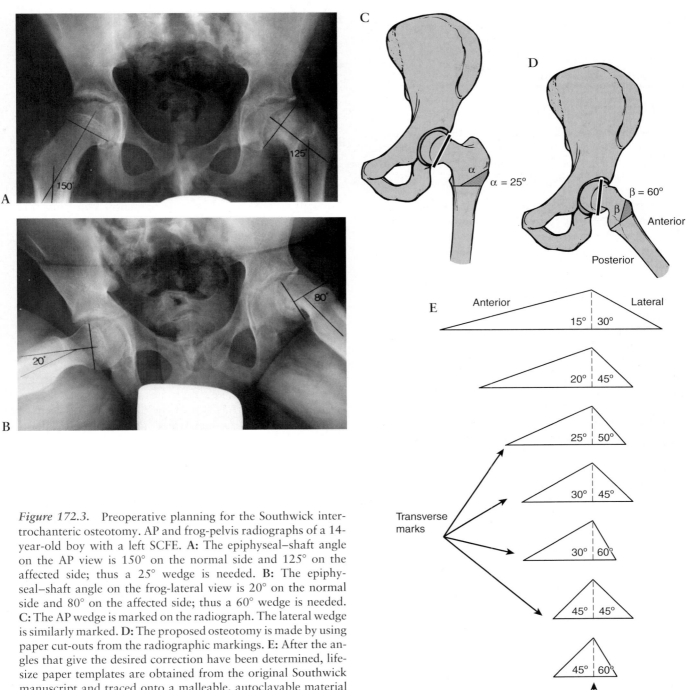

Figure 172.3. Preoperative planning for the Southwick intertrochanteric osteotomy. AP and frog-pelvis radiographs of a 14-year-old boy with a left SCFE. **A:** The epiphyseal–shaft angle on the AP view is 150° on the normal side and 125° on the affected side; thus a 25° wedge is needed. **B:** The epiphyseal–shaft angle on the frog-lateral view is 20° on the normal side and 80° on the affected side; thus a 60° wedge is needed. **C:** The AP wedge is marked on the radiograph. The lateral wedge is similarly marked. **D:** The proposed osteotomy is made by using paper cut-outs from the radiographic markings. **E:** After the angles that give the desired correction have been determined, life-size paper templates are obtained from the original Southwick manuscript and traced onto a malleable, autoclavable material (e.g., tin or a metallic suture wrapper). This template is then sterilized at the time of surgery.

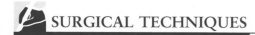

SURGICAL TECHNIQUES

STABLE SLIPPED CAPITAL FEMORAL EPIPHYSIS

IN SITU FIXATION

The most common stable SCFE surgical technique uses a cannulated screw system (3,48,62,87) (Fig. 172.4). In this technique, a single screw is placed into the center of the epiphysis in both AP and lateral planes.

- Position the patient supine on a fracture table, moving the image intensifier rather than the lower extremity. Take care when transporting the patient onto the fracture table; no reduction maneuvers are performed and forceful traction is not applied to the lower extremity. I use the fracture table only as a positioning device, allowing the involved limb to lie comfortably in its natural position of rotation.
- Place the opposite limb into abduction with the hip extended, and move the image intensifier into position between the two lower extremities.
- Prior to surgical draping, confirm the ability to obtain adequate AP and cross-table lateral images.
- Place a guide pin onto the skin overlying the proximal femur and obtain an AP image (48). Position the pin in the center of the epiphysis and perpendicular to the physis. Draw a line on the skin to record this guide pin position in the AP projection.
- Draw a similar skin line for the lateral image, again positioning the pin so that it is in the center of the epiphysis and perpendicular to the physis.

With an SCFE, the epiphysis is posteriorly displaced relative to the femoral neck, and the guide pin in the lateral projection angles from anterior to posterior. This is the opposite of femoral neck fractures, where it angles from posterior to anterior. Thus the two skin lines intersect on the anterolateral aspect of the thigh, and as the slip becomes more severe, the intersection point becomes more anterior. Because of the retroversion in the posteriorly displaced epiphysis in SCFE, the osseous entry point of the guide pin is on the anterior aspect of the femur. In mild SCFEs, it is often at the anterior intertrochanteric line; in severe SCFEs, it moves up onto the anterior femoral neck.

- Prepare and drape the anterolateral portion of the thigh. I prefer to use a transparent shower-curtain-type of isolation drape with multiple Kocher clamps on the base of the drape as weights; this allows movement of the image intensifier in both AP (Fig. 172.4*H*) and lateral (Fig. 172.4*I*) projections without violating surgical field sterility.

- Introduce the guide pin through the skin at the intersection of the skin lines; it may be introduced through either a stab wound or a small, 1–2 cm incision.
- Advance the guide pin onto the anterolateral cortex of the femur, keeping the drill and guide pin aligned according to the skin lines. Once the guide pin contacts the femoral cortex, its point of entry and angular direction is confirmed in both AP and lateral projections.
- When you are satisfied that the entry point and direction of the guide pin are correct, carefully advance the guide pin into the femoral neck, frequently checking the angle of entry on both AP and lateral images. Ideally, there should only be one entry point into the femoral cortex; extra holes act as stress risers and increase the risk of postoperative fracture. Do not advance the guide pin across the physis until you are certain that the pin will enter the center of the epiphysis perpendicular to the physis in both AP and lateral projections.
- After the pin has crossed the physis, advance the tip to the proper depth (no closer than 5 mm from the subchondral bone; any permanent pin position less than 5 mm from the subchondral bone increases the risk of joint penetration). This depth is determined on the lateral projection. Take care to ensure that the pin is not in the superior quadrant of the femoral head, because this position may jeopardize the epiphyseal blood supply.
- When the pin is in the appropriate position, determine screw length by placing another guide wire of identical length along the intraosseous guide wire and measuring the difference.
- Insert a cannulated screw in routine fashion after drilling and tapping. The screw should be at least 6.5 mm in diameter.
- While drilling and tapping, closely monitor the guide pin to ensure that it (a) does not break, (b) does not penetrate the joint and enter the abdominal cavity, or (c) does not withdraw from the femoral neck.
- After inserting the screw, remove the guide pin and confirm that the screw tip does not penetrate the joint. This can be done by one of several techniques: (a) move the limb in multiple directions in both AP and lateral views to confirm that it does not penetrate the joint, (b) use the approach-withdraw phenomenon, or (c) use intraoperative arthrography through the cannulated screw. My approach is a variation of the first technique. I obtain images of the hip every 10° to 15° while moving from a lateral to an AP projection, ensuring that the screw tip is no closer than 5 mm to the subchondral bone of the epiphysis. If it is closer than 5 mm, use a shorter screw.
- After confirmation of appropriate screw position and depth, close the incision.

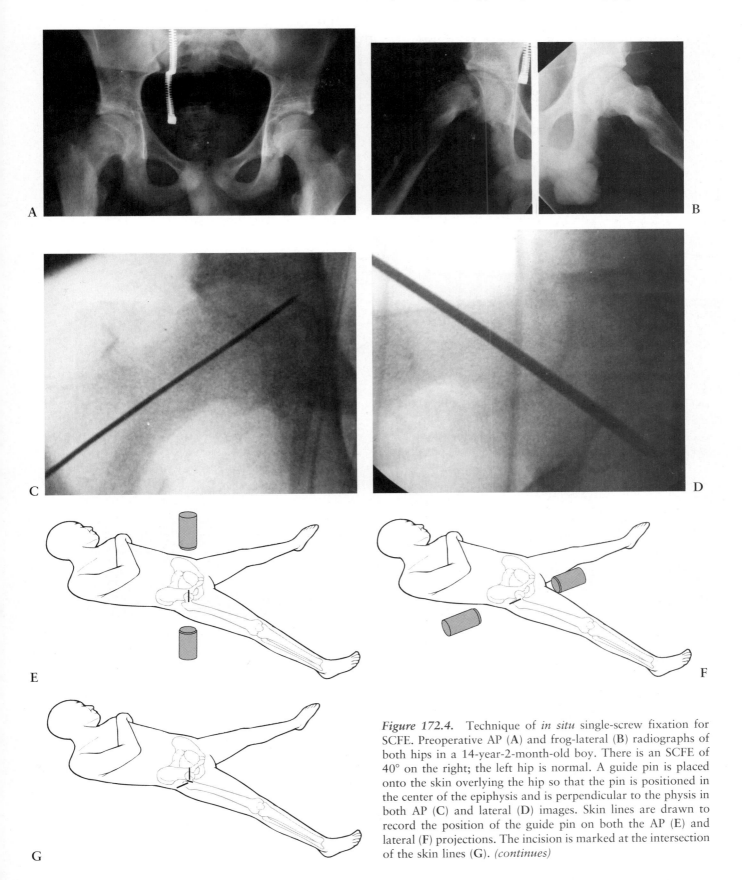

Figure 172.4. Technique of *in situ* single-screw fixation for SCFE. Preoperative AP (**A**) and frog-lateral (**B**) radiographs of both hips in a 14-year-2-month-old boy. There is an SCFE of 40° on the right; the left hip is normal. A guide pin is placed onto the skin overlying the hip so that the pin is positioned in the center of the epiphysis and is perpendicular to the physis in both AP (**C**) and lateral (**D**) images. Skin lines are drawn to record the position of the guide pin on both the AP (**E**) and lateral (**F**) projections. The incision is marked at the intersection of the skin lines (**G**). *(continues)*

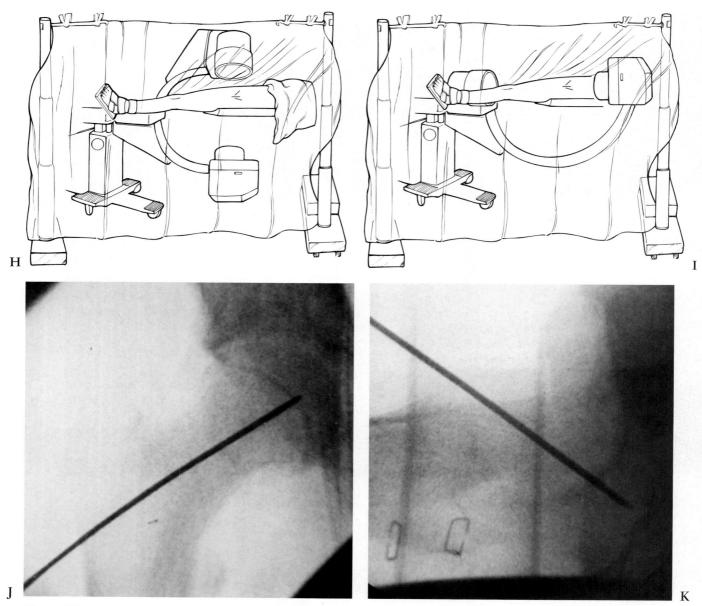

Figure 172.4.   (continued) After draping, multiple Kocher clamps are placed on the base of the drape to act as weights, which allows for movement of the image between AP (**H**) and lateral (**I**) images without violating surgical field sterility. The guide pin is advanced onto the anterolateral cortex of the femur so that the pin will enter the center of the epiphysis perpendicular to the physis. The guide pin is then advanced across the physis, and its tip is advanced no deeper than 5 mm from the subchondral bone [AP (**J**) and lateral (**K**) views]. *(continues)*

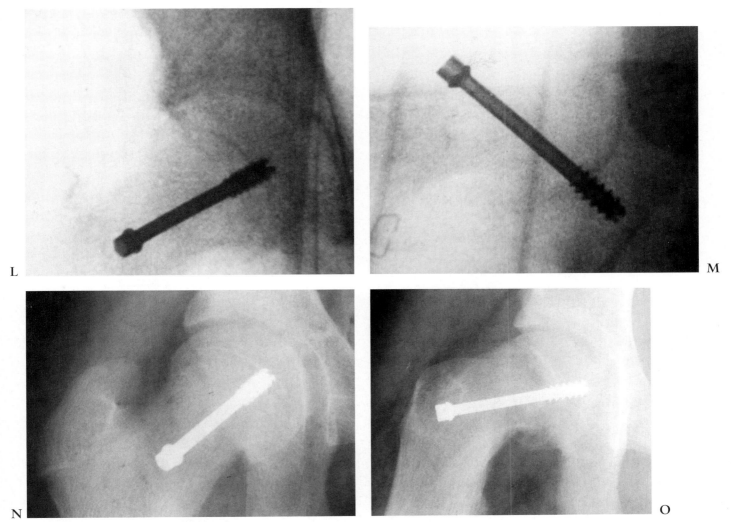

Figure 172.4. *(continued)* The appropriate depth of the pin tip is checked using the lateral image. A cannulated screw is inserted in routine fashion after drilling and tapping the hole (**L,M**). Postoperative radiographs demonstrate ideal screw position in the center of the epiphysis perpendicular to the physis in both AP (**N**) and lateral (**O**) projections.

EPIPHYSIODESIS

Open Autograft Technique with an Anterolateral Approach

The following technique is the Weiner (60) modification of the Hoyt-Heyman-Herndon procedure. The anterolateral approach (91) (Fig. 172.5) is now used instead of the older anterior iliofemoral approach (32). The advantages of this approach compared to the anterior approach are shorter operating time, less blood loss, easier instrument insertion, avoidance of lateral femoral cutaneous nerve injury, and fewer wound complications.

■ Position the patient supine on a radiolucent table.
■ Bump up the affected hip, and be sure you can obtain adequate AP and lateral images prior to surgical draping.

■ Prepare and drape free the entire lower extremity, hip, and iliac crest, as for a total hip arthroplasty.
■ Make a mid-lateral incision starting 4 inches below the level of the greater trochanter in the lateral midline of the upper thigh, continue the incision proximally to the greater trochanter, and then angle it obliquely to the anterior superior iliac spine.
■ Split the tensor fascia femoris proximally to the level of the anterior superior iliac spine.
■ Retract the tensor anteriorly and posteriorly, exposing the underlying gluteal musculature.
■ Retract the anteriormost fibers of the gluteus medius posteriorly to view the capsule.
■ Perform an H capsulotomy (Fig. 172.5A) and use retractors (large Cobra type) to expose the femoral head and neck; the area of slipping is now directly in view.

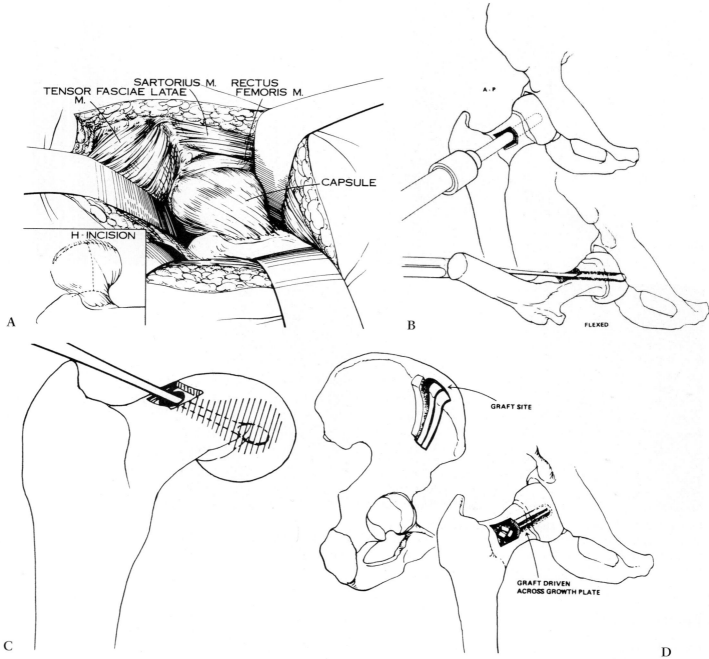

Figure 172.5.   Technique of open autograft epiphysiodesis. **A:** The exposure of the capsule and the H-shaped capsulotomy. **B:** The hollow mill drill used to create a tunnel across the physis. **C:** A curet is used to further enlarge the opening in the physis. **D:** Iliac crest bone graft is made into a sandwich and driven across the physis. (Parts A,C from Melby A, Hoyt WA Jr, Weiner DS. Treatment of Chronic Slipped Capital Femoral Epiphysis by Bone-Graft Epiphysiodesis. *J Bone Joint Surg Am* 1980;62:119, with permission. Parts B,D from Weiner DS, Weiner S, Melby A, Hoyt WA Jr. A 30-Year Experience with Bone Graft Epiphysiodesis in the Treatment of Slipped Capital Femoral Epiphysiodesis. *J Pediatr Orthop* 1984;4:145, with permission.)

■ Make a rectangular or square window in the femoral neck and insert a large hollow mill drill through this window. Under image control, drill the hollow mill across the physis into the epiphysis (Fig. 172.5*B*).

■ Remove a cylindrical core consisting of metaphyseal bone, physis, and epiphyseal bone.

■ Enlarge the cylindrical tunnel further by curettage, removing more of the physis (Fig. 172.5*C*).

■ Expose the outer table of the ilium, removing sections of corticocancellous bone, which are packaged together in sandwich fashion and driven into the epiphysis across the physis as a composite peg (Fig. 172.5*D*).

■ Perform routine closure.

■ In unstable cases, apply a bilateral hip spica cast with the epiphysis in the reduced position.

Percutaneous Allograft Technique

This technique, known as the Schmidt procedure, is similar to that of *in situ* fixation using a single central screw (76).

■ Position the patient supine on a fracture table with the involved hip in the neutral position and the knee extended.

■ Determine stability of the SCFE radiographically before sterile draping.

■ Gently mobilize the hip through internal rotation under the image intensifier. If the epiphysis moves relative to the metaphysis, the slip is considered to be unstable.

■ At this point, gently position the involved hip in 10° to 15° of abduction and with internal rotation such that the femoral neck is parallel to the floor. This position allows for a true anterior and lateral view with the image intensifier. A forced reduction maneuver is never performed.

■ After prepping and draping using an isolation drape, determine the guide pin entry point by the intersection of two skin lines using the same technique as *in situ* single-screw fixation.

■ Introduce the guide pin through a stab incision at the intersection of the skin lines, and advance it onto the anterolateral cortex of the femur. The ideal bone entry position for the guide pin is just below the greater trochanteric physis and above the thick cortical bone of the femoral shaft to avoid creating a stress riser in the subtrochanteric region.

■ Confirm the point of entry and angular direction of the guide pin in both AP and lateral views.

■ Carefully advance the guide pin into the femoral neck; it should not be advanced across the physis until confirmation that it will enter the center of the epiphysis perpendicular to the physis in both AP and lateral projections. Avoid placement of the pin into the anterolateral region of the epiphysis or traversing the posterior or inferior cortex of the femoral neck; either of these may injure the vascular supply of the proximal epiphysis and result in AVN.

■ After the pin has crossed the physis, advance the tip to the proper depth, stopping within 2 mm of the subchondral bone but not penetrating the joint. This depth is determined on the lateral projection.

■ Now place a second guide pin parallel to the first. This second guide pin secures the femoral epiphysis during subsequent reaming. Place it in a position that does not interfere with reaming, usually inferior to the first pin. A series of movements of the lower extremity in combination with movements of the image intensifier through its full arc of motion ensures no aberrantly placed pins.

■ Measure the centrally placed guide pin, and place a 10 mm cannulated reamer over it.

■ Drill the femoral neck over the guide pin to a depth of about 10 mm beyond the physis, but no closer than 2 mm to the subchondral bone.

■ Set the drill on reaming speed to avoid thermal necrosis. Drills more than 10 mm in diameter are not recommended; a 10 mm diameter is adequate to incite physeal closure.

■ Fashion a piece of freeze-dried irradiated cortical strut allograft to the appropriate dimensions using a high-speed burr. The approximate size of prepared allograft is $10 \times 5 \times 85$ mm. This strut graft should pass through the tissue protector apparatus of the 10 mm drill with some resistance.

■ Remove the guide pin, and pass the allograft through the hole and across the physis at least 1 cm.

■ Trim any allograft protruding beyond the drill hole in the femoral cortex flush with the cortex.

■ Remove the second guide pin stabilizing the epiphysis, and close the wound in routine fashion.

■ If the SCFE is deemed to be unstable, apply a spica cast.

PROXIMAL FEMORAL OSTEOTOMY

Physeal Osteotomy

I have had no experience with any of the physeal osteotomies, but two procedures are included here for the sake of completeness. With either the open reduction procedure of Dunn or the cuneiform osteotomy of Fish, a complete anatomic reduction can be achieved, although coxa breva will occur. Note that there is a high risk of AVN with these procedures.

Dunn Procedure The Dunn procedure, an open reduction of the severe SCFE, is popular in the United Kingdom and other countries with a British orthopaedic influence (13,22). An absolute prerequisite for this procedure is an open physis. The indications for this procedure in Dunn's original paper were a chronic SCFE of more than one-third the diameter of the physis, or an acute-on-chronic SCFE radiographically demonstrated by the presence of new bone along the posterior aspect of the metaphysis.

- Place the patient in the lateral decubitus position with the involved extremity up.
- Prepare and drape free the entire lower extremity, hip, and iliac crest area as for a total hip arthroplasty.
- Make an incision over the proximal part of the lateral femoral shaft, across the greater trochanter, and into the buttock.
- Incise the fascia lata and gluteus maximus in line with the skin incision.
- Define the anterior margin of the gluteus medius and drive a Jones bone spike between the glutei and the hip capsule.
- Similarly, define the posterior margin of the gluteus medius and drive a Jones bone spike between the abductors and the capsule.
- Divide the vastus lateralis 1.5 cm distal to its origin and elevate the greater trochanter through the trochanteric physis.
- Use sharp dissection to separate the muscles from the hip capsule.
- Retract the abductor muscles and attached greater trochanter proximally.
- Incise the hip capsule in the long axis of the neck and extend it around the anterior and posterior edges of the acetabulum (Fig. 172.6). The anterior capsular flap may be mobilized distally, but this must not be done with the posterior flap because the base of the posterior flap carries the blood supply to the femoral epiphysis.

- At this point, the subluxated femoral head is seen, as is the posterior surface of the femoral neck, which has a red, velvety appearance. The anterior femoral neck is pale and avascular (Fig. 172.6A).
- Incise the synovial membrane on the neck just anterior to the vascular area and around the anterior margin of the head.
- Strip off the posterior covering to the margin of the head down to the base of the neck. This dissection must be done sharply and without electrocautery.
- Slip a wide gouge into the plane between the physis and the femoral metaphysis. With gentle motion it will cut the physis, making it possible to lever the epiphysis off the neck. Once the epiphysis is detached from the metaphysis, it spontaneously reduces from its subluxated position and disappears back into the acetabulum (Fig. 172.6B).
- Now make two osteotomies. The first is in the long axis of the neck to remove the bony beak. The second is to shorten the neck a few millimeters (Fig. 172.6C).
- Make the second osteotomy with a slightly curved sweep, transverse to the top of the neck. This osteotomy removes the remains of the physis from the neck (Fig. 172.6D).
- Draw the femoral neck to one side and use a wide gouge to curet the remains of the physis from the epiphysis.
- Make a trial fit of the metaphysis onto the epiphysis; if there is any difficulty, further shorten the metaphysis

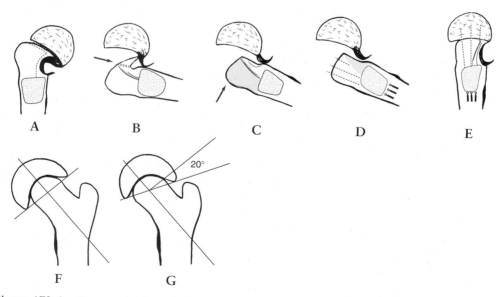

Figure 172.6.   Dunn procedure. See text above for a description of the technique. (From Dunn DM, Angel JC. Replacement of the Femoral Head by Open Operation in Severe Adolescent Slipping of the Upper Femoral Epiphysis. *J Bone Joint Surg Br* 1978;60:394, with permission.)

by another 1–2 mm and fashion it to fit the concave surface of the epiphysis.

- At this point, drill three threaded pins up the metaphysis, so that when the epiphysis is reduced they will engage the epiphysis in different parts (Fig. 172.6E).
- Now reduce the epiphysis and advance the pins into the epiphysis. After reduction, the epiphysis should sit squarely on the neck in the lateral view, and in 20° of valgus in the AP view (Figs. 172.6F,G).
- After radiographic confirmation of reduction and internal fixation, lightly suture the synovial membrane over the femoral neck and close the capsule.
- Reattach the greater trochanter with a screw and close the wound in a routine manner.

Cuneiform Osteotomy (Fish Procedure)   The indications for this procedure according to Fish (24,25) are an SCFE greater than 30° with an open physis.

- Position the patient on a radiolucent table in the supine position with a small bump under the involved hemipelvis.
- Drape the entire limb, hip, and iliac crest area as for a total hip arthroplasty.
- Approach the hip through an anterolateral exposure. Dissect between the sartorius and tensor fascia femoris muscles, exposing the anterior capsule. The capsule must be generously exposed proximal to the acetabular rim for adequate visualization (Fig. 172.7A).
- Make a longitudinal incision in the anterior capsule, and extend it in an H fashion both proximally and distally. Carefully retract the capsule; no retractors should be placed around the femoral neck either medially or laterally.
- Identify the proximal femoral epiphysis; it usually is barely visible at the acetabular rim. The anterior projection of the metaphysis is quite obvious and can be mistaken for the capital femoral epiphysis. In a very severe SCFE, it may be necessary to remove a portion of the metaphysis to visualize the epiphysis.
- Next, identify the location of the physis and determine its plane by gentle probing with a Keith needle.
- Determine the size of wedge to be removed by the degree of the slip and position of the epiphysis (Fig. 172.7B).
- Remove enough bone to allow an effortless anatomic reduction of the epiphysis on the metaphysis. A larger wedge is needed in a more severe SCFE. The base of the wedge must be in the plane of anticipated correction of the epiphysis, and the curved contour of the physis should match the corresponding curved metaphyseal neck.
- Gently remove the wedge in small pieces with an osteotome and mallet. Maintain continuous identification of the physis.

- Use extreme caution when approaching the posterior aspect of the neck. The posterior periosteum must be protected and preserved to avoid vascular damage.
- Remove the posterior bone (a curet is usually used), and use a large curet to remove any remaining physis (Fig. 172.7C). Once sufficient posterior bone has been removed, the epiphysis will effortlessly reduce with flexion, abduction, and internal rotation of the limb. If inadequate posterior bone has been removed, undue tension will be placed on the posterior periosteum, potentially compromising epiphyseal vascularity.
- Once an anatomic reduction has been obtained, achieve fixation with three or four threaded pins directed toward the center of the femoral head and only deep enough to obtain firm epiphyseal fixation (Fig. 172.7D).
- Confirm the position of the pins and epiphysis radiographically and perform routine closure.

Basilar Neck Osteotomy

The basilar neck osteotomy is theoretically safer than at the physis because it is performed just distal to the entry of the posterior retinacular vessels. It may be either intracapsular (the Kramer technique) (45) or extracapsular (the Barmada/Abraham technique) (2,6). The maximum amount of correction is less than with a physeal osteotomy, usually no more than 55°.

Intracapsular Osteotomy (Kramer Technique)   Kramer's indications are an SCFE greater than 40° on either the AP or the lateral radiographic view.

- Approach the hip laterally with an incision starting 2 cm distal and lateral to the anterosuperior iliac spine, curving distally and posteriorly over the greater trochanter and lateral femoral shaft to a point 10 cm distal to the base of the greater trochanter.
- Incise the fascia lata longitudinally and develop the interval between the gluteus medius and the tensor fascia lata. This dissection should be carried proximally to the inferior branch of the superior gluteal nerve, which innervates the tensor fascia lata.
- Open the hip capsule anteriorly along the anterosuperior surface of the femoral neck, and widely release it along the anterior intertrochanteric line.
- Reflect the vastus lateralis distally, exposing the base of the greater trochanter and the proximal femoral shaft.
- The margin between the articular cartilage of the femoral epiphysis and the callus, as well as the junction of the callus with the normal cortex of the femoral neck, can now be seen. Compare the distance between these two junctions with the amount calculated preoperatively from the radiographs. The widest part of the wedge will be in line with the widest portion of the slipped epiphysis, in the anterior and superior aspects

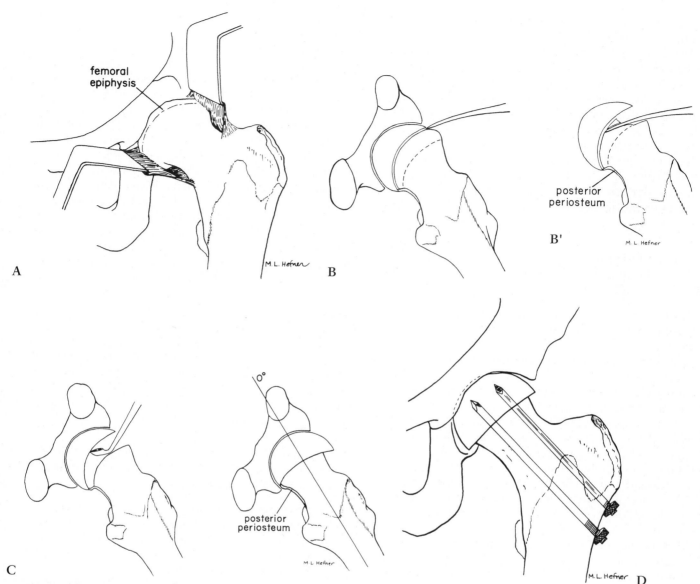

Figure 172.7.   Cuneiform osteotomy of Fish. **A:** Exposure of the femoral metaphysis. Note the minimal amount of the epiphysis that is initially seen. **B:** Location of the physis using a small curved osteotome. **B′:** The osteotomy is made by removing small pieces of bone with a sharp osteotome and mallet. The fragments are wiped away while being removed to ensure continuous identification of the physis. **C:** Further removal of the physeal cartilage with a curet, and then reduction of the epiphysis on the metaphysis. The diameter of the head is larger than that of the neck after removal of the bone wedge; thus the epiphysis overlaps the neck. **D:** After reduction of the epiphysis, it is fixed with three or four threaded pins. Note how much more of the articular surface is now visible compared to the preoperative situation (**A**). (From Fish JB. Cuneiform Osteotomy of the Femoral Neck in the Treatment of Slipped Capital Femoral Epiphysis. *J Bone Joint Surg Am* 1984;66:1153, with permission.)

of the neck. The most common mistake is to make the superior portion of the wedge too small, resulting in incomplete correction of the varus; if the anterior wedge is too wide, overcorrection of retroversion occurs.

- Make the distal osteotomy first, perpendicular to the femoral neck and following the anterior intertrochanteric line from proximal to distal. The cut should reach the posterior cortex but leave it intact.
- Direct the second osteotomy obliquely so that the cutting edge of the osteotome remains distal to the posterior retinacular blood supply. Anteriorly the capsule reaches the intertrochanteric line, but posteriorly the lateral third of the femoral neck is extracapsular; thus an osteotomy done at this level does not violate the posterior capsule and its retinacular supply.
- Before completing the osteotomy, drill one or two 5 mm, threaded Steinmann pins into the proximal fragment to ensure control of the osteotomy. The osteotomy is completed without penetrating the posterior cortex.
- Remove the bone wedge, and "greenstick" the posterior cortex, closing the osteotomy.
- Insert several 5-mm-diameter Steinmann pins from the outer cortex of the femoral shaft through the neck, across the osteotomy and into the epiphysis.
- Cut the pins to the appropriate length after radiographic confirmation of the osteotomy position and fixation.
- Close the wound in routine fashion.

Extracapsular Osteotomy (Barmada/Abraham Technique) The indication for an extracapsular osteotomy, according to Abraham, is an SCFE greater than 50°.

- Position the patient supine on the fracture table.
- Rotate the involved limb maximally internally by gently positioning the foot plate; abduct it approximately 5°.
- Widely abduct the contralateral limb, and place the image intensifier between the two lower extremities.
- Outline the patella with a marking pen and estimate the degree of fixed external rotation; most patients with a moderate or severe SCFE lack at least 15° of internal rotation.
- Prepare and drape the entire hip, thigh, and knee area.
- Make an anterolateral approach to the hip (Fig. 172.8A). Begin the incision at the anterosuperior iliac spine, and extend it distally and posteriorly to the anterior aspect of the greater trochanter and then distally along the proximal lateral femoral shaft.
- Longitudinally incise the fascia lata and develop the interval between the gluteus medius and tensor fascia lata.
- Locate the anterior joint capsule at the intertrochanteric line between the gluteus medius and the vastus lateralis.
- Using a periosteal elevator, elevate the anterior iliofem-

oral ligament from the anterior aspect of the femoral cortex (Fig. 172.8A).
- Gently place a narrow-tip Hohmann retractor around the superior aspect of the femoral neck superior and deep to the iliofemoral ligament; place another deep to the iliofemoral ligament proximal to the lesser trochanter.
- Plan the two-plane wedge osteotomy on the anterior surface by delineating a triangle based anteriorly and superiorly. The triangle base is usually 15–20 mm wide.
- Locate the proximal osteotomy by placing a 3-cm-long Kirschner wire (K-wire) on the anterior femoral surface from the lesser trochanter to the greater trochanter at the base of the neck and along the edge of the hip capsule (Fig. 172.8B).
- Confirm the position radiographically and mark the bone along the wire edge with an osteotome.
- After externally rotating the limb, drill a second K-wire just distal to the first wire in the AP plane, vertical to the femoral neck.
- Then internally rotate the limb and take a lateral image to confirm proper wire placement.
- The second, distal osteotomy line again starts from the lesser trochanter and goes to the physis of the greater trochanter. The angle this line makes with the first varies according to the amount of correction needed. A 15-mm-wide superiorly based wedge is usually needed.
- Make the osteotomy cuts with an oscillating saw (Fig. 172.8C), converging posteriorly to a single cortical cut.
- For maximal correction, remove the entire wedge of bone (Fig. 172.8D), especially superiorly.
- Internally rotate and abduct the lower extremity to close the osteotomy; maintain traction to prevent proximal femoral migration. Adequate correction is achieved when the patella can be internally rotated 15°. If the correction is inadequate, further bone may be removed from the metaphyseal side, but 20 mm of width anterosuperiorly is the maximum that should be removed.
- Now fix the osteotomy with three or four cannulated screws; only one screw need cross the physis to stabilize the slipped epiphysis (Fig. 172.8E). Avoid the superolateral quadrant of the femoral head when placing the transphyseal screw.
- Obtain permanent radiographs to confirm correction and internal fixation and then close the wound routinely.
- Reattach the iliofemoral ligament and capsule only if excessively elevated from the bone.

Intertrochanteric Osteotomy
The intertrochanteric osteotomy is the safest with regard to the risk of AVN, but it has an increased risk of chondrolysis in some studies (26,35,74,78,79). It is a compensatory osteotomy because of its distance from the level of pathology. This makes future total hip arthroplasty more

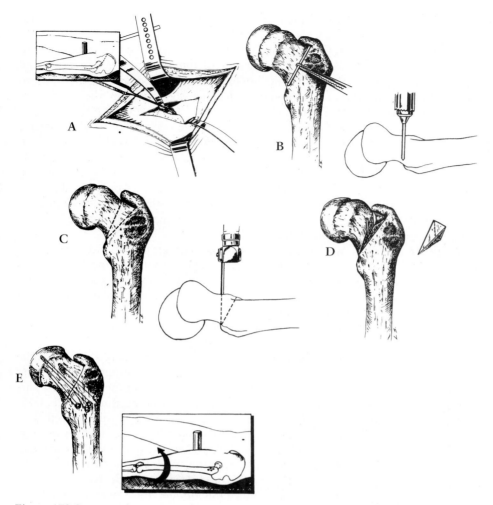

Figure 172.8. Extracapsular basilar neck osteotomy of Barmada and Abraham. **A:** A periosteal elevator is used to elevate the anterior iliofemoral ligament. *Inset:* The incision of the anterolateral exposure. **B:** The proximal osteotomy cut is determined by placing a 3 cm K-wire along the base of the neck. The correct site is scored with an osteotome after fluoroscopic confirmation. A vertically placed K-wire is drilled vertical to the femoral neck at the scored line. **C:** The distal osteotomy starts at the base of the neck inferiorly and extends obliquely along the intertrochanteric line to the greater trochanter. The proximal osteotomy starts at the same position distally and extends proximally so that a proximally based triangle is formed. **D:** The bone wedge is removed. **E:** The lower extremity is internally rotated and abducted to close the osteotomy site. Fix with three to four screws. (From Abraham E, Garst J, Barmada R. Treatment of Moderate to Severe Slipped Capital Femoral Epiphysis with Extracapsular Base of Neck Osteotomy. *J Pediatr Orthop* 1993;13:294, with permission.)

difficult (19). Because it is in the inter- and subtrochanteric areas, the risk of delayed union may be increased (69,74, 79); internal fixation is more difficult because of the zigzag deformity that is present after osteotomy. According to Southwick (79), the maximal amount of correction that can be achieved is 70°.

Biplane Trochanteric Osteotomy (Southwick Technique)
The indication for this procedure according to Southwick is an SCFE greater than 30°. This osteotomy corrects all three planes of deformity (varus, rotation, and flexion). The biplane osteotomy corrects the varus and adduction; rotation of the distal fragment relative to the proximal corrects the rotational deformity. Meticulous preoperative planning is essential (78,79).

- Position the patient supine on the fracture table with the affected limb draped free.
- Make a lateral incision 15–20 cm long along the posterior border of the greater trochanter.

- Incise the tensor fascia lata and vastus lateralis, and expose the femoral shaft subperiosteally.
- Identify the lesser trochanter; it can be brought into prominence by abduction and external rotation of the hip.
- Detach the psoas insertion from the lesser trochanter, taking care not to injure the nearby vessels or sciatic nerve.
- Identify the junction between the flat anterior surface and the slightly curved lateral surface of the femur; make a longitudinal mark along this junction using a sharp osteotome or oscillating saw. This mark identifies the anterolateral edge of the femur. It corresponds to the lateral (AP radiograph) and anterior edge of the femur (frog-lateral radiograph) used to make the intraoperative template.
- Next, make a transverse mark at the level of the lesser trochanter (Fig. 172.9A).
- Bend the previously made template, which consists of two right angles, at 90° and superimpose it on the

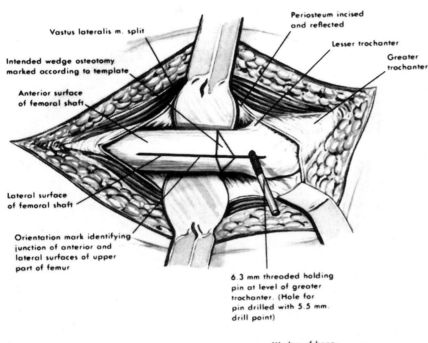

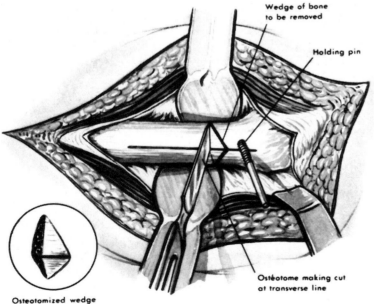

Figure 172.9. Operative technique of the Southwick intertrochanteric osteotomy. **A:** The osteotomy site is marked as shown. **B:** The osteotomy is made and the bone wedge removed. *(continues)*

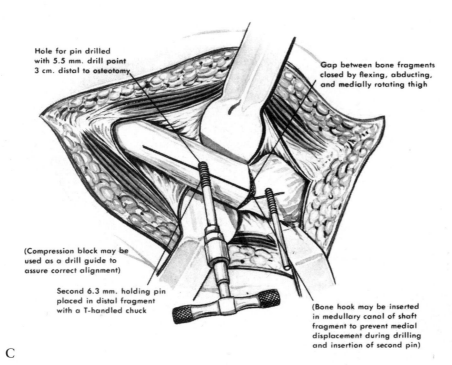

Hole for pin drilled
with 5.5 mm. drill point
3 cm. distal to osteotomy

Gap between bone fragments
closed by flexing, abducting,
and medially rotating thigh

(Compression block may be
used as a drill guide to
assure correct alignment)

Second 6.3 mm. holding pin
placed in distal fragment
with a T-handled chuck

(Bone hook may be inserted
in medullary canal of shaft
fragment to prevent medial
displacement during drilling
and insertion of second pin)

C

Figure 172.9.   (continued) **C:** The remainder of the medial and posterior transverse cut is made and, while controlling the proximal fragment with the pin attached to a T-handle chuck, the distal fragment is abducted and flexed, bringing the osteotomy surfaces together. The osteotomy is then internally fixed.

Postoperative radiographs (D,E) of the child in Figure 172.2 demonstrate fixation with a Southwick plate. The AP radiograph (**D**) demonstrates equal epiphyseal–shaft angles of 147°; the lateral radiograph (**E**) demonstrates a residual epiphysis–shaft angle on the left of 17° (34° − 17°). *(continues)*

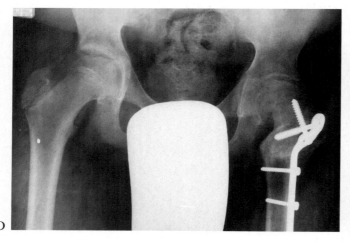

D

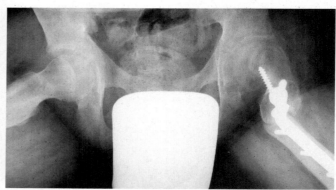

E

femur, with the hypotenuse of each triangle based proximally; they intersect at the longitudinal orientation mark.

- Wrap the template around the anterior and lateral surfaces of the femur and the outlines marked (Fig. 172.9B).
- Drill a 5.6 mm Haynes pin (or Schanz screw) into the greater trochanter parallel to the hypotenuse of the anterior triangle, starting about 6 mm proximal to the hypotenuse and directed toward the lesser trochanter. This pin is attached to a T-handled chuck and used to control the proximal fragment.
- Make the osteotomy following the template outline.
- Remove the wedge of bone, which consists of the lateral

and anterior femoral cortices. The proximal oblique surface is flat and angled by the amounts previously calculated in both sagittal and frontal planes (Fig. 172.9C).

- Make the remaining transverse cut of the osteotomy through the posterior and medial cortices at the level of the lesser trochanter.
- While stabilizing the proximal fragment with the pin, abduct the distal fragment and flex it to place the proximal oblique surface in contact with the transverse surface of the distal fragment (Fig. 172.9D). The orientation marks on both fragments should meet. As the osteotomy is closed, the two halves of the lesser trochanter separate, adding length to the limb. The combi-

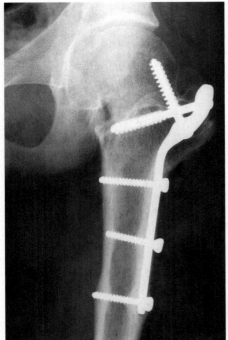
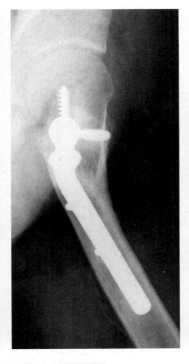
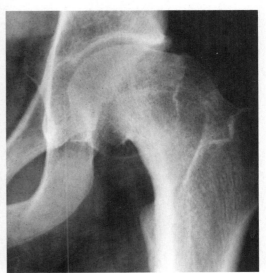

F,G
H

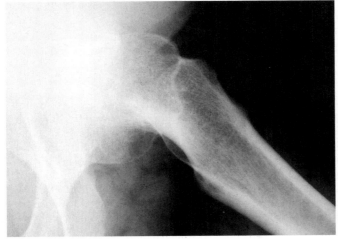

I

Figure 172.9. *(continued)* Radiographs at last follow-up (**F,G**) (child now 16 years old) demonstrate union of the osteotomy; note the remodeling at the osteotomy seen on the lateral views.

Fixation of a Southwick osteotomy with the more customary intertrochanteric lag/compression hip screw system (**H–M**). This 20-year-old man presented with a longstanding SCFE as shown on the AP (**H**) and lateral (**I**) views. The old SCFE deformity measured 82° using the lateral epiphysis–shaft angles (94° − 12°). *(continues)*

nation of posterior tilting and external rotation are related, so that internal rotation of the shaft relative to the proximal fragments is rarely necessary except in a very severe deformity. If the posterior SCFE is greater than 60°, then the distal fragment may need some additional internal rotation.

■ Now fix the osteotomy with the special side plate discussed by Southwick (79) (Fig. 172.9E), or with more typical intertrochanteric fixation (57,93) (either blade plate, compression hip screw, or dynamic compression plate) (Fig. 172.9F). Whatever method is selected, it must be appropriately templated out preoperatively using paper tracings and implant drawings. The operat-

ing room is not the place to first consider the method of fixation.

■ If the Southwick plate is used, apply it first to the posterolateral aspect of the greater trochanter using cancellous bone screws at least 5 cm long. The calcar should be engaged with at least one of the screws, and another one should be placed up into the femoral neck.

■ Next, attach the distal portion of the plate.

■ Apply compression at the osteotomy; use of a temporary compression device with pins while attaching the plate is often necessary.

■ If an AO blade plate is used, insert at least one of the

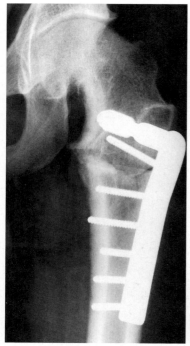
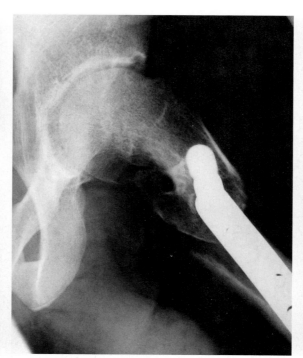
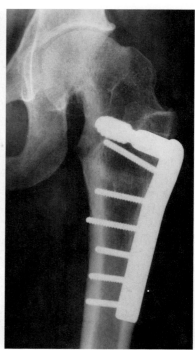

J,K

L

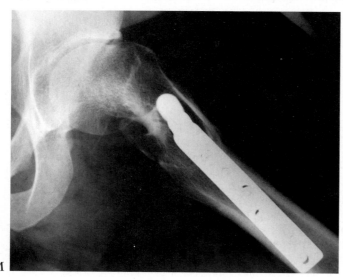

M

Figure 172.9. (continued) Immediate postoperative radiographs [AP (**J**) and lateral (**K**) views] demonstrate fixation with a hip screw system using a 95° dynamic compression plate. Note the short lag screw: It does not penetrate into the femoral head but rather into the proximal femoral metaphysis and neck, stopping just short of the calcar. The amount of correction achieved was 34°, with a final lateral epiphysis–shaft angle of 48°. The radiographs at last follow-up, at age 22.7 years, demonstrate osteotomy union [AP (**L**) and lateral (**M**) views]; again note the remodeling of the osteotomy in the lateral view. (Parts A–C from Tachdjian MO. *Pediatric Orthopaedics*, vol. 2, 2nd ed. Philadelphia: Saunders, 1990:1057, plate 37, with permission.)

screws attaching the distal fragment in compression mode using a standard AO technique.

■ Take final radiographs to confirm correction and fixation, and close the wound in routine fashion.

Biplane Trochanteric Osteotomy (Clark Modification of the Southwick Technique)

■ Use the standard exposure; make the transverse mark at the level of the lesser trochanter and the longitudinal mark at the junction of the anterior and lateral femoral cortices.

■ Mark the wedge to be cut using length measurements (18). Measure 15 mm proximal from the transverse mark along the longitudinal orientation mark and draw a line across the anterior shaft; this represents the anterosuperior wedge of bone to be removed (Fig. 172.10*A*). On the lateral surface of the shaft, measure 13 mm posteriorly along the transverse mark and draw a line from this point to the superior proximal line (Fig. 172.10*B*). This completed wedge is nearly the entire anterior surface and between a half to two thirds of the lateral surface of the shaft along the transverse line.

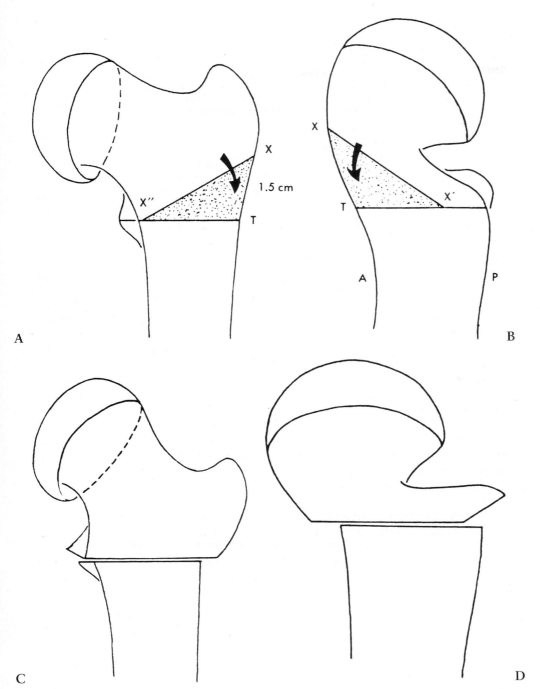

Figure 172.10. Clark modification of the Southwick intertrochanteric osteotomy. **A:** The transverse line is inscribed on the anterior and lateral surfaces of the femur at the level of the lesser trochanter (line $X'' - T$). Then a point X is measured 15 mm proximal from the transverse line along the longitudinal orientation mark. The line from X'' to X is then drawn, and the triangle $X''XT$ denotes the anterior wedge to be removed. **B:** Next, the point X' is measured 13 mm posterior to the longitudinal mark at the level of the transverse mark. The line from X to X' is drawn. The triangle $X'XT$ denotes the posterior wedge to be removed. The osteotomy is then made in standard Southwick fashion and the osteotomy closed. **C:** AP view after osteotomy. **D:** Lateral view after osteotomy. (From Clark CR, Southwick WO, Ogden JA. Anatomic Aspects of Slipped Capital Femoral Epiphysis and Correction by Biplane Osteotomy. *Instr Course Lect* 1980;29:90, with permission.)

- Then continue with the osteotomy in standard Southwick fashion, first making the oblique osteotomy, then the transverse cut, removing the wedge of bone, and then completing the transverse cut. The bone wedge that is removed should be large enough so that the upper oblique surface squarely fits on the lower transverse surface.
- Close the osteotomy (Fig. 172.10C,D) and perform internal fixation as previously described.

SURGICAL TECHNIQUES

UNSTABLE SLIPPED CAPITAL FEMORAL EPIPHYSIS

INTERNAL FIXATION

- Gently transfer the child from the bed to the fracture table after anesthesia induction. The induction of anesthesia removes the child's muscle spasm and guarding. This often results in a spontaneous, unintentional reduction of the slip with simple positioning of the child on the fracture table. I do not employ any intentional reduction maneuver unless the deformity is so severe that adequate internal fixation is not possible because of inadequate osseous contact between the epiphysis and metaphysis.
- Then proceed with cannulated screw fixation in the usual fashion. Place the first screw just as you would for a stable SCFE. The use of a second screw is controversial. Some authors advocate a second screw to control rotation and increase stability. Biomechanical studies do not show a two-fold increase in strength, and any screw off center axis has a much higher chance of joint penetration (38,41). Therefore, if a second screw is used, place it inferior to the first screw and with the final tip position at least 1 cm from the subchondral bone to reduce the risk of intraarticular penetration.

EPIPHYSIODESIS

The surgical technique is the same as that for a stable SCFE; the only difference is the application of a spica cast.

INTERTROCHANTERIC AND BASILAR NECK OSTEOTOMY

Intertrochanteric and basilar neck osteotomy procedures are contraindicated in the unstable SCFE.

CUNEIFORM OSTEOTOMY

Both Fish (24,25) and Dunn (22) will undertake their procedures in an acute-on-chronic SCFE as long as the other operative indications are met. There is no difference in the operative technique from that for a stable SCFE.

PROPHYLACTIC FIXATION OF THE OPPOSITE HIP

Prophylactic fixation of the opposite hip is controversial in North America, although it is more commonly accepted in Europe (31). In children with underlying endocrine or metabolic disorders (e.g., renal failure), prophylactic fixation of the uninvolved hip should be strongly considered (51,53). However, these types of SCFE are infrequent compared to the idiopathic SCFE.

In the idiopathic SCFE, the prevalence of bilaterality is 20% to 35% (49), with simultaneous presentation of bilaterality of 10% to 20%. Thus, if all children with unilateral SCFE have the opposite hip prophylactically fixed, 65% to 80% of these fixations will be unnecessary. This high rate of unnecessary surgery makes it difficult to recommend prophylactic fixation. There might be justification for prophylactic fixation to prevent an asymptomatic SCFE when patient follow-up is unreliable. The true incidence of asymptomatic SCFEs is unknown, as is the potential for the development of degenerative arthritis later in life. Also, it is not known if prophylactic fixation of these asymptomatic SCFEs will prevent the development of degenerative arthritis. Until this information is known, prophylactic fixation in the idiopathic situation should be approached with caution.

REHABILITATION AND POSTOPERATIVE PRINCIPLES

STABLE SLIPPED CAPITAL FEMORAL EPIPHYSIS

In Situ Fixation

Toe-touch weight bearing is allowed immediately after *in situ* fixation with stable SCFE (3,87). Discharge is often the same evening for a morning surgery, or the next day for an afternoon surgery. I recommend toe-touch weight bearing for 4–6 weeks; however, many children have no postoperative discomfort and it is not uncommon to see them return for their first postoperative visit 1–2 weeks later carrying their crutches! At the first postoperative visit, check the incision and obtain radiographs to ensure no change in fixation. The next visit is 4–6 weeks after surgery; obtain radiographs then also. Obtain both AP and frog-lateral radiographs of the pelvis so as to follow the opposite hip. After this time, allow normal activities except for running, jumping, and contact sports.

Counsel the child and parents to return immediately if there is any pain or loss of motion in either hip. Otherwise, return visits occur every 3 or 4 months, with repeat AP and frog-lateral radiographs of the pelvis, until complete physeal closure (50). After physeal closure, all physical activities are allowed. Screw removal is controversial. The morbidity and complications (incision, operative time, blood loss, fracture risk) for screw removal are much greater than for insertion.

Epiphysiodesis

Allow the child out of bed 48–96 hours after epiphysiodesis surgery and keep the child non-weight-bearing until physeal closure ensues. Full weight bearing is usually achieved by the tenth postoperative week (70,76,91).

Proximal Femoral Osteotomy

Dunn Procedure   Dunn (22) originally recommended 4 weeks of postoperative skin traction, with active range of motion exercises starting on the first postoperative day. Hip flexion to 90° should be achieved by 4 weeks. Then mobilize the patient with crutches; do not allow full weight bearing until radiographic union of the osteotomy, usually 2–3 months after surgery.

Fish Cuneiform Osteotomy   Keep the child in bed until comfortable and then allow the child up with crutches, with toe-touch weight bearing (25). Permit full weight bearing when there is radiographic evidence of osteotomy union, at an average of 5 months. Fish recommends pin removal; allow full activity 2 months after pin removal.

Basilar Neck Osteotomy   Kramer et al. (45) recommend partial weight bearing with crutches starting in the eighth postoperative week. Progression to full weight bearing varies according to the patient's weight, reliability, and generalized hip osteopenia.

Abraham et al. (2) recommend partial weight bearing with crutches for 6 to 8 weeks. Full weight bearing is allowed at 8 weeks. In the case of bilateral osteotomies, permit weight bearing as tolerated.

Intertrochanteric Osteotomy   Southwick (78) recommends bed rest with the limb in balanced suspension for 2 to 4 weeks. Keep the hip at 30° flexion. On the second or third postoperative day, allow the patient to sit at the bedside with support. Encourage mild active flexion of the hip and knee; when this flexion is comfortable and the wound is healed, allow non-weight-bearing with crutches.

Rao et al. (69) allow the patient to get out of bed on the first postoperative day and to walk with crutches without bearing weight on the third postoperative day. Start active range of motion exercises of the hip and knee on the seventh postoperative day. Permit full weight bearing when there is radiographic evidence of osteotomy union; physeal closure is not necessary for full weight bearing.

Müller (64) keeps the patient at bed rest for the first postoperative week. The limbs are held in abduction and internal rotation with the aid of boots and bars. On the tenth postoperative day, allow crutch walking with minimal weight bearing. Allow full weight bearing after 6 months.

UNSTABLE SLIPPED CAPITAL FEMORAL EPIPHYSIS

Screw Fixation

Allow the child to get up with crutches once she is comfortable (5,82). If there is any question regarding compliance or stability of fixation, I recommend the use of a wheelchair for the first 6 weeks. Maintain non-weight-bearing until early callus is seen at the slip. Once there is evidence of early healing, allow gradual and progressive weight bearing. This typically begins at 8–12 weeks. Progression to full weight bearing is usually achieved by 3–4 months after fixation. These children must be closely observed for the development of AVN; it will usually occur within the first 12 months after the slip. The remainder of the postoperative rehabilitation is no different from that of a stable SCFE.

Epiphysiodesis

In epiphysiodesis, a spica cast is applied, usually for 6–8 weeks. After cast removal, recommend non-weight-bearing until there is physeal closure. Full weight bearing is usually achieved 10 weeks after surgery (76,91,92).

Proximal Femoral Osteotomy

Dunn Procedure and Fish Cuneiform Osteotomy   The postoperative protocol is the same as for the stable SCFE.

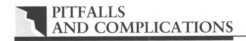

PITFALLS AND COMPLICATIONS

Table 172.1 shows the results, including complications, of treatment methods for SCFE.

AVASCULAR NECROSIS

Avascular necrosis usually occurs within the first year after an SCFE (52). AVN has not been reported in an untreated chronic stable SCFE. Its iatrogenic occurrence may be due to either realignment procedures (either closed reduction or proximal femoral osteotomy) or intraosseous vascular injury from internal fixation. Fixation that posteriorly exits the neck and reenters the epiphysis may dam-

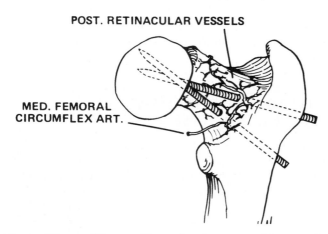

Figure 172.11.   Diagram illustrating the potential for vascular injury when internal fixation is placed posteriorly through the neck in an SCFE. (From Riley PM, Weiner DS, Gillespie R, Werner SD. Hazards of Internal Fixation in the Treatment of Slipped Capital Femoral Epiphysis. *J Bone Joint Surg Am* 1990; 72:1500, with permission.)

age the posterior retinacular vessels (Fig. 172.11) (71). Also, the superior weight-bearing quadrant of the femoral head is supplied by an artery that can be potentially injured by fixation devices (12). This may explain the high incidence of AVN when the fixation device is in this portion of the femoral head (Fig. 172.12). In the unstable SCFE, AVN is common and a result of the disease itself.

The long-term prognosis for AVN from SCFE is variable; many patients do reasonably well for some time. Degenerative changes gradually develop, but reconstructive surgery can usually be delayed until adulthood (44). In one series of 24 hips with AVN after an SCFE at 31 year follow-up, reconstructive surgery was required in four hips during adolescence and in five during adulthood. The remainder had not required reconstructive surgery but did show degenerative changes on recent radiographs. AVN from an acute unstable SCFE appears to be worse than that from a stable SCFE.

Avascular necrosis may either be segmental or complete (55). Treatment is difficult and there is no perfect solution. The first goals are to maintain joint motion and, as much as possible, to prevent further collapse. Relief from weight bearing is initially recommended. Unfortunately, healing of the necrotic areas may require a prolonged time, and most adolescents will not be compliant with prolonged non-weight-bearing.

Internal fixation may penetrate the joint and require removal if the collapse is in the area of the pin (Fig. 172.13). If the physis is still open, the epiphysis needs to be restabilized with appropriately redirected internal fixation. Further progression of a slip with concomitant AVN after hardware removal is a difficult problem that should be avoided.

After healing of the necrotic area, hip motion may be reasonably good if the AVN is segmental with no gross joint deformity present. With more extensive involvement, poor motion and pain may persist. In this case, there are multiple options to consider when medical therapy fails [e.g., nonsteroidal anti-inflammatory drugs (NSAIDs),

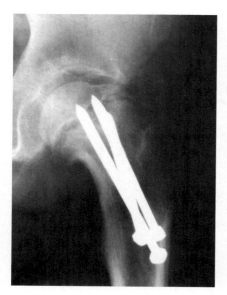
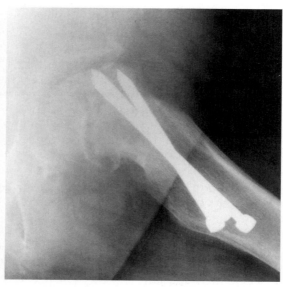

Figure 172.12.   The radiographs of a 12-year-old girl with avascular necrosis after pinning of a left SCFE. Note cluster of pins placed anteriorly.

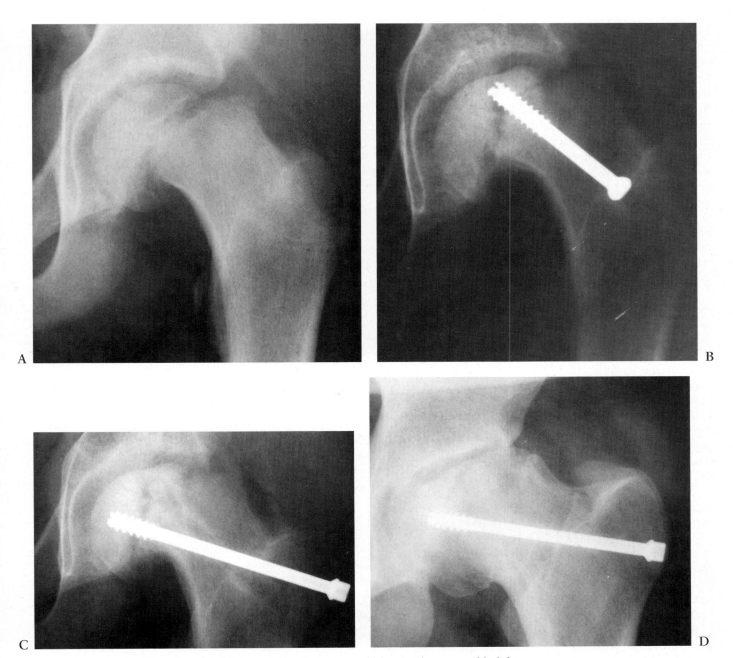

Figure 172.13. **A:** AP radiograph of the pelvis of a 14-year-old boy with an unstable left SCFE. **B:** Four months after fixation, the onset of avascular necrosis is apparent, and there is a concern for intraarticular screw penetration. **C:** The screw was removed and redirected in a different position. **D:** The last follow-up, 4 years after the initial SCFE, demonstrates physeal closure, partial joint incongruity, and a healed necrotic segment.

range-of-motion exercises, activity modification]. If hip motion can be improved by redirecting a noninvolved area of the femoral head to a more congruent weight-bearing position, then proximal femoral osteotomy may be considered. Another alternative is bone grafting the collapsed area to improve joint congruity (42,75) and

to provide further containment by femoral and/or pelvic osteotomy. Arthrodesis or total joint arthroplasty are considered if the hip is not salvageable. It must be remembered that these patients are young and heavy, which is a concern regarding the longevity of a total hip arthroplasty.

CHONDROLYSIS

Chondrolysis is an acute loss of articular cartilage in association with increasing joint pain and stiffness (54,58,89). Unlike AVN, chondrolysis can occur in the untreated stable SCFE. It may be aggravated by persistent intraarticular fixation or with spica casts. In the past, it was thought that black children and those of Hawaiian ancestry were more susceptible to its development (58,85); recent reports question this view (4,40,80). The exact etiology is unknown, although it may be an autoimmune process aggravated by the persistent pin penetration and secondary mechanical joint damage (63). Chondrolysis does not occur in all joints with pin penetration; however, its incidence is higher as the number of pins increases or they become closer to the subchondral bone (10). Transient intraoperative pin penetration that is corrected at surgery does not increase the risk of chondrolysis (96).

Chondrolysis usually appears within 1 year after diagnosis of the SCFE. Its clinical hallmark is severe loss of motion and pain in relation to slip magnitude. It is radiographically defined as a loss of more than 50% of the width of the weight-bearing portion of the articular space in children with unilateral SCFE (Fig. 172.14), or less than 3 mm width of the articular space in children with bilateral SCFE. When the diagnosis is suspected but there is no plain radiographic evidence, a technetium-99 methylenediphosphonate bone scan may be helpful (57). Marked periarticular uptake and premature closure of the greater trochanteric physis are highly predictive of future chondrolysis.

Once chondrolysis is diagnosed, it is incumbent on the surgeon to prove that there is no intraarticular hardware penetration (Fig. 172.15). If there is, the fixation must be removed and repositioned if the physis is still open. Occult sepsis must also be ruled out. The initial treatment for chondrolysis is rest, NSAIDs, and maintenance of joint motion by physiotherapy, traction, and protected weight bearing. In the refractory case, aggressive capsulotomy has been advocated (73).

The long-term outcome is variable. Up to 60% may do well with at least partial reconstitution of the articular cartilage and restoration of a clinically useful range of motion. In other cases, spontaneous ankylosis may occur. If spontaneous ankylosis occurs in an acceptable position, nothing further needs to be done. If spontaneous ankylosis occurs in an unacceptable position, then a femoral osteotomy below the ankylosis may be necessary to appropriately reposition the lower extremity in space. A painful, malpositioned hip often requires a formal hip arthrodesis (Fig. 172.14).

OTHER COMPLICATIONS

Other complications include slip progression, hardware complications beside joint penetration, femoral fracture, nerve palsy/injury, and nonunion or delayed union of an osteotomy or epiphysiodesis (71).

The incidence of slip progression in the stable SCFE is approximately 1% with *in situ* single-screw fixation; the incidence after epiphysiodesis is approximately 7% (Tables 172.1, 172.2).

If the internal fixation is left prominent from the cortical bone entry point, loosening of the screw due to a "windshield-wiper effect" can occur (56). A false aneurysm has also been reported with retained prominent hardware (33). Because of this, the screw head should not be more than 1.5 cm from the cortical surface. Sciatic nerve injury and septic arthritis are rare but described complications with internal fixation of SCFE.

Hardware breakage before removal was more common when smaller, multiple pins were used, especially when they entered the femoral neck posteriorly and reentered the epiphysis (Fig. 172.16) (71). It is less common with the single-cannulated screw and anterolateral placement. The hardware may also strip or break during removal, making complete removal impossible. This is much more common with titanium cannulated screws; in the young child with SCFE and hard bone, no titanium implants should be used (47,86).

Fracture of the femur may occur at the subtrochanteric, intertrochanteric, or neck level. Holes after hardware removal act as a stress riser and may lead to an intertrochanteric or subtrochanteric fracture. Fracture may also occur immediately after internal fixation if multiple starting points are made on the femur, even in the region of the femoral neck (7).

The Southwick osteotomy has a slight risk of delayed union or nonunion (69,74,79). This is not surprising when considering the low intertrochanteric position of the osteotomy in these obese children. With bone graft epiphysiodesis, there is a low but persistent incidence of epiphysiodesis failure.

SALVAGE PROCEDURES

Most salvage procedures are adequately discussed elsewhere [e.g., hip arthrodesis (8,11,14,67,81), total hip arthroplasty (19)]. Also see Chapters 105 and 106. For the rare case in which a trap door or other bone grafting procedure is needed for AVN, the reader is referred to the original manuscripts (42,75).

There are certain considerations regarding these procedures peculiar to children with SCFE. The most important is their young age and obesity. Union of an arthrodesis is more difficult because of obesity; a postoperative hip spica cast is recommended, even if rigid internal fixation is used. Arthrodesis after AVN is also more difficult, because of the lack of blood supply. If possible, both an intra- and an extraarticular arthrodesis should be performed.

The difficulties with arthrodesis in this patient popula-

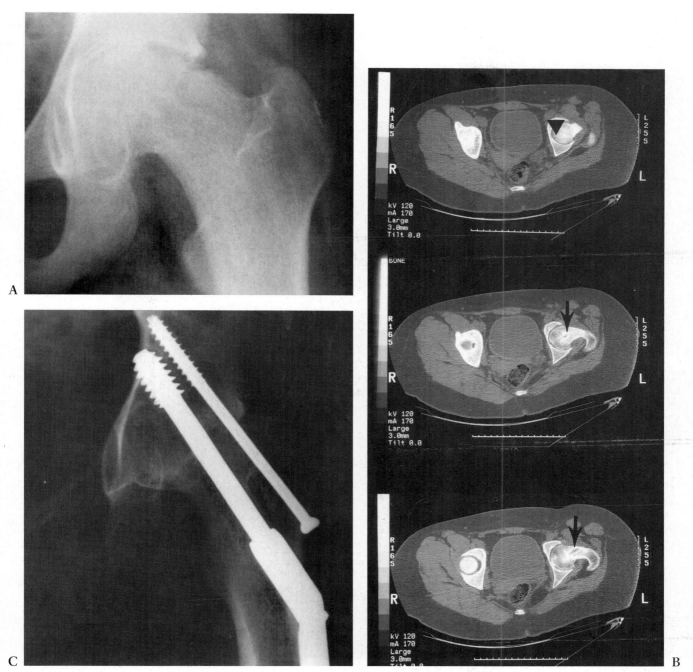

Figure 172.14. **A:** AP radiograph of the pelvis of a 13-year-old girl, 13 months after *in situ* fixation of a left SCFE. The radiographs with the fixation present were not available, and the single screw had since been removed. **B:** CT scan demonstrates the old screw track (*arrow*), with the tip being extremely close to the cartilage surface (*arrowhead*). The hip was painful and in an unacceptable position due to a marked flexion contracture. Conservative therapy was not beneficial and an arthrodesis was performed at age 14 years. **C:** Last follow-up at age 16 years demonstrated no pain, excellent ambulation ability, and a solid arthrodesis.

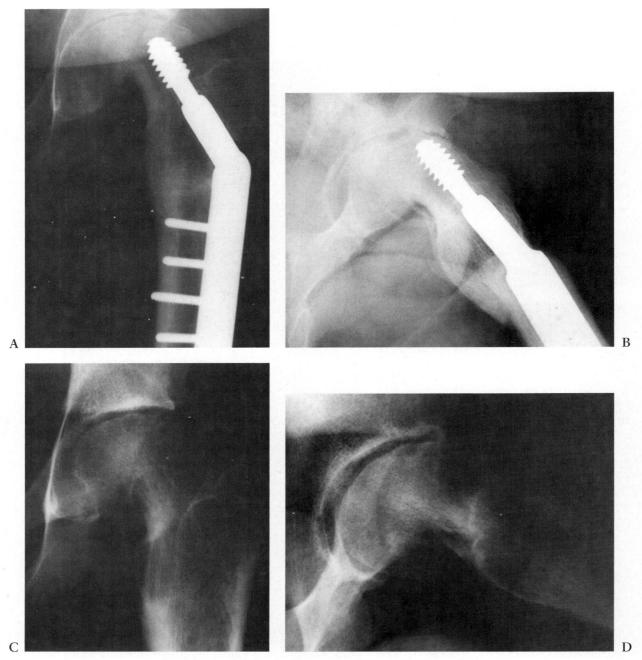

Figure 172.15. The AP (**A**) and lateral (**B**) radiographs of a 15-year-old boy who had undergone an osteotomy for a left SCFE 5 months before. He presented with increasing pain and stiffness. Note the joint narrowing and proximity of the lag screw tip to the joint. A CT scan confirmed intraarticular penetration by the lag screw. The hardware was removed. At last follow-up at age 18, his pain was completely gone and joint motion had improved. Note partial reconstitution of the joint space on both AP (**C**) and lateral (**D**) radiographs.

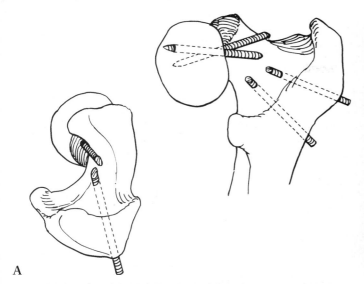

A

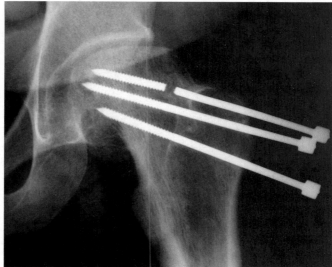

B

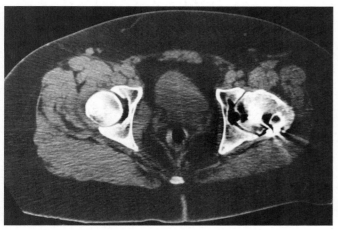

C

Figure 172.16. Broken pins in SCFE. **A:** Diagram showing how pins can break when they exit the femoral neck and then reenter the femoral head. **B:** The AP radiograph of the pelvis of a 23-year-old man who had an SCFE treated as a teenager with multiple-threaded Steinmann pins. Note the broken pin. **C:** The CT scan demonstrates the pin exiting the femoral neck and then reentering the femoral head. (Part A from Riley PM, Weiner DS, Gillespie R, Werner SD. Hazards of Internal Fixation in the Treatment of Slipped Capital Femoral Epiphysis. *J Bone Joint Surg Am* 1990;72:1500, with permission.)

tion makes arthroplasty more appealing. However, the risk of loosening and need for revision arthroplasty is likely to be quite high in these patients. Unfortunately, there are no published series specifically addressing the outcomes of total hip arthroplasty as the treatment for associated complications of SCFE.

REFERENCES

Each reference is categorized according to the following scheme: *, classic article; #, review article; !, basic research article; and +, clinical results/outcome study.

* 1. Aadelen RJ, Weiner DS, Hoyt W, Herndon CH. Acute Slipped Capital Femoral Epiphysis. *J Bone Joint Surg Am* 1974;56:1473.
+ 2. Abraham E, Garst J, Barmada R. Treatment of Moderate to Severe Slipped Capital Femoral Epiphysis with Extracapsular Base of Neck Osteotomy. *J Pediatr Orthop* 1993;13:294.
* 3. Aronson DD, Carlson WE. Slipped Capital Femoral Epiphysis: A Prospective Study of Fixation with a Single Screw. *J Bone Joint Surg Am* 1992;74:810.
+ 4. Aronson DD, Loder RT. Slipped Capital Femoral Epiphysis in Black Children. *J Pediatr Orthop* 1992;12:74.
# 5. Aronson DD, Loder RT. Treatment of the Unstable (Acute) Slipped Capital Femoral Epiphysis. *Clin Orthop* 1996;322:99.
+ 6. Barmada R, Bruch RF, Gimbel JS, Ray RD. Base of the Neck Extracapsular Osteotomy for Correction of Deformity in Slipped Capital Femoral Epiphysis. *Clin Orthop* 1978;132:98.
+ 7. Baynham GC, Lucie RS, Cummings RJ. Femoral Neck Fracture Secondary to *in Situ* Pinning of Slipped Capital Femoral Epiphysis: A Previously Unreported Complication. *J Pediatr Orthop* 1991;11:187.
+ 8. Benaroch TE, Richards BS, Haideri N, Smith C. Interme-

diate Follow-Up of a Simple Method of Hip Arthrodesis in Adolescent Patients. *J Pediatr Orthop* 1996;16:30.

+ 9. Betz RR, Steel HH, Emper WE, et al. Treatment of Slipped Capital Femoral Epiphysis: Spica Cast Immobilization. *J Bone Joint Surg Am* 1990;72:587.

! 10. Blanco JS, Taylor B, Johnston CE II. Comparison of Single Pin vs Multiple Pin Fixation in Treatment of Slipped Capital Femoral Epiphysis. *J Pediatr Orthop* 1992;12:384.

! 11. Blasier RB, Holmes JR. Intraoperative Positioning for Arthrodesis of the Hip with Double Beanbag Technique. *J Bone Joint Surg Am* 1990;72:766.

! 12. Brodetti A. The Blood Supply of the Femoral Neck and Head in Relation to the Damaging Effects of Nails and Screws. *J Bone Joint Surg Br* 1960;42:794.

+ 13. Broughton NS, Todd RC, Dunn DM, Angel JC. Open Reduction of the Severely Slipped Capital Femoral Epiphysis. *J Bone Joint Surg Br* 1988;70:435.

* 14. Callaghan JJ, Brand RA, Pedersen DR. Hip Arthrodesis. *J Bone Joint Surg Am* 1985;67:1328.

+ 15. Carlioz H, Vogt JC, Barba L, Doursounian L. Treatment of Slipped Upper Femoral Epiphysis: 89 Cases Operated on over 10 Years. *J Pediatr Orthop* 1984;4:153.

! 16. Carney BT, Weinstein SL, Noble J. Long-Term Follow-up of Slipped Capital Femoral Epiphysis. *J Bone Joint Surg Am* 1991;73:667.

! 17. Chung SMK, Batterman SC, Brighton CT. Shear Strength of the Human Femoral Capital Epiphyseal Plate. *J Bone Joint Surg Am* 1976;58:94.

18. Clark CR, Southwick WO, Ogden JA. Anatomic Aspects of Slipped Capital Femoral Epiphysis and Correction by Biplane Osteotomy. *Instr Course Lect* 1980;29:90.

+ 19. DeCoster TA, Incavo S, Frymoyer JW, Howe J. Hip Arthroplasty after Biplanar Femoral Osteotomy. *J Arthroplasty* 1989;4:79.

+ 20. DeRosa GP, Mullins RC, Kling TF Jr. Cuneiform Osteotomy of the Femoral Neck in Severe Slipped Capital Femoral Epiphysis. *Clin Orthop* 1997;322:48.

+ 21. Dietz FR. Traction Reduction of Acute and Acute-on-Chronic Slipped Capital Femoral Epiphysis. *Clin Orthop* 1994;302:101.

+ 22. Dunn DM, Angel JC. Replacement of the Femoral Head by Open Operation in Severe Adolescent Slipping of the Upper Femoral Epiphysis. *J Bone Joint Surg Br* 1978;60:394.

* 23. Fahey JJ, O'Brien ET. Acute Slipped Capital Femoral Epiphysis: Review of the Literature and Report of Ten Cases. *J Bone Joint Surg Am* 1965;47:1105.

* 24. Fish JB. Cuneiform Osteotomy of the Femoral Neck in the Treatment of Slipped Capital Femoral Epiphysis. *J Bone Joint Surg Am* 1984;66:1153.

+ 25. Fish JB. Cuneiform Osteotomy of the Femoral Neck in the Treatment of Slipped Capital Femoral Epiphysis. A Follow-up Note. *J Bone Joint Surg Am* 1994;76:46.

+ 26. Frymoyer JW. Chondrolysis of the Hip Following Southwick Osteotomy for Severe Slipped Capital Femoral Epiphysis. *Clin Orthop* 1974;99:120.

+ 27. Gage JR, Sundberg AB, Nolan DR, et al. Complications after Cuneiform Osteotomy for Moderately or Severely Slipped Capital Femoral Epiphysis. *J Bone Joint Surg Am* 1978;60:157.

! 28. Galbraith RT, Gelberman RH, Hajek PC, et al. Obesity and Decreased Femoral Anteversion in Adolescence. *J Orthop Res* 1987;5:523.

! 29. Gelberman RH, Cohen MS, Shaw BA, et al. The Association of Femoral Retroversion with Slipped Capital Femoral Epiphysis. *J Bone Joint Surg Am* 1986;68:1000.

+ 30. Goodman WW, Johnson JT, Robertson WW Jr. Single Screw Fixation for Acute and Acute-on-Chronic Slipped Capital Femoral Epiphysis. *Clin Orthop* 1996;322:86.

+ 31. Hägglund G. The Contralateral Hip in Slipped Capital Femoral Epiphysis. *J Pediatr Orthop* 1996;5B:158.

* 32. Herndon CH, Heyman CH, Bell DM. Treatment of Slipped Capital Femoral Epiphysis by Epiphysiodesis and Osteoplasty of the Femoral Neck. A Report of Further Experiences. *J Bone Joint Surg Am* 1963;45:999.

+ 33. Herndon WA, Yngve DA, Janssen TP. Iatrogenic False Aneurysm in Slipped Capital Femoral Epiphysis. *J Pediatr Orthop* 1984;4:754.

+ 34. Irani RN, Rosenzweig AH, Cotler HB, Schwentker EP. Epiphysiodesis in Slipped Capital Femoral Epiphysis: A Comparison of Various Surgical Modalities. *J Pediatr Orthop* 1985;5:661.

+ 35. Ireland J, Newman PH. Triplane Osteotomy for Severely Slipped Upper Femoral Epiphysis. *J Bone Joint Surg Br* 1978;60:390.

! 36. Jones JR, Paterson DC, Hillier TM, Foster BK. Remodelling after Pinning for Slipped Capital Femoral Epiphysis. *J Bone Joint Surg Br* 1990;72:568.

* 37. Kallio PE, Paterson DC, Foster BK, Lequesne GW. Classification in Slipped Capital Femoral Epiphysis. Sonographic Assessment of Stability and Remodeling. *Clin Orthop* 1993;294:196.

! 38. Karol LA, Doane RM, Cornicelli SF, et al. Single versus Double Screw Fixation for Treatment of Slipped Capital Femoral Epiphysis: A Biomechanical Analysis. *J Pediatr Orthop* 1992;12:741.

* 39. Kelsey JL, Keggi KJ, Soutwick WO. The Incidence and Distribution of Slipped Capital Femoral Epiphysis in Connecticut and Southwestern United States. *J Bone Joint Surg Am* 1970;52:1203.

+ 40. Kennedy JP, Weiner DS. Results of Slipped Capital Femoral Epiphysis in the Black Population. *J Pediatr Orthop* 1990;10:224.

! 41. Kibolski LJ, Doane RM, Karol LA, et al. Biomechanical Analysis of Single versus Double Screw Fixation in Slipped Capital Femoral Epiphysis at Physiological Load Levels. *J Pediatr Orthop* 1994;14:627.

+ 42. Ko J-Y, Meyers MH, Wenger DR. "Trapdoor" Procedure for Osteonecrosis with Segmental Collapse of the Femoral Head in Teenagers. *J Pediatr Orthop* 1995;15:7.

* 43. Koval KJ, Lehman WB, Rose D, et al. Treatment of Slipped Capital Femoral Epiphysis with a Cannulated Screw Technique. *J Bone Joint Surg Am* 1989;71:1370.

+ 44. Krahn TH, Canale ST, Beaty JC, et al. Long-term Follow-up of Patients with Avascular Necrosis after Treatment of Slipped Capital Femoral Epiphysis. *J Pediatr Orthop* 1993;13:154.

+ 45. Kramer WG, Craig WA, Noel S. Compensating Osteotomy at the Base of the Femoral Neck for Slipped Capital Femoral Epiphysis. *J Bone Joint Surg Am* 1976;58:796.

+ 46. Kulick RG, Denton JR. A Retrospective Study of 125 Cases of Slipped Capital Femoral Epiphysis. *Clin Orthop* 1982;162:87.

+ 47. Lee TK, Haynes RJ, Longo JA, Chu JR. Pin Removal in Slipped Capital Femoral Epiphysis: The Unsuitability of Titanium Devices. *J Pediatr Orthop* 1996;16;49.

* 48. Lindaman LM, Canale ST, Beaty JH, Warner WC. A Fluoroscopic Technique for Determining the Incision Site for Percutaneous Fixation of Slipped Capital Femoral Epiphysis. *J Pediatr Orthop* 1991;11:397.

! 49. Loder RT, and 47 Coinvestigators from 33 Orthopaedic Centers and 6 Continents. The Demographics of Slipped Capital Femoral Epiphysis. *Clin Orthop* 1996;322:8.

! 50. Loder RT, Aronson DD, Greenfield ML. The Epidemiology of Bilateral Slipped Capital Femoral Epiphysis. *J Bone Joint Surg Am* 1993;75:1141.

! 51. Loder RT, Hensinger RN. Slipped Capital Femoral Epiphysis Associated with Renal Failure Osteodystrophy. *J Pediatr Orthop* 1997;17:205.

* 52. Loder RT, Richards BS, Shapiro PS, et al. Acute Slipped Capital Femoral Epiphysis: The Importance of Physeal Stability. *J Bone Joint Surg Am* 1993;75:1134.

! 53. Loder RT, Wittenberg B, DeSilva G. Slipped Capital Femoral Epiphysis Associated with Endocrine Disorders. *J Pediatr Orthop* 1995;15:349.

+ 54. Lowe HG. Necrosis of Articular Cartilage after Slipping of the Capital Femoral Epiphysis. *J Bone Joint Surg Br* 1970;52:108.

55. Lubicky JP. Chondrolysis and Avascular Necrosis: Complications of Slipped Capital Femoral Epiphysis. *J Pediatr Orthop* 1996;5B:162.

+ 56. Maletis GB, Bassett GS. Windshield-Wiper Loosening: A Complication of in Situ Screw Fixation of Slipped Capital Femoral Epiphysis. *J Pediatr Orthop* 1993;13:607.

+ 57. Mandell GA, Keret D, Harcke HT, Bowen JR. Chondrolysis: Detection by Bone Scintigraphy. *J Pediatr Orthop* 1992;12:80.

+ 58. Maurer RC, Larsen IJ. Acute Necrosis of Cartilage in Slipped Capital Femoral Epiphysis. *J Bone Joint Surg Am* 1970;52:39.

+ 59. Meier MC, Meyer LC, Ferguson RL. Treatment of Slipped Capital Femoral Epiphysis with a Spica Cast. *J Bone Joint Surg Am* 1992;74:1522.

* 60. Melby A, Hoyt WA Jr, Weiner DS. Treatment of Chronic Slipped Capital Femoral Epiphysis by Bone-Graft Epiphysiodesis. *J Bone Joint Surg Am* 1980;62:119.

! 61. Mirkopulus N, Weiner DS, Askew M. The Evolving Slope of the Proximal Femoral Growth Plate Relationship to Slipped Capital Femoral Epiphysis. *J Pediatr Orthop* 1988;8:268.

* 62. Morrissy RT. Slipped Capital Femoral Epiphysis: Technique of Percutaneous in Situ Fixation. *J Pediatr Orthop* 1990;10:347.

! 63. Morrissy RT, Kalderan AE, Gerdes MH. Synovial Immunofluorescence in Patients with Slipped Capital Femoral Epiphysis. *J Pediatr Orthop* 1981;1:55.

64. Müller ME. Intertrochanteric Osteotomy: Indication, Pre-operative Planning, Technique. In: Schatzker J, ed. *The Intertrochanteric Osteotomy.* Berlin: Springer-Verlag, 1984;25.

+ 65. Nishiyama K, Sakamaki T, Ishii Y. Follow-up Study of the Subcapital Wedge Osteotomy for Severe Chronic Slipped Capital Femoral Epiphysis. *J Pediatr Orthop* 1989;9:412.

+ 66. Pearl AJ, Woodward B, Kelly RP. Cuneiform Osteotomy in the Treatment of Slipped Capital Femoral Epiphysis. *J Bone Joint Surg Am* 1961;43:947.

* 67. Price CT, Lovell WW. Thompson Arthrodesis of the Hip in Children. *J Bone Joint Surg Am* 1980;62:1118.

! 68. Pritchett JW, Perdue KD. Mechanical Factors in Slipped Capital Femoral Epiphysis. *J Pediatr Orthop* 1988;8:335.

+ 69. Rao JU, Francis AM, Siwek CW. The Treatment of Chronic Slipped Capital Femoral Epiphysis by Biplane Osteotomy. *J Bone Joint Surg Am* 1984;66:1169.

+ 70. Rao SB, Crawford AH, Burger RR, Roy DR. Open Bone Peg Epiphysiodesis for Slipped Capital Femoral Epiphysis. *J Pediatr Orthop* 1996;16:37.

+ 71. Riley PM, Weiner DS, Gillespie R, Werner SD. Hazards of Internal Fixation in the Treatment of Slipped Capital Femoral Epiphysis. *J Bone Joint Surg Am* 1990;72:1500.

+ 72. Ross PM, Lyne ED, Morawa LG. Slipped Capital Femoral Epiphysis Long-Term Results after 10-38 Years. *Clin Orthop* 1979;141:176.

+ 73. Roy DR, Crawford AH. Idiopathic Chondrolysis of the Hip: Management by Subtotal Capsulectomy and Aggressive Rehabilitation. *J Pediatr Orthop* 1988;8:203.

+ 74. Salvati EA, Robinson HJ Jr, O'Dowd TJ. Southwick Osteotomy for Severe Chronic Slipped Capital Femoral Epiphysis: Results and Complications. *J Bone Joint Surg Am* 1980;62:561.

+ 75. Scher MA, Jakim I. Intertrochanteric Osteotomy and Autogenous Bone-Grafting for Avascular Necrosis of the Femoral Head. *J Bone Joint Surg Am* 1993;75:1119.

+ 76. Schmidt TL, Cimino WG, Seidel FG. Allograft Epiphysiodesis for Slipped Capital Femoral Epiphysis. *Clin Orthop* 1996;322:61.

+ 77. Siegel DB, Kasser JR, Sponseller P, Gelberman RH. Slipped Capital Femoral Epiphysis: A Quantitative Analysis of Motion, Gait, and Femoral Remodeling after in Situ Fixation. *J Bone Joint Surg Am* 1991;73:659.

* 78. Southwick WO. Osteotomy through the Lesser Trochanter for Slipped Capital Femoral Epiphysis. *J Bone Joint Surg Am* 1967;49:807.

* 79. Southwick WO. Compression Fixation after Biplane Intertrochanteric Osteotomy for Slipped Capital Femoral Epiphysis. A Technical Improvement. *J Bone Joint Surg Am* 1973;55:1218.

+ 80. Spero CR, Masciale JP, Tornetta P III, et al. Slipped Capital Femoral Epiphysis in Black Children: Incidence of Chondrolysis. *J Pediatr Orthop* 1992;12:444.

+ 81. Sponseller PD, McBeath AA, Perpich M. Hip Arthrodesis in Young Patients. *J Bone Joint Surg Am* 1984;66:853.

82. Stanitski CL. Acute Slipped Capital Femoral Epiphysis:

Treatment Alternatives. *J Am Acad Orthop Surg* 1994; 2:96.

+ 83. Szypryt EP, Clement DA, Colton CL. Open Reduction or Epiphysiodesis for Slipped Upper Femoral Epiphysis. A Comparison of Dunn's Operation and the Heyman-Herndon Procedure. *J Bone Joint Surg Br* 1987;69:737.

84. Tachdjian MO. *Pediatric Orthopaedics*, 2nd ed. Philadelphia: Saunders, 1990.

+ 85. Tillemma DA, Golding JSR. Chondrolysis following Slipped Capital Femoral Epiphysis in Jamaica. *J Bone Joint Surg Am* 1971;53:1528.

+ 86. Vresilovic EJ, Spindler KP, Robertson WW Jr, et al. Failures of Pin Removal after *in Situ* Pinning of Slipped Capital Femoral Epiphysis: A Comparison of Different Pin Types. *J Pediatr Orthop* 1990;10:764.

* 87. Ward WT, Stefko J, Wood KB, Stanitski CL. Fixation with a Single Screw for Slipped Capital Femoral Epiphysis. *J Bone Joint Surg Am* 1992;74:799.

+ 88. Ward WT, Wood K. Open Bone Graft Epiphyseodesis for Slipped Capital Femoral Epiphysis. *J Pediatr Orthop* 1990;10:14.

+ 89. Warner WC Jr, Beaty JH, Canale ST. Chondrolysis after Slipped Capital Femoral Epiphysis. *J Pediatr Orthop* 1996;5B:168.

90. Weiner D. Pathogenesis of Slipped Capital Femoral Epiphysis: Current Concepts. *J Pediatr Orthop* 1996;5B:67.

* 91. Weiner DS, Weiner S, Melby A. Anterolateral Approach to the Hip for Bone Graft Epiphysiodesis in the Treatment of Slipped Capital Femoral Epiphysis. *J Pediatr Orthop* 1988;8:349.

* 92. Weiner DS, Weiner S, Melby A, Hoyt WA Jr. A 30-Year Experience with Bone Graft Epiphysiodesis in the Treatment of Slipped Capital Femoral Epiphysiodesis. *J Pediatr Orthop* 1984;4:145.

+ 93. Whiteside LA, Schoenecker PL. Combined Valgus Derotation Osteotomy and Cervical Osteoplasty for Severely Slipped Capital Femoral Epiphysis. *Clin Orthop* 1978; 132:88.

! 94. Wong-Chung J, Strong ML. Physeal Remodeling after Internal Fixation of Slipped Capital Femoral Epiphysis. *J Pediatr Orthop* 1991;11:2.

+ 95. Zahrawi FB, Stephens TL, Spencer GE Jr, McClough JM. Comparative Study of Pinning *in Situ* and Open Epiphysiodesis in 105 Patients with Slipped Capital Femoral Epiphysis. *Clin Orthop* 1983;177:160.

+ 96. Zionts LE. Transient Penetration of the Hip Joint During in Situ Cannulated Screw Fixation of Slipped Capital Femoral Epiphysis. *J Bone Joint Surg Am* 1991;73:1054.

## CHAPTER 173

LEGG-CALVÉ-PERTHES DISEASE

John A. Herring

INTRODUCTION

Legg-Calvé-Perthes disease is a form of idiopathic avascular necrosis of the femoral head. Although the exact etiology of the disorder is not known, the association of Legg-Calvé-Perthes disease with delayed skeletal maturation suggests a systemic susceptibility to the problem. Some children have abnormalities of coagulation with decreases in the factors involved in thrombolysis, which may predispose them to avascular necrosis.

The clinical course is quite variable, making it difficult for the clinician to know for certain which patients need and will benefit from treatment. Current use of the lateral pillar radiographic classification has improved our ability to assess severity and prognosis in an individual case. Children younger than 6 years of age at onset usually have a benign course, and major treatment is not often necessary because they have a longer growing time to remodel abnormalities. Children between 6 and 9 years of age at onset have more symptoms and often benefit from surgical treatment. Children older than 9 years of age have a more severe course, and their response to treatment is less predictable. In the long run, 50% of patients have no disability as adults and the other half develop degenerative hip disease by the fifth or sixth decade of life.

Treatment has been based on the containment principle, which means positioning the femoral head within the acetabulum in such a way as to reduce lateralization and collapse of the softened head. In the past, this was done with braces, but at present, femoral or pelvic osteotomies are preferred.

COURSE OF DISEASE AND NATURAL HISTORY

The initial events in the course of Legg-Calvé-Perthes disease are well established. The femoral head becomes ischemic for reasons unknown and for an unknown period of time. Several studies suggest that at least two episodes of ischemia are necessary to produce the typical changes of Legg-Calvé-Perthes disease (7,27). More recent studies have shown that a number of children have deficiencies of proteins S and C and hypofibrinolysis (8,9). The original studies suggested that the majority of children were deficient in these factors, but subsequent reports have found only a small proportion patients with Legg-Calvé with these coagulopathies (14).

J. A. Herring: Chief of Staff, Department of Orthopaedics, Texas Scottish Rite Hospital for Children, Dallas, Texas, 75219.

Following the ischemic episode, the femoral head becomes radiodense, then appears fragmented radiographically as dead bone is resorbed, and finally reossifies with new bone formation. These sequential phases have been classified by Waldenström (30) as increased density, fragmentation, reossification, and residual stages. No treatment to date has been shown to either accelerate or delay the healing process, although it was initially thought that femoral osteotomy resulted in more rapid healing. This was disproved in studies by Clancy and Steel (4) and Kendig and Evans (15). During the fragmentation phase in more severe disease, the head loses height, enlarges, and may flatten. As the head enlarges, the anterior and lateral portions of the head extrude from the acetabulum. Over several years, the femoral head completely reossifies and may remain round in mild cases, become ovoid in moderate cases, and become flattened in severe cases. Stulberg and colleagues (29) classified these groups according to femoral head status as:

- group I   normal head
- group II   round head
- group III   ovoid head and acetabulum
- group IV   flattened head and acetabulum
- group V   head collapsed and acetabulum failed to remodel

The prognosis for a child with Legg-Calvé-Perthes disease can be estimated to some degree. The most frequently reported prognostic factor is the age of the child at the onset of the disease. Most, but not all, children presenting at younger than 6 years of age have a good prognosis, whereas those between 6 and 9 years of age have a variable course. Children older than 9 years of age presenting with Legg-Calvé-Perthes disease have a worse prognosis than those with an earlier onset. Within these general guidelines, the disease is quite variable, and individual prognostication is difficult.

There are several classifications of severity of Legg-Calvé-Perthes disease. The Catterall classification delineates four groups based on areas of femoral head involvement (2):

- group I   anterior head involvement
- group II   central head involvement
- group III   lateral and central head involvement
- group IV   total head involvement

In addition, the presence of two or more risk factors (extrusion, Gage's sign, lateral calcification, and a horizontal growth plate) suggests a worse prognosis.

Because of problems with reproducibility of this classification, a newer system—the lateral pillar classification—has come into general use (Table 173.1 and Figs. 173.1 to 173.3) (12). In this scheme, the lateral portion of the femoral head is evaluated on the anteroposterior (AP) radiograph in the early fragmentation stage of the disease.

The natural history of Legg-Calvé-Perthes disease has been well studied, and all reports state that the majority of individuals with the disorder do well through most of their adult lives (6,10,23). McAndrew and Weinstein (17) have shown that with follow-up studies of 48 years, about 50% of the patients will develop severe enough hip disability to require a total hip replacement by their fifth or sixth decade of life. In these studies, those with onset of disease after 9 years of age had the highest incidence of poor results. These studies demonstrate that long-term prognosis is closely related to the roundness of the femoral head and the congruity of the hip joint.

Table 173.1.   *Lateral Pillar Classification*

Lateral pillar group	Classification criteria	Prediction of outcome
Group A (Fig. 173.1)	No radiolucency No loss of height	All children's hips are expected to remain round.
Group B (Fig. 173.2)	Some lucency in the lateral segment Loss of height not greater than half the original height	Younger children's hips do very well; most have a good result. One third of older children develop flattening of the femoral head.
Group C (Fig. 173.3)	Considerable lucency in lateral segment Loss of height greater than half the original height	Half of children's hips develop a flattened femoral head.

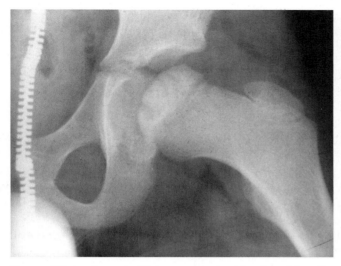

Figure 173.1. Lateral pillar group A classification. AP radiograph of the left hip showing well-demarcated lateral pillar. There is no loss of height in the lateral segment of the femoral head in spite of some changes in radiodensity.

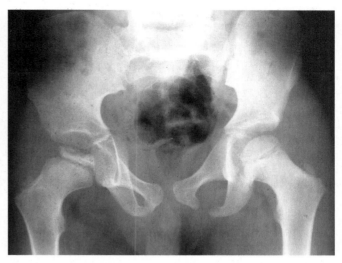

Figure 173.2. Lateral pillar group B classification.

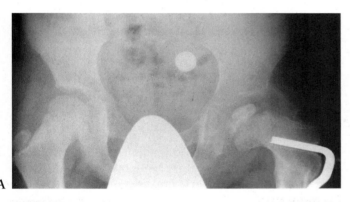

A

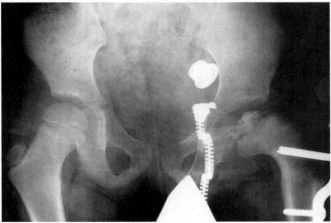

B

Figure 173.3. Lateral pillar group C classification. AP radiograph of the pelvis of a boy who has had a varus osteotomy for Legg-Calvé-Perthes disease. **A:** The lateral portion of the femoral head is lucent and collapsed relative to the central portion. **B:** AP radiograph 9 months later showing further collapse of the lateral pillar. **C:** AP radiograph several years later showing flattening of the femoral head.

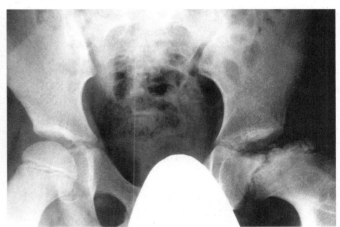

C

TREATMENT CONCEPTS

The earliest treatment efforts for Legg-Calvé-Perthes disease were directed at relief from weight bearing (16). This was a natural evolution, because in those early days, the disorder had just been distinguished from tuberculosis, and weight relief was the mainstay of treatment for tuberculous hips. With time, the concept of maintaining abduction along with bed rest became the basis for containment therapy (20). Subsequent studies showed good results with weight-bearing abduction devices, and ambulatory containment was born (11,19).

Salter (24) produced avascular necrosis in pigs and found that those animals whose hips were kept in abduction had femoral heads that remained round, whereas the femoral heads of the untreated animals flattened. Based on this work, surgical containment, either with femoral or pelvic osteotomy, has been commonly performed for Legg-Calvé-Perthes disease.

INDICATIONS FOR CONTAINMENT TREATMENT

Today there is considerable disagreement among different centers concerning indications for treatment of Legg-Calvé-Perthes disease. Our current approach is based on preliminary data from a long-term multicenter study that compared the treatment methods of range of motion, bracing, femoral osteotomy, and Salter osteotomy.

We recommend containment treatment for those children who meet the following criteria:

1. Age at onset of disease between 6 and 10 years
2. Lateral pillar group B involvement with bone age at onset of more than 6 years
3. Lateral pillar group C involvement
4. Hips with a reasonable range of motion

We recommend symptomatic treatment for the following:

1. All lateral pillar group A hips
2. Lateral pillar group B hips with a bone age at onset of 6 years or less
3. Any children younger than 6 years of age at the onset of the disease

Symptomatic treatment consists of reduction of activities when pain and limp worsen, and occasional periods of rest or traction when necessary for loss of range of motion. Anti-inflammatory medications are used when necessary. If persistent loss of motion occurs, a period of a few months of ambulatory abduction bracing may help the patient maintain range of motion.

The treatment of children older than 10 years of age at onset is difficult. Many surgeons perform containment surgery, with the caution that all may not go well. These children often lose range of motion after surgery and may even need abduction casting or bracing postoperatively. The combination of femoral and pelvic osteotomy may be appropriate in this age group.

RESTORATION OF MOTION

It is essential to regain range of motion before instituting containment treatment. In the child who has had recent onset of Legg-Calvé-Perthes disease and presents in the early radiographic stages, motion is usually relatively easily regained. Often a few days of bed rest are sufficient to regain enough abduction to "cover" the femoral head radiographically. If the hip is more resistant to loosening up, then a program of night traction in abduction may be helpful. After this, bracing or surgical containment may be instituted.

The child who has had symptoms for many months and who has reached the fragmentation stage may require more vigorous methods to regain motion. Try full-time traction and bed rest and, if these measures are insufficient, institute a period in Petrie plasters. The usual procedure is to evaluate the patient under anesthesia and perform an arthrogram to assess femoral head flattening. If the hip can be abducted sufficiently to cover the cartilaginous head, apply long-leg plasters with an abduction bar. If the hip will not abduct, decide whether "hinge abduction" is occurring. This is a condition in which the head levers out of the acetabulum with abduction instead of moving within the socket. If there is hinge abduction, containment surgical procedures are contraindicated because severe hip stiffness may ensue. If the head abducts but motion is limited by tight adductor muscles, an adductor tenotomy may be helpful, followed by the Petrie casts.

SURGICAL CONTAINMENT TREATMENTS

FEMORAL OSTEOTOMY

Some surgeons attempt to obtain sufficient range of motion to cover the hip before femoral osteotomy, but others perform the procedure even when there is reduced motion (Fig. 173.4). Because there is the occasional very stiff hip after the operation, I recommend that the surgery be performed only in children with at least 30° of hip abduction. In those patients who lack this motion, I regain range of motion by using Petrie casts for 6 weeks before performing femoral osteotomy. If the patient has had Legg-Calvé-Perthes disease for many months, there may be flattening of the femoral head, and thus I perform an arthrogram be-

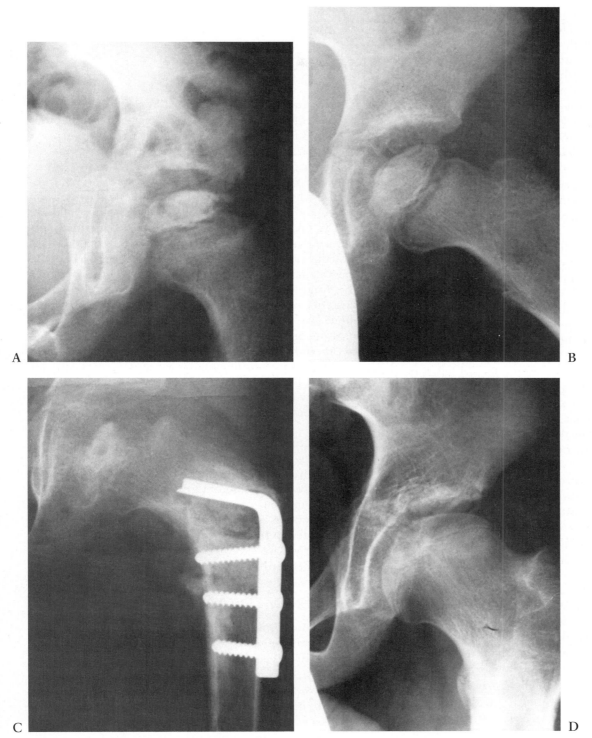

Figure 173.4. A 7 1/2-year-old boy with recent onset of symptoms. **A:** An anteroposterior radiograph of the left hip showing the risk signs of lucency of the lateral portion of the femoral head, metaphyseal lucency, and lateral widening of the joint space. **B:** An abduction-internal rotation radiograph of the left hip. There is adequate coverage of the femoral head on this view. Note the subchondral lucency over two thirds of the femoral head, classifying this as a Salter-Thompson type B. There is also lateral calcification, another of Catterall's risk signs. **C:** An AP radiograph following a varus proximal femoral osteotomy fixed with a blade plate. The neck-shaft angle is 118°. **D:** An AP radiograph 4 years after osteotomy showing satisfactory roundness of the femoral head. The blade plate was removed 1 year postoperative.

fore osteotomy. If the femoral head levers out of the joint with abduction (hinge abduction), a varus osteotomy is contraindicated. Instead, a trial period of Petrie casts may be instituted with repeat arthrogram to determine if the hinge abduction has resolved, in which case the osteotomy may be performed. Otherwise, other procedures such as valgus osteotomy may be appropriate in these late cases.

The osteotomy is usually performed at the subtrochanteric level. There are a variety of opinions as to how much varus and derotation should be used. Some surgeons estimate the amount of varus based on the amount of abduction required to cover the lateral portion of the femoral head under the acetabulum. Most surgeons, however, seek a certain neck-shaft angle regardless of the estimated coverage. A commonly used angle is 115° to 120°. A greater amount of varus will result in an abductor limp that may persist. Some remodeling of the neck-shaft angle will occur in younger children with lesser involvement, but older children and those with severe disease may not have the growth capacity to remodel the neck-shaft angle. Rab (22) has published a review of preoperative radiographic evaluation for osteotomies about the hip, which is helpful in the planning stage.

Some surgeons also derotate the femur, based on the concept that this will improve anterior coverage of the femoral head. This may cause the patient to out-toe and probably should be done minimally, if at all. Other surgeons perform a proximal osteotomy, and extend or anteriorly angulate the osteotomy to improve anterior coverage.

Rigidly fix these osteotomies with one of the blade plates or screw plate devices specifically designed for children. Immobilize in a cast those patients requiring muscle releases and those who cannot cooperate with limited weight bearing. (Remember that these children tend to be extremely active.) See Chapter 166 for more details on the operative technique.

Complications often occur because of inadequate fixation with these active children. Malunion into varus is a serious problem, which will result in a poor gait. Nonunion, however, is uncommon. The more severely involved hips may become progressively stiffer following the osteotomy. When this occurs, the varus of the osteotomy results in adduction of the thigh. It may be necessary to return the patient to the operating room for adductor muscle releases and placement of Petrie casts for a period of time to restore hip range of motion. We have even had to return patients to brace wear for 6 to 8 weeks to maintain abduction postoperatively.

Remove the fixation plate a year after the osteotomy. At that time, if there is excessive varus (perhaps less than 110° neck-shaft angle), an arrest of the greater trochanter may be appropriate to keep the trochanter below the femoral head. Occasionally, when excessive varus has been introduced, it may be necessary to perform a valgus femoral osteotomy subsequently to restore a normal gait.

SALTER INNOMINATE OSTEOTOMY

The prerequisites for an innominate osteotomy are similar to those of the femoral osteotomy but are more rigorous (Fig. 173.5). Salter has recommended that a full range of motion be obtained and that an arthrogram show no flattening of the femoral head as a prerequisite to his operation (25,26). In practice, many surgeons perform the procedure when an adequate range of motion has been obtained and the flattening of the femoral head is mild.

The operation is usually performed as originally described. Salter has emphasized lengthening the iliopsoas to reduce the pressure on the hip. Some surgeons prefer the Kalamchi modification of the procedure, which moves the distal fragment of the osteotomy into a notch in the posterior part of the pelvis (13). The purpose of this technique is to avoid lengthening the pelvis and increasing the pressure on the femoral head. Other surgeons add a shelf of cancellous bone over the femoral head to add to coverage. Most surgeons immobilize the hips in spica casts for 6 weeks, but some use screw fixation for the osteotomy and allow partial weight bearing until the osteotomy has healed. See Chapter 166 for details on operative technique.

An occasional complication of the procedure is hip stiffness, which at times can be severe. As with the femoral osteotomy, it may be necessary to perform muscle releases and use Petrie casts and braces postoperatively to regain range of motion. As with any osteotomy, it is important to position the osteotomy fragments properly and obtain secure internal fixation. If the fixation pins or screws are improperly placed, the osteotomy will displace posteriorly and be ineffective.

VALGUS OSTEOTOMY

A valgus osteotomy of the femur is occasionally indicated for the patient who presents late with well-established head deformity and hinge abduction (3,21). The purpose of the osteotomy is to reduce the adduction of the thigh and allow better weight-bearing alignment. At times, the femoral head will remodel after this procedure. This should be considered a late, reconstructive operation and is not appropriate as primary treatment. See Chapters 29, 104, and 166 for details on the operation.

COMBINED FEMORAL AND PELVIC OSTEOTOMY

The use of combined femoral varus and pelvic osteotomy (either Salter type or Chiari) has been advocated for se-

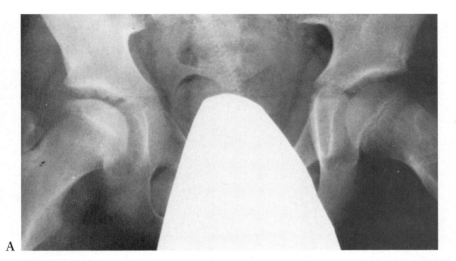

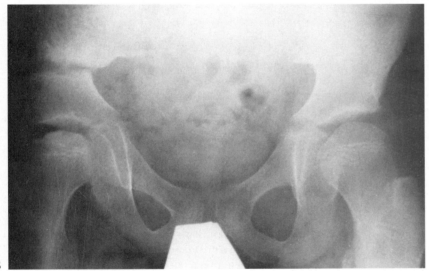

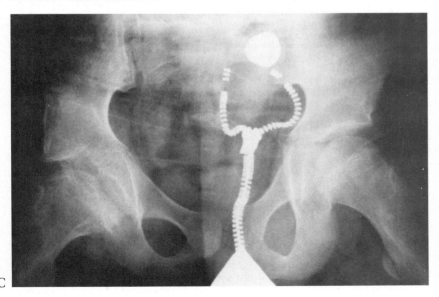

Figure 173.5. An 11-year-old boy with a history of 4 months of right hip discomfort and limp. Children of this age often have the poorest results regardless of treatment. **A:** An abduction-internal rotation radiograph showing adequate coverage of the right femoral head. The head is in the phase of increased density, and risk factors have not yet appeared. **B:** An anteroposterior radiograph 3 months after Salter innominate osteotomy. The pins have been removed, and the osteotomy is healed. The femoral head is showing signs of flattening. **C:** An AP radiograph 20 months after osteotomy. The femoral head has healed and is reasonably round. *(continued)*

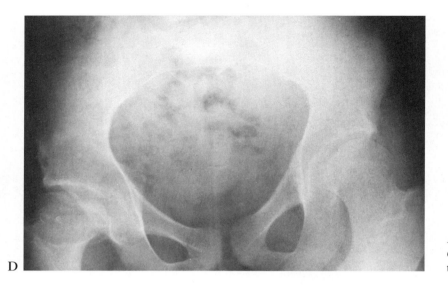

D

Figure 173.5. (continued) **D:** An AP radiograph 6 years after osteotomy. The femoral head has further flattened over the intervening years.

verely involved hips, especially in children older than 9 years of age at the onset of the disease. The current reports of this approach suggest that there is an improvement in outcome, but more evaluation is necessary before this procedure should be done commonly (5,18).

REMOVAL OF LOOSE BODY

Occasionally, a patient with Legg-Calvé-Perthes disease will develop an osteochondritic lesion, usually many years after the onset of the disorder. The symptoms of locking and popping suggest the diagnosis, which then may be confirmed with arthrography or computed tomography (CT) scanning. Arthroscopy may allow removal of either a loose body or, more commonly, a softened area in the center of the femoral head (1,28). Sometimes an anterior arthrotomy to locate the loose body is appropriate, but it may be necessary to dislocate the hip to find the loose body.

 ## AUTHOR'S PERSPECTIVE

My current approach to the treatment of a patient with Legg-Calvé-Perthes disease who presents when the disease is in the phase of increased density or early fragmentation follows: For a child whose bone age is six years or less, I institute conservative treatment (rest, anti-inflammatory agents) until there is enough fragmentation to determine lateral pillar classification. If the patient's hip is determined to be class A, I perform no further treatment. If the hip is determined to be class B, I continue symptomatic

treatment, and if it is Class C, I prefer containment surgery, usually a Salter osteotomy.

For a child whose bone age is greater than six years, if clinical signs are minimal, I observe the patient until I am certain of a significant degree of disease beyond class A. If significant clinical signs are present, I allow the patient to regain range of motion conservatively and consider containment surgery (I prefer Salter osteotomy).

In a child older than age 10, decision making is difficult. I consider containment surgery if the disease is in the early phase. Usually a Salter osteotomy is performed, sometimes combined with a proximal femoral varus osteotomy. In children in this age group, one must recognize that the overall prognosis is poor.

REFERENCES

Each reference is categorized according to the following scheme: *, classic article; #, review article; !, basic research article; and + , clinical results/outcome study.

+ 1. Bowen JR, Kumar VP, Joyce JD, Bowen JC. Osteochondritis Dissecans following Perthes' Disease. Arthroscopic-operative Treatment. *Clin Orthop Relat Res* 1986;209:49.

* 2. Catterall A. The Natural History of Perthes' Disease. *J Bone Joint Surg* 1971;53B:37.

* 3. Catterall A. *Legg-Calvé-Perthes Disease.* London: Churchill-Livingston, 1982.

! 4. Clancy M, Steel HH. The Effect of an Incomplete Intertrochanteric Osteotomy on Legg-Calvé-Perthes Disease. *J Bone Joint Surg* 1985;67A:213.

+ 5. Crutcher JP, Staheli LT. Combined Osteotomy as a Salvage Procedure for Severe Legg-Calvé-Perthes disease. *J Pediatr Orthop* 1992;12:151.

* 6. Eaton G. Long-term Results of Treatment in Coxa Plana: A Follow-up Study of Eighty-eight Patients. *J Bone Joint Surg* 1967;49A:1031.

! 7. Freeman MAR, England JPS. Experimental Infarction of the Immature Canine Femoral Head. *Proc R Soc Med* 1969;62:431.

! 8. Glueck C, Crawford A, Roy D, et al. Association of Antithrombotic Factor Deficiencies and Hypofibrinolysis with Legg-Perthes Disease. *J Bone Joint Surg* 1996;78A:3.

! 9. Glueck C, Glueck H, Greenfield D, et al. Protein C and S Deficiency, Thrombilia, and Hypofibrinolysis: Pathophysiologic Causes of Legg-Perthes Disease. *Pediatr Res* 1994;35:383.

* 10. Gower WE, Johnston RC. Legg-Perthes Disease: Long-term Follow-up of Thirty-six Patients. *J Bone Joint Surg* 1971;53A:759.

* 11. Harrison MH, Menon MP. Legg-Calvé-Perthes Disease. The Value of Roentgenographic Measurement in Clinical Practice with Special Reference to the Broomstick Plaster Method. *J Bone Joint Surg* 1966;48A:1310.

! 12. Herring JA, Neustadt JB, Williams JJ, et al. The Lateral Pillar Classification of Legg-Calvé-Perthes Disease. *J Pediatr Orthop* 1992;12:143.

+ 13. Kalamchi A. A Modified Salter Osteotomy. *J Bone Joint Surg* 1982;64A:183.

! 14. Kasser JR, Hresko T, McDougall PA, et al. Prospective Re-evaluation of the Association between Thrombotic Diathesis and Legg-Calvé-Perthes Disease. *Pediatric Orthopaedics Society of North America (POSNA) 1998 Annual Meeting.* Cleveland, 1998, p 96.

! 15. Kendig RJ, Evans GA. Biologic Osteotomy in Perthes Disease. *J Pediatr Orthop* 1986;6:278.

* 16. Legg AT. An obscure affection of the hip joint. *Boston Med Surg J* 1910;162:202.

* 17. McAndrew MP, Weinstein SL. A Long-term Follow-up of Legg-Calvé-Perthes Disease. *J Bone Joint Surg* 1984;66:860.

+ 18. Olney BW, Asher MA. Combined Innominate and Femoral Osteotomy for the Treatment of Severe Legg-Calvé-Perthes Disease. *J Pediatr Orthop* 1985;5:645.

* 19. Petrie JG, Bitenc I. The abduction weight-bearing treatment in Legg-Perthes's disease. *J Bone Joint Surg* 1971;53B:54.

* 20. Pike MM. Legg-Perthes Disease: A Method of Conservative Treatment. *J Bone Joint Surg* 1950;32A:663.

+ 21. Quain S, Catterall A. Hinge Abduction of the Hip: Diagnosis and Treatment. *J Bone Joint Surg* 1986;68B:61.

* 22. Rab G. Preoperative Roentgenographic Evaluation for Osteotomies about the Hip in Children. *J Bone Joint Surg* 1981;63A:306.

* 23. Ratliff AH. Perthes' Disease: A Study of Thirty-four Hips Observed for Thirty Years. *J Bone Joint Surg* 1967;49B:102.

! 24. Salter R. Experimental and Clinical Aspects of Perthes' Disease. *J Bone Joint Surg* 1966;48B:393.

* 25. Salter RB. Legg-Perthes Disease: The Scientific Basis for the Methods of Treatment and Their Indications. *Clin Orthop Relat Res* 1980;150:8.

* 26. Salter RB. The Present Status of Surgical Treatment for Legg-Perthes Disease. *J Bone Joint Surg* 1984;66A:961.

! 27. Sanchis M, Zahir A, Freeman MA. The Experimental Stimulation of Perthes Disease by Consecutive Interruptions of the Blood Supply to the Capital Femoral Epiphysis in the Puppy. *J Bone Joint Surg* 1973;55A:335.

+ 28. Schindler A, Lechevallier J, Rao N, Bowen J. Diagnostic and Therapeutic Arthroscopy of the Hip in Children and Adolescents: Evaluation of Results. *J Pediatr Orthop* 1995;15:317.

* 29. Stulberg SD, Cooperman DR, Wallensten R. The Natural History of Legg-Calvé-Perthes disease. *J Bone Joint Surg* 1981;63A:1095.

* 30. Waldenström H. On Coxa Plana. *Acta Chir Scand* 1923;55:557.

CHAPTER 174
CONGENITAL LOWER LIMB DEFICIENCY

William L. Oppenheim, Hugh G. Watts, Robert M. Bernstein, and Yoshio Setoguchi

W. L. Oppenheim: Division of Pediatric Orthopedics, University of California–Los Angeles School of Medicine; Shriners' Hospital, Los Angeles, California, 90095.
H. G. Watts: Shriners' Hospital; Department of Orthopedics, University of California–Los Angeles School of Medicine, Los Angeles, California, 90020.
R. M. Bernstein: Shriners' Hospital; Department of Orthopedics, University of California–Los Angeles School of Medicine, Los Angeles, California, 90020.
Y. Setoguchi: Shriners' Hospital; Department of Pediatrics, University of California–Los Angeles School of Medicine, Los Angeles, California, 90020.

This chapter focuses on a group of diverse congenital anomalies affecting the lower extremities of children. Many involve a failure of formation of various tissues, as well as leg-length discrepancy. The general approach to these patients is to evaluate their limbs in terms of potential function, to estimate the projected leg-length discrepancy at maturity, and then to address the situation either by standard leg-length equalization techniques or through the use of a prosthesis that can be adjusted in length as the child grows. When amputation is indicated as part of the overall solution, one must identify a key joint for salvage and then convert the tissue distal to that joint into a usable weight-bearing organ. The key joint is the most distal joint with sufficient function to power a prosthesis. Complicating the technical problems are psychological feelings of helplessness, anxiety, and frustration among parents and physicians alike.

The concept of sacrificing a body part to facilitate prosthetic fitting is initially poorly accepted by most parents, particularly if the part proposed for sacrifice appears quite normal. The parents rightly question why modern technology cannot be called upon to salvage their child's limb. Physicians faced with this scenario must improvise based on their combined expertise in prosthetics and reconstructive surgery. Although some of the procedures may initially appear radical to parents, with education and counseling the child and parents can accept them as simply reconstructive. Experience has shown that it is frequently preferable to convert a limb to a logical prosthetic level rather than embark on a prolonged operative reconstruction that, even when modestly successful, frequently precludes participation in normal childhood activities (41). Treatment thus requires an understanding of the natural history of the specific defect as well as a thorough knowledge of any associated abnormalities.

Because of the complicated nature of these conditions, evaluation and treatment are best carried out at special clinics where appropriate psychological, social, and pediatric support is available. Surgical procedures are not easily undertaken and rely on the parents' informed judgment based on a balanced medical presentation and the experience gained through the consultation process. An opportunity to associate with other families in similar circumstances who have already gone through the process is a reassuring influence and should be part of the family's decision-making process.

ETIOLOGY

The period during which a developing embryo is most susceptible to malformations being perpetuated in subsequent cell lines is between the fourth and eighth weeks postfertilization, the so-called period of organogenesis. Both the axial and appendicular skeletons form at this time. A single cell gives rise to billions of descendants, so the surprising thing is not that congenital anomalies occur, but that they do not occur even more frequently. Some conditions have a familial origin and hence a preordained genetic derivation. For example, congenital dislocation of the knee may occur sporadically or in association with Larsen's syndrome, an autosomal dominant condition in which dislocations of other joints and anomalies of the cervical spine also occur. Whatever the cause, once a defect is present, with the limb bud developing in a proximal

to distal progression, areas "downstream" from the initial insult may also be affected. For example, proximal femoral focal deficiency is frequently associated with a more distal fibula deficiency, and absence of the fibula in turn may be associated with absence of lateral foot rays.

Because other organ systems also differentiate during this gestational period, limb defects frequently are seen in the presence of anomalies exclusive of the musculoskeletal system. The VACTERLS syndrome refers to the association of vertebral, anal, cardiac, tracheoesophageal, renal or radial flaws, associated with limb defects and a single umbilical artery. In the amniotic band syndrome, the insult is thought to take place after limb bud development during the fetal period of gestation. Multiple bands may be present, predisposing to autoamputations. From this brief discussion, it is clear that limb reduction defects often present as part of a more general syndrome.

DIFFERENCES BETWEEN CHILD AND ADULT AMPUTEES

Amputation surgery in children differs from that in adults. In adults, amputation is frequently related to peripheral vascular disease or diabetes; healing is delayed and rehabilitation is difficult and prolonged. Adults are concerned about their body image, time lost from work, and their livelihood in general. Children, on the other hand, usually heal promptly and completely; conversion to an amputation at an early age is not ordinarily difficult or prolonged, and potential employability is not an immediate concern (see Chapter 175). Phantom pain and neuromas, which can significantly impact on the results in adults, do not appear as clinically significant in children and present only an occasional problem in adolescents. Gait training takes place spontaneously under the guidance of a prosthetist or physical therapist, and psychological acceptance of the limb is natural and not elaborate.

However, one problem peculiar to growing children is frequent overgrowth following transdiaphyseal amputations, particularly in the humerus, tibia, and fibula. This can result in a need for serial surgical revisions throughout growth (see section on Terminal Overgrowth at the end of this chapter). Where possible, perform amputation through an adjacent joint to avoid this problem, but this consideration must in turn be tempered by the concomitant goal of maintaining length. Through-joint amputations not only preserve length, but, by preservation of the adjacent growth plate, add to the length throughout childhood, preventing an initial adequate length from becoming a proportionately shorter stump as adult stature is attained.

ASSESSMENT AND GOAL SETTING

When assessing an infant with a limb deficiency, identify possible etiologic factors. Consider the influence of teratogenic agents such as thalidomide, maternal risk factors such as diabetes, and environmental factors such as radiation exposure. A genetics consultation is recommended to assess the risks for additional pregnancies and to offer counseling. Despite the gravity of the situation, the professional staff should maintain an optimistic demeanor. Nearly all children with lower extremity anomalies gain functional mobility, attend regular school, and lead quality lives, participating in sports such as swimming, skiing, tennis, and horseback riding. Schools may restrict participation in contact sports such as football and hockey because of the risk of injury to other children from prosthetic parts. The role of the parents and grandparents cannot be underestimated. Acceptance of the child as he is and the avoidance of overprotection, which can lead to an overly dependent and submissive personality, facilitates the child's development, sense of self worth, and eventual integration into the workplace.

CONGENITAL DEFICIENCY OF THE FIBULA

Congenital malformations of the fibula usually are not associated with classic modes of genetic transmission and thus likely result from embryonic insults occurring during the development of the limb bud. The severity ranges from simple hypoplasia to total absence of the fibula. Experimental evidence suggests that the earlier the insult occurs in embryonic development, the more likely is concurrent involvement of the proximal femur. Later insults involve the fibula and foot to a greater degree (46). Fibular deficiency thus may be accompanied by proximal femoral focal deficiency, shortening and/or bowing of the tibia, general limb growth retardation, delayed epiphyseal ossification, absence of rays, tarsal coalitions, residual fibrous bands, deficiencies of various muscles, genu valgum, and loss of ankle integrity (2,18,30,31,59,68). Upper extremity anomalies are also seen in some cases. Although rare compared to diseases such as developmental dysplasia of the hip or clubfeet, the fibula is the most common congenitally absent long bone (18).

Clinically, the most important issues are the stability and function of the ankle and foot and the overall length of the limb. To better characterize the variability, Achterman and Kalamchi (2) refined a classification originally utilized by Coventry and Johnson (18) (Fig. 174.1). In type IA, the entire fibula is present but shortened, leaving the proximal fibular epiphysis distal to the upper physis of the tibia, and the distal fibular physis proximal to the dome of the talus. In type IB, there is a partial absence of

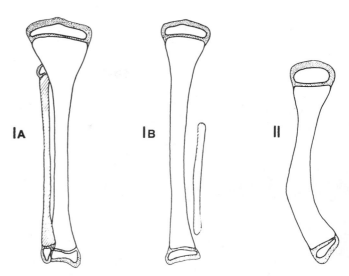

Figure 174.1. Achterman-Kalamchi classification of fibula hemimelia. See text for explanation.

the upper fibula, and the lower fibular epiphysis is likewise elevated above the talar dome and thus not buttressing the ankle. In type I deformities, the foot usually remains plantigrade but may be associated with a ball and socket ankle joint, and either equinovalgus or equinovarus may be present. In type II, by contrast, the entire fibula is absent, tibial bowing is frequent, and ankle instability is the rule. A residual lateral fibrous band may contribute to the type II deformity.

Some surgeons have used the absence of rays to predict ankle stability (e.g., a four-toed foot can be salvaged, but a three-toed foot should be sacrificed), but we have found that stability can be directly assessed and that a three-toed foot can often be serviceable. The degree of tibial shortening increases with advanced stages, although associated femoral shortening is maximal in type I. Children with type I feet will not require conversion to an amputation, but conversion is usually performed for the majority of children with type II deformities.

The literature abounds with ankle stabilization procedures for the treatment of type II deformities, but the test of time has not supported this approach (4,7,11,15). Stabilization by arthrodesis is complicated by delayed ossification of the epiphyses, as well as by potential inadvertent injury to the distal tibial physis. Kruger and Talbott (41) have pointed out that whereas the goal of preserving the foot might be laudable, in fact many children who undergo repetitive operations eventually undergo amputation, and that upon honest review there is good evidence that conversion should have been offered as a primary treatment rather than a secondary salvage procedure. In addition, we have found a higher incidence of complications when Syme amputation was performed as a salvage

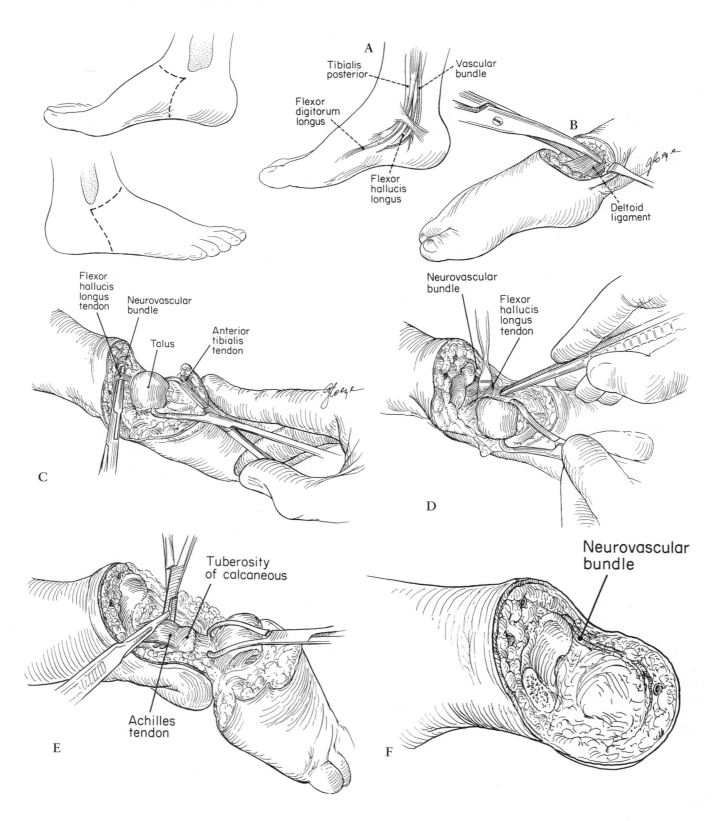

A Tibialis posterior   Vascular bundle   Flexor digitorum longus   Flexor hallucis longus

B Deltoid ligament

C Flexor hallucis longus tendon   Neurovascular bundle   Talus   Anterior tibialis tendon

D Neurovascular bundle   Flexor hallucis longus tendon

E Tuberosity of calcaneous   Achilles tendon

F Neurovascular bundle

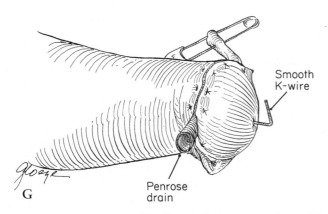

G

Figure 174.2. Syme's ankle disarticulation as performed in children. Make skin incisions from a point 1 cm distal to the medial malleolus to the tip of what would have been the fibula malleolus, as illustrated. **A:** Schematic of the anatomy posterior to the medial malleolus. **B:** Divide the collateral ligaments to facilitate hyper plantarflexion of the ankle. **C:** Location of the flexor hallucis longus posterior to the talus. **D:** Protect the neurovascular bundle by retraction of the flexor hallucis longus muscle tendon. **E:** Divide the Achilles tendon, taking care to include excision of the apophysis of the calcaneus. **F:** Preserve the neurovascular bundle to the end of the flap; avoid injury to the bundle at the level of the ankle joint. **G:** Close the wound over a drain, and stabilize the heel pad with a stout K-wire or smooth Steinmann pin inserted into the tibia from the plantar aspect of the heel.

procedure in multiply operated limbs rather than as a primary procedure (6). In areas where cultural concerns do not allow amputation, or in lesser developed areas where surgery is not available, it is feasible to fit a prosthesis around the foot.

In instances where the ankle is relatively stable and the overall length can be made acceptable, leg lengthening using Ilizarov techniques, in which the ankle is stabilized during lengthening, is an acceptable approach.

INDICATIONS FOR ANKLE DISARTICULATION IN CHILDREN

The indications for conversion to a below-knee amputation are (a) a deformity of the foot so severe that any surgery to make the foot plantigrade and functional is likely to fail (70) and (b) an estimated leg-length discrepancy at maturity of 7.5 cm or more (60). The value of 7.5 cm is arbitrary and tends to vary among physicians (46, 59,60). We now base our decision more on the stability of the ankle than the leg-length discrepancy, per se, provided the overall limb-length discrepancy at maturity is not projected to exceed 12 cm.

TECHNIQUE OF SYME'S AMPUTATION

- Begin the procedure of Syme's ankle disarticulation (Fig. 174.2) by making a fish-mouth incision with anterior and posterior skin flaps. The apex begins 1 cm distal to the medial malleolus and parallels the anterior ankle joint to a point estimated to be the level where the fibular tip would ordinarily be palpable.
- Carry the dissection down through the subcutaneous tissue to the level of the medial and lateral collateral ligaments of the ankle, ligating larger vessels and controlling smaller ones with electrocautery.
- Identify the nerves. Gently tension, sharply divide, and allow the nerves to retract away from potential subcutaneous positioning.
- Divide the collateral ligaments so that the talar dome can be pulled forward away from the distal tibia.
- In the interval between the talus and tibia, identify the flexor hallucis longus tendon. It is the key to locating and protecting the neurovascular bundle posteromedially. By protecting this tendon and drawing it medially with a retractor, the dissection can be continued with the neurovascular bundle shielded so that the actual division of the posterior tibial artery will be at the most distal portion of the posterior flap.
- Excise the calcaneus from the heel pad in a subperiosteal fashion so that the periosteum remains intact, maintaining the structural integrity of the fat pad, which has a hydraulic-like function during weight bearing. Be sure that the entire calcaneal apophysis is excised so that it will not form a persistent ossicle later (Fig. 174.3). Two centimeters of the distal Achilles tendon can be resected to ensure there will be no tendency to reattach and pull the heel pad posteriorly. Shave the distal tibia only in older children, because smoothing and remodeling occur spontaneously in younger children once the talus no longer occupies the mortise.
- Finally, stabilize the heel pad underneath the tibia by inserting a stout Kirschner wire (K-wire) through the pad into the tibia, and close the skin over a Penrose drain with absorbable subcutaneous sutures and interrupted nylon sutures for the skin. In approximating the heel pad to the tibia, take care to avoid crimping the posterior tibial artery.

After skin repair, apply Xeroform (Sherwood Medical, Markham, Ontario) gauze, fluffs, sterile cast padding, and a spica cast for short stumps (as when the amputation is combined with a knee fusion for proximal femoral focal deficiency). A long-leg cast can be applied when the knee can be effectively flexed to prevent the cast from sliding off. Remove the drain at 2 days and allow 6 weeks for soft-tissue healing in the cast. An elastic wrap is occasionally necessary for several additional weeks to control any re-

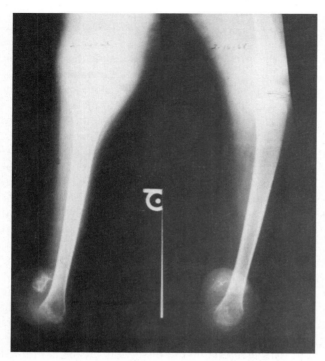

Figure 174.3.   In performing Syme's amputation, be certain to excise the entire apophysis, otherwise it will persist and complicate later prosthetic fitting. This one required removal during adolescence.

sidual stump edema. The stump is ready for prosthetic fitting between the tenth and twelfth weeks.

Associated tibial bowing ordinarily corrects spontaneously after a Syme's amputation, but in those cases accompanied by bowing in excess of 30°, perform a tibial osteotomy simultaneously, and extend the K-wire to act as intramedullary fixation.

TECHNIQUE OF BOYD AMPUTATION

Some authors have reported problems with stabilization of the heel pad in the Syme's amputation and thus prefer the Boyd amputation, in which the calcaneus is displaced anteriorly in an effort to fuse it into the distal tibia or at least to stabilize it under the tibial plafond (8,10,70). Modest additional length can also be maintained by this approach. Alternatively, the distal tibial physis can be excised at the time of calcaneal tibial fusion, so that the bulbous self-suspending stump gradually "ascends" to the level of the opposite calf. In deformities with severely displaced equinus hind feet, repositioning of the calcaneus under the tibia may not be possible, and Syme's procedure is preferred. No shaping of the malleoli is necessary in young children in either the Boyd or the Syme ankle con-

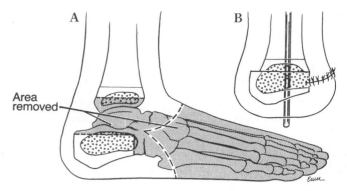

Figure 174.4.   Boyd's amputation. A: Scheme of bony resection. B: Final position, emphasizing anterior displacement of the calcaneus to provide a rounded stump.

version. Without the talus occupying the mortise, the malleoli remodel to a satisfactory shape. Either procedure yields a pleasing stump because the prominent malleoli atrophy after talar excision.

- Boyd amputation (8) utilizes an approach similar to the Syme procedure just described. However, excise only the talus and forefoot, leaving the calcaneus attached to the fat pad (Fig. 174.4).
- Carefully shave the articular cartilage of the distal tibia with a knife until the ossific nucleus is encountered; take care to breech neither the distal tibial physis nor its surrounding perichondrium, unless shortening of the stump is desired.
- Osteotomize the anterior portion of the calcaneus, if necessary, just distal to the peroneal tubercle; shave the superior surface flat, allowing it to sit congruously under the prepared distal tibia.
- Divide the Achilles tendon through the space left by the enucleation of the talus. When performed properly, the heel pad can be positioned in its normal weight-bearing attitude but slightly displaced anteriorly.
- Use a smooth Steinmann pin to secure the final position, extending it through the calcaneus across the distal tibial physis into the medullary canal of the tibia.
- Close the skin over a drain.

The postoperative management is similar to that described for the Syme's amputation.

RESULTS OF ANKLE DISARTICULATION

With the exception of one patient who died of unrelated causes, in our series of 61 patients with Syme amputations (6), all were ambulatory, and patient satisfaction was excellent. Patients participated in sports activities, including bicycling, swimming, football, soccer, and roller skating.

Although some did report occasional problems, such as calluses and rashes, on closer inspection these problems seemed to be related to prosthetic fit rather than to the stump per se, and they were easily addressed with minor prosthetic accommodations in the socket. Posterior heel pad migration was commonly encountered, although it rarely required surgical intervention. Hypertrophy of the skin over the distal tibia and prosthetic adjustment were usually enough to compensate for changes in heel pad position. Of these patients, 40% felt that they had no functional restriction at all, and all of the adults reviewed were employed.

In an alternate study evaluating the physical and psychological function in young patients after Syme's amputation, the results documented a surprisingly easy adjustment process (6). The age of amputation may be important, and it seemed preferable that the procedure be performed prior to the age of 18 months to 2 years, because at this time the infant has an incompletely developed body image and adapts to the new physical status quite quickly. It seems that a missing foot compensated by a functional prosthesis is more acceptable to a child or teenager than a significantly deformed foot that compromises activities and gait.

COMPLICATIONS OF ANKLE DISARTICULATION

Posterior heel pad migration, wound sloughs, and damage to the distal tibial physis are seen in both the Boyd and the Syme conversions. In addition, an occult retained calcaneal apophysis and later pencilling of the distal tibia may complicate Syme's amputation. Careful attention to the indications and surgical details will limit the problems encountered. Displacement of the heel pad, although frequent, is rarely an indication for reoperation.

PROCEDURES TO STABILIZE THE ANKLE

In the past, many attempts have been made to create a lateral buttress to replace the fibula. The Bardenhauer procedure (7) involved inserting the talus into a sagittal split in the tibia, clearly breaching the growth plate. The Albee procedure (4) involved buttressing by autogenous bone grafted into the tibial metaphysis in an effort to replace the fibular malleolus. Lacking a growth plate, the buttress would quickly rise above the level of the ankle, mitigating its effectiveness.

More recent attempts at ankle stabilization have centered on the Gruca procedure (28,54). In a review of this technique by Thomas and Williams (60) at the Royal Children's Hospital in Melbourne, patients were considered for the procedure only if they exhibited minimal shortening of the tibia and had a foot that comfortably reached

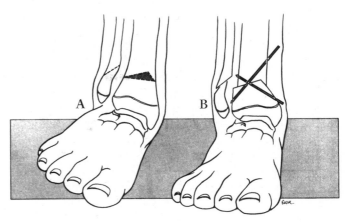

Figure 174.5. The Wiltse osteotomy reduces the medial prominence of the ankle following correction of a residual valgus ankle deformity, as might accompany lesser degrees of fibula deficiency. **A:** Plan of wedge resection. **B:** After closure and fixation of the osteotomy.

the ground with no gross deformity. Of seven attempts reported, three had been converted to an amputation, three were awaiting amputation, and the remaining patient had embarked on a program of leg-length equalization. Thus, this procedure is not definitive for most patients and can be regarded only as an interim procedure to be followed by an amputation beause of the progressive leg-length inequality that develops. With rare exception, it appears that Syme's or Boyd's amputations are the preferred primary treatment for type II (complete) fibular deficiencies.

WILTSE OSTEOTOMY

While stabilization procedures in the absence of a fibula have not been very successful, for specific cases of partial absence resulting in a mild leg-length discrepancy and a valgus but stable ankle, Wiltse (69) proposed a supramalleolar osteotomy designed to minimize the prominence of the medial malleolus. The osteotomy is performed toward the end of growth through an anterior approach to the ankle (Fig. 174.5).

CONGENITAL DEFICIENCY OF THE TIBIA

Unlike most other longitudinal deficiencies, congenital deficiency of the tibia, the rarest form of lower extremity deficiency, may be sporadic or inherited. Both autosomal dominant and recessive patterns have been reported. The anomaly is frequently associated with other system deficits such as herniae, gonadal malformations, hypospadias, cleft palate, imperforate anus, and congenital heart disease. Associated vascular abnormalities may underlie the malformations (32). Always search for absent or duplicated rays, ipsilateral proximal femoral focal deficiency (PFFD), contralateral clubfoot, hemivertebra, hip dysplasia, coxa valga, syndactyly, and lobster claw deformities (53). In contrast to fibular deficiencies, the foot is in a varus position, and the knee may be unstable due to an associated absence of collateral or cruciate ligaments.

There are two classification systems available in the literature. The Kalamchi classification is perhaps simpler and more straightforward (Fig. 174.6), but the classification of Jones et al. (35) is the most widely accepted. It separates the deficiencies radiographically into five types: 1a, 1b, 2, 3, and 4 (Table 174.1). Both classifications are helpful in formulating treatment.

The distinction is whether a proximal portion of the

tibia remains, and whether this portion is meaningfully powered by a quadriceps mechanism. Usually the fragment is palpable, and active knee extension is easily discerned. However, this is not always a simple distinction in a chubby uncooperative infant, so the cartilaginous remnant may need to be sought by arthrography, ultrasonography, magnetic resonance imaging (MRI), or direct observation during surgery. Radiographically, a marked reduction in width and delayed ossification of the distal femur are also suggestive of an absent or nonfunctional proximal segment. When this tibial fragment is present and powered, surgery is warranted to fuse the fibula into the fragment and then to perform a Syme's amputation, which produces a functional below-knee amputation (Fig. 174.7). When the proximal fragment is absent (Jones type 1a), knee disarticulation is warranted, resulting in a functional above-knee amputee. Try to avoid above-knee amputation in treating congenital tibial deficiency because of problems with bony overgrowth, skin problems associated with the residual limb, not to mention the loss of the major growth physis of the femur and resultant shortening (36).

The Brown procedure (12,13) (described in the following section), which centralizes the fibula under the femur, is an alternative that allows the child to function as a below-knee prosthetic user rather than as an above-knee amputee. Most authors report disappointing results, in part because of recurring knee flexion contractures, which result from an imbalance between the hamstrings and a weak, albeit present, quadriceps musculature (35,42,58). The Brown procedure (12) may nevertheless be offered if a functioning quadriceps mechanism of grade 3 strength or better is present, because some patients can achieve a functional below-knee stump that allows active knee flexion and extension, according to Simmons et al. (55). Residual ligamentous laxity following Brown centralization can be controlled by an appropriately designed prosthetic socket. Keep in mind that if the Brown procedure proves unsuccessful, the limb may be salvaged and a perfectly acceptable result obtained by performing a knee disarticulation, which would have been the alternative operation anyway. In some severe cases of concomitant femoral shortening, fusion of the fibula into the femur may be desirable to add length to an otherwise short above-knee stump. Unfortunately, 20% to 30% of tibial deficiencies occur bilaterally with an additional compromise of the final functional ability of the patient, regardless of the treatment approach.

When the proximal tibial anlage is present and powered (Jones types 1b and 2), surgery is warranted to fuse the fibula into the fragment when it is sufficiently ossified. Simultaneously, Syme's amputation is performed and the result is a functional below-knee amputee.

De Sanctis et al. (22) presented another strategy and reported three cases treated with Jones type 2 deformities

Table 174.1.   *Jones Classification of Tibial Dysplasia*

Type	Radiologic description	Treatment possibilities
1a	Tibia not seen at infancy	Knee disarticulation
	Hypoplastic lower femoral epiphysis	Brown fibula centralization
	Tibia does not appear with growth	
1b	Tibia not seen at infancy	Syme's or Boyd's amputation with or without tibiofibula synostosis
	Normal lower femoral physis	
	Proximal tibia appears later with growth	
2	Proximal tibial anlage seen early	Syme's or Boyd's amputation
	Distal tibia absent	
3	Distal tibia present Proximal tibia not seen	Syme's amputation
4	Distal tibial diastasis	Syme's amputation versus ankle salvage and limb lengthening

From Jones D, Barnes J, Lloyd-Roberts GC. Congenital Aplasia and Dysplasia of the Tibia with Intact Fibula. Classification and Management. *J Bone Joint Surg Br* 1978;60:31, with permission.

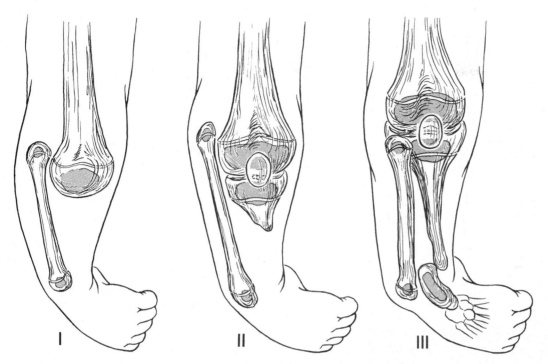

Figure 174.6. The Kalamchi classification for congenital tibial deficiency. Type I, no tibial anlage. Type II, tibial anlage present. Type III, tibial fibula diastasis.

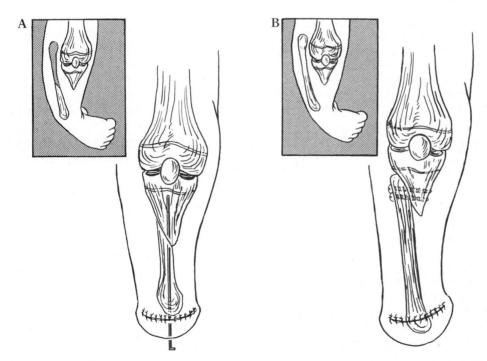

Figure 174.7. **A:** Transfer of the fibular into the tibial anlage in Kalamchi type II deformities of the tibia. **B:** Side-to-side fixation of the fibula into the tibia after resection of the upper portion of the fibula.

(tibial anlage present) by correction of the foot deformity shortly after birth through a combination of casting and soft-tissue release followed by fibulotibial diaphyseal reconstruction, alignment of the axis of the leg with the foot (talofibular arthrodesis), and leg-length equalization by the Ilizarov method. In a preliminary report, two of the patients achieved satisfactory ambulation, whereas the other sustained recurrence of deformity during the lengthening process.

The Jones type 3 tibial deficiency, characterized by a deficiency of the proximal tibia with a distal, abnormally formed tibial remnant, is extremely rare. This has been adequately treated with a Syme's or Chopart's amputation. The Jones type 4 deformity, with diastasis of the distal tibia and fibula, may be treated by Syme's amputation, or an ankle reconstruction may be attempted (53).

TOTAL ABSENCE OF THE TIBIA

Brown Fibula Centralization

■ Create an anterior U-shaped incision that parallels the distal femoral condyles (Fig. 174.8A), and develop a skin flap proximally that allows access to the quadriceps expansion.

■ Make a lateral parapatellar longitudinal incision through the expansion that, based on the radiograph, will allow exposure of the upper fibula, which is displaced proximally from its normal position. Now incise and excise the tissue between the upper fibula and the femoral epiphysis as necessary to allow transposition of the fibular head to a point under the midportion of the femoral epiphysis (Fig. 174.8B). Brown excised the upper $\frac{3}{8}$ inch of the fibula to provide a flat surface to oppose to the distal femur.

■ Fix the fibula in position with cross K-wires (Fig. 174.8C) and leave intact the insertion of the patella ligament; reattachment to the fibula itself is not necessary. If the fibula is too high to be brought distally, remove a segment of bone from the upper third of the fibula to facilitate positioning under the femur.

■ Fix the reconstituted fibula with a smooth Steinmann pin placed intramedullary. A Syme's or Boyd's ankle disarticulation can be done simultaneously or at a later time.

■ Close the skin over a hemovac drain, and immobilize the limb from toe to groin in a maximal, but comfortable, degree of extension.

Change the cast at monthly intervals up to the third or fourth month, at which time remove the K-wires and immediately apply a prosthesis. We prefer to attempt the operation at the age of walking, between 1 and 2 years of age, rather than keeping the patient in a cast until the time when a prosthesis can be applied.

Complications include ligamentous instability, dislocation or subluxation of the fibula from under the femur, stiffness, and recurrent knee flexion contracture. The latter can be treated by hamstring release, but after one or two attempts at making this procedure work, consider knee disarticulation or tibial fibula fusion.

Knee Disarticulation

The mainstay of treatment for Kalamchi type I tibial deformity, in which there is no meaningful tibial remnant, is a knee disarticulation with prosthetic fitting as an above-knee amputee. The distal femoral growth plate is preserved by this technique and therefore considerable growth potential is salvaged. Take care during the procedure not to inadvertently breech the growth plate or the surrounding perichondrium. The following description assumes a nonfunctional tibial anlage, so the usual structures are described. In the actual situation, modifications may be necessary depending on what is actually encountered.

■ With the patient in a supine position and under tourniquet control, make an anterior transverse skin incision commencing 1–2 cm distal to the tibial tubercle (or where it should be), sloping upward medially and laterally toward the joint line to a point slightly posterior to the mid-coronal plane (Fig. 174.9). Carry the incision posteriorly 2–3 cm distal to the popliteal crease. Any extraneous flap tissue can always be trimmed later, but too short a flap may necessitate shortening the femur, potentially injuring the physis.

■ Incise the deep fascia in line with the fish-mouth skin incision. If present, divide the patellar ligament and excise the patella to prevent later chondromalacia.

■ With the knee flexed to 90°, divide the medial and lateral collateral ligaments and anterior and posterior cruciate ligaments as distally as feasible.

■ Isolate and ligate the popliteal artery and accompanying veins individually.

■ Gently pull the posterior tibial nerve distally and divide it proximally; if it is accompanied by large veins, ligate these before they are allowed to retract proximally. Treat the peroneal nerve similarly.

■ Next, divide the sartorius, gracilis, semimembranosus, and semitendinosus tendons at their insertions into the tibia, and the biceps femoris at its fibular insertion. Section the iliotibial band transverse to its fibers, and incise the capsule of the knee at the joint line, eventually circumferentially.

■ Finally, divide the gastrocnemius muscle heads at their origins on the femur, and pass the leg off the table.

■ Close by approximating the hamstring tendons and the patellar ligament to the cruciate ligaments, trimming any excess skin and closing the skin flaps over a drain.

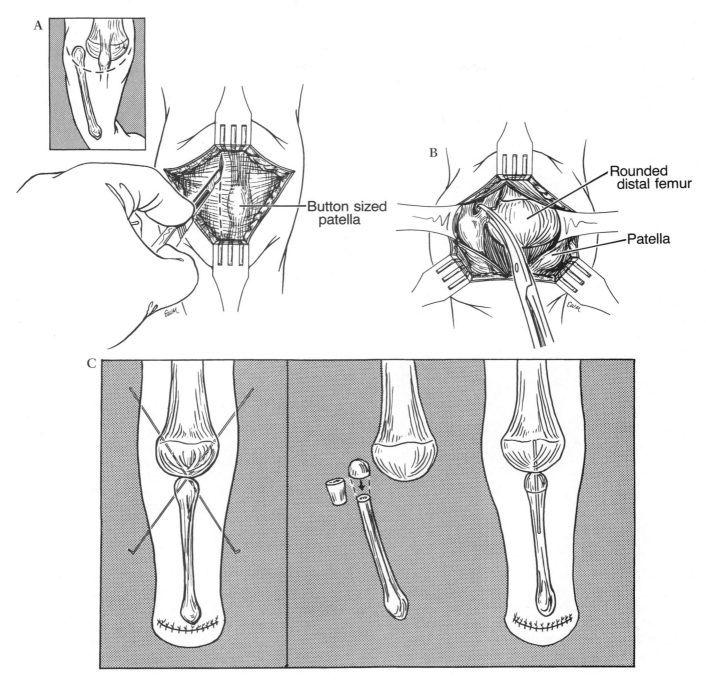

Figure 174.8. The Brown procedure. **A:** Incision utilized for the Brown procedure. **B:** Release of fibular tethering; note roundness of distal femur. **C:** Cross K-wire fixation. If the fibula cannot be relocated distally under the femur, a segmental resection of the upper part of the fibula may help.

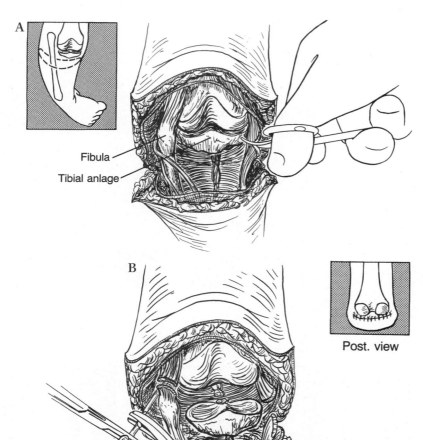

Fibula
Tibial anlage

Peroneal nerve

Post. view

Figure 174.9.   Knee disarticulation for severe tibial deficiency. **A:** Expose the distal femur through a transverse incision. The patellar and tibial anlage shown here for clarity are usually absent in those cases requiring knee disarticulation. **B:** Divide the collateral ligaments, ligate the neurovascular bundle, and divide the peroneal nerve. We routinely resect the patella to prevent later chrondromalacia.

It is unnecessary and meddlesome to trim the femoral condyles, as might be attempted for an adult.

■ Apply a rigid plaster dressing that will remain for 4–6 weeks; in small children, a single hip spica may be necessary to keep the cast in position.

PARTIAL ABSENCE OF THE TIBIA

Transfer of the Fibula into the Proximal Tibial Anlage

The transfer of the fibula into the proximal tibial anlage can be done in an end-to-end fashion with intramedullary pins, or by side-to-side approximation with interfragmentary screw fixation. Fusion must await the development of a bony tibial diaphysis, if it is not initially present.

■ Make a longitudinal anterior incision centered over the distal portion of the tibial remnant (Fig. 174.7).

■ Approach the fibula through a separate lateral incision and dissect the peroneal nerve free where it crosses the fibula.

■ Transect the fibula at the level of the distal tibial anlage, and excise the proximal portion. Transpose the distal fibula by incising intervening tissue as necessary. Align the distal transected fibula with the tibial anlage and secure the final alignment with the tibia with a K-wire or smooth intramedullary Steinmann pin.

■ Alternatively, if the anlage is very short, a side-to-side fusion may be performed by fixation with small screws or cross K-wires. Apply a long-leg or single-hip spica cast until healing is assured (2–3 months).

Perform prosthetic fitting shortly after cast removal. At

times, the union can appear tenuous, especially if considerable residual cartilage was encountered in the tibial anlage, but progressive ossification of the fibrous union does mature over time. A simultaneous Syme's amputation is usually performed, although some surgeons continue to attempt preservation of the foot by tibiofibular fusion. The Ilizarov apparatus can be used to align and fuse the foot, but the results of such an approach are thus far unreported.

CONGENITAL DISLOCATION OF THE KNEE

Congenital dislocation of the knee (CDK) is a rare condition encompassing a continuum from mild subluxation to frank dislocation. According to Parsch (48), Koptis reported a frequency of about 1.7 per 100,000 live births. Breech presentation occurs in 30% to 40% (44). CDK is easily recognized in the neonatal period, with the knee fixed in hyperextension. The femoral condyles may be palpable in the popliteal region. The patella may not be easily located, often being displaced laterally.

Table 174.2 presents the associated anomalies and syndromes of CDK. Accompanying musculoskeletal anomalies occur in more than 50% of cases, the most common being dislocated hips and clubfeet (37). In association with Larsen's syndrome, abnormalities of the cervical spine are frequent and should be sought (9).

Thus, CDK might better be characterized as a syndrome rather than an isolated entity. Pathologic findings at surgery include quadriceps fibrosis, ablation of the suprapatellar pouch, anterior dislocation of the hamstring tendons, femoral and tibial articular surface dysplasia, and anterior cruciate elongation and attenuation (19). Children seen in the first few months of life can be treated with biweekly casting or traction until reduction is ob-

Table 174.2.   Congenital Dislocation of the Knee: Associated Anomalies and Syndromes

Talipes equinovarus
Talipes equinovalgus
Developmental dislocation of the hip
Larsen's syndrome
   Multiple joint dislocations
   Cervical or other spine abnormalities
   Typical facies and spatulate thumbs and toes
Arthrogryposis
   Multiple contractures
   Fusiform joints
   Extensor dimpling

tained or progress toward reduction is deemed to have failed. Parsch (48) found conservative treatment to be successful in two thirds of patients.

Should conservative treatment fail, open reduction is necessary. A failure is defined by persistent subluxation of the tibia on the femur, as visualized on a lateral radiograph, or the inability to obtain 45° of flexion after a trial of closed reduction and serial casting. Obliteration of the suprapatellar pouch may be seen when arthrography is performed in nonresponsive patients. Accompanying congenital hip dislocation can be difficult to treat by conventional closed methods until the knee deformity has been controlled. This is due to a tight quadriceps becoming even tighter with knee reduction and in turn precluding reduction of the hip. The Pavlik harness in such cases, aside from being difficult to apply, may actually be counterproductive unless knee flexion has been obtained prior to application. Some authors have reported its successful use in such instances (33,45).

OPEN REDUCTION

Given the pathologic findings in CDK, direct surgery toward lengthening the contracted quadriceps mechanism by V-Y advancement or Z-plasty, and releasing the tight medial and lateral capsular structures; after that, reduction can be accomplished (Fig 174.10). Anterior cruciate ligament augmentation or advancement, meniscectomy, and posterior capsule reefing are rarely necessary.

- Use an anterior midline incision curving distally and laterally. Enter the joint through a parapatellar approach. If the iliotibial band is tight anteriorly to the lateral femoral condyle, release it with a diagonal incision that can later be reapproximated in a lengthened position.
- The quadriceps tendon must be lengthened. Employ a V-Y technique (Fig. 174.10E). This release allows inspection of the joint prior to repair of the quadriceps, so that any remaining adhesions in the suprapatellar pouch area can be released, and reduction can then be obtained and secured by flexion of the knee.
- The collateral ligaments of the knee may need to be carefully released to facilitate knee flexion. The hamstring tendons ordinarily spontaneously retreat from an anterior position to one posterior to the femoral epicondyles.
- After quadriceps repair and closure, immobilize the knee in a long-leg cast flexed to 45° for 6–8 weeks.

Most children spontaneously move their knees following cast removal without the need for formal physical therapy. The goal is 90° of active flexion. Bilateral cases, however, do not seem to recover as much motion as unilateral cases (34).

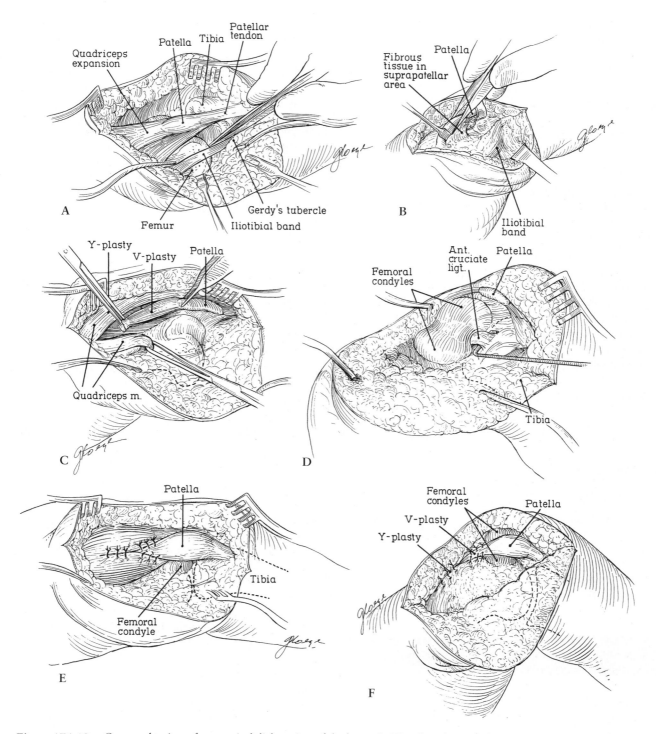

Figure 174.10.   Open reduction of congenital dislocation of the knee. **A:** Visualize the pathology through a lateral approach. The iliotibial band and quadriceps tendon are usually contracted, the hamstring tendons may be subluxed anterior to the femoral epicondyles, and the anterior cruciate often is attenuated, stretched, or absent. **B:** A condensation of fibrous tissue may connect the distal quadriceps expansion to the distal femur and should be released. **C:** Perform a V-Y quadriceps plasty. **D:** With the quadriceps divided, flexion of the knee promotes spontaneous reduction and the anterior cruciate can be inspected. Do not repair the cruciate, even if attenuated. **E:** Repair the quadriceps with the knee located. **F:** Position of immobilization postoperatively. *(continued)*

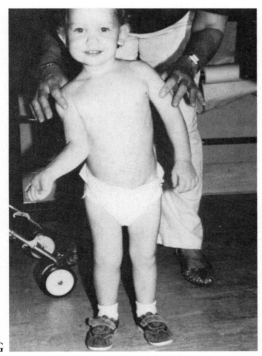
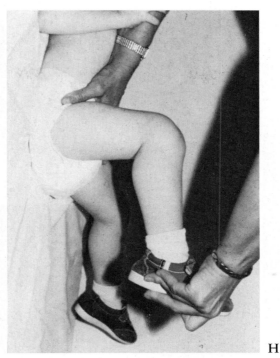

G

H

Figure 174.10. *(continued)* **G,H:** Result at 3-year follow-up. From Johnson EJ, Audell R, Oppenheim WL. Congenital Dislocation of the Knee. *J Pediatr Orthop* 1987;7:194, with permission.

CONGENITAL DISLOCATION OF THE PATELLA

Congenital dislocation of the patella (CDP) presents a challenge to the orthopedist. Not only is the patella small and misshapen, but the femoral groove is often shallow, and the entire quadriceps musculature is displaced laterally and contracted. In longstanding cases, the tibia may be laterally rotated, subluxated, and in mild valgus because of the abnormal pull of the quadriceps. The tibial tubercle appears lateral to its usual position, resulting in an increased Q angle. The diagnosis can be made by direct palpation and confirmed by radiography, ultrasonography, or MRI. Keep in mind that the patella does not normally ossify until 4–6 years of age. It is thus easy to miss the diagnosis if relying on radiography alone. The keys to diagnosis are a high level of suspicion in addition to the clinical findings of a knee flexion contracture associated with an external rotation deformity of the tibia, lack of full extension, and weakness. Because of this, the diagnosis is rarely made before the age of walking.

Congenital dislocation of the patella may be familial, occur sporadically, or be associated with Down syndrome or arthrogryposis. It frequently occurs bilaterally. The natural history of untreated patellar dislocation is early degenerative arthritis, pain, and disability. Conservative therapy is futile; surgery is indicated once the diagnosis becomes clear. Most operative techniques have stressed a soft-tissue release of the quadriceps associated with a V-Y-plasty of the quadriceps tendon, with realignment of the patellar ligament insertion. The operative technique must not breach the tibial physis in skeletally immature individuals, but realignment of the patellar ligament can be performed utilizing the Roux Goldthwait procedure (split patellar tendon transfer), or alternatively, the patellar ligament, in its entirety, can be medially transposed into the periosteum over the proximal tibia. We routinely perform a Galleazzi semitendinosus tenodesis of the patella. In skeletally mature individuals, the tibial tubercle itself may be translocated medially.

TECHNIQUE OF REDUCTION

There are several techniques to correct a congenitally dislocated patella (26,27,56). We prefer the following technique.

■ Begin with a straight lateral incision at the junction of the middle and upper thirds of the thigh and extend it distally lateral to the dislocated patella across the femoral condyle, and then swing medially across but 2 cm distal to the tibial tubercle (Fig. 174.11).

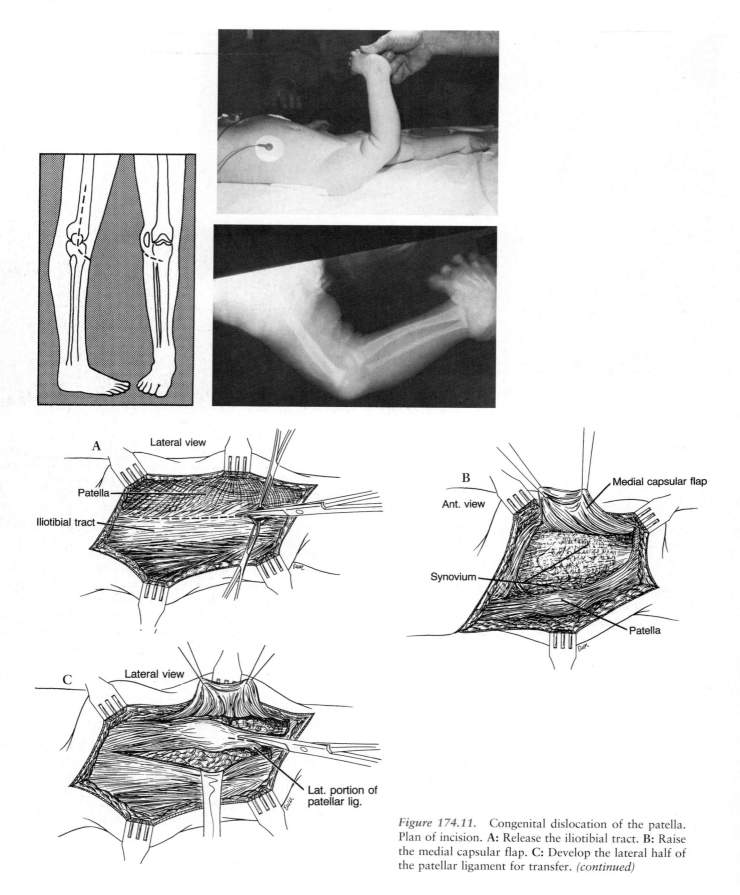

Figure 174.11.   Congenital dislocation of the patella. Plan of incision. **A:** Release the iliotibial tract. **B:** Raise the medial capsular flap. **C:** Develop the lateral half of the patellar ligament for transfer. *(continued)*

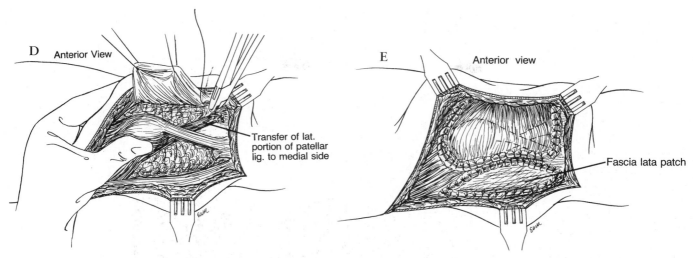

Figure 174.11. *(continued)* **D:** Transfer the lateral patellar ligament to the medial aspect of the tibia. **E:** Repair the medial capsular flap over the patella and advance the vastus medialis insertion. The resulting lateral capsular defect may be patched with a piece of harvested fascia lata.

- Dissect down to the iliotibial band, and divide it obliquely so it may later be repaired in a lengthened position if necessary. Follow the band posteriorly to its insertion on the femur by separating it from the adherent fibers of the vastus lateralis; this portion of the band is known as the lateral intermuscular septum.
- Elevate the quadriceps extraperiosteally off the femur and up the lateral aspect of the femur to the proximal one-quarter.
- Lateral to the patella, make an incision through the capsule and connect it to the main release along the vastus lateralis.
- On the medial side of the patella, incise the large flap of attenuated capsule for later plication, and separate the vastus medialis from the quadriceps expansion distally.
- Relocate the patella in the femoral groove. If flexion cannot be accomplished to 90° with the patella in the groove, lengthen the quadriceps in a V-Y fashion and/or release any fibrotic bands.
- Now sew the semicircular flap over the patella and anchor it to the tissue along its lateral aspect. Advance the vastus medialis as necessary to produce stable tracking of the patella. Flex the knee at each stage to see if the patella is becoming more stable in the femoral groove; if not, adjust the tension of the suturing accordingly.
- The patellar ligament almost always appears to be attached too laterally on the tibia, so split the patellar ligament longitudinally and detach the lateral portion just proximal to its insertion. Then transfer this detached free stump under the medial portion of the ligament and suture it into the periosteum along the medial

aspect of the tibia near the insertion of the tibial collateral ligament. Take care not to make the attachment so tight that the patella becomes rotated around its longitudinal axis. A piece of tensor fascia lata may be used to close the lateral capsular defect, if desired, although we do not routinely do this.

GALLEAZZI PROCEDURE

As mentioned, we routinely perform the Galleazzi semitendinosus transfer procedure to keep the patella relocated.

- First, identify the semitendinosus tendon at its insertion into the pes anserinus. Through the main incision or through a separate incision, release the tendon at its musculotendinous junction and free the tendon to its distal insertion into the pes anserina, which can be partially released to allow the insertion of the tendon to move more medially on the tibia.
- Make an oblique drill hole from inferomedially to superolaterally through the lower medial patella, parallel to the articular surface.
- Then pass the semitendinosus stump through the drill hole and suture it to itself or to the dorsal periosteum of the patella to complete the tenodesis.
- After wound closure, apply a long-leg cast for 4–6 weeks.

Commence active and passive exercises of the knee when the cast is removed if the child does not exhibit spontaneous motion and improvement. In older children, the hamstrings may occasionally need to be lengthened to correct a residual fixed flexion deformity. We have not employed prolonged bracing following cast removal.

CONGENITAL COXA VARA

Congenital or developmental coxa vara occurs perinatally and is characterized by a decreased femoral neck shaft angle in association with a primary femoral neck defect. This defect involves both the inferior portion of the capital physis and the adjacent metaphysis. Histologically, it represents a defect in enchondral ossification (16,51). Some authors have commented on a hereditary tendency, but there is no predilection for sex or race (5,16,46,67). Radiographs confirm the decreased neck shaft angle as well as a shallow acetabulum and widened teardrop. Because of the varus, the center–edge angle may appear to be normal, which can cause the examiner to underestimate the true dysplasia of the acetabulum.

Although the etiology is unknown, studies of the natural history suggest the early onset of degenerative arthritis and increasing disability for those cases that progress (5). Because of this, the mainstay of treatment has been proximal valgus osteotomy. Most cases are diagnosed because of a limp or waddling gait in children 3–12 years of age. Only a few children present with leg or back pain. Coxa vara can also present in association with syndromes such as coxa vara with femoral shortening, coxa vara as part of PFFD, multiple epiphyseal dysplasia, cleidocranial dysostosis, achondroplasia, or hypothyroidism. In addition, coxa vara can be acquired as a sequella of Legg-Perthes disease, infection, trauma, or as a complication of treatment for developmental hip dysplasia or other diseases. For the true developmental or congenital cases with only mild shortening or femoral bowing, Weinstein et al. (67) utilized Hilgenreiner's epiphyseal angle to help define treatment indications. This is the angle formed between Hilgenreiner's line and a line drawn on the anteroposterior (AP) radiographic projection parallel to the capital physis. In the study by Weinstein et al., when the angle was in excess of 60°, progression was the rule; if it was less than 45°, the deformities spontaneously corrected. In the 46° to 59° range, the natural history was not predictable so the patients were observed for signs of progression prior to undergoing surgery. The goal of surgical correction was to restore the Hilgenreiner epiphyseal angle to less than 45° (Fig. 174.12).

In our practice, we simply utilize the neck–shaft angle on standing AP radiographs with both knees in the same position and pointing as anteriorly as possible. Deformities associated with a neck–shaft angle of 110° or better are followed with the expectation of resolution. Those less than 100° are operated early to avoid continued shear stress on the physis. The group between 100° and 110°

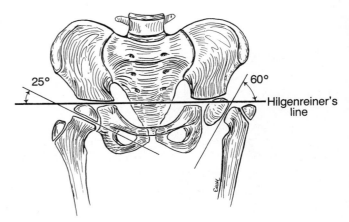

Figure 174.12. The Hilgenreiner epiphyseal angle. This measurement is helpful in predicting which cases of coxa vara should be observed and which should be operated on.

are observed for 6 months to 1 year to see whether they will spontaneously resolve.

The goal of surgery is to restore a normal neck–shaft angle while avoiding damage to the capital physis and greater trochanteric apophysis. However, Schmidt and Kalamchi (52) have noted premature closure of the capital physis in 90% of operated case, even when direct injury was avoided. In addition, they carefully studied the acetabular development, noted it to be deficient, and concluded that unless correction to 140° or better was achieved at surgery, the acetabular dysplasia did not improve. Thus the goal is correction of the neck–shaft angle to at least 140°.

VALGUS OSTEOTOMY

Determine the amount of correction to be obtained on the preoperative radiograph. Use an image intensifier prior to commencing the actual surgery to obtain a final check on the true neck–shaft angle. Rotate the hip until the femoral neck appears the longest, and then measure the neck–shaft angle on that particular projection. If necessary, perform a percutaneous adductor tenotomy to facilitate later closure of the bony osteotomy. Because of the incidence of premature physeal closure of the capital physis, and the possibility that this may be related to tight musculature, consider lengthening the iliopsoas as well.

- Approach the hip laterally through a longitudinal skin incision and split the iliotibial band. Elevate the vastus lateralis subperiosteally from the proximal femur. Use a pediatric osteotomy screw (or, alternatively, a pediatric blade plate and matching instrument set) (Fig. 174.13).
- Place a guide wire along the front of the femoral neck to locate its axis, and introduce a guide pin through the lateral cortex up to but not through the capital physis.

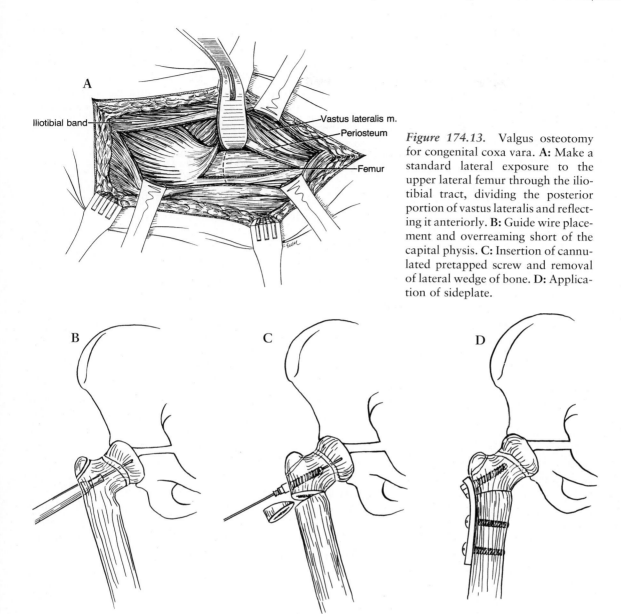

Iliotibial band

Vastus lateralis m.
Periosteum

Femur

Figure 174.13. Valgus osteotomy for congenital coxa vara. **A:** Make a standard lateral exposure to the upper lateral femur through the iliotibial tract, dividing the posterior portion of vastus lateralis and reflecting it anteriorly. **B:** Guide wire placement and overreaming short of the capital physis. **C:** Insertion of cannulated pretapped screw and removal of lateral wedge of bone. **D:** Application of sideplate.

- Ream over this wire, then tap the hole under image intensifier control, and finally introduce a screw of appropriate length. Attach the spanner to the femoral neck screw to control the proximal portion while removing with an oscillating saw a wedge of bone based laterally at the level of the lesser trochanter.
- Now close the osteotomy and apply a two-hole side plate bent with the bending irons to accommodate the new shape of the lateral cortex.
- Check the position with the image intensifier or plain radiographs, and then secure the plate to the proximal femoral shaft using 4.5 mm screws.
- Then irrigate the wound and close it over a hemovac drain, which is removed at 48 hours.

Immobilize the child in a one-and-one-half hip spica cast for 6 weeks or until the osteotomy is radiographically united. Treat residual leg-length discrepancy by a lift and, if necessary, by an appropriately planned epiphysiodesis of the opposite femur.

Complications include continued acetabular dysplasia, premature closure of the capital physis, overgrowth of the greater trochanteric, leg-length discrepancy, recurrence of varus, malunion, nonunion, failure of fixation, avascular necrosis, and infection. These problems may be treated as necessary by techniques described in Chapters 29, 166, 170, 171, and 173. Repeat valgus osteotomy is sometimes required if the enchondral neck defect has not healed within a year.

CONGENITAL DEFICIENCIES OF THE FEMUR

Congenital deficiencies of the femur form a continuum from simple hypoplasia to total absence. The deficiencies may be diffuse or limited to the upper or lower portions, and they are often associated with other limb deficits and other organ anomalies. Many classification schemes have been proposed to aid in selecting proper treatment. Most focus on PFFD. Some include congenital short femur as the least affected category in the spectrum. However, a child with a congenital short femur is most frequently amenable to lengthening, whereas few with PFFD are. Hence, we prefer to think of these deformities as separate entities.

Treatment can range from observation to amputation and fitting with a prosthesis, so a general treatment protocol is not easy to describe. Subtleties of hip, knee, or ankle strength and motion, along with the wishes of the family regarding cosmesis, may play pivotal roles in the final plan, and no one treatment will ever be correct for every child.

CONGENITAL SHORT FEMUR

For children with congenital shortness of the femur who have a stable hip and knee (including those instances in which a stable knee and hip have resulted through surgical intervention), limb lengthening may be indicated. Children whose limbs are predicted to have a discrepancy at maturity in the range of 5–15 cm can be considered for lengthening. We prefer to lengthen using Ilizarov's biology (i.e., lengthening of a healing callus) while utilizing a unilateral half-pin fixator (such as the Wagner) (64) for its safety and convenience. For less than 5 cm of predicted leg-length discrepancy, we perform percutaneous epiphysiodesis.

Leg equalization of up to 5 cm can usually be gained by epiphysiodesis. For example, a child with a predicted discrepancy of 7.5 cm would be left with a 2.5 cm discrepancy after epiphysiodesis. The parents need to decide whether the potential complications associated with lengthening are worth it to correct the remaining discrepancy.

Keep in mind that the need to equalize the length of the extremities does not have to be accomplished by a single technique. A difference of 10 cm could, for example, be made up with an acceptance of a 2 cm difference, the addition of a 1 cm lift inside the shoe, and an epiphysiodesis of 7 cm, resulting in a final lengthening of 10 cm. A lengthening of 10 cm is within reason, whereas a lengthening of 20 cm would be beyond the margin of current practice. For discrepancies predicted to be in excess of 20 cm, seriously consider amputation and prosthetic fitting.

In general, the milder forms of femoral dysplasia are associated with coxa vara, whereas the more serious forms, normally classified under the banner of PFFD, are associated with subtrochanteric bowing. Subtrochanteric bowing may be corrected prior to consideration of limb-length equalization. However, coxa vara can help stabilize the hip joint during femoral lengthening and is better corrected after the lengthening is complete.

PROXIMAL FEMORAL FOCAL DEFICIENCY

The management of children with PFFD has been confused by an array of classification systems that have focused on the radiographic appearance of the hip. The major decisions in caring for a child with PFFD concern primarily the marked limb shortening and depend very little on the anatomy of the hip.

Classification

Clearly, children with PFFD are not all the same. Classification systems can be used to organize clinical material for presentation in the medical literature, or they can be used to help the orthopedic surgeon make clinical decisions for an individual child; sometimes they serve both functions. Aitken's (3) classification of PFFD is an example of the first use. It focuses entirely on the radiographic appearance of the bones of the upper end of the femur and the pelvis (Fig. 174.14). This classification plays a moderately small role in the overall decision making. The classifications of Pappas (47), Fixen (24), and Amstutz (5) are similarly constrained. By contrast, the classification by Torode and Gillespie (62) is concise and practical: "short" (i.e., lengthenable) or "very short" (extend with a prosthesis). This useful classification scheme focuses on the real problem—the marked limb shortening.

Clinical Decision Issues

Initially, help the family decide whether their child has a useful extremity that can be lengthened, or whether lengthening is unrealistic and the leg needs to be shortened and the difference to the ground made up with a prosthesis.

Amstutz (5) made a significant contribution by pointing out that the length of the short leg compared to the normal leg at infancy remains in the same proportion at maturity. This allows prediction, while the child is still an infant, of what the ultimate leg-length difference will be at the end of growth. The parents can become accustomed to the problems that need to be faced, which usually makes their decisions easier. Orthopedic surgeons have differed between stating leg-length differences as absolute numbers of centimeters versus percentages of the bone length. There is no agreement currently. An average male femur at maturity is approximately 46 cm, and an average female femur is 43 cm. A leg-length difference anticipated to be

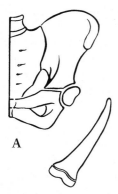
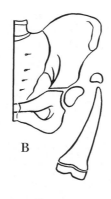
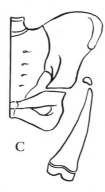
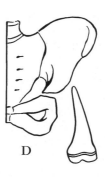

Figure 174.14.   The Aitken classification for proximal femoral focal deficiency. Types A and B generally have a well-developed acetabulum and by implication a femoral head anlage, even when not initially visualized. Types C and D are usually shorter and the acetabular landmarks are ill defined. Types B and C are characterized on early radiographs by a tufted appearance of the upper femur, which most likely is an ossified portion of femur above a nonossified area.

greater than 40% to 50% of the normal length at maturity will not likely leave a child with a good functioning extremity even if lengthened.

The options for making up for the marked leg-length difference are to (a) lengthen; (b) remove the foot and fit the child as a below-knee amputee, accepting the huge difference in knee heights; (c) remove the foot, fuse the knee, and shorten the limb so that the child can be fitted as an above-knee amputee; or (d) perform a Van Nes rotationplasty.

Lengthen the Short Bone   If children with a congenitally short femur are excluded from the category of PFFD, relatively few children with a PFFD would have limbs that can be equalized by lengthening.

The hip needs to be stable before lengthening can proceed, although rarely the proximal arm of the lengthening device can be fixed to the pelvis.

Even though the diagnosis is described as a proximal femoral deficiency, most children have deformity in the distal femoral condyles and the ligaments about the knee, as well as deficiencies of the fibula and foot. Lengthening a femur that has a congenital deficiency is much more likely to result in anterior subluxation of the femur on the tibia, ultimately resulting in poor knee function. Lengthening should not be performed by surgeons who do not do it on a frequent basis.

Fit as a Below-Knee Amputee   Remove the foot by Syme's or Boyd's amputation (discussed previously) and use an extra-long below-knee prosthesis. This is a simple solution, but it is cosmetically unappealing due to the great difference in knee heights, which is especially ob-

vious when the child is sitting. This choice is less frequently taken now than in years past.

Shorten and Fit at the Above-Knee Level   If lengthening is not a realistically practical option, consider shortening the limb sufficiently that the child will be able to function well as an above-knee amputee. King (38) initially suggested the concept of a single skeletal lever, and he fused the knee joint in an effort to improve hip function and to facilitate prosthetic fitting. As a part of this procedure, the foot must be removed. This can be done either as Syme's or as Boyd's amputation. Many surgeons favor Syme's amputation because of its simplicity. However, Syme's amputation done in infancy has more of a tendency to "pencil-point thinning" of the distal tibia. The worries about heel-pad migration are probably overstated, because the skin of children will modify to the pressures applied, as witnessed in children with untreated clubfeet who are able to walk on the dorsum of their feet without skin breakdown. However, there is not good scientific evidence to enable an informed choice between these two procedures, so the choice tends to be one of personal preference of the surgeon.

Ultimately, the end of the stump on the deficient side should be sufficiently short to allow room for a standard mechanical knee joint in the prosthesis to be at the level of the opposite, normal knee. Although orthopedic surgeons have often focused on the end of the bony stump as seen on a scanogram, remember that there is soft tissue beyond that as well as room needed for the socket padding and the thickness of the socket itself—a total of almost 3 cm. An ideal to aim for is that the end of the bone of the stump be 10 cm proximal to the knee joint on the opposite side.

Most children with PFFD have a tibia on the short side that is approximately 90% or more of the normal length (i.e., in boys about 37 cm and in girls about 35 cm, or about 10 cm shorter than the average normal femur). This means that if the tibia is left intact and there is any segment of femur remaining, the probability is overwhelming that the stump will be excessively long. There should therefore be plans to either excise one or both physes around the knee if considering a knee fusion or, alternatively, be a plan for epiphysiodesis at the appropriate time.

Knee Fusion   Most children with PFFD live with the anatomic knee held in flexion. They will often sit on the thigh section of their prosthesis. This gives decreased control and power over the prosthesis and aligns the vertical axis of the prosthesis lateral to the center of gravity, producing a lateral lurch in the stance phase of gait. Function can be greatly enhanced if the femur is fused to the tibia. When this is done, the fusion must be done with the knee in full extension. Initially, there may be enough of a hip flexion contracture that the residual extremity will not come to neutral at the hip, but this stretches out in short order (38). In the past, this procedure was not frequently performed, but it is now routine. Delay knee fusion until the proximal tibial center of ossification is easily visualized by plain radiography, usually between 18 months and 2 years of age.

■ Use an anterolateral approach. Section the patellar ligament and remove the patella along with the menisci and cruciate ligaments. Perform the femoral resection just proximal to the distal physis; divide the gastrocnemius at the level of the insertions to the posterior femoral condyles. Protect the peroneal nerve and posterior neurovascular bundle throughout the resection.

■ Use a knife or micro–air saw to resect the articular cartilage of the tibia, carefully exposing the ossification nucleus to its widest diameter.

■ Introduce a Rush rod retrograde through the intercondylar notch of the femur, exiting along the lateral aspect of the proximal femur. Then withdraw it and drive it antegrade across the knee to fix the fusion in good alignment. The Rush rod should be centralized in the proximal tibial physis as much as possible. We have not observed growth arrest, but cross K-wire fixation above the tibial physis is an alternative method of fixation.

■ Use the resected distal femur for supplemental bone graft, if needed.

■ Close the wound over suction drainage.

Syme's amputation may be performed at the same time, although some surgeons delay this stage for 6 weeks.

Van Nes Procedure   An alternative to the knee fusion just described and the fitting as an above-knee amputee is the Van Nes rotationplasty (63), in which the leg is rotated 180° so that the ankle functions as a substitute for the knee (25,29,39,40,63) (Fig. 174.15). A special prosthesis is used that uses the ankle as the knee and the foot as the leg, similar to a standard below-knee prosthesis. (The socket usually has an additional thigh support attached with outside hinges.) For this to be successful, there are three requirements:

• The length must be appropriate. Ultimately, the reversed ankle should be at approximately the level of the opposite knee joint. Plantar flexion and dorsiflexion of the foot is a composite of the motion at the ankle and the subtalar joints. The axis of rotation for the purposes of prosthetic fitting is at the tip of the lateral malleolus. The limb can be shortened an appropriate amount at the time of rotation and/or knee fusion. It is rare to have the extremity too short, because that would be due to a considerable deformity in the tibia and would probably be associated with an inadequately functioning ankle joint.

• The ankle must be sufficiently normal to function as a substitute knee. It must have an appropriate range of motion and sufficient strength to power a prosthesis. A foot with all five rays usually has these requirements, but not invariably.

• The psychological acceptance of the procedure needs to be within the tolerable limits of the patient, the family, and the medical personnel looking after the child. Concerns may vary from age to age and culture to culture. In medical centers where the Van Nes procedure is frequently performed, there are usually other children and families who can act as models and counsel potential patients and their parents. The psychology of the medical staff cannot be ignored. If the medical personnel feel that such procedures are bizarre, it is clear that they will not be offered, or they will be presented in such a manner that no patient would accept the choice. As a consequence, some centers in the United States have moderately large numbers of children who have had the procedure and other centers have none.

Additionally, prosthetic facilities must be considered. The prosthesis that is required following a Van Nes procedure is difficult to fit. If good prosthetic facilities are not available, avoid this operation.

■ Perform the knee fusion as previously described, but use the soft-tissue redundancy obtained from the femoral resection to derotate the limb.

■ Secure the knee derotation with an oblique K-wire across the fusion site, supplementing the Rush rod fixation (61).

■ Either extend the knee wound along the tibial crest or use an additional incision over the mid tibia. Incise the periosteum and resect and discard at least 1 inch of the tibia.

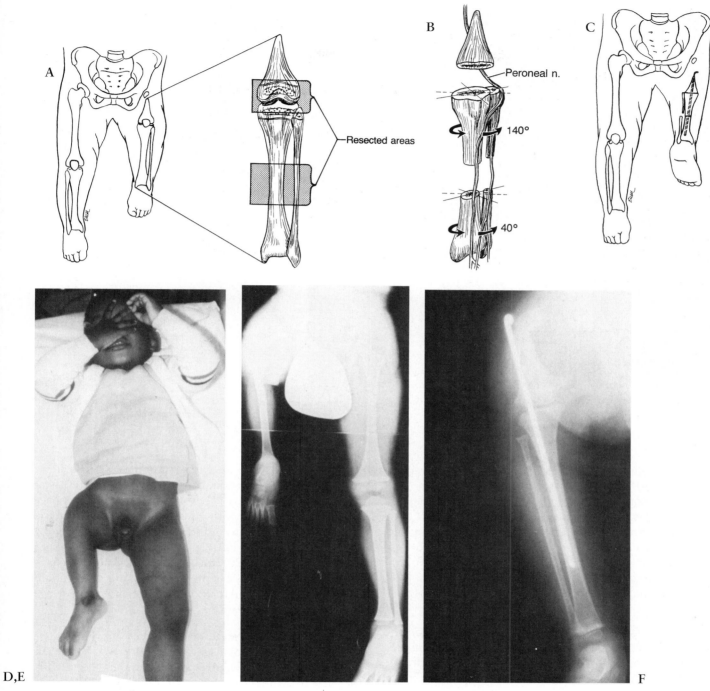

Figure 174.15.   The Van Nes turnaround procedure. **A:** Area of bony resection. **B:** Plan for derotation. The removal of bone leads to soft-tissue redundancy and the ability to rotate without injuring the muscle or neurovascular bundles. **C:** After derotation, the ankle is 180° from its usual orientation. **D,E:** Preoperative clinical appearance. **F:** Radiographs show the knee fusion and the tibial turnaround osteotomy. *(continued)*

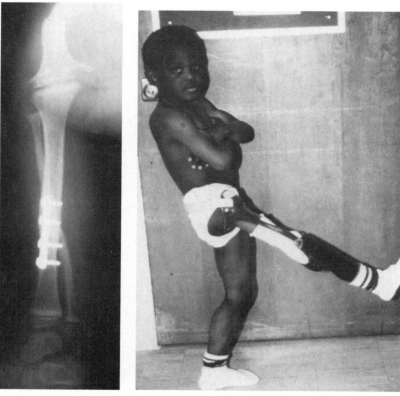

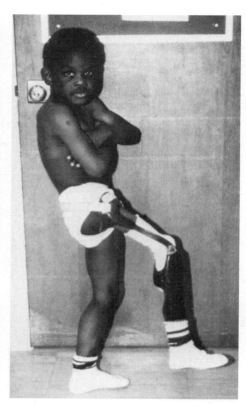

G,H

I

Figure 174.15. *(continued)* **G:** Radiographs show the knee fusion and the tibial turnaround osteotomy. **H,I:** Postoperative clinical appearance.

- Further rotate the limb laterally until the ankle is repositioned 180° with respect to the hip.
- Fix the tibia with a four-hole semitubular AO plate, or use a long enough intramedullary Rush rod to fix both the knee and the hip, and another oblique K-wire to secure rotation.
- Perform an anterior compartment release prior to closure, and use a spica cast until radiographic consolidation of the osteotomies, which usually requires 6–8 weeks.

Complications   Late fractures at the end of the intramedullary fixation device occurred in two of our patients but healed uneventfully in a spica cast. Although Hall and Bochman (29) have stated that the procedure should not be performed until maturity because remodeling and derotation of the limb require further surgery, we perform the procedure at about 2 years of age. We are content with rerotating the limb as necessary. In our experience, approximately half the patients required one repeat surgery to rerotate the limb, but only one patient of 13 required a third surgery.

Other Issues
Length of the Stump   As discussed, most children who have had conversion of their PFFD extremity to an above-

knee amputation end up with a stump that is too long. At the time of knee fusion, consider excision of the distal femoral and/or the proximal tibial physis. Some orthopaedic surgeons are wary of doing this for fear that the extremity will be much too short; however, proper application of growth data using the Green-Anderson-Mesner charts (see Chapter 170) can alleviate that fear. Moseley's straight line graph (see Chapter 170) does not differentiate between the femur and the tibia and does not provide the answer for this calculation.

Before the Definitive Surgery   Regardless of what the decision is for ultimate management, there is a period when the difference in leg lengths can be considerable, yet it is too early to do anything definitive surgically. Lifts greater than 5 cm in height tend to lead to ankle sprains, but ankle–foot prostheses can be used to decrease this likelihood. However, when the difference gets to 8 or 9 cm, an extension prosthesis (sometimes called an extension orthosis or even a prosthosis) can be made that has a hole in the front of the prosthesis distally through which the forefoot extends. If tried at too young an age, when the length difference is less than 5 cm, however, there is not room enough below the socket to fit a foot on the end of such a prosthesis.

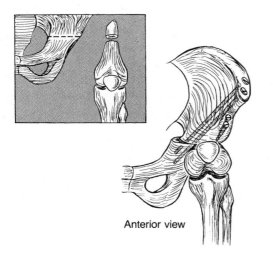

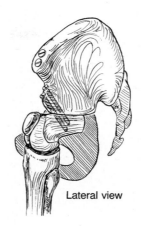

Anterior view   Lateral view

Figure 174.16. In rare cases, the knee can be used as a surrogate hip in conjunction with a Chiari osteotomy combined with fusion of the femoral remnant into the pelvis.

Reconstruction of the Hip Joint In the past, there has been a great deal of focus on the radiograph of the upper end of the femur. What is seen by the radiograph, however, is only the bone. What is going on with the cartilage, let alone the muscles, is not seen. If there is absolutely no acetabulum, the decisions regarding the management of limb length given in this chapter apply. If, on the other hand, the acetabulum is satisfactorily formed and there is some element of a femoral head in the acetabulum and some segment of upper femur that are not joined, consider surgery. Wait until there is sufficient ossification of the two fragments that they can be fused together, bone to bone. There is certainly no rush to do this, and more complications occur from proceeding too soon, before there is adequate bone stock.

Fusion of the Distal Femur to the Pelvis The distal femur can be fused to the pelvis in order to use the knee joint as a replacement for the hip joint (Fig. 174.16). This has the theoretical advantage of providing a stable hip. However, the knee joint does not allow reasonable rotation. Once it is fused to the pelvis, the distal femur has some capacity to grow, and the hip joint will grow to a point that is mechanically disadvantageous, depending on the orientation of the distal femur at the time of fusion to the pelvis. Although there have been a small number of reports of such cases (24,57), most surgeons feel that this is not an advantageous procedure and avoid it (23,25).

MISCELLANEOUS ITEMS

TERMINAL OVERGROWTH

"Overgrowth" of amputation stumps in children has always been a problem and can occur even in congenital amputees. It is particularly a problem in the humerus, the fibula, and the tibia. Pellicore et al. (1,49) found that 15% of their juvenile patients who had amputations before 12 years of age required revision, whereas none did if the amputations were done at a later age. Yet, if children required stump revisions and they were older than 12 years, overgrowth could still occur.

This overgrowth is not a result of stimulation of the physis proximally but of the development of appositional new bone on the end of the stump (see Chapter 175). The easiest way to manage the problem is to avoid it by performing amputations through a joint, where possible, so that the end of the bone is covered by its normal cartilage. If this is not possible, a number of maneuvers have been used with varying success. Silastic end pieces (either as a stemmed plug that fits into the medullary cavity or as a cap that fits over the end of the diaphyseal bone) have been tried, but frequent breakage and dislodgement of the plug or cap have led to their abandonment. Surgical procedures that provide a smooth periosteal surface around the end of the bone appear to be successful in many cases. The Marquardt method (50) (Fig. 174.17) introduced the use of autogenons epiphyseal caps. Davids et al. (21) recently reviewed their patients. Apophyseal cartilage from the iliac crest can be used. Our preference is to use the proximal fibula and invert its diaphysis into the tibial or humeral medullary canal. This cartilage cap is not expected to grow but only to provide a smooth nonosseous surface to prevent osteoblastic reaction. This has been very effective. Keep this technique in mind for situations in which transosseous amputations are required. It may be possible to salvage an epiphysial cap from part of the discarded specimen (e.g., the first metatarsal head, the talar head, or the os calcis), which could then be attached to the end of the cut bone.

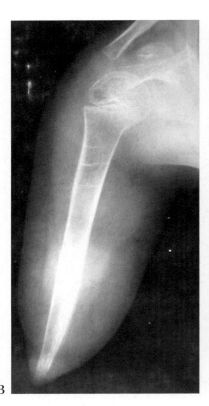
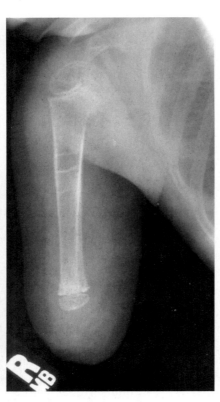

A,B

Figure 174.17. Modified Marquardt method of capping bony overgrowth in a transdiaphyseal amputation in a growing child. **A:** Preoperative radiograph showing terminal overgrowth of an above-elbow amputation. **B:** Postoperative appearance after transfer of a epiphyseal cartilage graft onto the revised distal humerus.

In children who have had amputations for tumors and who receive postoperative chemotherapy, bone protrusion at the end of the stump may be caused by soft-tissue retraction rather than terminal overgrowth. In such children, the chemotherapy adversely influences the healing of the fascia, so that the muscles draw proximally, leaving the bone protruding subcutaneously. If a stump revision is done while the child is still receiving chemotherapy, the complication is likely to recur. Several revisions may lead to an unfortunately short stump. It is better to wait until 3–6 months after the cessation of the chemotherapy to do a definitive procedure.

CONSERVATION OF PARTS FOR TOE-TO-THUMB TRANSFER

Not infrequently in treating lower extremity defects, there are concurrent hand abnormalities. Toe-to-hand transfers are now well-established procedures, so before any lower extremity parts are discarded, search for possible uses for the reconstruction of the upper extremities. We have assisted the hand surgeon with harvesting the parts prior to Syme's or Boyd's amputation, with very gratifying results.

LENGTHENING OF SHORT AMPUTATION STUMPS

For children who have amputation stumps that are very short (acquired or congenital), the gain of even a small amount of length may provide an adequate lever to use a more functional prosthesis. The advantages are decreased energy consumption, improved prosthetic control, decreased heat retention, increased comfort from the lesser weight of the prosthesis, and fewer components requiring repairs, as well as decreased cost.

Children with loss of an upper extremity, especially if the loss is congenital, frequently choose not to wear prostheses. However, longer residual limbs may allow for grasping objects in the midline between the stumps for "bimanual" activity without a prosthesis. Additionally, a longer distal segment can permit objects to be grasped between a lengthened humeral stump and the chest, or between a lengthened forearm and the upper arm.

Watts (66) reported lengthening 32 short amputation stumps in 27 patients. All were lengthened by gradual distraction using Ilizarov techniques (see Chapters 32 and 171). The 16 children who completed lengthening of their femurs or tibias achieved sufficient length to be fitted with a prosthesis at one level more distal than previously possible (Fig. 174.18). Children who underwent lengthening of their upper extremities were more difficult to assess. Three patients were lengthened with the anticipation that a prosthesis would not be used after lengthening. All became "users," in that they became able to grasp objects between the lengthened stump and trunk. Of the remaining patients—all with upper extremity lengthenings—all

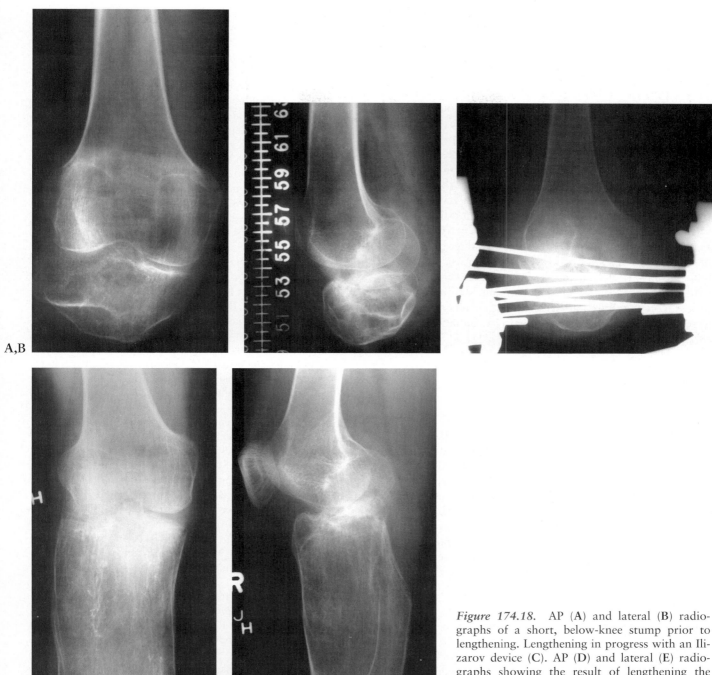

A,B

C

D,E

Figure 174.18. AP (**A**) and lateral (**B**) radiographs of a short, below-knee stump prior to lengthening. Lengthening in progress with an Ilizarov device (**C**). AP (**D**) and lateral (**E**) radiographs showing the result of lengthening the stump. The patient was converted from a functional above-knee prosthesis to a below-knee prosthesis.

but one are "wearers" of their prostheses but not constantly.

A WORD ABOUT PROSTHESES

Modern prosthetic methods help make the surgeon look good. Of less importance today than previously is the exact placement of the surgical scar, the nature of the skin, or even such complications as a displaced fat pad. Further enhancing the activities of these amputees are recent advances in prosthetic feet utilizing newer space-age energy-storing materials that have the ability to absorb and store energy at the beginning of stance, only to redeliver the energy at toe-off (14,43,65). This results in a livelier feel to the limb, and it may enhance certain activities such as running. Amputees now compete in athletic activities previously felt to be beyond their capabilities. A cottage industry has arisen that caters to amputees who are high-grade athletes in such sports as running, swimming, and skiing. Young children growing up with such conversions have a better chance than ever to enjoy an enhanced physical and psychological environment (6,21).

 AUTHORS' PERSPECTIVE

This is a very rewarding group of patients to treat surgically. Patients with these complex problems are frequently beyond the capabilities of most community orthopaedic surgeons and hospitals and are cared for at specialized centers. The long-term physician–patient relationship that develops is gratifying. The children are otherwise healthy and their zest for living and full participation in life is admirable. Early medical intervention is important for them to develop early independence and to reach their maximal potential. It is a privilege to care for them.

REFERENCES

Each reference is categorized according to the following scheme: *, classic article; #, review article; !, basic research article; and +, clinical results/outcome study.

+ 1. Abraham E, Pellicore RJ, Hamilton RC. Stump Overgrowth in Juvenile Amputees: *J Pediatr Orthop* 1986;6:66.
+ 2. Achterman C, Kalamchi A. Congenital Deficiency of the Fibula. *J Bone Joint Surgery Br* 1979;61:133.
* 3. Aitken GT. Amputation as a Treatment for Certain Lower-Extremity Congenital Anomalies. *J Bone Joint Surg Am* 1959;41:1267.
# 4. Albee F. *Orthopaedic and Reconstruction Surgery*. Philadelphia: WB Saunders, 1921:914.

5. Amstutz HC. The Morphology, Natural History, and Treatment of Proximal Femoral Focal Deficiencies. In: Aitken GT, ed. *Proximal Femoral Focal Deficiency. A Congenital Anomaly*. Washington, DC: National Academy of Sciences, 1969:50.
+ 6. Anderson L, Westin GW, Oppenheim WL. Syme Amputation in Children: Indications, Results, and Long-Term Follow-up. *J Pediatr Orthop* 1984;4:550.
+ 7. Bardenhauer. Reported by Rincheval. Ein Neues Operations Verfahren zur Behandlung Congenitaler Deffecte Eines Unterarm und Unterschenkelknochens. *Arch Klin Chir* 1894;48:802.
+ 8. Blum CE, Kalamchi A. Boyd Amputations in Children. *Clin Orthop* 1982;165:138.
+ 9. Bowen JR, Ortega K, Ray S, MacEwen GD. Spinal Deformities in Larsen's Syndrome. *Clin Orthop* 1985;197:159.
* 10. Boyd HB. Amputation of the Foot with Calcaneotibial Arthrodesis. *J Bone Joint Surg* 1939;21:997.
* 11. Braun H. Ueber Die Intrauterinen Frakturen der Tibia. *Arch Klin Chir* 1886;34:668.
+ 12. Brown FW. Construction of Knee Joint in Congenital Total Absence of the Tibia (Paraxial Hemimelia Tibia). *J Bone Joint Surg Am* 1965;47:695.
+ 13. Brown FW, Pohnert WH. Construction of a Knee Joint in Meromelia Tibia (Congenital Absence of the Tibia). A Fifteen Year Follow-up Study. *J Bone Joint Surg Am* 1972;54:1333.
+ 14. Burgess EM, Hittenberger DA, Forsgren SM, Lindh D. The Seattle Prosthetic Foot—A Design for Active Sports: Preliminary Studies. *Orthotic Prosthetics* 1983;37:25.
+ 15. Choi BI, Kumar SJ, Bowen RJ. Amputation or Limb Lengthening for Partial or Total Absence of the Fibula. *J Bone Joint Surg Am* 1990;72:1391.
! 16. Chung SMK, Riser WH. The Histological Characteristics of Congenital Coxa Vara. A Case Report of a Five Year Old Boy. *Clin Orthop* 1978;132:71.
* 17. Conn HR. A New Method for Operative Reduction for Congenital Luxation of the Patella. *J Bone Joint Surg Am* 1925;7:370.
+ 18. Coventry MB, Johnson EW. Congenital Absence of the Fibula. *J Bone Joint Surg Am* 1952;34:941.
+ 19. Curtis BH, Fisher RL. Congenital Hyperextension with Anterior Subluxation of the Knee. *J Bone Joint Surg Am* 1969;51:255.
+ 20. Dal Monte A, Donzelli O. Tibial Lengthening According to Ilizarov in Congenital Hypoplasia of the Leg. *J Pediatr Orthop* 1987;7:135.
+ 21. Davids JR, Meyer LC, Blackhurst DW. Operative Treatment of Bone Overgrowth in Children Who Have an Acquired or Congenital Amputation. *J Bone Joint Surg Am* 1995;77:1490.
+ 22. De Sanctis N, Razzano E, Scognamiglio R, Rega AN. Tibial Agenesis: A New Rationale in Management of Type II—Report of Three Cases with Long-Term Follow-Up. *J Pediatr Orthop* 1990;10:198.
# 23. Epps CH. Proximal Femoral Focal Deficiency. Current Concepts Review. *J Bone Joint Surg Am* 1983;65:867.

George T. Rab

Amputations in children, while following many of the same principles as in adults, require special considerations and techniques because of continuing growth (1). This chapter reviews the general disorders requiring amputation and specific techniques useful in the skeletally immature patient.

GENERAL PRINCIPLES

Skeletal growth and remodeling have an enormous effect on the ultimate success of a pediatric amputation, particularly in the younger child. For example, a 6-year-old child who has a successful above-knee amputation will have an extremely short stump at maturity because of loss of the distal femoral physis. In addition, stumps in children tend to become narrow and conical with growth, and this may subsequently lead to poor rotational control of a prosthesis.

A problem unique to pediatric amputations is terminal overgrowth. Overgrowth probably results from distal ap-

position of bone by the active periosteum, although the exact mechanism is not understood. Overgrowth is not dependent on the physis, and epiphysiodesis will not arrest it. Overgrowth never occurs after disarticulation. Terminal overgrowth is most severe before 6 years of age, and several revisions (three or more) may be required during the growing years. Overgrowth is not seen after about 12 years of age. The bones most likely to exhibit overgrowth are the humerus, fibula, and tibia. The exact incidence depends on the diagnostic categories of the reported series (congenital or traumatic). Many surgical remedies for overgrowth, such as capping, osteotomy, and surgical cross-union, have been attempted and discarded; the only effective treatment seems to be surgical revision of the pointed distal bone and its overlying bursa.

Emotional issues are generally far less troublesome for the pediatric amputee than for the adult amputee. The congenital amputee, born without the limb segment, accepts the condition as normal. Children who lose a limb traumatically generally rehabilitate quickly when a prosthesis is fitted. The main requirement of the child is function and durability, often with little concern for appearance or body image. However, parental acceptance of congenital or acquired amputations may be difficult. Feelings of guilt or inappropriate fears may require specialized

G. T. Rab: Department of Orthopaedics, University of California–Davis, Sacramento, California, 95817.

counseling. Phantom limb and phantom pain, common in the adult amputee, are rare in children and generally absent in the congenital amputee.

The unique congenital disorders of children, special surgical techniques, and the special aspects of prosthetic fittings during growth have led to multidisciplinary child amputee clinics in centers throughout the country (6). The value and success of this approach has been documented, and the surgeon should consider referral to a regional center if one is available.

Standard surgical principles for amputation in the child include the following:

- Preserve the physis. Amputations through the metaphysis (such as above-knee or distal forearm level) or diaphysis are not recommended in children because of the progressive relative shortening of the residual limb. This is most critical in the femur, but it is applicable to other long bones as well.
- Disarticulate when possible. Disarticulation completely eliminates the problem of terminal overgrowth and subsequent revision surgery.
- Preserve stump shape. The pediatric amputation stump becomes conical with growth, so preservation of bony architecture such as a short segment of proximal fibula or the distal condyles of the humerus will assist in subsequent rotational control of the prosthesis.
- Be creative with soft-tissue coverage. Pediatric amputees rarely suffer from the wound-healing problems that commonly affect dysvascular adult amputees. Split-thickness skin can often be successfully used in the child to preserve an otherwise satisfactory stump without adequate skin coverage. The split-thickness skin graft can hypertrophy and become sufficiently strong to withstand the shear forces of prosthesis use.

DISORDERS REQUIRING AMPUTATION IN CHILDREN

CONGENITAL AMPUTATIONS

The child born with a single or multiple limb deficiency knows no other body image and has a remarkable ability to use a prosthesis to enhance function (5,8). Although the child automatically accepts the limb deficiency as normal, parents are often emotionally overwhelmed by depression and guilt. Early referral of the family to a regional child amputee clinic facilitates the counseling and acceptance by the family that is as necessary for a satisfactory outcome as orthopaedic or prosthetic management.

Many congenital amputees require no surgical conversion to a different level, but revision of stumps for terminal overgrowth is common, particularly for the humerus. Conversion of the upper extremity is rarely necessary. It is usually unnecessary to remove upper extremity nubbins,

which the child may find useful for holding small objects or activating powered prostheses. Lower extremity conversion should be done to enhance prosthetic fitting if it facilitates ambulation, but durability and function, not cosmesis, are the goals. In general, useful deformities should be retained.

Prosthetic fitting of the upper extremity is done when the child is sitting independently, usually at about 6 months. Initial upper extremity terminal devices are passive, but they can be activated when grasping becomes important (1.5 to 2 years of age). Lower extremity prostheses are fitted when the child begins pulling to stand or cruising. A fixed knee with waistband suspension is used for above-knee amputees. Frequent length adjustments of the prosthesis will be required with growth. Children will discard upper-limb prostheses if they perceive them to be nonfunctional, and children with multiple limb deficiencies often reject prostheses because they interfere with the specialized movements required by daily living activities.

TRAUMATIC AMPUTATIONS

While traumatic injuries can occur to any child, there is considerable evidence that the typical child with a traumatic amputation comes from a socially dysfunctional background. Most are boys from single-parent homes who are rebellious or running away from home. The psychological ability of these patients to undergo extensive treatment, revision of level, and rehabilitation is often very limited. Be sensitive to these psychosocial issues and obtain consultation early from appropriate professionals.

Set surgical and rehabilitation goals early. Often it is necessary to consider amputation at a more proximal level rather than subject the child to an emotionally draining series of heroic procedures to preserve length. Traumatic amputees may not tolerate multiple procedures or extensive rehabilitation efforts if they do not have the emotional base of support of a functioning family system.

Most traumatic amputations involve the lower extremity, and terminal overgrowth, particularly of the tibia, is often a problem. Many of these patients will wait until they can no longer tolerate their prosthesis before presenting for a revision of the overgrown stump, making smooth coordination of surgery and prosthetic fitting difficult.

A special problem arises when the traumatic amputee has lost soft tissue from a degloving injury proximal to the bony amputation level. Occasionally, it is appropriate to sacrifice bone length if considerations warrant it. However, other options include extensive use of split skin graft (much better tolerated in children than in adults), tissue expanders, or microvascular free tissue transfer. Skin traction (Fig. 175.1) over a 1- to 2-week period can add several centimeters of full-thickness circumferential skin and al-

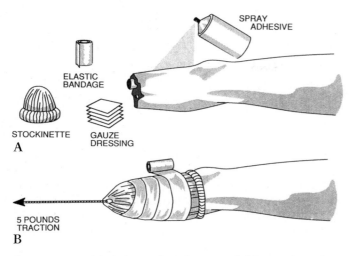

Figure 175.1. Technique of application of skin traction after traumatic amputation.

lows inspection of the open wound for appropriate care in the interim.

If the wound allows it, a rigid plaster dressing permits rapid mobilization of the trauma patient, while minimizing pain and reducing the tendency to form contractures.

BURN AMPUTATIONS

Burn amputations present a dilemma: how to obtain skin coverage while salvaging the most distal amputation level possible. Extensive use of split-thickness skin is often successful in the child. Stump breakdown is less of a problem in the child than in the adult. Attempt to preserve length if at all possible. Proximal joint stiffness seems to be more of a problem in burn amputees than in other amputees, and it should be addressed early and aggressively in the rehabilitation effort.

AMPUTATIONS FOR MALIGNANT TUMORS

Limb salvage for malignant bone and soft-tissue tumors has become technically feasible in older children, but amputation is still often necessary for local control of tumors. Amputation also may be the treatment of choice for malignant tumors in children younger than 10 years because skeletal growth is disturbed by limb-sparing techniques. Amputation is usually indicated when a pathologic fracture occurs through a malignant lesion.

Amputation for a tumor requires the same technical care as any tumor procedure, with the goal being complete local control of the lesion for cure or palliation. Adjuvant chemotherapy or radiation therapy may be appropriate.

Because of the possibility of a short lifespan, and the added psychological stress to the family and child of adjuvant treatments in the addition to limb loss, these children should receive aggressive, early rehabilitation. Rigid dressings and immediate pylons can ease the immense emotional strain of the diagnosis and treatment. Use interim prostheses early, as chemotherapy and weight loss may postpone definitive fitting.

SPECIFIC AMPUTATION TECHNIQUES FOR CHILDREN

The surgical techniques (e.g., handling of soft tissues, division of bones, and treatment of sectioned nerves) for amputations in children are generally the same as the techniques in adults (see Chapters 120–122). However, amputations in skeletally immature patients present special considerations.

UPPER EXTREMITY

Above-Elbow Amputation
Very short above-elbow amputations preserve the cosmetic contour of the shoulder girdle, but most children reject prosthetic fitting attempts. Mid-humerus and longer levels allow artificial limb function, but the stump will become thin and conical, so every attempt should be made to maintain its shape by preserving the distal humeral condyles if possible. Marquardt (7) has described a right-angle osteotomy 5 cm proximal to the end of the above-elbow stump to assist with prosthesis suspension and rotational control. Above-elbow amputees have a high incidence of terminal overgrowth, and parents should be warned of the likelihood of multiple revisions.

Elbow Disarticulation
Elbow disarticulation, while rarely performed, is an excellent amputation option for children. It eliminates the problem of overgrowth, and the preservation of the distal humeral condyles aids in prosthetic fitting. As puberty approaches, consider epiphysiodesis of the distal humeral epiphysis. This provides shortening of the amputated limb in comparison to the contralateral limb, allowing internal prosthetic elbow hinges.

Below-Elbow Amputation
Overgrowth is generally not a problem in the below-elbow stump. Preserve as much length as possible. Even short below-elbow stumps, distal to the biceps insertion on the radius, can aid with prosthetic stabilization and internal prosthetic control.

Wrist Disarticulation
Wrist disarticulation is an excellent amputation level in the child. It does not restrict pronation–supination, and overgrowth does not occur.

LOWER EXTREMITY

The same techniques described for adult amputation for hemipelvectomy and hip disarticulation are applicable to children. As in adults, the prosthetic rejection rate after hemipelvectomy or hip disarticulation is high (see Chapters 120 and 122).

Above-Knee Amputation

Except in adolescents, the above-knee amputation level is a poor option for children because of loss of the distal femoral physis. The relative shortening of the leg with growth is dramatic and is worsened by the problem of terminal overgrowth.

Knee Disarticulation

The long stump, preservation of growth, muscle control, and lack of terminal overgrowth make knee disarticulation an ideal amputation level in the child. The patella may be retained. Suture the hamstrings to the cruciate stump and oversew the quadriceps tendon to them. This tenodesis preserves the strength of the muscles for walking and prevents their slippage around the distal bone end.

As maturity (bone age 10–11 years in girls and 12–13 years in boys) approaches, do a distal femoral epiphysiodesis to allow slight shortening, which facilitates prosthetic design using an internal hinge. Consult a prosthetist to determine the optimal amount of shortening for prosthetic fitting.

Below-Knee Amputation

In adult amputees, preserving the knee joint enhances prosthetic ambulation potential, because above-knee amputees require more energy for prosthetic ambulation than do below-knee amputees. As most pediatric amputees will become geriatric amputees, it is desirable to salvage the knee joint in pediatric amputation surgery if possible. However, below-knee amputations have specific problems in children. Terminal overgrowth of the tibia and fibula are almost inevitable, and multiple revisions are the rule. Varus angulation in younger children occurs often and may be severe enough to require tibial osteotomy. The thin, conical stump makes rotational control difficult. Patellar-tendon-bearing prosthesis is a misnomer in the growing child, because the rapid change in length makes nearly all prostheses essentially end-bearing. For all of these reasons, ankle disarticulation is preferable to below-knee amputation if at all possible.

Surgical techniques for the below-knee amputations are the same for the child as for the adult, except that the skin flaps can be widely variable because the vascular supply in children is so rich. If possible, avoid scars directly over the end of the stump. Split-thickness skin is remarkably well tolerated in the child and may hypertrophy to give good results in maturity, even at this weight-bearing level.

Preserve the fibula if at all possible, even if it is very short. The broad shape of the combined proximal tibia and fibula enhances rotational prosthetic control. Surgical cross-union and other techniques to prevent terminal overgrowth do not work and may lead to proximal migration of the fibula.

Ankle Disarticulation (Pediatric Syme Amputation)

Although the classic Syme amputation is not done in children, the similar procedure of ankle disarticulation carries the same name by popular usage (Fig. 175.2). The pediatric Syme amputation, while having the benefits of a disarticulation, can be difficult to perform well because of the late problem of posterior heel-pad migration (2). Modern prosthetic technique allows fitting of bulbous stumps, which often taper with maturation. The main use of the Syme amputation is in congenital anomalies, especially fibular hemimelia and proximal femoral focal deficiency. I prefer the Boyd amputation, described in the next section, over the Syme.

- Perform surgery with a pneumatic tourniquet. Between points just distal to the medial and lateral malleoli, connect an anterior incision dorsally and a plantar incision directly inferiorly (Fig. 175.2). Carry the incisions, without extensive subcutaneous undermining, straight down to bone, ligating vascular structures and tagging the anterior tibial and toe extensor tendons.
- Grab the talus with a towel clip and plantar-flex it to its extreme. With a scalpel directed toward the bone, carefully dissect out first the talus and then the os calcis

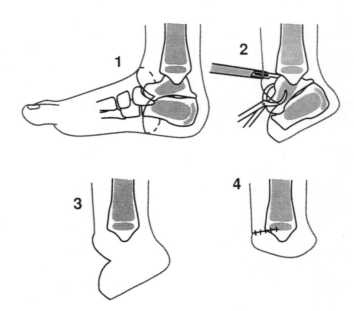

Figure 175.2. Technique of pediatric Syme amputation. See text for details.

in a similar manner. Avoiding any injury to the subcutaneous tissue is critical to the success of the operation. Ensure that the excision includes the cartilaginous apophysis of the posterior os calcis.

■ Sever the Achilles tendon and allow it to retract into the leg. Trim the cartilaginous malleoli transversely to the level of the tibial plafond with a scalpel. Suture the anterior tibial and toe extensor tendons to the anterior edge of the heel pad to prevent posterior migration. Avoid the temptation to trim the dog-ears over the malleoli: They will remodel. Trimming may jeopardize the vascular supply to the heel flap.

■ Close the skin and subcutaneous tissue with fine absorbable suture over a suction drain, and apply an above-knee rigid plaster dressing with molding over the femoral condyles.

Boyd Amputation

The Boyd amputation, while similar to the pediatric Syme amputation, preserves the posterior os calcis and thus stabilizes the heel pad (Fig. 175.3) (3). Take care to place the heel in a plantigrade position and to divide the Achilles tendon, so that the heel does not drift into plantar flexion. If properly done, the Boyd produces an excellent end-bearing stump without the problem of terminal overgrowth. Boyd amputations produce a bulbous stump that may improve with growth.

■ Make a skin incision in a fashion similar to that for the pediatric Syme amputation. Tagging the anterior tendons is unnecessary. Disarticulate the midfoot and

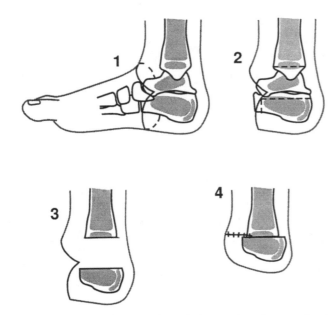

Figure 175.3. Technique of Boyd amputation. See text for details.

forefoot from the talus and calcaneus. Grab the talus with a towel clip and carefully shell it out by plantar-flexing it and releasing soft-tissue attachments to the talus with a small scalpel. The subcutaneous tissue must not be damaged during this procedure.

■ Shave the distal tibial articular surface transversely until the ossific nucleus of the distal tibial epiphysis is exposed, using a scalpel or fine osteotome (usually just held by hand; a mallet is unnecessary). Similarly, shave the superior surface of the os calcis down to cancellous bone, making it flat parallel to the weight-bearing surface of the heel. Shorten the anterior end of the os calcis. Sever the Achilles tendon and allow it to retract; this prevents late plantar flexion drift of the os calcis.

■ Approximate the raw surfaces of the tibial epiphysis and os calcis while bringing the os calcis forward (anterior) slightly. Hold them together with one or more smooth Kirschner wires inserted through the heel pad. If the Boyd amputation is being combined with a knee fusion for proximal femoral focal deficiency, the heel can be fixed with a longitudinal Rush rod passed up the heel, tibial canal, and through the knee fusion site. Use bone graft from discarded bones if desired. Ensure that the weight-bearing surface of the heel is plantigrade; avoid even slight plantar flexion.

■ Close the wound over a suction drain using fine absorbable stitches for all layers (I use 4-0 polyglycolic acid), and bend the pin(s) externally to avoid migration. Immobilize the limb in a spica cast or long-leg cast, depending on age.

■ Remove the pins at 4–6 weeks and continue immobilization in a long-leg cast (molded over the femoral condyles) until radiographic union.

Foot Amputation

Midfoot amputations at the Lisfranc or Chopart level are usually traumatic; this is not a desirable level for an elective amputation. In managing these injuries, sever the Achilles tendon to help prevent equinus contracture, and anchor extensor tendons, if available, to the anterior bony structures. Conversion to a higher-level (Boyd or pediatric Syme) amputation is often required (4).

Distal partial foot amputations, usually at a metatarsal level, are very well tolerated by children and require only a space-filling prosthetic shoe insert.

PITFALLS AND COMPLICATIONS

The primary pitfalls and complications unique to the management of pediatric amputations come from the improper applications of adult amputation principles to the child. Adult principles fail to take into account the need to preserve epiphyses for normal growth, to preserve distal shape for prosthetic control, or to be creative with skin coverage so that length is not traded for simplicity of initial wound closure. The complication of terminal overgrowth following through-bone amputations in children is predictable and requires surgical revision at 2- to 4-year intervals until growth ceases. Painful neuromas and phantom pain are very rare and generally occur only when the amputation is acquired in adolescence. Management is the same as adults (see Chapters 120 and 121).

REFERENCES

Each reference is categorized according to the following scheme: *, classic article; #, review article; !, basic research article; and +, clinical results/outcome study.

+ 1. Aiken GT. Surgical Amputation in Children. *J Bone Joint Surg Am* 1963;45:1735.

+ 2. Anderson L, Westin GW, Oppenheim WL. Syme Amputations in Children: Indications, Results, and Long-term Follow-up. *J Pediatr Orthop* 1984;4:550.

+ 3. Blum CE, Kalamchi A. Boyd Amputations in Children. *Clin Orthop* 1982;165:135.

+ 4. Green WB, Carey JM. Partial Foot Amputations in Children: A Comparison of the Several Types with the Syme Amputation. *J Bone Joint Surg Am* 1982;64:438.

5. Kaimchi A, ed. *Congenital Lower Limb Deficiencies.* New York: Springer-Verlag, 1989.

+ 6. Lambert CN, Hamilton RC, Tellicore RJ. The Juvenile Amputee Program: Its Social and Economic Value. A Follow-up Study after the Age of 21. *J Bone Joint Surg Am* 1969;51:1135.

7. Marquardt E. In: Bowker JH, Michael JW, eds. *Atlas of Limb Prosthetics: Surgical, Prosthetic, and Rehabilitation Principles.* St. Louis, MO: Mosby-Year Book, 1992: 852.

8. Setoguchi Y, Posenfelder R. *The Limb-Deficient Child.* Springfield, IL: Charles C. Thomas, 1982.

CHAPTER 176

BONE AND JOINT INFECTIONS IN CHILDREN

Paul P. Griffin

Septic arthritis and osteomyelitis in children are similar in their clinical presentation, diagnosis, and treatment. Both are usually secondary to bacteremia, but they may occur simultaneously, or the septic arthritis may be secondary to the osteomyelitis. When the two are present, the problems of diagnosis, treatment, and sequelae are greater than when either occurs alone. Although there are similarities between them, subtle differences occur in the physical findings, pathology, treatment, and prognosis. These differences make it important that they be viewed as separate problems.

P. P. Griffin: Department of Orthopaedic Education, Medical University of South Carolina, Greenville Memorial Hospital, Greenville, SC, 29690.

ACUTE HEMATOGENOUS OSTEOMYELITIS

Acute hematogenous osteomyelitis occurs in all age groups but is more common in children than in adults. The peak age for occurrence is 18 to 24 months, and the mean age about 6 years. Since the development of antibiotics, prognosis and results of treatment have dramatically improved so that acute hematogenous osteomyelitis should no longer be a life-threatening disease. Sequelae from the infection, if diagnosed early and treated appropriately, are minimal and chronic osteomyelitis is now rare. In older children, osteomyelitis is usually monostotic, but in the neonate, it is not uncommon to find multiple sites of infection.

PATHOLOGY

Acute hematogenous osteomyelitis is a blood-borne infection that begins in the metaphysis of long bones and in the metaphyseal equivalent areas of the remainder of the skeleton. In 1911, Koch (25) demonstrated that the intravenous injection of bacteria frequently caused infection that began in the metaphyses of long bones near the physis. The metaphyseal location of infection is related to the vascular anatomy in the region, where the terminal nutrient vessels enter large sinusoidal vessels. The blood flow velocity in these vessels is slow, which encourages the bacteria to settle. In addition, the host defense mechanism is compromised because of the paucity of monocytic cells in the sinusoidal spaces.

More recently, Morrissy and Haynes (29) demonstrated in the rabbit model that the inflammatory response and bone destruction are slightly more distal to the physis than the area where the bacteria are found. It is in the area of this inflammatory response that the destruction of the bone trabeculae occurs as a response to the inflammatory process. By injuring the metaphyseal area of the rabbit's extremity just before intravenous injection of a bolus of bacteria, Morrissy found that the development of osteomyelitis was much more predictable than when there was no preceding injury. This correlates with the clinical finding that there is frequently a history of injury before the onset of osteomyelitis. Trauma may cause thrombosis of the sinusoidal vessels, and the thrombus serves as a culture medium for the bacterial growth.

The inflammatory process begins with edema and a cellular influx that will evolve into an abscess if the response is not altered by appropriate treatment. The purulent exudate spreads through the thin porous cortex of the metaphysis and elevates the periosteum, which causes subperiosteal reactive bone formation.

If the infection is untreated, the periosteum eventually is destroyed. Loss of the periosteum severely interferes with the healing of a fracture should one occur in the course of the disease. Before the development of antibiotics, the exudate, if it was not surgically released, would eventually drain through the skin, as described by Smith in 1874 (39). The elevation of the periosteum interrupts the periosteal blood supply to the cortex. Loss of the periosteal blood supply, along with vascular thrombosis caused by the pus passing through the haversian system, renders the cortex ischemic. The ischemic bone becomes a cortical sequestrum.

In children younger than 2 years of age, it is rare that a cortical sequestrum is produced. The reason for this is not clear, but it may be that the increased porosity of the metaphyseal cortex in the young child allows the exudate to exit through the metaphyseal cortex and decompresses the bone before it is forced through the haversian system of the diaphysis. Where the metaphysis of the long bone is partially intracapsular, as in the proximal femur, humerus, and ankle, secondary septic arthritis can result from the spontaneous decompression of the metaphysis.

In newborns, Trueta (42) demonstrated that metaphyseal vessels transverse the proximal femoral physis. These vessels passing from the metaphysis to the epiphysis apparently allow bacteria and the inflammatory process to cross the physis into the epiphysis. In this age group, the physis and the epiphysis can be severely damaged from the infection (Fig. 176.1). The vessels that cross the physis in the neonate progressively disappear beginning at 8 months of age (42). By 18 months, the epiphyseal and metaphyseal circulations are completely separate. Once the physis becomes a barrier to the metaphyseal vessels, inflammatory destruction of the physis and epiphysis is rare.

CLINICAL PICTURE

The presenting symptoms of osteomyelitis depend on the severity of the infection, its location, and the age of the patient. Approximately 30% of the patients with osteomyelitis are not ill and have few systemic symptoms. In patients who are not ill, the initial diagnosis is frequently in error, with the most common misdiagnosis being some type of malignancy. Except for an elevated sedimentation rate, which is almost always present, the laboratory data may be normal in this subgroup of patients.

Regardless of the severity of the infection, the most constant symptom is localized pain that causes the child to limp or not use the extremity. Swelling is usually present, and its extent reflects the severity of the infection. Local tenderness is always present. The more superficial the bone, the more easily this can be demonstrated. Why 30% of patients have a mild presentation of osteomyelitis is not clear. In some instances, it reflects the use of antibiotics to treat fever of undetermined etiology or other infections in other areas of the body. It may also reflect the prevalence of the use of antibiotics in the production of meat for consumption.

In acutely unaltered hematogenous osteomyelitis, the signs and symptoms are an elevated temperature in an anorexic, irritable child with significant pain and limitation of function of an extremity. Swelling, tenderness, and sometimes redness are common and impressive. In the infant, swelling may extend throughout the entire segment of the extremity (Fig. 176.2). Motion in the adjacent joint is limited and causes protective muscle spasm. Infants may present with pseudoparalysis, and older children will limp or refuse to walk if the lower extremity is affected. Pain with localized tenderness and swelling in the metaphysis of a long bone is sufficient to make a presumptive diagnosis of osteomyelitis in an ill child.

The peripheral blood changes vary with the severity of the infection. The white blood cell count is usually ele-

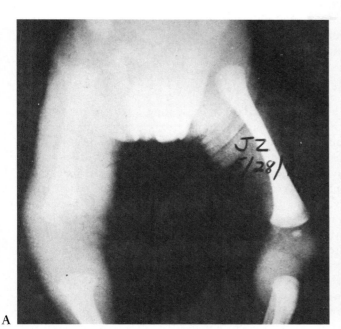

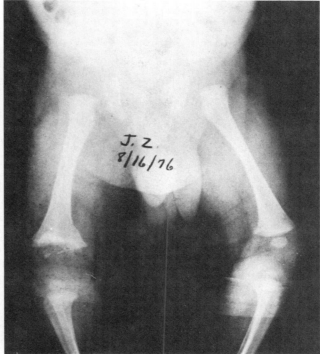

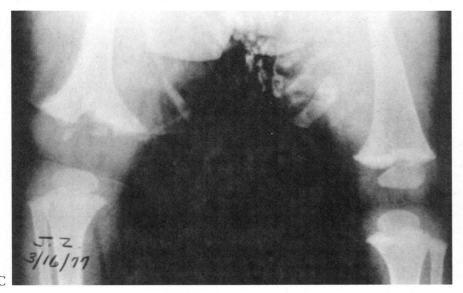

Figure 176.1. **A:** Two-month-old infant with osteomyelitis in the right femur. Note the soft-tissue swelling. **B:** Three months later, there is widening of the metaphysis with cupping as well as resorption of the ossified epiphysis. **C:** Seven months later, the femur was already shorter than the opposite femur.

vated, with a shift to the left. If infection has been present for several days, the red blood cell count, hemoglobin, and hematocrit will be lower than normal. Sedimentation rate is almost always elevated. Blood cultures should always be taken when osteomyelitis is suspected; a positive culture is usually found in 60% to 65% of patients.

RADIOGRAPHS

Initial radiographic evidence of osteomyelitis is not in the bone but in the deep soft tissues, where swelling is the

initial radiographic sign (Fig. 176.3). The swelling occurs within the first 2 days of symptoms and obliterates the lucent muscle planes progressively from the bone to the subcutaneous tissue. With this pattern of soft-tissue swelling, the diagnosis of osteomyelitis must be considered. When osteomyelitis is suspected, take radiographs with the appropriate exposure and anatomic position. It is important that both extremities have radiographs in the identical position for comparison. Ask the radiographic technician to use soft-tissue technique for the first radio-

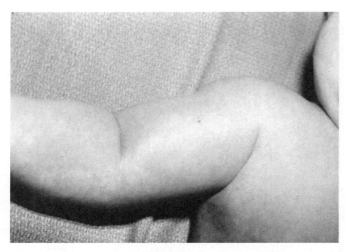

Figure 176.2.   Osteomyelitis of the humerus. Swelling extends both proximal and distal to the humerus.

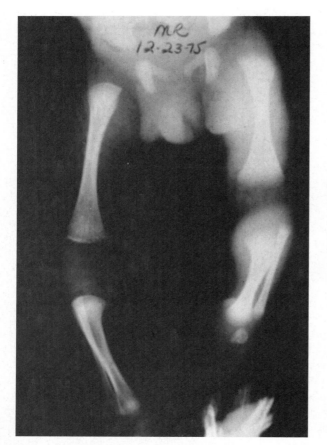

Figure 176.3.   Soft-tissue swelling of the left thigh in a neonate with osteomyelitis.

graph and bone technique for a second. After 10 days of uncontrolled infection, radiolucent areas can be seen in the metaphysis. New periosteal bone is another late radiographic manifestation of osteomyelitis. This periosteal bone is a result of the elevation of the periosteum by the exudate that has passed through the cortex.

BONE IMAGING

The current standard in evaluating a patient for possible early osteomyelitis includes the option of imaging with radionuclides. An increase in uptake may be present in the area of infection as early as 24 hours after onset, but an increase in uptake is not diagnostic of osteomyelitis; it only reflects increased blood flow and osteoblastic activity, which may also occur in the presence of tumors and trauma. The value of the radionuclear studies is in localization of the area of infection and in identifying multiple sites of infection. The greatest help from a bone scan is in a patient who has been partially treated; when the clinical signs are poorly defined, as in infection of the pelvis or spine; and in managing a patient with subacute osteomyelitis. False-negative bone scans and gallium scans do occur (1). This is particularly true in osteomyelitis of the pelvis and in the neonate. It is probably related to the decreased blood flow from thrombosis. In the neonate, the bone scan is accurate in only 30% to 40% of patients (2). However, if both technetium and gallium scans are positive, the diagnosis is almost always infection. This is particularly helpful in patients with suspected osteomyelitis in the pelvis and will facilitate an early diagnosis (12). Because gallium has more radioactivity than technetium, it should not be used except in very difficult cases (5). Computed tomography (CT) scan and magnetic resonance imaging (MRI) can be of benefit when the clinical facts are not sufficient to make the diagnosis. Mazur et al. (27) reported a sensitivity of 97% and a specificity of 92% for MRI. However, these imaging modalities are seldom needed and should be used only in difficult cases. Their routine use is not justified. A particularly valuable area for the use of CT is in osteomyelitis of the pelvis, in which early swelling can be identified as well as very early bone changes that are seldom seen on routine radiographs made early in the course of the infection.

DIAGNOSIS

The diagnosis of acute hematogenous osteomyelitis is made from the history, physical examination, and laboratory studies, and is confirmed by radiographs, bone scan, MRI if needed, and aspiration of the bone. Although 30% of the patients are not acutely ill, the remainder are ill and give a history of the fairly rapid onset of pain accompanied by swelling, localized tenderness, and impaired function such as a limp, refusal to walk, or pseudoparalysis. In those who are ill, the temperature is elevated, and the young child is irritable and anorexic. An exception is in the neonate who may not show an elevated temperature and who may have minimal laboratory changes. Neonates frequently present with failure to thrive. The neonate may be moribund and respond poorly to physical stimulation. Because of these differences, the diagnosis is frequently delayed until destruction of the physis and epiphysis has occurred. In the neonate who shows failure to thrive, osteomyelitis should be considered as a possible cause. The most dramatic physical finding in the neonate usually is swelling of an entire extremity (Fig. 176.2). Radiographs should show the characteristic soft-tissue swelling.

With these findings, always aspirate metaphysis in the area of maximum tenderness with a large-bore needle. Use fluoroscopic control to make certain that the needle enters the metaphysis near but not in the physis. If pus is not obtained from beneath the periosteum, push the needle through the cortex. Culture any aspirate, pus, or blood obtained. In addition to culturing the aspirate, culture the blood, nose, throat, and any skin lesions. Perform peripheral blood studies, including a white blood cell count, hematocrit, and sedimentation rate.

TREATMENT

Early effective treatment is the most important factor that influences the results in osteomyelitis (43). Two significant sequelae arise with osteomyelitis. One is physeal and epiphyseal destruction in the neonate and infant; the other is chronic osteomyelitis with a cortical sequestrum in the older child. Prevention of these two problems depends on early diagnosis and effective treatment. When these two sequelae are prevented, the results from treatment of osteomyelitis is uniformly good.

Conservative treatment with systemic antibiotics plus rest and protection of the involved limb is successful in most patients. Surgical treatment is indicated if pus is obtained on bone aspiration or if the response to conservative treatment is not favorable within 48 hours. A favorable response is one in which the temperature elevation rapidly diminishes, and the pain and swelling is decreased. If no abscess is present and the correct antibiotic is delivered in an adequate dose, pain, fever, and even swelling should be significantly reduced by 48 hours.

Start antibiotics immediately after the aspiration. The choice of antibiotics is made from the statistics concerning the most likely pathogen as influenced by age, presence of chronic disease, and any organisms found on the Gram stain. After culture results and sensitivities are known, change the antibiotic to a more appropriate one, if necessary.

In the neonate, *Staphylococcus aureus,* group B Streptococcus, and gram-negative bacilli are frequent pathogens. Therefore, in the neonate a semisynthetic penicillin will be effective for the staphylococcal and streptococcal infections, but an aminoglycoside should be added because of the possible presence of a gram-negative organism.

In the child between 2 months and 3 years of age who has not been vaccinated for *Haemophilus influenzae,* this organism can be the pathogen in as many as 10% of the cases. For these patients, cefuroxime may be the drug of choice because it is effective against Staphylococcus, Streptococcus, and *H. influenzae.* If *H. influenzae* is the pathogen, the possibility of secondary meningitis is always present.

After 3 years of age, Staphylococcus and Streptococcus organisms are the most common pathogens causing osteomyelitis. In this age group, a semisynthetic penicillin or a first-generation cephalosporin is the antibiotic of choice. Both give adequate bone levels and are effective. The advantage of the cephalosporins over semisynthetic penicillins is that if the treatment is changed from parenteral to oral antibiotics, the oral cephalosporins are more palatable than either cloxacillin or dicloxacillin. If the pathogen cultured is a methicillin-resistant *S. aureus,* vancomycin is the drug of choice.

Administer the initial antibiotics parenterally. After 2 or 3 days, if the response to treatment has been favorable with a decrease in the fever, pain, and swelling, oral antibiotics may be the preferred route of delivery in a selected group of patients. To use oral antibiotics, there should be a positive culture to ensure that the appropriate antibiotic is being administered. Compliance must be ensured by knowing the dependability of the patient and family. Tolerance of the oral antibiotic at the required dosage must be shown. The dose of antibiotic must be sufficient to give a bactericidal level as determined by measurement of the antibiotic level or by the dilution technique. In the dilution method, a 1 to 8 dilution at the peak and a 1 to 2 in the trough should be bactericidal. The required dose of a semisynthetic penicillin to obtain these bactericidal levels can be reduced by the addition of probenecid in children of 2 years and older (33).

Among the controversies that surround the treatment of osteomyelitis, the duration of the antibiotic treatment is the greatest. Dich et al. (10) reported data on a series of patients with staphylococcal osteomyelitis treated for less than 21 days compared with a group treated for more than 21 days. The rate of recurrence of development of chronic osteomyelitis was 19% in those treated for less than 21 days and only 2% in those treated for more than 21 days. I prefer to judge the need for extended treatment on the patient's response and on the presence of bone changes on routine radiographs. In all patients, antibiotics for 21 days should be the rule, extending this to 6 weeks or more in selected cases. In the patient who presents early and responds rapidly and in whom no abscess is demonstrated by aspiration, the shorter period of antibiotic therapy may be adequate. When pus is present or radiographic evidence of bone destruction or a sequestrum is present, give antibiotics for longer periods of time. Before antibiotics are discontinued, the sedimentation rate should be declining and near normal.

SURGICAL TREATMENT

There are three indications for surgical drainage: if pus is obtained on the initial aspiration, if the clinical response is not significant after 48 hours of antibiotics, or if there is radiographic evidence of bone destruction requiring removal of a metaphyseal sequestrum or granulation tissue. This latter indication is controversial, and it may be preferable to depend on conservative treatment before undertaking surgical curettage.

The surgical treatment is to remove pus, dead bone, and granulation tissue. Even though antibiotics may have been started, the material removed at surgery should always be cultured. Make the opening in the cortex small but large enough to insert a curet for removal of granulation tissue and to irrigate the metaphysis thoroughly. Place the hole near the physis in the area of maximum tenderness (Fig. 176.4), taking care to protect the physis. This

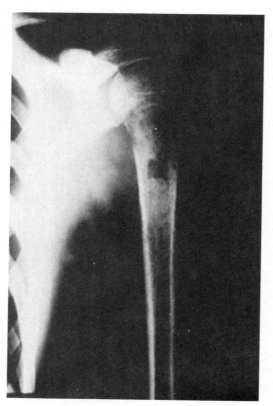

Figure 176.4.   The surgical opening in this proximal humerus is too distal to the epiphysis. The patient had a recurrence of symptoms 2 months later.

is best done under fluoroscopy or by a marker placed at the level of the physis and confirmed by a radiograph.

Close the wound over drains. I prefer a suction drain. Controversy exists as to whether irrigation with saline is helpful. If it is done well, it should be of some benefit. Drains should be removed after 48 hours.

Protection of the extremity in a splint in a functional position is important to prevent a fracture. It usually increases the patient's comfort level as well. Unprotected weight bearing after surgical decompression or where there is extensive cortical destruction with or without a sequestrum may result in a fracture.

SUBACUTE OSTEOMYELITIS

The host defense against pathogen virulence frequently results in a standoff, with local bone destruction that is limited compared with that of acute osteomyelitis. This results in a subacute infection. In 1969, King and Mayo (24) reported data on a series of patients diagnosed as having subacute osteomyelitis. In all of these patients, radiographic changes were seen at the time the patients were first evaluated. They described eight types of subacute osteomyelitis based on the radiographic appearance. Others have added to this clinical description (14,15).

CLINICAL PICTURE

The onset of subacute osteomyelitis is insidious. The child is not ill, and little or no functional impairment is present. The most constant complaint is a localized pain that may have periods of exacerbation and remission. The pain frequently is exacerbated following a period of unusual activity. If the involvement is in a subcutaneous bone, local swelling is occasionally present. Like the pain, the swelling seems to increase and subside with activity. Symptoms may be present for weeks or months before the child is brought to a physician for evaluation. Laboratory studies may be normal, including the sedimentation rate, although it is elevated in some patients.

The diagnosis is made on the radiographic appearance of the lesion. The most common type of subacute osteomyelitis is a well-circumscribed lytic lesion with sclerotic borders, which is known as Brodie's abscess. Such lesions may be found in the metaphysis, epiphysis, and rarely, in the diaphysis. Metaphyseal lesions frequently extend across the physis and into the epiphysis (Fig. 176.5). Fortunately, this appears to be a response that does not injure the physis. A second type exhibits a lytic area in the cortex with little or no bone response. In others, the cortex becomes very sclerotic but without onion skin—like periosteal new bone. However, there is a subperiosteal new bone type that has an onion skin appearance. Rarely, the in-

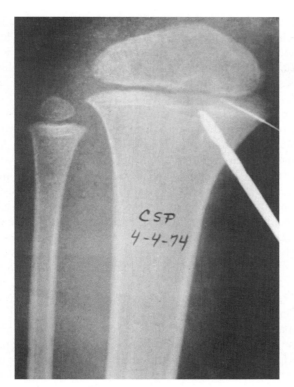

Figure 176.5. Brodie's abscess extended from the metaphysis to the epiphysis. Normal growth continued after curettage of the lesion.

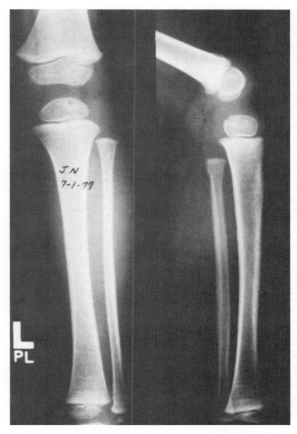

Figure 176.6. Lesion in the proximal epiphysis of the tibia.

volvement in the metaphysis may be diffuse without a clear border.

DIAGNOSIS

As many as 50% of patients with subacute osteomyelitis have an initial incorrect diagnosis. Subacute osteomyelitis should be the diagnosis until proven otherwise if there is local swelling, with local pain, and one of the classic radiographic appearances, along with an elevated sedimentation rate. Bone scans are almost always positive, although they are not diagnostic. MRI is frequently the most useful imaging and should be used in those with a destructive lesion or in any patient with radiographic changes suggestive of a malignancy.

TREATMENT

The initial step in treatment of the lytic type is surgery. If the diagnosis is established by the pathology, both gross and microscopic, curet and culture the granulation tissue present in the lesion. Start antibiotics immediately after surgery. In most of these lesions, *S. aureus* is the pathogen; therefore, a semisynthetic penicillin or a first-generation cephalosporin is the drug of choice. If the diagnosis is

made without biopsy, some lesions will respond to antibiotics without surgery (35). If the lesion is in the epiphysis and a surgical approach is potentially harmful, the initial treatment should be antibiotics for several weeks (Fig. 176.6). However, most epiphyseal lesions can be drained without harm to the articular surface or to the physis if the surgical approach is appropriately planned (15). In the subperiosteal, cortical, sclerotic, and diffuse metaphyseal types, surgical treatment has less to offer. In these patients, the clinical picture is more likely to resemble a neoplasm, and a surgical biopsy will be necessary for diagnosis. These types usually respond to adequate antibiotic therapy.

CHRONIC OSTEOMYELITIS

Chronic osteomyelitis is seen much less frequently today than before the antibiotic era. It usually results from a delay in diagnosis or inadequate treatment. It is seen more often today in North America in immigrants from underdeveloped countries. The delay in controlling the infection results in the formation of a cortical sequestrum, which is due to ischemia from the cortical, intramedullary, and subperiosteal spread of pus. The antibiotic cannot adequately reach the bacteria located within dead bone, so surgical removal of the infected tissue must be done.

TREATMENT

In chronic osteomyelitis, start antibiotics immediately after deep tissue cultures of the wound are made. Continue the antibiotics for an extended period of time until the sedimentation rate is normal and the wound is benign. The indication for surgical treatment in chronic osteomyelitis is the presence of local pain and swelling, with or without drainage, in a bone with an area of lysis or a sequestrum, or both. Removal of the sequestrum and granulation tissue is the goal of the surgical exploration. Care must be taken not to jeopardize the integrity of the diaphysis by excessive removal of bone. The sequestrum should be removed, preferably after the involucrum is mature. Wide saucerization of the cortex should not be done because bone regeneration in chronic osteomyelitis may be severely limited. This is particularly true when there is no involucrum.

The removal of all dead tissue is the first step in surgical treatment. If possible, the wound should be closed and drains placed in the wound. Suction drainage and irrigation should be done for several days postoperatively. An antibiotic irrigation solution may be preferable to saline. The insertion of antibiotic-impregnated methylmethacralate beads in the defect after debridement should be considered in the patient who has had repeated surgical procedures. The absence of an involucrum indicates an inadequate periosteum. Periosteal healing is then unlikely. In such a patient, a cancellous bone graft should be placed in the defect after there is healing from the initial debridement and the infection is under control. If the bone cannot be covered by local skin, a local muscle should be transferred to cover the defect. In large uncovered areas, a myocutaneous flap may be required to cover the bone and fill the defect adequately (41). In some locations, a free microvascularized flap may be necessary. Good full-thickness and soft-tissue skin coverage will accelerate and improve the quality of healing (see Chapters 8 and 35). After surgical debridement, protect the extremity to prevent pathologic fracture.

SPECIAL CONDITIONS

SICKLE CELL DISEASE

In the patient with sickle cell disease, differentiation between an infarct and acute osteomyelitis can be difficult (23,26,31,32). Both produce fever, bone pain, tenderness, erythema, and swelling. An increase in the white cell count and an elevated sedimentation rate are also present. The presence of swelling and tenderness in the shaft of a long bone is more typical of osteomyelitis in a patient with sickle cell disease, whereas in a patient who does not have sickle cell disease, osteomyelitis has its onset in the metaphysis.

To distinguish an infarct from infection requires an astute evaluation of the degree of clinical signs and symptoms. The bone should be aspirated and cultured, and blood cultures should made if there is a strong possibility of infection. The pathogen in sickle cell osteomyelitis may be *S. aureus*, salmonella, or any other organism. Staphylococcus and salmonella are the two most common organisms cultured in osteomyelitis in a patient with sickle cell disease. In 15 patients with sickle cell disease with osteomyelitis, Epps et al. (11) reported that *S. aureus* was culture in eight, salmonella in six, and *Proteus mirabilis* in one.

Treatment of osteomyelitis is surgical (11) with the addition of antibiotics for 6 weeks. Chronic osteomyelitis in the patient with sickle cell disease is more common than in those who do not have sickle cell disease. Repeat surgical debridement may be needed in those patients who are not free of symptoms by 6 weeks. As in all patients with sickle cell disease, good hydration and transfusion are preoperative requirements.

CHRONIC RECURRENT MULTIFOCAL OSTEOMYELITIS

This is a rare condition of unknown etiology. It is more common in Europe than in the United States. In some reports, many patients have pustulosis palmaris et plantaris as well as recurrent multiple osteomyelitis (3,6,22). However, Yu and associates (45) reported on seven patients, none of whom had pustulosis palmaris et plantaris. Benhamou and associates (3) found some patients who in addition to pustulosis palmaris et plantaris also had Crohn's disease and some others had polyarthritis. They suggested that this condition was linked with seronegative spondyloarthritis.

The onset of chronic recurrent multifocal osteomyelitis is gradual and usually without significant temperature elevation. Pain is commonly reported. Lesions are most common in the femur, tibia, and spine, but other bones may be involved. There may be swelling and erythema over the lesions. Pressure over the involved part is painful, and if the spine is affected, flexion and extension and pressure over the involved vertebra causes pain.

The diagnosis is one of exclusion. Radiographs may show sclerosis, hyperostosis, or lysis. The radiographic changes have the appearance of bacterial osteomyelitis or of a sarcoma. Peripheral blood changes are minimal. A technetium-99 scan may show increased uptake or may be normal. Changes of inflammation suggestive of osteomyelitis are seen on biopsy material. Cultures of the lesions are negative.

The symptoms usually last between 1 and 4 years. When the patient has polyarthritis, symptoms generally last longer. Vertebra plana may result if a vertebra is involved. The height of the vertebra is not restored with time (45). Carr et al. (6) reported one patient with progressive kyphosis that required spinal fusion. Treatment is symptomatic with a nonsteroidal anti-inflammatory drug. Carr et al. (6) found that antibiotics may be helpful, and I have used cefalexin in one patient during recurrent episodes with possible benefits; however, antibiotics are not generally recommended.

INFECTION IN THE SPINE

The meaning of the "discitis" has been a source of confusion for many years. In 1964, Menelaus (28) gave credit to Eric Price for coining the word discitis for an infection of the disc space with little or no bone involvement. For many years, this remained a common concept of spinal infection in children. However, with the use of tomography it became apparent that osteomyelitis of the adjacent vertebrae always was present when the disc was infection. Ring et al. (34) labeled this condition pyogenic infectious spondylitis. The nomenclature for discitis from a bacterial infection should no longer be confusing. Pyogenic infectious spondylitis is not common but must be considered as a possible cause of back pain in a child and particularly in the very young child. The most frequent etiologic agent cultured is staphylococcus; however, streptococcus and, to a lesser extent, salmonella may be cultured (19,37).

The gradual onset of back pain is the most consistent symptom. Small children refuse to sit or walk. Leg pain and weakness may cause the child to not walk or to limp. The classic picture is a child sitting with the spine in extension and hands resting on the bed behind the trunk for support. Percussion over the affected vertebrae is painful even before changes on routine radiographs are present. When the clinical picture of bacterial spondylitis is present, blood cultures should be done. Hoffer et al. (19) recommended computer-guided biopsy if cultures were negative. I believe with the predominate bacteria known to cause this condition being staphylococcus and streptococcus that it is reasonable to assume that one of these organisms is present and to treat the child with the appropriate antibiotic. A response should be noted within 3 days, and if not, an additional antibiotic added or biopsy done. Patients who are not treated with antibiotics do recover when the spine is immobilized; however, this approach may prolong the time to recovery and can increase the need for surgical drainage (34). I prefer to administer an antibiotic for the infection and to provide symptomatic treatment to relieve back pain.

OSTEOMYELITIS OF THE PELVIS

Infection of the pelvis is rare, and the diagnosis is difficult (18). The ilium is the most frequent pelvic bone affected, but the ischium and pubis may be involved. Pain about the hip and a limp or refusal to walk are commonly reported. Most patients have a fever. The white cell count is elevated, as is the sedimentation rate.

Symptoms may be localized to the hip, the abdomen, the buttocks or low back, with sciatica-like symptoms. The location of the infection determines the location of pain. The hip is the most common area for pain, and when this is the presentation, an infection has to be considered. This pain occurs when the ilium is involved near the innominate bone, and osteomyelitis near the acetabulum can decompress in the hip joint and infect the joint. Buttock pain occurs if the ilium outer table is eroded, usually near the sacroiliac joint. Decompression through the inner wall may cause sciatica-like symptoms if the pus goes into the true pelvis and irritates the sciatic nerve or the pus may ascend and cause abdominal pain.

The diagnosis of osteomyelitis is made from the laboratory changes, the physical examination, and the use of the bone scan, CT, and MRI (30,40). Initial imaging with any of these modalities may be normal early in the course of the disease, but all tests will become positive eventually. The MRI will ordinarily be the first to show the swelling and bone involvement. It can distinguish soft-tissue swelling and show whether it is from bone or has a nonosseous origin. The MRI cannot differentiate infection from a tumor or infarction (40).

Physical evaluation includes observing the gait if the patient can walk. Perform range-of-motion examination of the hip gently. Passive motion of the infected hip is usually quite painful and limited whereas in infection of the pelvis more motion is present and less painful. Pressure on the pelvis is painful. Pressure over the buttock is painful if the ilium has decompressed through the outer table.

Administer appropriate antibiotics parenterally then orally. If treatment is started before an extraosseous abscess develops, antibiotic treatment is the only treatment required. When an abscess is present, surgical drainage is appropriate. Drain gluteal abscess posterior through the gluteus maximus, and a pelvic abscess through the abdomen but stay retroperitoneally. Chronic osteomyelitis of the pelvis is very rare, and most patients recover without residual problems (30).

SEPTIC ARTHRITIS

Septic arthritis occurs in all age groups but primarily affects the very young child. The peak incidence is between the age of 1 and 2 years of age (16). In neonates and other infants, the hip is the joint most commonly affected, but the knee is more commonly involved in older children. Infection in the hip joint is frequently secondary to osteomyelitis of the proximal femur, particularly in the infant. Septic arthritis of the shoulder and ankle may be secondary to spontaneous decompression of pus from the proximal humerus and distal fibula, respectively. Residual effects from septic arthritis are related to a delay in diagnosis and treatment, and to the presence of osteomyelitis.

BACTERIOLOGY

Over the last 20 years, the pathogens common in septic arthritis have changed. In the 1950s and 1960s, *S. aureus* was the organism most commonly cultured from septic joints. In a 1967 study of 116 infected joints in children with a mean age of 3 years, *S. aureus* was the most frequent organism cultured and 8% had *H. influenzae* (14). In the 1970s, the incidence of *H. influenzae* increased and was the most common organism cultured in children younger than 4 years of age (17). Jackson and Nelson (20) reported *S. aureus* in 30%, group B streptococcus in 21%, and gram-negative organisms in 28% in children aged 1 month to 5 years. However, in the infant younger than 3 months of age who acquires a joint infection while in the hospital, staphylococcus is the most common organism cultured. Approximately two thirds of hospital-acquired joint infections were found by Dan (8) to have *S. aureus* and one fifth Candida species as the pathogen. Since the development of the vaccine for *H. influenzae,* this organism is rarely the pathogen in septic arthritis.

PATHOPHYSIOLOGY

Septic arthritis in children is usually acquired by a hematogenous route. This may be either direct inoculation into the synovium or secondary to hematogenous osteomyelitis that decompresses into the joint. Osteomyelitis with secondary septic arthritis of the hip is common in the neonate but can occur in children of all ages. The ankle and shoulder, where the metaphysis may be partially intracapsular, occasionally is infected secondary to osteomyelitis. In the infant, in whom there are vessels that transverse the physis from the metaphysis to the epiphysis, the infection can spread from the metaphysis to the epiphysis and the adjacent joint. Bacteria are deposited in the synovium, and an inflammatory reaction develops. The inflamed synovium allows blood products and bacteria to enter the synovial fluid, including large numbers of leukocytes. The inflamed synovium, the white blood cells, and the bacteria contribute to the enzymatic destruction of the articular cartilage by the release of collagenase and proteases. Even the chondrocyte may contribute to cartilage destruction; Jasin (21) has shown that the chondrocyte may be stimulated to release chondrolytic enzymes by the action of either bacterial liposaccharide or interleukin 1 (IL-I). The depletion of

glycoaminoglycans in the cartilage matrix begins rapidly. Within 24 hours there is a significant loss. The loss of collagen follows (38). It is because of the multiple sources of these enzymes (bacteria, white blood cells, and synovial cells) that antibiotics alone cannot prevent destruction of the cartilage. Thorough cleansing of the joint is essential to successful treatment.

CLINICAL SIGNS AND SYMPTOMS

The onset of septic arthritis is characterized by the rapid development of joint pain and a fever of 100° to 104°F (38° to 40°C). Although the rapid onset of pain is variable, it is usually severe within 24 to 48 hours so that the child refuses to use the extremity. Irritability and malaise may precede the onset of pain. Pseudoparalysis is common in the very young. The physical examination is dramatic in the severity of the limitation of motion of the affected joint. Even with the gentlest attempt to move the extremity passively, there is extreme pain and spasm, and little motion is obtained. The joint is swollen, hot, and globally tender. The affected joint assumes a resting position that maximizes the capsular volume to reduce the tension in the joint. The hip is held flexed abducted and externally rotated. The most comfortable position for most other joints is some degree of flexion. In the neonate, minimal spontaneous movement, swelling of the joints, slight fever, and irritability may be the only changes present.

DIAGNOSIS

The clinical features of acute septic arthritis are usually, but not always, dramatic enough to exclude other diagnoses. However, always aspirate a joint when infection is considered to be a possibility, even when the child does not have the classic severe pain of septic arthritis. Infected joint fluid is cloudy, and mucin is diminished. A drop of fluid rubbed between the thumb and a finger will feel watery and will not string as the opposed fingers are separated. The most important studies of the fluid are a culture, Gram stain, white blood cell count, and differential. If sufficient fluid is available, other valuable measurements that should be obtained are glucose and lactic acid levels. The white cell count is usually between 50,000 and 200,000. More important, the differential is greater than 90% polymorphonuclear leukocytes. A joint fluid sugar of 50 mg/dl less than the blood sugar is common. In nongonococcal arthritis, the lactic acid level is elevated. It is important that the specimen for cell count is anticoagulated; if this is not done, the fluid will quickly coagulate. This makes the cell count incorrect. Aspiration of the hip and shoulder should be done under fluoroscopic control. If no fluid is aspirated, injection of a radiopaque dye into the joint will confirm that the needle is intra-articular.

In addition to the joint aspiration, peripheral blood

studies should be done to include a complete blood count and sedimentation rate. The white blood cell count is generally elevated with an increase in polymorphonuclear leukocytes, and the sedimentation rate is elevated. If the child is seriously ill and the infection present for several days, the erythrocyte count and hematocrit will be low.

Counterimmunoelectrophoresis of the synovial fluid can be helpful when the cultures are negative; it is particularly helpful when there has been partial treatment by antibiotics. This test can identify the presence of *H. influenzae, Streptococcus pneumoniae,* and meningococcus (9). A gallium scan has some use when the diagnosis is difficult. Bowman et al. (5) used gallium and reported accuracy in diagnosis of 91% in 34 patients with septic arthritis. The radiation dose from gallium is higher than from technetium, and it should be used only in difficult cases.

DIFFERENTIAL DIAGNOSIS

In the patient with the classic onset of fever, severe joint pain, and limited motion, there is little to confuse the diagnosis. However, conditions such as toxic synovitis, monarticular rheumatoid arthritis, and osteomyelitis can at times present a diagnostic problem. The child with toxic synovitis can usually be excluded by the clinical findings. The child is not ill, pain is not severe, and motion is only slightly limited. Acute-onset monoarticular rheumatoid arthritis may have many of the features of sepsis, and in such a patient, joint fluid analysis may be the only way to differentiate between these two diseases early in the course of the disease. In rheumatoid arthritis, pain can be severe, motion very limited, and the child febrile and ill. The synovial fluid may have as many as 70,000 cells, but on the differential, there will be less than 80% polymorphonucleocytes, unlike the 90% to 100% found in septic arthritis. In rheumatoid arthritis, the joint sugar level is similar to that in the blood sugar. The mucin in rheumatoid synovial fluid is diminished, as it is in septic fluid. The leukocyte differential and the glucose levels may be the only differentiating feature between these two diseases.

Osteomyelitis can be difficult to differentiate from septic arthritis. In both conditions, the child may be febrile and have the peripheral blood changes of infection. In both conditions, the patient exhibits limited joint motion, but in osteomyelitis, the adjacent joint will generally have a moderate range of motion if the examiner is gentle and protects the extremity from sudden motion. By careful palpation, tenderness will be found over the infected metaphysis and not the joint. Swelling is also different. In osteomyelitis, the swelling begins over the metaphysis and spreads to include much of the extremity segment (Fig. 176.2). The adjacent joint may be swollen from a sympathetic effusion, but it is not particularly tender. The swelling in septic arthritis is confined to the intracapsular space.

If there is swelling over the bone and also joint effusion, it is important to aspirate both the joint and the bone, with aspiration first at the most unlikely site for the infection, followed by aspiration of the suspected site. Radiographs will show the typical deep soft-tissue swelling if osteomyelitis is present. When soft-tissue swelling is present in the thigh and the hip joint space is wide on the radiograph, the patient has osteomyelitis plus a secondary septic arthritis until proven otherwise (Fig. 176.7).

TREATMENT

The objectives of treatment are to sterilize the joint, evacuate the debris associated with infection, relieve pain, and prevent deformity. Since the discovery of antibiotics, controversy has arisen as to the most effective way to cleanse the joint of the products of infection. This has centered mainly on whether or not aspiration and irrigation are as effective as arthrotomy and irrigation. There are no adequate studies to evaluate the superiority of one method over the other, and because of the many variables, it is unlikely that a comparative study will ever be done.

What we do know is that early diagnosis and treatment with the appropriate antibiotic are the most important aspects of treatment (17). There is little argument that the hip is special and needs to be decompressed to prevent dislocation as well as a tamponade of the circulation to the femoral head. Arthrotomy is necessary for the hip to be cleansed adequately of the debris and intra-articular pressure relieved. Intermittent or continuous irrigation for 48 to 72 hours through catheters has been used in the past (16). There is little proof that it affects the outcome, but it is not to be condemned. However, antibiotic solution should not be used for irrigation. Antibiotics reach the synovium and synovial fluid sufficiently to deliver the necessary bactericidal concentration of the antibiotic into the joint. If postarthrotomy intermittent irrigation is used, extreme care to maintain sterile technique is important to prevent a nosocomial infection through the irrigation system. I no longer use postarthrotomy irrigation.

The first step in treatment of septic arthritis is aspiration of the joint to confirm the diagnosis. If pus is obtained, the joint should be irrigated with saline until the irrigation fluid returns clear. The hip and shoulder should be immediately opened and irrigated after aspiration and joint fluid analysis confirms the diagnosis. In other joints, if infection has been present for 4 or 5 days, the large amount of fibrin and debris that has accumulated may be difficult to remove by needle. In these patients, arthrotomy or irrigation by arthroscopy is the preferred method of joint debridement. I do not recommend arthroscopic irrigation because I believe the motions of the arthroscope necessary to remove the debris adequately irritates the inflamed synovium. I have seen several failures when this

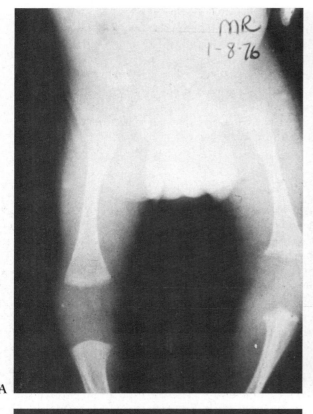

A

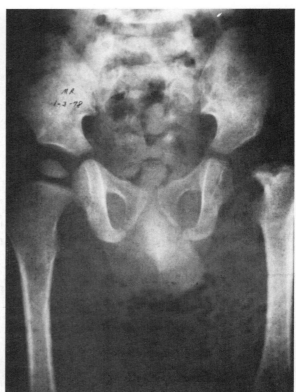

B

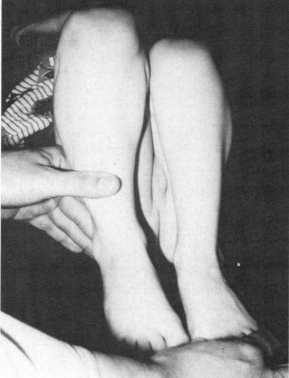

C

Figure 176.7.   **A:** Soft-tissue swelling in a neonate. Notice the hip joint space. **B:** Two years later, the metaphysis is subluxated, the acetabulum is dysplastic, and there is no ossified femoral head. **C:** This image demonstrates the shortening of the left femur.

technique is used in a joint that by all rights should have had a successful outcome.

Decompression/Debridement of the Hip

I prefer the anterior approach to the hip to the posterior approach. In the anterior approach the posterior superior epiphyses vessels are less likely to be damaged, and the anterior arthrotomy does not leave a posterior defect in the capsule where the hip can dislocate.

- Make an anterior approach (see Chapter 3).
- Then make a 1 cm capsulotomy through which the joint is irrigated.
- I do not drill the femoral neck. In the infant, only a small portion of the neck within the capsule is ossified, so drilling is likely to injure the physis. If the septic hip is secondary to osteomyelitis, the femoral neck has already decompressed itself.
- Although I no longer use irrigation postoperatively, I do leave a drain near the opening in the capsule and remove it at 48 hours.
- Take a synovial biopsy for culture and close the skin. Synovial tissue cultures may be positive when the aspiration is negative.

After either the aspiration, arthroscopic drainage, or arthrotomy, I place the extremity in balance suspension traction for several days in the older child. If properly applied, traction protects the joint and relieves pain, separates the joint surfaces, and allows motion. Protective use of the joint can begin shortly after the joint is no longer painful. If the hip appears unstable or it is dislocated, it should be held in the reduced position with a spica cast. Salter et al. (36) has shown that in the rabbit, continuous passive motion is beneficial to the articular cartilage. Its value in septic arthritis in children has not been established, however.

Immediately after the aspiration, the appropriate systemic parenteral antibiotic should be started. It should be one that is effective for the most likely pathogen. Age, environment, and the Gram stain determine the initial choice of antibiotic. In the neonate, multiple organisms are not uncommon. A semisynthetic penicillin for the staphylococci and streptococci plus an aminoglycoside for the gram-negative organisms should be used in the neonate. Between the age of 1 month and 5 years, *H. Influenzae* is as common as staphylococcus and streptococcus infection if the child has not been vaccinated for *H. influenzae*. In this age group, cefuroxime or ceftriaxone may be the drug of choice because they are effective against both the gram-positive cocci and *H. influenzae*. After age 5 years, a semisynthetic penicillin or a first-generation cephalosporin is the drug of choice. Both are effective against streptococcus and staphylococcus organisms. The oral cephalosporins taste better than the oral synthetic

penicillin, and for that reason, a cephalosporin may be preferable.

The use of oral antibiotics after 2 to 3 days of intravenous antibiotics can be effective in selected patients. The prerequisite for the use of oral treatment is a rapid clinical response to treatment, a positive culture, an available laboratory to measure serum levels, a reliable family, and proof that the child can tolerate the oral antibiotic. A positive culture is beneficial for proving the effectiveness of the blood level of the agent being used. The dosage has to be sufficient to give a peak serum bactericidal level at a dilution of between 1 to 8 and 1 to 16, and a dilution of 1 to 2 at the trough or a bactericidal concentration present in the trough for those antibiotics that have a bactericidal level. In a patient who does not have a positive culture but who has shown a rapid response to the parenteral antibiotic, it is not unreasonable to continue treatment with an oral antibiotic. The duration for antibiotic treatment is not absolute. In uncomplicated cases without osteomyelitis, 2 to 3 weeks should be sufficient. Be sure the patient is symptomatically doing well and that the sedimentation rate is reduced before discontinuing the antibiotic.

The residual effects from septic arthritis diagnosed and treated within 2 days and in some cases even longer are minimal. In the infant, a delay in diagnosis and treatment is more likely than in older children. The hip is more commonly affected in the infant, and osteomyelitis with secondary septic arthritis is more common in the proximal femur. Until the physis becomes a barrier to the metaphyseal vessels crossing into the epiphysis, the physis and epiphysis are in jeopardy. This anatomic fact and the frequent delay in diagnosis in the infant are the reasons that the poorest results from septic arthritis are in infants and in the hip. The physis and the epiphysis may both be completely destroyed by osteomyelitis with associated septic arthritis. Spontaneous decompression of the pus into the hip joint may cause damage to the epiphyseal blood supply by tamponade, and the intracapsular pressure may cause a dislocation of the hip. In my report in 1967, 15% of infected hips had a poor result and 75% of poor results were patients with septic arthritis of the hip secondary to osteomyelitis (16).

Significant sequelae to septic arthritis are rare except in the hip, where delay in treatment of the infant has allowed the partial or complete destruction of the physis and epiphysis. If the hip is dislocated, closed reduction is superior to open reduction (44). When the residual femoral head is inadequate to be effective as a functioning hip; attempts at surgical reconstruction should be avoided. Following total destruction of the head and neck, trochanteric arthroplasty has been done in an attempt to improve function and to maintain length (7). This procedure has many problems. With time, dislocation gradually occurs. A varus osteotomy delays the subluxation, but with time, the varus gradually straightens and subluxation occurs (13). Betz et al. (4) reported that the long-term functional results in the patient in whom the head is destroyed is better if reconstruction is not attempted.

If coxa vara, coxa valga, or acetabular dysplasia is the sequela to hip infection, it can be successfully treated by the appropriate osteotomy. The prerequisite to an osteotomy about the hip is a femoral head that is stable and sufficient to function effectively. If this is not possible, reduction of the head should not be attempted.

TUBERCULOUS ARTHRITIS

Tuberculosis of the bones and joints is uncommon in the countries of the developed world, particularly in North America. But it remains a common scourge in underdeveloped countries. Over the past decade, there has been a substantial increase in migration to developed countries from underdeveloped areas, such that tuberculosis is now more common and must always be suspected in children who present with chronic infections, particularly if their families have recently immigrated from underdeveloped countries. Tuberculosis is a chronic granulomatous infection caused by *Mycobacterium tuberculosis*. In countries where raw milk is consumed, bovine transmission can cause infection by *Mycobacterium bovi*. Tuberculosis is a localized destructive disease that spreads by the hematogenous route from a primary focus, most commonly located in the lungs and infected mediastinal lymph nodes.

As with pyogenic infections, tuberculous infections of joints can occur by direct hematogenous infection of the synovium or by invasion of the joint from an adjacent osteomyelitis involving the epiphysis or metaphysis. A tuberculous focus in bone spreads by centrifugal destruction of bone, producing increasing amounts of exudate and caseous necrotic material. Increasing pressure and bone destruction results in perforation of the bony cortex, forming a soft-tissue "cold abscess" so named because of the absence of acute inflammation. The infection spreads along tissue planes and may present as a subcutaneous abscess or fistula.

Primary joint tuberculosis or secondary spread from adjacent bone involvement results in the proliferation of tuberculous granulation tissue in the joint, which produces a pannus that rapidly covers articular cartilage, destroying the cartilage and underlying subchondral bone. Destruction is most extensive around the periphery of the joint at the attachments of the synovial membrane.

The clinical presentation of a chronically ill child with a history of easy fatigability and weight loss. The evolution of the disease is insidious, and involvement is usually monoarticular or in a single site. It is important to seek a family history of tuberculosis. With lower extremity involvement, the patients limp and the affected joint is stiff.

Crying at night is typical, because the pain seems to increase because protective muscle spasm relaxes at night. Physical findings depend on the anatomic area involved. Infection is most frequent in the spine, followed in order of frequency by the hip, knee, ankle, sacroiliac joint, shoulder, and wrist. Tuberculous spondylitis in the child is characterized by a painful, stiff back and a protective gait in which the child keeps the back hyperextended. Infection in the thoracic spine and the thoracolumbar junction is common. Kyphosis develops as bone destruction progresses. In the extremities, muscular atrophy is usually marked.

Characteristic laboratory findings are a hypochromic anemia, normal or only a slight increase in the peripheral white blood cell count, a modestly elevated erythrocyte sedimentation rate, and positive tubercular skin test. Synovial fluid analysis shows a white blood cell count averaging 20,000 cells/mm³ (range 3,000 to 100,000 cells), with 40% lymphocytes and monocytes, which is much more than that seen in pyogenic infections. Cultures are usually positive, but diagnosis can be quickly confirmed by histologic examination of tissue obtained by biopsy of the synovium of infected joints or sites of bone involvement.

Plane film radiography is usually adequate to demonstrate the changes from tuberculous arthritis, although it is often indistinguishable from monoarticular rheumatoid arthritis. Characteristic findings are the triad of Phemister, which consists of periarticular osteoporosis, gradual narrowing of the joint space, and erosions of the bone peripherally at the synovial attachments. In the late stage of tuberculosis, there may be complete destruction of joints, with dense sclerotic changes in adjacent bone. The disease is typically monoarticular, as opposed to juvenile arthritis, which is usually polyarticular. In the spine, the initial presentation shows disk space narrowing and destruction of the adjacent endplates of the vertebrae. With progression of the disease, a paraspinal mass is common. Subsequent collapse of involved vertebra and extension of the infection to adjacent levels leads to kyphosis and formation of a gibbous. Infection often extends along the psoas muscle sheaths and can present as abscesses in the flanks or groin. Paraplegia can occur due to tuberculous involvement of the meninges or due to mechanical pressure from the infection and collapse of the vertebral elements. This is known as Pott's disease.

Treatment is primarily with multiple antituberculous drugs. General medicine measures to treat other focuses of the disease and to ensure good health habits and adequate nutrition are important. Orthopaedic care consists of conservative measures to preserve motion and strength, and to prevent deformity. Surgery is performed when necessary to debride necrotic bone and soft tissue, and to eliminate abscess. Today, surgery is most commonly required to correct spinal deformity and treat paraparesis. For treatment, three drugs are preferred, and because of the large percentage of drug-resistant infections in certain areas, four drugs may be advisable. Drugs include isoniazid, rifampin, streptomycin, ethambutol, and pyrazinamide, as well as others. Pyridoxine supplementation may be necessary when treating with isoniazid. Monitor patients for hepatotoxicity, impaired renal infection, eighth cranial nerve toxicity, serum sickness–like syndromes, and thrombocytopenia.

REFERENCES

Each reference is categorized according to the following scheme: *, classic article; #, review article; !, basic research article; and +, clinical results/outcome study.

+ 1. Ang JG, Gelfand MJ. Decreased Gallium Uptake in Acute Hematogenous Osteomyelitis. *Clin Nucl Med* 1983;8:301.

+ 2. Ash JM, Gilday DL. The Futility of Bone Scanning in Neonatal Osteomyelitis: Concise Communication. *J Nucl Med* 1980;21:417.

+ 3. Benhamou L, Chamot AM, Kahn MF. Synovitis-Acne-Pustulosis Hyperostosis-Osteomyelitis Syndrome (SAPHO) A new Syndrome Among the Spondyloarthritis. *Clin Exp Rheumatol* 1988;6:109.

+ 4. Betz RR, Cooperman DR, Wopperer JM, et al. Late Sequelae of Septic Arthritis of the Hip in Infancy and Childhood. *J Pediatr Orthop* 1990;10:365.

+ 5. Bowman TR, Johnson RA, Sherman FC. Gallium Scintigraphy for Diagnosis of Septic Arthritis and Osteomyelitis in Children. *J Pediatr Orthop* 1986;6:317.

+ 6. Carr AJ, Cole WG, Roberton DM, Chow CW. Chronic Multifocal Osteomyelitis. *J Bone Joint Surg* 1993;75-B:582.

+ 7. Choi IH, Pizzutillo PD, Bowen JR, et al. Sequelae and Reconstruction after Septic Arthritis of the Hip in Infants. *J Bone Joint Surg* 1900;72-A:1150.

+ 8. Dan M. Septic Arthritis in Young Infants: Clinical and Microbiologic Correlations and Therapeutic Implications. *Rev Infect Dis* 1984;6:174.

+ 9. DeLucas PA, Gutman LT, Ruderman RS. Counterimmunoelectrophoresis of Synovial Fluid in the Diagnosis of Septic Arthritis. *J Pediatr Orthop* 1985;5:167.

+ 10. Dich VQ, Nelson JD, Haltalin KC. Osteomyelitis in Infants and Children: A Review of 163 Cases. *Am J Dis Child* 1975;129:1278.

+ 11. Epps CH, Bryant DD, Coles MJM. Osteomyelitis in Patients Who Have Sickle Cell Disease. *J Bone Joint Surg* 1991;73:A:1281.

+ 12. Farley T, Conway J, Shulman ST. Hematogenous Pelvic Osteomyelitis in Children. Clinical Correlates of Newer Scanning Methods. *Am J Dis Child* 1985;139:946.

+ 13. Freeland AE, Sullivan DJ, Westin GW. Greater Trochanter Hip Arthroplasty in Children with Loss of the Femoral Head. *J Bone Joint Surg* 1980;62-A:1351.

+ 14. Gledhill RB. Subacute Osteomyelitis in Children. *Clin Orthop* 1973;96:57.

+ 15. Green NE, Beauchange RD, Griffin PP. Primary Subacute Epiphyseal Osteomyelitis. *J Bone Joint Surg* 1981;63-A:107.

16. Griffin PP. Bone and Joint Infections in Children. *Pediatr Clin North Am* 1967;14:533.

+ 17. Herndon WA, Knauer S, Sullivan, Gross RH. Management of Septic Arthritis in Children. *J Pediatr Orthop* 1986;6:576.

+ 18. Highland TR, LaMont RL. Osteomyelitis of the Pelvis in Children. *J Bone Joint Surg* 1983;65A:230.

+ 19. Hoffer FA, Strand RD, Gebhardt MC. Percutaneous Biopsy of Pyogenic Infection of the Spine in Children. *J Pediatr Orthop* 1988;8:442.

+ 20. Jackson MA, Nelson JD. Etiology and Medical Management of Acute Suppurative Bone and Joint Infections in Pediatric Patients. *J Pediatr Orthop* 1982;2:313.

! 21. Jasin HE. Bacterial Lipopolysaccharides Induce In Vitro Degradation of Cartilage Matrix through Chondrocyte Activation. *J Clin Invest* 1983;72:2014.

+ 22. Jurik AG, Hehnig O, Ternowitz T, Muller BN. Chronic Recurrent Multifocal Osteomyelitis: A Follow-up Study. *J Pediatr Orthop* 1988;8:49.

+ 23. Keely K, Buchanan GR. Acute Infarction of Long Bone in Children with Sickle Cell Anemia. *J Pediatr* 1982;101:170.

+ 24. King DM, Mayo KM. Subacute Hematogenous Osteomyelitis. *J Bone Joint Surg* 1969;51-B:458.

* 25. Koch J. Undersuchangen uber die Lokalisation der Bakteries das Verhalten des Knochen Markes und die Verenderungen der Knochen, inc besondere der Epiphysen bei Infekuouskrankheiten. *Z Hyg Infectionskr* 1911;69:436.

+ 26. Mallouk A, Talab Y: Bone and Joint Infections in Patients with Sickle Cell Disease. *J Pediatr Orthop* 1985;5:158.

+ 27. Mazur JH, Ross G, Cumming J, et al. Usefulness of Magnetic Resonance Imaging for the Diagnosis of Acute Musculoskeletal Infections in Children. *J Pediatr Orthop* 1995;15:144.

+ 28. Menelaus MB. Discitis: An Inflammation Affecting the Intervertebral Discs in Children. *J Bone Joint Surg* 1964;46:B:16.

! 29. Morrissy RT, Haynes DW. Acute Hematogenous Osteomyelitis: A Model with Trauma as an Etiology. *J Pediatr Orthop* 1989;9:447.

+ 30. Mustafa MM, Saez-Llorens X, McCracken GH Jr, Nelson JD. Acute Hematogenous Pelvic Osteomyelitis in Infants and Children. *Pediatr Infect Dis J* 1990;9:416.

+ 31. Piehl FC, Davis RJ, Pugh SI. Osteo in Sickle Cell Disease. *J Pediatr Orthop* 1993;13:225.

+ 32. Pugh CA, Hughes JK, Abrams BC. Osteo in Patients with Sickle Cell Disease. *J Bone Joint Surg* 1971;53-A:1.

+ 33. Prober CG, Yeager AS. Use of the Serum Bactericidal Titer to Assess the Adequacy of Oral Antibiotic Therapy in the Treatment of Acute Hematogenous Osteomyelitis. *J Pediatr* 1979;96:131.

+ 34. Ring D, Johnston CE, Wenger DR. Pyogenic Infectious

Spondylitis in Children. *J Pediatr Orthop* 1995;15(5): 652.

+ 35. Roberts JM, Drummond DS, Breed AL, Chesney J. Subacute Hematogenous Osteomyelitis in Children: A Retrospective Study. *J Pediatr Orthop* 1982;2:249.

! 36. Salter RB, Bell RS, Keeley FM. The Protective Effect of Continuous Passive Motion on Living Articular Cartilage in Acute Septic Arthritis: An Experimental Investigation in the Rabbit. *Clin Orthop* 1981;159:223.

+ 37. Silverthorn KG, Gillespie WJ. Pyogenic Spinal Osteomyelitis. *N Z Med J* 1986;99:62.

! 38. Smith RL, Schurman DJ, Kajiyania G, et al. The Effect of Antibiotics on the Desctruction of Cartilage in Experimental Infectious Arthritis. *J Bone Joint Surg* 1987;69-A:1063.

* 39. Smith T. On the Acute Arthritis of Infants. *St. Bartholemew's Hospital Report* 1874;10:189.

+ 40. Stutley JE, Conway WF. Magnetic Resonance Imaging of the Pelvis and Hips. *Orthopedics* 1994;17:1053.

+ 41. Tong Y, Wei XR, Qiu GX, et al. The Treatment of Chronic Hematogenous Osteomyelitis. *Clin Orthop* 1987;215:72.

* 42. Trueta J. The Normal Vascular Anatomy of the Human Femoral Head During Growth. *J Bone Joint Surg* 1957; 39-B:358.

+ 43. Vaughan PA, Newman NM, Rosman MA. Acute Hematogenous Osteomyelitis in Children. *J Pediatr Orthop* 1987;7:652.

+ 44. Wopperer JM, White JS, Gillespie R, et al. Long Term Follow-up of Infantile Hip Sepsis. *J Pediatr Orthop* 1988;8:322.

+ 45. Yu L, Kasser JR, O'Rourke E, Kozakowich H. Chronic Recurrent Multifocal Osteomyelitis Associated with Vertebra Plana. *J Bone Joint Surg* 1989;71A:105.

Cerebral palsy (CP) is a disorder of movement or posture caused by a nonprogressive lesion of the brain acquired at or around the time of birth (3). Although musculoskeletal deformities and imbalances are usual, and certain clinical patterns are relatively common, the condition is extremely heterogeneous. The brain lesions tend not to be highly localized and therefore usually produce more than an isolated deficit. At least five basic movement disorders—spasticity, athetosis, ataxia, rigidity, and tremor—are described; various possibilities for distribution include monoplegia, hemiplegia, diplegia, and total body involvement.

Although spasticity is most common, many patients have more than one movement disorder. It is important

to identify the primary movement disorder because, in general, operations are designed for patients with spasticity. Because the brain lesion is often diffuse, deficits in proprioception, stereognosis, and perceptual integration can result. Keeping cognizant of these other deficits will remind the orthopaedic surgeon to set reasonably modest goals for treatment.

Specific deformities and functional losses are seen repetitively in patients with CP, depending on the pattern of neurologic involvement. For example, the combination of windblown hips and scoliosis is typically seen in the total-body-involved spastic quadriplegia patient. Valgus feet and mild crouch gait are typically seen in spastic diplegia. By applying basic principles of surgical correction, the orthopaedist may improve positioning, function, and appearance of the extremities in selected patients.

L. A. Rinsky: Palo Alto, California, 94304.

GOALS OF TREATMENT

Many CP patients will need and benefit from lower extremity surgery. The goals vary depending on the overall functional ability of the patient (i.e., nonambulator, "therapy" or nonfunctional ambulator, household ambulator, community ambulator with assistive devices, or independent community ambulator). Goals for lower extremity surgery in nonambulators are often limited to improving comfort and easing nursing care, or decreasing contractures sufficiently to allow deformed feet to be fitted with shoes. Assisted transfers of a nonambulator in and out of a wheelchair can be facilitated if the patient can be stood on plantigrade feet with fairly straight hips and knees. For household or community walkers, the goal should be to improve the efficiency of gait (i.e., decrease the energy cost) by minimizing contractures and balancing spasticity. However, the basic ability to walk is dictated by the patient's brain and is not affected by the orthopaedic surgeon. Because the prognosis for independent walking can be established by 2 or 3 years of age (depending on the equilibrium and primitive reflexes), the surgeon should have realistic goals in mind by the time surgery is undertaken (3).

A far smaller percentage of CP patients will need or truly benefit from upper extremity surgery. The goals of upper extremity reconstructive surgery usually relate to improvement in function, occasionally for ease of hygiene or personal care (such as pulling a long sleeve shirt over a wrist and hand that is locked in flexion), and rarely for improvement in cosmesis. Coexistent deficits in stereognosis and motor planning limit the goals that should be expected when trying to rebalance motor control about the wrist and hand. Additionally, any cognitive problems further minimize the ability of the CP patient to cooperate in a postoperative therapy program. In general, this will mean that most upper extremity surgery *for functional improvement* will be performed on children who are spastic hemiplegics with only mild or no cognitive deficits.

For the sake of clarity, it is important to discuss only one anatomic deformity at a time. However, it is vital always to think of the joints and muscles above and below the target deformity. Make repeated examinations before deciding on surgical intervention. Consideration must be given not only to the effects of other deformities on the index deformity, but also to the effects that any proposed surgery will have on the neighboring joints. A classic example of this is the increased lordosis that occurs after an apparently appropriate hamstring lengthening because of a lack of attention to preexisting increased hip flexor spasticity. Similarly, a mild tendency toward crouch gait will often worsen following a heel cord lengthening done in isolation.

I have found the gait analysis laboratory to be helpful in planning surgical procedures in CP, especially when several procedures must be performed simultaneously. By using combinations of dynamic gait electromyographic (EMG) analysis and video monitoring of joint range during gait, I have found that in more than half the cases the preoperative gait analysis affects my decision as to which operative procedures are necessary.

Most surgery designed for gait improvement should probably be delayed until the pattern of gait is fairly well established (usually between 4 and 8 years of age) with a goal of finishing surgical intervention (if possible) by the first or second grade of school. Similarly, surgery for upper extremity functional improvement usually is most appropriate at about the same age. It often takes a series of examinations on a young child to accurately assess the motor, sensory, and cognitive resources of a not-always-cooperative child.

The procedures described here represent my preferences for treating the most common lower-extremity deformities in spastic CP. Keep in mind that even with well-planned and carefully executed surgery, deformities occasionally recur or progress in children with CP, and salvage or reconstructive procedures may later become necessary.

FOOT AND ANKLE DEFORMITIES

EQUINUS DEFORMITY

Indications for Surgery

Equinus deformity is very common and is one of the few deformities that may actually exist in isolation in spastic CP, especially in hemiplegics. The indications for surgical correction are simple: fixed equinus such that the ankle cannot be dorsiflexed to neutral, with the hindfoot locked in varus in a walking or potentially ambulatory patient. In diplegics, equinus helps in transferring the weight-bearing line anteriorly, which assists in extending the knee. Thus, when crouching is present in diplegia, the surgeon should not lengthen the triceps surae in isolation; usually, hamstring or hip flexor surgery must be combined with it. Not all tiptoeing CP patients have fixed equinus. For a dynamic deformity, it is best to try an extended period of bracing with a rigid plastic ankle–foot orthosis or a series of short-leg walking casts for 2–3 weeks at a time.

An additional alternative for the patient with dynamic equinus is an injection of botulinum-A toxin (1–2 μm/kg body weight per calf), which will fairly reliably temporarily relieve spasticity and tone for a period of up to 6 months (16).

Tendo-Achilles Lengthening through the Posteromedial Approach

In an older patient with a severe, longstanding equinus contracture (e.g., a 10-year-old hemiplegic who has always walked on his toes), heel cord lengthening through a standard posteromedial longitudinal incision with a Z-type tendon lengthening is recommended, because there is likely to be a fixed capsular contracture of the ankle requiring capsulotomy as well. The amount of lengthening should be approximately enough that with the foot in neutral, half the available excursion of the tendo-Achilles is set. An additional check for the amount of lengthening is the so-called geometric method, in which the amount of lengthening is half the perpendicular distance that the first metatarsal head protrudes inferiorly to the heel during maximal passive dorsiflexion (10). Once the amount of lengthening is determined, perform the suture repair with the foot in equinus so as to minimize tension during the repair. After the repair, check the foot in the neutral position to make sure that there is still some residual tension on the muscle–tendon unit.

Hoke Procedure

- In most patients, a Hoke procedure is preferred for heel cord lengthening (Fig. 177.1). This can be accomplished in a number of ways. The method involves three opposing cuts, each one halfway through the tendon. Make two medial cuts proximally and distally, with one lateral cut halfway between the two, or vice versa. Then dorsiflex the foot just to neutral, thus causing a sliding lengthening. No sutures are necessary.
- The best visualization of the procedure is accomplished through a medial longitudinal incision 4–6 cm in length. It is rare to need a posterior capsulotomy of the ankle in CP. By placing the incision slightly further anteriorly, the posterior tibial tendon or toe flexors may also be approached, if desired. However, occasionally the longitudinal scar may be prominent. Alternatively, use two small transverse incisions, with two of the ten-

don cuts through one incision and one tendon cut through a second incision. With a subcuticular closure, the scar is essentially invisible.

- Finally, the entire procedure can be performed percutaneously. This is now my preferred technique if a heel cord lengthening is the only procedure needing to be done. Make the same three cuts in the tendon using a #15-C scalpel blade through three tiny percutaneous incisions. The proximal cut should be at about the level of the musculotendinous junction. It is essential to dorsiflex the foot to only 10° or 15° above neutral, with the knee slightly flexed.

Gastrocnemius Recession

In the occasional ambulatory, tiptoeing child with a dramatic and consistently positive Silfverskiöld test (in which the amount of dorsiflexion is much improved with the knee flexed as compared to the degree in full knee extension), I perform a simple gastrocnemius recession (24).

- Make a longitudinal incision in the lower middle calf slightly medially over the palpable lower border of the gastrocnemius muscle belly. Separate the gastrocnemius aponeurosis from the underlying soleus; this plane is easier to find proximally.
- Divide transversely only the gastrocnemius aponeurosis and dorsiflex the foot to 5° to 10° above neutral. I will usually tack down the aponeurosis with a few absorbable stitches. Occasionally, it is also necessary to divide a few fibers of the underlying soleus aponeurosis to obtain adequate dorsiflexion. No muscle fibers, however, are divided. This has the theoretical advantage that overcorrection is very unlikely, although recurrence of equinus may be slightly more likely.

Postoperative Care

The postoperative care is the same whatever type of equinus correction is chosen. Apply an above-knee cast with the knee in 5° or 10° of flexion. At 2–3 weeks, cut the cast down to a below-knee walking cast. Allow ambulation immediately after surgery if no other contraindications are present. If no other simultaneous surgery was performed requiring immobilization above the knee (e.g., hamstring or iliopsoas release), a below-knee walking cast can be used following any type of heel cord lengthening. The child will tend to flex the knees with only a below-knee cast, but within 24 hours she can be coaxed into extending her knees to near neutral. Using a below-knee cast facilitates the rehabilitation. Remove all casts at 6–8 weeks. A plastic, right angle, or articulated ankle–foot orthosis (AFO) is frequently used part-time for at least 3–6 months. Patients who have no selective control of dorsiflexion will often require the orthosis on a more or less permanent basis. Use nighttime splinting in neutral in those patients who tend to drift back into equinus.

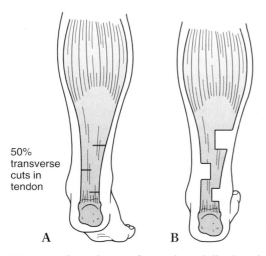

50% transverse cuts in tendon

A   B

Figure 177.1.   Hoke technique for tendo-Achilles lengthening.

Complications

If fixed equinus recurs, lengthen the tendon by the Z technique a second time. Forewarn parents that recurrence of some equinus does occur in perhaps 10% of children who undergo tendo-Achilles lengthening (TAL); however, many children who do not make heel contact at foot strike do so more because of flexed knees than because of fixed equinus. Overlengthening is far worse than a recurrence of the original equinus. There is no universally successful management for postoperative calcaneus deformity. The first rule is to avoid overlengthening. Some tension should always remain on the tendon unit after lengthening. If calcaneus deformity does occur, tendon reconstructions have not always been satisfactory. Reshortening of the tendo-Achilles may be tried, or tenodesis of the Achilles to the posterior tibia or fibula, but these are unlikely to restore true muscle function.

A dynamic gait analysis may demonstrate which muscles are active in stance. The anterior tibial tendon can be transferred posteriorly to the heel, and theoretically the peroneus brevis and half the posterior tibial tendon can also be transferred to the os calcis. However, restoration of fully satisfactory plantar flexor strength is unlikely. Should postoperative calcaneus deformity occur, a rigid AFO with a wide proximal anterior tibial restraint ("floor reaction" AFO) will have to be used in addition to attempts at reinforcing plantar flexor strength.

VARUS DEFORMITY

Indications for Surgery

Varus deformity may be either dynamic or fixed. It appears most often in hemiplegics, compared with the more typical valgus deformity seen in diplegics. Dynamic gait EMG analysis is most helpful in determining the phasic nature of the tibialis anterior and posterior muscles and the peroneals. Generally, patients under 4 years of age have not fully established a gait pattern and can be managed with orthotics. The indications for surgery then depend on the age of the patient, whether the varus is mild or severe, and which muscles are most "at fault" on the EMG.

For the milder, flexible varus deformities, a posterior tibial myotendinous lengthening (25) is the simplest approach, but it is rarely appropriate to perform it as an isolated procedure. This is often combined with a TAL. For more significant, but still flexible, varus deformities, a split anterior tibial tendon (SPLATT) procedure (13) can be combined with the posterior tibial myotendinous lengthening, or the posterior tibial tendon can be split and transferred laterally to the peroneus brevis (15,23).

If any of these procedures are being considered, preoperative gait EMG, if available, should demonstrate excessive or even continuous phasic firing of the anterior and posterior tibial muscles throughout the gait cycle. One

should not expect postoperative changes in the phasic pattern of muscle firing after transfer (11). Currently, I favor the split posterior tibial tendon transfer (usually along with TAL) in patients with dynamic varus and equinus deformity, because plantar flexor strength is not sacrificed quite as much, and only the muscle direction is changed. It is important to realize that spastic muscles, although overactive, are still weakened. In fact, I frequently split both the anterior and the posterior tibial tendons with lateral transfer of both in cases of dynamic varus. Others perform just the SPLATT transfer with TAL for the same dynamic varus deformity. The postoperative regimen in either case is the same as described for TAL.

I would caution against ever transferring the entire posterior tibial tendon anteriorly through the interosseous membrane in a patient with spastic CP. I have abandoned that technique because of the occurrence of late calcaneovalgus deformity. I would also caution against complete tenotomy of the posterior tibial tendon in the spastic foot, because late valgus is likely.

If a fixed varus deformity is present in the hindfoot, as determined by the block test, add a bony reconstruction to the soft-tissue releases or transfer. Perform the block test by having the patient stand with a 1–2 cm block under the heel and lateral border of the foot. If the heel varus resolves, then it is compensatory and results from forefoot pronation of the first ray. If heel varus persists on the block, it is fixed (see the section on cavus in Chapter 167). In the case of a younger patient, the choices are either a sliding lateral displacement osteotomy or a Dwyer-type of laterally based closing wedge of the calcaneus. In a patient older than 12 years with significant fixed varus deformity, perform a triple arthrodesis.

Posterior Tibial Tendon Lengthening

■ Through a longitudinal supramalleolar posteromedial incision, approach the posterior tibial muscle. At least 2–4 cm proximal to the most distal muscle fibers, divide the tendinous portion of the posterior tibial muscle obliquely. Passively evert the foot under direct visualization to observe the tendon slide. This produces an aponeurotic lengthening that leaves the muscle fibers in continuity. No sutures are needed.

■ Alternatively, a supramalleolar Z-lengthening of the posterior tibial tendon can be performed, but this is a more complex procedure and requires suture repair.

I prefer the first method, usually in combination with a TAL and SPLATT. Use a postoperative short-leg walking cast for 6 weeks.

SPLATT Procedure

■ Isolate the anterior tibial tendon at its insertion as far distally as possible through a 1-inch (2.5 cm) incision over the first cuneiform bone. Split the tendon in half longitudinally and free the lateral half (see Chapter 167).

- Make a second incision over the anterior compartment of the leg 3–4 inches (7.5–10.0 cm) above the ankle. Pass the lateral half of the tendon proximally into the second incision. It is helpful to have a Bunnell-type suture through the free end of the tendon.

- Then make a third incision laterally over the cuboid bone. Pass the lateral half of the anterior tibial tendon subcutaneously, deep to the extensor retinaculum to the third incision. Suture the tendon either to the periosteum of the cuboid or, better, route it through a small bony vertical tunnel in the cuboid. I prefer using an absorbable pullout stitch over a padded plantar button or splint. On subsequent removal of the cast, the pullout suture can simply be cut flush with the skin.

- Prior to closure, tension on the tendon proximally should tend to dorsiflex the foot in a neutral position. That is, a yoke has been created and the tension in each limb both medially and laterally should be fairly similar. Use a short-leg cast for 6 weeks.

Split Posterior Tibial Tendon Transfer

Usually four small 1- to 1.5-inch (2.5 to 3.4 cm) incisions are used, although the entire procedure can readily be performed through the Cincinnati horizontal transverse incision commonly used for clubfoot (31) (see Chapter 167).

- Begin with a 1-inch (2.5 cm) medial longitudinal incision over the navicular tuberosity. Isolate the posterior tibial tendon at its insertion and split it distally, detaching the plantar half. Tag this with a heavy nonabsorbable suture. (Fig. 177.2).

- Make the second incision medial and longitudinal, 1 cm posterior to the medial border of the tibia. Using a curved tendon passer, pass the tagged suture with the plantar half of the posterior tibial tendon through the sheath directly posterior to the tibia. Tease this backward to propagate the split. Deliver the tendon into the medial proximal incision.

- Place a third incision just posterior to the distal fibula. Then pass the tagged tendon laterally just posterior to the tibia and fibula to the peroneal tendon sheath. Pass the split tendon within the sheath to the area of the fifth metatarsal–cuboid articulation, where the fourth short incision is made. Then suture the split tendon to the peroneus brevis under moderate tension with the foot in neutral. Apply a short-leg cast.

Calcaneal Osteotomy (Lateral Displacement, or Dwyer)

- Expose the lateral calcaneus subperiosteally through an oblique lateral incision immediately behind the peroneal tendons. Use an oscillating saw to cut through the calcaneus more or less parallel to the posterior calcaneal facet. Temporarily open the osteotomy laterally to use a curved Freer or small elevator to medially strip subperiosteally. Unless this step is done, it will be impossible to displace the tuberosity fragment. I caution against hammering an osteotome to complete the osteotomy medially because of the danger to the neurovascular bundle and flexor tendons, which are directly apposed medially (Fig. 177.3).

- When the tuberosity has been sufficiently mobilized, displace it laterally enough (0.5–1.2 cm) to put the heel in neutral or slight valgus. Make sure that the tuberosity fragment does not slide proximally. Insert a single smooth pin from the plantar surface of the calcaneus across the osteotomy to hold the reduction. Leave it in place for 3 or 4 weeks.

- The Dwyer technique is perhaps simpler because no medial dissection is necessary; however, it mildly decreases the heel height and theoretically also decreases plantar flexor strength. Make the first bony cut as described previously, but then remove an oblique laterally based wedge (Fig. 177.3) sufficient to correct the hind-

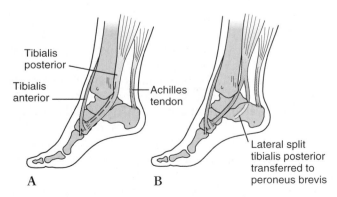

Figure 177.2. Split posterior tibial tendon transfer.

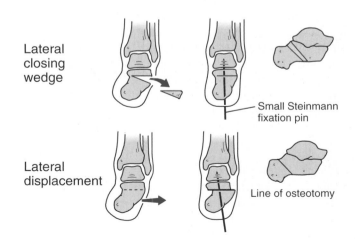

Figure 177.3. Calcaneal osteotomy for fixed hindfoot varus.

foot varus, bringing the heel directly in line with the long axis of the tibia. Close the bony surfaces and stabilize with either a smooth Steinmann pin (which is removed in 3 weeks) or a staple. I prefer pins. Allow weight bearing after 3 weeks.

Triple Arthrodesis

The technique for triple arthrodesis is fairly standard (see Chapter 115).

- Make an oblique incision over the sinus tarsi and expose the sinus by maintaining a distally based flap of the extensor brevis muscle and overlying fat pad. Instead of continuing distally in the subperiosteal plane toward the calcaneal–cuboid joint, I use a 2 cm osteotome to cut across the joint dorsally in the longitudinal plane. This creates a small myo-osseous flap, but more important, it nicely exposes the calcaneal–cuboid articulation.
- Depending on the degree of varus, take laterally based wedges from the subtalar and calcaneocuboid joints. I use a micro-oscillating or sagittal saw. In general, the wedges should probably be taken smaller than you initially think is necessary, so that an excessive amount of bone is not removed.
- I usually use two pins, both placed axially: one to hold the calcaneocuboid joint and the other the talonavicular joint. A third pin, vertically placed across the talocalcaneal articulation, is optional. Apply a heavily padded, above-knee cast.

Allow no weight bearing until the pins are removed at 6 weeks. Then apply a short-leg walking cast and maintain it until the fusion is solid, which usually takes an additional 6–8 weeks.

VALGUS DEFORMITY

Valgus feet are common in CP and are especially frequent in spastic diplegia and quadriplegia. Although, at first glance, predominant spasticity of the peroneal muscles would seem to be the primary cause, the etiology usually is multifactorial and includes excessive external tibial torsion, knee flexion deformity, and calcaneal equinus. The deformity usually remains flexible until adolescence. Secondary callosities develop over the talar head and the first metatarsal head, and hallux valgus develops. Initially, manage the deformity with an AFO; however, if the deformity becomes severe, brace fitting is increasingly difficult.

Indications for Surgery

Subtalar stabilization is indicated before the valgus deformity becomes fixed, usually by 6–10 years of age. Traditionally, some modification of the Grice extra-articular arthrodesis procedure was most commonly performed, using internal fixation (3,7). Depending on calcaneal position, a TAL is often necessary as well. The deformity must be passively correctable (at least with the foot in equinus) for the Grice procedure to work. More recently, one of several types of calcaneal osteotomies has become preferred because it maintains subtalar mobility while correcting the valgus (18,23,27). Although correction can be obtained by a simple opening lateral wedge osteotomy in the tuberosity using a cortical graft (bank or autogenous), I prefer either a medial calcaneal slide, or, occasionally, a lateral column lengthening. This latter technique of Evans, popularized by Mosca (18), has the advantage that it can partially correct the lateral subluxation at the midfoot. All of these also require reasonably supple feet that are passively correctable to neutral, or that can be made so with a simple heel cord lengthening.

The Grice procedure should not be performed in children less than 4 years of age because the bones are too small and cartilaginous. After age 12, a triple arthrodesis is usually more appropriate unless the valgus remains totally flexible. Occasionally, all or much of the apparent valgus is built into the tibiotalar joint with a relatively short fibula. A preoperative standing anteroposterior radiograph of the ankle should always be taken before the Grice procedure is performed. Do not attempt to correct the subtalar joint into varus to make up for ankle valgus. True ankle valgus must be corrected by a supramalleolar osteotomy or, rarely, a medial growth arrest, depending on age. Of course, the patient should be at least a household assisted ambulator (or have a reasonable prognosis for attaining that level of function) before considering foot reconstructive surgery.

Calcaneal Osteotomy (Medial Displacement or Lengthening)

- Use the same lateral oblique incision (posterior and parallel to the peroneal tendons) as for a Dwyer osteotomy. Use an oscillating saw to cut the tuberosity parallel to and below the posterior facet. If only the hindfoot is in valgus, then there is a choice of either using a laterally based opening wedge (held with an allograft cortical wedge), or sliding the distal fragment medially (Fig. 177.4).
- To successfully displace medially, it is necessary to carefully subperiosteally dissect medially from the lateral approach to mobilize the distal fragment. After medial displacement sufficient to place the heel in neutral alignment, accomplish fixation with a smooth Steinmann pin placed vertically from the plantar surface.
- I do not have long-term experience with distal calcaneal lengthening, but I have used it in cases of mild to moderate, very flexible valgus, and early results have been excellent. In this technique, make a transverse vertical osteotomy in the calcaneal neck, parallel to the calcaneal–cuboid joint. After mobilizing the distal fragment, use a lamina spreader to open the osteotomy, and simul-

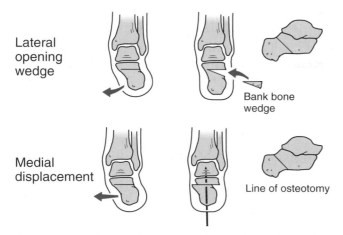

Figure 177.4. Calcaneal osteotomy for fixed hindfoot valgus.

taneously reduce the lateral talonavicular subluxation. Insert a trapezoidal cortical cancellous graft (I prefer allograft). It may be wise to provisionally fix the calcaneocuboid joint with a smooth Kirschner wire before lengthening; this prevents subluxation. A longitudinally placed K-wire, from distally across the calcaneal–cuboid joint, is optional if needed to maintain stability, and once it is passed through the calcaneocuboid joint, the original wire is removed. If a TAL has not been performed prior to the osteotomy, recheck after completion of the osteotomy to make sure that there is not a fixed ankle equinus deformity.

Grice Procedure

- Through an oblique incision extending from the lateral talonavicular joint to the peroneal tendons, sharply elevate the contents of the sinus tarsi from proximal to distal. Clean the lateral body and neck of the talus and the calcaneal floor of the sinus tarsi of all soft tissue. Ideally, expose no articular surfaces.
- Pack the sinus tarsi with corticocancellous graft taken from the iliac crest. Iliac graft rather than tibial or fibular is preferred because it is incorporated readily, it is abundantly available, there is enough graft from one crest to fuse both feet simultaneously, and the iliac crest graft does not carry the risks of donor site fatigue fracture after surgery (as do tibial grafts) or later valgus deformity (as with fibular grafts). Unlike "structural" grafts of tibial or fibular cortex, iliac graft is not used to correct deformity, only to obtain fusion. Because the iliac graft itself does not provide fixation, supplemental internal fixation is mandatory.
- Some surgeons insert a screw through the neck of the talus into the calcaneus, and this has the advantage of earlier weight bearing. However, I prefer to use a percutaneous Steinmann pin, inserted under direct vision

from the lateral plantar aspect of the calcaneus proximally across the sinus tarsi into the talus, because there is no retained hardware that can either back out or impinge against the anterior ankle structures (Fig. 177.5).

- Apply a long-leg cast for 4 weeks postoperatively, and then remove the pin. Weight bearing may be allowed in a short-leg cast for the next 4–6 weeks.

Complications

Failure to deal with fixed equinus of the hindfoot will make reduction of the calcaneus under the talus difficult or impossible. The heel will remain in valgus despite posi-

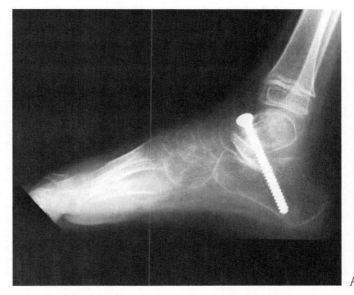

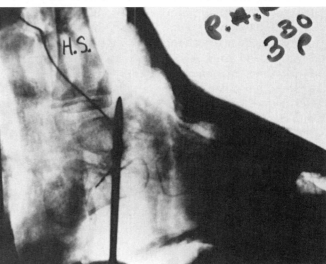

Figure 177.5. **A:** Subtalar arthrodesis with screw fixation. **B:** Temporary fixation using a Steinmann pin for subtalar arthrodesis.

tioning the graft. Another potential complication is that the graft may "melt away." This is especially likely when excessive external tibial torsion is present. Occasionally, sufficient fibrous stability may remain even with graft resorption so that further treatment is not necessary. If significant valgus recurs, triple arthrodesis may be considered as a salvage procedure.

Overcorrection into varus may appear to develop gradually, but it is usually the direct result of intraoperative overcorrection. If the extra-articular arthrodesis is solid, correction of a postoperative varus can be obtained with a closing lateral wedge osteotomy of the heel.

Triple Arthrodesis

The basic technique for triple arthrodesis is described in Chapter 115; however, for spastic valgus feet, additional principles are important. It is critical to ascertain before surgery that the ankle itself is in relatively normal alignment. If there is excessive external tibial torsion, correct this before performing the triple arthrodesis. Although flexible valgus feet can be corrected by the simple removal of joint surfaces, possibly with an inlay graft, most spastic valgus feet in older patients are rigid and require extensive bony wedge resection to obtain correction. Additionally, poor correction can be caused by inadequate exposure of the talonavicular joint.

- Use an additional 1-inch (2.5 cm) medial longitudinal incision over the talonavicular joint if the medial aspect is not well visualized from the main incision. This will allow excellent visualization when a Chandler retractor is passed from the main lateral incision out through the medial incision to protect the dorsal soft-tissue structures.
- If the foot is passively correctable to neutral before surgery, only the cartilaginous joint surfaces must be removed. However, in more severe valgus feet, remove medially based wedges of bone. Pack the sinus tarsi with cancellous bone from either the wedges or the iliac crest.
- I recommend using at least two smooth Steinmann pins for fixation. Pass one distally through the center of the exposed navicular and pass a second distally through the center of the cuboid. Then drive them retrograde into the talus and calcaneus, respectively. A third vertical pin through the talocalcaneal joint is optional. Take intraoperative radiographs; it is surprising how misplaced the pins can be. I usually place a small suction drain.
- Use an above-knee (or patellar tendon bearing) non-weight-bearing cast for 6 weeks postoperatively, and then remove the pins and apply a short-leg walking cast.

EXCESSIVE TIBIAL TORSION

Indications for Surgery

Excessive external tibial torsion is commonly seen in diplegia and quadriplegia, apparently as a compensation for excessive medial femoral torsion. This malalignment will contribute to valgus foot deformities, bunions, and other problems. Tibial osteotomy is indicated when it is necessary to keep the foot pointed correctly forward, especially following femoral derotation (external) osteotomy, or as part of correction for severe valgus feet.

Tibial Osteotomy

- Make a 5–10 cm longitudinal incision proximally over the lateral anterior compartment. Always perform a fasciotomy of both the anterior and the peroneal compartments.
- By following the intermuscular septum, make a limited subperiosteal exposure of the fibula somewhat more distal than the tibial site to avoid the peroneal nerve. Osteotomize the fibula with a micro power saw.
- Expose the tibia circumferentially subperiosteally just distal to the tibial tubercle. To avoid anterior growth arrest, the osteotomy site must be distal to the anterior extension of the physis. The operation can also be performed in the supramalleolar metaphysis, where the risk of compartment syndrome and peroneal palsy is less. I recommend operating distally if correction of an ankle valgus is also desired.
- Insert half-pins from medial to lateral through separate incisions prior to the osteotomy. Place one pin proximal to the incision and one distal, with both pins going through two cortices but only through the medial skin. Perform the osteotomy with an oscillating power saw, and control rotation with the pins. It is helpful to insert the pins so that the angle between them is the same as the angle of rotation you want. Then, when rotation is complete, the pins will be exactly parallel to each other.
- Immobilize the limb in a long-leg cast, incorporating the pins in plaster. If no additional tendon work has been done, an external fixator could be used, but this does not seem worth the expense. Clinical union occurs within 2 months in children. Weight bearing is usually allowed after 4 weeks, at which time the pins are pulled out through the cast.

See Chapter 168 for the alternative technique of supramalleolar tibial rotational osteotomy.

KNEE DEFORMITIES

FLEXION DEFORMITY

Indications for Surgery

Although the most common knee deformity in spastic CP is flexion contracture, the knees may be neutral or even hyperextended during the midstance phase of gait (3,8, 21,23). The knees (like every other joint in CP) cannot be evaluated in isolation. The cause of severe knee flexion—whether dynamic or fixed—is rarely as simple as excessive hamstring spasticity. Overlengthened or weak plantar flexors, fixed hip flexion contracture, and poor equilibrium all contribute to crouch. We can do little about faulty equilibrium, and we certainly recognize that a small knee flexion deformity is usually preferable to recurvatum. Therefore, not all knee flexion deformities (even fixed ones) require surgical release.

I divide spastic knee flexion deformity into two types. In the more common and familiar "crouched" type, the knee flexion is associated with feet that are flat on the floor or the heels are only slightly elevated (often in valgus). There is usually a fixed hip flexion deformity with increased iliopsoas spasticity, which must be released. The worst thing to do in these cases is a TAL, because it will increase the crouch.

In the "jumped" type of knee flexion deformity, the ankles are in marked fixed equinus. This type of patient needs a modest TAL, in addition to lengthening of the hamstrings and probably the iliopsoas.

In ambulators or potential ambulators, perform distal hamstring lengthening when the knees cannot be straightened during ambulation to less that 15° of flexion, and when other causes of crouch gait (at the hips or ankles) are absent or can be dealt with simultaneously. Knee flexor release is also indicated in older patients who are crouched and have knee pain during transfers or limited ambulation. If the degree of fixed contracture of the knee is greater than 20°, posterior knee capsulotomy is occasionally needed, but usually this is not needed in a walking CP patient with crouch.

In nonambulators, distal hamstring release is occasionally performed to decrease extreme flexor spasticity at the knee; this facilitates sitting and dressing. The hamstrings may also be released proximally through the same medial incision used for adductor and psoas release. However, the only time I use a proximal release of the hamstrings is in the patient who has not only tight hamstrings but also severe hip extension deformity. Such a patient stands with an absent or reversed lumbar lordosis. She tends to slide out of a wheelchair because the hamstring spasticity extends the hips. When proximal release is performed, the sciatic nerve must be avoided; it can be confused with the tendinous origin—a potential catastrophe.

Distal Hamstring Lengthening

- Place the patient supine and make a short, midaxial, longitudinal incision on the back of the knee. This allows repeated intraoperative assessments of the degree of improvement of straight-leg raising. In a typical patient with either no fixed-knee flexion contracture or only a mild one (10° to 20°), the contracture can be stretched out by wedging casts after hamstring release.
- Perform a Z-lengthening or simple tenotomy of the semitendinosis. The gracilis may also be tenotomized at your discretion. Perform an aponeurotic lengthening of

the semimembranosus and biceps tendon by oblique division of the tendon within the muscle belly. The lengthening should be sufficient to allow 70° of straight-leg raising. This is easily determined in the supine position.

- I always lengthen the biceps last because it is often not as tight as the medial hamstrings. In such cases, if adequate straight-leg raising is present after lengthening only medially, leave the biceps intact.

After surgery, apply a cylinder or long-leg cast. Mobilize the patient immediately with a walker or crutches if equilibrium is satisfactory. Mobilize more severely equilibrium-impaired patients in a standing frame chosen by the physical therapist.

Recently, if no additional surgery has been performed simultaneously at the ankles, I have used only a knee immobilizer postoperatively, again allowing immediate mobilization. If a joint capsule contracture was present preoperatively, do not apply the cast fully straight, but only at the limits of the maximal preoperative degree of extension. Begin wedging in 2 days.

In the rare, walking CP patient who actually needs a posterior capsulotomy, a better exposure is obtained by operating with the patient prone. In such cases, I prefer short posterior medial and posterior lateral incisions to better visualize the capsule. After a simple hamstring release, 3 weeks of immobilization is usually sufficient, although a little extra time may be needed if the casts have to be progressively wedged into extension following a capsulotomy.

Proximal Hamstring Lengthening

If you elect to release the hamstrings proximally (21), perform the operation through an oblique adductor approach or through a short medial transverse incision just below the buttocks.

- Make certain that this operation is performed without the use of anesthetic paralyzing agents, so that stimulation of the sciatic nerve with the cautery can warn you if the sciatic nerve is in close proximity to the hamstring origins.
- After choosing which skin incision to use, make a longitudinal incision in the fascia. Use blunt finger dissection in the plane posterior to the adductor magnus tendon. Start with the knee in flexion to relax the sciatic nerve, which is deep in the incision, near the femoral shaft. Intermittently extend the knee while flexing the hip to aid in defining and delivering the hamstring origins. Use a nerve stimulator if there is any confusion between the nerve and tendon.
- Do not divide the proximal hamstrings until you are certain that the nerve is safe from harm; use the cautery. Gently retest the range of knee extension with the hip flexed; after satisfactory release, knee extension should

markedly increase. Never forcefully extend the knee maximally while the hip is flexed.

■ Base postoperative immobilization on whatever other releases are carried out. If only hamstrings are released, then knee immobilizers for 2–3 weeks is sufficient, and mobilization can begin immediately.

Complications

Failure to fully assess the cause of the knee flexion deformity before surgery may lead to a poor result. The crouch gait will persist if a hip flexion deformity is ignored or if hyperdorsiflexed ankles are not braced. If preoperative quadriceps spasticity is severe, recurvatum may occur following overly generous hamstring weakening. Myotendinous (aponeurotic) lengthening, when performed too far distal (close to the junction of the tendon with the most distal muscle fibers), may result in complete transverse separation. The key here is simply to get enough proximal exposure so that there are plenty of muscle fibers distally to allow the slide after the intramuscular release of the tendon.

The popliteal artery and sciatic nerve are limiting structures about the knee. When applying the cast, do not try to forcibly straighten the knee if the patient is under anesthesia. A sciatic stretch palsy is difficult to detect acutely in a CP patient with severe involvement but is still a very undesirable complication. If the preexisting fixed contracture is significant (i.e., more than 20°), plan to correct it gradually after surgery using wedged casts with the patient awake.

EXTENSION DEFORMITY

Indications for Surgery

Knee hyperextension is not a fixed deformity in CP. It usually occurs dynamically at midstance and is secondary to fixed ankle equinus or excessive quadriceps spasticity, especially of the rectus femoris. The heel cord contracture, if present, must be corrected, but weakening of the quadriceps remains a problem. There is a natural reluctance to weaken the quadriceps, because it is necessary to maintain upright posture. However, many CP patients, even with mild degrees of crouch, will have excessive cospasticity of the rectus femoris. The simultaneous, excessive rectus femoris and hamstring spasms lead to a stiff-kneed, short-stride gait (8). However, I do not believe that every ambulatory patient who undergoes a hamstring lengthening needs a simultaneous rectus femoris procedure.

If knee hyperextension is associated with a hip flexion deformity, it is simple to release and recess a small section of the origin of the rectus femoris tendon at the time of the iliopsoas recession or lengthening. This produces minimal quadriceps weakening, but it is safe. Unfortunately, a tenotomized rectus may spontaneously reattach to the anterior inferior iliac spine.

Do not release the rectus origin routinely at the time of hip flexor release in CP. Release it only if there is a hyperextended knee gait, or occasionally in nonwalkers if the fixed flexion contracture is very severe.

For the patient with a rigid stiff-knee gait without much of a hip flexion deformity, the usual indication for rectus surgery is inadequate knee flexion late in the swing phase. Such extensor spasticity interferes with foot clearance. In such cases, it is reasonable to selectively transfer the rectus femoris either medially to the semitendinosis or laterally to the iliotibial band. If a laboratory analysis of the gait is available, the rectus will usually be found to fire excessively or throughout swing phase on dynamic gait EMG. The rectus femoris transfer can be performed simultaneously with hamstring lengthening without fear of increasing crouch, or it can be performed some time later if the knee tends toward recurvatum.

Distal Rectus Femoris Transfer

■ Make an anterior incision transversely or longitudinally about 6 cm proximal to the patella (8). Undermining proximally allows identification and separation of the interval between the vasti and the rectus. Proximally, this can easily be done bluntly, but distally the rectus tendon blends with the common quadriceps tendon. Further separation must be done sharply, while avoiding entry into the knee joint, to a level near the superior pole of the patella.

■ If a slight correction of gait into external rotation is desired (i.e., in cases where there is excessive inturning at the knee), isolate the rectus tendon and bluntly separate proximally. Then transfer the distal stump through a subcutaneous tunnel to the semitendinosis medially. If the hamstrings have been lengthened sometime previously, and the distal stump of the semitendinosis is not available, the transfer can be into the sartorius. If there is preexisting excessive external rotation at the knee, then transfer the distal stump of the rectus through a subcutaneous tunnel to the iliotibial band or the biceps femoris. There should be no tendency toward increased crouch as long as the vastus medialis, lateralis, and intermedius remain intact, because they provide the bulk of quadriceps strength.

■ Postoperatively, use removable extension knee immobilizers part time for 3–4 weeks.

HIP DEFORMITIES

Hip deformities in CP span a spectrum from mild hip dynamic flexion deformity to complete painful dislocation. The three most common components are adduction, flexion, and internal rotation. Although these components will be considered separately, usually all three coexist to some degree.

ADDUCTION DEFORMITY

Some degree of excessive adductor spasticity is seen in most patients with CP. Primary abduction deformity is rare and usually the result of overzealous adductor release and neurectomy of both the anterior and the posterior branches of the obturator nerve.

Indications for Surgery

Adductor release is indicated in ambulators when scissoring occurs or when passive abduction (in extension) is less than 20°. It is also indicated in limited walkers or sitters as part of the surgery for early hip subluxation. Occasionally, in the patient with severe total body involvement, the adductor release is necessary to facilitate perineal care. Adductor release is nearly always a part of the treatment for more severe degrees of hip subluxation, which require sufficient release to obtain a satisfactory range of abduction (1). Patients must be assessed individually because the extent of release required and the need for adductor transfer or neurectomy varies. In general, there is a trend away from anterior branch neurectomy except in the severely involved, nonwalking patient.

As an alternative procedure, the longus and gracilis may be recessed (sutured more distally to the underlying adductor magnus or brevis) or transferred posteriorly to the ischium (3,6,22). To accomplish a posterior transfer, the lithotomy position is best. The theoretical advantage of posterior adductor transfer is improvement in hip extensor tone. The brevis may also be transferred; however, its entire origin is a fleshy muscle belly that does not hold sutures well. In at least two of the adductor transfers I have performed, the transferred origins pulled off the bony ischium. Postoperative radiographs proved this, as I placed radiopaque markers in the origin of the longus. Others have also noted the tendency for posteriorly transferred adductors to migrate postoperatively back to their origins (17). The extra dissection necessary for adductor transfer hardly seems worthwhile in most patients, and I have abandoned it. I simply perform a release without anterior neurectomy in the majority of cases. The extent of the release depends on the degree of deformity.

Bilateral adductor release should be performed in most diplegic and quadriplegic patients when both hips are adducted or have limited passive abduction. This is the most common situation. Even when one is less adducted than the other, both hips should usually be released in these patients, because when only a unilateral soft-tissue release is performed, there is a tendency for the nonoperated hip to subsequently become unstable (4).

However, an occasional severe quadriplegic CP patient will have true windblown hips. This is especially common with severe neurogenic scoliosis and pelvic obliquity (the pelvis is "down" on the abducted side). The abducted hip will be well covered and should not have an adductor release if the abduction is fixed. Of course, the hemiplegic patient with adductor limitation will also need only a unilateral release. The posterior branch of the obturator nerve should very rarely be divided. Only following failure of a prior extensive adductor release and anterior branch obturator neurectomy with recurrence or persistence of adduction deformity would one consider a posterior branch or intrapelvic obturator neurectomy.

Adductor Release

Under most circumstances, other surgery will be performed simultaneously on the hip (e.g., iliopsoas recession, open reduction). Therefore, my preferred technique is to simply extend the anterior bikini incision slightly medially. (The bikini incision is oblique, just distal and parallel to the inguinal ligament.) The skin incision also may be made longitudinally or obliquely over the adductor longus origin. Through the Ludloff-type approach (Chapter 3), the psoas tendon can be tenotomized, but it cannot easily be recessed or divided above the pelvic brim.

- Whichever skin incision is chosen, define the adductor tendons, including the longus and gracilis, by blunt dissection after longitudinally opening the fascia. Completely release the longus and gracilis at their origins as proximally as possible. Next, assess the range of passive abduction. If this is not at least 40°, further release is necessary, including the brevis and pectineus. If still it is tight, the medial hip capsule may need to be divided transversely.

- Because the anterior branches of the obturator nerve lie on the anterior surface of the adductor brevis, always identify the nerve before releasing much of the brevis. Only in the nonwalking patient with severe involvement is a segment of the nerve (usually two or three branches) removed. I often use a small suction drain for the rather considerable dead space.

- Maintain postoperative abduction for 2–3 weeks, using two long-leg casts with a bar between them. Recently, I have used just two knee immobilizers with an abduction pillow, allowing immediate weight bearing and mobilization if there was no simultaneous bony surgery requiring a cast.

Complications

The most common problem with adductor release is expecting too much and doing too little. If there is a pelvic obliquity from scoliosis and the "higher" femoral head is luxating, adductor release alone will not maintain hip reduction unless the structural scoliosis and obliquity are controlled. If there is any evidence of early hip subluxation (even with a level pelvis), the iliopsoas must be lengthened.

FLEXION DEFORMITY

A mild degree of fixed hip flexion deformity is normal in neonates. In the spastic CP patient, this flexion deformity may persist or gradually worsen, especially if the patient is a nonwalker. Spasticity of the iliopsoas is the main cause of the deformity, although every muscle that passes anterior to the transverse axis of the hip contributes to hip flexion. Clinical measurement of hip flexion deformity is best performed by the prone-lying Staheli test (28). The better-known Thomas test is affected more by spasticity of the contralateral side, which tends to roll the pelvis as the opposite limb is flexed. This makes it difficult to ascertain the neutral position of the pelvis.

Radiographic assessment of hip flexion deformity is made by measuring the lateral sacrofemoral angle on films taken with the patient prone or supine and the hips maximally extended. The sacrofemoral angle is that formed between the top of the sacrum and the axis of the extended femoral shaft. The normal angle is 40° to 60°, which decreases with hip flexion deformity. Fixed hip flexion deformity causes the patient to stand with either a lordotic spine and fairly straight knees or a flat back and crouched knees. In either case, the sacrofemoral angle is reduced (3).

Indications for Surgery

Iliopsoas weakening is indicated in walkers with radiographically normal hips if fixed hip flexion is greater than 15°. Release or lengthening of the psoas is also a part of correction of any degree of hip subluxation in CP. Usually, whenever a derotation osteotomy is performed for excessive anteversion, the iliopsoas should be lengthened or recessed. In nonwalkers, a simple complete distal tenotomy (usually performed with an adductor release) can be made through either a Ludloff incision or an anterior bikini incision. In patients with bilateral flexion deformities but fixed, windblown hips, adductor release is performed only on the adducted (high) side. The iliopsoas is released bilaterally. In the rare case when there is truly limited adduction on the abducted side of the pelvis (the down hemipelvis), the origins of the tensor and the gluteus medius and minimus are also released on the abducted side.

In most cases of ambulatory CP patients, I prefer a simple oblique tenotomy of the psoas tendon as far proximally as possible, where there are still abundant investing iliacus muscle fibers. This has the net effect of markedly weakening the psoas while only moderately weakening the iliacus portion. No sutures are required, making it simpler than the formal recession, as no suture repair is necessary. This is similar to what most surgeons usually do in performing open reduction of congenitally dislocated hips in otherwise normal children.

Iliopsoas Recession or Lengthening

■ I perform an iliopsoas recession or lengthening through the usual bikini anterior incision by identifying the interval between the sartorius and the iliacus, assuming no acetabular procedure or open reduction is necessary (Fig. 177.6). Visualize and protect the lateral femoral cutaneous nerve deep to the enveloping fascia exiting the pelvis on the anterior surface of the sartorius just medial to the anterosuperior iliac spine. Do not detach the sartorius. On the other hand, if the psoas lengthening is a part of an open reduction or acetabular procedure, use the more extensile standard Smith-Peterson anterior interval between the sartorius and the tensor fascia muscle.

■ Locate the femoral nerve on the anterior surface of the iliacus but deep to the iliacus fascia, and retract it gently medially with a blunt retractor. The psoas tendon is deep in the iliacus muscle fibers and tightly applied to the anterior medial hip capsule. Isolate the tendon proximally, separating it from the muscle fibers of the iliacus, and divide it at the pelvic brim (30).

■ In performing a formal recession, flex and externally rotate the hip so that the tendon can be followed distally to the lesser trochanter where the entire tendon is detached. Free the conjoined muscle–tendon unit from the anterior hip capsule and reattach it with two heavy sutures more proximally on the anterior capsule (2). The net effect is to decrease the mechanical advantage of the iliopsoas muscle by placing the insertion closer to the axis of hip flexion.

Postoperative Care

Postoperatively, avoid prolonged hip flexion for 3 weeks. This is most easily accomplished by applying two long-leg casts. If bilateral adductor release has also been done, place a broomstick bar between the casts to maintain abduction. The patient is cared for in the prone, the supine, or even a standing position as long as hip flexion is avoided, except briefly for meals, transport, and so forth. If the patient underwent an open reduction, some type of spica cast will be necessary for at least 6 weeks. If the hips were windblown before surgery, two long-leg casts with

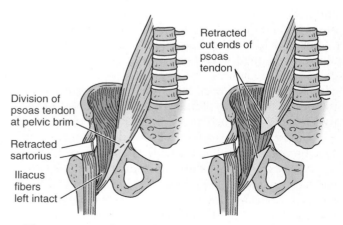

Figure 177.6. Iliopsoas lengthening at the pelvic brim.

a spreader bar can be used, but instruct the parents to maintain the hips windblown to the opposite direction. If the pelvis is level and only soft-tissue procedures have been done, I now prefer to mobilize the patient immediately postoperatively, so I use just knee immobilizers and an abduction pillow at night.

Complications

There should not be any confusion between the femoral nerve and the psoas tendon. Distal tenotomy of the entire psoas tendon severely weakens hip flexion and should not be done in a child who can or potentially might be an independent, crutch-free walker. One should expect that in most patients younger than 7 years without severe scoliosis or pelvic obliquity, a psoas and adductor release performed in the presence of no more than mild hip dysplasia will prevent subsequent dislocation. There is not universal agreement as to whether postoperative nighttime abduction bracing is necessary. However, I recommend at least 3–6 months of abduction bracing using a foam wedge or abduction brace if there is any radiographic evidence of dysplasia (14).

When there is severe preexisting pelvic obliquity, severe acetabular dysplasia, or another type of secondary bony change (typically in patients older than 8–10 years), correction of the scoliosis or acetabular reconstruction must be performed to maintain hip reduction; muscle release alone will be insufficient in such cases. Most commonly, for patients 6 years or older, with mild to moderate degrees of acetabular dysplasia, I will add a Dega-type pelvic osteotomy (19) or Staheli acetabular augmentation (shelf)-type procedure (32).

INTERNAL ROTATION DEFORMITY

Indications for Surgery

Excessive medial femoral torsion (increased femoral anteversion) is very common in spastic CP. It manifests as internal rotation deformity, mainly in walkers. In spastic patients who are only sitters, the excess anteversion contributes to hip dysplasia and dislocation, but the internal rotation is not so apparent with the patient in the sitting position. The cause of the increased anteversion is probably muscle imbalance of more than just the psoas; the iliopsoas is nearly always contracted in patients with excessive hip anteversion and internal rotation gait. In normal patients, the anterior fibers of the gluteus medius and minimus and the tensor are the main hip internal rotators. This fact has encouraged Steel (29) to perform anterior transfer of the trochanteric insertion of the gluteus medius and minimus for internal rotation gait, converting abductors to external retractors. In general, I do not favor this operation because it carries the risk of weakening the abductor mechanism, thus possibly trading an internal

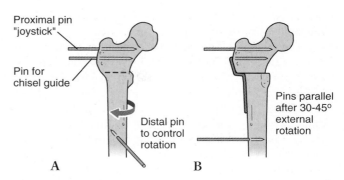

Figure 177.7. Use of pins to control rotation.

rotation deformity for a Trendelenburg limp. Furthermore, the operation is indicated only in patients with no flexion contracture (i.e., a normal iliopsoas) and spastic abductors—a situation seldom encountered.

My preferences for correction of internal rotation gait are based on patient age and ambulator status. In patients 4–8 years of age, I usually perform adductor release and iliopsoas intramuscular lengthening or recession, and I follow the patient for a number of years. In most patients, the excessive internal rotation will gradually improve as the hip flexion contracture and adduction tendency improve and the anteversion decreases. After 8–10 years of age, if the patient is still ambulating with an excessive internal rotation gait, I usually prefer subtrochanteric derotation osteotomy using the AO-ASIF (Association for the Study of Internal Fixation) technique. In many cases, little varusization is needed because the "coxa valga" seen on radiographs is more apparent than real, and it will disappear with derotation alone.

Subtrochanteric Derotation Osteotomy

- Perform the operation on the image intensifier table with the patient supine and the leg draped free. Place a small folded blanket or towel under the buttocks so that the prep and exposure will be sufficiently proximal and posterior.
- Make a standard lateral approach to the proximal femur and insert three guide pins: one for the chisel alignment, one more proximal in the greater trochanter to be used as a joy stick to control the proximal fragment, and one distal to the end of the plate to control rotation. Typically, the distalmost pin will be inserted at an angle of 30° to 45°, internally rotated in relation to the proximalmost pin (Fig. 177.7).
- Make sure that the femur is circumferentially exposed subperiosteally in the area of the planned osteotomy. Insert the appropriate child or adolescent blade chisel into the greater trochanter along the course of the first pin so that the osteotomy can be cut through the middle of the lesser trochanter. Always use the chisel guide;

otherwise, there is a tendency to angle the blade so that the shaft of the plate is placed in flexion.

▪ Confirm the chisel position with the image intensifier; remove the chisel halfway through, and complete the osteotomy with an oscillating saw. Rotate the distal fragment externally using the preplaced pins as a guide. If increased varus is desired, remove a small wedge medially, which is one half of the shaft diameter after derotating. Insert the blade plate using the bone-holding forceps to maintain reduction. I use the dynamic compression feature of the plate to close the osteotomy further. At least 20° to 30° of residual internal rotation should be left after the derotation (i.e., the distal fragment should not be excessively externally rotated). Varus should be added to the osteotomy only when there is a true valgus deformity of the femoral neck, and when there is an abundant range of abduction. Each added degree of varus is equivalent to adding 1° of adduction and subtracting 1° of abduction.

If hamstring lengthening is contemplated, the femur may easily be derotated through the lateral hamstring exposure incision. Use a six-hole plate, as described in Chapter 168.

If preoperatively there was no subluxation, and neither acetabular reconstruction nor capsulorrhaphy has been performed, then no cast is needed. Manage the patient in a wheelchair for 4–6 weeks, allowing gentle motion. Then allow partial weight bearing with crutches or a walker until healing of the bone is secure, usually at about 3 months. Most commonly in CP, some other acetabular work will have been done, so a spica cast will be necessary. The spica cast should usually be placed in nearly full hip extension and moderate abduction. Iliopsoas recession or release is usually performed prior to or simultaneously with the subtrochanteric osteotomy.

One potential pitfall is failure to consider concomitant excessive external tibial torsion. In such a case, following femoral derotation, the foot will point excessively laterally unless a simultaneous internal derotation is performed on the tibia (3).

SUBLUXATION AND DISLOCATION OF THE HIP

Hip dislocation generally occurs in nonwalkers with total body involvement, whereas in those patients who walk with crutches, the deformity more often progresses only to subluxation. However, even patients who are independent ambulators may develop complete dislocations. The etiology of the dislocation is a combination of excessive femoral anteversion with persistent spastic adduction and flexion, often associated with pelvic obliquity secondary to structural scoliosis. Dislocation has been alleged to cause scoliosis, seating problems, decubiti, fractures, and diffi-

culties with perineal care (5,12,14,19,20,26). Although hip dislocation is associated with all these problems, they are in fact caused not by the dislocation but by the muscle imbalance and the rigidity of the hip contracture. Furthermore, for CP adults, the status of hip location per se is not as important a determinant of walking ability as having reasonable cognitive function, balance, and a level pelvis with mobile hips.

Indications for Surgery

Not all severely subluxated or dislocated spastic hips will cause pain, although probably at least half will be symptomatic. The ability for a severely involved patient to sit comfortably probably has as much to do with the enthusiasm and motivation of the people caring for him as it does with whether his hip is radiographically reduced. Thus, it is not always necessary to treat older patients with spastic dislocated hips (20).

On the other hand, it is always desirable to maintain range of motion and prevent subluxation by appropriate early soft-tissue release and bracing in younger patients. The following guidelines and prerequisites are suggested for decision making for surgical correction of spastically dislocated hips:

1. Prevention of hip dislocation by early soft-tissue release is easier and more effective than late reconstructions (14).

2. The degree of reconstruction is determined by the degree of dysplasia. That is, to relocate a completely dislocated hip in an 8-year-old CP patient will usually require at least a femoral osteotomy, possibly a pelvic osteotomy, as well as soft-tissue release.

3. Soft-tissue release is always necessary whenever bony reconstruction is planned.

4. Femoral varus osteotomy, although still useful in maintaining reduction, cannot be counted on to induce acetabular development in patients older than 8 years. The femoral neck–shaft angle should not be placed in excessive varus (i.e., leave at least 110°).

5. Femoral shortening is a useful adjunct to relocating a high-riding dislocation without tension. This is far preferable to any type of traction, which is generally poorly tolerated by CP patients.

6. For patients older than 8 years with hip dysplasia and dislocation, acetabular reconstruction usually will be necessary (3,9,19,32). Although nearly all types of pelvic osteotomies have been performed in the past, including Salter and Pemberton procedures, the most useful include the Dega and Chiari osteotomies and the shelf procedure (acetabular augmentation). The shelf procedure can be added to any other pelvic osteotomy should additional femoral head coverage be necessary.

7. A severely deformed femoral head with absent cartilage should not be relocated. A painful located hip is

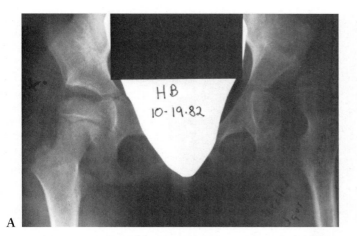

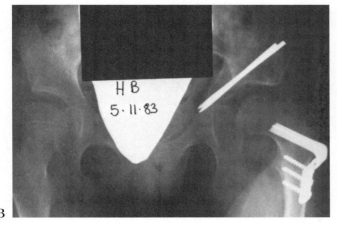

Figure 177.8. **A:** A 9-year-old child with spastic cerebral palsy and severe dislocation of left hip. **B:** The same child after Chiari osteotomy and varus osteotomy.

probably no better than a painful dislocated hip. This is common in patients older than 10 years with a chronically subluxated hip.

8. Always try to keep spica cast immobilization to a minimum.

9. Finally, do not attempt relocation of a unilateral hip dislocation using hip surgery alone if a severe scoliosis with fixed pelvic obliquity is present. The pelvis should probably be leveled first.

In those patients 8 years or older with a fully dislocated spastic hip, my typical correction would consist of, in one stage, a femoral shortening and Chiari osteotomy with a supplemental shelf. Very little varus would be added to the femur, and appropriate soft-tissue release (e.g., adductors, psoas) and anterior branch obturator neurectomy would also be performed (Fig. 177.8). In the more common 6- to 10-year-old spastic patient with moderate dysplasia but without frank dislocation, I do extensive soft-tissue release and a Dega osteotomy, or possibly an acetabular augmen-

tation. I find the advantages to be no retained hardware, technical simplicity, the possibility of doing both hips simultaneously, and consistently satisfactory results (Fig. 177.9). In a patient under 6 years with a unilateral dislocation, a soft-tissue release with femoral derotation and shortening is performed, with the occasional addition of a pelvic osteotomy or shelf procedure (Fig. 177.10).

The Dega procedure is similar to a Pemberton osteotomy in that both are periacetabular incomplete innominate osteotomies that bend down the superior portion of the acetabular roof. The main difference is that the hinge for acetabular roof redirection is medial with the Dega (so that the added coverage is more superolateral), whereas with Pemberton's osteotomy the hinge is more posteriomedial (so that the coverage is more anterolateral). I prefer the Dega procedure in cases of CP because it more adequately deals with the usual elongated acetabulum with superolateral deficiency.(Fig. 177.11).

Dega Osteotomy

Usually, a medial adductor and psoas release is performed first, often with a femoral shortening and/or varus osteotomy if necessary for reduction (19). Use an image intensifier with the leg draped free.

■ Perform the Dega osteotomy through the standard anterior bikini incision with the iliac apophysis split and the iliac wing exposed both medially and laterally. I usually do not separately detach the sartorius but leave it attached to the medial half of the apophysis and abdominal muscles. Release the origin of the direct head of the rectus tendon and peel off the reflected head from the superior capsule. Place blunt retractors superior and inferior to the capsule for a wide exposure.

■ If there is dysplasia but no significant subluxation, the capsule does not have to be opened. However, subluxated or dislocated hips require a standard acetabular debridement and capsulorrhaphy.

■ The Dega osteotomy itself is performed from directly lateral, on a line from the middle of the anterior inferior iliac spine to the sciatic notch. Use a series of curved osteotomes after initiating the cut with a saw or high-speed cutting tool. Aim the osteotomy cuts medially and inferiorly, extending to but not through the medial cortex near the triradiate cartilage, as monitored on the image intensifier. Both anterior and posterior corners of the osteotomy need to be completed to the medial wall. Anteriorly, this is easy to do, as it is under direct visualization. Posteriorly, place a blunt Hohmann retractor in the notch, and use a 45° Kerrison rongeur to complete the posterior corner of the osteotomy from lateral.

■ Next, insert a wide, curved osteotome into the osteotomy and lever the superior portion of the acetabulum in a caudal direction until the relatively vertical lateral

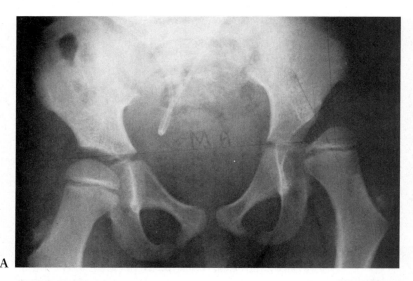

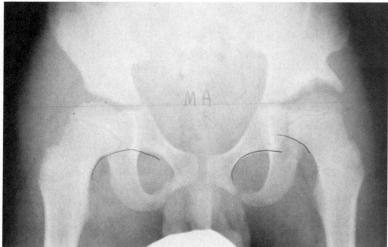

Figure 177.9.   **A:** A 7-year-old with spastic cerebral palsy and a unilateral dysplastic left hip. **B:** The same child after acetabular augmentation and iliopsoas and adductor release.

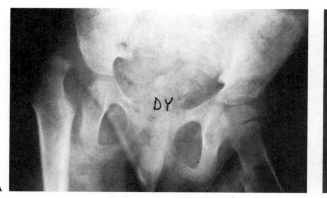

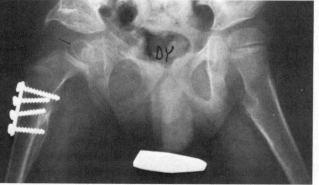

Figure 177.10.   **A:** A 4-year-old child with spastic cerebral palsy and complete dislocation of the right hip. **B:** Following open reduction, femoral osteotomy, Pemberton procedure, and adductor and psoas release.

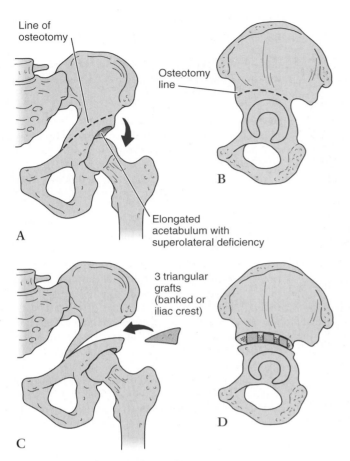

Line of
osteotomy

Osteotomy
line

Elongated
acetabulum with
superolateral deficiency

A

B

3 triangular
grafts
(banked or
iliac crest)

C

D

Figure 177.11. Dega osteotomy.

acetabulum has been brought to a more horizontal position. There will now be a lateral gap at the osteotomy site of 1–1.5 cm. To hold the osteotomy open, use two or three bicortical triangular grafts from the anterior crest (or occasionally from the femoral varus osteotomy, if done). No internal fixation is necessary. When performed correctly, the osteotomy will be remarkably stable because of the intact medial column.

■ After routine closure, apply a hip spica cast and leave it in place for 6 weeks.

Shelf Procedure
The technique for a shelf procedure is as follows (32):

■ Make a standard anterior approach to the hip using a slightly extended bikini incision. Expose subperiosteally the entire outer wing of the ilium. Isolate the direct head of the rectus tendon but leave it intact; detach and tag the reflected head where it veers off the direct head just below the anterior inferior spine.

■ Perform a proximal psoas lengthening or tenotomy simultaneously with any other necessary adductor re-

lease. Expose the hip capsule extensively, as for an open reduction. Tease the reflected head of the rectus femoris tendon as far posteriorly as possible, at least to a position of approximately 1 or 2 o'clock. This can be done easily more anteriorly, but it will require sharp dissection from where the origin of the reflected head blends with the capsule posteriorly.

■ Thin the superior capsule near the bone of the lateral wall of the ilium using a scalpel and curet. Make a series of drill holes or use a high-speed burr to create a gently curved slot over the superior dome of the acetabulum. Either plain film radiographic control or image intensification is mandatory to confirm that the slot is created far enough inferiorly. Ideally, the slot should be just proximal to the acetabular cartilage; there is always a tendency to create the slot several millimeters too far superiorly. (*Hint*: Continue thinning the superior capsule against the lateral iliac cortex until a fine line of cartilage is just visible.) The hip joint itself is usually not entered despite the ease with which the femoral head may be palpated thorough the capsule.

■ After creating the slot, harvest abundant corticocancellous strips with a gouge from the outer wall of the ilium. It is perfectly acceptable to take a full-thickness graft from the crest in the area just behind and including the anterior superior spine. This will facilitate closure, although it will diminish the normal pelvic contours. It is important, however, that the bone graft be no thicker than unicortical when placed, so that it will mold to the convexity of the femoral head.

■ Pack the grafts into the slot, first in a radial direction and then perpendicularly. Bring the previously tagged reflected head of the rectus back over the entire mass of bone graft, helping to seat it, and anchor it on the superior capsule. Tie the reflected head of the rectus back to the original straight head of the rectus. The purpose of retying the reflected head is simply to hold the graft in place.

■ Closure is routine. A single spica cast may be used if the patient is hemiplegic or if the opposite hip has a fixed abduction contracture. However, it is usually preferable in patients with CP to use a one-and-a-half spica or a double spica cast if both hips are done simultaneously.

Pitfalls
The graft for a shelf must be placed at least part way posterior as well as superior. It is easier to pack grafts superiorly and anteriorly, but it is probably more important in a sitting patient to cover the posterosuperior femoral head. It is possible to pack too much graft over the femoral head. In this situation, abduction will be limited, although one would expect remodeling to eventually occur. An acetabular augmentation is usually not needed in a very young patient, 4 years or younger. If it is placed,

one cannot expect the augmented portion of the acetabulum to enlarge because there is no growth cartilage in the shelf itself. Therefore, the femoral head as it grows may gradually "outgrow" its socket.

Salvage Procedures

If the femoral head is severely deformed and the patient is skeletally mature with a high-riding dislocation, the alternatives are arthrodesis, resectional arthroplasty, or total hip arthroplasty. None of these procedures is highly desirable for the majority of patients (3,12). All are salvage procedures, and all have considerable complications. Femoral head and neck resection usually improves perineal care in the adult patient with a severe high-riding dislocation and severe contracture. However, subsequent heterotopic ossification is common, and some of the patients still have pain despite femoral head and neck resection. In such cases, it is desirable to interpose some type of soft tissue, such as by closing the hip capsule or by sewing the psoas tendon to the stump of the proximal femur. There is no agreement as to how much of the femur to resect, but it should certainly be enough to allow a full range of motion. This usually means that the resection must be down to the level above, at, or just below the lesser trochanter. This is certainly much more bone resection than would be done in any other Girdlestone-type resection. The patient should not be immobilized in a spica cast but may be placed in skeletal traction for 2 weeks. If the patient will tolerate it, an articulated external fixator is a reasonable alternative. As femoral head and neck resection is a salvage procedure, perform it only in total-care, severely involved patients to improve nursing care and comfort.

REFERENCES

Each reference is categorized according to the following scheme: *, classic article; #, review article; !, basic research article; and +, clinical results/outcome study.

* 1. Banks HH, Green WT. Adductor Myotomy and Obturator Neurectomy for the Correction of Adduction Contracture of the Hip in Cerebral Palsy. *J Bone Joint Surg Am* 1960;42:11.

* 2. Bleck EE. Postural and Gait Abnormalities Caused by Hip-Flexion Deformity in Spastic Cerebral Palsy: Treatment by Iliopsoas Recession. *J Bone Joint Surg Am* 1971; 53:1468.

3. Bleck EE. *Orthopaedic Management in Cerebral Palsy.* London: MacKeith Press, 1987.

+ 4. Carr C, Gage GR. The Fate of the Nonoperated Hip in Cerebral Palsy. *J Pediatr Orthop* 1987;7:262.

+ 5. Cooperman DR, Bartucci E, Dietrick E, Millar EA. Hip Dislocation in Spastic Cerebral Palsy: Long-Term Consequences. *J Pediatr Orthop* 1987;7:268.

+ 6. Couch WH, DeRosa GP, Throop FB. Thigh Adductor Transfer for Spastic Cerebral Palsy. *Dev Med Child Neurol* 1977;19:343.

+ 7. Dennyson WG, Fulford GE. Subtalar Arthrodesis by Cancellous Grafts and Metallic Internal Fixation. *J Bone Joint Surg Br* 1976;58:507.

8. Gage JR. Surgical Treatment of Knee Dysfunction in Cerebral Palsy. *Clin Orthop* 1990;253:45.

9. Gamble JG, Rinsky LA, Bleck EE. Established Hip Dislocations in Children with Cerebral Palsy. *Clin Orthop* 1990;253:90.

! 10. Garbarino JL, Clancy M. A Geometric Method of Calculating Tendoachilles Lengthening. *J Pediatr Orthop* 1985;5:573.

+ 11. Green NE, Griffin PP, Shiavi R. Split Posterior Tibial Tendon Transfers in Spastic Cerebral Palsy. *J Bone Joint Surg Am* 1983;65:748.

+ 12. Hoffer MM, Abram E, Nickel VL. Salvage Surgery at the Hip to Improve Sitting Posture of Mentally Retarded, Severely Disabled Children with Cerebral Palsy. *Dev Med Child Neurol* 1972;14:51.

+ 13. Hoffer MM, Barakat G, Koffman M. Ten-Year Followup of Split Anterior Tibial Tendon Transfer in Cerebral Palsied Patients with Spastis Equinovarus Deformity. *J Pediatr Orthop* 1985;5:432.

+ 14. Kalen V, Bleck EE. Prevention of Paralytic Dislocation of the Hip. *Dev Med Child Neurol* 1985;27:17.

+ 15. Kling TF, Kauffer H, Hensinger RN. Split Posterior Tibial Tendon Transfers in Children with Cerebral Spastic Paralysis and Equinovarus Deformity *J Bone Joint Surg Am* 1985;67:186.

+ 16. Koman LA, Mooney JF, Smith BP, et al. Management of Spasticity in Cerebral Palsy with Botulinum-A Toxin: Report of a Preliminary, Randomized, Double-Blind Trial. *J Pediatr Orthop* 1994;14:299.

+ 17. Loder RT, Harbuz A, Aronson DD, Lee CL. Postoperative Migration of the Adductor Tendon after Posterior Adductor Transfer in Children with Cerebral Palsy. *Dev Med Child Neurol* 1992;34:787.

+ 18. Mosca VS. Calcaneal Lengthening for Valgus Deformity of the Hindfoot: Results in Children Who Had Severe, Symptomatic Flatfoot and Skewfoot. *J Bone Joint Surg Am* 1995;77:500.

+ 19. Mubarak SJ, Valencia FG, Wenger DR. One-Stage Correction of the Spastic Dislocated Hip. *J Bone Joint Surg Am* 1992;74:1347.

+ 20. Pritchett JW. The Untreated Unstable Hip in Severe Cerebral Palsy. *Clin Orthop* 1983;173:169.

* 21. Reimers J. Contracture of the Hamstrings in Spastic Cerebral Palsy: A Study of Three Methods of Operative Correction. *J Bone Joint Surg Br* 1974;56:102.

+ 22. Reimers J, Poulsen S. Adductor Transfer versus Tenotomy for Stability of the Hip in Spastic Cerebral Palsy. *J Pediatr Orthop* 1984;4:52.

23. Renshaw TS, Green NE, Griffin PP, Root L. Cerebral Palsy: Orthopaedic Management. *Instr Course Lect* 1996;45:475.

24. Rosenthal RK, Simon SR. The Vulpius Gastrocnemius-Soleus Lengthening. In: Sussman M, ed. *The Diplegic*

Child. Rosemont, IL: American Academy of Orthopaedic Surgeons, 1992:355.

* 25. Ruda R, Frost HM. Cerebral Palsy: Spastic Varus and Forefoot Adductus, Treated by Intramuscular Posterior Tibial Tendon Lengthening. *Clin Orthop* 1971;79:61.

26. Sherk HH, Pasquariello PD, Doherty J. Hip Dislocation in Cerebral Palsy: Selection for Treatment. *Dev Med Child Neurol* 1983;25:738.

* 27. Silver CM, Simon SD, Lichtman HM. Long-term Follow-up Observations on Calcaneal Osteotomy. *Clin Orthop* 1974;99:181.

* 28. Staheli L. The Prone Hip Extension Test. *Clin Orthop* 1977;123:1215.

+ 29. Steel HH. Gluteus Medius and Minimus Insertion Advancement for Correction of Internal Rotation Gait in Spastic Cerebral Palsy. *J Bone Joint Surg Am* 1980;62:919.

+ 30. Sutherland DH, Silberfarb JL, Kaufman KR, et al. Psoas Release at the Pelvic Brim in Ambulatory Patients with Cerebral Palsy: Operative Technique and Functional Outcome. *J Pediatr Orthop* 1997;17:563.

+ 31. Townsend DR, Wells L, Lowenberg D. The Cincinnati Incision for the Split Posterior Tibial Tendon Transfer: A Technical Note. *J Pediatr Orthop* 1990;10:667.

+ 32. Zuckerman JD, Staheli LT, McLaughlin JF. Acetabular Augmentation for Progressive Hip Subluxation in Cerebral Palsy. *J Pediatr Orthop* 1984;4:436.

CHAPTER 178

MUSCLE AND NERVE DISORDERS IN CHILDREN

William G. Mackenzie and J. Richard Bowen

The hallmark of a muscle or nerve problem is weakness, but signs such as delayed motor development, fatigability, muscle cramps during activity, muscle wasting, and orthopaedic conditions such as cavus feet, claw hands or toes, a long C-shaped scoliosis, and dynamic scapular winging are often seen (111). Most muscle and nerve disorders can be diagnosed by a careful history and physical examination, and by specific laboratory tests, electromyography, nerve conduction studies, muscle and nerve biopsies, and genetic evaluation.

DIAGNOSIS OF MUSCLE AND NERVE DISORDERS

HISTORY AND PHYSICAL EXAMINATION, LABORATORY TESTS

Each symptom in the patient's history must be pursued to determine its onset, duration, exacerbating or relieving factors, and response to any treatment. The history can provide important clues to help in the diagnosis. Was the weakness present at birth or of recent onset and is it progressive? Weakness present at birth but not progressive may describe a child with a congenital myopathy, whereas onset of weakness in a young boy with gradual worsening is typical of muscular dystrophy. Detecting muscle weakness, usually by observation or muscle testing, is a major component of the clinical examination. Generalized muscle weakness results in hypotonia (floppiness), ptosis, a tent shaped mouth (bouche de tapir) and delayed motor development. Localized muscle atrophy is often observed at the shoulder girdle and the quadriceps muscle.

Strength can be evaluated by observing activities such as walking, dressing or undressing, and by testing individual muscles. Grading of activity-related muscle strength is a good screening method, especially in young, uncooperative patients. The activities are considered by regions: the hips, legs, shoulders, arms, and bulbar area (ie, respiratory function). Weakness can result in delayed development of the motor milestones (e.g., head control, sitting, crawling, standing, walking, running), Meryon's sign (i.e., reduced muscle resistance of the shoulder against the examiner's hand when lifted under the arms), Gowers' sign (i.e., use of the hands to "climb up the legs" to a standing position when rising from a sitting position on the floor), and difficulty in climbing steps or rising from a chair (117,137, 229). A 5-year-old boy with Duchenne muscular dystrophy may have a normal walk but when asked to run, the pelvic girdle and quadriceps weakness is quickly unmasked.

Evaluation of muscle strength is an excellent means of localizing the distribution of weakness, but it requires patient cooperation and can be difficult if there are associated fixed deformities. Agonist muscles (ie, prime movers) and antagonist muscles (ie, stabilizers) are graded for strength through the range of joint mobility. For example, the muscles controlling the foot may be tested for strength in dorsiflexion, plantar flexion, inversion, and eversion.

Although individual muscle testing is time consuming, tedious, and almost impossible in young, uncooperative children, it is essential as a baseline study for patients with suspected muscle or nerve disease. Muscle testing often is better performed in a special therapy session in which adequate time can be allotted. The Medical Research Council scale is generally accepted and grades muscle power as follows: 0, no contraction; 1, flicker or trace of contraction; 2, active motion with gravity eliminated; 3, active motion against gravity; 4, active motion against gravity and resistance; and 5, normal power (226). Myometric (dynamometric) methods are also useful in quantitating muscle strength, especially in evaluating therapeutic techniques (97).

Deep tendon reflexes of the biceps, triceps, knee, and ankle should be tested, along with the superficial reflexes of the abdomen and the great toe plantar response. The quality of reflex is judged by the briskness of muscle contracture and is best graded as absent, hypoactive, normal, or hyperactive. Children with spinal muscular atrophy and peripheral neuropathies typically have absent reflexes, whereas myopathic disorders such as muscular dystrophy have reflexes until later in the course of the disease.

The sensory examination includes the evaluation of pain, light touch, deep touch, two-point tactile, vibration, and temperature. Self-mutilation and Charcot joint changes are almost always manifestations of sensory loss. In neuropathies, multiple modalities may be affected, producing a "glove" or "stocking" distribution of loss, paresthesia, "pins and needles" sensation, and dysesthesia. Bulbar involvement is evaluated by cranial nerve testing. Cerebellar testing, particularly the Romberg sign for ataxia, is important when the differential diagnosis includes Friedreich's ataxia.

Muscle fasciculation, best seen by looking at the tongue or hands, is common in neuropathic disorders such as spinal muscular atrophy.

INVESTIGATION

Serum Enzymes

The serum enzymes elevated in muscle disorders include the aminotransferases (transaminases), aldolase, lactate dehydrogenase, and creatine phosphokinase (CPK). The serum CPK level is a sensitive and valuable screening test

W. G. Mackenzie: Assistant Professor, Jefferson Medical College, Wilmington, Delaware, 19899.

J. R. Bowen: Professor, Jefferson Medical College; Surgeon in Chief of duPont Hospital for Children, Wilmington, Delaware, 19899.

to demonstrate disease of striated muscle (343). Skeletal muscle, heart muscle, and brain tissue contain CPK, which catalyzes the release of phosphate from creatine phosphate. The high CPK level seen in Duchenne's muscular dystrophy (50 to 100 times normal) and other muscle disorders represents leakage from the muscle cell during necrosis. Aldolase and serum glutamic-oxaloacetic transaminase levels also may be elevated in muscle disease but are not as sensitive as the CPK level (352) and are also elevated by hepatic dysfunction.

GENETIC ANALYSIS

Recent advances in molecular genetics have greatly enhanced our knowledge of the gene abnormalities causing neuromuscular diseases (Table 178.1). This information should eventually result in more effective management of these disorders.

Molecular genetic techniques have been used to define other rare neuromuscular disorders in children. Metabolic myopathies, which are caused by abnormalities of glycogen, glucose, or lipid metabolism, have been well characterized. Mitochondrial DNA defects or mutations cause a broad spectrum of mitochondrial encephalomyopathies, which feature variable weakness with encephalopathic, cardiac, and visceral manifestations.

Cardiac and Pulmonary Evaluation

Cardiac and pulmonary abnormalities are very common in children with neuromuscular disease. Careful evaluation allows optimal daily management and an assessment of preoperative risks.

Electrocardiography and echocardiography are used to evaluate cardiac function (66). Patients with muscular dystrophy may develop cardiomyopathy or mitral valve prolapse secondary to papillary muscle weakness. Children with Friedreich's ataxia, Emery-Dreifuss dystrophy, and infantile myasthenia gravis may have arrhythmias (99,113,166,288,295,378).

Pulmonary compromise so commonly seen in these patients can be assessed by questions about shortness of breath, frequency of pulmonary infections, and more objectively, by pulmonary function or sleep studies.

ELECTROMYOGRAPHY

Electromyographic (EMG) studies can differentiate a neuropathy from a myopathy but are seldom specific. A normal muscle is silent at rest and produces an interference pattern at maximal activity. In neuropathies, fibrillations and fasciculations occur at rest and the interference pattern is reduced at maximal activity. In myopathies, the muscle is silent at rest and has polyphasic individual po-

---

Table 178.1. *Gene Location of Some Neuromuscular Disorders*

Chromosomal disorder	Location	Reference
Duchenne and Becker's muscular dystrophy	Xp21.2	Cell 50:509, 1987 Ann Rev Genet 1988 Proc Jap Acad 1988 Neuron 2:1019, 1989 Nature 344:60, 1990
Emery-Driefuss dystrophy	Xq28	Am Acad Neur Course 240
Facioscapulohumeral dystrophy	4q35	Lancet 336:651, 1990
Myotonic dystrophy	19q13	Proc Natl Acad Sci 1982 Neurology 36:1146, 1986

Charcot-Marie-Tooth
  Type I
  Type II
	
	17p11.2
	1p35–p36
		Hum Genet 34:388, 1982
		Ann Neurol 14:679, 1983
		Exp Neurol 104:186, 1989

Spinal muscular atrophy
  Bulbar type
  Chronic childhood
	
	Xq21.3-12
	5q11.2–13.3
		
		Science 237:120, 1987
		Nature 344:540, 1990

Friedreich's ataxia	9q21	Am Acad Neur Course 240
Huntington's disease	4	Nature 306:234, 1983
McArdle's disease	11	Nature 1987
Wilson's disease	13	Am Acad Neur Course 240

tentials of low amplitude and short duration during activity. Myotonia frequently presents as a classic pattern of spontaneous bursts of potentials that wax and wane and give an acoustic pattern resembling a dive bomber. Muscle evaluation should include the areas of the body involved in the weakness, and examination of four muscles is usually sufficient. The deltoid and vastus lateralis are good muscles to study in children, because they are frequently involved in neuromuscular diseases of childhood. In myopathies, there may be no correlation between the severity of the muscle weakness and the electromyography.

NERVE CONDUCTION STUDIES

Nerve conduction velocities depend on the degree of myelination and the diameter of the neuron. The median, ulnar, peroneal, and posterior tibial nerves most commonly are studied, and normal adult values are 45 to 65 m/sec. In infants, the velocity is about half that of the adult level, which is reached by 3 to 5 years of age (235). Motor conduction velocity typically is delayed in demyelinating neuropathies but is normal in anterior horn cell disease, root disease, or myopathies. Repetitive stimulation of the motor nerve can reveal pathologic fatigability, as in myasthenia gravis (34). Sensory conduction velocities are delayed and occasionally are helpful in diagnosing the mixed neuropathies, such as peroneal muscle atrophy or Friedreich's ataxia.

MALIGNANT HYPERTHERMIA

Malignant hyperthermia is characterized by muscle rigidity and necrosis associated with a rapid rise in body temperature (82,219,274). One in about 15,000 people in the general population develops malignant hyperthermia during general anesthesia. Although it has been reported to be associated with many disorders including the congenital myopathies, muscular dystrophy, osteogenesis imperfecta, myelomeningocele, and King's syndrome (ie, short stature, scoliosis, cryptorchidism, pectus carinatum, characteristic facial features) (82,174,175,189,225,328,336, 360), it is mainly associated with central core myopathy, with which it is closely linked. There is an abnormality of the ryanodine receptor gene at the 19q13.1 locus (121).

These reactions of malignant hyperthermia can be triggered by the administration of depolarizing muscle relaxants (e.g., succinylcholine chloride) or inhalational anaesthetics (e.g., halothane). If possible, these medications should be avoided in patients at known risk. Patients with previous episodes or a positive family history (transmitted as an autosomal dominant trait) of malignant hyperthermia may be treated prophylactically with sodium dantrolene. Preoperative assessment of risk is difficult (315). In vitro muscle contraction tests to various triggering agents are available but require a muscle biopsy. There are pres-

ently no commercially available means of establishing the presence of the malignant hyperthermia gene.

Prompt treatment of malignant hyperthermia is imperative at the earliest signs of tachycardia, tachypnea, or a rigid masseter muscle, because survival is unlikely after significant hyperthermia. Treatment consists of termination of all anesthetic agents, ventilation with 100% oxygen, cooling (e.g., ice packs, iced intravenous fluids, gastric irrigation, cooling blankets), intravenous sodium bicarbonate for metabolic acidosis, and administration of sodium dantrolene (1 mg/kg/min, up to 10 mg/kg total dose) (187,193). Treatment is continued for as long as 6 hours after an attack. In patients at high risk for malignant hyperthermia, the recommended local anesthesia is procaine, and for general anesthesia, narcotics, barbiturates, or neuroleptic drugs, and prophylactic dantrolene sodium are used (239).

MUSCLE BIOPSY

A muscle biopsy is often valuable for a definitive diagnosis of muscle disorder (140). Three issues are important: selection of the muscle, technique of the biopsy, and specimen care. Muscles with mild involvement should be selected in chronic disease, but severely involved muscle should be chosen in acute disease. The histology of severely involved muscle in chronic disease may show only secondary changes and not be diagnostic. Commonly selected muscles are the vastus lateralis, rectus femoris, deltoid, gastrocnemius, and biceps brachii. Obtain an adequate specimen from the belly of the muscle. Avoid areas of musculotendinous junction, scar from previous surgery, immunization sites, and electrode insertion sites for EMG (103).

Obtain an adequate specimen, and either give it directly to the technologist or have it transported quickly to the laboratory. Traditional techniques of maintaining muscle length are not needed for routine muscle biopsy. A moderate volume (250 mg) is needed to assay for enzyme systems to characterize metabolic myopathies. Part of the specimen is sent for genetic and protein analysis, and part of the specimen is frozen rapidly in liquid nitrogen to preserve the enzymes and prevent. Histochemical evaluation includes staining with hematoxylin and eosin, Verhoeff–van Gieson, periodic acid–Schiff (PAS) stain for glycogen, Gomori trichrome, oil red O for lipids, and methylene green–pyronine for RNA. Staining for adenosine triphosphatase (ATPase) at selected pH determines fiber types. In skeletal muscle, the ratio of muscle fiber types I and II is 1 to 2. Type I fibers have low ATPase activity and glycogen and high oxidative activity, and type II fibers have the opposite relative amounts. At present, fibers are subtyped based on ATPase activity (88).

Open biopsy technique offers the advantages of a large sample and proper orientation and length of the specimen fibers, but it has the disadvantage of unsightly scars. Needle biopsy is cosmetically better but has the disadvantage of producing a small sample with disoriented fibers (63,96). Coordinate the method of specimen handling and biopsy technique with the pathologist to ensure adequate results.

Open Muscle Biopsy Technique

Open muscle biopsy usually is performed with local anesthesia (1% Xylocaine without epinephrine) and sedation. The muscle must not be infiltrated with Xylocaine. Make a 2.5 cm incision, preferably following the skin lines, over the belly of the selected muscle. Expose a 2×0.5 cm cylinder of muscle (the long axis parallel to the muscle fibers), and excise the specimen with a scalpel. Electrocautery should not be used before removing the specimen. Sutures at either end of the specimen tied over a tongue blade or muscle biopsy forceps can be used to maintain specimen length. The procedure is usually performed on an outpatient basis, and complications are uncommon.

Needle Muscle Biopsy Technique

The vastus lateralis muscle is commonly used as the site of needle biopsy. The Bergstrom needle, consisting of a cannula and sliding trocar with cutting blade, typically obtains a specimen of about 200 fibers. After administration of local anesthesia (1% Xylocaine without epinephrine), make a stab incision over the belly of the muscle. Insert the needle into the muscle, and activate the cutting blade to obtain the specimen. Suction can be applied to the needle hub to improve the biopsy size (239). Several repeat specimens may be obtained through the same skin incision by changing the direction of the needle. Close the skin by a single stitch or adhesive strip and apply pressure over the muscle for several minutes to reduce the risk of hematoma formation.

NERVE BIOPSY

A nerve biopsy may aid in the diagnosis of a peripheral neuropathy but is rarely required. The sural nerve, which is entirely sensory, usually is selected because it innervates only a small area of the skin over the dorsolateral aspect of the foot, and the sensory loss is not usually a functional problem. Light and electron microscopy, the latter of which requires glutaraldehyde fixation are used for specimen evaluation. Preparation of the specimen needs to be coordinated with the pathologist before the biopsy (327).

To biopsy the sural nerve, make a 3-cm longitudinal incision over the posterolateral aspect of the leg parallel to the interval between the tendo Achilles and the peroneus brevis muscle. The nerve courses beside the lesser saphenous vein. Isolate 2.5 cm of the nerve in the interval and cut it sharply (not with scissors). If less than 1 cm of the nerve is taken, the ends can be reapproximated with mi-

crovascular sutures, but this repair is very time consuming for such a mild sensory loss and not usually done. If the nerve is not resutured, secure the proximal end in the deep layer of the subcutaneous fat, which helps to protect against painful neuroma formation.

COMMON MUSCLE DISORDERS WITH ORTHOPAEDIC DEFORMITIES

Muscle diseases (myopathies) are inherited or acquired and constitute a diverse group of conditions that include structural congenital myopathies, diseases that typically present as a floppy infant, with muscle biopsy demonstrating structural abnormalities within the muscle cell; dystrophies, conditions in which the muscle initially develops and functions normally but then progressively degenerates and atrophies; myotonias, syndromes characterized by the delayed relaxation of muscle; and metabolic conditions, considered to include diseases with specific metabolic abnormalities and acquired myopathies, such as those secondary to infections, autoimmune disorders, and conditions related to toxins (62).

BENIGN CONGENITAL MYOPATHIES OF CHILDHOOD

Congenital myopathies are a group of clinically similar illnesses that present with hypotonia and weakness from birth; muscle biopsy demonstrates structural abnormalities in the muscle cell. Most myopathies have an autosomal dominant transmission, are nonprogressive, and are characterized by symmetric proximal muscle weakness. Serum enzyme levels are normal or mildly elevated, and an EMG may show myopathic changes. The types of myopathies are differentiated by genetic studies, histochemical, or electron microscopic evaluation of the muscle biopsy specimen and include nemaline myopathy (rod body), central core disease, myotubular myopathy (central nuclear), congenital fiber-type disproportion, minicore disease, and nonspecific congenital myopathies (4,15,36, 50,70,88,101,102,104,134,241,303,321). Myotubular myopathy has a gene abnormality at the xq28 locus, central core disease at 19q13.1, and nemaline myopathy at 1q21 (2-tropomyosin gene).

Orthopaedic problems include contractures, postural foot deformities, dislocation of the hip, and scoliosis (11, 36,53,127,197,222,261,298,306). A potential life-threatening complication of treatment in patients with central core myopathy is malignant hyperthermia (82,101,174, 175,189,238).

Contractures and Foot Deformities

The contractures and foot deformities in patients with congenital myopathies are caused by hypotonia with abnormal posturing and are usually controlled with stretching therapy, periodic serial stretching casts, supportive orthoses, or occasionally, tendon lengthenings.

Hip Dislocation

Dislocated hips can occur at birth or develop later in children with congenital myopathies. They are usually easily reducible in early infancy but require prolonged treatment to achieve stability. Any lax-jointed, low-toned infant or any older child who presents before walking with an easily reducible dislocated hip without contractures should be suspected of having a myopathy. The hips are treated in the early stages similar to those in infants with typical congenitally dislocated hips, except that the total time of treatment is often prolonged and stability of the hip is difficult to achieve.

The Pavlik harness is excellent for maintaining reduction in newborns and young infants. The hips reduce initially in flexion of about 110° and mild abduction of 45°. Instruct caregivers not to dislocate a hip inadvertently by positioning it in adduction. These hips tend to redislocate easily, requiring frequent (initially, almost daily) adjustment of the Pavlik harness. Prone positioning in the Pavlik harness is helpful. It is important not to allow the hip to remain persistently posteriorly dislocated in the Pavlik harness, because this creates a severe treatment complication. After the hip is stable, maintain the harness in about 90° of flexion and 45° of abduction until adequate bony and cartilaginous support develops. There is no time-honored rule for the length of treatment, but the total course should be long enough to allow joint stability and formation of a normal cartilaginous acetabulum.

Treat an older child who has developed contracture of the hip or whose hip does not easily reduce initially in skin traction until the femoral head approaches the area of the acetabulum. With the patient under general anesthesia, gently reduce the hip and apply a cast to maintain stability. Cast treatment may be necessary for as long as 6 months. Hip dysplasia after treatment for dislocation from hypotonia and joint laxity may improve with abduction bracing. Use an abduction brace and a standing frame with the legs in abduction for these children, in whom the development of walking skills is usually delayed. After ambulation is achieved, an abduction brace is helpful, but most children have difficulty walking in the brace. If dysplasia persists despite brace therapy in an ambulating child, perform a varus derotation proximal femoral osteotomy and, if needed, an acetabular redirectional osteotomy.

Scoliosis

Scoliosis that presents at a young age tends to be progressive, often has a long C-shaped or double-curve pattern, and is most difficult to treat in a hypotonic patient with respiratory compromise. The orthopaedic dilemmas include poor tolerance from respiratory compromise in a thoracolumbosacral orthosis or spinal fusion with subsequent inhibition of spinal growth in a young child, resulting in a short trunk. As soon as scoliosis is recognized, institute treatment by linearly posturing the spine on pads when supine and, if respiratory capacity permits, by a thoracolumbosacral orthosis with abdominal relief. Pulmonary function studies of the patient in and out of the orthosis are necessary to determine the safety of orthotic treatment. If the orthosis cannot be used, a wheelchair can be modified with asymmetric lateral supports, a slightly reclined back, and a firm seat.

Indications for Spinal Fusion   If the scoliosis progresses despite orthotic treatment, posterior spinal fusion is necessary, unless cardiopulmonary incapacity is life threatening, even though this fusion inhibits longitudinal growth of the spine if performed before skeletal maturity. Internal fixation is essential, preferably with segmental instrumentation. The fusion extends from the high thoracic area to the sacrum. The Luque technique has been performed without fusion to allow spinal growth in the young child, but this remains an unproven technique because of certain obvious risks, such as wire breakage, rod breakage, and growth over the upper ends of the rods, with subsequent kyphoscoliosis. We recommend a posterior spinal fusion with the unit rod, a modification of the Luque technique, from the first or second thoracic vertebra to the sacrum, and we discourage the use of anterior spinal procedures in patients with respiratory compromise. The unit rod is preferred because it prevents cephalad-caudad movement of the rods, spinal rotation, and pelvic obliquity without the use of rod interconnecting devices. In nonambulatory patients with progressive scoliosis, we recommend stabilization to the sacrum.

Segmental Posterior Spinal Fusion with Unit Rod or Luque Rod Instrumentation
- Place the patient in the prone position on a four-poster scoliosis operative frame so that the abdomen is free of pressure (6,25,37,77,110,213,214,218,231,247).
- Make a dorsal longitudinal skin incision over the spinous processes of the vertebrae to be fused, and forcibly retract the skin margins with Weitlander retractors to reduce the bleeding.
- Incise the subcutaneous tissue to the dorsolumbar fascia, exposing the tips of the spinous processes from T1 to the sacrum.
- Slit the cartilaginous caps of the spinous processes longitudinally, and interconnect them by splitting the supraspinous ligament.
- With a Cobb elevator, retract the cartilaginous caps laterally, perform a subperiosteal dissection down each side of the lamina, and pack gauze between the bone and paraspinous muscle to maintain hemostasis.

- Then expose each vertebra subperiosteally laterally from inferiorly to superiorly to the tips of the transverse processes in the thoracic area and to the base of the transverse processes in the lumbar area.
- Place the self-retaining Weitlander retractors progressively deeper in the wound, and spread them widely against the paraspinous muscles to minimize bleeding.
- Promptly electrocauterize soft-tissue bleeding and control bone bleeding with small quantities of bone wax.
- Expose the posterior superior iliac spines and adjacent iliac crest by elevating the erector spinae off the sacrum
- Expose the outer table of the ilium subperiosteally down to the greater sciatic notch. With the drill guide developed for the unit rod, drill holes in the ilium from the bottom of the posterior superior spines to pass 1 to 2 cm above the sciatic notch (Fig. 178.1). Be very careful

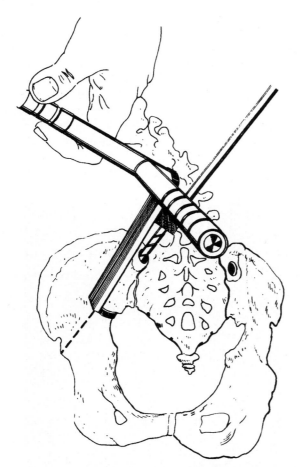

Figure 178.1. The holes in the ilium are drilled by using a drill guide that hooks into the sciatic notch. The hole enters at the posterior superior iliac spine and is drilled 2 cm past the sciatic notch. (From Dias RC, Miller F, Dabney K, et al. Surgical Correction of Spinal Deformity Using a Unit Rod in Children with Cerebral Palsy. *J Pediatr Orthop* 1996;16:734, with permission.)

to stay within the intraosseous area, and probe the hole to confirm this.
- Carefully remove the ligamentum flavum from the midline for sublaminar wire passage.
- Pass dual stainless steel wire strands under each lamina, except at the top of the fusion and at L5, where two dual strands are used for strength. Be extremely cautious not to cause neural damage while passing the wires.
- With a rongeur, osteotome or power burr, decorticate and perform facetectomies of the vertebrae in the area to be fused. Corticocancellous allograft is typically used in these children (150 to 250 g).
- If instrumentation with the unit rod is required, select the appropriate length of rod.
- Place a flexible measuring rod along the lamina on the concave side of the scoliosis. The unit rods are prebent to the contour of the normal spine, which corresponds to the desired postoperative spinal posture. The unit rod is available in 1/4- and 3/8-inch sizes, the smaller being used in children weighing less 30 to 40 pounds or in very osteopenic children.
- Secure the unit rod to the pelvis in a manner similar to the Galveston technique for Luque segmental spinal fusion (6,77).
- Cross the pelvic legs of the rod, and insert them into the pelvis, being careful to be in line with the drilled holes. Rod holders can be used to guide the legs during gradual alternate side impaction (Fig. 178.2).
- Then tighten the sublaminar wires by twisting at each level starting at L5 and moving proximally. Push the rod to the spine at each level, resulting in gradual correction of the deformity.
- Close the fascia with interrupted and overlying continuous suture with no drains. Perform subcutaneous and skin closure.

If Luque rod instrumentation is desired, contour two Luque rods, one for the concave side of the scoliosis and one for the convex side. The Luque rods are available in the same sizes as the unit rods, and the suggestions for use are outlined above. Before the operative procedure, obtain lateral bending radiographs to determine the flexibility of the scoliosis, and bend the Luque rods to achieve no more than 10° additional correction beyond the preoperative bending radiographs. Bend the superior end of the convex rod and the inferior end of the concave rod into the shape of an L. Apply the rod on the concave side of the scoliosis first, and place the L portion between spinous processes or through a drill hole in the spinous process to prevent migration of the rod. If stabilization to the pelvis is required, bend the inferior end of the Luque rods as described for the Galveston technique (6). As described for the unit rod instrumentation, secure the rod to the lamina using the sublaminar wires. Apply the convex wires in similar manner, and cut and carefully tighten all

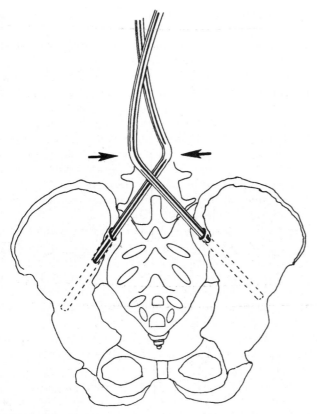

Figure 178.2. The rod is inserted into the pelvis by crossing the pelvic legs, keeping them aligned with the orientation of the drilled holes. (From Dias RC, Miller F, Dabney K, et al. Surgical Correction of Spinal Deformity Using a Unit rod in Children with Cerebral Palsy. *J Pediatr Orthop* 1996;16:734, with permission.)

wires. The two rods are connected inferiorly and superiorly to provide additional stability. We prefer to interconnect the rods securely to prevent cephalad-caudad shifting, spinal rotation and loss of pelvic obliquity correction. Rod connectors can prevent shifting of the rods. The fusion technique, bone grafting, and wound closure are identical to that described earlier for the unit rod.

MUSCULAR DYSTROPHY

The muscular dystrophies constitute a group of inherited muscle disorders characterized by progressive muscle weakness due to primary degeneration of muscle fibers. It has become apparent that these disorders are caused by specific gene abnormalities (301,340).

The muscular dystrophies are classified by age at onset, groups of muscles first affected, genetic transmission, and areas of body with progressive weakness (301).

Duchenne Muscular Dystrophy

Duchenne muscular dystrophy occurs in about 3 of 100,000 boys and usually has an early childhood onset, leading to loss of ability to walk and eventual death (128, 229). It is transmitted genetically as a sex-linked recessive trait and is due to a mutation or deletion of DNA at a locus (Xp21) on the short arm of the X chromosome (106, 120,163,164,200,312). About two thirds of the boys inherit the gene abnormality from the mother, and one third are thought to be due to new mutations. The onset is initially insidious, often with delayed motor milestones, with weakness clinically apparent by 3 years age (385). The weakness first involves the pelvic-girdle musculature, followed by the shoulder girdle musculature, and then distal musculature of the upper and lower extremities (2,387).

By 4 years of age, the boy stumbles, falls frequently, and has difficulty climbing steps and running. Pseudohypertrophy of the gastrocsoleus (Fig. 178.3), deltoid, and serratus anterior muscles is secondary to the dystrophic process and accumulation of fat within the muscles and fibrous tissue. The weakness results in a wide-based waddling gait associated with increased lumbar lordosis (Fig. 178.4). Gowers' sign (Fig. 178.5) is a characteristic way for a child with this type muscular dystrophy to rise from the floor to a standing position (137). This maneuver may be demonstrated by placing the boy prone on the floor. First, he crawls into the knee-elbow position; then, with hands and feet on the floor, he raises his hands consecu-

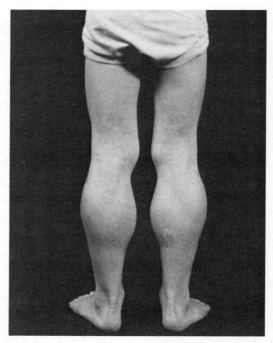

Figure 178.3. Pseudohypertrophy of the calf muscles in a boy with Duchenne muscular dystrophy.

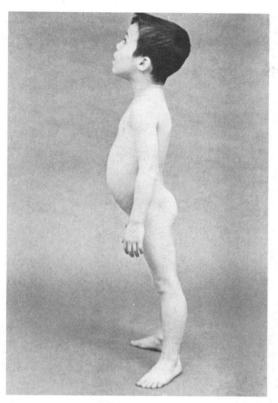

Figure 178.4. A boy with Duchenne muscular dystrophy who stands with lordotic spinal posture and has pseudohypertrophy of the calf muscles.

tively to the knees and pushes to an upright posture. The knee reflexes are diminished and sensation is normal. Progressive weakness is unremitting, and ambulation becomes more difficult, until between ages 9 and 12 years, the boy loses the ability to walk. Scoliosis and increasing contractures of the lower extremities develop. The weakness progresses until total care is required and severe cardiopulmonary compromise occurs between ages 17 and 22 years (5,14,44,49,173,201,314,319,387).

The diagnosis can often be made on the basis of family history, clinical presentation, and an elevation of serum creatinine phosphokinase (often 100 times normal in young children). Traditionally, muscle biopsy has been used to confirm the diagnosis but modern techniques of DNA analysis using peripheral blood can provide a definitive diagnosis, help to identify carriers, and allow prenatal diagnosis for 70% to 80% of the children (298). The molecular basis of Duchenne and Becker's muscular dystrophy is the absence or abnormality of dystrophin (a subsarcolemmal protein) and dystrophin-associated glycoproteins (found in the sarcolemma or muscle cell membrane) (106,120,163,164,200,312). These proteins are found in skeletal, smooth and cardiac muscle, and

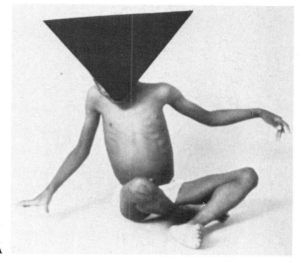

A

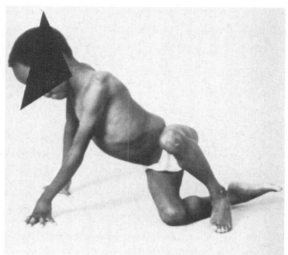

B

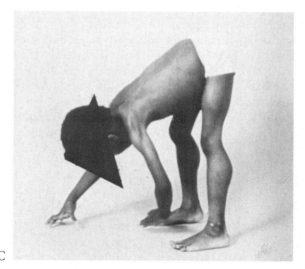

C

Figure 178.5. Gowers' sign is a characteristic way for a child with Duchenne muscular dystrophy to rise from the floor (**A** to **C**) by first using the hands to crawl into the knee-elbow position *(continued)*

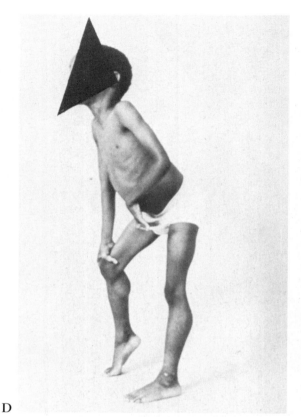
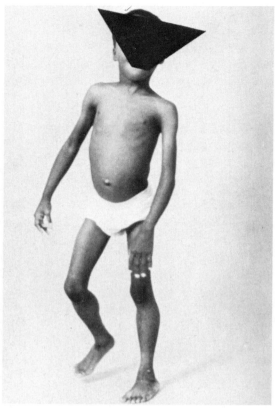

D   E

Figure 178.5.   (continued) (**D** to **E**) and then to push on the knees to achieve an upright
position. Gowers' maneuver demonstrates weakness in the shoulder and pelvic muscles.

brain. In the 20% of children who do not have a diagnosis
by DNA analysis, muscle biopsy can be diagnostic. The
biopsy typically from the vastus lateralis shows muscle
fiber degeneration, regeneration, fibrosis, fatty infiltration, central nuclear migration and hypertrophic muscle
cells (86). Absence of dystrophin is diagnostic. EMG,
rarely required, shows myopathic changes with muscle action potentials of reduced amplitude and brief duration.
The nerve conduction velocities are normal.

Orthopaedic treatment is aimed at maintenance of
strength and walking ability for as long as practical and prevention of deformities (144,179,309,353,356,367,381,
382). The single most important factor in maintaining
strength is prevention of prolonged immobilization. If a
boy with Duchenne muscular dystrophy is immobilized by
any method, functional losses tend to be permanent. Therefore, make every reasonable effort to maintain strength by
resistive muscle exercises. The patient should perform
stretching exercises, especially of the muscles most subject
to contractures (e.g., tensor fasciae latae, hip and knee flexors, and ankle plantar flexors) several times each day.

Prednisone and other steroids have been used successfully in these children from about 5 years of age to improve

muscle strength (142). Complications from this treatment
include weight gain, hypertension, behavior disturbances,
increased appetite, cushingoid features, and osteopenia.
Take into account chronic steroid useage when administering general anesthesia.

Myoblast transfer therapy to induce dystrophin production has not been successful (206). Attempts are being
made to use viral vectors to transfer functional parts of
the dystrophin gene to affected individuals.

Fractures

Muscle weakness predisposes the patient with Duchenne
muscular dystrophy to falls, and relative inactivity results
in osteopenic bone (162). Fractures of long bones occur
in 20% of children with Duchenne muscular dystrophy,
typically occurring with falls during daily activity or physical therapy (26,162,305,320). These fractures often her-
ald the end of the ambulatory stage. Treat nondisplaced
fractures of the femur and tibia in lightweight long-leg
casts or splints. Encourage weight bearing on the noninvolved leg immediately and within days on the fractured
leg. Bed rest and traction are contraindicated. Displaced
fractures of the lower limbs require prompt surgical stabi-

lization. Apply a lightweight orthosis to the leg over the area of internal fixation and begin ambulation. The family should be aware that fracture complications are higher with early mobilization but that the added risk is necessary to avoid even more serious problems.

Contractures

Contractures are inevitable in these patients, but controlling the severity greatly enhances the quality of life. Toe walking, caused by contractures of the tendo Achilles, can sometimes be detected in patients as young as 3 years of age, and it responds to stretching therapy or serial plaster casts. Tendon lengthening in young ambulatory patients is discouraged because of resulting weakness. For the ambulatory patient, a nighttime ankle-foot orthosis helps eliminate the typical equinus posturing of the foot during sleep, and muscle stretching therapy delays progression of contractures (320). Despite aggressive therapy, the ability to walk becomes threatened between 8 and 12 years of age from quadriceps muscle weakness (331); contractures of the hip flexors (Thomas test), hamstring muscles, and iliotibial tract (Ober test); and equinovarus deformities of the feet. As these children lose the ability to walk independently, surgical releases of lower extremity contractures and long-leg bracing can prolong standing and ambulation for several years (9,26,29,64,73,156,265,272,279, 310,316,320,354,355,367). When surgical releases are delayed until the children have almost stopped walking, the severity of weakness usually means that standing or walking is possible only with knee-ankle-foot orthoses. Earlier surgery followed by physical therapy and limited bracing (ankle-foot orthoses) can be just as effective (13, 108,179,266).

Procedures used to treat contractures in Duchenne muscular dystrophy include Yount fasciotomy of the iliotibial tract, Ober release of the iliotibial band, distal hamstring lengthening, transfer of the posterior tibialis tendon to the dorsum of the foot, percutaneous lengthening of the tendo Achilles, and open lengthening of the tendo Achilles.

The iliotibial tract is released by a combination of the Yount (380) fasciotomy distally and the Ober (245) release proximally. The hamstrings are released distally, and the tendo Achilles is lengthened by a percutaneous method (Fig. 178.6). The late weakness of the posterior tibialis muscle often causes a varus deformity of the foot, which is sometimes treated by a posterior tibialis tendon transfer through the interosseous membrane of the tibia and fibula to the dorsum of the foot, which maintains a plantigrade foot. If, however, the varus is not severe and the posterior tibialis muscle is weak, a tenotomy can be performed easily just posterior to the medial malleolus (308). The tenotomy is often the treatment of choice, because the child must wear an orthosis in any case.

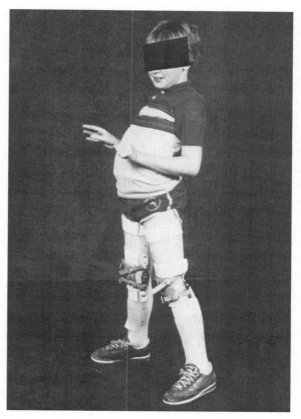

Figure 178.6. A boy with Duchenne muscular dystrophy who has undergone operative release of the iliotibial tract, distal hamstring muscle release, and percutaneous tendo Achilles lengthening. He now ambulates with long-leg braces.

Yount Fasciotomy of the Iliotibial Tract

- Expose the iliotibial tract through a 2 cm lateral longitudinal incision, located proximal to the lateral femoral condyle.
- Incise the iliotibial tract, fascia lata, and intramuscular septum transversely at a level 2.5 cm proximal to the patella. Protect the biceps tendon and the common peroneal nerve posteriorly.
- A segment of the iliotibial tract and septum may be removed in patients with severe contractures to prevent recurrence.

Ober Release of the Iliotibial Band

- With the patient in a lateral decubitus position, make an incision from 3 cm posterosuperior to the greater trochanter of the femur obliquely to 2 cm inferior to the anterosuperior iliac spine.
- Incise the iliotibial band from the anterior portion of the gluteus maximus muscle anteriorly to the anterosuperior spine.
- Incise the fascia surrounding the tensor fasciae latae transversely.

Transfer of the Posterior Tibialis Tendon to the Dorsum of the Foot

- Through a 2 cm medial longitudinal incision centered over the talonavicular joint, free the posterior tibialis tendon from its distal insertions.
- Make a second 2 cm incision midlongitudinally at the musculotendinous junction of the posterior tibialis tendon just posteromedial to the tibia, and isolate the posterior tibialis tendon.
- Place a blunt, smooth elevator beneath the tendon and lift it medially, drawing the tendon into the proximal wound. Elevate the muscle origin from the tibia and interosseous membrane for several centimeters proximally.
- Make a third incision of 1 cm anterolaterally between the tibia and the fibula, 2.5 cm above the ankle joint.
- Direct a long, curved tendon passer from the second incision posterior to the tibia, through the interosseous membrane, to the third incision.
- Open the jaws of the tendon passer to create an opening in the interosseous membrane. Some surgeons fashion a 2-cm long window in the membrane using a scalpel; this reduces the chance of adhesions between the tendon and membrane (although this is not a major consideration in patients with Duchenne muscular dystrophy).
- Place a heavy, nonabsorbable suture in the distal end of the tibialis posterior tendon. Using a suture, draw the posterior tibial tendon forward through the interosseous membrane to the third incision.
- Make a fourth 2 cm incision over the dorsal surface of the third cuneiform or the third metatarsal.
- Retract the extensor tendons and incise the periosteum in a cruciate fashion.
- Drill a 0.6 cm hole plantarly through the bone.
- Direct the tendon passer subcutaneously from the fourth incision to the third incision, and deliver the tendon subcutaneously to the fourth incision. During passing, be careful to allow no twisting or kinking of the tendon. Some surgeons prefer to pass the tendon beneath the extensor retinaculum, but in our experience, this procedure is unnecessary, and it may become the site of tendon adhesion that restricts motion.
- Pass the sutures attached to the tendon end through the plantar surface of the foot with long, straight needles. The needles and sutures should exit the plantar surface of the foot in a non-weight-bearing area.
- Direct the tendon into the drill hole, hold the foot in a neutral position, and anchor the sutures snugly over a heavily padded button. The tendon can also be fixed to the midfoot using one of the available anchor systems.
- Further secure the tendon to the drill hole site by interrupted sutures to the periosteum.
- Close the incision and apply a well-padded long-leg cast with the foot in a slightly dorsiflexed position. Particular attention should be directed toward padding the proximal fibula, where the peroneal nerve is most cutaneous.

Postoperatively, remove the long-leg cast after 2 weeks, and apply a short-leg walking cast for an additional 4 weeks. After cast removal, remove the button, place the extremity in a brace, and begin active exercises.

Percutaneous Lengthening of the Tendo Achilles

- Perform a percutaneous tenotomy with the patient in a prone position.
- Dorsiflex the foot to maintain the tendo Achilles in a taut position.
- Palpitate the posterior tibial artery in the neurovascular bundle, and protect it during the procedure. The tendo Achilles rotates 90° on the longitudinal axis between its origin and insertion, and the medial fibers proximally are posterior at the insertion.
- Make a longitudinal 3 mm stab wound medial to the tendo Achilles and 1 cm superior to the calcaneus, and divide the anterior two thirds of the tendon fibers.
- Make a second stab wound incision dorsally 2 cm below the palpable musculotendinous junction and divide the medial two thirds of the tendon fibers.
- Dorsiflex the foot and the tendo Achilles lengthens.
- Close the stab wounds, and apply a well-padded cast at 5° dorsiflexion for 4 weeks.

Open Lengthening of the Tendo Achilles

- With the patient in a prone position, make a 5 cm longitudinal incision from the superomedial aspect of the calcaneus proximally along the medial border of the tendo Achilles.
- Divide the subcutaneous tissue and tendon sheath, and evacuate the rotation of the tendo Achilles.
- Incise the midposterior area of the tendon longitudinally by a stab wound. Place a clamp in the stab wound incision, and open it so that the tendon splits in the longitudinal direction of the fibers.
- Cut one part of the split tendon transversely distally and the other proximally, creating a Z-plasty tenotomy.
- Dorsiflex the foot to 5° above neutral and suture the tendon in the lengthened position. Apply a well-padded cast for 6 weeks, followed by a brace.

Postoperative Care   Most surgery is performed bilaterally in one operative procedure, and lightweight long-leg casts are applied with the knees in extension and the feet neutral.

Standing is begun the day after surgery, and a rapid return to walking is encouraged. We incorporate a strip of polyurethane foam (7.5 × 1.5 cm) for padding dorsally under the standard long-leg cast. Ten days later, the casts are removed, long-leg orthoses are measured, and casts are reapplied until the orthoses are fabricated. The knee-ankle-foot orthosis prescription should include lightweight materials (usually plastics), contouring proximally to allow the buttocks to rest on the brace, drop-lock hinges at the knee, solid ankles in the neutral position, tarsal straps, and extension beyond the metatarsal heads (377).

Equinovarus Deformity

Later in the disease process, the child becomes confined to a wheelchair. At this stage, contractures of the knees and hips are inevitable. Surgical releases usually are not required; instead, a program to maintain motion is indicated to prevent the progression of contracture that would hinder a good sitting position in the wheelchair. Occasionally, a patient, especially one who earlier refused surgery to prolong walking or refused orthotics, develops a severe, rigid equinovarus deformity of the foot that causes pain on the anterolateral aspect of the foot or the inability to wear shoes. Multiple tenotomies (tendo Achilles, tibialis posterior, and flexor digitorum longus) and postoperative casting can achieve a satisfactory foot position. Severe, stiff longstanding deformity can be corrected operatively with a tarsal medullostomy, but postoperative foot edema may persist for at least 6 months.

Tarsal Medullostomy

- Place the patient in the supine position, and control hemostasis during the procedure with a pneumatic tourniquet.
- Make a 3 mm stab wound skin incision obliquely over the sinus tarsi.
- Introduce a 3 mm oval curette into the sinus tarsi. Curette the talonavicular, calcaneocuboid, and subtalar joints, leaving the outer cortical margins intact. Carefully avoid injuring the neurovascular structures.
- Close the stab wound incision with a single stitch, and place the leg in a well-padded long-leg cast with the knee flexed and the foot in neutral position.

After surgery, elevate the foot to control edema. Use a long-leg cast for 1 month, and a short-leg cast for an additional 2 months (Fig. 178.7).

Spinal Deformities

Scoliosis occurs in almost all boys with Duchenne muscular dystrophy (49,168,212,313). During the period that

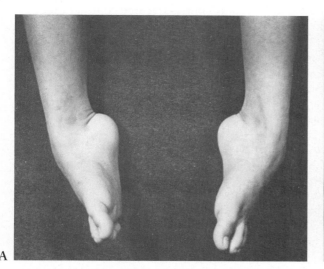
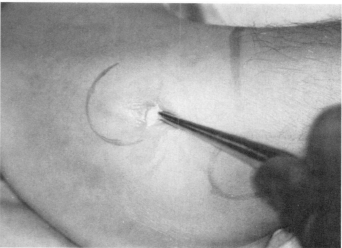
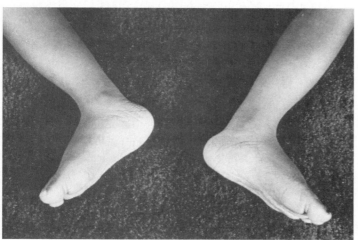

Figure 178.7. A: A boy with Duchenne muscular dystrophy and a severe equinovarus foot deformity. B: The deformity was corrected by a tarsal medullostomy. C: After surgery, the foot has maintained a neutral position.

a boy with Duchenne muscular dystrophy is able to walk, spinal lordosis develops to compensate for weakness of the trunk and pelvic muscles. By the time the child must use a wheelchair, a functional kyphosis typically develops. Wilkins hypothesized that the kyphosis unlocks the posterior facet joints, causing an unstable spin and progressive scoliosis (269,366). For whatever reason, scoliosis typically becomes apparent during the last months of walking or soon after confinement to a wheelchair (41,78,230, 307). The peak rate of progression occurs between 13 and 15 years, with up to 3° of progression per month. The scoliosis is typically a long C-shaped thoracolumbar curve that progresses steadily until a severe deformity results (Fig. 178.8*A, B*). The scoliosis eventually involves the pelvis, leading to severe pelvic obliquity and difficulty in sitting, back pain, skin breakdown, pulmonary compromise, and loss of hand function because of obligatory use of the hands for support of the trunk (313). A few patients do not develop the spinal kyphosis but persist with the lordotic posture after ambulation ceases. They develop a less progressive scoliosis, but by 6 to 8 years after ambulation ceases, severe scoliosis usually develops. Various spinal orthoses and wheelchair adaptations have been used to control the scoliosis, but none has been totally successful, and at best, they only delayed the progression of curvature.

Posterior spinal fusion and instrumentation is indicated for progressive scoliosis of 30° or greater. Preoperative cardiac and pulmonary evaluation must be done to determine the anesthetic risk. A vital capacity of less than 35% normal indicates that pulmonary complications are more likely (178,232,270).

We prefer segmental spinal instrumentation and posterior fusion with the unit rod or Luque instrumentation with Galveston pelvic fixation from T2 to the sacrum (37, 115,284,329,330,332,362). The unit rod technique is described earlier in this chapter. The patients are ventilated for the first 24 hours in the intensive care unit and then quickly mobilized to return muscle strength and to avoid pulmonary and gastrointestinal complications. No postoperative bracing is required.

If the preoperative pelvic obliquity is 10° or less and the scoliosis is 40° or less, fusion to L5 will provide a good result (240,330) (Fig. 178.8*C, D*).

Vertical shifting of independent Luque rods has been reported and can be avoided by crosslinking the rods (37, 126,232,240).

Intraoperative blood loss can be extensive (37,232,240, 284,296,332,362). Careful intraoperative hemostasis, use of allograft, and speed will reduce blood loss. Preoperative autologous blood donation, intraoperative cell-saver techniques, and reinfusion of postoperative drainage will reduce the need for homologous transfusion.

Becker's Muscular Dystrophy

Becker's muscular dystrophy is an X-linked disorder with a clinical pattern similar to that of the Duchenne type, but it is milder and with slower progression (22,23,31). It results from a deletion in the same gene that causes the Duchenne type. Dystrophin is present but in reduced amounts, typically above 20% (164,199). Proximal girdle muscle weakness and pseudohypertrophy are apparent by 7 years of age, with maintenance of walking ability until age 16 and death occurring in middle adult life after cardiopulmonary failure (100). Clinically, the patient with Becker's muscular dystrophy resembles a "strong" patient with Duchenne muscular dystrophy in the juvenile years. The CPK level is markedly elevated, with levels similar to those seen in Duchenne muscular dystrophy, and the results of muscle biopsy resemble those in Duchenne muscular dystrophy. Orthopaedic problems include equinus, cavus, and scoliosis (186). The early major orthopaedic problem is progressive contracture of the tendo Achilles, which may be controlled by muscle-stretching therapy and by a nighttime ankle-foot orthosis to prevent the typical equinus posturing of the foot during sleep. Periodic serial stretching casts usually control the mild contractures, and tendo Achilles lengthening has occasionally been necessary.

Progressive proximal muscle weakness causes a wide-based gait and exaggerated spinal lordosis. In the teenage years, ambulation can be facilitated by canes for balance and a knee-ankle-foot orthosis. Scoliosis can occur and is managed as for the Duchenne type (186).

Limb Girdle Muscular Dystrophy

The term limb girdle muscular dystrophy represents a group of patients with muscle weakness in a girdle distribution and autosomal inheritance. Leyden (209) described a type with predominantely pelvic girdle weakness, and Erb (105) described a shoulder girdle type. Typical findings include elevation of the CPK level, myopathic changes on EMG, and dystrophic changes on muscle biopsy. Recent advances in molecular genetics have established several syndromes with different gene abnormalities that had been classified as limb girdle dystrophies (87). There is a wide range of clinical severity. For example, severe autosomal recessive muscular dystrophy of childhood is characterized by absence of a sarcoglycan called adhalin (87) and can present with a clinical course similar to that of Duchenne's muscular dystrophy or with a later onset, milder type.

Orthopaedic problems are similar to those seen in other types of muscular dystrophies, and the principles of management are the same.

Facioscapulohumeral Dystrophy

Facioscapulohumeral dystrophy (Landouzy-Déjérine dystrophy) is transmitted by an autosomal dominant gene,

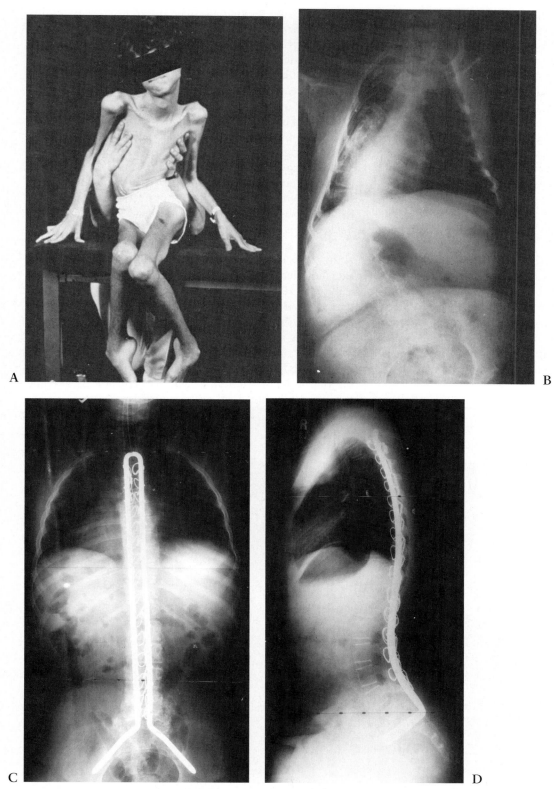

Figure 178.8. A: After becoming nonambulatory from Duchenne muscular dystrophy, this boy developed a severe scoliosis, which led to pelvic obliquity and difficulty sitting. B: The radiograph demonstrates a long C-shaped pattern of scoliosis. AP (C) and lateral radiographs obtained after a posterior spinal fusion with Unit rod instrumentation (D).

has an onset usually in adolescence, involves the facial and then the shoulder girdle muscles, and has a slow progression, with an expected average to long life span (87, 148,204,349). The disease is uncommon, with a prevalence of about 1 in 20,000 (249,250). The early weakness results in a lack of facial mobility, sloping of the shoulders, and difficulty in raising the arms above the head. The upper arm and scapular muscles are involved earlier than the deltoid and forearm muscles. In longstanding, severe cases, the wrist extensor muscles are more involved than the flexors, producing a wrist drop called the praying mantis posture. The CPK level is normal to slightly elevated, and muscle biopsy shows only slight changes, such as isolated atrophic fibers and variation in fiber size. The gene abnormality has been localized to 4Q35, but no gene product has been identified (114,365).

Facioscapulohumeral dystrophy presents as four clinical variations: typical, as described; late exacerbation type, which may consist of only mild facial weakness for years and then rapid deterioration in midlife; infantile type, which has an onset before age 1 year and is severely crippling, requiring a wheelchair by age 9 years (38); and scapuloperoneal syndrome, in which the peroneal and tibialis anterior muscles are involved early in the illness (16, 109).

The faciohumeral pattern of muscle weakness occurs in several diseases that must be differentiated, including myotubular myopathy, nemaline central cord disease. and mitochondrial myopathy (34).

Orthopaedic problems include a dropped wrist and foot, scapular instability, and back pain. The dropped wrist is treated by a splint and the dropped foot by an ankle-foot orthosis with a rigid ankle in neutral position. Lordosis (Fig. 178.9*A, B*), which is initially flexible, usually develops in the lumbar spine but may become so severe and rigid that the sacrum becomes horizontal. The lordosis produces severe back pain that may be treated by a lumbosacral orthosis. In ambulatory patients, the orthosis should support the back but not necessarily correct the lordosis, which may be necessary for walking. Surgery for back pain is almost never indicated.

Weakness of the serratus anterior, rhomboid, trapezium, and latissimus dorsi muscles limits elevation of the shoulder by allowing scapular winging and rotation (Fig. 178.10*A, B*). If the deltoid muscle is strong and scapular winging inhibits function so that the arm cannot be raised above the horizontal level, a scapulothoracic arthrodesis may be effective in improving shoulder flexion and abduction (42,43,61,177,188,207,321) (Fig. 178.10*C*). The operation initially should be performed on one side; if helpful, it can be considered for the contralateral side.

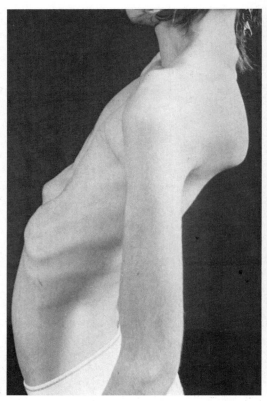
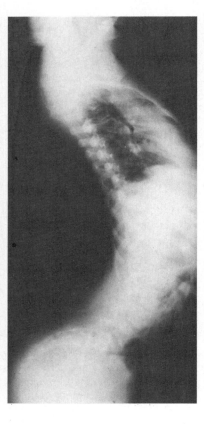

A,B

Figure 178.9. Photograph (**A**) and radiograph of a boy with facioscapulohumeral dystrophy and severe spinal lordosis (**B**). The lordosis frequently results in disabling back pain.

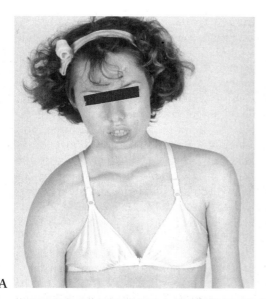

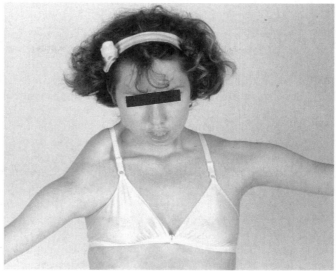

A

B

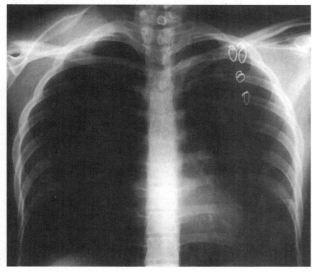

C

Figure 178.10. Facioscapulohumeral dystrophy in a young woman with shoulders in neutral (**A**) and abduction (**B**). Note the improved abduction and appearance of left shoulder after scapulothoracic arthrodesis. Radiograph (**C**) demonstrates the wiring technique and preoperative position of the right scapula.

Scapulothoracic Arthrodesis

- Place the patient prone on bolsters. Free drape the shoulder and arm to allow shoulder motion and access to the brachial and radial pulses.
- Make a 6 cm incision along the medial border of the scapula, with the scapula in a reduced position.
- Divide the insertion of the rhomboids into the vertebral border of the scapula to provide access to the thoracic surface of the scapula.
- Elevate subperiosteally the medial 2 cm of the subscapularis and the supra and infraspinatus. The medial origin of subscapularis needs to be resected to allow scapulothoracic contact.
- Position the vertebral end of the scapular spine at rib 3 or 4. Expose ribs 3,4,5, and 6 subperiosteally (avoid damaging the parietal pleura).
- Drill two sets of holes at the scapular spine and one set at the vertebral border of the scapula over each of the lower three ribs.
- Harvest a corticocancellous iliac graft, and fashion three 2 cm cortical pieces, and space two drill holes 1 cm apart in each piece.
- Place two 18-gauge stainless steel wires under rib 3 and one under the lower ribs, and thread them through the scapula and the pieces of autograft. Position the scapula so there is a 20° angle between the medial border of the scapula and the spine.
- Decorticate the ribs and undersurface of the scapula, apply cancellous autograft, and tighten the wires.
- Check for normal pulses in the arm and for desired shoulder range of motion. Use a shoulder immobilizer for postoperative immobilization.

Congenital Muscular Dystrophy

The term "congenital muscular dystrophy" is used to describe an autosomal recessive group of disorders that present with muscle weakness at birth or shortly thereafter and a dystrophic pattern on muscle biopsy. Neonatal hypotonia is typical, but some children present with joint contractures (which may be an arthrogrypotic picture). The condition tends to remain static, but there can be slow progression or, alternatively, functional improvement and achievement of walking ability. Respiratory and swallowing problems depend on the severity of the weakness. The CPK may be slightly elevated, EMG reveals a myopathic pattern, and the muscle biopsy indicates severe dystrophic changes (87,224,384).

A number of syndromes of congenital muscular dystrophy in association with central nervous system involvement have been described: Fukuyama-type congenital muscular dystrophy, muscle-eye-brain disease, and the Walker-Warburg syndrome (87,124,125,190). Children with congenital muscular dystrophy have severe mental retardation and guarded prognoses. A subgroup of children with classical congenital muscular dystrophy with white matter changes in the brain lack laminin M (merosin), an extracellular protein (87,345).

Orthopaedic care includes obtaining a muscle biopsy, treating contractures, and correcting deformities (182, 251,370). Mild contractures respond to therapy and splinting but tend to recur. Rigid and recurrent deformities are difficult and are treated as described in the section on arthrogryposis.

MYOTONIC SYNDROMES

Pathology

Myotonia is characterized by a sustained contraction or delayed relaxation of skeletal muscle after cessation of voluntary contracture or mechanical stimulation. It does not occur spontaneously but is initiated by voluntary contracture or stimulation and is usually accentuated by cold or periods of rest (74). Myotonia is seen in a number of illnesses, such as myotonic dystrophy, myotonia congenita, paramyotonia congenita, Schwartz-Jampel syndrome, drug-induced myotonia, and muscle contracture induced by exercise (80,227,344,372). Significant orthopaedic deformities occur in myotonic dystrophy and in Schwartz-Jampel syndrome, which is rare.

Myotonia is best demonstrated clinically by muscle contracture after a blow to the muscle belly by a reflex hammer or by a hand-grasp test, in which the patient grasps the observer's hand, tries to release, but immediate relaxation fails and an unwinding motion of the fingers must occur to unclasp the hand (34). In infants, myotonia may be manifest by delayed opening of the eyes after closure with crying. EMG demonstrates a characteristic pattern and confirms the clinical myotonia. The frequency

of discharge is initially increased, followed by a gradual decrease and cessation, which produces an acoustic pattern that sounds like a dive bomber.

Myotonic Dystrophy

Myotonic dystrophy (Steinert's disease) is an autosomal dominant disorder characterized by myotonia, a progressive dystrophic process of muscle leading to weakness and atrophy and various endocrine and systemic abnormalities (48,60,75,374). The molecular abnormality is an unstable expansion of DNA with a variable number of trinucleotide repeats in the myotonia protein kinase gene on chromosome 19 (12,35,45,123,151,152,157,216,291,298).

This disorder is classified into congenital and adult forms, which are very distinct.

Congenital Myotonic Dystrophy Congenital myotonic dystrophy occurs almost entirely in children born to mothers with myotonic dystrophy (Fig. 178.11A). Myotonic mothers usually have premature onset of labor, postpartum hemorrhage, and poor uterine tone, which predisposes the infant to cerebral damage and static encephalopathy (ie, cerebral palsy). The pregnancy is frequently complicated by poor fetal movements and hydramnios. In children with severe encephalopathy, an underlying myotonia can be overlooked. The child appears to have only a complex form of cerebral palsy, but evaluation of the mother demonstrates the characteristics of myotonia, and the diagnosis in the child can be suspected. In the neonatal period, the main characteristic features are hypotonia with difficulty in sucking and respiratory distress (27). The neonate frequently has facial paresis and a triangular, fish-shaped mouth, with the upper lip forming an inverted V. Mental retardation is common, and the mean IQ is approximately 66 (51). There is marked wasting of the sternocleidomastoid and trapezium muscles, and in most patients, muscle function improves in the first decade of life. Most of these children walk by age 4 or 5 years. Cataracts usually do not occur until about 14 years of age. Conduction abnormalities and myocardial dysfunction are common, and these children routinely require electrocardiograms and echocardiograms routinely (118).

Almost all children with congenital myotonic dystrophy have orthopaedic problems, including talipes equinovarus, congenital dislocation of the hip, severe truncal weakness, and contractures of the extremities (167). Children with congenital myotonic dystrophy should be treated aggressively orthopaedically because their conditions improve for several years after birth (24,51,153,154, 246,351,386).

About half of the children with congenital myotonic dystrophy have talipes equinovarus (262) (Fig. 178.11B). The talipes equinovarus is not a typical clubfoot. The equinus is the most dramatic component of the deformity. The forefoot is usually plantarflexed on the hind foot, and the

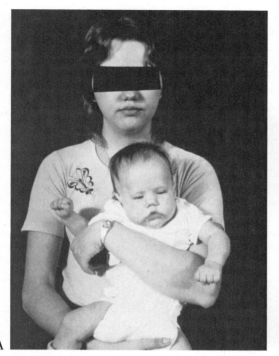
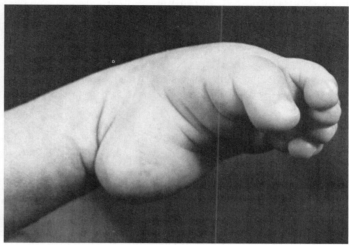

Figure 178.11. **A:** A mother with the adult type of myotonic dystrophy and her daughter with the congenital type of myotonic dystrophy. **B:** A foot with talipes equinovarus from congenital myotonic dystrophy. The equinus is severe, the forefoot is plantar flexed on the hindfoot, and the first toe is more flexed than the other toes.

first toe is usually more plantarflexed than the other toes. There is usually a wide space between the first and second toes. In the newborn, the clubfoot is best treated by serial casting, gradually bringing the foot to the neutral position. There is considerable variation in the stiffness of the foot, from a rigid foot to a hypotonic positional deformity. In most patients, the foot can be casted to a neutral position. Careful attention should be given to the toe plate on the cast to maintain a neutral position; otherwise, the toes curl around the end of the cast, resulting in an increasingly severe toe deformity. The most resistant component of the clubfoot is usually the equinus deformity; therefore, attention should be directed toward molding the cast at the longitudinal arch of the foot, so that a breach of the arch will not occur. After the foot is casted to a neutral position, it must be maintained until ambulation begins. Frequently, these patients are severely hypotonic, and walking may be delayed until they are 3 to 4 years old, making prolonged maintenance a difficult orthopaedic problem. Bivalved casts are most useful, although they have a tendency to slip distally on the foot, and orthoses require frequent modifications to accommodate growth.

A few patients develop severely rigid equinovarus feet that cannot be corrected with serial casting and thus require surgical correction. We recommend that surgical procedures not be performed before the child is 1 year of age, because the children are exceedingly hypotonic, and the risks of anesthesia and subsequent surgical complications are high. A posteromedial lateral release usually corrects the deformity (52,223,311,347,348). Overzealous correction should not be performed, because a severe valgus deformity of the foot may occur. The foot must be maintained in a neutral position after surgery, which may require an orthosis for several years.

Structural hyphoscoliosis develops slowly over the childhood years in some children (67). An orthosis typically prevents progression in the childhood years until the pubertal growth spurt, when progression occurs. Spinal fusion and instrumentation is effective, but mesenteric artery syndrome has been reported and experienced by the authors (67).

Adult Myotonic Dystrophy   In the adult form of myotonic dystrophy, symptoms become noticeable in late adolescence or early adult life, although myotonia may be present in childhood. Muscle cramps, nasal voice character, and progressive weakness are observed first. The facial muscle atrophy of the temple, jaw, and neck muscles produces a lower lip droop called an inverted smile and a characteristic "hatchet-face" or "swan-neck" facies. The muscle weakness is more prominent distally, especially in the calf muscles and forearms, but the intrinsic muscles of the hands and feet frequently are spared until later in the disease. Smooth muscle may be involved, resulting in dysphasia, recurrent pulmonary infections, and lower gastrointestinal tract dysfunction (135). Cataracts, frontal baldness, mild mental retardation, and cardiac abnormalities are seen. The endocrine abnormalities result in abnormal glucose tolerance and insulin release, with frank diabetes mellitus, hypothyroidism, and gonadal dysfunction (171). Deep tendon reflexes are usually absent or diminished in the distal muscles, and the disease is progressive until death in the fifth to sixth decade of life from cardiorespiratory compromise.

Laboratory tests frequently show a slightly elevated CPK level, hypogammaglobulinemia with low IgA, and a glucose tolerance test of the diabetic type (143). The EMG demonstrates typical myotonia. The muscle biopsy shows changes that include internal nuclei and type I fiber atrophy.

Orthopaedic problems are associated with weakness of the neck muscles, pain, or mild subluxation that usually responds symptomatically to a soft cervical collar. Equinus deformity of the foot may be controlled by an ankle-foot orthosis. Occasionally, a pes cavovarus or pes planus deformity develops, and orthotic inserts typically resolve painful callosities. If a rigid foot deformity causes pain and instability, a triple arthrodesis to realign the hind foot and midfoot is helpful. Toe deformities consist of a flexion and a valgus deformity of the hallux, which may curl under the second toe. The second to fifth toes develop flexion contractures of the distal interphalangeal joints with dorsal callus formation. If these deformities are severe, the hallux is treated by an osteotomy of the middle phalanx with realignment and Steinmann pin fixation, and the second through fifth toes are treated by partial phalangectomy of the distal aspect of the proximal phalanx and internal fixation with Kirschner wires. These surgical techniques are described later in the section on peripheral neuropathies.

Anesthetic complications are common, and careful preoperative evaluation is important (220).

COMMON NERVE DISORDERS WITH ORTHOPAEDIC DEFORMITIES

PERIPHERAL NEUROPATHIES

A neuropathy is a condition of a peripheral nerve that may have motor signs manifested as weakness or decreased deep tendon reflexes; sensory abnormalities, which are usually more severe distally than proximally; or autonomic changes, resulting in impaired sweating, atrophy of the skin, or loss of hair.

The neuropathies are categorized as mononeuropathy, which is limited to a nerve, nerve root, or plexus (e.g., entrapment syndrome, brachial plexus injury, Bell's palsy); mononeuropathy multiplex, which involves multiple peripheral nerves (e.g., polyarteritis nodosa); and acquired polyneuropathies (e.g., diabetes, vitamin deficiencies, alcoholic neuropathy, drug-induced neuropathy, collagen vascular disease, genetic polyneuropathies such as Charcot-Marie-Tooth disease). Peripheral neuropathy, demyelinating polyneuropathy, myositis, encephalopathy, and recurrent infection are associated with acquired immunodeficiency syndrome (AIDS) (17,71,208). The incidence of neuromuscular disease in AIDS patients is unknown, but the diagnosis must be considered in inflammatory polyneuropathy or myopathy. Complex orthopaedic problems occur in many of the neuropathies.

The hereditary neuropathies are a group of genetically determined diseases with nerve fiber degeneration or segmental demyelinization. The pathology of nerve fiber degeneration involves a "dying-back" phenomenon that usually begins peripherally in the longest nerve fibers. Segmental demyelinating diseases involve inadequate peripheral myelinization by the Schwann cells and result in slowed nerve conduction velocities.

The hereditary neuropathies are classified as hereditary motor and sensory neuropathies (e.g., Charcot-Marie-Tooth disease), hereditary sensory neuropathy (e.g., congenital absence of pain), spinocerebellar degeneration (e.g., Friedreich's ataxia), and metabolic defects with neuropathy. The hereditary metabolic neuropathies are rare and include metachromatic leukodystrophy (ie, sulfatide lipidosis), Bassen-Kornzweig syndrome (ie, beta-lipoproteinemia), infantile and juvenile amaurotic idiocy, globoid cell leukodystrophy (ie, Krabbe's disease), angiokeratoma corporis diffusum (ie, Fabry's disease), Chédiak-Steinbrinck-Higashi syndrome, Tangier disease (ie, alpha-lipoproteinemia), and Cockayne's syndrome.

Hereditary Motor and Sensory Neuropathy

The hereditary motor and sensory neuropathies are an inherited group of diseases of peripheral nerves with sensory and motor involvement. The general clinical characteristics include distal symmetric muscle weakness, manifested by equinus feet, steppage gait, cavus feet, and loss of fine motor function in the hands; there is a mild sensory abnormality, usually causing poor balance and clumsiness and decreased deep tendon reflexes. Evaluate any patient with distal muscle weakness and cavus deformity of the feet for hereditary sensory-motor neuropathy. The disorders have been classified according to clinical manifestations, pathology, heredity, and electrophysiologic changes (72, 92, 94, 95, 98, 130, 141, 149, 185, 263, 264, 277, 278, 324) (Table 178.2).

Hereditary sensory and motor neuropathy types I and II are most common and constitute the classic forms of

Table 178.2. *Classification of Hereditary Sensory-Motor Neuropathies*

Type	Other names	Nerve heredity	Conduction	Orthopaedic problems
I	Hypertrophic form of Charcot-Marie-Tooth disease Peroneal muscular atrophy Roussy-Levy syndrome (277, 288)	Autosomal dominant	Delayed	Pes cavus Claw hands Hip dysplasia Scoliosis Claw toes
II	Neuronal form of Charcot-Marie-Tooth disease Peroneal muscular atrophy (93)	Autosomal dominant	Near normal	Pes calcaneovarus Claw toes Claw hands Scoliosis Hip dysplasia
III	Déjérine-Sottas disease (72) Hereditary neuropathy of infancy (130) Peroneal muscular atrophy	Autosomal dominant	Very delayed	Trunk ataxia Delayed motor milestones Scoliosis Pes cavus Dropped foot
IV	Refsum's disease (34, 185, 263, 264, 324) Phytanic acid storage neuropathy	Autosomal dominant	Delayed	Epiphyseal dysplasia Shortened metacarpals Pes cavus Pes equinus Scoliosis
V	Neuropathy with spastic paraplegia	Autosomal dominant	Slightly delayed	Spastic paraplegia Contractures

Charcot-Marie-Tooth disease, which is also called peroneal muscular atrophy (54,346). The hypertrophic form of Charcot-Marie-Tooth disease (type I) is associated with segmental demyelinization, reduced nerve conduction velocity, and an enlarged palpable superficial nerve with an insidious onset in the first or second decade of life. There is a broad range of clinical severity. The progression is slow, although a wheelchair is often required in middle to late adult life. Type IA is usually caused by a duplication of a gene on chromosome 17 for peripheral myelin protein 22 (PMP-22), a glycoprotein expressed in the myelin sheath. Type IB, which has a similar presentation to type IA, is caused by a mutation of the Po gene on chromosome 1n41. The neuronal form of Charcot-Marie-Tooth disease (type II) is clinically similar to the hypertrophic form, except that the pathogenesis involves axonal degeneration and not demyelination, nerve conduction velocities are near normal, the nerves are not enlarged, and leg atrophy is severe, producing a stork-leg appearance. Type II has been linked to chromosome 1p35-p36. An X-linked type

has an abnormality in the connexin gene at xq13. The orthopaedic problems of Charcot-Marie-Tooth disease include pes cavus, claw toes, drop feet, hip dysplasia, and scoliosis (69,358).

Other types of hereditary motor and sensory neuropathy are type III, or Déjérine-Sottas disease, which is similar to type I but more severe; and type IV, or Refsum's disease (92). Of interest to the orthopaedic surgeon is hereditary neuropathy with a liability to pressure palsies (HNPP) (371). The onset is in adolescence, and nerve palsies can occur with minor trauma to the peripheral nerves. Extreme care must be taken during surgery to avoid traction on peripheral nerves and, if possible, to avoid the use of a tourniquet.

Cavus Feet
Cavus feet (Fig. 178.12A) are commonly seen in peripheral neuropathies, spina bifida, poliomyelitis, Friedreich's ataxia, spinal cord lesions, and several less common neurologic illnesses. The pathogenesis involves muscle imbal-

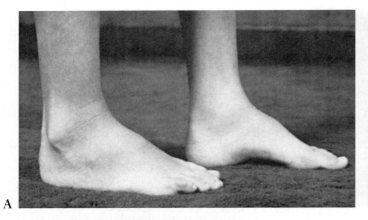

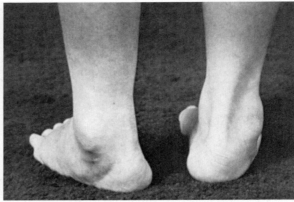

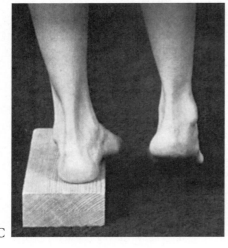

Figure 178.12. **A:** A cavus foot in a patient with Charcot-Marie-Tooth disease. **B:** A cavus foot, demonstrating heel varus during stance. The depression of the first metatarsal forces the foot into varus. **C:** The Coleman block test, demonstrating the flexibility of the hindfoot. When the depressed first metatarsal is allowed to hang off the block, the heel is no longer forced into varus during stance.

ance, but the specific mechanism is unknown (32,33,252, 283,287). A cavus foot has a pathologic elevation of the longitudinal arch of less than 150° on the lateral radiograph at the intersection of the axis of the first metatarsal and the calcaneus (169). There are three forms of pes cavus, as determined by the orientation of the os calcis during stances: pes cavovarus if the os calcis is inverted; pes calcaneocavus if the os calcis pitch (long axis of the os calcis to the floor) is greater than 30° or the long axis of the tibia to the long axis of the os calcis is greater than 130°, and pes equinocavus if the os calcis pitch is less than 20° (287).

In Charcot-Marie-Tooth disease, a pes cavovarus deformity combined with decreased proprioception results in difficulty in walking, lack of balance, and painful callosities. The peripheral neuropathy initially causes weakness of the intrinsic muscles of the foot and peroneal muscles, resulting in a forefoot drop, relative shortening of the long toe extensors because of the forefoot drop, and hyperextension at the metatarsophalangeal joints. Hyperextension leads to a secondary tightening of the long toe flexor tendons and to flexion of interphalangeal joint and a claw

toe deformity. The posterior tibialis muscle initially remains strong, and the first metatarsal droops more than the remainder of the forefoot. During stance, the plantarflexed first metatarsal forces the foot into supination, and contracture of the relatively strong posterior tibialis tendon holds the heel in varus (Fig. 178.12*B*). Initially, the foot is flexible, but the plantar fascia also shortens, contributing to the depression of the first metatarsal and a fixed varus deformity of the heel. The rigidity of the heel varus is determined by the Coleman lateral block test (Fig. 178.12*C*), in which a plantarflexed first metatarsal is allowed to hang over a 2.5 cm block, eliminating the forced forefoot pronation (negating the tripod effect); if the heel returns to a neutral position with this maneuver, the hindfoot deformity is not fixed (58,59,252). Therefore, attention may be directed toward the midfoot and forefoot.

The patient progressively becomes more clumsy, and as the cavovarus deformity becomes more rigid, painful calluses develop over the heel, the base of the fifth metatarsal, and the head of the first metatarsal (tripod foot). Subsequent bony adaptations result in a rigid equinocavovarus foot deformity (Fig. 178.13).

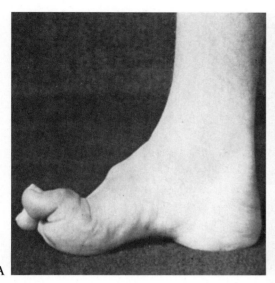
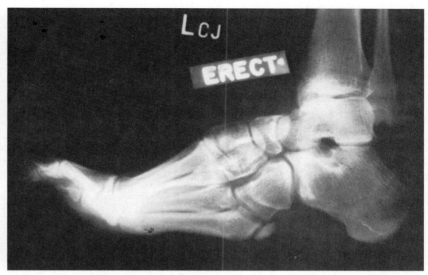

Figure 178.13. **A:** A rigid cavus foot caused by Charcot-Marie-Tooth disease in a skeletally mature patient. **B:** Radiograph of a rigid cavus foot, demonstrates the elevated longitudinal arch, heel varus, hypertrophy of the fifth metatarsal, and claw toes.

Treatment of the cavus foot depends on the patient's age, flexibility of the foot, bony deformity, and muscle imbalance. In the early stages, the whole foot may be slightly supinated, the arch moderately elevated, and the great toe slightly cocked upward. As soon as the diagnosis is confirmed, begin daily manipulation of the foot to resist the depression of the first metatarsal, stretching of the plantar fascia and tendo Achilles, and extension of the toes. A nighttime ankle-foot orthosis in a neutral ankle position is recommended to prevent the foot from dangling into the equinus posture during sleep and to delay the onset of a fixed deformity. A supple foot can be treated nonoperatively by manipulation followed by serial stretching in a short walking cast, followed by an ankle-foot orthosis with a rigid ankle in neutral position and a lateral heel extension to resist varus.

If fixed soft-tissue or bony deformity develops, surgery becomes necessary to maintain a plantigrade foot. The goals of surgery are to correct deformity, restore muscle balance, and if necessary, stabilize the foot. Rigid deformities, usually consisting of a heel varus and a plantarflexed first metatarsal, must be corrected before tendon transfers are performed.

In children younger than 12 years of age, triple arthrodesis is contraindicated (364). Other procedures that can be performed include a plantar medial release to reduce the midfoot contracture; extension osteotomy of the first metatarsal to correct a rigid plantarflexed first metatarsal; transfer of the extensor hallucis longus tendon to the neck of the first metatarsal and interphalangeal fusion (Jones procedure); transfer of the extensor digitorum longus ten-

dons to the third cuneiform (Hibbs procedure); transfer of the posterior tibialis tendon through the tibiofibular interosseous membrane to the dorsum of the foot to remove a deforming force and achieve dorsiflexion of the ankle; Dwyer or medial translation calcaneal osteotomy to correct heel varus if the heel does not correct with the Coleman block test; and a metatarsal osteotomy to correct the forefoot (90,91,161,181,273,297,302,333,359,361). In children younger than 8 to 10 years of age, the heel and first ray are usually flexible and will correct with soft-tissue releases and serial casting. Hindfoot equinus and tendo Achilles contracture are often present. Tendo Achilles lengthening should not be performed simultaneously with the plantar medial release because it is important to have a stable hindfoot to allow correction of the longitudinal arch with serial casting. In the older child with greater weakness, a rigid hindfoot, and fixed plantar flexion of the first metatarsal, the plantar medial release is combined with an extension osteotomy of the first metatarsal (and adjacent metatarsals if required), calcaneal osteotomy, and a posterior tibialis tendon transfer to the dorsum of the foot (Fig. 178.14*A*, *B*). In the skeletally immature, avoid damage to the first metatarsal physis when performing proximal osteotomies.

In the rigid, skeletally mature foot, definitive procedures include radical plantar fascial release (Steindler plantar flexor tenotomy) to relieve midfoot cavus; transfer of the posterior tibialis tendon through the tibiofibular interosseous membrane to the dorsum of the foot to achieve dorsiflexion of the ankle; transfer of the extensor hallucis longus tendon to the neck of the first metatarsal

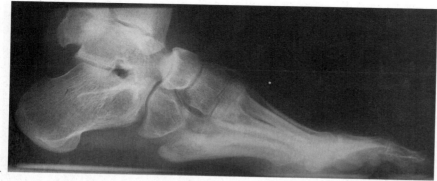

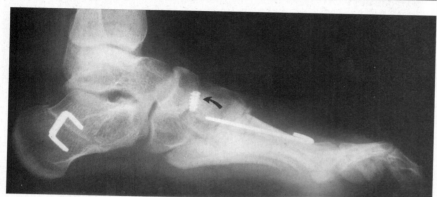

Figure 178.14. Preoperative (**A**) and postoperative radiographs of a cavovarus foot (**B**). Surgery included a plantarmedial release; extension osteotomy of the first metatarsal, Dwyer calcaneal osteotomy, and anterior transfer of the tibialis posterior tendon (note method of fixation of tendon at arrow).

and interphalangeal fusion (Jones procedure); correction of claw toes by interphalangeal joint arthrodesis; and extensor tendon release or transfer, calcaneal and metatarsal osteotomies to correct a rigid cavus foot; or as a salvage procedure for severe deformity, triple arthrodesis to correct severe heel varus and severe midfoot deformity and achieve hind foot stability (7,10,57,90,91,176,181,210, 281,325,361,376) (Fig. 178.15A, B). Tendon transfer is rarely indicated in the adult foot without an associated bone realignment.

Long-term review of patients with triple arthrodesis indicates satisfactory results, but there is a high incidence of radiologic ankle and midfoot arthritis (289,364). A study of triple arthrodesis using force plate analysis demonstrates increased midfoot load bearing and load concentration under the metatarsal heads (318). The incidence of pseudarthrosis, typically in the talonavicular joint, is reported to occur up to 25% of the time. This can be symptomatic and require revision surgery (289).

Transfer of the Common Extensor Tendon to the Third Cuneiform for Claw Toe Deformities (Hibbs Procedure)

■ Make a slightly curved, longitudinal incision on the dorsum of the common extensor tendons, centered over the third cuneiform (126).

■ Incise the subcutaneous tissue by sharp dissection, and protect any neurovascular structures.

■ Divide the common extensor tendons as far distally as possible.

■ Drill a 6.3 mm diameter hole in the third cuneiform from dorsal to plantar.

■ With a pullout suture, draw the proximal ends of the common extensor tendons into the drill hole, and secure the pullout suture on the plantar surface over a padded button.

■ Close the wound, and apply a well-padded short-leg cast for 6 weeks.

Midanterior Tarsal Wedge Osteotomy for Cavus Deformity (Cole Procedure)

■ Make a dorsolongitudinal skin incision over the extensor tendons to the third and fourth toes, beginning just proximal to the midtarsal joints and extending distally through the middle of the metatarsals (57).

■ Separate the extensor tendons to the third and fourth toes, and excise the periosteum overlying the tarsal bones.

■ Identify the tarsal bones radiographically.

■ Perform a dorsally based wedge osteotomy centered over the navicular medially and the cuboid laterally to include the navicular cuneiform joints. The width of the

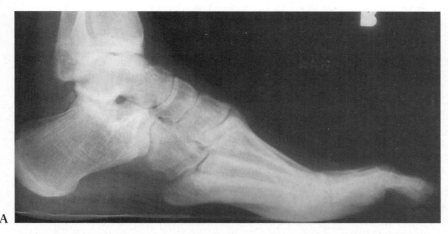

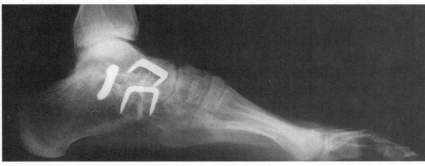

Figure 178.15. Pre- (**A**) and postoperative radiographs of a cavovarus foot treated by a triple arthrodesis (**B**).

wedge is determined by the severity of the deformity to be corrected.

- Remove the dorsal wedge, and elevate the forefoot to close the wedge osteotomy. Be sure to correct for rotation deformities (e.g., pronation, supination) of the forefoot at this time.
- Close the periosteum with interrupted sutures, and approximate the skin. Apply a short-leg plaster cast from the toes to the knee. Adequate healing is usually obtained within 4 weeks.

Calcaneal Osteotomy for Pes Cavovarus Deformity (Dwyer Procedure)

- Expose the lateral area of the calcaneus through an incision parallel, posterior, and inferior to the peroneus longus tendon (89).
- Strip the periosteum of the lateral area of the calcaneus superiorly and inferiorly.
- Remove a laterally based wedge of bone from the calcaneus just posterior, inferior, and parallel to the peroneus longus tendon. The medial edge of the wedge should not penetrate the medial cortex of the calcaneus.
- Correct the varus deformity of the calcaneus by closing the osteotomy and fracturing its medial cortex. Dorsiflex the forefoot against the pull of the tendo Achilles to stabilize the osteotomy. The varus deformity should

be corrected with the heel in neutral or slight valgus position.

- Close the wound and immobilize the foot in a short-leg cast until the osteotomy is healed in about 6 weeks.

Jones Procedure

- A Jones procedure is transfer of the extensor hallucis longus tendon to the neck of the first metatarsal and fusion of the interphalangeal joint.
- Make a dorsolongitudinal 1.5 cm incision over the interphalangeal joint of the hallux (181).
- Expose the extensor hallucis longus tendon, and cut it transversely 1 cm proximal to the interphalangeal joint.
- Cut the dorsal capsule of the interphalangeal joint transversely, and excise the cartilaginous surfaces of the interphalangeal joint.
- Insert a Kirschner wire from distal to proximal across the interphalangeal joint; cut the wire approximately 3 mm from the cutaneous margin, and bend it to prevent migration.
- Close the skin by interrupted sutures.
- Expose the neck of the first metatarsal through a dorsomedial 2.5 cm incision, dissect the extensor hallucis longus tendon, and protect the short extensor tendon.
- Periosteally expose the neck of the first metatarsal and drill a hole transversely through the longitudinal axis

of the bone approximately 1 cm proximal to the metarsophalangeal joint.

- Pass the extensor hallucis longus tendon through the hole, and suture it on itself with interrupted sutures.
- Close the wounds, and apply a well-padded short-leg cast, with a plantar extension to protect the toes.

Postoperatively, allow weight bearing after 2 weeks, and remove the cast and Kirschner wire 6 weeks after surgery.

Plantar Medial Release (Modified Steindler Procedure)

- Make a longitudinal 4 cm incision along the medial side of the foot from the calcaneal tuberosity distally (325). Separate the plantar aponeurosis from the plantar foot muscles, and incise the plantar fascia transversely at the plantar surface of the calcaneus.
- With a blunt periosteal elevator, lift the origins of the abductor hallucis muscle, the flexor digitorum brevis muscle, and the abductor digitiminimi muscle from the periosteum of the calcaneus. Avoid removal of cortical bone or periosteum with the fascia and muscle attachments.
- Carry the dissection to the calcaneocuboid joint, releasing the quadratus plantae and the long plantar ligament. The entire dissection should be carried out near the periosteum of the calcaneus, avoiding neurovascular structures.
- Then dorsiflex the foot to the corrected position and close the skin.
- Apply a well-padded short-leg cast with particular attention to adequate padding over the metatarsal heads and dorsum of the foot to prevent pressure necrosis of the skin.

Postoperatively, maintain the cast for 6 weeks. Apply serial stretching casts on a weekly basis to obtain adequate correction, if desired, beginning about 1 week after surgery.

Triple Arthrodesis

- Make a straight 5 cm incision obliquely over the sinus tarsi, extending from the peroneus brevis tendon to the extensor tendons.
- Dissect the subcutaneous tissue sharply, and distally reflect the tendinous origin of the extensor brevis tendon.
- Incise the capsule of the calcaneocuboid joint, and remove the articular surfaces with an osteotome.
- Then incise the lateral capsule of the talonavicular joint, and remove the articular surfaces of this joint with an osteotome. A small incision over the medial aspect of the talonavicular joint allows better visualization for cartilage removal.
- Incise the capsule of the subtalar joint. With an osteotome, excise the surfaces of the anterior, medial, and posterior articular facets of the subtalar joint. Carefully

remove the medial borders of the subtalar joint so that the neurovascular bundle and tendons are not damaged.

- Remove wedges of bone as necessary to correct any deformity, and position the foot in the neutral position. Maintain the foot in the neutral position, and suture the reflected flap of the extensor digitorum brevis in the sinus tarsi. Fixation can be achieved with staples, Steinman pins, or cannulated screws.
- Close the wound and overlay it with a gauze dressing. Apply a well-padded long-leg cast as the foot is maintained in neutral position.

Postoperatively, triple arthrodesis typically requires 12 weeks to heal. In patients in whom continued ambulation and standing are necessary for maintenance of function, walking may begin as soon as tolerable, but periodic radiographs are necessary to verify proper foot position.

Claw Toes

The claw toe deformity (Fig. 178.16) is caused by intrinsic muscle weakness that allows the long toe flexor muscles to continue to flex the interphalangeal joint and the long toe extensor muscles to extend the metatarsophalangeal joint without stability provided by the weak intrinsic muscles. Callosities develop over the heads of the proximal phalanges from contact in the shoes and under the metatarsal heads. Initially, clawing is flexible and should receive daily manipulative therapy. Fixed clawing requires operative treatment, which is usually performed simultaneously with other procedures for the cavus foot. Our choice of treatment of the second to fifth toes includes a tenotomy of the long extensor tendons, dorsal capsulotomy of the metatarsophalangeal joint, and arthrodesis of the interphalangeal joint if the toes cannot come down into 20° of passive flexion.

- Stabilize the interphalangeal arthrodesis with intramedullary Kirschner wire fixation.
- Transfer the extensor tendons to the middorsal area of the foot to assist in active dorsiflexion of the foot, if desired (Hibbs procedure).
- For clawing of the hallux, transplant the long extensor tendon to the neck of the first metatarsal (Jones procedure), and perform interphalangeal joint fusion. Take care not to damage the extensor brevis tendon, or the hallux will droop.

Extensor Tendon Tenotomy, Dorsal Capsulotomy of the Proximal Interphalangeal Joint, and Interphalangeal Fusion

- Make a 1 cm dorsolongitudinal incision over the proximal interphalangeal joint of the toe.
- By sharp dissection, identify the common extensor tendon, and incise it transversely.
- Then incise the dorsal capsule of the proximal interpha-

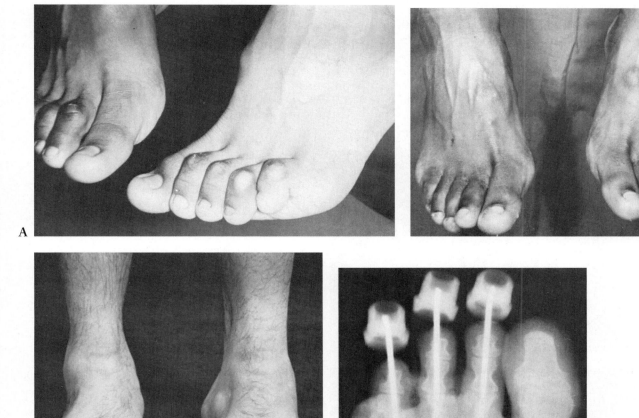

Figure 178.16. **A:** Preoperative photograph of flexible claw toes in a patient with Charcot-Marie-Tooth disease. **B:** The toes corrected. **C:** Preoperative photograph of rigid claw toes in a patient with Charcot-Marie-tooth disease. **D:** Postoperative radiograph demonstrates straightening of the toes by an interphalangeal fusion with Kirschner wires.

langeal joint transversely, and expose the articular surface by flexing the toe.

- With an osteotome, excise the articular surfaces of the interphalangeal joint, and then close the incision.
- Extend the toe to a neutral position, and place a smooth Kirschner wire from the tip of the distal phalanx through the distal phalangeal joint and proximal interphalangeal joint to the proximal phalanx.
- Cut the Kirschner wire 0.5 cm from the tip of the phalanx and bend it at least 45° to prevent proximal migration.

After surgery, the toes are protected by a well-padded short-leg cast with the plantar surface extending well past the phalanges, or have the patient wear a hard-sole wooden shoe until interphalangeal arthrodesis has occurred in about 4 weeks.

Scoliosis

There is a 10% incidence of scoliosis in hereditary motor and sensory neuropathy types I and II (157). The other types of hereditary sensory-motor neuropathy also have associated scoliosis, but the incidence is unknown. Progressive curves between 20° and 40° in immature patients are treated by a thoracolumbosacral orthosis until maturity. The amount of progression after treatment is unknown. Progressive curves greater than 40° to 50° in immature patients are treated by a posterior spinal fusion and instrumentation. The patterns are similar to those seen in idiopathic scoliosis. The fusion should include the measured curve (i.e., Cobb method) and additional vertebrae as necessary to achieve adequate truncal balance because of the associated truncal weakness. No patients in our series have required fusion to the sacrum or to the cervical area. Because there is a high incidence of failure of somatosensory-evoked potential monitoring, preparation must be made for a wake-up test (195).

Claw Hands

Intrinsic muscle weakness (Fig. 178.17) interferes with fine motor coordination, as in writing, and wrist weakness makes sports and carrying heavy objects difficult. Most patients tolerate the weakness by adjusting their lifestyle or by using simple adaptive equipment. In some patients with type I hereditary sensory-motor neuropathy and moderate weakness, opponensplasty with intrinsic muscle reconstruction is helpful (234,375). Kling and Drennan (192) reported on a small group of patients with type II

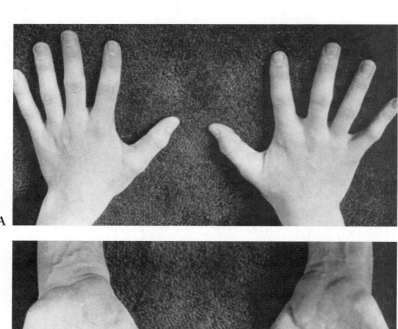

A

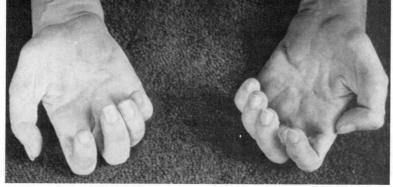

B

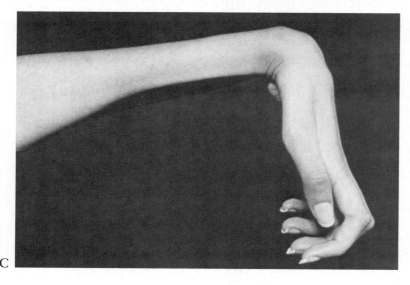

C

Figure 178.17. **A:** Hands with intrinsic muscle weakness caused by Charcot-Marie-Tooth disease. **B:** Claw hands caused by muscle weakness and contractures from Charcot-Marie-Tooth disease. **C:** A functionless hand with severely atrophic muscles from Charcot-Marie-Tooth disease.

hereditary sensory-motor neuropathy who developed severe upper extremity atrophy, which leads to a functionless hand. An orthosis may help to maintain a neutral posture.

Hip Dysplasia

Severe bilateral hip dysplasia has been reported in patients with onset of neuropathy in the first decade of life (198, 357). The dysplasia can be asymptomatic or minimally symptomatic and may remain undetected until early adolescence. Children with Charcot-Marie-Tooth disease need to be evaluated radiographically to detect early dysplasia. Typically, the femur has mild coxa valga and anteversion, and the superolateral corner of the acetabulum is deficient, which allows lateral subluxation during ambulation (Fig. 178.18). The acetabular dysplasia is treated by redirection of the acetabulum by single, double, or triple innominate osteotomies or shelf arthroplasty, depending on the severity of the deformity (286,323). The Chiari procedure may be necessary if severe changes in the acetabulum prevent the femoral head from being fully reduced into the true acetabulum.

Hereditary Sensory Neuropathies

Hereditary sensory neuropathies are characterized by decreased specific sensory perceptions, painless ulcerations, and Charcot joints. There are four major hereditary sensory neuropathies: autosomal dominant hereditary sensory neuropathy, autosomal recessive hereditary sensory neuropathy, familial dysautonomia (Riley-Day syndrome), and familial sensory neuropathy with anhidrosis (248,259).

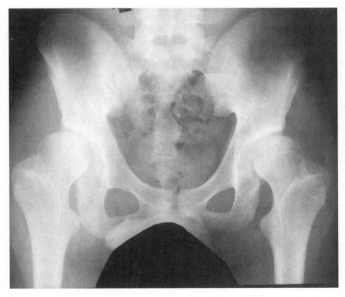

Figure 178.18. Hip dysplasia in a 16-year-old boy with CMT IA.

Patients with autosomal dominant hereditary sensory neuropathy have marked loss of sensation to pin prick and temperature in the lower extremities that can result in severe trophic changes. The upper extremities are less involved. A nerve biopsy shows a decreased number of myelinated sensory fibers. In autosomal recessive hereditary sensory neuropathy, the sensation of touch is more severely affected than those of pain and temperature, but the upper and lower extremities are severely affected, and nerve biopsy shows a total absence of myelinated sensory nerve fibers.

Familial dysautonomia, a disease of the peripheral nervous system secondary to a gene defect at the 9q31-33 locus, is characterized by a reduction in small and large myelinated nerve fibers. Clinical manifestations include a labile blood pressure, insensitivity to pain, abnormal gastrointestinal mobility, lack of fungiform papillae on the tongue, ataxia, areflexia and kyphoscoliosis. It occurs in Ashkenazi Jews with a prevalence of 1/3600. The children develop a progressive kyphoscoliosis, and death usually occurs in infancy or childhood from chronic pulmonary insufficiency and aspiration (267,268,379). Familial sensory neuropathy with anhidrosis is characterized by decreased temperature perception, intact touch sensation, absent axon reflex to histamine, below-normal intelligence, and anhidrosis.

Orthopaedic problems in patients with hereditary sensory neuropathy include Charcot joints, joint dislocations, fractures, chronic osteomyelitis, and severe kyphoscoliosis (215,256). Treatment of spinal deformity is difficult because of the typical high rigid kyphosis, osteopenia, labile autonomic nervous system, and insensitivity to pain. Spinal fusion and instrumentation have a high incidence of complications but is beneficial (280).

Charcot Joints   A Charcot joint is characterized by a painless arthropathy in which the synovium is hypertrophic, ligamentous laxity causing joint instability, and eventual joint surface destruction. The lack of protective sensation allows unrestricted repetitive trauma, and large weight-bearing joints are most frequently and severely involved. Recurrent microtrauma causes synovial inflammation, hemarthrosis, periosteal elevation with subsequent cortical bone thickening, physeal widening, osteonecrosis, and osteochondritis dissecans. Minor trauma can lead to undetected dislocations and fractures (1,180, 194).

Treatment initially involves protecting the joint from trauma by patient training, adaptive tools to reduce traumatic exposure, and protective orthoses. Joint instability usually can be treated by an orthosis, or if it is severe, a fusion can be attempted. Fusions are difficult to achieve and require prolonged immobilization; because delayed union and pseudarthrosis are common, augmentation with a bone graft is often required. A fusion also tends to transfer stress to adjacent joints, which can become deformed. Periodic radiographic spinal evaluation should be performed to detect early Charcot changes of vertebrae and to allow treatment by a spinal fusion to prevent neurologic damage. Osteomyelitis by hematogenous or contiguous spread occurs frequently in Charcot joints. Cutaneous ulcers should be protected to eliminate repetitive trauma and should be treated aggressively with local care to obtain healing. After a joint is infected, the prognosis is poor. Antibiotic therapy, protection of the extremity, and excision of infected or necrotic bone may contain the infection, but uncontrolled infection may require amputation (136).

Neuropathic Ulcers   Neuropathic ulcers are caused by repetitive trauma to an anesthetized area. In children, the hands may be mutilated by repetitive biting or other trauma, causing ulceration, osteomyelitis, and autoamputation of the phalanges. In childhood, ulcerations of the feet are most common (Fig. 178.19). The only effective therapy is to teach the patient protective techniques and to use protective orthoses.

Friedreich's Ataxia

Friedreich's ataxia (i.e., hereditary spinocerebellar ataxia) is the most common spinocerebellar degenerative disease. It usually is autosomal recessive, although it may be autosomal dominant or sex linked (20). The gene abnormality is on chromosome 9 (55). The onset is at the end of the first decade and is characterized by progressive ataxia of the limbs and of gait, the presence of Romberg's sign, absent knee and ankle reflexes, extensor plantar responses, dysarthria, scoliosis, pes cavus, weakness, loss of

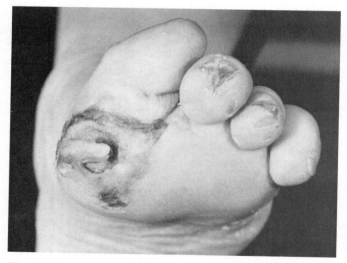

Figure 178.19. Neuropathic ulcer in a patient with hereditary sensory neuropathy.

position and vibration sense in the legs, cardiomyopathy, and diabetes (30,131,202).

By the age of 15 years, most patients are severely ataxic; by 20 years of age (average, 15.8 years), most are confined to a wheelchair; and by 40 years of age (average, 36 years), death occurs from cardiopulmonary failure (47,160,338). Sural nerve biopsies show axonal degeneration; the central nervous system exhibits changes in the posterolateral columns of the spinal cord and cell loss in the deep cerebellar nuclei. Muscle biopsy reveals fiber group atrophy characteristic of denervation (88).

Although there is no known cure for Friedreich's ataxia, treatment of the orthopaedic deformities of pes cavus and scoliosis substantially enhances the quality of life, especially in the less severely involved patient.

Foot Deformities   The foot deformities of Friedreich's ataxia are an equinus foot, pes cavovarus, tripod stance, and claw toes. As in Charcot-Marie-Tooth disease, the intrinsic muscles are weak, with the foot everters and dorsiflexors being weaker than the foot inverters and plantar flexors, unlike the usual Charcot-Marie-Tooth disease, the severe ataxia causes a markedly unstable foot.

The goals of treatment are achieving a stable plantigrade foot, balancing muscle function, and correcting deformity. In the immature foot, which is almost always flexible, an ankle-foot orthosis and stretching exercises are usually sufficient. More rigid foot deformities occur during the adolescent years. Our preference for treatment of the cavus foot and instability is a triple arthrodesis; for the muscle imbalance, a transfer of the posterior tibialis tendon through the interosseous membrane to the dorsum of the foot is indicated; and for claw toes, an interphalangeal joint arthrodesis is preferred (217). These surgical techniques were previously described under peripheral neuropathies.

Scoliosis   Severe scoliosis occurs in more than 80% of patients presenting between ages 9 and 21 years and is relentlessly progressive, even after skeletal maturity (47, 66,112,157,160,203). Scoliosis in this disorder is not a collapsing spine disorder, such as that seen in poliomyelitis. It is very similar to idiopathic scoliosis in its behavior. A thoracolumbar orthosis may be prescribed for a curve between 20° and 40°, but there is insufficient evidence to support the efficacy of this treatment, and at best, it only slows progression (47,66). The orthosis is poorly tolerated in ataxic, unstable ambulatory patients, because it eliminates trunk motion used to correct imbalance during gait. Nighttime bracing often is an acceptable compromise. For progressive scoliosis greater than 40° to 60°, extension of the fusion to the sacrum is not always required. A posterior spinal fusion from the high thoracic area is indicated. Segmental instrumentation should be used, which allows for rapid postoperative mobilization without a brace. A thorough cardiopulmonary evaluation and ongoing monitoring are mandatory because virtually all patients have cardiomyopathy.

SPINAL MUSCULAR ATROPHY

Spinal muscular atrophy is a group of hereditary illnesses with proximal muscle weakness caused by degeneration of the anterior horn cells of the spinal cord and bulbar motor nuclei (337). The hypotonia is symmetric, the lower extremities are weaker than the upper extremities, there is no sensory loss or upper motor neuron signs, and fasciculations of the tongue and tremors of the hands are common (46,350). Cardiac function is not impaired. The prognosis for life expectancy depends on respiratory capacity. The spinal muscular atrophies are divided into several syndromes according to the severity of weakness, age at onset of symptoms, distribution of muscle weakness, and pattern of heredity (334) (Table 178.3). The clinical presentations of the syndromes vary and may overlap in the spectrum of syndromes (133). The most common forms are types I, II, and III (184,253,254).

Type I spinal muscular atrophy (i.e., Werdnig-Hoffmann disease) is the most severe illness. The onset occurs within the first 3 months of life, and the patient presents with progressive weakness and hypotonia with spontaneous movement confined to the toes, fingers, and hands. Infants with this disease are never able to develop head control or roll over, bulbar weakness results in difficulty in sucking, tendon reflexes are absent, and death usually occurs within the first year of life, before significant orthopaedic problems develop (40,165,363). Types I, II and III are caused by abnormalities of the survival motorneuron gene (SMN) on chromosome 5.

In Type II spinal muscular atrophy (i.e., intermediate to severe spinal muscular atrophy) the infant develops normally for the first 6 months of life and learns to sit, but symmetric proximal muscle weakness ensues (155). The children never stand or walk. Fasciculations of the tongue and a fine motor tremor of the hand are helpful diagnostic signs. The weakness is moderate, with survival until late adolescence or early adult life. The patients must use a wheelchair, and they develop postural contractures of hip flexion, knee flexion, and foot equinus. Scoliosis is common, progressing rapidly and markedly reducing respiratory ability. Prognosis is related to the progressive muscle weakness and spinal deformity, which eventually lead to respiratory failure.

Type III spinal muscular atrophy (i.e., Kugelberg-Welander disease, mild spinal muscular atrophy) has an insidious onset in children from 2 to 12 years of age with episodes of weakness. Patients have a waddling gait, with difficulty in climbing steps and getting up from the floor. The prognosis is good, and there is only a minimal respiratory deficit. Patients tend to have flat feet (eversion of the foot), pelvic girdle weakness, a mild hand tremor, and scoliosis (129,196).

Evans and Drennan (107) group patients with spinal muscular atrophy according to function. Group I children are unable to sit independently and usually die in infancy of pulmonary failure. Group II children develop head control, can sit independently, and usually survive until young adult life. Group III patients pull to stand and walk, and may live into the fourth decade. Group IV patients can walk, run and climb steps, but usually require wheelchairs by the third decade and have a long life expectancy (107, 383). The major orthopaedic problems are spinal deformities, contractures, and hip instability.

Spinal Deformities

Spinal deformities develop in virtually all patients who are poor ambulators and in about half of those who initially

Table 178.3.   Types of Spinal Muscular Atrophy

Form	Age at onset	Progression of disability	Inheritance
Type I	<3 mg	Rapid	Autosomal recessive
Type II	6 mos–3 yr	Moderately rapid	Autosomal recessive
Type III	1–15 yr	Moderate	Autosomal recessive
Adult (254)	18–50 yr	Slow	Probably recessive
Scapular Peroneal atrophy (184)	Variable	Slow	Autosomal dominant
Charcot-Marie-Tooth disease-neuronal (93)	Variable	Slow	Autosomal dominant
Facioscapulohumeral-neurogenic (109)	Variable	Slow	Autosomal dominant
Distal (235)	Variable	Slow	Autosomal recessive

learn to walk and run. The most common deformity is a long C-shaped scoliosis, and severe pelvic obliquity develops as the curve progresses. A kyphosis is usually associated with the scoliosis, and a progressive spinal deformity decreases pulmonary capacity and jeopardizes sitting posture (66,81,150,157,228,294). In a series of patients followed at the Alfred I. duPont Hospital for Children (Wilmington, DE), the average age at onset of scoliosis was 7.6 years (range, infancy to 13 years) (8). In a mild deformity, a soft thoracolumbosacral orthosis with a large abdominal relief provides trunk support and may delay progression of the curve, but the orthosis must not compress the chest and further compromise respiratory function (228). Pulmonary function evaluations before and after application of the orthosis are used to determine safe parameters, because often an orthosis decreases the tidal volume by as much as 20% (8). In severely compromised patients, the posterior half of an orthosis may be used alone, but this is less effective. Typically, scoliosis is progressive, and when the curve reaches 40° to 45°, a posterior spinal fusion from the high thoracic area to the sacrum with internal fixation is recommended. In a child younger than 10 years old with a progressive scoliosis greater than 60°, surgery is indicated.

Before any anticipated surgical procedure, pulmonary evaluation must be performed. Severe postoperative respiratory problems are seen with a vital capacity less than 25% normal (228). An intense respiratory rehabilitation program, emphasizing inhalation strength, coughing, and maintenance of good pulmonary hygiene, can temporarily improve respiratory ability by about 15% to help during the perioperative period. After surgery, the pulmonary function usually returns to the preoperative level and gradually declines, but one study suggests an improvement (271).

We prefer segmental fixation with the Luque rods and Galveston pelvic fixation or the unit rod in this group of patients because they allow rapid postoperative mobilization, which helps in the general care and especially in pulmonary care (39,258). Patients with spinal muscular atrophy typically have severely osteopenic bone, and supplementary bone grafts are necessary to achieve an adequate fusion mass. Loss of pelvic fixation due to the rods cutting out of the ilium anteriorly requires revision because colonic perforation can occur (228). In young children with a large deformity and osteopenic bone, do not attempt an extensive correction, and use the smaller $\frac{1}{4}$- or $\frac{3}{16}$-inch rods. Rod connectors when using Luque rods prevent rod shift and increasing deformity. For 3 to 4 months postoperatively, a thoracolumbosacral orthosis can be used when the patient is sitting or standing to give additional support and to prevent the wires of the Luque rod or unit rod from pulling loose from the osteopenic bone. In patients with severe respiratory compromise with a large curve, the usual methods of internal fixation may

be impossible, and halo-dependent traction followed by spinal fusion and limited instrumentation may be the only reasonable alternative. Anterior spinal fusions generally are not recommended in patients with spinal muscular atrophy because postoperative respiratory compromise is severe (8,228). Postoperative ventilation for 24 to 48 hours in an intensive care unit is often required. For all patients, the period of immobilization should be only a few days, and sitting or ambulation should be started as soon as tolerable, except for the rare problem requiring the halo-dependent technique. Even in this situation, the patient can be up in a wheelchair in overhead traction during the day.

Contractures

Contractures develop in the upper and lower extremities and are more frequently seen in the severely weak children. Flexion contractures of the elbow and adduction contractures of the shoulder are common but rarely a functional problem. Bedridden infants assume a frog-leg position, and lower extremity contractures occur with the hip in flexion abduction, the knee flexed, and the foot in equinus. Wheelchair-dependent patients develop flexion contractures of the hip and knee and equinovarus deformity of the foot (107). Ambulatory patients have only mild contractures, which seldom interfere with walking. A maintenance motion-therapy program with intermittent splinting can control most contractures, and surgery is seldom required. Soft-tissue procedures are effective in reducing contractures but are indicated only if a contracture inhibits some functional ability or becomes painful. Surgical releases are used to get these children into long-leg braces or a standing frame. Hip flexion contractures require release of the fascia lata, sartorius, rectus femoris, and iliopsoas. Knee flexion contractures require tenotomy of the medial and lateral hamstrings and iliotibial band. Foot deformities seldom require surgery, but a severe equinovarus contracture occasionally causes a skin ulceration on the foot. Tenotomy of the tendo Achilles and posterior tibialis tendon with manipulation and casting for 6 weeks with lightweight plastic material are usually adequate to correct the foot posture.

Hip instability is a common problem in the more severe types of spinal muscular atrophy (107,294,341). Hip dislocation was seen in 50% of the functional group I children, 39% of group II, 37% of group III, but it did not occur in group IV, according to an unpublished series. The highest incidence of hip pain occurred in the group II children. In children who are limited ambulators or confined to a wheelchair and have a mobile painless dislocated hip, nonoperative management is recommended.

POLIOMYELITIS

Poliomyelitis is an acute enteroviral illness that selectively involves the anterior horn cells of the spinal cord and the brain stem motor nuclei. New cases have been rare since prophylactic vaccines became available in the 1960s (282, 285). The virus is transmitted by the oropharyngeal-fecal route, and humans are the reservoir. The incubation period is 6 to 20 days, and an estimated 1% to 2% of infected people develop neural symptoms. Coxsackieviruses and echoviruses produce a similar illness and should be considered in sporadic cases.

The illness is divided into three stages: acute, convalescent, and chronic. The acute stage begins with gastrointestinal symptoms (e.g., nausea, vomiting, sore throat), a febrile illness (usually less than 103°F), followed by meningeal symptoms (e.g., headache, nuchal rigidity, back pain, pain on straight-leg raising), and severe muscle pain. An asymmetric paralysis occurs within 2 days of the meningeal symptoms and usually reaches its maximum within 48 hours. The legs are usually weaker than the arms, but weakness may occur in any muscle group, including the bulbar muscles. The most commonly involved muscles are the gluteal muscles, hip flexors, quadriceps, tibialis anterior, medial hamstrings, deltoid, triceps, and pectoralis major (299). There is no sensory loss, and the cerebrospinal fluid has a high protein level in the active stage. The EMG and muscle biopsy results show denervation. During the acute phase, patients should minimize activities (usually by bed rest), apply hot packs to painful muscles, position extremities in the anatomic position to prevent contractures, and perform general passive range of motion on all joints to the limits of tolerance (293). The acute stage ends when the temperature is normal for 48 hours and there is absence of progressive muscle involvement.

The convalescent stage begins 48 hours after the temperature has returned to normal and continues for as long as 2 years, during which time muscle strength improves spontaneously. The major recovery occurs in the first month, with the exception of the triceps surae and deltoid muscles, which improve much more slowly. Sharrard (300) reports recovery of muscle strength to average two grades above the level at 1 month and one grade above the level at 6 months. Orthopaedic treatment consists of restoring a full range of motion of joints, correcting contractures, and maximizing muscle strength. Overactivity of muscles in the early convalescent stage can inhibit functional return, and contractures of antagonistic muscles must be stretched before weaker muscles are exercised. Braces and orthoses may be used at night to prevent deformities and during therapy sessions to assist function. Equinus deformity of the foot requires a short-leg brace, and quadriceps weakness of grade IV or less requires a long-leg brace with knee-hinge locks.

The chronic stage begins 2 years after the onset of weakness, and no further muscle strength recovery is anticipated. Orthopaedic treatment consists of managing the chronic consequences of paralysis, muscle imbalance, and growth. Joint imbalance is classified into two types: flaccid joints (i.e., negative, static) and active joints with muscle imbalance (i.e., dynamic). Flaccid joints deform only if allowed to be postured in an abnormal position over prolonged periods (139). Deformity can be prevented by maintaining the joint in a neutral position by an orthosis and an exercise program. Active joints with muscle imbalance develop fixed deformities that begin as soft-tissue contractures and evolve into bony deformities that worsen with growth.

Orthopaedic treatment consists of prescribing orthoses, performing muscle-balancing procedures, and performing bony procedures (Tables 178.4 through 178.8). Orthoses can permanently stabilize a flaccid joint or augment function in a dynamically imbalanced joint. Spring-loaded orthoses are useful to counterbalance unopposed muscle tensions. Muscle-balancing procedures consist of tendon transfers, which produce joint stability and active motor power and eliminate deforming forces (292). The principles of tendon transfer demand that muscle of normal or good strength must be used because typically one grade of strength is lost after a transfer, and loss of function of the transferred muscle must be balanced or an iatrogenic deformity will occur (158,221,236,244). The joint to be moved by the transferred tendon must be free of deformity and have an acceptable range of motion, or the transferred tendon cannot overcome the deformity. The excursion and strength of the transferred muscle must be similar to those of the muscle being replaced, and good surgical technique is essential. The tendon must be routed straight from its origin to insertion, have a smooth gliding channel, and be placed under tension. Postoperative management of a transferred tendon usually includes immobilization for 4 weeks with the joint in a slightly overcorrected position, followed by guarded motion for an additional 3 to 4 weeks. Postoperative muscle training is important to obtain optimal function of transferred tendons.

Bony procedures are directed toward correcting fixed deformities and stabilizing joints (56,205,242,243). Residual growth and loss of joint function must be considered before performing a bony procedure. Ideally, bony procedures are not performed until the patient reaches about 12 years of age, when adequate growth has been achieved.

ARTHROGRYPOSIS

Arthrogryposis mutiplex congenita is a nonprogressive disorder associated with neurogenic and myopathic disease. It is characterized by rigid or dislocated joints, muscle atrophy or aplasia, fusiform or cylindrical extremities with thin subcutaneous tissue and lack of skin creases, and normal sensation and intelligence (3,19,79,119,255, 275,276,326). The pathogenesis involves severe weakness during early intrauterine life that restricts fetal mobility,

Table 178.4.   Selected Procedures for the Treatment of the Involved Hip in Poliomyelitis

Deformity	Treatment	References*
Flexion abduction, external rotation contractures	Ober fasciotomy Tachdjian, p. 1129	JBJS 18:105,936
	Young procedure JBJS 20:314, 1938 JBJS 31-A:141, 1941	JBJS 8:171, 926
Gluteus medius paralysis with hip instability	Mustard procedure JBJS 41-B:289, 1959	JBJS 34-A:64, 1952
	External oblique transfer to greater trochanter	JBJS 32-A:207, 1950 JBJS 45-A:199, 1963
	Posterior transfer of tensor	JAMA 80:242, 1923
	fasciae latae muscle	NEJM 209:61, 1933
Paralytic dislocation	Proximal femoral varus derotation osteotomy	JBJS 36-B:375, 1954 JBJS 44-B:573, 1962
	Open reduction	JBJS 41-B:279, 1959
	Arthrodeses	JBJS 32-A:904, 1950

* JBJS, Journal of Bone and Joint Surgery; Tachdjian, M. O. Tachdjian (ed.), Congenital Dislocation of the Hip, New York, Churchill Livingstone, 1982; JAMA, Journal of the American Medical Association; NEJM, New England Journal of Medicine.

Table 178.5.   Selected Procedures for the Treatment of the Involved Knee in Poliomyelitis

Deformity	Treatment	References*
Quadriceps femoris paralysis	Biceps femoris and semitendinosus transfer	JBJS 37-A:347, 1955 JBJS 13:515, 1931 JBJS 30-A:541, 1948
Flexion contracture	Soft-tissue release or femoral osteotomy	JBJS 20:839, 1938 JBJS 11:40, 1927
Genu recurvatum	Tibial osteotomy	JAMA 120:207, 1942 AOS 114:40, 1957
	Irwin technique	Ingram
	Soft-tissue tenodesis	JBJS 58-A:978, 1976
Flail knee	Orthosis with drop-lock knee and arthrodesis	AS 40:90, 1940

* JBJS, Journal of Bone and Joint Surgery; JAMA, Journal of the American Medical Association; AOS, Acta Orthopaedica Scandinavica; Ingram, A. T. Ingram, Paralytic disorders, In A. H. Crenshaw (ed.), Campbell's Operative Orthopaedics, p. 2979, St. Louis, C.V. Mosby Co., 1987; AS, Archives of Surgery.

Table 178.6. Selected Procedures for the Treatment of the Involved Shoulder in Poliomyelitis

Deformity	Treatment	References*
Partial deltoid paralysis	Anterior advancement of deltoid	Ingram
Extensive paralysis	Shoulder arthrodesis	
	Charnley	JBJS 46-B:614, 1964
	Gill	JBJS 13:287, 1931
	Watson-Jones	JBJS 15:862, 1933

* Ingram, A. T. Ingram, Paralytic disorders, In A. H. Crenshaw (ed.), Campbell's Operative Orthopaedics, p. 3002, St. Louis, C.V. Mosby Co., 1987; JBJS, Journal of Bone and Joint Surgery.

with subsequent loss of muscle mass and contractures of joints. All extremities are involved in 46% of patients with arthrogryposis, only lower extremities in 43%, and only upper extremities in 11% (335). Serum CPK, chromosomal analysis, EMG, and nerve conduction studies are rarely helpful in diagnosis, but a muscle biopsy may show neuropathic or myopathic changes. More than 90% of these patients have neurogenic illnesses, and 7% have myogenic disorders (18,342).

Although more than 150 conditions have been associated with congenital contractures, amyoplasia congenita or arthrogryposis multiplex congenita accounts for the classic form of arthrogryposis that is characterized by symmetric contractures; internally rotated shoulders, extended elbows, markedly flexed hands and wrists, flexed or extended knees, severe talipes equinovarus, frequently dislocated hips, and a port-wine stain over the forehead area (122,146). Even though these patients are severely disabled, many develop ambulatory potentials; 46.6% have independent ambulation, 33.3% walk with braces, and 20% use wheelchairs (322). Another infrequent form

of arthrogryposis is distal arthrogryposis, which has autosomal dominant transmission with variable penetrance. The hands and feet are primarily involved, but knees and hips occasionally are affected (147).

The combination of weakness and stiffness of joints in arthrogrypotic patients produces severe disabilities, and the goals of orthopaedic treatment are to obtain the maximum range of motion of joints and maintain the extremities in a functional position. Twenty-five percent of infants with multiple congenital contractures sustain birth fractures (usually of the femoral shaft) or epiphyseal separation, which are attributed to difficult deliveries. If they are not displaced, these fractures heal rapidly with splint immobilization (76).

Contractures

Initial therapy for all contractures consists of passive stretching and serial splinting to improve joint motion (132,251). Passive stretching exercises are performed at least four times daily and are guided by the patient's parents, who are trained and supervised by physical thera-

Table 178.7. Selected Procedures for the Treatment of the Involved Elbow in Poliomyelitis

Deformity	Treatment	References*
Paralysis of flexion	Steindler flexorplasty	AAOS 1:276, 1944
		JBJS 45-A:513, 1963
	Clark pectoralis major transfer	JBJS 34:180, 1946
	Carol triceps transfer	JBJS 52-A:239, 1970

* AAOS, American Academy of Orthopaedic Surgeons Instructional Course Lectures; JBJS, Journal of Bone and Joint Surgery.

Table 178.8. Selected Procedures for the Treatment of the Involved Foot and Ankle in Poliomyelitis		
Deformity	**Treatment**	**References***
Paralysis of peroneal muscle	Lateral transfer of anterior tibial tendon to bone of second or third metatarsal	Ingram
Paralysis of anterior tibial muscle	Anterior transfer of peroneal longus	SGO 86:717, 1948
Paralysis of triceps surae	Transfer of peroneus longus and brevis posterior tibial, flexor hallucis longus, tibialis anterior	JBJS 38-A:751, 1956 JBJS 48-A:1541, 1966 JBJS 40-A:911, 1958
Paralysis of tibialis anterior, toe extensors, and peronei	Anterior transfer of tibialis posterior to bone of third metatarsal	JBJS 37-A:396, 1955 JBJS 36-A:1 181, 1954
Instability or deformity	Triple arthrodesis	
	Ryerson	JBJS 5:453, 1923
	Lambrinudi	PRSM 26:788, 1933
	Hoke	AJOS 3:494, 1921
	Subtalar arthrodesis-Grice	JBJS 34-A:927, 1952
	Pantalar arthrodesis	JBJS 47-A: 1315, 1965
	Calcaneal osteotomy	JBJS 59-B:233, 1977
	Dwyer	JBJS 41-B:80, 1959
	Evans	JBJS 57-B:270, 1975
Flexible claw toes	Girdlestone-Taylor transfer	JBJS 33-B:539, 1951
	Jones procedure	BMJ 1:749, 1916
Pes cavus	Steindler stripping	AJOS 2:8, 1920
	Cole dorsal tarsal wedge	JBJS 22:895, 1940

* Ingram, A. T. Ingram, Paralytic disorders, In A. H. Crenshaw (ed.), Campbell's Operative Orthopaedics, p. 2931, St. Louis, C.V. Mosby Co., 1987; SGO, Surgery, Gynecology and Obstetrics; JBJS, Journal of Bone and Joint Surgery; PRSM, Proceedings of the Royal Society of Medicine; AJOS, American Journal of Orthopaedic Surgery; BMJ, British Medical Journal.

pists. Avoid rigid cast fixation for most patients. Many parents tend to exercise the extremity as a unit, and this should be discouraged; specific attention should be directed to passive stretching of independent joints. After each joint is passively stretched, apply thermoplastic splints between sessions to maintain position. The thermoplastic splints require frequent modifications as the patient grows and the joint mobility increases. In the knee and elbow, the contractures may be so severe that radiographs are occasionally necessary to determine the proper plane for passive flexion and extension exercises.

Upper Extremity Deformities

The goals of treatment of the upper extremity in children with arthrogryposis are to provide an extremity that can be brought to the mouth and stabilized for feeding and to provide for toilet care or pulling up from sitting (370).

Passive stretching exercises have been the most successful to obtain motion, but the wrist, shoulder, and fingers are the most resistant. The elbow achieves the most significant benefit from the stretching therapy, and mild changes substantially improve the ability to dress, self-feed, and care for personal hygiene. Defer most surgery until the patient is old enough to demonstrate functional achievements (211).

A derotation osteotomy of the humerus is occasionally useful if the hand is in a nonfunctional position from shoulder rotation. Perform the derotation osteotomy at the proximal third of the humerus, and immobilize the site in a shoulder spica cast until healing occurs. Tricepsplasty (i.e., lengthening of the triceps tendon and posterior capsulotomy of the elbow joint) is recommended by Williams (369) to restore motion to the extended elbow (235). Unfortunately, some motion is lost with growth. Flexor muscle power to the elbow can be facilitated by triceps tendon transfer, but this is done at the expense of active extension. In our experience, the pectoralis transfer by fascia lata extension through to the ulna has been most desirable. The maintenance of the triceps function is very helpful for the mobility of the patient. Transfer of function can be successful only if an adequate range of motion has been obtained by conservative or, if necessary, surgical methods.

The wrist flexion deformity can be managed by a proximal row carpectomy or wrist fusion toward the end of growth. Surgery of small joints of the hand has not been successful in achieving motion or improving function (21).

Tricepsplasty and Posterior Capsulotomy of the Elbow (Williams Procedure).

■ Make a posterolongitudinal incision from the distal third of the triceps tendon to 2 cm inferior to the olecranon.
■ Expose the triceps tendon, and incise it as an inverted V just below the musculotendinous junction.
■ Reflect the insertion of the triceps tendon distally, and incise the capsule between the humerus and olecranon. Gently flex the elbow. Tight collateral ligaments and occasionally the radiohumeral capsule may require division to obtain adequate flexion.
■ Protect the ulnar nerve by removing it from its sheath and allowing it to prolapse forward if any tension develops. The elbow should flex to at least 90°.
■ Repair the triceps tendon in the lengthened position by the V-Y technique, and close the wound.
■ Postoperative immobilization is necessary for 10 days, after which physical therapy is instituted to maintain the increased range of motion.

Steindler Flexorplasty of the Elbow

A Steindler flexorplasty of the elbow to restore active elbow flexion is indicated if there are active, strong forearm pronator and flexor muscles (e.g., pronator teres, flexor carpi radialis, palmaris longus, flexor digitorum sublimis, flexor carpi ulnaris), the elbow has adequate motion, the triceps muscle extends the elbow, and the elbow flexor muscles are paralyzed.

■ Make an approximately 9 cm curved longitudinal incision over the medial side of the elbow, beginning about 7 cm proximal to the medial epicondyle, extending over the posterior aspect of the medial epicondyle, and ending distally on the volar surface of the forearm along the pronator teres muscle. Identify the ulnar nerve.
■ Remove the common attachment of the flexors to the medial epicondyle with an osteotome.

■ Free the muscles distally for about 4 cm.
■ Flex the elbow, and reattach the excised medial epicondyle with its muscles to the humerus with a screw or strong sutures 5 cm proximally at the intermuscular septum between the brachialis and triceps.
■ Close the wound, and apply a cast with the elbow flexed and the forearm supinated.

Postoperatively, the cast is worn for about 6 weeks, after which begin active training.

Transfer of the Pectoralis Major Muscle to the Ulna with Fascial Graft

■ Place the patient in a supine position, with the arm held in mild abduction and the elbow extended.
■ Use two incisions. Make the first incision from the inferior half of the axillary crease distally to the level of the middle third of the humerus. Expose the insertion of the pectoralis major muscle, and free it from the humerus.
■ Make a transverse incision at the anterior aspect of the elbow. Carry dissection down bluntly to the anterior surface of the ulna.
■ Using the tip of the olecranon as a guide, expose the ulna anteriorly about 2 cm distal to this point.
■ Incise the periosteum and drill a hole in the ulna from anterior to posterior. Leave the drill in place.
■ Make an incision along the lateral aspect of the thigh from the greater trochanter to just above the knee.
■ Dissect free a strip of fascia lata as long and wide as possible, and remove it.
■ Close the wound in a routine manner, with no attempt to close the defect in the fascia lata.
■ Sew the fascia lata into a tube with interrupted stitches. Then pass the rolled-up fascia lata subcutaneously between the wounds on the forearm.
■ Crisscross a strong absorbable suture along the lower end of the fascia lata, and thread it onto two straight needles that are placed through the hole in the ulna after the drill point has been removed. Pull the end of the fascia lata down in to the ulna, and tie the free ends of the suture over a sponge and button.
■ Flex the elbow 70° to 90°, and drape the other end of the fascia lata around and suture it under slight tension to the pectoralis major.
■ Close the wounds, and apply a splint to hold the elbow at 90°.

At 2 to 3 weeks postoperatively, replace the cast by a dial lock brace to allow flexion and block extension just below a right angle. Gradually increase the extension over the next month, and have the patient exercise the elbow into flexion several times daily.

Anterior Transfer of the Triceps Muscle for Restoration of Elbow Flexion (Bunnell-Williams Procedure)

■ Make a posterolongitudinal incision over the distal

fourth of the triceps tendon, extending distally midway between the radius and ulna, over the proximal third of the forearm.

■ Dissect the triceps tendon off the olecranon with a strip of periosteum from the upper shaft of the ulna.

■ Mobilize the triceps off the humerus to the midhumeral level.

■ Flex the elbow 90°, and separate the interval between the brachioradialis and pronator teres muscles.

■ Roll the periosteal elongation of the triceps and tendon into a tube, pass it around the lateral side of the arm superficial to the radial nerve, and attach it to the bicipital tubercle of the radius through drill holes.

■ Secure the tendon under tension with the elbow almost fully flexed.

■ Close the wound.

Postoperatively, hold the arm in the flexed position for 1 month, after which general physical therapy can begin.

Carpectomy for Severe Flexion Deformity of the Wrist (White and Stubbins Procedure)

■ Expose the carpal bones through a transverse posterior incision.

■ Retract the extensor tendons medially and laterally to expose the dorsal area of the proximal row of carpal bones.

■ Excise the proximal row of carpal bone, and dorsiflex the wrist to test the position. If inadequate dorsiflexion is achieved, all carpal bones except the pisiform may be excised to obtain adequate dorsiflexion. Dorsiflex the wrist to about 20°, and hold the forearm in a neutral position.

After surgery, use a long-arm cast for 3 weeks, followed by a short-arm cast for an additional 2 to 3 weeks. After removal of the cast, have the patient wear a wrist splint part time, usually at night, to prevent recurrence of the flexion deformity.

Wrist Arthrodesis

■ Make a 6-cm incision dorsally, extending midway from the base of the second and third metacarpals, across Lister's tubercle proximally, and up the dorsal radial surface.

■ Dissect the interval between the extensor pollicis longus and the extensor digitorum communis.

■ Denude the dorsal surface of the radius, carpal bones, and proximal area of the second and third metacarpals of fibrous or granulation tissue to expose the distal radius, dorsal carpal bone, and proximal area of the second and third metacarpals.

■ Cut a 1 cm wide bony slot in the dorsal radius across the carpal bones (i.e., lunate, scaphoid, capitate, trapezoid) into the bases of the second and third metacarpals.

■ Place a corticocancellous iliac bone graft in the slot,

and close the wound. A Steinman pin placed down the third metacarpal into the radius provides some fixation.

After surgery, place the wrist in neutral, and apply a long-arm cast. This cast is worn until the arthrodesis is firm, usually 10 to 12 weeks.

Knee Deformities

The knee deserves early aggressive attention, because most patients with arthrogryposis can walk or stand if the knee is in a suitable position (317). Motion from at least 15° to 45° of flexion is desirable but may not be obtained in rigid extremities. Rigid knees that have 35° to 40° of flexion are stable for standing and sitting; full extension makes sitting awkward, and excessive flexion makes standing impossible. Knee flexion contractures (65% of patients) are more common than extension contractures (6%). Daily passive stretching with thermoplastic maintenance splinting is the most effective treatment to increase motion in infants and young children. Forty percent of patients can be managed by nonoperative treatment programs (339).

Recurrence of a knee deformity is common, and in juvenile and adolescent patients, recalcitrant contractures, often with posterior subluxation of the tibia, respond to two-pin traction. Place the proximal pin in the proximal metaphysis of the tibia, so that the anterior traction reduces the knee subluxation, and place the distal pin in the distal metaphysis of the tibia, so that longitudinal traction can reduce the flexion contracture of the knee. The two-pin traction method requires prolonged hospitalization and may be combined with hamstring lengthening and posterior capsulotomy. Recurrence of the flexion deformities may occur in growing children because the joint capsule and rigid periarticular soft tissues do not stretch adequately during growth.

A few patients develop marked bony and cartilaginous joint deformities, making joint motion impossible. An osteotomy, usually of the distal femur, is used to reposition the knee to 35° of flexion, which allows adequate sitting and standing. The angulation of the distal femur causes a mild iatrogenic cosmetic deformity.

In the extended knee, the joint is often rigid and resistant to therapy. The patella may be dislocated laterally, and the tibia may be dislocated anteriorly. A radiograph of the knee may be necessary for orientation before initiating to stretching therapy. For the dislocated knee in the infant, apply longitudinal skin traction to the tibial area of the legs, initially at 1 lb (0.45 kg) and progressing to a maximum of 5 lb (2.25 kg). Continue traction until the tibial plateau is beneath the femoral condyle, and then initiate flexion therapy. As soon as the knee can be flexed to about 30° in the reduced position, discontinue traction and apply splints to maintain reduction. If reduction cannot be achieved by traction, open reduction, consisting of a quadriceps lengthening, release of the lateral patellar retinaculum, and occasionally, knee ligament lengthening is necessary (65). After flexion is acquired, prolonged orthotic management is necessary to maintain motion.

Hip Deformities

In patients with arthrogryposis, the hip joint is frequently contracted (82%) and dislocated (58%) (290). The absolute treatment goal for hip contractures is to obtain a functional position of motion in the flexion–extension plane, which is a major benefit. At birth, the hips are frequently in a nonfunctional position of abduction, flexion, and external rotation (i.e., Buddha-like position) and should be passively stretched and sprinted. In the newborn, a cloth band can be wrapped around the proximal part of the leg to reduce the abduction contracture. In patients between 1 and 3 years of age, casts are applied to the legs, with a bar incorporated between the casts to control abduction and rotation, and the hips are passively stretched, placing the patient in a prone position. A hip flexion contracture of 30° is acceptable, because the lumbar spine can provide adequate compensatory motion. If adequate correction has not been obtained in the patient by 2 years of age, a soft-tissue release is helpful, or a varus extension intertrochanteric osteotomy may allow the desired position without producing additional muscle weakness. If a rigid contracture prevents ambulation, trochanteric osteotomies can reposition the extremity at about 35° of hip flexion and bring the hip out of the abducted position to allow adequate sitting and standing (290).

Hip dislocation is typically teratogenic and can be bilateral or unilateral. Occasionally, there is a reasonably mobile, nonteratogenic dislocated hip that can be treated in a manner similar to a typical congenitally dislocated hip if treatment is initiated before 3 months of age. Bilateral hip dislocations are best left untreated and attention directed toward obtaining adequate motion (172). A teratogenic unilateral hip dislocation was formerly thought to cause severe contractures, pelvic obliquity, and secondary scoliosis, but this is not always the case in arthrogryposis (84). An ipsilateral knee flexion contracture should be corrected before reduction is attempted, because knee therapy can redislocate the hip. Skin traction (i.e., a home traction program) and passive stretching therapy are used to obtain as much hip motion as possible (183). Occasionally, the femoral head reduces to the level of the acetabulum, and a closed reduction can be performed similar to that done for a typical congenitally dislocated hip, but postoperative casting should not allow the hip to contract in a nonfunctional position.

By the time a child is 1 year old, most teratogenic unilateral dislocations of the hip require open reduction through an anterior approach, extensive soft-tissue release, and possibly femoral shortening to obtain an adequate reduction. After surgery, a maximum of 6 weeks of casting from the thorax to the toes, followed by prolonged orthotic control, is necessary for adequate joint remodeling. Inadequate reduction with subsequent redislocation or subluxation does occur. if the hip cannot be reduced adequately, the pelvic obliquity is treated by an intertrochanteric femoral osteotomy to position the leg functionally, and a shoe lift is used to accommodate the limb length discrepancy until a properly timed ipsilateral epiphysiodesis is performed (28,257). If there is any question about obtaining good motion, it is better to leave the unilateral hip dislocation unreduced. A stiff hip produces a more significant problem than the other possible related conditions.

Foot Deformities

The most common (84%) foot deformity in arthrogryposis is talipes equinovarus. Convex pes valgus, calcaneovalgus, and cavovarus deformities are seen occasionally. These severely deformed feet are often extremely stiff, and the goal of treatment is to obtain a pain-free plantigrade foot at maturity.

At birth, the talipes equinovarus is treated by serial taping and passive stretching therapy. The passive stretching is performed four times each day, and the taping is changed every other day to reflect changes in position. Thirty-one of the 80 patients in our series have had successful nonsurgical treatment, even though a perfect result was not obtained (251). In patients with nonplantigrade feet but reasonable motion, a posteromediolateral release was satisfactory in 15 of 20 feet. After a posteromediolateral release, prolonged orthotic care and extensive passive stretching are necessary.

Recurrence in patients older than 10 years of age is best treated by a triple arthrodesis. In the rigid foot, a talectomy performed when the child is between 1 and 2 years old gives the most satisfactory plantigrade foot (84, 138,145,170,191). Recurrence after the age of 10 years is best treated by a triple arthrodesis.

Talectomy

- Make a skin incision from just distolateral to the head of the talus, extending obliquely inferoposteriorly to 1 inch (2.5 cm) inferior to the lateral malleolus (Ollier approach).
- Retract the peroneus longus and brevis tendons inferiorly, and incise the talocalcaneal portion of the bifurcate ligament.
- Turn the foot medially to expose the talar neck. The talus may be excised as one piece or in fragments.
- Strip the ligaments from both the medial and lateral aspects of the malleolus, and displace the foot posteriorly on the tibia so that the medial malleolus is in contact with the navicular and the lateral malleolus is at the calcaneocuboid joint.
- Align the foot to the desired rotation (i.e., long axis of the foot is perpendicular of the anterior tibia), and

reshape the malleoli to fit the calcaneus in the new position. Any tight tendons or ligaments may be lengthened to allow proper orientation of the foot. The foot should align without tension.

■ Close the wound, and apply a long-leg cast with the knee flexed and the foot in the corrected position. If the knee motion is inadequate to achieve cast support, place a Steinmann pin through the tibia and incorporate it into a short leg cast.

Postoperatively, change the long-leg cast at 2 weeks to a short-leg cast for an additional 10 weeks. Allow weight bearing about 1 month after surgery. After the cast is removed, use a solid ankle-foot orthosis to maintain position.

Scoliosis

The reported incidence of scoliosis varies from 0% to 42%, but a figure of about 20% seems acceptable (159, 260). Noncongenital scoliosis may be present at birth or may develop in early childhood; it is progressive, becomes rigid, and is associated with pelvic obliquity (83,116,304). Congenital scoliosis is far less common. A thoracolumbosacral orthosis is preferred in curves between 20° and 40°, and a posterior spinal fusion and instrumentation is preferred in progressive curves of more than about 40°. Because the scoliosis tends to be rigid, the fusion should not be delayed in progressive curves, or a severe deformity will develop. Arthrodesis is difficult to achieve, and a high incidence of pseudarthrosis is reported.

In severe curves with pelvic obliquity, an anterior release followed by a posterior spinal fusion to the sacrum with instrumentation enhances correction of the curve and pelvic obliquity (233).

REFERENCES

Each reference is categorized according to the following scheme: *, classic article; #, review article; !, basic research article; and +, clinical results/outcome study.

+ 1. Abell JM Jr, Hayes JT. Charcot Knee Due to Congenital Insensitivity to Pain. *J Bone Joint Surg* 1964;46-A: 1287,.

2. Aberion G, Alba A, Lee MH, Solomon M. Pulmonary Care of Duchenne Type Muscular Dystrophy. *NY State J Med* 1973;73:1206.

3. Adams RD, Denny-Brown D, Pearson CM. *Disease of Muscles.* New York: Paul B. Hoeber, 1953:229.

+ 4. Afifi AK, Smith JW, Zellweger H. Congenital Nonprogressive Myopathy. Central Core Disease and Nemaline Myopathy in One Family. *Neurology* 1965;15: 371.

+ 5. Alexander MA, Johnson EW, Petty J, Stauch D. Mechanical Ventilation of Patients with Late Stage Du-

chenne Muscular Dystrophy: Management in the Home. *Arch Phys Med Rehabil* 1979;60:289.

* 6. Allen BL Jr, Ferguson RL. The Galveston Technique for LRod Instrumentation of the Scoliotic Spine. *Spine* 1982;7:276.

+ 7. Angus PD, Cowell HR. Triple Athrodesis—A Critical Long-Term Review. *J Bone Joint Surg* 1986;68-B:260.

+ 8. Aprin H, Bowen JR, MacEwen GD, Hall JE. Spine Fusion in Patients with Spinal Muscular Atrophy. *J Bone Joint Surg* 1982:64-A:1179.

+ 9. Archibald DC, Vignos PJ Jr. A Study of Contractures in Muscular Dystrophy. *Arch Phys Med Rehabil* 1959; 40:150.

+ 10. Arendar GM, Canelo SB, Arenda T. *Long-term Follow-up of 148 Triple Arthrodesis Functional Results.* Presented at SICOT 90, XVIII, World Congress, Montreal, 1990.

+ 11. Armstro RM, Koenigsberger R, Mellinger J, Lovelace RE. Central Core Disease with Congenital Hip Dislocation: Study of Two Families. *Neurology* 1971;21:369.

! 12. Aslandis C, Jansen G, Amenmiya C, et al. Cloning of the Essential Myotonic Dystrophy Region and Mapping of the Putative Defect. *Nature* 1992;355:548.

+ 13. Bach JR, McKeon J. Orthopedic Surgery and Rehabilitation for the Prolongation of Brace-free Ambulation of Patients with Duchenne Muscular Dystrophy. *Am J Phys Med Rehabil* 1991;70:323.

14. Bach JR, O'Brien J, Krolenberg R, Alba AS. Muscular Dystrophy. A Management of End Stage Respiratory Failure in Duchenne Muscular Dystrophy. *Muscle Nerve* 1987;10:177.

+ 15. Badurska B, Fidziansia A, Kamieniecka Z, et al. Myotubular Myopathy. *J Neurol Sci* 1969;8:563.

+ 16. Bailey RO, Marzulo DC, Hans MB. Muscular Dystrophy. Infantile Facioscapulohumeral Muscular Dystrophy: New Observations. *Acta Neurol Scand* 1986;74: 51.

17. Bailey RO, Turok DI, Jaufmann BP, Singh JK. AIDS. Myositis and Acquired Immunodeficiency Syndrome. *Hum Pathol* 1987;18:749.

+ 18. Banker BQ. Neuropathologic Aspects of Arthrogryposis Multiplex Congenita. *Clin Orthop* 1985;194: 30.

+ 19. Banker BQ, Victor M, Adams RD. Arthrogryposis Multiplex Due to Congenital Muscular Dystrophy. *Brain* 1957;80:319.

20. Barbeau A. Friedreich's Ataxia 1978. An Overview. *Can J Neurol Sci* 1978;15:161.

+ 21. Bayne LG. Hand Assessment and Management of Arthrogryposis Multiplex Congenita. *Clin Orthop* 1985;194:68.

+ 22. Becker PE. Two New Families of Benign Sex-Linked Recessive Muscular Dystrophy. *Rev Can Biol Exp* 1962;21:551.

+ 23. Becker PE, Kiener F. Eline Neue X-Chromosale Muskeldystrophies *Arch Psychiatr Nervenkr* 193:427, 1955.

+ 24. Bell DB, Smith DW. Myotonic Dystrophy in the Neonate. *J Pediatr* 1972;81:83.

+ 25. Bell DF, Moseley CF, Koreska J. Unit Rod Segmental

Spinal Instrumentation in the Management of Patients with Progressive Neuromuscular Spinal Deformity. *Spine* 1989;14:1301.

+ 26. Bonnet I, Burgot D, Bonnard C, Glorion B. Surgery of the Lower Limbs in Duchenne Muscular Dystrophy. *French J Orthop Surg* 1991;5:160.

+ 27. Bossen EH, Shelburne JD, Verkauf BS. Respiratory Muscle Involvement in Infantile Myotonic Dystrophy. *Arch Pathol* 1974;97:250.

+ 28. Bowen JR, Johnson WJ. Percutaneous Epiphysiodesis. *Clin Orthop* 1984;190:170.

+ 29. Bowker JH, Halpin PJ. Factors Determining Success in Reambulation of the Child with Progressive Muscular Dystrophy. *Orthop Clin North Am* 1978;9:431.

30. Bradley WG. *Disorders of Peripheral Nerves.* Oxford: Blackwell Scientific, 1974.

+ 31. Bradley WG, Jones MZ, Mussini JM, Fawcett PR. Becker Type Muscular Dystrophy. *Muscle Nerve* 1978; 1:111.

+ 32. Brewerton DA, Sandifer PH, Sweetnam DR. "Idiopathic" Pes Cavus. *Br Med J* 1963;2:659.

+ 33. Brewster AH, Larson CB. Cavus Feet. *J Bone Joint Surg* 1940;22:361.

34. Brooke MH. *A Clinician's View of Neuromuscular Disease.* Baltimore: Williams & Wilkins, 1977.

! 35. Brook JD, McCurrach ME, Harley HG, et al. Molecular Basis of Myotonic Dystrophy: Expansion of a Trinucleotide (CTG) Repeat at the 3' End of a Transcript Encoding a Protein Kinase Family Member. *Cell* 1992; 68:799.

36. Brooke MH. A Neuromuscular Disease Characterized by Fibre Type Disproportion. In: Kakulas BA, ed. *Clinical Studies in Myology.* Proceedings of the Second International Congress on Muscle Diseases. Part 2, Perth, Australia, 1971. Amsterdam: Excerpta Medica, 1973.

+ 37. Brooria MJ, Banta JV, Renshaw TS. Spinal Fusion Augmented by Luque Rod Segmental Instrumentation for Neuromuscular Scoliosis. *J Bone Joint Surg* 1989;71-A:132.

+ 38. Brouwer OF, Padberg GW, Wijmenga C, Frants RR. Facioscapulohumeral Muscular Dystrophy in Early Childhood. *Arch Neurol* 1994;51:387.

+ 39. Brown JC, Zeller JL, Swank SM, et al. Surgical and Functional Results of Spine Fusion in Spinal Muscular Atrophy. *Spine* 1989;14:763.

+ 40. Buchthal F, Olsen PZ. Electromyography and Muscle Biopsy in Infantile Spinal Muscular Atrophy. *Brain* 1970;93:15.

41. Bunch WH. Muscular Dystrophy. In: Hardy JH, ed. *Spinal Deformity in Neurological and Muscular Disorders.* St. Louis: C.V. Mosby, 1974.

* 42. Bunch WH. Scapulo-thoracic Fusion for Shoulder Stabilization in Muscular Dystrophy. *Minn Med* 1973;56: 391.

+ 43. Bunch WH, Siegel IM. Scapulothoracic Arthrodesis in Facioscapulohumeral Muscular Dystrophy. *J Bone Joint Surg* 1993;75-A:372.

+ 44. Burke SS, Grove NM, Houser CR, Johnson, DM. Respiratory Aspects of Pseudohypertrophic Muscular Dystrophy. *Am J Dis Child* 1971;121:230.

! 45. Buxton J, Shelbourne P, Davies J, et al. Detection of an Unstable Fragment of DNA Specific to Individuals with Myotonic Dystrophy. *Nature* 1992;355:547.

+ 46. Byers RK, Banker BQ. Infantile Muscular Atrophy. *Arch Neurol* 1961;5:140.

+ 47. Cady RB, Babechko WP. Incidence, Natural History and Treatment of Scoliosis in Friedreich's Ataxia. *J Pediatr Orthop* 1984;4:673.

+ 48. Calderon R. Myotonic Dystrophy: A Neglected Cause of Mental Retardation. *J Pediatr* 1966;68:423.

+ 49. Cambridge W, Drennan JC. Scoliosis Associated with Duchenne Muscular Dystrophy. *J Pediatr Orthop* 1987;7:436.

+ 50. Campbell MJ, Rebeiz JJ, Walton JN. Myotubular Centronuclear or Pericentronuclear Myopathy. *J Neurol Sci* 1969;8:425.

+ 51. Carroll JE, Brooke MH, Kaiser K. Diagnosis of Infantile Myotonic Dystrophy. *Lancet* 1975;2:608.

52. Carroll NC. Pathoanatomy and Surgical Treatment of the Resistant Clubfoot. *Instr Course Lect* 1988;37:93.

+ 53. Cavanagh NPC, Lake BD, McMeniman P: Congenital Fibre Type Disproportion Myopathy. *Arch Dis Child* 1979;54:735.

* 54. Charcot J, Marie P. Sur une Forme Particuliere d'Atrophic Musculaire Progressive, Souvent Familiale, Debutant par les Pieds et les Jambes et Atteignant Plus Tard les Mains. *Rev Med* 1886;6:97.

! 55. Chamberlain S, Shaw J, Rowland A, et al: Mapping of Mutation Causing Friedreich's Ataxia to Human Chromosome 9. *Nature* 1988;334:248.

* 56. Chiari K. Medial Displacement Osteotomy of the Pelvis. *Clin Orthop* 1974;98:55.

+ 57. Cole WH. The Treatment of Claw-Foot. *J Bone Joint Surg* 1940;22:895.

58. Coleman SS. *Complex Foot Deformities in Children.* Philadelphia, Lea & Febiger, 1983.

* 59. Coleman SS, Chesnut WJ. A Simple Test for Hindfoot Flexibility in the Cavovarus Foot. *Clin Orthop* 1977; 123:60.

+ 60. Cook AW, Bird TD, Spence AM, et al. Myotonic Dystrophy, Mitral Valve Prolapse, and Stroke. *Lancet* 1978;1:335.

+ 61. Copeland SA, Howard RC. Thoracoscapular Fusion for Facioscapulohumeral Dystrophy. *J Bone Joint Surg* 1978;60-B:547.

62. Cowell HR. Genetic Aspects of Orthopaedic Disease. *Clin Orthop* 1975;107:36.

+ 63. Curless RG, Nelson MB. Needle Biopsies of Muscle in infants for Diagnosis and Reserch. *Dev Med Child Neurol* 1975;17:592.

64. Curtis BH. Orthopaedic Management of Muscular Dystrophy and Related Disorders. *Instr Course Lect* 1970;19:78.

+ 65. Curtis BH, Fisher RL. Congenital Hyperextension and Anterior Subluxation of the Knee. *J Bone Joint Surg* 1969;51-A:255.

+ 66. Daher YH, Lonstein JE, Winter RB, Bradford DS: Spinal Deformities in Patients with Friedreich's Ataxia: A Review of 19 Patients. *J Pediatr Orthop* 1985;5:553.

+ 67. Daher Y, Lonstein J, Winter R, Bradford DS. Spinal

Deformities in Patients with Muscular Dystrophy Other Than Duchenne—A Review of 11 Patients Having Surgical Treatment. *Spine* 1985;10:614.

+ 68. Daher YH, Lonstein JE, Winter RB, Bradford DS. Spinal Surgery in Spinal Muscular Atrophy. *J Pediatr Orthop* 1985;5:391.

+ 69. Daher YH, Lonstein JE, Winter RB, Bradford DS. Spinal Deformities in Patients with Charcot-Marie-Tooth Disease. A Review of 12 Patients. *Clin Orthop* 1986;202:219.

+ 70. Dahl DS, Klutzow FW. Congenital Rod Disease. Further Evidence of Innervational Abnormalities as the Basis for the Clinicopathologic Features. *J Neurol Sci* 1974;23:371.

+ 71. Dalakas MC, Pezeshkpour GH. Neuromuscular Diseases Associated with Human Immunodeficiency Virus Infection. *Ann Neurol* 1988;38:375.

* 72. Dejerine J, Sottas J. Sur la Neurite Interstitielle Hypertrophique et Progressive de l'Enfance. *Coll R Soc Biol* 1893;45:63.

+ 73. Demos J. Early Diagnosis and Treatment of Rapidly Developing Duchenne de Boulogne Type Myopathy (Type DDB1). *Am J Phys Med* 1971;50:271.

74. Denny-Brown D, Nevin S. The Phenomenon of Myotonia. *Brain* 1941;64:1.

+ 75. DeWind LT, Jones RJ. Cardiovascular Observations in Dystrophia Myotonica. *JAMA* 1950;144:299.

+ 76. Diamond LS, Alegado R. Perinatal Fractures in Arthrogryposis Multiplex Congenita. *J Pediatr Orthop* 1981;1:189.

+ 77. Dias CD, Miller F, Dabney K, et al. Surgical Correction of Spinal Deformity Using a Unit rod in Children with Cerebral Palsy. *J Pediatr Orthop* 1996;16:734.

+ 78. Dorando C, Newman MK. Bracing for Severe Scoliosis of Muscular Dystrophy Patients. *Phys Ther Rev* 1957;37:230.

+ 79. Drachman DB, Banker BQ. Arthrogryposis Multiplex Congenita. A Case Due to Disease of the Anterior Horn Cells. *Arch Neurol* 1961;5:77.

+ 80. Drager GA, Hammill JF, Shy GM. Paramyotonia Congenita. *Arch Neurol Psychiatry* 1958;80:1.

+ 81. Drennan JC. Skeletal Deformities in Spinal Muscular Atrophy. [Abstract.] *Clin Orthop* 1978;133:266.

82. Drennan JC. *Orthopedic Management of Neuromuscular Disorders*. Philadelphia: J.B. Lippincott, 1983:61.

+ 83. Drummond DS, Mackenzie DA. Scoliosis in Arthrogryposis Multiplex Congenita. *Spine* 1978;3:146.

84. Drummond DS, Siller TM, Cruess RL. Management of Arthrogryposis Multiplex Congenita. *Instr Course Lect* 1974;23:79.

+ 85. Dubowitz V. The Floppy Infant. *Clin Dev Med* 1969;31:41.

86. Dubowitz V. *Muscle Biopsy*, 2nd ed. London: Bailliere Tindall, 1985.

87. Dubowitz V. *Muscle Disorders in Childhood*. Philadelphia: W.B. Saunders Company, 1995.

88. Dubowitz V, Brooke MH. *Muscle Biopsy: A Modern Approach*. Philadelphia: W.B. Saunders, 1973.

* 89. Duchenne GB. Recherches sur le Paralysie Musculaire

Pseudohypertrophique ou Paralysie Myosclerosique. *Arch Gen Med* 1868;11:5.

* 90. Dwyer FC. Osteotomy of the Calcaneum for Pes Cavus. *J Bone joint Surg* 1959;41-B:80.

91. Dwyer FC. The Present Status of the Problem of Pes Cavus. *Clin Orthop* 1975;106:254.

92. Dyck PJ. Inherited Neuronal Degeneration and Atrophy Affecting Peripheral Motor Sensory and Autonomic Neurons. In: Dyck PJ, Thomas PK, Lambert EH, eds. *Peripheral Neuropathy*. Philadelphia: W.B. Saunders, 1975:825.

93. Dyck PJ, Chance PF, Lebo RV, Carney JA. Hereditary Motor and Sensory Neuropathies. In: Dyck PJ, Thomas PJ, Griffin JW, et al, eds. *Peripheral Neuropathy,* 3rd ed. Philadelphia: WB Saunders, 1993:1094.

94. Dyck PJ, Lambert EH. Lower Motor and Primary Sensory Neuron Diseases with Peroneal Muscular Atrophy. Part 1: Neurologic, Genetic and Electrophysiologic Findings in Hereditary Polyneuropathies. *Arch Neurol* 1968;18:603.

95. Dyck PJ, Lambert EH. Lower Motor and Primary Sensory Neuron Diseases with Peroneal Muscular Atrophy. Part II: Neurologic, Genetic, and Electrophysiologic Findings in Various Neuronal Degenerations. *Arch Neurol* 1968;18:619.

+ 96. Edwards RHT. Percutaneous Needle-Biopsy of Skeletal Muscle in Diagnosis and Research. *Lancet* 1971;2:593.

+ 97. Edwards RHT, McDonnell M. Hand-held Dynamometer for Evaluating Voluntary Muscle Function. *Lancet* 1974;2:757.

+ 98. Eldjarn L, Try K, Stokke O, et al. Dietary Effects on Serum Phytanic-Acid Levels and on Clinical Manifestations in Heredopathia Atactica Polyneuritiformis. *Lancet* 1966;1:691.

* 99. Emery AE. X-Linked Muscular Dystrophy with Early Contractures and Cardiomyopathy (Emery-Dreifuss Type). *Clin Genet* 1987;32:360.

+ 100. Emery AEH, Skinner R. Clinical Studies in Benign (Becker Type) X-Linked Muscular Dystrophy. *Clin Genet* 1976;10:189.

+ 101. Eng GD, Epstein BS, Engel WK, et al. Malignant Hyperthermia and Central Core Disease in a Child with Congenital Dislocating Hips. *Arch Neurol* 1978;35:189.

+ 102. Engel AG. Late Onset Rod Myopathy (a New Syndrome?): Light and Electron Microscopic Observations in Two Cases. *Mayo Clin Proc* 1966;41:713.

+ 103. Engel WK. Focal Myopathic Changes Produced by Electromyographic and Hypodermic Needles. *Arch Neurol* 1967;16:509.

+ 104. Engel WK, Foster JM, Hughes BP, et al: Central Core Disease: An Investigation of a Rare Muscle Cell Abnormality. *Brain* 1961;84:167.

+ 105. Erb W. Uber die "Juvenile Form" progressiven Muskelatrophie ihre Beziehunger zur sogennanten Pseudohypertrophie der Muskeln. *Dtsch Arch Klin Med* 1884;34:467.

! 106. Ervasti JM, Ohlendieck K, Kahl SD, et al. Deficiency of a Glycoprotein Component of the Dystrophin Complex in Dystrophic Muscle. *Nature* 1990;345:315.

107. Evans GA, Drennan JC. Functional Classification and

Orthopaedic Management of Spinal Muscular Atrophy. *J Bone Joint Surg* 1981;63-B:516.

+ 108. Eyring EJ, Johnson EW, Burnett C. Surgery in Muscular Dystrophy. *JAMA* 1972;222:1056.

+ 109. Fenichel GM, Emery ES, Hunt P. Neurogenic Atrophy Simulating Facioscapulohumeral Dystrophy: A Dominant Form. *Arch Neurol* 1967;17:257,.

110. Ferguson RL, Allen BL. Segmental Spinal Instrumentation for Routine Scoliotic Curve. *Contemp Orthop* 1980;2:450.

+ 111. Fiddian NJ, King RJ. The Winged Scapula. *Clin Orthop* 1984;185:228.

+ 112. Filla A, DeMichele G, Caruso G, et al. Genetic Data and Natural History of Friedreich's Disease: A Study of 80 Italian Patients. *J Neurol* 1990;237:345.

+ 113. Fiorista F, Brambilla G, Saviotti M, et al. Myocardial Infarction in a Child Aged Ten with Duchenne Muscular Dystrophy. *Z Kardiol* 1981;70:784.

! 114. Fisher J, Upadhaya M. Molecular Genetics of Facioscapulohumeral Dystrophy. *Neuromuscul Disord* 1997;7:55.

+ 115. Fisk JR, Bunch WH. Scoliosis in Neuromuscular Disease. *Orthop Clin North Am* 1979;10:863.

+ 116. Fitti RM, D'Auria TM. Arthrogryposis Multiplex Congenita. *J Pediatr* 1956;48:797.

117. Florence JM, Brooke MH, Carroll JE. Evaluation of the Child with Muscular Weakness. *Orthop Clin North Am* 1978;9:49.

+ 118. Fossberg H, Olofsson BO, Eriksson A, Andersson S. Cardiac Involvement in Congenital Myotonic Dystrophy. *Br Heart J* 1990;63(2):119.

+ 119. Fowler M. A Case of Arthrogryposis Multiplex Congenita with Lesions in the Nervous System. *Arch Dis Child* 1959;3:505.

! 120. Franco A, Lansman JB. Calcium Entry Through Stretch Inactivated Ion Channels in MDX Myotubes. *Nature* 1990;344:670.

+ 121. Frank J, Yadollah H, Butler I, et al. Central Core Disease and Malignant Hyperthermia Syndrome. *Arch Neurol* 1980;7:11.

+ 122. Friedlander HL, Westin GW, Wood WL Jr. Arthrogryposis Multiplex Congenita. *J Bone Joint Surg* 1968; 50-A:89.

! 123. Fu Y-H, Pizzuti A, Fenwick RG Jr, et al. An Unstable Triplet Repeat in a Gene Related to Myotonic Muscular Dystrophy. *Science* 1992;255:1256.

! 124. Fukuyama Y, Osawa MA. A Genetic Study of the Fukuyama Type Congenital Muscular Dystrophy. *Brain Dev* 1983;6:373.

+ 125. Fukuyama Y, Osawa M, Suzuki H. Congenital Progressive Muscular Dystrophy of the Fukuyama Type—Clinical, Genetic, and Pathological Considerations. *Brain Dev* 1981;3:1.

+ 126. Galasko CSB, Delaney C, Morris P. Spinal Stabilization in Duchenne Muscular Dystrophy. *J Bone Joint Surg* 1992;74-B:210.

+ 127. Gamble JG, Rinsky LA, Lee JH: Orthopaedic Aspects of Central Core Disease. *J Bone Joint Surg* 1988;70-A: 1061.

+ 128. Gardner-Medwin D. Mutation Rate in Duchenne Type of Muscular Dystrophy. 1. *Med Genet* 1970;7:334.

+ 129. Garvie JM, Woolf AL. Kugelberg-Welander Syndrome (Hereditary Proximal Spinal Muscular Atrophy). *Br Med J* 1966;1:1458.

* 130. Gee S. Hereditary Infantile Spastic Paraplegia. *St Bartholomew's Hosp Rep* 1889;25:81.

* 131. Geoffroy G, Barbau A, Breton G, et al. Clinical Description and Roentgenologic Evaluation of Patients with Friedreich's Ataxia. *Can J Neurol Sci* 1976;3:279.

+ 132. Gibson DA, Urs NDK. Arthrogryposis Multiplex Congenita. *J Bone Joint Surg* 1970;52-B:483.

+ 133. Gilliam TC, Brzustowicz LM, Castilla LH, et al: Genetic Homogeneity between Acute and Chronic Forms of Spinal Muscular Atrophy. *Nature* 1990;345:823.

134. Goebel H. Congenital Myopathies. In: Adachi M, Scher J, eds. Current Trends in Neurosciences—Neuromuscular Disease. New York: Igaku-Shoin, 1990:197.

+ 135. Goldberg HI, Sheft DJ. Esophageal and Colon Changes in Myotonia Dystrophica. *Gastroenterology* 1972;63: 134.

+ 136. Goodman MA, Swartz W. Infection in a Charcot Joint. *J Bone Joint Surg* 1985;67-A:642.

* 137. Gowers WR. *Pseudohypertrophic Muscular Paralysis.* London: J & A Churchill, 1879.

+ 138. Green ADL, Fixsen JA, Lloyd-Roberts GC. Talectomy for Arthrogryposis Multiplex Congenita. *J Bone Joint Surg* 1984;66-B:697.

139. Green WT, Grice DS. The Management of Chronic Poliomyelitis. *Instr Course Lect* 1952;9:85.

+ 140. Greenfield JG, Cornman T, Shy GM. The Prognostic Value of the Muscle Biopsy in the "Floppy Infant." *Brain* 1958;81:461.

! 141. Griffiths LR, Swi MB, McLeod JG, Nicholson GA. Chromosome I Linkage Studies in Charcot-Marie-Tooth Neuropathy Type 1. *Am J Hum Genet* 1988;42: 756.

+ 142. Griggs RC, Moxley RT, Mendell JR, et al. Prednisone in Duchenne Muscular Dystrophy—A Randomized, Controlled Trial Defining the Time Course and Dose Response. *Arch Neurol* 1991;48:383.

+ 143. Grove DI, O'Callaghan SJ, Burston TO, Forbes IJ. Immunological Function in Dystrophia Myotonica. *Br Med J* 1973;3:81.

+ 144. Gucker T III: The Orthopaedic Management of Progressive Muscular Dystrophy. *J Am Phys Ther Assoc* 1964;44:243.

+ 145. Guidera KJ, Drennan JC. Foot and Ankle Deformities in Arthrogryposis Multiplex Congenita. *Clin Orthop* 1985;194:93.

146. Hall JG. Genetic Aspects of Arthrogryposis. *Clin Orthop* 1985;194:44.

147. Hall JG, Reed SD, Greene G. The Distal Arthrogryposis: Delineation of New Entities-Review and Nosologic Discussion. *Am J Med Genet* 1982;11:185.

+ 148. Hanson PA, Rowland LP. Mobius Syndrome and Facioscapulohumeral Muscular Dystrophy. *Arch Neurol* 1971;24:31.

149. Harding AE, Thomas PK. Genetically Determined Neu-

ropathies. In: Asbury AK, Gilliatt RW, eds. *Peripheral Nerve Disorders*. London: Butterworths, 1984:347.

\# 150. Hardy JH, ed. *Spinal Deformity in Neurological and Muscular Disorders*. St. Louis: C.V. Mosby, 1974.

! 151. Harley HG, Brook JD, Rundle SA, et al. Expansion of an Unstable DNA Region and Phenotypic Variation in Myotonic Dystrophy. *Nature* 1992a;35:545.

\# 152. Harper P. *Myotonic Dystrophy*, 2nd ed. Philadelphia: W.B. Saunders, 1989.

+ 153. Harper PS. Congenital Myotonic Dystrophy in Britain. 1: Clinical Aspects. *Arch Dis Child* 1975;50:505.

\# 154. Harper PS. *Myotonic Dystrophy*, 12th ed. Philadelphia: W.B. Saunders, 1979.

+ 155. Hausmanowa-Petrusewicz I. Infantile and Juvenile Spinal Muscular Atrophy. In: Walton JN, Conal N, Scarlatto G, eds. *Muscle Diseases: Proceedings of International Congress, Milan, 1969*. Amsterdam: Excerpta Medical, 1970:558.

+ 156. Heckmatt J, Dubowitz V, Hyde S, et al. Prolongation of Walking in Duchenne Muscular Dystrophy with Lightweight Orthoses: Review of 57 Cases. *Dev Med Child Neurol* 1985;27:149.

+ 157. Hensinger RN, MacEwen GD. Spinal Deformity Associated with Heritable Neurological Conditions: Spinal Muscular Atrophy, Friedreich's Ataxia, Familial Dysautonomia, and Charcot-Marie-Tooth Disease. *J Bone Joint Surg* 1976;58-A:13.

\# 158. Herndon CH. Tendon Transplantation at the Knee and Foot. *Instr Course Lect* 1961;18:145.

+ 159. Herron LD, Westin GW, Dawson EG. Scoliosis in Arthrogryposis Multiplex Congenita. *J Bone Joint Surg* 1978;60-A:293.

+ 160. Hewer RL. A Study of Fatal Cases of Friedreich's Ataxia. *Br Med* 1968;3:649.

* 161. Hibbs RA. An Operation for "Claw-Foot." *JAMA* 1919;73:1583.

+ 162. Hirotani H, Doko S, Fukunaga H, et al. Fractures in Patients with Myopathies. *Arch Phys Med Rehabil* 1979;60:178.

* 163. Hoffman EP, Brown RH Jr, Kunkull AN. Dystrophin: The Protein Product of the Duchenne Muscular Dystrophy Locus. *Cell* 1987;51:919.

+ 164. Hoffman EP, Kunkull AN, Angelini C, et al. Improved Diagnosis of Becker Muscular Dystrophy by Dystrophin Testing. *Neurology* 1989;39:1011.

* 165. Hoffman J. Uber chronische spinale Muskelatrophie im Kindersalter, auf familiarer Bases. *Dtsch Z Nervenheilk* 1893;3:427.

+ 166. Hopkins LC, Jackson JA, Elsas LJ. Emery-Dreifuss Humeroperoneal Muscular Dystrophy: An X-Linked Myopathy with Unusual Contractures and Bradycardia. *Ann Neurol* 1981;10:230.

* 167. Howard R. A Case of Congenital Defect of the Muscular System (Dystrophia Muscularis Congenita) and Its Association with Congenital Talipes Equinovarus. *Proc R Soc Med* 1908;1:157.

+ 168. Hsu JD. The Natural History of Spine Curvature Progression in the Nonambulatory Duchenne Muscular Dystrophy Patient. *Spine* 1983:8:771.

\# 169. Hsu JD, Imbus CE. Pes Cavus. In Jahss MH, ed. *Disorders of the Foot*, Vol 1. Philadelphia: W.B. Saunders, 1982:463.

+ 170. Hsu LC, Jaffray D, Leong JCY. Talectomy for Clubfoot in Arthrogryposis. *J Bone Joint Surg* 1984;66-B:694.

+ 171. Huff TA, Horton ES, Lebovitz HE. Abnormal Insulin Secretion in Myotonic Dystrophy. *N Engl J Med* 1967; 277:837.

+ 172. Huurman WW, Jacobsen ST. The Hip in Arthrogryposis Multiplex Congenita. *Clin Orthop* 1985;194: 81.

+ 173. Inkley SR, Oldenburg FC, Vignos PJ. Pulmonary Function in Duchenne Muscular Dystrophy Related to Stage of Disease. *Am J Med* 1974;56:297.

+ 174. Isaacs H, Barlow MB. Malignant Hyperpyrexia during Anesthesia: Possible Association with Subclinical Myopathy. *Br Med J* 1970;1:275.

\# 175. Isaacs H, Barlow MB. Malignant Hyperpyrexia. *J Neurol Neurosurg Psychiatry* 1973;36:228.

+ 176. Jacobs JE, Carr CR. Progressive Muscular Atrophy of the Peroneal Type (Charcot-Marie-Tooth Disease), Orthopaedic Management and End Result Study. *J Bone Joint Surg* 1950;32-A:27.

+ 177. Jakab E, Gledhill RB. Simplified Technique for Scapulocostal Fusion in Fascioscapulohumeral Dystrophy. *J Pediatr Orthop* 1993;13:749.

+ 178. Jenkins JG, Bohn D, Edmonds JF, et al. Evaluation of Pulmonary Function in Muscular Dystrophy Patients Requiring Spinal Surgery. *Crit Care Med* 1982;10:645.

\# 179. Johnson EW, Kennedy JH. Comprehensive Management of Duchenne Muscular Dystrophy. *Arch Phys Med Rehabil* 1971;52:110.

\# 180. Johnson JTH. Neuropathic Fractures and Joint Injuries. *J Bone Joint Surg* 1967;49-A:1.

* 181. Jones R. The Soldier's Foot and the Treatment of Common Deformities of the Foot. *Br Med J* 1916;1:749.

+ 182. Jones R, Khan R, Hughes S, Dubowitz V. Congenital Muscular Dystrophy, The Importance of Early Diagnosis and Orthopaedic Management in the Long-term Prognosis. *J Bone Joint Surg* 1979;61-B:13.

+ 183. Joseph K, MacEwen GD, Boos ML. Home Traction in the Management of Congenital Dislocation of the Hip. *Clin Orthop* 1982;165:83.

+ 184. Kaeser HE. Scapulo-peroneal Muscular Atrophy. *Brain* 1965;88:407.

! 185. Kahlke W, Wagener H. Conversion of H3-Phytol to Phytanic Acid and Its Incorporation into Plasma Lipid Fractions in Heredopathia Atactica Polyneuritiformis. *Metabolism* 1966;15:687.

+ 186. Kaneda RR. Becker's Muscular Dystrophy: Orthopaedic Implications. *J Am Osteopath Assoc* 1980;79:332.

\# 187. Kaus S, Rockoff M: Malignant Hyperthermia. *Pediatr Clin North Am* 1994;41(1):221.

+ 188. Ketenjian AY. Scapulocostal Stabilization for Scapula Winging in Facioscapulohumeral Muscular Dystrophy. *J Bone Joint Surg* 1978;60-A:476.

+ 189. King JO, Denborough MA, Zapf PW. Inheritance of Malignant Hyperpyrexia. *Lancet* 1972;1:365.

! 190. Kinoshita M, Iwasaki Y, Wada F, Segawa M. A Case of Congenital Polymyositis—A Possible Pathogenesis of "Fukuyama Type Congenital Muscular Dystrophy." *Rinsho Shinkeigaku* 1980;20:911.

+ 191. Kite JH. Arthrogryposis Multiplex Congenita. *South Med J* 1955;48:1141.

+ 192. Kling TF Jr, Drennan JC. *Orthopaedic Management of Hereditary Motor and Sensory Neuropathies.* Presented at the 34th Annual Meeting of the American Academy for Cerebral Palsy and Developmental Medicine, October 1980.

+ 193. Kolb ME, Hom ML, Martz R. Dantrolene in Human Malignant Hyperthermia. *Anesthesiology* 1982;56:254. (Facioscapulohumeral Dystrophy Presenting in Infancy with Facial Diplegia and Sensorineural Deafness. *Ann Neurol* 1985;17:513.)

+ 194. Krettek C, Gluer S, Thermann H, et al. Non-union of the Ulna in a 10-month-old Child Who Had Type IV Hereditary Sensory Neuropathy. *J Bone Joint Surg* 1997;79A:1232.

+ 195. Krishna M, Taylor JF, Brown MC, et al: Failure of Somatosensory-evoked Potential Monitoring in Sensoriomotor Neuropathy. *Spine* 1991;16:479.

+ 196. Kugelberg E, Welander L. Heredofamilial Juvenile Muscular Atrophy Stimulating Muscular Dystrophy. *Arch Neurot Psychiatry* 1956;75:500.

+ 197. Kumano K: Congenital Non-progressive Myopathy, Associated with Scoliosis—Clinical, Histological, Histochemical and Electron Microscopic Studies of Seven Cases. *J Jpn Orthop Assoc* 1980;54:381.

+ 198. Kumar SJ, Marks HG, Bowen JR, MacEwen GD. Hip Dysplasia Associated with Charcot-Marie-Tooth Disease in the Older Child and Adolescent. *J Pediatr Orthop* 1985;5:511.

! 199. Kunkel LM, Mejmancik JF, Caskey CT. Analysis of Deletions in DNA From Patients with Becker and Duchenne Muscular Dystrophy. *Nature* 1986;322:73.

! 200. Kunkel LM, Monaco AP, Hoffman E, et al. Molecular Studies of Progressive Muscular Dystrophy (Duchenne). *Enzyme* 1987;38:72.

+ 201. Kurz LT, Mubarak SJ, Schultz P, et al. Correlation of Scoliosis and Pulmonary Function in Duchenne Muscular Dystrophy. *J Pediatr Orthop* 1983;3:347.

202. Labelle H, Duhaime M, Allard P: Spinal Deformities in Friedreich's Ataxia. In: Weinstein SL, ed. *The Pediatric Spine: Principles and Practice.* New York: Raven Press, 1994:999.

+ 203. Labelle H, Tohmie S, Duhaime M, Allard P. Natural History of Scoliosis in Friedreich's Ataxia. *J Bone Joint Surg* 1986;68-A:564.

* 204. Landouzy L, Dejerine J. De la Myopathie Atrophique Progressive (Myopathic Hereditaire), Debutant, Dans l'Enfance, par le Face, sans Alteration du Systeme Nerveux. *Coll R Acad Sci Paris* 1884;98:53.

+ 205. Lau JHK, Parker JC, Hsu LCS, Leong JCY. Paralytic Hip Instability in Poliomyelitis. *J Bone Joint Surg* 1986;68-B:528.

! 206. Law PK, Bertorini TE, Goodwin TG, et al. Dystrophin Production Induced by Myoblast Transfer Therapy in Duchenne Muscular Dystrophy. [Letter.] *Lancet* 1990;14:114.

+ 207. Letournel E, Fardeau M, Lytle JO, et al. Scapulothora-cic Arthrodesis for Patients Who Have Facioscapulo-humeral Muscular Dystrophy. *J Bone Joint Surg* 1990;72-A:78.

208. Levy RM, Bredesen DE, Rosenblum ML. Neurological Manifestations of the Acquired Immunodeficiency Syndrome (AIDS): Experience at UCSF and Review of the Literature. *J Neurosurg* 1985;62:475.

* 209. Leyden E. *Klinik der Ruckenmarks-Krankheiten,* Vol 2. Berlin: Hirschwalk, 1876.

+ 210. Lipscomb PR, Sanchez JJ. Anterior Transplantation of the Posterior Tibial Tendon for Persistent Palsy of the Common Peroneal Nerve. *J Bone Joint Surg* 1961;43-A:60.

+ 211. Lloyd-Roberts GC, Lettin AWF. Arthrogryposis Multiplex Congenita. *J Bone Joint Surg* 1970;52-B:494.

+ 212. Lord J, Behrman B, Varzos N, et al. Scoliosis Associated with Duchenne Muscular Dystrophy. *Arch Phys Med Rehabil* 1990;71:13.

* 213. Luque ER. The Anatomic Basis and Development of Segmental Spinal Instrumentation. *Spine* 1982;7:256.

+ 214. Luque ED, Cardoso A. Sequential Correction of Scoliosis with Rigid Internal Fixation. [Abstract.] *Orthop Trans* 1977;1:136.

215. MacEwen GD, Floyd GC. Congenital Insensitivity to Pain and Its Orthopaedic Implications. *Clin Orthop* 1970;68:100.

! 216. Mahadevan M, Tsilfidis C, Saboourin L, et al. Myotonic Dystrophy Mutation: An Unstable CTG Repeat in the 3' Untranslated Region of the Gene. *Science* 1992;255:1253.

+ 217. Makin M. The Surgical Treatment of Friedreich's Ataxia. *J Bone Joint Surg* 1953;35-A:425.

+ 218. Maloney WJ, Rinsky LA, Gamble JG: Simultaneous Correction of Pelvic Obliquity, Frontal Plane and Sagittal Plane Deformities in Neuromuscular Scoliosis Using a Unit Rod with Segmental Sublaminar Wires: A Preliminary Report. *J Pediatr Orthop* 1990;10:742.

219. Marhidon MB. Malignant Hyperthermia: Current Concepts. *Arch Surg* 1982;117:349.

+ 220. Mathieu J, Allard P, Goberl G, et al. Anesthetic and Surgical Complications in 219 Cases of Myotonic Dystrophy. *Neurology* 1997;49(6):1646.

221. Mayer L. The Physiologic Method of Tendon Transplants: Review after Forty Years. *Instr Course Lect* 1956;13:116.

+ 222. McComb RD, Markesbery WR, O'Connor WN. Fatal Neonatal Nemaline Myopathy with Multiple Congenital Anomalies. *J Pediatr* 1979;94:47.

* 223. McKay DW. New Concept of and Approach to Clubfoot Treatment: Section 2—Correction of the Clubfoot. *J Pediatr Orthop* 1983;3:10.

+ 224. McManamin JB, Becker LE, Murphy EG. Congenital Muscular Dystrophy: A Clinicopathologic Report of 24 Cases. *J Pediatr Orthop* 1982;100:692.

+ 225. McPherson EW, Taylor CA Jr. The King Syndrome: Malignant Hyperthermia, Myopathy, and Multiple Anomalies. *Am J Med Genet* 1981;8:159.

226. Medical Research Council. *Aids to the Investigation of Peripheral Nerve Injuries.* London: Her Majesty's Stationery Office, 1943.

+ 227. Mereu TR, Porter LH, Hug G. Myotonia, Shortness of Stature and Hip Dysplasia: Schwartz-Jampel Syndrome. *Am J Dis Child* 1969;117:470.

+ 228. Merlini L, Granata C, Bonfiglioli S, et al. Scoliosis in Spinal Muscular Atrophy: Natural History and Management. *Dev Med Child Neurol* 1989;31:501.

* 229. Meryon E. On Granular or Fatty Degeneration of the Voluntary Muscles. *Trans Med Chir Sec Edinb* 1852; 35:72.

+ 230. Miller F, Moseley CF, Koreska J, Levison I. Pulmonary Function and Scoliosis in Duchenne Dystrophy. *J Pediatr Orthop* 1988;8:133.

231. Miller F, Moseley C, Koreska J: Pelvic Anatomy Relative to Lumbosacral Instrumentation. *J Spinal Disord* 1990;3(2):169.

+ 232. Miller F, Moseley CF, Koreska J. Spinal Fusion in Duchenne Muscular Dystrophy. *Dev Med Child Neurol* 1992;34:775.

+ 233. Miller LS, Gray JM, Ashley RK, Skinner SR. *The Surgical Management of Scoliosis in Poliomyelitis.* (Shriners Hospital for Crippled Children, University of California) Presented at SICOT 90, XVIII, World Congress, Montreal, 1990.

+ 234. Miller MJ, Williams LL, Slack SL, Nappi JF. The hand in Charcot-Marie-Tooth Disease. *J Hand Surg [Br]* 1991;16(2):191.

+ 235. Moosa A, Dubowitz V. Postnatal Maturation of Peripheral Nerves in Preterm and Full-term Infants. *J Pediatr* 1971;79:915.

236. Mortens J, Pilcher MF. Tendon Transplantation in the Prevention of Foot Deformities after Poliomyelitis in Children. *J Bone Joint Surg* 1956;38-B:633.

237. Morton NE, Chung CS. Formal Genetics of Muscular Dystrophy. *Am J Hum Genet* 1959;11:360.

+ 238. Moulds RFW, Denborough MA. Procaine in Malignant Hyper-pyrexia. *Br Med J* 1972;4:526.

+ 239. Mubarak SJ, Chambers HG, Wenger DR. Percutaneous Muscle Biopsy in the Diagnosis of Neuromuscular Disease. *J Pediatr Orthop* 1992;12:191.

+ 240. Mubarak SJ, Morin WD, Leach J. Spinal fusion in Duchenne Muscular Dystrophy—Fixation and Fusion to the Sacropelvis? *J Pediatr Orthop* 1993;13:752.

+ 241. Munsat TL, Thompson LR, Coleman RF. Centronuclear ("Myotubular") Myopathy. *Arch Neurol* 1969; 20:120.

* 242. Mustard WT. Iliopsoas Transfer for Weakness of the Hip Abductors: A Preliminary Report. *J Bone Joint Surg* 1952;34-A:647.

+ 243. Mustard WT. A Follow-up Study of Iliopsoas Transfer for Hip Instability. *J Bone Joint Surg* 1959;41-B:289.

* 244. Ober FR. Tendon Transplantation in the Lower Extremity. *N Engl J Med* 1933;209:52.

+ 245. Ober FR. The Role of the Iliotibial Band and Fascia Lata as a Factor in the Causation of Lowback Disabilities and Sciatica. *J Bone Joint Surg* 1936;18:105.

+ 246. O'Brien TA, Harper PS. Course, Prognosis and Complications of Childhood-Onset Mytonic Dystrophy. *Dev Med Child Neurol* 1984;26:62.

+ 247. Oheneba B, Lonstein JE, Winter RB, et al. Management of Neuromuscular Spine Deformities with Luque Segmental Instrumentation. *J Bone Joint Surg* 1989;71-A: 548.

+ 248. Okuno T, Inoue A, Izumo S. Congenital Insensitivity to Pain with Anhidrosis. *J Bone Joint Surg* 1990;72-A: 279.

* 249. Padberg G. *Facioscapulohumeral Disease.* Thesis, University of Leiden, 1982.

+ 250. Padberg G, Eriksson AW, Volkers WS, et al. Linkage Studies in Autosomal Dominant Facioscapulohumeral Muscular Dystrophy. *J Neurol Sci* 1984;65:261.

+ 251. Palmer PM, MacEwen GD, Bowen JR, Matthews PA. Passive Motion Therapy for Infants with Arthrogryposis. *Clin Orthop* 1985;184:54.

+ 252. Paulos L, Coleman SS, Samuelson KM. Pes Cavovarus. *J Bone Joint Surg* 1980;62-A:942.

+ 253. Pearn J, Hudgson P. Distal Spinal Muscular Atrophy. *J Neurol Sci* 1979;43:183.

+ 254. Pearn JH, Hudgson P, Walton JN. A Clinical and Genetic Study of Spinal Muscular Atrophy of Adult Onset. *Brain* 1978;101:591.

+ 255. Pearson CM, Fowler WG. Hereditary Nonprogressive Muscular Dystrophy Inducing Arthrogryposis Syndrome. *Brain* 1963;86:75.

+ 256. Petrie JG. A Case of Progressive Joint Disorders Caused by Insensitivity to Pain. *J Bone Joint Surg* 1953;35-B: 399.

* 257. Phemister DB. Operative Arrestment of Longitudinal Growth of Bones in the Treatment of Deformities. *J Bone Joint Surg* 1933;15:1.

+ 258. Piasecki JO, Mahinpour A, Levine DB: Long-term follow-up of spinal fusion in spinal muscular atrophy. *Clin Orthop* 1986;207:44.

+ 259. Pinsky L, DiGeorge AM. Congenital Familial Sensory Neuropathy with Anhidrosis. *J Pediatr* 1966;68:1.

260. Poznanski AK, La Rowe PC. Radiographic Manifestations of the Arthrogryposis Syndrome. *Radiology* 1970;95:353.

+ 261. Ramsey PL, Hensinger RN. Congenital Dislocation of the Hip Associated with Central Core Disease. *J Bone Joint Surg* 1975;57-A:648.

+ 262. Ray, S, Bowen JR, Marks HG. Foot Deformity in Myotonic Dystrophy. *Foot Ankle* 1984;5:125.

* 263. Refsum S. Heredopathia Atactica Polyneuritiformis: A Familial Syndrome Not Hitherto Described. *Acta Psychiatr Neurol Suppl* 1946;38:1.

* 264. Refsum S, Salmonsen L, Skatvedt M. Heredopathia Atactica Polyneuritiformis in Children. *J Pediatr* 1949; 35:335.

+ 265. Rideau Y, Duport G, Delaubier A. Premieres remissions reproductibles dans l'evolution de la dystrophie musculare de Duchenne. *Bull Acad Natl Med* 1986;170:605.

+ 266. Rideau Y, Glorion B, Duport G. Prolongation of Ambulation in the Muscular Dystrophies. *Acta Neurol [Napoli]* 1983;5:390.

+ 267. Riley CM, Day RL, Greeley DM, Langford WS. Central Autonomic Dysfunction with Defective Lacrimation. *Pediatrics* 1949;3:468.

268. Riley CM, Moore RH. Familial Dysautonomia Differentiated from Related Disorders. *Pediatrics* 1966;37: 435.

+ 269. Robin GC, Brief LP. Scoliosis in Childhood Muscular Dystrophy. *J Bone Joint Surg* 1971;53-A:466.

+ 270. Robin JC. Scoliosis in Duchenne's Muscular Dystrophy. *Isr J Med Sci* 1977;13:203.

+ 271. Robinson D, Galasko CS, Delaney C, et al. Scoliosis and Lung Function in Spinal Muscular Atrophy. *European Spine Journal* 1995;4:268.

+ 272. Rodillo EB, Fernandez-Bermejo E, Heckmatt JZ, Dubowitz V. Prevention of Rapidly Progressive Scoliosis in Duchenne Muscular Dystrophy by Prolongation of Walking with Orthoses. *J Child Neurol* 1988;3 9.

+ 273. Roper BA, Tibrewal SB. Soft Tissue Surgery in Charcot-Marie-Tooth Disease. *J Bone Joint Surg* 1989;71(B):17.

+ 274. Rosenberg H. Clinical Presentation of Malignant Hyperthermia. *Br J Anaesth* 1981;60:268.

* 275. Rosenkranz E. Uber kongenitale Kontrakturen der oberen Extremitaten: Im Anschluss an die Mitteilung eines einschlagigen Falles. *Z Orthop* 1905;14:905.

+ 276. Rossi E. Le Syndrome Arthromyodysplasique Congenital. *Helv Paediatr Acta* 1947;2:82.

* 277. Roussy G, Levy G. Sept Cas d'une Maladie Familiale Particuliere: Troubles de la Marche, Pieds, Bets et Areflexie Tendineuse Generalisee, avec Accessoirement, Legere Maladresse des Mains. *Rev Neurol* 1926;54:427.

* 278. Roussy G, Levy G. A Propos de la Dystasie Areflexique Hereditaire. *Rev Neurol* 1934;62:763.

+ 279. Roy L, Gibson DA. Pseudohypertrophic Muscular Dystrophy and Its Surgical Management: Review of 30 Patients. *Can J Surg* 1970;13:13.

+ 280. Rubery PT, Spielman JH, Hester P, et al. Scoliosis in Familial Dysautonomia. *J Bone Joint Surg* 1995;77A:1362.

* 281. Ryerson EW. Arthrodesing Operations on the Feet. *J Bone Joint Surg* 1923;5:453.

282. Sabin AB. Oral Poliovirus Vaccine: History of Its Development and Prospects. Eradication of Poliomyelitis. *JAMA* 1965;194:872.

+ 283. Sabir M, Lyttle D. Pathogenesis of Pes Cavus in Charcot-Marie-Tooth Disease. *Clin Orthop* 1984;184:223.

+ 284. Sakai DN, Hsu JD, Bonnett CA, Brown JC. Stabilization of the Collapsing Spine in Duchenne Muscular Dystrophy. *Clin Orthop* 1977;128:256.

* 285. Salk JE. Studies in Human Subjects on Active Immunization Against Poliomyelitis. *JAMA* 1953;151:1081.

+ 286. Salter RB, Dubos JP. The First Fifteen Years' Personal Experience with Innominate Osteotomy in the Treatment of Congenital Dislocation and Subluxation of the Hip. *Clin Orthop* 1974;98:72.

287. Samilson RL, Dillon W. Cavus, Cavovarus, and Calcaneocavus. *Clin Orthop* 1983;177:125.

+ 288. Sanjal SK, Leung RK, Tierney RC, et al. Mitral Valve Prolapse Syndrome in Children with Duchenne's Progressive Muscular Dystrophy. *Pediatrics* 1979;63:116.

+ 289. Santavirta S, Turunen V, Ylinen P, et al. Foot and Ankle Fusions in Charcot-Marie-Tooth Disease. *Arch Orthop Trauma Surg* 1993;112:175.

290. Sarwark JF, MacEwen GD, Scott CI Jr. Amyoplasia (A Common Form of Arthrogryposis). *J Bone Joint Surg* 1990;72-A:465.

! 291. Schonk D, Coerwrankel-Driessen M, vanDalen I, et al. Definition of Subchromosomal Intervals Around the Myotonic Dystrophy Gene Region at 19q. *Genomics* 1989;4:384.

+ 292. Schottsdaedt ER, Larsen LJ, Bost FC. Complete Muscle Transposition. *J Bone Joint Surg* 1955;37-A:897.

+ 293. Schuch CP, Farmer TW. Physical Therapy in Acute Infectious Polyneuritis. *Phys Ther Rev* 1955;35:238.

+ 294. Schwentker EP, Gibson DA. The Orthopaedic Aspects of Spinal Muscular Atrophy. *J Bone Joint Surg* 1976;58-A:32.

+ 295. Seay AR, Ziter FA, Thompson JA. Cardiac Arrest during Induction of Anesthesia in Duchenne Muscular Dystrophy. *J Pediatr Orthop* 1978;93:88.

+ 296. Shapiro F, Sethna N, Colan S, et al. Spinal Fusion in Duchenne Muscular Dystrophy: A Multidisciplinary Approach. *Muscle Nerve* 1992;15:604.

297. Shapiro F, Specht L. Current Concepts Review: The Diagnosis and Orthopaedic Treatment of Childhood Spinal Muscular Atrophy, Peripheral Neuropathy, Friedreich Ataxia and Arthrogryposis. *J Bone Joint Surg* 1993;75(A):1699.

298. Shapiro F, Specht L: Current Concepts Review. The Diagnosis and Orthopaedic Treatment of Inherited Muscular Diseases of Childhood. *J Bone Joint Surgery* 1993;75(A):439.

+ 299. Sharrard WJW. The Distribution of the Permanent Paralysis in the Lower Limb in Poliomyelitis. *J Bone Joint Surg* 1955;37-B:540.

+ 300. Sharrard WJW. Muscle Recovery in Poliomyelitis. *J Bone Joint Surg* 1955;37-B:63.

301. Sher JH. Neuromuscular Disease. In: Adachi M, Sher JH, eds. *Muscular Dystrophy*. New York: Igaku-Shoin, 1990:122.

+ 302. Sherman FC, Westin W. Plantar Release in the Correction of Deformities of the Foot in Children. *J Bone Joint Surg* 1981;63-A:1382.

+ 303. Shy GM, Engel WK, Somers JE, Wanko T. Nemaline Myopathy. A New Congenital Myopathy. *Brain* 1963;86:793.

+ 304. Siebold RM, Winter RB, Moe JH. The Treatment of Scoliosis in Arthrogryposis Multiplex Congenita. *Clin Orthop* 1974;103:191.

+ 305. Siegel I. Fractures of Long Bones in Duchenne Muscular Dystrophy. *J Trauma* 1977;17:219.

+ 306. Siegel I. Foot Deformity in Myotubular Myopathy: Pathology of Intrinsic Foot Musculature. *Arch Neurol* 1983;40:589.

+ 307. Siegel IM. Scoliosis in Muscular Dystrophy. *Clin Orthop* 1973;93:235.

+ 308. Siegel IM. Prolongation of Ambulation through Early Percutaneous Tenotomy and Bracing with Plastic Orthoses. *Isr J Med Sci* 1977;13:192.

309. Siegel IM. The Management of Muscular Dystrophy: A Clinical Review. *Muscle Nerve* 1978;1:453.

+ 310. Siegel I, Miller JE, Ray RD. Subcutaneous Lower Limb Tenotomy in the Treatment of Pseudohypertrophic

Muscular Dystrophy. *J Bone Joint Surg* 1968;50(A): 1437.

+ 311. Simons GW. Complete Subtalar Release in Clubfeet. Part 1. A Preliminary Report. *J Bone Joint Surg* 1985; 67-A:1044.

! 312. Slater GR. The Missing Link in Duchenne Muscular Dystrophy. *Nature* 1987;330:693.

+ 313. Smith AD, Koreska J, Moseley CF. Progression of Scoliosis in Duchenne Muscular Dystrophy. *J Bone Joint Surg* 1989;71-A:1066.

+ 314. Smith PE, Claverley PM, Edwards RH. Hypoxemia during Sleep in Duchenne Muscular Dystrophy. *Am Rev Respir Dis* 1988;137:884.

315. Smith RJ. Malignant Hyperthermia. Preoperative Assessment of Risk Factors. *Br J Anaesth* 1988;60:317.

+ 316. Smith SE, Green NE, Cole RJ, et al. Prolongation of Ambulation in Children with Duchenne Muscular Dystrophy by Subcutaneous Lower Limb Tenotomy. *J Pediatr Orthop* 1993;13:336.

+ 317. Sodergard J, Ryoppy S. The Knee in Arthrogryposis Multiplex Congenita. *J Pediatr Orthop* 1990;10:177.

+ 318. Southwell RB, Sherman FC. Triple Athrodesis: A Long-Term Study with Force Plate Analysis. *Foot Ankle* 1981;1:15.

319. Spencer GE Jr. Orthopaedic Care of Progressive Muscular Dystrophy. *J Bone Joint Surg* 1967;49-A:1201.

+ 320. Spencer GE Jr, Vignos PJ Jr. Bracing for Ambulation in Childhood Progressive Muscular Dystrophy. *J Bone Joint Surg* 1962;44A:234.

+ 321. Spira E. The Treatment of Dropped Shoulder—A New Operative Technique. *J Bone Joint Surg* 1948;30(A): 229.

+ 322. St Clair HS, Zimbler S. A Plan of Management and Treatment Results in the Arthrogrypotic Hip. *Clin Orthop* 1985;194:74.

* 323. Steel HH. Triple Osteotomy of the Innominate Bone. *J Bone Joint Surg* 1973;55-A:343.

+ 324. Steinberg D, Vroom FQ, Engel WK, et al.: Refsum's Disease—A Recently Characterized Lipidosis Involving the Nervous System. *Ann Intern Med* 1967;66:365.

* 325. Steindler A. Stripping of the Os Calcis. *J Orthop Surg* 1920;2:8.

+ 326. Stern WG. Arthrogryposis Multiplex Congenita. *JAMA* 1923;81:1507.

327. Stevens JC, Lofgren EP, Dyck PJ. Biopsy of Peripheral Nerves. In: Dyck PJ, Thomas PK, Lambert EH, eds. *Peripheral Neuropathy*, Vol 1. Philadelphia: W.B. Saunders, 1975:410.

+ 328. Stevenson AJ, Torkelson RD. King's Syndrome with Malignant Hyperthemia. Potential Outpatient Risks. *Am J Dis Child* 1987;141:271.

+ 329. Sullivan JA, Conner SB. Comparison of Harrington Instrumentation and Segmental Spinal Instrumentation in the Management of Neuromuscular Spinal Deformity. *Spine* 1982;7:299.

+ 330. Sussman MD. Advantage of Early Spinal Stabilization and Fusion in Patients with Duchenne Muscular Dystrophy. *J Pediatr Orthop* 1984;4:532.

331. Sutherland DH, Olshen R, Cooper L. The Pathomechanics of Gait in Duchenne Muscular Dystrophy. *Dev Med Child Neurol* 1981;23:3.

+ 332. Swank SM, Brown JC, Perry R. Spinal Fusion in Duchenne's Muscular Dystrophy. *Spine* 1982;7:484.

+ 333. Swanson AB, Brown HS, Coleman JD. The Cavus Foot Concept of Production and Treatment by Metatarsal Osteotomy. *J Bone Joint Surg* 1966;48A:1019.

334. Swash M, Schwartz MS. *Neuromuscular Disease.* New York: Springer-Verlag, 1981.

335. Swinyard CA, Mayer V. Multiple Congenital Contractures: Public Health Considerations of Arthrogryposis Multiplex Congenita. *JAMA* 1963;183:23.

+ 336. Tello CA, de Tello AM. *Malignant Hyperthermia and Congenital Lordo Scoliosis.* Poster 34, presented at EPOS and POSNA combined meeting, Montreal, CA, September 1990.

+ 337. Thieffry S, Arthuis M, Bargeton E. Werdnig-Hoffman: 40 Cases with 11 Autopsies. *Rev Neurol* 1955;93:621.

+ 338. Thilenius OG, Grossman BJ. Friedreich's Ataxia with Heart Disease in Children. *Pediatrics* 1961;27:246.

+ 339. Thomas B, Schopler S, Wood W, Oppenheim WL. The Knee in Arthrogryposis. *Clin Orthop* 1985;194:87.

! 340. Thomas NS, Williams H, Eisas LJ, et al. Localization of the Gene for Emery-Dreifuss Muscular Dystrophy to the Distal Long Arm of the X-Chromosome. *J Med Genet* 1986;23:596.

+ 341. Thompson CE, Larsen LJ: Recurrent hip dislocation in intermediate spinal atrophy. *J Pediatr Orthop* 1990; 10:638.

342. Thompson GH, Bilenker RM. Comprehensive Management of Arthrogryposis Multiplex Congenita. *Clin Orthop* 1984;194:6.

+ 343. Thomson WH, Leyburn P, Walton JN. Serum Enzyme Activity in Muscular Dystrophy. *Br Med J* 1960;2: 1276.

+ 344. Thrush DC, Morris CJ, Salmon MV. Paramyotonia Congenita: A Clinical, Histochemical and Pathological Study. *Brain* 1972;95:537.

+ 345. Tome FMS, Evangelista T, Lecleric A, et al. Congenital Muscular Dystrophy with Merosin Deficiency. *Life Sci* 1994;317:351.

* 346. Tooth HH. The Peroneal Type of Progressive Muscular Atrophy. London: H.K. Lewis, 1886.

* 347. Turco VJ. Surgical Correction of the Resistant Clubfoot: One-Stage Posteromedial Release with Internal Fixation. A Preliminary Report. *J Bone Joint Surg* 1971;53-A:466.

* 348. Turco VJ. Resistant Congenital Clubfoot—One-Stage Posteromedial Release with Internal Fixation. A Follow-up Report of a 15-Year Experience. *J Bone Joint Surg* 1979;61-A:805.

+ 349. Tyler FH, Stephens FE. Studies in Disorders of Muscle. II: Clinical Manifestations and Inheritance of Facioscapulohumeral Dystrophy in a Large Family. *Ann Intern Med* 1950;32:640.

+ 350. Van Wijngaarden GK, Bethlem J. Benign Infantile Spinal Muscular Atrophy: A Prospective Study. *Brain* 1973;96:163.

+ 351. Vanier TM. Dystrophia Myotonia in Childhood. *Br Med J* 1960;2:1284.

+ 352. Vignos PJ Jr. Diagnosis of Progressive Muscular Dystrophy. *J Bone Joint Surg* 1967;49-A:1212.

+ 353. Vignos PJ Jr, Spencer GE Jr, Archibald KC. Management of Progressive Muscular Dystrophy in Childhood. *JAMA* 1963;184:89.

+ 354. Vignos PJ Jr, Wagner MB, Kaplan JS, Spencer GE. Predicting the Success of Reambulation in Patients with Duchenne Muscular Dystrophy. *J Bone Joint Surg* 1983;65-A:719.

+ 355. Vignos PJ, Wagner MB, Karlinchak B, Katirji B. Evaluation of a Program for Long-Term Treatment of Duchenne Muscular Dystrophy. Experience at the University Hospitals of Cleveland. *J Bone Joint Surg* 1996; 78A:1844.

+ 356. Vignos PJ Jr, Watkins MP. The Effect of Exercise in Muscular Dystrophy. *JAMA* 1966;197:843.

+ 357. Walker JJ, Nelson KR, Heavilon JA, et al. Hip Abnormalities in Children with Charcot-Marie-Tooth Disease. *J Pediatr Orthop* 1994;14(1):54.

+ 358. Walker JJ, Nelson KR, Stevens DB, et al. Spinal Deformity in Charcot-Marie-Tooth Disease. *Spine* 1994; 19(9):1044.

+ 359. Wang GJ, Shaffer LW. Osteotomy of the Metatarsals for Pes Cavus. *South Med J* 1977;70:77.

+ 360. Wang JM, Stanley TH. Duchenne Muscular Dystrophy and Malignant Hyperthermia—Two Case Reports. *Can Anesth Sec J* 1986;33:492.

+ 361. Watanabe RS. Metatarsal Osteotomy for the Cavus Foot. *Clin Orthop* 1990;252:217.

+ 362. Weimann R, Gibson DA, Moseley CF, et al. Surgical Stabilization of the Spine in Duchenne Muscular Dystrophy. *Spine* 1983;8:776.

* 363. Werdnig G. Zwen fruhintantile hereditare Falle von progressiver Muskelatrophie unter dem Bilde der Dystrophic, aber auf Neurotischer. *Grundlage Arch Psychiatr Nervenkrankh* 1891;22:437.

+ 364. Wetmore RS, Drennan JC. Long-term Results of Triple Arthrodesis in Charcot-Marie-Tooth Disease. *J Bone Joint Surg* 1989;71-A:417.

! 365. Wijmenga C, Frants RR, Brouwer OF, et al. The Facioscapulohumeral Muscular Dystrophy Gene Maps to Chromosome 4. *Lancet* 1990;2:651.

+ 366. Wilkins KE, Gibson DA. The Patterns of Spinal Deformity in Duchenne Muscular Dystrophy. *J Bone Joint Surg* 1976;58-A:24.

+ 367. Williams EA, Read L, Ellis A, Morris P, Galasko CSB. The Management of Equinus Deformity in Duchenne Muscular Dystrophy. *J Bone Joint Surg* 1984;66-B: 546.

368. Williams P. The Management of Arthrogryposis. *Orthop Clin North Am* 1978;9:67.

+ 369. Williams PF. The Elbow in Arthrogryposis. *J Bone Joint Surg* 1973;55B:834.

+ 370. Williams PF. Management of Upper Limb Problems in Arthrogryposis. *Clin Orthop* 1985;194:60.

371. Windebank AJ. Inherited Recurrent Focal Neuropathies. In: Dyck PJ, Thomas PJ, Griffin JW, et al. eds. *Peripheral Neuropathy*, 3rd ed. Philadelphia: W.B. Saunders, 1993:1137.

+ 372. Winters JL, McLaughlin LA. Myotonia Congenita. *J Bone Joint Surg* 1970;52-A:1345.

373. Wirth CR, Jacobs RL, Rolander SD. Neuropathic Spinal Arthropathy: A Review of the Charcot Spine. *Spine* 1980;5:558.

+ 374. Wolintz AH, Sonnenblick EH, Engel WK. Stokes-Adams Syndrome and Atrial Arrythmias as the Presenting Symptoms of Myotonic Dystrophy, with Response to Electrocardioversion. *Ann Intern Med* 1966;65: 1260.

+ 375. Wood VE, Huene D, Nguyen J. Treatment of the Upper Limb in Charcot-Marie-Tooth Disease. *J Hand Surg [Br]* 1995;20(4):511.

+ 376. Wukich DK, Bowen JR. A Long-term Study of Triple Arthrodesis For Correction of Pes Cavovarus in Charcot-Marie-Tooth Disease. *J Pediatr Orthop* 1989;9: 433.

377. Yates G. Molded Plastics in Bracing. *Clin Orthop* 1974; 102:46.

+ 378. Yazawa Y. Mitral Valve Prolapse Related to Geometrical Changes of the Heart in Cases of Progressive Muscular Dystrophy. *Clin Cardiol* 1984;7:198.

+ 379. Yoslow W, Becker MH, Bartels J, Thompson WAL. Familial Dysautonomia Review of Sixty-Five Cases. *J Bone Joint Surg* 1971;53-A:1541.

* 380. Yount CC. The Role of the Tensor Fasciae Femoris in Certain Deformities of the Lower Extremities. *J Bone Joint Surg* 1926;8:171.

+ 381. Zatz M, Betti RT. Benign Duchenne Muscular Dystrophy in a Patient with Growth Hormone Deficiency: A Five-Year Follow-up. *Am J Med Genet* 1986;24:567.

+ 382. Zatz M, Betti RT, Frota-Pessoa O. Treatment of Duchenne Muscular Dystrophy with Growth Hormone Inhibitors. *Am J Med Genet* 1986;24:549.

+ 383. Zerres K, Rudnik-Schoneborn S, Forrest E, et al. A Collaborative Study on the Natural History of Childhood and Juvenile Onset Proximal Spinal Muscular Atrophy. J Neurosci 1997;146:67.

+ 384. Zetlweger H, Afifi A, McCormick WF, Mergner W. Severe Congenital Muscular Dystrophy. *Am J Dis Child* 1967;114:591.

+ 385. Zellweger H, Antonik A. Newborn Screening for Duchenne Muscular Dystrophy. *Pediatrics* 1975;5:30.

+ 386. Zellweger J, Lonasescu V. Early Onset of Myotonic Dystrophy in Infants. *Am J Dis Child* 1973;125:601.

+ 387. Ziter FA, Allsop KG, Tyler FH. Assessment of Muscle Strength in Duchenne Muscular Dystrophy. *Neurology* 1977;27:981.

## CHAPTER 179

THE ORTHOPAEDIC MANAGEMENT OF MYELODYSPLASIA AND SPINA BIFIDA

Nigel S. Broughton and Malcolm B. Menelaus

Myelodysplasia and spina bifida are congenital anomalies characterized by abnormality of the closure of the neural tube. They constitute a group of disturbances including failure of full development of structures derived from the neural tube and the meninges. These disturbances result in abnormal neural control of organs innervated by the affected part of the spinal cord. This abnormal innervation gives rise to multiple organ involvement, including effects on bladder and bowel, as well as denervation of muscles resulting in paralysis.

The orthopaedic management of spina bifida is aimed at allowing children to fulfill their maximum physical and social potential within the limitations imposed by the congenital anomaly.

N. S. Broughton: Consultant Orthopaedic Surgeon, Department of Orthopaedics, Frankston Hospital, Victoria, Frankston, Australia.

M. B. Menelaus: Chief Orthopaedic Surgeon, Emeritus, Royal Children's Hospital, Melbourne, Australia.

ASSESSMENT OF NEUROSEGMENTAL LEVEL

Assessment of the neurosegmental level is important because it allows us to predict the functional status of the child. Assessment should be performed as early as possible and repeated annually, using the grading indicated in Table 179.1 with accurate recording of muscle power. Neurosegmental level can be confirmed and any significant deterioration in neurologic status requiring investigation for a tethered cord or cord syrinx is easily detected (Fig. 179.1). Assessment of the level becomes more accurate after the age of 5 years, when the child is more cooperative.

We use a classification based on Sharrard's original description of nerve root innervation to define a precise level and code the power in the muscle as shown in Table 179.2.

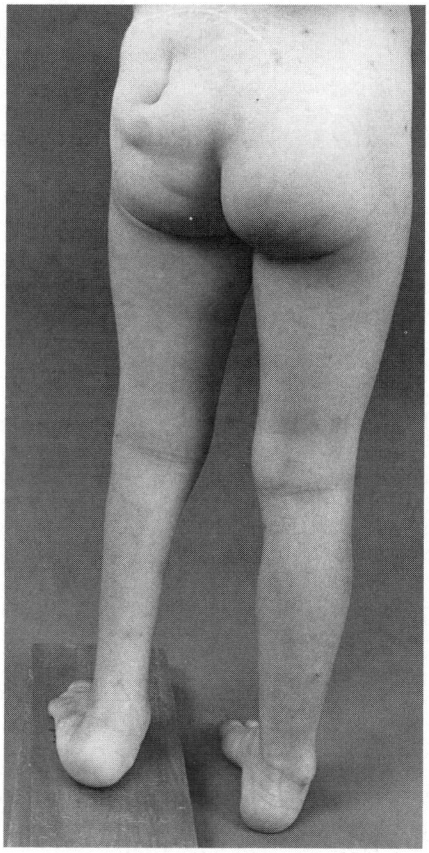

Figure 179.1. In hemimyelodysplasia, there is gross asymmetry of the neurosegmental level, often resulting in leg-length discrepancy. The difference in leg lengths can usually be managed by epiphyseodesis in the long limb, but when there is gross discrepancy, leg lengthening may be more appropriate. (Reproduced with permission from Menelaus MB. *Orthopaedic Management of Spina Bifida Cystica,* 2nd ed. Edinburgh: Churchill Livingstone, 1980.).

Table 179.1. Coding of Muscle Strength

0—none	No contraction felt in the muscle
1—trace	Can see, or feel, muscle belly flicker but no visible movement
2—poor	Movement possible with gravity eliminated
3—fair	Movement possible against gravity but takes no resistance
4—good	Movement possible and takes resistance to break test
5—normal	Movement possible and muscle cannot be "broken" in shortened range

Table 179.2. Assessment of Neurosegmental Level

Thoracic	No active movement at the hip
L-1	Iliopsoas grade 2 or better
L-2	Iliopsoas, sartorius, and adductors all grade 3 or better
L-3	Quadriceps grade 3 or better and meet criteria for L-2
L-4	Medial hamstring or tibialis anterior grade 3 or better and meet criteria for L-3
L-5	Lateral hamstrings grade 3 or better and meet criteria for L-4 plus one of the following three: gluteus medius grade 2 or better, peroneus tertius grade 4 or better, tibialis posterior grade 3 or better.
S-1	Two of the following three: gastrocnemius or soleus grade 2 or better, gluteus medius grade 3 or better, gluteus maximus grade 2 or better and meet criteria for L-5.
S-2	Gastrocnemius or soleus grade 3 or better and gluteus medius and gluteus maximus grade 4 or better and meet criteria for S-1.
No loss	All leg muscles normal strength

Assessment of quadriceps and hip abductor power provide a reasonable estimate of walking ability. Community ambulation is unlikely if the quadriceps and hip abductors have no power; community ambulation with splints and aids is likely if quadriceps are innervated but hip abductors are not; and community ambulation is probable if both quadriceps and hip abductors have power. The prediction of walking ability is important in determining the type and extent of surgical treatment required to correct deformity in childhood.

Recent work has suggested that the hip abductors are innervated at the same or higher level than the tibialis anterior and has confirmed that the medial hamstrings are innervated at a higher level than was originally described (15). However, further work is necessary to determine the significance of these findings.

CAUSES OF DEFORMITY

MUSCLE IMBALANCE DUE TO LOWER MOTOR NEURON LESIONS

In large part, the lowest innervated segment is determined by the developmental defect. However, further lower motor neuron lesions may be caused by postnatal drying and infection of the neural plate. If the child is expected to survive, this should be avoided by closure of the defect within 24 hours. Shurtleff has also demonstrated that trauma to the exposed neural plate at vaginal delivery can produce further lower motor neuron lesions; this problem can be prevented by electing to deliver known spina bifida fetuses by cesarean section at 36 weeks' gestation (20). Lower motor neuron lesions can also be produced in childhood when growth produces traction on a tethered cord, damaging nerve roots.

Various patterns of paralysis are seen according to the lowest innervated myotome. The resulting muscle imbalance can, in some cases, predict the likely deformity. For example, in a limb where there is innervation down to and including L-5, indicated by activity in the tibialis anterior, peroneus tertius, and the extensor digitorum longus with no activity in soleus or gastrocnemius, a calcaneus or calcaneovalgus deformity of the foot commonly occurs.

Sharrard stated that hip flexion contracture was greatest where the muscle imbalance was greatest, that is, with innervation to L-2, L-3, and L-4 (19). However, our findings have been that hip flexion contracture is most common in children with a thoracic level lesion where there is no muscle activity at the hip. There is no evidence of spasticity in patients with the most severe flexion contracture at the hip (2,21). Fixed hip deformity is not predictable from the state of muscle activity around the hip.

Dislocation of the hip in spina bifida has been considered to be due to muscle imbalance (19), but our studies have shown that about 30% of hips with no muscle imbalance dislocate, whereas 70% of hips with innervation to L-4 and presumed to have the greatest muscle imbalance neither dislocate nor require any operation. Dislocation of the hip in spina bifida is not inevitable when there is muscle imbalance across the hip (2).

Studies on the natural history of deformity at the knee also raise doubts about the role of muscle imbalance in producing fixed deformity (24).

MUSCLE IMBALANCE DUE TO UPPER MOTOR NEURON LESIONS

Upper motor lesions resulting in spasticity of muscles are present in two thirds of children with myelomeningocele (Fig. 179.2*A*, *B*, *C*).

Three patterns can be recognized. In the first pattern, flaccid paralysis is present, but in levels more distal, there is a spastic paralysis with exaggerated reflex activity. In the second pattern, there is only a narrow segment of flaccid paralysis (resembling spinal cord transection) and purely reflex activity below the level. In the third pattern, there is incomplete transection and hence myotomes can show spasticity with increased reflexes, but there is also a degree of voluntary movement.

Because muscles across a joint may be flaccid, normally innervated, or spastic, various degrees of imbalance may be produced. Although muscle imbalance between flaccid and spastic muscles can give rise to severe deformity of the foot, the argument for this is less convincing at the hip or knee, and other explanations for severe deformity should be sought.

INTRAUTERINE POSTURE

The average hip flexion contracture, in all children with myelomeningocele at birth, is about 20°, and this angle decreases with lesions at all levels up to the age of 1 year. In children with a lesion at the thoracic level, this decrease is less than in other levels. Intrauterine pressure causes various patterns of foot deformity at birth in paralyzed feet.

HABITUALLY ASSUMED POSTURE

Children with thoracic level lesions often develop external rotation and abduction deformities of the hips if they are allowed to lie for long periods in this position. Prolonged sitting may be a factor in the development of flexion deformity at the hips and knees in high-level lesions.

ARTHROGRYPOSIS-LIKE DEFORMITIES

Some children with significant deformity at birth resemble patients with arthrogryposis multiplex congenita, with ri-

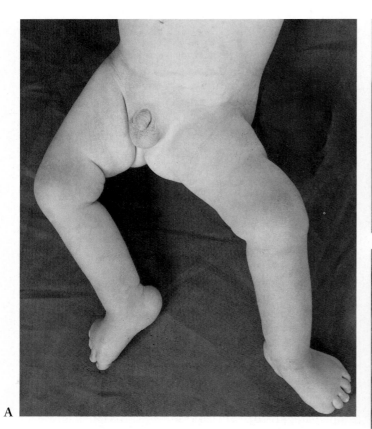

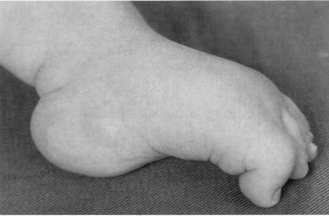

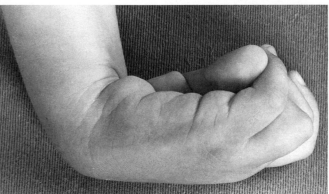

Figure 179.2.   Spasticity has resulted in deformity in the upper and lower limbs of this child. **A:** An abduction contracture has developed at the hip. This was corrected by a lateral release. **B:** Spasticity of flexor hallucis longus. **C:** Spasticity of wrist flexors and the intrinsics in the hand. (B and C reproduced with permission from Menelaus MB. *Orthopaedic Management of Spina Bifida Cystica,* 2nd ed. Edinburgh: Churchill Livingstone, 1980.)

gidity of joints and absence of normal creases. These deformities may be present at one or more joints, are resistant to standard management, and require radical surgery for their correction.

UNKNOWN FACTORS

We simply do not know why most patients with thoracic level lesions develop deformity, including all possible foot deformities.

GOAL OF ORTHOPAEDIC MANAGEMENT

The goal of orthopaedic management is to produce a stable posture for sitting or walking. Hip flexion contractures and knee flexion contractures give rise to difficulties in standing and walking, as well as increased energy expenditure. Successful treatment of these deformities ensures a stable posture.

Conservative treatment of deformity in the child with spina bifida is ineffective and gives rise to cast sores and pathologic fractures; therefore, in general, surgical intervention is preferable.

The goals of surgical management are to avoid unnecessary operations that confer no benefit on the patient, to perform multiple operations at the same time, and to use the minimum period of postoperative immobilization possible. We plan surgery with an awareness of what the child is likely to achieve in walking in the long term so that the surgical goals are realistic (11–13).

Children with thoracic neurosegmental levels are unlikely to continue effective walking into adolescence. Until then, we encourage them to walk and they enjoy standing.

As their condition progresses, we use reciprocating gait orthoses or hip-knee-foot orthoses (HKFOs). They will require increasing use of a wheelchair with time. Surgery aims at a trouble-free wheelchair existence. We correct foot deformity of a degree that precludes normal footwear, generally by soft-tissue release. Extensive hip surgery is not indicated, but we aim to correct excessive flexion contracture by soft-tissue release to prevent excessive lumbar lordosis.

Children with L-1 and L-2 neurosegmental levels are rarely community ambulators as adolescents, but the time spent walking in braces may be longer than in children with thoracic level lesions, so surgery to improve brace fitting should be considered.

Children with L-3, L-4, and L-5 neurosegmental levels with strong quadriceps are usually good walkers. They usually require an ankle-foot orthosis to stabilize the ankle. The need for crutches or walking aids depends on the strength of the abductors at the hip. The surgeon should assume that the child will achieve worthwhile walking, and therefore, extensive surgery to correct deformities at the hip, knee, and foot may be justified. Furthermore, soft-tissue surgery is justified for these patients during childhood, recognizing that bony surgery, such as triple arthrodesis, may be necessary at maturity.

The child may start walking with extensive bracing, including hip control orthoses, but as confidence builds up, the extent of the bracing can be reduced to below the knee.

Most children with sacral lesions are effective community ambulators until adulthood, when some deteriorate and cease walking. Hip deformity is uncommon, but surgery is often necessary for foot and toe deformities.

SURGICAL CORRECTION OF DEFORMITIES OF THE HIP

Hip flexion contracture and hip dislocation were previously thought to be due entirely to muscle imbalance across the hip (19). We have now shown that the hip flexion contracture is most common and most severe in children with thoracic neurosegmental level (2). Dislocation of the hip is also common in thoracic neurosegmental level, whereas in children with innervation to L-4, who presumably have maximum muscle imbalance, only a third develop hip dislocation or require hip surgery (2). Therefore, muscle imbalance is one of a number of factors implicated in the development of hip flexion contracture and hip dislocation. Prophylactic surgery to correct muscle imbalance is no longer undertaken because many children with muscle imbalance develop no deformity or dislocation at the hip.

RELEASE OF HIP FLEXION CONTRACTURE

Hip flexion contracture is commonly seen in normal neonates and in neonates with spina bifida with all neurosegmental levels. The deformity decreases during the first year of life but improves least in thoracic neurosegmental levels (2,21), and in these patients, it has a strong tendency to increase again with advancing years.

If hip flexion deformity is interfering with the child's ability to walk (generally this occurs when the deformity is greater than 20°), we perform a soft-tissue release.

- Drape the patient so that Thomas' test can be performed throughout the procedure.
- The procedure is best performed through the incision described by Salter for innominate osteotomy (see Chapter 166).
- Sweep the muscles off both the inner and the outer surfaces of the ilium, divide the psoas tendon, release the sartorius and rectus femoris, and if necessary, divide the anterior capsule of the hip joint transversely.
- At the conclusion of this procedure, the anterior superior iliac spine and adjacent portions of the iliac crest will protrude forward and should be removed.

Our results of long-term follow-up are satisfactory (8). If the hip is also dislocated, consider reducing the hip along the lines described in the next section. In a thoracic-level nonwalker, correction of the hip flexion contracture is commonly attempted without reduction of a dislocated hip (Fig. 179.3A, B, C).

Postoperatively, the child should be nursed alternately prone and supine, with the hips extended for 6 weeks. We also use low trolleys on casters so the child can lie prone on these and move around the house using the arms.

CORRECTION OF HIP DISLOCATION

The presence of hip dislocation is not an indication to attempt reduction. Reduction should be attempted only when the child will derive considerable benefit from this procedure (6,7,10). Attempts at operative reduction are not always successful, may result in stiff painful hips, are sometimes associated with heterotopic calcification, and generally reduce the child's ability to walk. An untreated dislocated hip is rarely painful, but if the dislocation is unilateral, it may give rise to limb-length discrepancy, which is troublesome for walkers and can cause seating difficulties for wheelchair users. Most specialists would agree that there is little difference in walking ability of children with high neurosegmental levels who have located or dislocated hips (Fig. 179.4A, B).

Children with hip dislocation who would benefit from surgery to reduce the hip are those with low-level lesions

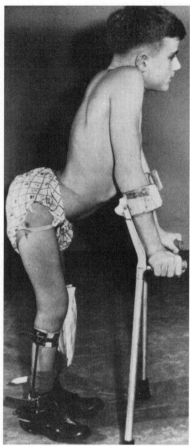
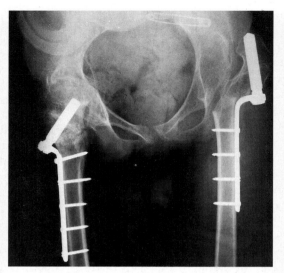
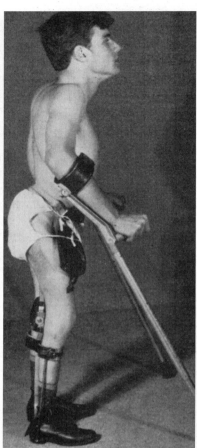

A,B   C

Figure 179.3.   **A:** Undesirable flexion posture in a boy with L-4 lesion. He has strong psoas and quadriceps muscles but gluteal weakness and has developed fixed flexion deformity of both hips. Note the gross lumbar lordosis and that his center of gravity is in front of rather than directly over his feet. **B:** We are usually able to correct the deformity with an extensive soft-tissue anterior hip release. However, on this occasion, because of the severity of the deformity, extension femoral osteotomies have been performed. No attempt was made to reduce the left hip; he remains a community ambulator. **C:** Postoperatively he has a much better extension posture, although some of his lumbar lordosis is fixed. The operation was performed 25 years ago and the patient is still walking. (Reproduced with permission from Menelaus MB. *Orthopaedic Management of Spina Bifida Cystica,* 1st ed. Edinburgh: Churchill Livingstone, 1971.)

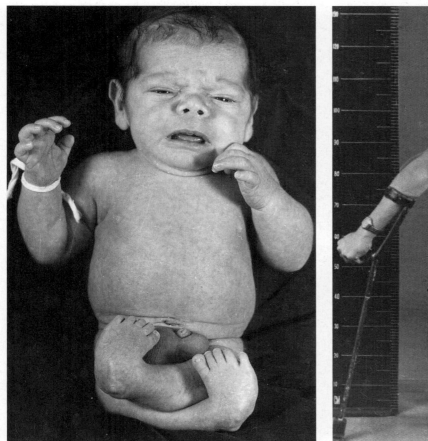
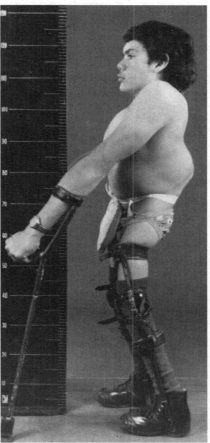

Figure 179.4. **A:** This child was born with severe arthrogrypotic deformities of the lower limbs. He was treated by soft-tissue releases on one occasion, but his bilateral hip dislocations were not reduced. **B:** Same child at the age of 17 years demonstrating a satisfactory extension posture in KAFOs. He is now 32 years old and remains a household ambulator. (Reproduced with permission from Menelaus MB. *Orthopaedic Management of Spina Bifida Cystica*, 2nd ed. Edinburgh: Churchill Livingstone, 1980.)

at L-3 and below. They usually have strong quadriceps, do not require bracing above the knee, and will probably be good walkers. In this group, unilateral hip dislocations should generally be reduced (Figs. 179.5A, B, C, D and 179.6A, B). In general, bilateral hip dislocations in this group do not benefit from attempts at reduction, but reduction is occasionally performed if the dislocated hips are not high and surgery is necessary in any case for hip flexion contracture. In children with high-level lesions (thoracic, L-1, and L-2) and therefore weak quadriceps, bilateral hip dislocations should not be reduced. Children with unilateral hip dislocations may benefit from reduction if the dislocation is not gross, the other leg has a low lesion, and surgery is necessary anyway to correct hip flexion deformity. We have seen few problems from leaving a unilateral hip dislocation untreated in a child with a high-level lesion (Table 179.3).

If the hip dislocation is present at birth and is irreducible, attempts at reduction should not be made because it will lead to stiffness. If the hip is unstable but can be easily reduced by Ortolani's test and the lesion is low, it is worthwhile using abduction bracing to encourage acetabular development. However, the brace should not interfere with closure of the spinal defect and its postoperative management.

Operative reduction should aim for correction with the minimum of postoperative immobilization. The principles of the operation are

- to achieve a concentric reduction of the femoral head with capsulorrhaphy and excision of intra-articular structures (see Chapter 166).
- correction of muscle imbalance by flexor and adductor releases.

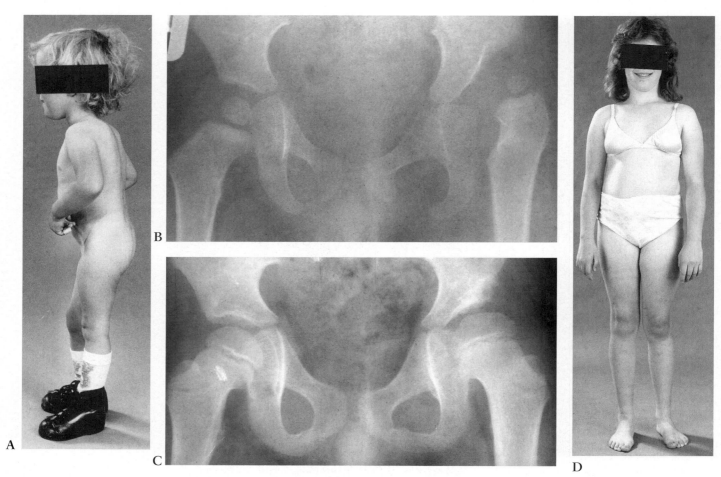

Figure 179.5.   **A:** This child had normal muscle power in her right leg but an L-5 lesion on the left. **B:** A radiograph demonstrates dislocation of the left hip. **C:** Same child treated by open reduction, psoas lengthening, and a Pemberton osteotomy. The follow-up radiograph shows a concentric reduction. **D:** At the age of 15 years there is little leg-length discrepancy, but note the left calf is slightly smaller. (**A** and **B** reproduced with permission from Williams PF, Cole WG. *Orthopaedic Management in Childhood.* London: Chapman and Hall, 1991).

Table 179.3. *Indications for Reduction of Hip Dislocation in Spina Bifida*		
	Unilateral	*Bilateral*
High-level lesion Weak quadriceps Require above-knee bracing Probably short-term walkers	Occasionally reduce if dislocation is not gross, the other leg has a low lesion, or surgery is required in any case for flexion deformity	Never reduce
Low-level lesion Strong quadriceps Short bracing Lifetime walkers	Usually reduce	Occasionally reduce if dislocation is not gross and surgery is required in any case for flexion contracture

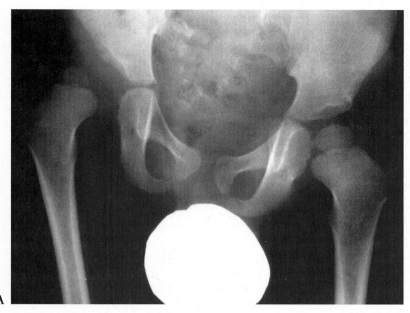

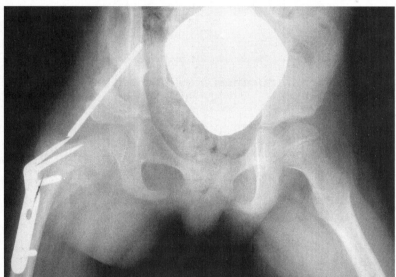

Figure 179.6. **A:** Unilateral hip dislocation in a low-level lesion. **B:** This dislocation has been treated by open reduction, Pemberton osteotomy, and a femoral osteotomy.

- improvement in acetabular coverage, generally by a Pemberton osteotomy. This is performed through an approach similar to that described for a soft-tissue release of the hip (see the previous section).

Plaster immobilization is necessary for only 6 weeks postoperatively.

PROVISION OF ABDUCTOR AND EXTENSOR POWER AT THE HIP

Muscle transfers about the hip were popular for spina bifida (4) when it was thought that muscle imbalance caused hip dislocation and contractures. Because we now know that the relationship between muscle imbalance and hip deformity is less clear, we believe that there is no place for the use of prophylactic muscle transfers, because prediction of development of deformity is not possible from muscle strengths.

Some surgeons believe that muscle transfers are appropriate in selected circumstances, but there is general agreement now against the use of posterior iliopsoas transfer (19) because gait analysis has established that the energy cost following this procedure is unacceptably high.

If the surgeon believes that there is a specific patient with a low lumbar lesion who might have a better gait following muscle transfer (gait analysis may facilitate the decision-making process), then the triple transfer, described by Yngve and Lindseth (25), or external oblique transfer alone would seem to be the most logical, considering our present state of knowledge. The triple transfer consists of external oblique transfer to the greater trochanter, transfer of the adductor origin posteriorly, and posterior transfer of the origin of tensor fascia lata, often in combination with a varus derotation femoral osteotomy to improve gait and reduce the risk of dislocation. Transfer of the iliopsoas to the anterior greater trochanter, as described by Mustard (16), frequently leads to fixed flexion deformity. The indications for muscle transfers at the hip are now few.

CORRECTION OF DEFORMITIES OF THE KNEE

KNEE FLEXION CONTRACTURE

Flexion deformity of the knee and limitation of flexion of the knee are most common in children with thoracic neurosegmental lesions and not in children in whom there is muscle imbalance at the knee (24).

Flexion of up to 20° is common at birth and generally improves spontaneously. If there is a fixed flexion deformity of greater than 20° in the neonate, then serial casting may be necessary. If a fixed flexion deformity is found in a child older than 3 years of age who has the potential for walking, we perform a soft-tissue release. Knee flexion correction often occurs with hip flexion contracture, and both should be corrected at the same time. Knee flexion is corrected by releasing all of the hamstring tendons at the knee. Posterior capsulotomy of the knee is usually necessary to achieve full correction (14) (Fig. 179.7A, B, C). It is important that a full correction of the flexion deformity is obtained at operation because recurrence follows incomplete correction and further correction with serial plaster casts is usually incomplete. Transfers of the hamstrings into the patella or lower femur have generally been disappointing and are not advised. An extension supracondylar osteotomy is infrequently used for flexion deformity in the child approaching skeletal maturity.

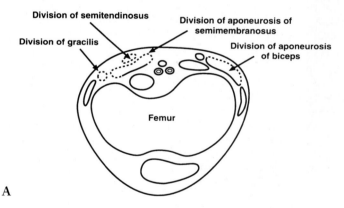

Minimum Procedure

A

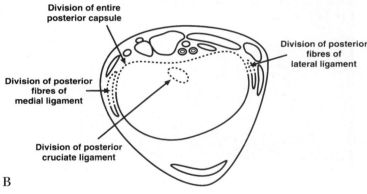

Additional Optional Procedures at Joint Level

B

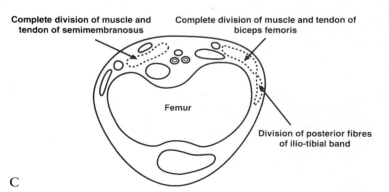

Additional Optional Procedures Above Joint Level

C

Figure 179.7. **A:** Transverse section at the distal femur showing the minimum procedure for soft-tissue release. **B:** Additional procedures at the knee level that may be necessary to achieve a full correction. **C:** Additional procedures above the joint level that may be necessary to achieve a full correction. (Reproduced with permission from Marshall PD, Broughton NS, Menelaus MB, Graham HK. Surgical Release of Knee Flexion Contractures in Myelomeningocele. *J Bone Joint Surg* 1996;78B:912.)

EXTENSION DEFORMITY

Some neonates present with a recurrent extension deformity of the knee, but this usually responds to serial casting. The knee may be held rigidly in extension and have the featureless appearance of arthrogryposis multiplex congenita. Tenotomy of the ligamentum patella (18) is best performed at about 6 years of age, when the extension deformity becomes troublesome as the legs grow. At this age the child can manage knee locks on a long-leg brace without assistance. Walking in a knee-ankle-foot orthosis can begin a few days after the operation. The child uses night splints at 90° of flexion for 2 months. Quadricepsplasty is usually not indicated because there is usually insufficient voluntary power in the muscle to make the procedure worthwhile.

VALGUS DEFORMITY

Valgus deformity is uncommon. It can generally be managed by medial growth plate stapling, and it seldom requires lower femoral or upper tibial osteotomy.

CORRECTION OF TORSIONAL DEFORMITIES OF THE TIBIA

EXTERNAL ROTATION OF THE TIBIA

External rotation of the tibia is commonly associated with a valgus ankle. It should be treated after the age of 8 years by supramalleolar rotational osteotomy of the tibia, which can be combined with correction of the valgus ankle at the supramalleolar level (see later).

INTERNAL ROTATION OF THE TIBIA

Although minor degrees of internal rotation of the tibia can be corrected by transfer of the semitendinosus to the biceps femoris, we have now largely abandoned the procedure because such an indication is seldom present. Gross degrees of the deformity are corrected in the first 3 years of life by osteoclasis of the tibia and fibula (Fig. 179.8) or at a later age by supramalleolar external rotation osteotomy.

CORRECTION OF DEFORMITIES OF THE FOOT

Deformities of the foot in spina bifida are common at all levels of neurosegmental defect. In patients with high-level lesions, 89% of feet are deformed despite the absence of

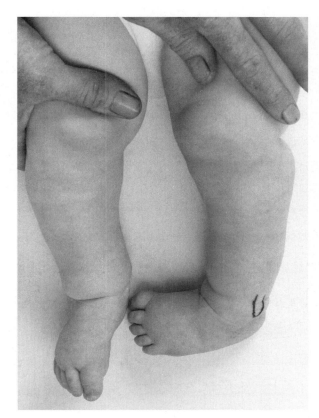

Figure 179.8. Internal tibial torsion of the left leg. This problem was treated by tibial osteoclasis.

muscle imbalance (3). Of those with low-level lesions, 76% are deformed, and the incidence of various deformities are similar to those encountered in high-level lesions (9). Those with calcaneus deformity have a higher incidence of activity of the tibialis anterior with calf weakness but calcaneus is common in the absence of this muscle imbalance. Spasticity is present in a high percentage of patients with high-level lesions but in none of those with undeformed feet. Spasticity is much less common (ratio of 1:2) in patients with low-level lesions.

TRIPLE ARTHRODESIS

The goal of the management of foot deformity is to achieve a plantargrade and mobile foot. However, there are occasions when triple arthrodesis is the most appropriate method to correct a complex deformity. The lateral inlay technique (23) has proved particularly valuable in patients with spina bifida (Fig. 179.9*A, B, C*). Long-term follow-up has confirmed this impression (17). Triple arthrodesis must be used with caution in the older ambulatory patient because of the risk of plantar pressure sores in a rigid foot that is devoid of sensation.

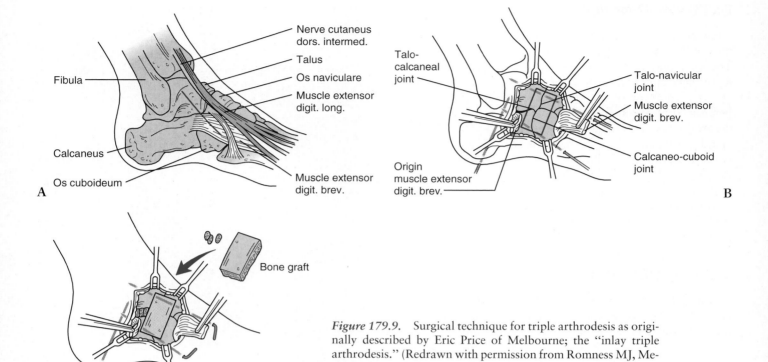

Figure 179.9. Surgical technique for triple arthrodesis as originally described by Eric Price of Melbourne; the "inlay triple arthrodesis." (Redrawn with permission from Romness MJ, Menelaus MB. Inlay Triple Arthrodesis: A Technique for the Undeformed or Valgus Foot. *Orthop Traumatol* 1995;4:114.)

- Make a straight incision centered over the junction of the four bones to be fused (Fig. 179.9*A*).
- Lift the extensor digitorum brevis distally and retract the extensors medially to allow exposure of the talonavicular, calcaneocuboid, and subtalar joints. Excise the capsules and expose the sinus.
- Hold the foot in the desired position and insert 4.5 mm wires through the talonavicular, the calcaneocuboid, and the subtalar joints (Fig. 179.9*C*). Cut a trough as shown and decorticate the sinus tarsi. Take an oblong-shaped graft from the upper third of the ipsilateral tibia and punch it into the trough to give a tight fit. Insert chips of bone graft into the subtalar joint.

EQUINOVARUS DEFORMITY

The rigidity of the equinovarus deformity varies from that seen in the usual form of talipes equinovarus to the more commonly seen rigid, "arthrogrypotic" deformity, which has a high rate of recurrence despite apparent adequate correction initially. In general, a varus deformity requires operative correction to establish a plantigrade foot; otherwise, pressure sores due to weight bearing on a small area of the sole are inevitable.

Initially, the treatment consists of serial correction in well-padded plaster casts that are changed frequently while the baby is still hospitalized after birth, and later at 2- to 4-week intervals as circumstances demand. Although it may not be apparent at birth, the tendo Achillis is usually short, and a closed tenotomy should be performed when convenient, between 3 and 6 months of age.

If a child older than 3 months of age is thriving and does not require surgery for concomitant conditions in other systems, we perform a posteromedial release. The Cincinnati surgical approach for this technique is described in Chapter 167. Because recurrence is likely, excision of portions of the tendo Achillis, tibialis anterior, tibialis posterior, and the long toe flexors is necessary rather than lengthening. If the deformity recurs, we perform a repeat soft-tissue release.

In some patients for whom demands on the foot are high, trophic ulceration is likely, so in cases in which repeat soft-tissue release is not controlling the deformity, further procedures are necessary. Although we have used talectomy for this situation in the past, we now prefer variations of the Vereberlyi-Ogston procedure with decancellation of the talus and cuboid to allow collapse of these bones and correction of deformity (22). Tendon transfers have no part in the management of this deformity (see Chapter 167).

If deformity recurs between the ages of 7 and 14 years, it is wise to accept the deformity, provide appropriate footwear, and aim to correct the deformity by triple arthrodesis at skeletal maturity.

Pure Equinus Deformity

A pure equinus deformity can be present in patients with any neurosegmental level. It responds well to open or closed tenotomy, depending on the severity of the deformity and the age of the child.

CALCANEUS DEFORMITY

Calcaneus deformity is common in spina bifida patients, most commonly seen in children with an L-5 neurosegmental lesion but also commonly seen in the absence of muscle imbalance. The major problem with calcaneus deformity is the development of pressure sores because large forces are transmitted through a small area of insensitive heel. This deformity is usually left untreated until muscle power can be properly assessed at the age of about 3 years.

If the deformity is progressing and the tibialis anterior is of normal strength, a transfer of the tibialis anterior through the interosseous membrane to the heel is appropriate, although some surgeons simply lengthen it. If extensor hallucis longus, extensor digitorum longus, or peroneus tertius are active, they should be divided at the same time. If the calcaneus deformity is fixed, we combine this procedure with a full anterior ankle capsulotomy to allow correction of the deformity (1).

If the anterior muscles are weak or spastic, we perform a tenodesis of the tendo Achillis to the lower fibular metaphysis. This procedure may stimulate growth at the lower end of the fibula and correct any tendency to develop ankle valgus.

In a late-presenting severe fixed calcaneus deformity with a "pistol-grip" heel, an osteotomy of the calcaneus removing a wedge based posteriorly improves the weight-bearing area. Concomitant valgus of the heel may be corrected by adding varus to the osteotomy. This can be performed in combination with tendon transfers and tenodesis as appropriate. A plantar release may be required as well in the treatment of concomitant cavus deformity.

VALGUS DEFORMITY

In general, valgus feet create less trouble than varus feet and can usually be controlled by orthoses until adolescence. The precise site of bony deformity should be identified; it may be at the ankle, at the subtalar joint, or at both these sites. Clinical examination and weight-bearing radiography enable the precise site of deformity to be identified.

Ankle Valgus

Ankle valgus can be recognized clinically because the distal end of the fibula can be palpated proximal to the tip of the medial malleolus. On the radiograph, the distal fibular growth plate lies proximal to the dome of the talus, as opposed to the normal relationship for that age. This appearance is associated with a wedge-shaped distal tibial epiphysis.

The relative shortening of the fibula can be reduced by tendo Achillis tenodesis to the fibula if this procedure is indicated for coexisting calcaneus deformity. The valgus effect of the wedge-shaped distal tibia epiphysis can be corrected by a medial arrest of the distal tibial growth plate either by the insertion of a screw from the tip of the medial malleolus across the growth plate or by the Phemister technique. To be effective, this procedure must be performed before the child is 7 to 8 years of age. After this age, a supramalleolar osteotomy is indicated if the deformity is sufficiently severe to be producing undue pressure on the skin over the medial malleolus, where its excessive prominence rubs on ankle-foot orthoses or footwear. This is done 1 cm above the growth plate with excision of a medially based wedge, together with an oblique distal fibular osteotomy. The tibial osteotomy is fixed with two crossed K-wires. Any rotational deformity can be corrected at the same time. We have experienced a 5% incidence of wound breakdown and delayed union following this procedure.

Subtalar Valgus

Subtalar valgus can usually be controlled by orthoses in children younger than the age of 10 years, but division of spastic peroneal muscles may be necessary. If an orthosis fails to control this problem, we would now avoid subtalar fusion and perform a calcaneal osteotomy by excising a medially based wedge and also shifting the distal calcaneus medially. The position is held by a Steinmann pin. If the presentation is close to skeletal maturity, it is commonly associated with a planoabductus deformity, which is best treated by a lateral inlay triple fusion (23).

Ankle Plus Subtalar Valgus

Each deformity should be addressed separately and corrected as described in the previous section. If the patient is nearly mature, this may well necessitate a supramalleolar osteotomy with a lateral inlay triple fusion.

CAVUS DEFORMITY

Management of a cavus deformity depends on the degree and rigidity of the deformity and the age of the child. Minor deformity can be observed and any pressure effects minimized with an appropriate insole. Treat progressive deformity for children up to the age of 5 years by a plantar release procedure. For children older than 5 years, soft-tissue release may have to be combined with osteotomies at the bases of all metatarsals. If there is an element of supination in the forefoot deformity and the hindfoot is mobile, the osteotomies may be limited to the first or first and second metatarsal bases to improve the weight-bearing area of the foot. Osteotomy of the calcaneus is indicated if there is an associated varus deformity of the heel. Triple arthrodesis is indicated if there is a significant varus and cavus deformity in the child close to skeletal maturity.

PARALYTIC CONVEX PES VALGUS (VERTICAL TALUS)

Paralytic convex pes valgus (vertical talus) occurs in less than 2% of children with spina bifida. It can present at birth and is then similar to the congenital vertical talus that is not associated with spina bifida. It can also occur in a less rigid form, which develops slowly over the first years of life (5).

Surgical correction is necessary and involves reduction of the talonavicular (and sometimes the calcaneocuboid) joint and correction of the ankle equinus and heel valgus. These objectives can be achieved through a Cincinnati surgical approach (see Chapter 167). The operation is best performed in the first year of life.

- Section the tibialis anterior, extensor digitorum longus, and the peroneal muscles, and lengthen the tendo Achillis.
- Perform a lateral release of the subtalar joint and, if the valgus deformity is gross, insert a lateral bone block into the subtalar joint.
- Maintain correction with longitudinal and vertical K-wires for 4 to 6 weeks, as well as immobilization in a cast for 3 months postoperatively.
- Use a carefully molded ankle-foot orthosis to control planus, heel valgus, and the flail ankle.

FLAIL ANKLE

We treat the flail ankle with an ankle-foot orthosis until maturity. Ankle fusion in children has a high failure rate, as does pantalar fusion.

CLAW TOES

Claw toes are common in patients with L-5 and sacral lesions. In the second to fifth toes, open flexor tenotomy and closed extensor tenotomy generally corrects the mobile deformity sufficiently to prevent pressure effects on the tip or dorsum of the affected toe. Rigid deformity requires interphalangeal arthrodesis and extensor tenotomy, as well as dorsal release at the metatarsophalangeal joint.

Clawing of the hallux can give rise to pressure sores over the first metatarsal head and over the dorsum of the interphalangeal joint. If the deformity is correctable in the younger child, tenodesis of flexor hallucis longus to the proximal phalanx corrects the deformity but may have to be combined with a dorsal capsulotomy of the first

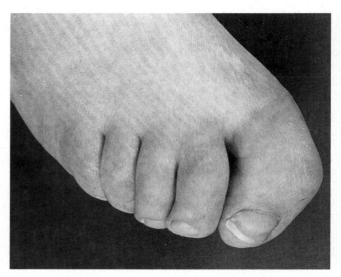

Figure 179.10. Interphalangeal valgus and pronation of the hallux. This problem was treated by interphalangeal arthrodesis. (Reproduced with permission from Menelaus MB. *Orthopaedic Management of Spina Bifida Cystica,* 2nd ed. Edinburgh: Churchill Livingstone, 1980.)

metatarsophalangeal joint. In the older child, when the interphalangeal joint deformity is fixed, we perform a Robert Jones procedure with fusion of the interphalangeal joint and transfer of the extensor hallucis longus to the neck of the first metatarsal (Fig. 179.10).

REFERENCES

Each reference is categorized according to the following scheme: *, classic article; #, review article; !, basic research article; and +, clinical results/outcome study.

+ 1. Bliss DG, Menelaus MB. The Results of Transfer of the Tibialis Anterior to the Heel in Patients Who Have a Myelomeningocele. *J Bone Joint Surg* 1986;68-A:1258.
* 2. Broughton NS, Menelaus MB, Cole WG, Shurtleff DB. The Natural History of Hip Deformity in Myelomeningocele. *J Bone Joint Surg* 1993;75-B:760.
+ 3. Broughton NS, Graham G, Menelaus MB. The High Incidence of Foot Deformity in Patients with High-level Spina Bifida. *J Bone Joint Surg* 1994;76-B:548.
+ 4. Buisson JS, Hamblen DL. Eectromyographic Assessment of the Transplanted Iliopsoas Muscle in Spina Bifida Cystica. *Dev Med Child Neurol Suppl* 1972;27:29.
+ 5. Duckworth T, Smith TW. The Treatment of Paralytic Convex Pes Valgus. *J Bone Joint Surg* 1974;56-B:305.
* 6. Feiwell E, Sakai D, Blatt T. The Effect of Hip Reduction on Function in Patients with Myelomeningocele. *J Bone Joint Surg* 1978;60-A:169.

+ 7. Fraser RK, Bourke HM, Broughton NS, Menelaus MB. Unilateral Dislocation of the Hip in Spina Bifida—A Long-term Followup. *J Bone Joint Surg* 1995;77-B:615.

+ 8. Frawley PA, Broughton NS, Menelaus MB. Anterior Release for Fixed Flexion Deformity of the Hip in Spina Bifida. *J Bone Joint Surg* 1996;78-B:299.

+ 9. Frawley PA, Broughton NS, Menelaus MB. Incidence and Type of Foot Deformities in Patients with Low-level Spina Bifida. *J Pediatr Orthop* 1998;18:312.

+ 10. Heeg M, Broughton NS, Menelaus MB. Bilateral Dislocation of the Hip in Spina Bifida. A Long Term Follow-up Study. *J Pediatr Orthop* 1998;18:434.

11. Hoffer MM, Feiwell E, Perry J, Bonnett C. Functional Ambulation in Patients with Myelomeningocele. *J Bone Joint Surg* 1973;55A:137.

12. Menelaus MB. Orthopaedic Management of Children with Myelomeningocele: A Plea for Realistic Goals. Dev Med Child Neurol 1976;37(Suppl):18.

* 13. Broughton NS, Menelaus MB. *Menelaus' Orthopaedic Management of Spina Bifida Cystica,* 3rd ed. London: Saunders, 1998.

+ 14. Marshall PD, Broughton NS, Menelaus MB, Graham HK. Surgical Release of Knee Flexion Contractures in Myelomeningocele. *J Bone Joint Surg* 1996;78-B:912.

15. McDonald CM, Jaffe KM, Shurtleff DB. *Functional Patterns of Innervation in the Lower limb Musculature of Children with Myelomeningocele: Implications for Ambulation.* Presented at International Society for Research into Hydrocephalus and Spina Bifida, New Castle, Northern Ireland, 1987.

+ 16. Mustard WT. A Follow-up Study of Iliopsoas Transfer for Hip Instability. *J Bone Joint Surg* 1959;41-B:289.

+ 17. Olney BW, Menelaus MB. Triple Arthrodesis in Spina Bifida Patients—A Long-Term Followup. *J Bone Joint Surg* 1988;70-B:234.

+ 18. Sandhu PS, Broughton NS, Menelaus MB. Tenotomy of the Ligamentum Patellae in Spina Bifida: Management of Limited Flexion Range at the Knee. *J Bone Joint Surg* 1995;77-B:832.

* 19. Sharrard WJW. Posterior Iliopsoas Transplantation in the Treatment of Paralytic Dislocation of the Hip. *J Bone Joint Surg* 1964;46-B:426.

20. Shurtleff DB. Myelomeningocele: A New or a Vanishing Disease? *Z Kinderchir* 1986;1(Suppl):5.

+ 21. Shurtleff DB, Menelaus MB, Stahlei LT, et al: Natural History of Flexion Deformity of the Hip in Myelodysplasia. *J Pediatr Orthop* 1986;6:666.

+ 22. Spires TD, Gross, RH, Low W, Barringer W. Management of the Resistant Myelodysplastic or Arthrogrypotic Clubfoot with the Vereberlyi-Ogston Procedure. *J Pediatr Orthop* 1984;4:705.

+ 23. Williams PF, Menelaus MB. Triple Arthrodesis by Inlay Grafting—A Method Suitable for the Undeformed or Valgus Foot. *J Bone Joint Surg* 1977;59B:333.

+ 24. Wright JD, Menelaus MB, Broughton NS, Shurtleff DB. Natural History of Knee Contractures in Myelomeningocele. *J Pediatr Orthop* 1991;11:725.

+ 25. Yngve DA, Lindseth RE. Effectiveness of Muscle Transfers in Myelomeningocele Hips Measured by Radiographic Indices. *J Pediatr Orthop* 1982;2:121.

## CHAPTER 180

BONE DYSPLASIAS, METABOLIC BONE DISEASES, AND GENERALIZED SYNDROMES

Lori A. Karol

SKELETAL DYSPLASIAS

The skeletal dysplasias are a diverse group of disorders in which the structure of the bone is inherently abnormal, thus altering the growth of affected individuals. The trunk and extremities are abnormally sized, leading to disproportionate short stature, defined as a height less than the third percentile for the individual's chronologic age. Some of the dysplasias are genetically transmitted, whereas others occur sporadically.

The diagnosis in skeletal dysplasias can most often be made clinically. Short stature should be noted when present, and body proportion and trunk and limb shortening may be helpful. The various definitions of skeletal dyspla-

sias are shown in Table 180.1. If limb shortening is most notable in the proximal segments (i.e., humerus or femur), the term *rhizomelic* can be applied. Shortening of the midportion of the limb is termed *mesomelic*, and *acromelic* describes distal shortening. The area of the bone most disturbed by the dysplasia can help establish the diagnosis. For example, multiple epiphyseal dysplasia (MED) affects the epiphyses, whereas the metaphysis is most involved in the various forms of metaphyseal chondrodysplasia. The presence or absence of spinal involvement also is helpful in reaching a diagnosis.

Associated medical findings, such as precocious puberty in fibrous dysplasia, may aid in the diagnosis. In addition, identifying a specific dysplasia may lead to the identification and, therefore, treatment of associated medical conditions. For example, patients with nail-patella syndrome are at increased risk for renal failure, the onset

---

L. A. Karol: Orthopaedic Department, Texas Scottish Rite Hospital for Children, Dallas, Texas, 75219.

Table 180.1.	Definitions
rhizomelic	shortening in the proximal segments of the extremity
mesomelic	affecting the midportions of the limb
acromelic	distal shortening

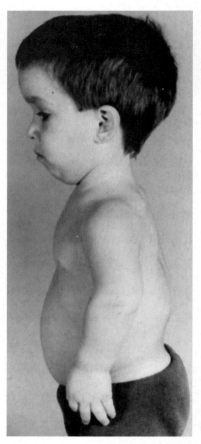

Figure 180.1.   Four-year-old boy with achondroplasia. Note the prominent forehead, flexion contractures of the elbow, trident hand, and thoracolumbar kyphosis.

of which is insidious and would go unnoticed if not for the proper surveillance due to the known association with the syndrome (94).

Collaboration with a geneticist can facilitate making the diagnosis in difficult cases. Genetic counseling may be of interest to the patient and family. Some dysplasias are unclassifiable and should be treated on an individual basis.

Advances in molecular genetics have furthered understanding of the mechanisms of bony abnormalities in these conditions. Although gene replacement treatment is not yet possible, research is progressing rapidly in this direction. See Dietz and Mathews (65) for an excellent review of the genetic basis of the inherited skeletal dysplasias.

ACHONDROPLASIA

Achondroplasia is the most common form of dwarfism, with a prevalence of 1.3 per 100,000 live births (3). It is inherited in an autosomal dominant pattern, although most cases are the result of spontaneous mutations. Molecular genetic research has found that there is a point mutation in the gene that encodes fibroblast growth factor receptor 3 (19,32,229), located on the short arm of chromosome 4 (183). Achondroplasia is characterized by a rhizomelic pattern of involvement, with the humerus and femur affected more than the distal extremities. Prenatal diagnosis is possible by monitoring the growth of the femur during the second trimester (165).

Histology reveals disturbed endochondral ossification. Intramembranous bone formation is not affected. Pathologic study of the growth plate shows marked abnormalities in the zone of hypertrophy, with loss of normal columnation of chondrocytes and accumulation of excess matrix (171). Periosteal bone formation is histologically normal. Additionally, the epiphysis itself is not affected by the dysplasia; therefore, there is no predisposition toward early degenerative arthritis.

The clinical appearance of achondroplasia is recognizable at birth. The baby is short limbed and has a disproportionately large head. Trunk length is normal. Facial features include a flattened nasal bridge, prominent mandible, and enlarged forehead. The hands characteristically have a space between the long and ring fingers, referred to as the "trident hand." Elbow flexion contractures and radial head dislocation may be present. The lower limbs may be bowed, and the musculature appears enlarged. Thoracolumbar kyphosis may be present in infants (Fig. 180.1).

Radiographic findings in achondroplasia include an inverted V-shaped growth plate, best seen in the distal femur (Fig. 180.2). The metaphysis is widened, and the epiphysis is relatively normal. The long bones of the leg may be bowed. The pelvis is wide but short, with small sciatic notches. The shape of the inner pelvis has been described as a "champagne glass" appearance. The radiographic hallmark of the achondroplastic spine is progressive narrowing of the transverse interpedicular distance as one measures from cephalad to caudad in the lumbar spine (Fig. 180.3). The pedicles are thickened, and there may be posterior scalloping of the vertebral bodies.

Orthopaedic concerns most frequently focus on the spine (25,237). In infancy, compression of the brain stem and cervical cord secondary to stenosis of the foramen

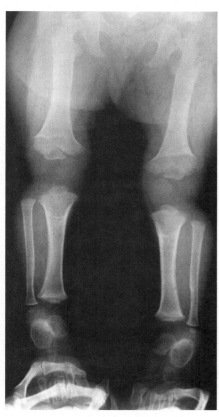

Figure 180.2. One-year-old girl with achondroplasia. The physis of the distal femur appears as an inverted V.

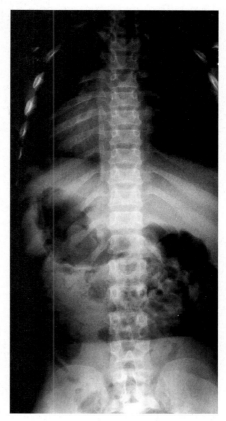

Figure 180.3. Progressive interpedicular narrowing in the lumbar spine of a 5-year-old girl with achondroplasia.

magnum has been described (127,167,265). Symptoms include sleep apnea (more specifically, central hypoapnea), and neurologic examination may reveal hypotonia (which is common in all infants with achondroplasia) or clonus. When compression is noted, posterior surgical decompression of the foramen magnum is recommended to prevent sudden death (265,269). Other neurosurgical concerns include Chiari malformations at the craniocervical junction and hydrocephalus, which occasionally requires shunting (76). Sleep apnea can also occur because of upper airway obstruction, and sleep studies may be able to identify those children whose respiratory compromise is due to craniocervical abnormalities and those due to obstructive airway problems (254,255,272). Because the orthopaedist often is involved in the care of the infant with achondroplasia, awareness of these conditions is imperative if appropriate neurosurgical referral is to be made.

Thoracolumbar kyphosis occurs in the slightly older infant with achondroplasia (Fig. 180.4). Kyphosis occurs nearly universally in the young baby. Possible causes include ligamentous laxity, hypotonia, enlarged head size, and hip flexion contractures. In most cases, the kyphosis resolves as the child begins to walk. A recent theory, pop-

ularized by Hall (100) and Pauli et al. (168), proposes that unsupported sitting by the hypotonic infant leads to the development of thoracolumbar kyphosis. The authors advocate prohibiting unsupported sitting to prevent the kyphosis from occurring, and early brace treatment with a thoracolumbosacral orthosis (TLSO) for those babies who do develop kyphosis. Other authors have recommended using a brace if kyphosis persists beyond 2 years of age. For refractory cases, surgical treatment consisting of anterior and posterior fusion without instrumentation may be necessary. Progressive kyphosis and kyphosis measuring greater than 40° at 5 years of age are indications for surgery (237). Fusion is generally obtained without instrumentation, because the narrowed canal and kyphotic deformity predispose the patient to neurologic injury and paraplegia if hardware is introduced (see Chapters 158 and 161).

Spinal stenosis is the most common orthopaedic problem in achondroplasia (237) and may become symptomatic in patients in their early teen years (119). Symptoms include leg and back pain (neurogenic claudication), lower extremity weakness, and loss of endurance during ambulation. The patient attempts to relieve pain during walking by hunching over to reduce the lumbar lordosis, which

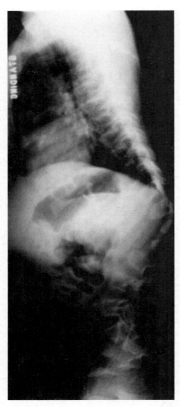

Figure 180.4.   Persistent thoracolumbar kyphosis in a 4-year-old boy with achondroplasia.

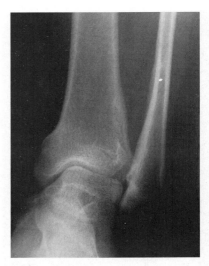

Figure 180.5.   Relative fibular overgrowth in a 13-year-old girl with achondroplasia.

produces more space within the spinal canal. The decreased space within the spinal canal is due to narrowing and thickening of the pedicles, hypertrophy of the facets, and enlargement of the laminae (132). Magnetic resonance imaging (MRI) is useful in visualizing the extent of the stenosis. The condition is treated by posterior decompression, with wide laminectomy. The surgeon should attempt to preserve the facets, but this may not be possible if the stenosis is severe. Primary fusion usually is not necessary.

Angular deformity may occur in the lower limbs in childhood (18), and may be due in part to overgrowth of the fibula in relation to the tibia (171) (Fig. 180.5). Tibial osteotomy remains the treatment of choice for patients with symptomatic or cosmetically objectionable varus. Epiphysiodesis of the fibula has had mixed results (see Chapter 169).

Treatment of the patient's short stature remains controversial. There has been enthusiasm, particularly in Europe, for the application of the Ilizarov technique for lengthening the limbs in children with achondroplasia (88,267) (see Chapter 171). Treatment with recombinant growth hormone has been investigated and found to increase growth in some individuals with achondroplasia (111, 156,257,266).

DIASTROPHIC DYSPLASIA

Diastrophic dysplasia is a severe form of short-limbed dwarfism, which is inherited in an autosomal recessive pattern. Its gene, located on chromosome 5, is responsible for the sulfation of proteoglycans, a crucial component of cartilage (230). Prenatal DNA testing can establish the diagnosis. Histologic study of the growth plate shows abnormalities in collagen (221) and decreased numbers of chondrocytes.

Clinical features are striking at birth. The child has very short limbs. There is flattening of the nasal bridge and a puffy-cheeked appearance. Cleft palate is frequently present. Severe clubfoot deformities are always present, and joint contractures are common. The thumb, which is radially deviated and short, has been described as a "hitchhiker thumb." Within the first months of the child's life, the pinnae of the ears become swollen and ossify. The crumpled and enlarged pinnae have been termed "cauliflower ear" (249). In some affected children, tracheomalacia may be life-threatening during the neonatal period. The child's intelligence is normal.

Radiographic findings include the delayed appearance of the epiphyses. When the epiphyses do ossify, they are irregular and may be flattened (especially at the proximal femur) (244). Coxa vara is common and may result in hip dislocation. The long bones are short but appear thickened. Scoliosis is seen in older children (Fig. 180.6). The first metacarpal is short in relation to the rest of the hand and is triangular in shape, leading to the development of the hitchhiker deformity.

Orthopaedic concerns include the severe clubfeet, which are resistant to casting and are prone to early recurrence after surgical intervention. Postoperative bracing is

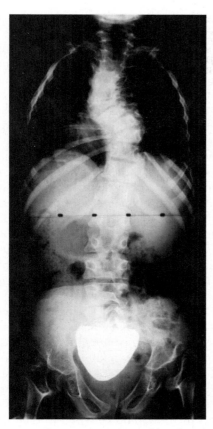

Figure 180.6.   Scoliosis in an 8-year-old girl with diastrophic dysplasia. Note the bilateral hip dislocations.

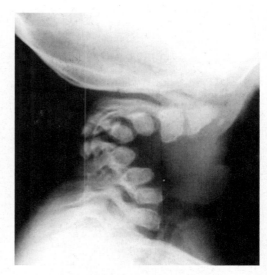

Figure 180.7.   Cervical kyphosis in a 2-year-old girl with diastrophic dysplasia.

used in these children. Repeated surgical releases of the feet are difficult but should be aggressive (see Chapter 167). Other foot deformities are also seen in patients with diastrophic dysplasia (190). Joint contractures of the hip and knee may not be treatable with soft-tissue release. Osteotomy is required for fixed deformity. Hip dislocation is common and is difficult to treat. Because of the epiphyseal abnormalities, premature degenerative arthritis does occur.

Scoliosis is common and frequently severe in children with diastrophic dysplasia (109,173,237). Surgical fusion is indicated for large curves. Cervical kyphosis may be severe and lead to neurologic compromise (80,173) (Fig. 180.7). Atlantoaxial instability has also been described with diastrophic dysplasia (180). Careful assessment of the child's neck before general anesthesia can prevent death due to neurological causes (24). Surgical atlantoaxial fusion is indicated in progressive cases.

METAPHYSEAL CHONDRODYSPLASIA

Metaphyseal chondrodysplasia is a group of diseases of autosomal dominant and recessive inheritances. The two most common forms are the Schmid and McKusick types. The McKusick form is also known as cartilage hair hypoplasia. The primary defect is an abnormality in the physis of the zone of primary calcification, with clusters of chondrocytes protruding into the metaphysis. The gene coding for type X collagen, which is present in hypertrophic chondrocytes located at the growth plate, is abnormal in Schmid metaphyseal chondrodysplasia (250,253).

Clinically, short stature is always present but varies in severity (182). Genu varum is common. Radiographs reveal widened physes and cupping of the epiphysis (Fig. 180.8), which may be mistaken for rickets. Serum chemistry, however, is normal in metaphyseal chondrodysplasia (77) (except for Jansen type, in which hypercalcemia may be present [197]). Coxa vara can be seen in the Schmid form, and cervical instability may be seen in the McKusick form. The long bones may be bowed, leading to angular deformities. The epiphyses are normal.

Orthopaedic treatment consists of osteotomies for symptomatic or progressive angular deformities. Patients with the McKusick form, which has been linked with immunodeficiency, have recently been treated by bone marrow transplantation (23,245).

MULTIPLE EPIPHYSEAL DYSPLASIA

Multiple epiphyseal dysplasia (MED) is one of the most common of the bone dysplasias. It is inherited by autosomal dominant transmission and has been found to be genetically variable among families (60).

The disorder is characterized by symmetric involvement of the epiphyses with a delay in their ossification. Radiographically, they appear mottled and irregular. The

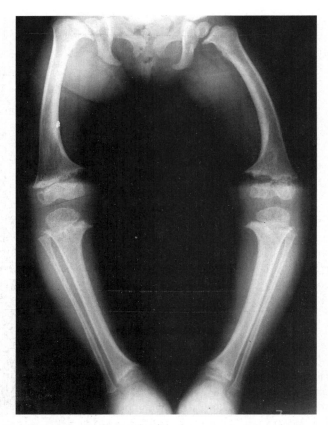

Figure 180.8.   Radiograph of the lower extremities of a 4-year-old girl with metaphyseal chondrodysplasia. Genu varum and widened physes are seen.

fragile, predisposing the patient to multiple fractures. Several classifications of the disease exist (124). In 1906, Looser divided OI into congenita and tarda forms, with the specific type determined by whether the patient developed fractures at birth or later. The most commonly applied classification is that by Sillence (208), who categorized patients based on how the condition was inherited (i.e., autosomal dominant or recessive) and on the presence of specific clinical features (Table 180.2).

The prevalence of OI is 21.8 per 100,000 live births, with Sillence type I being the most common form (3). Prenatal diagnosis of the congenital form of OI is possible with ultrasound (22), but milder forms of OI (e.g., Sillence types I and IV) do not have abnormal ultrasound findings (235). In families with known mutations, chorionic villous sampling may help establish the prenatal diagnosis (235).

The underlying genetic defect in OI is an abnormality in the gene that encodes for the alpha chain of type I collagen (45). Mutations are almost always present, involving either the COL1A1 or COL1A2 genes, which encode the procollagen. In affected individuals, the organization of type I collagen is in disarray. In type I OI, there is a quantitative abnormality in the amount of type I collagen; in the other forms of OI, there are both quantitative and qualitative anomalies in type I collagen (44). Abnormalities can be seen in dermal fibroblasts obtained from skin biopsies, in which the ratio of type I to type III collagen (which is uninvolved in patients with OI) is compared with age-matched normal specimens. Routine use of skin biopsy for diagnosis is discouraged, however, because the

hips, knees, and ankles are most frequently involved; in the upper extremity, the shoulder is most commonly affected (113). The spine is essentially normal. In the differential diagnosis of bilateral Legg-Calvé-Perthes disease, always include MED (2) and perform radiographs of the knees and ankles. An abnormal epiphyseal height-to-metaphyseal width ratio for the distal femur has been found in most children with MED and has been proposed as helpful in early diagnosis (246). Another characteristic finding is the double-layered appearance of the patella on lateral radiographs (205). Avascular necrosis of the femoral head frequently occurs in patients with MED (133).

Adult height usually is at the lower range of normal. Joint pain may appear in the first decade or remain quiescent until early adult life. Treatment is the same as that for osteoarthritis, consisting of joint replacement for advanced cases (238).

OSTEOGENESIS IMPERFECTA

Osteogenesis imperfecta (OI) is a group of genetically transmitted dysplasias in which the bones are extremely

Table 180.2.   Sillence Classification of Osteogenesis Imperfecta

Type	Inheritance	Clinical features
I	Autosomal dominant	Blue sclerae Fractures—variable Hearing loss—common ± Poor dentition
II	Autosomal recessive	Blue sclerae Intrauterine or early death Severe fractures
III	Autosomal recessive	Rare Fractures—multiple Extreme short stature Normal sclerae
IV	Autosomal dominant	Fractures—variable Normal sclerae Hearing-normal ± Poor dentition

history and physical examination usually are sufficient to establish the diagnosis (224).

Morphologic changes are seen in growth plate cartilage (193). Histologically, there is a relative increase in woven bone that does not mature to lamellar bone. The osteocyte number is increased. Trabeculae are thin and poorly arranged, and the haversian canal system does not develop. Bone mineral density is decreased on dual energy x-ray absorptiometry (DEXA) scans, even in milder forms of the disease (271).

Clinical manifestations vary, with the spectrum ranging from that of stillborn babies with numerous fractures and intracranial bleeds to active adolescents with a history of several fractures occurring at various times during their childhood. Musculoskeletal findings include short stature, bowing of the extremities, and scoliosis. Blue sclerae are seen in Sillence type I and II patients, and in some type III patients, with the color most intense and long-lasting in type I patients (209). Dentition may be poor due to defective dentin, a condition known as *dentinogenesis imperfecta*. Hearing loss may occur secondary to middle ear involvement. The face is trefoil shaped. Clinical findings

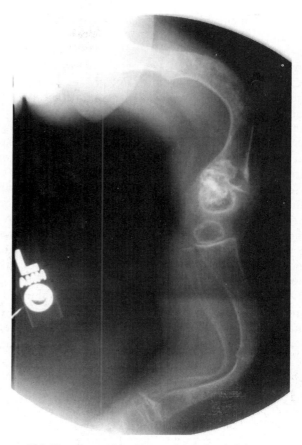

Figure 180.10. Severe bowing, multiple healed fractures, and epiphyseal calcifications in the lower extremity of a child with severe osteogenesis imperfecta.

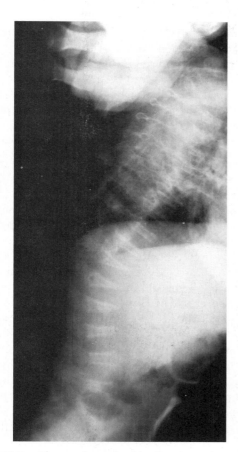

Figure 180.9. Flattened vertebral bodies throughout the spine of a 1-year-old boy with severe osteogenesis imperfecta.

in patients with type IV OI may be quite subtle, and the differential diagnosis between OI and child abuse can be vexing.

Radiographic findings vary with disease severity as well. Fractures may be seen throughout the skeletal system. Coxa vara is a common sequela of femoral neck fracture. Protrusio acetabuli can develop. *Wormian* bones are seen on skull radiographs. The vertebrae may be biconcave, and compression fractures may be present (Fig. 180.9). The long bones are thin and osteopenic. The femur may have a "concertina" appearance, that is, a crumpled shape due to multiple fractures. There is widening of the metaphyses, and growth arrests may occur. Irregular calcifications may extend into the metaphysis, a condition referred to as "popcorn epiphysis" (Fig. 180.10).

The motor development of children with severe OI is delayed. Physical therapy has been useful in helping the patient develop head and trunk control, and when therapy is used in combination with surgery and bracing, sitting and ambulation may be improved (27). The ability of the child to sit independently by age 10 months has been correlated with achieving walking as a primary means of mobility (55).

Orthopaedic management is required to treat fractures as well as to attempt to prevent fractures. Fractures usually heal within a normal time interval, but the tendency to refracture persists. Disuse osteopenia further weakens the bones, so immobilization should be kept to the minimum time necessary to ensure fracture healing. Orthoses may be needed on a long-term basis to assist in weight bearing and to reduce the incidence of fractures (89). Nonunions may occur (867).

Surgical intervention can help prevent fractures and maintain limb alignment. Intramedullary fixation for load sharing, in combination with multiple osteotomies, was popularized by Sofield and Miller (218). Telescoping rods are technically more challenging to insert, but because they grow with the child, the chances of refracture with growth are lessened (13,14) (Fig. 180.11). Gamble et al. (87) showed that although the Bailey-Dubow rod was difficult to insert properly, it was beneficial in providing internal support to growing bones. Other authors also have

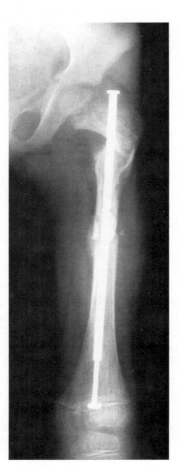

Figure 180.11. Bailey-Dubow elongating rod in the femur of a 7-year-old boy with osteogenesis imperfecta.

published favorable results using the Bailey-Dubow device but state that the hardware does require periodic revision during patient growth (154,270).

MULTIPLE FEMORAL OSTEOTOMIES AND INSERTION OF BAILEY-DUBOW RODS

The insertion of a Bailey-Dubow rod in the femur proceeds as follows (Fig. 180.12):

- Preoperatively, check available lengths of rods.
- Type and crossmatch blood.
- Position the patient in the lateral decubitus position on a radiolucent table and drape the lower extremity free.
- Perform a gentle subperiosteal exposure of the femur.
- Perform multiple osteotomies where needed to pass a straight rod.
- Ream the medullary canal to allow rod passage.
- Drill the female end of the rod into proximal fragment in a retrograde direction through the fracture or osteotomy, exiting just medial to the greater trochanter.
- Exchange the drill bit for a T-piece through the proximal skin incision.
- Crimp the T-piece onto the female end of the rod using pliers.
- Perform a perapatellar exposure of the femoral intercondylar notch at the knee.
- Insert the male solid rod up through the femoral notch.
- Engage the male rod into the female rod.
- Tap each rod in fully.
- Twist the male rod 90° within the femoral epiphysis to deter distal migration into the knee.
- Close and dress the incisions and apply a spica cast.

Rush and Sheffield rods also have been used to treat OI-related fractures (228). Intramedullary fixation has been recommended in the treatment of severely involved young children with type III OI (43). Motor development has been augmented in children with type III OI by performing surgery before 3.5 years of age (74).

Vertebral involvement leads to scoliosis and kyphosis in the severely affected groups of patients. Biconcave deformity of the vertebral bodies has been linked with the early onset of scoliosis (114). Chest cage deformity may result from bracing because of rib fragility (21), and curve progression is not halted by brace wear (102,268). Treatment is surgical but is fraught with technical problems. Fixation of the spine with conventional spinal hardware is difficult to achieve because of osteopenia. Methylmethacrylate augmentation and the use of mersilene tapes have been proposed as means to assist in fixation (21). Fusion *in situ* is the norm, because correction is very difficult to achieve.

Brain stem compression from basilar invagination has received recent attention (42). The condition has been

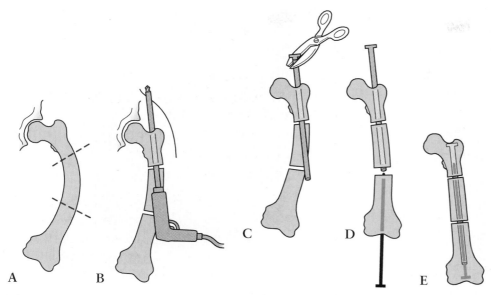

Figure 180.12. Surgical technique for inserting Bailey-Dubow elongation rod. **A:** Bowed femur and planned osteotomies. **B:** Hollow rod drilled into proximal fragment and out a small incision in buttock. **C:** Exchange of drill bit for T-piece; crimp with pliers. **D:** Solid rod inserted through knee. **E:** Rods engaged, advanced fully, and buried in femoral epiphysis.

found in as many as 25% of patients (210) and is often associated with macrocephaly and hydrocephalus. Clinical signs of basilar invagination include nystagmus, cranial nerve palsies, papilloedema, and facial spasm. Surgical treatment is difficult (104). In severely involved patients, basilar invagination may lead to early death due to respiratory arrest (143).

Anesthetic management of the child with OI can be complicated. There is a predisposition to hyperthermia that is biochemically different from the classic malignant hyperthermia (172). Blood loss during surgery may also be massive (219).

Medical treatment of OI is still experimental. Fluoride, vitamin therapy, and calcitonin have been tried in the past. Current research is aimed at treating OI at the molecular level (90,139).

MORQUIO'S SYNDROME

Morquio's syndrome, one of the mucopolysaccharidoses, is characterized by the lack of N-Ac-Gal-6 sulfate sulfatase, a lysosomal enzyme. Deficiency of this enzyme causes an increase in urinary keratan sulfate (112). The syndrome is inherited in an autosomal recessive pattern.

Clinically, affected patients appear normal when they are babies. The clinical features appear later, as glycosaminoglycans accumulate (Fig. 180.13). Signs of Morquio's syndrome include short-trunk dwarfism, ligamentous laxity, and genu valgum. Facial features are not striking. Ky-

phosis of the thoracic spine and pectus carinatum may be present. The patient's intelligence is normal. Hepatosplenomegaly is not associated with Morquio's syndrome.

Radiographs reveal tongue-shaped projections originating from the anterior vertebral body (Fig. 180.14). Platyspondyly is present. Odontoid hypoplasia, resulting in atlantoaxial instability, is common and the surgeon should look for it (152). The epiphyses are irregular and flattened, and may fragment in the weight-bearing joints. The bases of the metacarpals are pointed, and the bones of the hand are short and thick (196). The radiographic appearance is very similar to that seen in spondyloepiphyseal dysplasia.

Orthopaedic management of atlantoaxial instability often is necessary, with atlantoaxial fusion the recommended treatment (152,226) (Fig. 180.15) (see Chapter 158). Difficulty in walking is easily attributed to the genu valgum (Fig. 180.16), but the surgeon must be cautious and confirm that the cervical spine is not the cause of the changes in ambulation. Anesthesiology concerns are related to possible cervical instability. Life expectancy usually is normal.

MULTIPLE HEREDITARY OSTEOCHONDROMATOSIS

Multiple hereditary osteochondromatosis is one of the more common forms of dysplasia, occurring in 9 per million people. It is genetically transmitted as an autosomal

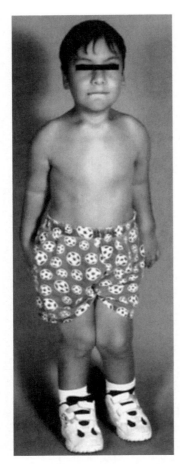

Figure 180.13. Clinical appearance of a 6-year-old boy with Morquio's syndrome.

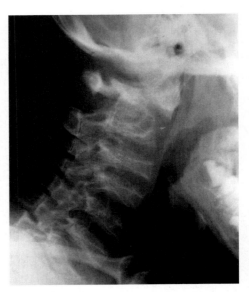

Figure 180.15. Odontoid hypoplasia and atlantoaxial instability in a 6-year-old boy with Morquio's syndrome.

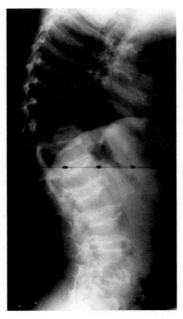

Figure 180.14. Platyspondyly and vertebral irregularities in a 6-year-old boy with Morquio's syndrome.

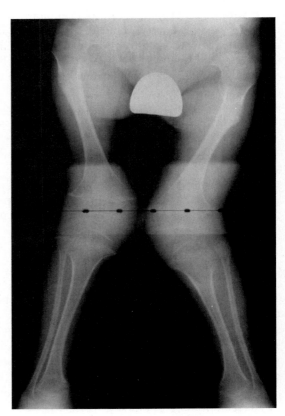

Figure 180.16. Genu valgum in a child with Morquio's syndrome.

dominant trait. Severity of involvement varies among family members, but penetrance is 100% (260). Masses develop in those bones that are formed by endochondral ossification, with a predisposition for the long bones, scapula, ribs, and pelvis.

Histologic examination reveals normal bone that is in continuity with the metaphysis of the parent bone. The exostosis is covered by a cap of hyaline cartilage, usually less than 3 mm in thickness. The deep surface of the cartilaginous cap is involved in endochondral ossification, leading to growth of the lesion.

The diagnosis normally is made during the patient's first decade of life. Multiple bumps, which are usually nontender, may be palpable throughout the skeleton. The patient tends to be short in stature. The spine is rarely affected (1,9,157). Limb-length discrepancy and angular deformity are common because of disturbance of normal longitudinal growth. Scapular lesions can lead to "winging" (56).

On radiographs, lesions can be seen around the metaphysis of the long bones, along the borders of the scapula, on the ribs, or originating from the iliac apophysis. The exostoses may be sessile, with a broad base or origin, or they may be pedunculated, arising from the bone on a bony stalk. The medullary canal of the mass is in continuity with the canal of the long bone. There is a predilection for the masses to appear at the end of the bone that grows fastest (e.g., the distal rather than the proximal radius) and for greater involvement of the smaller bone of two-bone limbs (e.g., the ulna more so than the radius) (Fig. 180.17). Pedunculated lesions typically point away from the epiphysis.

Orthopaedic management consists of excision of painful exostoses and observation of those that remain asymptomatic (40,264). Excision may be postponed until adolescence, when multiple symptomatic lesions can be excised under one anesthetic. Angular deformities may require correction, especially at the knee, where valgus is common (168). Genu valgum may lead to patellofemoral instability (151). Compression of surrounding structures may occur owing to the size of the osteochondromas. The peroneal nerve is particularly prone to compression from masses and is susceptible to injury during surgical excision of proximal fibular lesions (38,264). Proximal tibial lesions may irritate the pes anserinus (81). Large exostoses of the distal tibia can compress the adjacent fibula, leading to erosion and deformity (57,214).

Wrist involvement in hereditary osteochondromatosis is quite common, consisting of distal ulnar and radial osteochondromas, shortening of the ulna, tilt of the distal radial epiphysis, and ulnar translation of the carpus (Fig. 180.18). Dislocation of the radial head may occur because of the ulnar shortening (117). At present, treatment of osteochondromatosis of the forearm is controversial. Some authors advocate early excision of osteochondro-

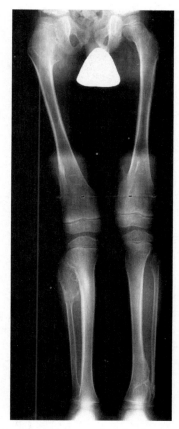

Figure 180.17. Multiple osteochondromatosis of the femur, tibiae, and fibulae in a 6-year-old boy.

mas around the wrist, believing that such treatment prevents subsequent deformity and radial head dislocation (169,170). However, a recent study comprising 78 patients with forearm osteochondromas found that function was not compromised and that cosmetic concerns were rare in those patients who did not have early, aggressive treatment of their exostoses (10). Outcome studies agree that deformities of the upper extremity in patients who have hereditary multiple exostoses are well tolerated and cause little loss of function as measured both objectively and subjectively (222). When osteochondromas result in progressive discrepancy in length between the radius and the ulna, and forearm rotation becomes painful, osteotomy of the bowed radius can be performed with satisfactory but not perfect results. Acute lengthening and gradual lengthening of the ulna (via the Ilizarov technique) have both been described (54,256). Radial head excision is reserved for pain relief in skeletally mature patients.

Malignant transformation of benign osteochondromas into chondrosarcoma occurs in less than 1% of affected individuals. The physician should become clinically suspicious when a lesion increases in size or becomes painful

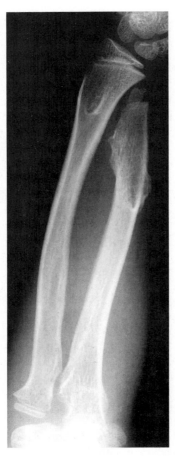

Figure 180.18. Shortening of the ulna and translation of the carpus due to multiple osteochondromatosis.

Pathology reveals clusters of chondrocytes within the lesions. Mitotic figures may be present but should be few in number. Grossly, the lesions appear as gray-white masses amid the bone and may feel gritty due to calcification.

Radiographic findings show lucent, streaky lesions within the metaphyses (134,194). Calcification can be seen within the lesion. The cortex of the bone may expand with the lesion, especially in the phalanges of the hand. The metaphysis becomes widened and trumpet shaped. Angular deformity and shortening are seen (179) (Fig. 180.19).

Orthopaedic management involves correcting angular deformity and equalizing limb length. Osteotomy addresses angulation, and lengthening procedures are useful for shortened extremities. Regenerate formation is adequate during lengthening despite the presence of enchondromas.

Malignant degeneration of enchondromas to chondrosarcoma does occur, and newly painful lesions should trigger suspicion. Maffucci's syndrome is associated with

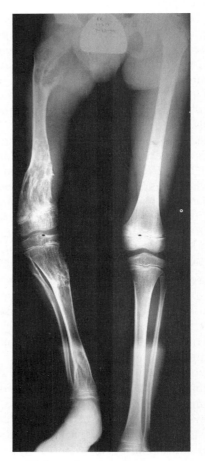

Figure 180.19. Unilateral enchondromatosis in an 8-year-old boy.

after skeletal maturity. The cartilage cap of a benign osteochondroma is quite thin; a cap greater than 1 cm in thickness suggests malignant transformation. Accurate measurements of cartilage cap thickness can be made using MRI or ultrasound scans (135). Even if a chondrosarcoma occurs, such malignancies are late to metastasize; usually respond well to wide resection; and have a good prognosis, particularly in long bone lesions (see Chapters 127 and 128).

ENCHONDROMATOSIS

Enchondromatosis is a noninherited bone dysplasia in which masses of cartilage form within the metaphyses of tubular bones and the pelvis. Lesions may be single or multiple and involve only a single extremity, or they may affect multiple extremities. Asymmetry is a hallmark of the disease, with one side of the body markedly more involved than the other side. Multiple enchondromatosis is known as Ollier's disease; enchondromatosis with multiple hemangiomas is known as Maffucci's syndrome.

nonskeletal malignancies at an alarming rate (199). See Chapters 127 and 128 for more detail.

FIBROUS DYSPLASIA

Fibrous dysplasia is a noninherited dysplasia in which bone is replaced by abnormal fibrous tissue. One bone (monostotic fibrous dysplasia) or multiple bones (polyostotic fibrous dysplasia) may be affected. In the polyostotic form, usually one side of the patient's body is involved to a greater degree than the other side. The disease can be associated with endocrine abnormalities and hyperpigmented skin lesions, known as McCune-Albright syndrome (41,126,129). Precocious puberty is the hallmark of the McCune-Albright variant.

Pathology reveals a fibrous stroma full of fibroblasts. Multiple immature fragments of woven bone are seen within the stroma, an appearance similar to that of alphabet soup. The bone has widened osteoid seams and does not mature into lamellar bone.

The clinical diagnosis usually becomes apparent within the patient's first two decades of life. Presenting signs include pain, limp, deformity, or pathologic fractures. Involvement of the skull and facial bones can occur in varying degrees. Leg-length discrepancy is common.

Radiographs reveal ill-defined, lucent lesions that have a ground-glass appearance because of the calcification of immature bone. The cortex is thinned, and the shaft of the involved bone may expand. Lesions are metaphyseal or diaphyseal in location. Coxa vara with "shepherd's crook" deformity of the proximal femur is a classic radiographic finding (Fig. 180.20). Isolated lesions may be mis-

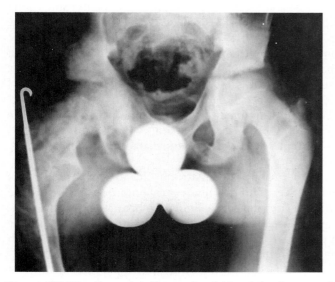

Figure 180.20. Extensive fibrous dysplasia of the femur and pelvis in a 13-year-old boy. Note the "shepherd's crook" deformity of the proximal femur.

taken for simple bone cysts, particularly in the humerus. Spinal involvement, usually associated with neurologic compromise, has been described (73,96,150,174). Because the diagnosis can usually be made from radiographs, biopsy is rarely necessary.

Orthopaedic treatment depends on the site of the lesions and on the biomechanical implications of the weakened bone. Pain, progressive deformity, and impending pathologic fracture are indications for surgery. Closed treatment of fractures due to fibrous dysplasia usually is sufficient for the upper extremities but is rarely successful for the lower extremities, for which the demands of weight bearing require strong bony support (225). Excision and curettage rarely work because bone graft is quickly replaced by the abnormal fibrous tissue (97). When bone grafting is necessary, cortical strut grafts (e.g., the fibula) take longer to resorb and thus provide more structural support (35,75).

Femoral neck lesions are particularly problematic. Osteotomy to correct coxa vara, combined with curettage and grafting of the femoral neck (usually with cortical bone), is performed when the calcar becomes progressively thin, leading to coxa vara and a painful limp. Internal fixation should be used, but extension of the lesion up into the femoral neck makes standard fixation tenuous (97). Osteotomies to correct deformity and intramedullary fixation, particularly using reconstruction nails, which provide fixation into the femoral head and neck, can help restore alignment and support in the femur and tibia (82). Because the medullary canal in fibrous dysplasia is less distinct and very vascular, the surgeon should anticipate difficulties when using closed techniques as well as increased blood loss during intramedullary fixation. Osteotomies tend to heal reasonably well, and nonunions are uncommon.

Leg-length discrepancy may be significant enough to require surgical equalization. For moderate discrepancies, contralateral epiphysiodesis is far simpler than lengthening procedures.

The activity of the disease usually regresses in adulthood (106). Malignant tumors have been described as having originated from both the monostotic and the polyostotic forms of fibrous dysplasia (105,189,195). A 3% rate of malignant transformation has recently been reported by the Mayo Clinic, with the majority of tumors being osteosarcomas (189). Degeneration of fibrous dysplasia into aneurysmal bone cysts has also been described (153) (see Chapter 127).

NEUROFIBROMATOSIS

Neurofibromatosis (von Recklinghausen's disease) is the most prevalent skeletal dysplasia transmitted by a single gene. It is inherited in an autosomal dominant pattern with variable expression, although the disease is believed to occur due to a new mutation in half of the affected individuals (248). The estimated prevalence is 1 per 1000 live births.

The disorder has two forms. Neurofibromatosis type I (NF-I) is the more common form and is characterized by peripheral neurofibromas, skeletal involvement, and "café au lait spots." The genetic locus for NF-I has been localized to chromosome 17q11.2, an area that encodes for the protein neurofibromin (98,206). This protein is present in several organ systems and is believed to be a tumor suppressor (249). Neurofibromatosis type II (NF-II) manifests as central neurofibromas with bilateral acoustic neuromas and usually presents in the third or fourth decade of life (142). The gene for NF-II has been localized to chromosome 22 and encodes for the protein schwannomin (131).

Histologic examination of neurofibromas has shown a palisading arrangement of densely packed fibrous bundles and spindle cells. Grossly, the masses are firm and pale.

There are numerous clinical features of neurofibromatosis. The National Institutes of Health has developed specific criteria for the diagnosis of neurofibromatosis (Table 180.3). The most common skin lesion is the café au lait spot, a hyperpigmented irregular area with a smooth border that varies in size and shape (Fig. 180.21). These spots usually are not present immediately after birth but appear and increase in number throughout childhood. More subtle skin findings in patients with neurofibromatosis include axillary or inguinal freckling. Fibroma molluscum are superficial, raised nodules that represent dermal neurofibromas. They are not seen in prepubertal children. Nevi are heavily pigmented lesions that may present unilaterally. The lesions may be hypersensitive and may overlie plexiform neurofibromas. Plexiform neurofibromas are large nerve tumors that are locally invasive,

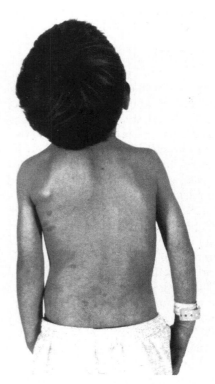

Figure 180.21. Multiple café au lait spots in a 3-year-old boy with neurofibromatosis and scoliosis.

feel like a "bag of worms," and have the potential for malignant transformation.

Skeletal lesions vary as well. Scoliosis is most common, occurring in up to 64% of patients with neurofibromatosis (50). Three types of scoliosis exist. The first is an idiopathic-appearing curve without significant bony changes or kyphosis. A second form is the dysplastic type, a short, sharp curve in which six or fewer vertebrae are involved. The dysplastic curve occurs in up to 72% of patients with neurofibromatosis and scoliosis (212). The vertebrae may assume a wedge shape, rotation usually is severe, and penciling of the apical ribs is characteristic. The neural foramen may be expanded owing to pressure from dumbbell neurofibromata. A third form of scoliosis is a dysplastic curve with associated hyperkyphosis (Fig. 180.22A,B).

Hypertrophy or hemiatrophy due to neurofibromatosis can be seen, and the physician should rule out the disease whenever evaluating a child with hemihypertrophy. Congenital pseudarthrosis of the tibia and forearm may be present. Protrusio acetabuli is also seen in patients with neurofibromatosis.

Orthopaedic treatment of the skeletal involvement of neurofibromatosis most often involves the spine. Treatment of the idiopathic-type curve is similar to the treatment of adolescent idiopathic scoliosis (see Chapters 155,

Table 180.3.   NIH Criteria for Diagnosis of Neurofibromatosis
Patients must have at least two of the following findings:
• Six or more café au lait spots, measuring 0.5 cm in diameter in prepubertal children or 1.5 cm in postpubertal individuals
• Two or more neurofibromas, or one plexiform neurofibroma
• Axillary or inguinal freckling
• Optic glioma
• Two or more Lisch's nodules (tan specks in the iris that represent hamartomas)
• A distinctive bony lesion, such as cortical thinning of a long bone without pseudarthrosis or frank pseudarthrosis
• A first-degree relative with neurofibromatosis

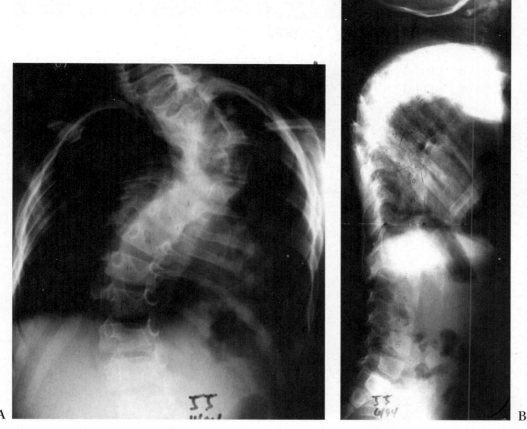

Figure 180.22. PA (**A**) and lateral (**B**) radiographs of a dysplastic kyphotic curve in a 3-year-old boy with neurofibromatosis.

156, and 158). Bracing is used for progressive curves in growing patients, with spinal fusion reserved for larger curves. Dysplastic curves have a more ominous prognosis, with rapid progression commonly seen. Those curves that are most prone to progression occur in younger patients, are greater in magnitude at presentation, are associated with kyphosis, and have vertebral and rib erosive changes (84). Spinal fusion was often complicated by pseudarthrosis (50,212), leading to the current recommendation of combined anterior and posterior spinal fusions to treat these curves (263). Surgery should not be delayed in young children with dystrophic curves (37). Even with anterior and posterior fusion, some dystrophic curves continue to progress, requiring difficult subsequent revision procedures (50,110,118,261).

Spinal surgery in patients with neurofibromatosis is technically challenging for several reasons. First, the bone itself is often soft due to erosion from neurofibromas. This compromises the purchase of hooks or screws used during instrumentation. Second, the surgical approach can be difficult owing to thoracic neurofibromas surrounding the

spine (198). Last, intradural lesions and outpouchings of dura (known as *dural ectasia*) are seen in patients with neurofibromatosis, increasing the risk of neurologic complications during surgical correction (72,108). Preoperative MRI studies of the spinal cord are imperative in patients with neurofibromatosis (50).

Cervical spine involvement in patients with neurofibromatosis has also been described (50,99). Severe cervical kyphosis has been seen in patients with plexiform neurofibromas (252) (Fig. 180.23). Neurologic compromise has been described in these patients (47,130).

Leg-length discrepancy may occur due to neurofibromatosis. The treatment of hemihypertrophy is individualized and ranges from epiphysiodesis for mild cases to ablative amputation for severely affected persons.

Congenital pseudarthrosis of the tibia is one of the most challenging disorders treated by pediatric orthopaedists. The condition usually, but not always, is associated with neurofibromatosis. Boyd (33) described four types of congenital pseudarthrosis of the tibia (Fig. 180.24; Table 180.4).

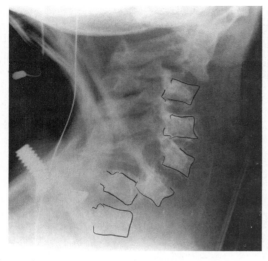

Figure 180.23.   Cervical kyphosis in a 3-year-old girl with neurofibromatosis.

Table 180.4.	Types of Pseudarthrosis of the Tibia
Type I	Increased density of the medullary canal Bowing present
Type II	Defect in tubulation of the medullary canal Bowing and constriction present
Type III	Cystic lesion at the apex of the bow; precursor to frank pseudoarthrosis
Type IV	True pseudoarthrosis, with tapering of the ends of the fracture

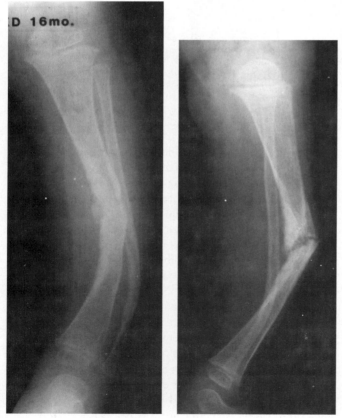

A,B

Figure 180.24.   AP (**A**) and lateral (**B**) views of the tibia of a 16-month-old girl with congenital pseudarthrosis of the tibia and neurofibromatosis.

A recently described variant of congenital anterolateral bowing of the tibia has been described in which the fibula is stout, and the bowing remodels without treatment and does not progress to pseudoarthrosis. This benign form does not occur in patients with neurofibromatosis (241).

Treatment of congenital pseudarthrosis of the tibia is controversial (166). Myriad methods have been employed to obtain union, but all have led to failures in some patients (15). The prepseudarthrosis should be treated with total contact clamshell orthoses. Once the tibia has fractured, closed treatment will not be successful (49). The traditional treatment for congenital pseudarthrosis of the tibia is intramedullary fixation of the tibia and fibula, with excision of the pseudarthrosis and bone grafting. The Williams rod can be inserted through the calcaneus into the tibia and usually is left protruding across the ankle joint. With growth, the rod migrates proximally into the tibia (4) (Fig. 180.25A,B).

Newer methods of treating congenital pseudarthrosis of the tibia have been recommended in response to the high rate of nonunion using intramedullary fixation. Advocates for Ilizarov fixation and bone transport as well as for vascularized fibula transfer find that union can be achieved in some, but not all, patients with congenital pseudarthrosis of the tibia (31,46,62,66,78,91,93,211, 242,258) (see Chapters 36, 169, and 171). The long-term ability to maintain union in these patients remains unknown. Amputation continues to be a feasible option for the patient who has undergone several operations and still fails to achieve union (115). A long-term study by Crossett et al. (52) found that approximately half of their patients with congenital pseudarthrosis of the tibia eventually were treated by amputation. Regardless of the method used to achieve union, precaution must be taken to prevent recurrent fractures. Protection of the tibia with ankle-foot orthoses is usually prescribed. Even when union is achieved, muscle weakness and gait disturbances are almost always present (122).

Leg-length discrepancy is nearly universal following congenital pseudarthrosis of the tibia, with the affected leg being shorter than the normal limb. Equalization surgery is often indicated.

Pseudarthrosis of the forearm is also associated with neurofibromatosis and likewise is difficult to treat (48, 141). Protrusio acetabuli may also result from neurofibromatosis (118) and usually is associated with contiguous neurofibromas (136).

Patients with neurofibromatosis are prone to developing malignancies of tissues of neural crest origin as well as others (49,204).

METABOLIC BONE DISEASES

Metabolic bone disease is caused by abnormalities in the metabolism of calcium and phosphate. Rickets and renal osteodystrophy are the most common forms of metabolic bone disease in children. A thorough understanding of calcium metabolism is required to evaluate affected patients properly (30,138).

The human body is very sensitive to calcium, particularly the cardiovascular and neurologic systems, in which irritability, conductivity, and contractility rely on the precise control of serum calcium levels. Nearly all of the body's calcium is stored in bone in the form of hydroxyapatite, with a small proportion circulating in the bloodstream. Serum calcium levels are regulated by vitamin D and parathyroid hormone (PTH) through their actions on the gut, kidneys, and bone. Calcium is absorbed in the distal duodenum and proximal jejunum by means of a transport mechanism that is activated by the active form of vitamin D (1,25-dihydroxy vitamin D) and by PTH.

Provitamin D is ingested as ergosterol or is produced by the liver as 7-dehydrocholesterol. When they are exposed to ultraviolet light, these compounds become calciferol and cholecalciferol. The first hydroxylation occurs in the liver and the second hydroxylation takes place in the kidney, with the end result being 1,25-dihydroxy

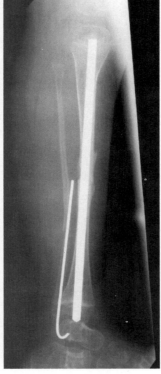

A,B

Figure 180.25.   **A:** Intramedullary fixation in congenital pseudarthrosis of the tibia. **B:** Note the proximal migration of the distal end of the rod.

vitamin D (233). Conversion to this dihydroxy form is stimulated by hypocalcemia and high levels of PTH.

PTH is produced in the parathyroid glands and is released in response to hypocalcemia. PTH allows for the absorption of calcium from the gut and renal tubules, frees calcium from hydroxyapatite in bone, and activates osteoclasts, an event that takes on importance in renal osteodystrophy.

NUTRITIONAL RICKETS

Nutritional rickets is caused by inadequate dietary intake of vitamin D in the growing child. Although the condition is uncommon in the United States (116), it remains a problem throughout the rest of the world. Children who are fed a vegetarian diet or who are breast fed for prolonged periods of time are at increased risk for nutritional rickets (188). Malabsorption of vitamin D due to celiac or hepatic disease results in gastrointestinal rickets, which is more commonly seen in developed countries. In either form, the lack of vitamin D results in the inability to absorb calcium or phosphorus. PTH is released in response to the hypocalcemia, but hypophosphatemia persists. Laboratory studies reveal normal or mildly decreased serum calcium, decreased serum phosphate, elevated PTH, and decreased vitamin D.

Histologic changes are most notable at the growth plate, where loss of columnation occurs in the zone of hypertrophy. Because there is insufficient calcium to mineralize bone, plump chondrocytes persist into the zone of provisional calcification and down into the metaphysis. There is sparse mineralization and elongation of the growth plates. Within trabecular bone, large amounts of unmineralized osteoid surround the fragile trabeculae.

Radiographic findings show marked widening of the growth plate due to the absence of the zone of provisional calcification (Fig. 180.26). The metaphyses are flared or cupped. The long bones may be abnormally bowed because they are unable to withstand mechanical stress. The trabecular pattern of the bone is indistinct. Osteopenia is present. Looser's lines (radiolucent lines extending transversely across the axis of the bone) are associated with rickets and are present in approximately 20% of patients with all forms of rickets (223).

Most children affected with nutritional rickets are quite young (188). Clinical features include short stature, muscular weakness, and ligamentous laxity. Genu varum and periarticular enlargement of the wrists, elbows, and ankles may be noted. The term "rachitic rosary" refers to the prominence of the costochondral cartilages along the chest wall. The abdomen may be protuberant. Neurologic involvement, such as listlessness and irritability, may be present.

Treatment of nutritional rickets, which should be supervised by a pediatric endocrinologist, consists of vitamin

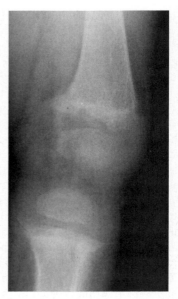

Figure 180.26. Osteopenia and growth plate widening in the knee of a 1-year-old girl with nutritional rickets.

D replacement. Osteotomies are rarely required for residual deformity following medical treatment.

NEONATAL RICKETS

A form of rickets has been described in which premature neonates in intensive care units sustain multiple fractures without antecedent trauma (125). Risk factors include hepatobiliary disease, total parenteral nutrition, diuretic therapy, physical therapy with passive motion, and chest percussion therapy. The fractures require minimal immobilization to heal. The patients are treated by the neonatal intensivists with supplemental feedings (53).

VITAMIN D–RESISTANT RICKETS

Vitamin D–resistant rickets, also known as familial hypophosphatemic rickets, is a group of diseases in which ordinary dietary intake of vitamin D is inadequate in maintaining normal mineral balance (251). The condition usually is inherited in an X-linked dominant pattern, although an autosomal dominant form also exists (69). The genetic locus for the disease has been identified (7,71,184,185). A renal tubular defect leads to the inability to reabsorb phosphate, resulting in phosphate diabetes and hypophosphatemia (39,71,101). Laboratory studies reveal near-normal levels of calcium, PTH, and vitamin D but low levels of serum phosphate. Urinary phosphate and serum alkaline phosphatase are elevated.

Affected children present with bowing of the lower extremities, short stature, bone pain, and dental caries (69).

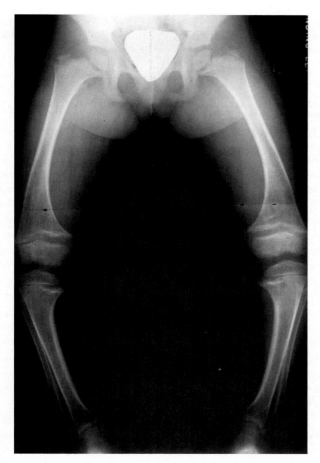

Figure 180.27. Bowing and physeal widening in the lower extremities of a 4-year-old girl with hypophosphatemic rickets.

The disease becomes clinically apparent after 12 months of age, but it can be diagnosed earlier by laboratory testing for urine phosphate levels in suspected infants (146).

Radiographic changes and histologic findings are similar to those seen in patients with nutritional rickets (Fig. 180.27).

Treatment of hypophosphatemic rickets is primarily medical, typically consisting of oral replacement of phosphate and large amounts of vitamin D (247). Nephrocalcinosis is a known complication of medical treatment (227). Growth hormone therapy has been used to improve phosphate metabolism and increase stature in these patients (164,191,262).

Orthopaedic management consists of osteotomies to treat residual deformities of the lower extremities (79,187) (see Chapters 168 and 169). Careful preoperative planning is required because the deformities are multiplanar and thus may benefit from external fixation that precisely corrects angulation in each plane (121). Bone healing is delayed after osteotomy and may take approximately twice as long as expected in metabolically normal chil-

dren. Calcification of ligaments and degeneration of articular cartilage may occur in affected adults (79).

MISCELLANEOUS FORMS OF RICKETS

On rare occasions, rickets may occur in patients with neurofibromatosis or fibrous dysplasia (137). Anticonvulsant drug therapy may also produce rickets (236). In addition, certain tumors may produce hypophosphatemic rickets. Patients with no family history of rickets should be suspect. Tumors usually are present in bone or skin (103).

RENAL OSTEODYSTROPHY

Renal osteodystrophy is a more common form of metabolic bone disease (29). Glomerular disease leads to retention of phosphate. The injured kidney is unable to perform the final hydroxylation of vitamin D. Hypocalcemia ensues, which stimulates secondary hyperparathyroidism. It is the secondary hyperparathyroidism that produces most of the skeletal manifestations of renal osteodystrophy.

PTH enables osteoclasts to resorb bone. In renal osteodystrophy, lysis of bone is extensive, resulting in the development of osteitis fibrosa (163). A small number of patients may develop osteosclerosis.

Laboratory studies show elevated levels of blood urea nitrogen (BUN), creatinine, alkaline phosphatase, and PTH. Serum calcium and vitamin D levels are low, whereas the serum phosphate level is high.

Children with renal osteodystrophy are short for their age. Bone pain may be present, and pathologic fractures can occur (11). Hip pain and limp, secondary to slipped capital femoral epiphysis, may be present (203). This occurs in children who are younger than those most often seen with slipped epiphyses, and the condition usually is bilateral. The previously described features of nutritional rickets may also be present. Bowing of the long bones and genu valgum are common.

Radiographic findings are striking. Resorption of bone can be seen at the terminal tufts of the distal phalanges, the symphysis pubis (Fig. 180.28), and the end of the clavicle. Metaphyseal resorption of bone leads to widened physes and slipped capital femoral epiphysis (SCFE; see Chapter 172) (Fig. 180.29). Disturbance of the proximal lateral tibial physis with associated genu valgum has been described (161). Brown tumors appear as large, lucent lesions with indistinct margins within the pelvis or long bones. These tumors can best be seen on MRI (158). "Rugger jersey" spine describes the sclerotic appearance of the vertebral endplates seen on a lateral radiograph. Periarticular soft-tissue calcification may be seen.

Treatment is primarily medical and is aimed at correcting the metabolic imbalance. Calcitriol, administered in high doses intravenously, orally, or by dialysis, has been

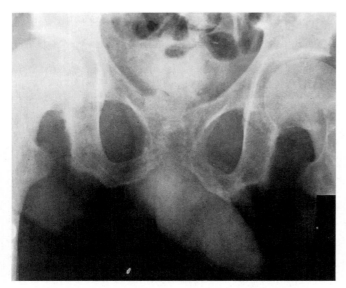

Figure 180.28. Resorption of the pubis due to renal osteodystrophy.

found to be helpful in the treatment of pediatric renal osteodystrophy by lowering PTH levels (192). Pinning of SCFEs may be necessary (107), but osteopenia and continued metaphyseal resorption may compromise fixation (see Chapter 172). The patient's hip pain may resolve simply with medical treatment. Osteolysis of the distal femoral physis has also been described, with cast immobilization and medical treatment sufficient to promote healing and remodeling (231). When an angular deformity of the lower extremities interferes with gait, osteotomy of the

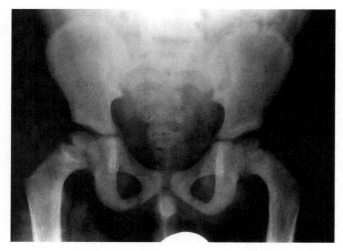

Figure 180.29. Physeal widening and slipped capital femoral epiphysis in a 7-year-old boy presenting with hip pain. A diagnosis of renal failure was made.

femur or tibia is indicated. Best results are obtained if the patient's metabolic state is optimized before surgery (58, 160).

GENERALIZED SYNDROMES

DOWN SYNDROME

Down syndrome is one of the most common genetically transmitted diseases, with a prevalence of 9.2 per 10,000 live births (5,159). It results from trisomy of chromosome 21 because of maternal nondisjunction, translocation, or mosaicism. One risk factor for Down syndrome is advancing maternal age. The most notable feature is mental retardation, but a variety of other congenital malformations, including heart defects, commonly occur (120). The IQs of children with Down syndrome vary considerably. About 30% of patients develop orthopaedic problems that require hospitalization (63).

Clinical features include a characteristic facies, with upslanting palpebral fissures, prominent epicanthal folds, mild microcephaly, and a protruding tongue. The child tends to be short. Ligamentous laxity is universal. Development is delayed, with the onset of ambulation usually not occurring until 2 to 3 years of age.

Radiographic findings include a characteristic appearance of the pelvis. The iliac wings are widened, the ischial rami are small and tapered, and the acetabulae are horizontal. Coxa valga is present. Hand radiographs show that all five metacarpals are equal in length, and there is clinodactyly of the small finger.

Orthopaedic concerns arise from the ligamentous laxity and its effects on the spine, hips, knees, and feet. Atlantoaxial instability, the most commonly recognized skeletal manifestation of Down syndrome, is caused by laxity in the transverse ligament. The radiographic definition of atlantoaxial instability is an increase in the atlanto-dens interval (ADI), as seen on flexion lateral cervical radiographs (Fig. 181.30). It has been reported to occur in 9% to 31% of persons with Down syndrome (177). Patients with atlantoaxial instability have a particularly high rate of associated congenital cervical spine anomalies (e.g., os odontoideum, hypoplasia of the posterior arch of C-1, and hypoplasia of the dens) that may have an impact on surgical treatment (140,176).

Children with Down syndrome are usually screened for cervical instability. The American Academy of Pediatrics Committee on Sports Medicine and Fitness conducted a review of the literature and concluded that greater effort should be directed toward "identification of those patients who already have or who later have complaints or physical findings consistent with symptomatic spinal cord injury" rather than obtaining routine radiographs (6). This report pointed out that almost all children who suffered

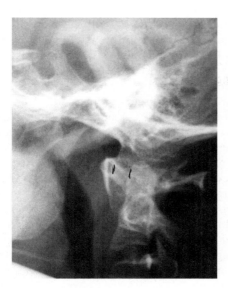

Figure 180.30.   The atlanto-dens interval is increased in flexion in this 12-year-old boy with Down syndrome.

catastrophic neurologic injury because of atlantoaxial instability had pre-existing neurologic symptoms, and that children rarely develop abnormal radiographic findings following normal films (147).

Activity modification to protect patients with increased ADI from head trauma by removing them from "at-risk" athletic activities is the traditional recommendation. A few authors have proposed that because neurologic abnormalities are so rare even in affected children, activity restriction may be unnecessary (51). Others have found that an equal proportion of patients have neurologic signs with and without radiographic instability of the cervical spine, and they question the need to screen all patients (186). Once atlantoaxial instability is documented radiographically, rarely does it increase significantly over time (175). Neurologic injury following nonspinal surgery has been described; thus, preoperative radiographic evaluation of the cervical spine in patients with Down syndrome is warranted (59,148,240).

Surgical treatment of atlantoaxial instability consists of posterior spinal fusion with halo immobilization (181). A high complication rate with major complications, including nonunion, loss of reduction, neurologic deterioration, late subaxial instability, infection, and wound dehiscence, should be anticipated after posterior arthrodesis of the upper cervical spine in patients with Down syndrome. Ligamentous laxity in patients with precarious preoperative neurologic status increases the neurologic mortality risk during surgery (213). Nonsurgical management is currently recommended for patients with Down syndrome who have atlantoaxial instability but no neurologic signs or symptoms (67,200).

Recent attention has also been directed at instability between the occiput and C-1. Posterior occipitoatlantal hypermobility (POAH), defined as subluxation of the occiput posteriorly during extension of the neck, has been identified in 8% to 63% of patients with Down syndrome (85,162). The discrepancy in prevalence is probably due to the difference in techniques used to measure motion at this level. Plain radiographs may suggest instability, but precise measurement of hypermobility is fraught with error and is best evaluated with MRI (123,259). POAH may be seen in patients with atlantoaxial instability (243). Treatment is based on the child's neurologic status and on the amount of space available for the spinal cord (239). Posterior occipital-cervical fusion has been recommended (145).

The lower cervical spine may also become symptomatic in patients with Down syndrome. Spondylolysis of the cervical spine and early degenerative arthritis have been described (239).

Ligamentous laxity may predispose the patient to instability of the joints of the lower extremities, resulting in hip dislocations and patellar subluxation and dislocation. Approximately 7.9% of patients with Down syndrome have some hip abnormality, including dysplasia, dislocation, avascular necrosis, or SCFE (202). Dislocation of the hip in patients with Down syndrome is rarely painful initially but may become so over time. Treatment is difficult, because redislocation is not uncommon. Nonoperative bracing is rarely successful, but prolonged spica casting may allow the hip to stabilize in a reduced position. Open reduction, capsulorrhaphy of the attenuated capsule, and femoral and pelvic osteotomy may result in a stable hip (20) (see Chapter 166).

SCFE is also associated with Down syndrome. Hypothyroidism may be a predisposing factor, so thyroid function tests should be ordered for children with both Down syndrome and SCFE. Treatment is *in situ* fixation, but hardware failure may occur (see Chapter 172).

Patellofemoral instability is present in more than one third of patients with Down syndrome, but it rarely affects their ability to walk (68). Surgery is advised in selected cases and consists of aggressive realignment and Galleazzi transfer of the semitendinosus to the patella (see Chapter 87).

Planovalgus of the feet is nearly universal in these patients.

ARTHROGRYPOSIS MULTIPLEX CONGENITA

Arthrogryposis multiplex congenita is a syndrome in which multiple joints are rigid at birth (100). The disorder is nonprogressive, and the cause is unclear. Abnormalities of muscles, joints, and nervous system; teratogens; infection; and environmental factors have all been implicated.

Many genetic syndromes include arthrogrypotic contractures and, thus, should be considered when evaluating a child with joint rigidity. The disease can resemble spinal muscular atrophy, and genetic associations between the two diseases have been proposed (36). Arthrogryposis usually is not genetically transmitted, but genetic research is being performed on the less common inherited forms (16,28,36,83,207,217).

Myopathic and neuropathic forms of arthrogryposis exist (178). The neuropathic type is more common (17). Muscle changes include replacement of skeletal muscle by fibrofatty tissue. Neuropathic findings include a decrease in the number of anterior horn cells, with sparing of the posterior columns. Sensation is not affected.

Clinically, most children have contractures of all four extremities. There is occasional sparing of the upper extremities and rare sparing of the lower extremities. There is a distal form of the disease that consists of hand and foot contractures, including clubfeet (16). Intelligence is usually normal to above normal (217).

The affected limbs appear smooth, without transverse creases at the joints. Muscle mass is decreased, but the atrophy may be difficult to appreciate in young infants. Motion in the joints is limited but painless, and a solid block is felt at the extremes of range of motion.

In patients with extensive involvement, the hips are flexed, abducted, and externally rotated. Dislocation is common. The knees may have flexion or hyperextension contractures. Rigid clubfeet usually are present, but vertical talus may occur. The upper extremities, when involved, are adducted at the shoulder and internally rotated. The elbows may have flexion or extension contractures. The wrist may be flexed and ulnarly deviated, with flexion of the fingers and thumb-in-palm deformity. Scoliosis may be seen in young children.

Orthopaedic treatment is individualized. The goal of surgery is to improve function and enable ambulation when possible. With surgery, it has been found that up to 85% of patients with amyoplasia can walk at least on a limited basis by 5 years of age (201). The prognosis for ventilator-dependent babies is less favorable (26). Recurrence of deformities is common following surgery, and orthoses are usually prescribed.

In the neonatal period, focus on establishing a correct diagnosis. Include examination by a geneticist and a pediatric neurologist. Muscle biopsy is occasionally needed. Initiate physical therapy for range-of-motion and developmental skills. Range of motion should always be performed with great care, because pathologic fractures may occur.

Surgery to address hip dislocation has been recommended in patients with arthrogryposis. Pavlik harness treatment is unsuccessful, so open reduction is the treatment of choice. The medial approach has been specifically advocated by Staheli et al. (220) for use in arthrogryposis.

Bilateral dislocations may be addressed medially during the same surgery, with good results reported in 80% of a series of 40 dislocated hips in arthrogrypotic children (232) (see Chapter 166).

Knee contractures are difficult to treat. Knee flexion contractures require surgery more often than hyperextension contractures (149,215). Surgery is indicated if physical therapy fails to attain less than 30° flexion contracture. Hamstring tenotomy and posterior capsulotomy, with or without femoral shortening osteotomy, are required (234). Sectioning of the cruciate ligaments and resection of intra-articular fibrous tissue often is necessary. Femoral extension osteotomy can increase extension at the knee, but flexion deformity of the distal femur recurs with growth of the child (61). Chronic contractures lead to bony changes, such as squaring off of the femoral condyles and joint incongruity (94). Ilizarov techniques have been used in difficult cases (34) (see Chapter 171). Many children who have undergone knee flexion contracture surgery stop walking in adolescence (149).

Surgical correction of clubfeet should be performed around the age when the child learns to walk, which is nearly always delayed in babies with arthrogryposis. Posteromedial release, with resection of tendons and capsules, and lateral column shortening, when needed, is the initial surgery of choice. Recurrence of deformity has been seen in 73% of children with arthrogryposis (155). Talectomy or tarsal medullostomy is usually reserved for recurrent severe deformity, but the procedure has been performed in primary releases by some surgeons (64,92,144,216) (see Chapter 167).

Upper extremity surgery should be delayed until a complete functional assessment can be performed. Optimally, one elbow should be extended for toileting and use of walking aids, and the contralateral elbow should be flexed to enable the child to self-feed (12). The ability of these intelligent children to adapt to their deformities can be surprising, so care should be taken not to intervene surgically when the child is functioning satisfactorily. Surgical procedures that may be useful for the upper extremities include rotational osteotomy of the humerus, triceps transfer to gain active elbow flexion, capsulotomies at the elbow, and wrist stabilization.

OSTEOPETROSIS

Osteopetrosis, otherwise known as Albers-Schönberg disease and "marble bone disease" is apparently a hereditary disease of bone characterized by abnormal function of osteoclasts. This results in varying degrees of bone remodeling deficiency, the skeleton being predominately composed of primary unremodeled trabecular bone and calcified cartilage. On electron microscopy, there are increased numbers of osteoclasts but their ruffled border is absent or diminished.

This is an exceedingly rare disorder. Most orthopaedic surgeons will not encounter a single case in their lifetime. Pediatric referral centers may see only a few cases at any given time. A recent review of the management of osteopetrosis by Armstrong, Newfield, and Gillespie based upon a review of the literature and a survey of the members of the Pediatric Orthopaedic Society of North America (10a), is highly recommended for readers interested in more details on this rare disorder. They provide an excellent summary of the characteristics of osteopetrosis, list 63 references, and provide clinical details on 79 patients found in their survey.

Osteopetrosis can be classified into an infantile malignant type. It is inherited by autosomal recessive transmission and a more benign adult form, which is autosomal dominant. The latter can be divided into Type I. This is characterized by marked thickening of the cranial vault, and a substantially lesser risk of fractures. Type II is characterized by vertebral end-plate thickening resulting in the classic appearance of "rugger jersey" spine and "endobones" in the pelvis. Type II has a higher incidence of fracture and delayed union as well. There is an extremely rare third form that is autosomal recessive. It is regarded as an "intermediate" form.

The underlying molecular abnormality, which results in dysfunction of the osteoclast, has not yet been established in humans. However, mutations have been found in the mouse and rat that produce an autosomal recessive type of osteopetrosis. In the *op* mouse and the *tl* rat, the production of colony-stimulating factor − 1 (CSF-1) appears to be deficient or the factor is inactive.

Patients with infantile malignant osteopetrosis are usually diagnosed during their first year of life and only 30% of patients survive past the age of 6 years, dying of complications resulting from myelophthisic anemia which is due to obliteration of their marrow spaces by unremodeled bone. Clinical characteristics include blindness, failure to thrive, seizures, repeated infections, pathologic fractures, hepatosplenomegaly, hypersplenism, hydrocephalus, mental retardation, cranial nerve palsies, and hemorrhagic diathesis.

The infants are lethargic and underdeveloped with macrocephaly, frontal bossing, hypertelorism, exophthalmos, and flattening of the nasal bridge with chronic rhinitis.

Radiographs show increased density in the bone of the entire skeleton and the complete absence of the medullary canal. There is metaphyseal widening producing club-shaped long bones, and the "bone within a bone" phenomenon is seen in the pelvis, vertebra, hands and feet. Transverse radiolucent bands can be seen in the metaphyseal regions of the long bones. The skull may progressively thicken and show a "hair-on-end" appearance. Transverse or short oblique pathologic-type diaphyseal and metaphyseal fractures are common.

The adult form is compatible with a normal lifespan although patients are prone to long-bone fractures. The age of presentation of these patients can be quite variable depending upon the severity of the disease. Up to 40% of patients may remain asymptomatic. There may be a family history of the disease or of multiple fractures. Laboratory studies show mild or moderate anemia and increased serum acid phosphatase. Bone involvement is less severe than in the infantile form but osteomyelitis of the jaw, progressive coxa vara, lateral bowing of the long-bones, spondylolysis and spondylolisthesis of L4 and L5 or both, and osteoarthritis of the hips and the knees may develop in adults. Dental malocclusion and caries can be problems. The diagnosis is usually obvious from the clinical presentation and characteristic radiographs. It can be confirmed by bone biopsy.

There is no treatment for osteopetrosis, although bone marrow transplantation (in selected patients) has been successful in reversing hematologic and skeletal defects of the disease. Variable results have been obtained with restriction of dietary calcium, splenectomy, high dose prednisone to increase bone marrow hematopoiesis, parathormone, calcitriol, and gamma-interferon.

Orthopaedic treatment is usually focused on management of their fractures (which usually respond to nonoperative closed treatment), and treatment for coxa vara. In the 79 patients reviewed by Armstrong et al. (10a) 20 were treated surgically for coxa vara, all of whom had complications. Valgus osteotomy provided the most consistent results. Fourteen subtrochanteric and 31 other fractures of the femur were treated with traction or casting, with good results in the majority. Twenty-nine tibial fractures, and upper extremity fractures healed well with closed reduction and cast immobilization. For the most part, spine problems were treated non-operatively.

The diaphyseal bone in osteopetrosis is quite hard, chalky, and brittle. It is difficult to drill. It is easily over heated causing necrosis, possibly leading to implant loosening or infection. When placing screws for pins in osteopetrotic bone, it is extremely important to use sharp, fresh drill points and pins. Clean these often and exchange them if necessary to maintain their sharpness. The drills must be cooled constantly by bathing them with sterile saline. The lack of a medullary canal makes drilling even more difficult. Intramedullary nailing is nearly always impossible and internal fixation with plates, because of the multiple screw holes required, is usually best avoided. The presence of a plate on the diaphysis often results in a stress riser, which leads to subsequent fractures at the ends of the plate. If rigid fixation is required for treatment than external fixation is probably the best choice. These patients seem to heal their fractures well in most cases of the adult form. The bone they heal with, however, is defective.

REFERENCES

Each reference is categorized according to the following scheme: *, classic article; #, review article; !, basic research article; and +, clinical results/outcome study.

+ 1. Albrecht S, Crutchfield JS, Se Gall GK. On Spinal Osteochondromas. *J Neurosurg* 1992;77:247.

2. Andersen PE Jr, Schantz K, Bollerslev J, Justesen P. Bilateral Femoral Head Dysplasia and Osteochondritis. Multiple Epiphyseal Dysplasia Tarda, Spondyloepiphyseal Tarda, and Bilateral Legg-Perthes Disease. *Acta Radiol* 1988;29:705.

* 3. Andersen PE Jr, Hauge M. Congenital Generalised Bone Dysplasia: A Clinical, Radiological, and Epidemiological Survey. *J Med Genet* 1989;26:37.

+ 4. Anderson DJ, Schoenecker PL, Sheridan JJ, Rich MM. Use of an Intramedullary Rod for the Treatment of Congenital Pseudarthrosis of the Tibia. *J Bone Joint Surg* 1992;74A:161.

5. Anonymous. Down Syndrome Prevalence at Birth—United States, 1983–1990. *MMWR Morb Mortal Wkly Rep* 1994;43:617.

* 6. Anonymous. Atlantoaxial Instability in Down Syndrome: Subject Review. American Academy of Pediatrics Committee on Sports Medicine and Fitness. *Pediatrics* 1995;96:151.

! 7. Anonymous. A Gene (PEX) with Homologies to Endopeptidases is Mutated in Patients with X-linked Hypophosphatemic Rickets. The HYP Consortium. *Nat Genet* 1995;11:130.

+ 8. Aprin H, Zink WP, Hall JE. Management of Dislocation of the Hip in Down Syndrome. *J Pediatr Orthop* 1985;5:428.

+ 9. Arasil E, Erdem A, Yuceer N. Osteochondroma of the Upper Cervical Spine: A Case Report. *Spine* 1996;21:516.

+ 10. Arms DM, Strecker WB, Manske PR, Schoenecker PL. Management of Forearm Deformity in Multiple Hereditary Osteochondromatosis. *J Pediatr Orthop* 1997;17:450.

10a. Armstrong DG, Newfield JT, Gillespie R. Orthopaedic Management of Osteopetrosis: Results of a Survey and Review of the Literature. *J Pediatr Orthop* 1999;122.

+ 11. Arvin M, White SJ, Braunstein EM. Growth Plate Injury of the Hand and Wrist in Renal Osteodystrophy. *Skeletal Radiol* 1990;19:515.

12. Axt MW, Niethard FU, Doderlein L, Weber M. Principles of Treatment of the Upper Extremity in Arthrogryposis Multiplex Congenita Type I. *J Pediatr Orthop B* 1997;6:179.

+ 13. Bailey RW. Further Clinical Experience with the Extensible Nail. *Clin Orthop* 1981;159:171.

* 14. Bailey RW, Dubow HI. Evolution of the Concept of an Extensible Nail Accommodating to Normal Longitudinal Bone Growth: Clinical Considerations and Implications. *Clin Orthop* 1981;159:157.

+ 15. Baker JK, Cain TE, Tullos HS. Intramedullary Fixation for Congenital Pseudarthrosis of the Tibia. *J Bone Joint Surg* 1992;74A:169.

16. Bamshad M, Jorde LB, Carey JC. A Revised and Extended Classification of the Distal Arthrogryposes. *Am J Med Genet* 1996;65:277.

17. Banker BQ: Neuropathologic Aspects of Arthrogryposis Multiplex Congenita. *Clin Orthop* 1985;194:30.

18. Bassett GS. Lower-extremity Abnormalities in Dwarfing Conditions. *Instr Course Lect* 1990;39:389.

! 19. Bellus GA, Hefferon TW, Ortiz de Luna RI, et al. Achondroplasia Is Defined by Recurrent G380R Mutations of FGFR3. *Am J Hum Genet* 1995;56:368.

+ 20. Bennet GC, Rang M, Roye DP, Aprin H. Dislocation of the Hip in Trisomy 21. *J Bone Joint Surg* 1982;64B:289.

+ 21. Benson DR, Newman DC. The Spine and Surgical Treatment in Osteogenesis Imperfecta. *Clin Orthop* 1981;159:147.

! 22. Berge LN, Marton V, Tanebjaerg L, et al. Prenatal Diagnosis of Osteogenesis Imperfecta. *Acta Obstet Gynecol Scand* 1995;74:321.

! 23. Berthet F, Siegrist CA, Ozsahin H, et al. Bone Marrow Transplantation in Cartilage-hair Hypoplasia: Correction of the Immunodeficiency but not of the Chondrodysplasia. *Eur J Pediatr* 1996;155:286.

+ 24. Bethem D, Winter RB, Lutter L. Disorders of the Spine in Diastrophic Dwarfism. *J Bone Joint Surg* 1980;62A:529.

25. Bethem D, Winter RB, Lutter L, et al. Spinal Disorders of Dwarfism: Review of the Literature and Report of Eighty Cases. *J Bone Joint Surg* 1981;63A:1412.

+ 26. Bianchi DW, Van Marter LJ. An Approach to Ventilator-Dependent Neonates with Arthrogryposis. *Pediatrics* 1994;94:682.

27. Binder H, Conway A, Hason S, et al. Comprehensive Rehabilitation of the Child with Osteogenesis Imperfecta. *Am J Med Genet* 1993;45:265.

! 28. Bingham PM, Shen N, Rennert H, et al. Arthrogryposis due to Infantile Neuronal Degeneration Associated with Deletion of the SMNT Gene. *Neurology* 1997;49:848.

29. Blockey NJ, Murphy AV, Mocan H. Management of Rachitic Deformities in Children with Chronic Renal Failure. *J Bone Joint Surg* 1986;68B:792.

30. Boden SD, Kaplan FS. Calcium Homeostasis. *Orthop Clin North Am* 1990;21:31.

+ 31. Boero S, Catagni M, Donzelli O, et al. Congenital Pseudarthrosis of the Tibia Associated with Neurofibromatosis I: Treatment with Ilizarov's Device. *J Pediatr Orthop* 1997;17:675.

! 32. Bonaventure J, Rousseau F, Legeai-Mallet L, et al. Common Mutations in the Fibroblast Growth Factor Receptor 3 (FGFR 3) Gene Account for Achondroplasia, Hypochondroplasia, and Thanatophoric Dwarfism. *Am J Med Genet* 1996;63:148.

* 33. Boyd HB. Pathology and Natural History of Congenital Pseudarthrosis of the Tibia. *Clin Orthop* 1982;166:5.

+ 34. Brunner R, Hefti F, Tgetgel JD. Arthrogrypotic Joint

Contracture at the Knee and the Foot: Correction with a Circular Frame. *J Pediatr Orthop B* 1997;6:192.

+ 35. Bryant DD, Grant RE, Tang D. Fibular Strut Grafting for Fibrous Dysplasia of the Femoral Neck. *J Natl Med Assoc* 1992;84:893.

! 36. Burglen L, Amiel J, Viollet L, et al. Survival Motor Neuron Gene Deletion in the Arthrogryposis Multiplex Congenita—Spinal Muscular Atrophy Association. *J Clin Invest* 1996;98:1130.

+ 37. Calvert PT, Edgar MA, Webb PJ. Scoliosis in Neurofibromatosis: The Natural History with and without Operation. *J Bone Joint Surg* 1989;71B:246.

+ 38. Cardelia JM, Dormans JP, Drummond DS, et al. Proximal Fibular Osteochondroma with Associated Peroneal Nerve Palsy: A Review of Six Cases. *J Pediatr Orthop* 1995;15:574.

39. Carpenter TO. New Perspectives on the Biology and Treatment of X-linked Hypophosphatemic Rickets. *Pediatr Clin North Am* 1997;44:443.

+ 40. Cates HE, Burgess RC. Incidence of Brachydactyly and Hand Exostosis in Hereditary Multiple Exostosis. *J Hand Surg* 1991;16:127.

+ 41. Cavanah SF, Dons RF. McCune-Albright Syndrome: How Many Endocrinopathies Can One Patient Have? *South Med J* 1993;86:364.

+ 42. Charnas LR, Marini JC. Communicating Hydrocephalus, Basilar Invagination, and Other Neurologic Features in Osteogenesis Imperfecta. *Neurology* 1993;43:2603.

+ 43. Cole WG. Early Surgical Management of Severe Forms of Osteogenesis Imperfecta. *Am J Med Genet* 1993;45:270.

+ 44. Cole WG, Dalgleish R. Perinatal Lethal Osteogenesis Imperfecta. *J Med Genet* 1995;32:284.

! 45. Cole WG. The Nicholas Andry Award—1996. The Molecular Pathology of Osteogenesis Imperfecta. *Clin Orthop* 1997;343:235.

+ 46. Coleman SS, Coleman DA. Congenital Pseudarthrosis of the Tibia: Treatment by Transfer of the Ipsilateral Fibula with Vascular Pedicle. *J Pediatr Orthop* 1994;14:156.

+ 47. Craig JB, Govender S. Neurofibromatosis of the Cervical Spine: A Report of Eight Cases. *J Bone Joint Surg* 1992;74B:575.

+ 48. Craigen MA, Clarke NM. Familial Congenital Pseudarthrosis of Ulna. *J Hand Surg* 1995;20:331.

* 49. Crawford AH Jr, Bagamery N. Osseous Manifestations of Neurofibromatosis in Childhood. *J Pediatr Orthop* 1986;6:72.

* 50. Crawford AH. Pitfalls of Spinal Deformities Associated with Neurofibromatosis in Children. *Clin Orthop* 1989;245:29.

+ 51. Cremers MJ, Bol E, de Roos F, van Gijn J. Risk of Sports Activities in Children with Down's Syndrome and Atlantoaxial Instability. *Lancet* 1993;342:511.

+ 52. Crossett LS, Beaty JH, Betz RR, et al. Congenital Pseudarthrosis of the Tibia: Long-term Follow-up Study. *Clin Orthop* 1989;245:16.

+ 53. Dabezies EJ, Warren PD. Fractures in Very Low Birth Weight Infants with Rickets. *Clin Orthop* 1997;335:233.

+ 54. Dahl MT. The Gradual Correction of Forearm Deformities in Multiple Hereditary Exostoses. *Hand Clin* 1993;9:707.

+ 55. Daly K, Wisbeach A, Sanpera I Jr, Fixsen JA. The Prognosis for Walking in Osteogenesis Imperfecta. *J Bone Joint Surg* 1996;78B:7.

+ 56. Danielsson LG, el-Haddad I. Winged Scapula due to Osteochondroma: Report of 3 Children. *Acta Orthop Scand* 1989;60:728.

+ 57. Danielsson LG, el-Haddad I, Quadros O. Distal Tibial Osteochondroma Deforming the Fibula. *Acta Orthop Scand* 1990;61:469.

+ 58. Davids JR, Fisher R, Lum G, Von Glinski S. Angular Deformity of the Lower Extremity in Children with Renal Osteodystrophy. *J Pediatr Orthop* 1992;12:291.

+ 59. De Leon SY, Ilbawi MN, Egel RT, et al. Perioperative Spinal Canal Narrowing in Patients with Down's Syndrome. *Ann Thorac Surg* 1991;52:1325.

! 60. Deere M, Blanton SH, Scott CI, et al. Genetic Heterogeneity in Multiple Epiphyseal Dysplasia. *Am J Hum Genet* 1995;56:698.

+ 61. Del Bello DA, Watts HG. Distal Femoral Extension Osteotomy for Knee Flexion Contracture in Patients with Arthrogryposis. *J Pediatr Orthop* 1996;16:122.

+ 62. Delgado-Martinez AD, Rodriguez-Merchan EC, Olsen B. Congenital Pseudarthrosis of the Tibia. *Int Orthop* 1996;20:192.

63. Diamond LS, Lynne D, Sigman B. Orthopedic Disorders in Patients with Down's Syndrome. *Orthop Clin North Am* 1981;12:57.

+ 64. Dias LS, Stern LS. Talectomy in the Treatment of Resistant Talipes Equinovarus Deformity in Myelomeningocele and Arthrogryposis. *J Pediatr Orthop* 1987;7:39.

65. Dietz FR, Mathews KD. Update on the Genetic Bases of Disorders with Orthopaedic Manifestations. *J Bone Joint Surg* 1996;78A:1583.

+ 66. Dormans JP, Krajbich JI, Zuker R, Demuynk M. Congenital Pseudarthrosis of the Tibia: Treatment with Free Vascularized Fibular Grafts. *J Pediatr Orthop* 1990;10:623.

+ 67. Doyle JS, Lauerman WC, Wood KB, Krause DR. Complications and Long-term Outcome of Upper Cervical Spine Arthrodesis in Patients with Down Syndrome. *Spine* 1996;21:1223.

+ 68. Dugdale TW, Renshaw TS. Instability of the Patellofemoral Joint in Down Syndrome. *J Bone Joint Surg* 1986;68A:405.

! 69. Econs MJ, Francis F. Positional Cloning of the PEX Gene: New Insights into the Pathophysiology of X-linked Hypophosphatemic Rickets. *Am J Physiol* 1997;273:F489.

! 70. Econs MJ, McEnery PT, Lennon F, Speer MC. Autosomal Dominant Hypophosphatemic Rickets is Linked to Chromosome 12p13. *J Clin Invest* 1997;100:2653.

71. Econs MJ, Samsa GP, Monger M, et al. X-linked Hypophosphatemic Rickets: A Disease Often Unknown to Affected Patients. *Bone Miner* 1994;24:17.

+ 72. Egelhoff JC, Bates DJ, Ross JS, et al. Spinal MR Findings in Neurofibromatosis Types 1 and 2. *AJNR Am J Neuroradiol* 1992;13:1071.

+ 73. Ehara S, Kattapuram SV, Rosenberg AE. Fibrous Dysplasia of the Spine. *Spine* 1992;17:977.

+ 74. Engelbert RH, Helders PJ, Keessen W, et al. Intramedullary Rodding in Type III Osteogenesis Imperfecta: Effects on Neuromotor Development in 10 Children. *Acta Orthop Scand* 1995;66:361.

* 75. Enneking WF, Gearen PF. Fibrous Dysplasia of the Femoral Neck: Treatment by Cortical Bone-grafting. *J Bone Joint Surg* 1986;68A:1415.

+ 76. Erdincler P, Dashti R, Kaynar MY, et al. Hydrocephalus and Chronically Increased Intracranial Pressure in Achondroplasia. *Childs Nerv Syst* 1997;13:345.

+ 77. Evans R, Caffey J. Metaphyseal Dysostosis Resembling Vitamin D Refractory Rickets. *Am J Dis Child* 1958;95:581.

+ 78. Fabry G, Lammens J, Van Melkebeek J, Stuyck J. Treatment of Congenital Pseudarthrosis with the Ilizarov Technique. *J Pediatr Orthop* 1988;8:67.

+ 79. Ferris B, Walker C, Jackson A, Kirwan E. The Orthopaedic Management of Hypophosphataemic Rickets. *J Pediatr Orthop* 1991;11:367.

+ 80. Forese LL, Berdon WE, Harcke HT, et al. Severe Midcervical Kyphosis with Cord Compression in Larsen's Syndrome and Diastrophic Dysplasia: Unrelated Syndromes with Similar Radiologic Findings and Neurosurgical Implications. *Pediatr Radiol* 1995;25:136.

+ 81. Fraser RK, Nattrass GR, Chow CW, Cole WG. Pes Anserinus Syndrome due to Solitary Tibial Spurs and Osteochondromas. *J Pediatr Orthop* 1996;16:247.

+ 82. Freeman BH, d Bray EW, Meyer LC. Multiple Osteotomies with Zickel Nail Fixation for Polyostotic Fibrous Dysplasia Involving the Proximal Part of the Femur. *J Bone Joint Surg* 1987;69A:691.

+ 83. Frijns CJ, Van Deutekom J, Frants RR, Jennekens FG. Dominant Congenital Benign Spinal Muscular Atrophy. *Muscle Nerve* 1994;17:192.

+ 84. Funasaki H, Winter RB, Lonstein JB, Denis F. Pathophysiology of Spinal Deformities in Neurofibromatosis: An Analysis of Seventy-one Patients Who Had Curve Associated with Dystrophic Changes. *J Bone Joint Surg* 1994;76:692.

+ 85. Gabriel KR, Mason DE, Carango P. Occipito-atlantal Translation in Down's Syndrome. *Spine* 1990;15:997.

+ 86. Gamble JG, Rinsky LA, Strudwick J, Bleck EE. Nonunion of Fractures in Children Who Have Osteogenesis Imperfecta. *J Bone Joint Surg* 1988;70A:439.

+ 87. Gamble JG, Strudwick WJ, Rinsky LA, Bleck EE. Complications of Intramedullary Rods in Osteogenous Imperfecta: Bailey-Dubow Rods Versus Nonelongating Rods. *J Pediatr Orthop* 1988;8:645.

+ 88. Ganel A, Horoszowski H. Limb Lengthening in Children with Achondroplasia: Differences Based on Gender. *Clin Orthop* 1996;332:179.

+ 89. Gerber LH, Binder H, Weintrob J, et al. Rehabilitation of Children and Infants with Osteogenesis Imperfecta: A Program for Ambulation. *Clin Orthop* 1990;251:254.

90. Gertner JM, Root L. Osteogenesis Imperfecta. *Orthop Clin North Am* 1990;21:151.

+ 91. Gilbert A, Brockman R. Congenital Pseudarthrosis of the Tibia: Long-term Followup of 29 Cases Treated by Microvascular Bone Transfer. *Clin Orthop* 1995;314:37.

+ 92. Greene ADL, Fixen JA, Lloyd-Roberts GC. Talectomy for Arthrogryposis Multiplex Congenita. *J Bone Joint Surg* 1984;66:697.

+ 93. Grill F. Treatment of Congenital Pseudarthrosis of Tibia with the Circular Frame Technique. *J Pediatr Orthop B* 1996;5:6.

+ 94. Guidera KJ, Kortright L, Barber V, Ogden JA. Radiographic Changes in Arthrogrypotic Knees. *Skeletal Radiol* 1991;20:193.

+ 95. Guidera KJ, Satterwhite Y, Ogden JA, et al. Nail Patella Syndrome: A Review of 44 Orthopaedic Patients. *J Pediatr Orthop* 1991;11:737.

+ 96. Guille JT, Bowen JR. Scoliosis and Fibrous Dysplasia of the Spine. *Spine* 1995;20:248.

+ 97. Guille JT, Kumar SJ, MacEwen GD. Fibrous Dysplasia of the Proximal Part of the Femur. *J Bone Joint Surg* 1998;80A:648.

! 98. Gutmann DH, Collins FS. The Neurofibromatosis Type I Gene and Its Product, Neurofibromin. *Neuron* 1993;10:335.

+ 99. Haddad FS, Williams RL, Bentley G. The Cervical Spine in Neurofibromatosis. *Br J Hosp Med* 1995;53:318.

100. Hall JG. Arthrogryposis Multiplex Congenita: Etiology, Genetics, Classification, Diagnostic Approach, and General Aspects. *J Pediatr Orthop B* 1997;6:159.

! 101. Hanna JD, Niimi K, Chan JC. X-linked Hypophosphatemia: Genetic and Clinical Correlates. *Am J Dis Child* 1991;145:86.

+ 102. Hanscom DA, Winter RB, Lutter L, et al. Osteogenesis Imperfecta: Radiographic Classification, Natural History, and Treatment of Spinal Deformities. *J Bone Joint Surg* 1992;74:598.

+ 103. Hanukoglu A, Chalew SA, Sun CJ, et al. Surgically Curable Hypophosphatemic Rickets: Diagnosis and Management. *Clin Pediatr* 1989;28:321.

+ 104. Harkey HL, Crockard HA, Stevens JM, et al. The Operative Management of Basilar Impression in Osteogenesis Imperfecta. *Neurosurgery* 1990;27:782.

+ 105. Harris NL, Eilert RE, Davino N, et al. Osteogenic Sarcoma Arising from Bony Regenerate Following Ilizarov Femoral Lengthening through Fibrous Dysplasia. *J Pediatr Orthop* 1994;14:123.

* 106. Harris WH, Dudley HR Jr, Barry RJ. The Natural History of Fibrous Dysplasia. *J Bone Joint Surg* 1962:44A:207.

+ 107. Hartjen CA, Koman LA. Treatment of Slipped Capital Femoral Epiphysis Resulting from Juvenile Renal Osteodystrophy. *J Pediatr Orthop* 1990;10:551.

+ 108. Helfen M, Gotzinger R, Lutke A, et al. Intrathoracic Dural Ectasia Mimicking Neurofibroma and Scoliosis: A Case Report. *Int Orthop* 1995;19:181.

* 109. Herring JA. The Spinal Disorders in Diastrophic Dwarfism. *J Bone Joint Surg* 1978;60A:177.

+ 110. Holt RT, Johnson JR. Cotrel-Dubousset Instrumentation in Neurofibromatosis Spine Curves: A Preliminary Report. *Clin Orthop* 1989;245:19.

+ 111. Horton WA, Hecht JT, Hood OJ, et al. Growth Hormone Therapy in Achondroplasia. *Am J Med Genet* 1992;42:667.

! 112. Humbel RC, Marchal C, Fall M. Diagnosis of Morquio's Disease: A Simple Chromatographic Method for the Identification of Keratosulfate in Urine. *J Pediatr* 1972;81:107.

+ 113. Ingram RR. The Shoulder in Multiple Epiphyseal Dysplasia. *J Bone Joint Surg* 1991;73B:277.

+ 114. Ishikawa S, Kumar SJ, Takahashi HE, Homma M. Vertebral Body Shape as a Predictor of Spinal Deformity in Osteogenesis Imperfecta. *J Bone Joint Surg* 1996;78A:212.

+ 115. Jacobsen ST, Crawford AH, Millar EA, Steel HH. The Syme Amputation in Patients with Congenital Pseudarthrosis of the Tibia. *J Bone Joint Surg* 1983;65A:533.

+ 116. Jacobsen ST, Hull CK, Crawford AH. Nutritional Rickets. *J Pediatr Orthop* 1986;6:713.

+ 117. Janelle C, Stanciu C. Relationship Between Osteochondromas of the Forearm in Children and Dislocation of the Radial Head. *Ann Chir* 1993;47:888.

+ 118. Joseph KN, Bowen JR, MacEwen GD. Unusual Orthopedic Manifestations of Neurofibromatosis. *Clin Orthop* 1992;278:17.

* 119. Kahanovitz N, Rimoin DL, Sillence DO. The Clinical Spectrum of Lumbar Spine Disease in Achondroplasia. *Spine* 1982;7:137.

120. Kallen B, Mastroiacovo P, Robert E. Major Congenital Malformations in Down Syndrome. *Am J Med Genet* 1996;65:160.

+ 121. Kanel JS, Price CT. Unilateral External Fixation for Corrective Osteotomies in Patients with Hypophosphatemic Rickets. *J Pediatr Orthop* 1995;15:232.

+ 122. Karol LA, Haideri NF, Halliday SE, et al. Gait Analysis and Muscle Strength in Children with Congenital Pseudarthrosis of the Tibia: The Effect of Treatment. *J Pediatr Orthop* 1998;18:381.

+ 123. Karol LA, Sheffield EG, Crawford K, et al. Reproducibility in the Measurement of Atlanto-occipital Instability in Children with Down Syndrome. *Spine* 1996;21:2463.

124. Kocher MS, Shapiro F. Osteogenesis Imperfecta. *J Am Acad Orthop Surg* 1998;6:225.

+ 125. Koo WW, Sherman R, Succop P, et al. Fractures and Rickets in Very Low Birth Weight Infants: Conservative Management and Outcome. *J Pediatr Orthop* 1993;13:577.

+ 126. Kupcha PC, Guille JT, Tassanawipas A, Bowen JR. Polyostotic Fibrous Dysplasia and Acromegaly. *J Pediatr Orthop* 1991;11:95.

127. Lachman RS. Neurologic Abnormalities in the Skeletal Dysplasias: A Clinical and Radiological Perspective. *Am J Med Genet* 1997;69:33.

+ 128. Li MH, Holtas S. MR Imaging of Spinal Neurofibromatosis. *Acta Radiol* 1991;32:279.

* 129. Lichenstein L, Jaffe HL. Fibrous Dysplasia of Bone: A Condition Affecting One, Several, or Many Bones, the Graver Cases of which May Present Abnormal Pigmentation of Skin, Premature Sexual Development, or Still Other Extraskeletal Abnormalities. *Arch Pathol* 1942;33:777.

+ 130. Lovell AT, Alexander R, Grundy EM. Silent, Unstable, Cervical Spine Injury in Multiple Neurofibromatosis [Letter]. *Anaesthesia* 1994;49:453.

! 131. Lutchman M, Rouleau GA. The Neurofibromatosis Type 2 Gene Product, Schwannomin, Suppresses Growth of NIH 3T3 Cells. *Cancer Res* 1995;55:2270.

! 132. Lutter LD, Longstein JE, Winter RB, Langer LO. Anatomy of the Achondroplastic Lumbar Canal. *Clin Orthop* 1977;126:139.

+ 133. Mackenzie WG, Bassett GS, Mandell GA, Scott CI Jr. Avascular Necrosis of the Hip in Multiple Epiphyseal Dysplasia. *J Pediatr Orthop* 1989;9:666.

+ 134. Mainzer F, Minagi H, Steinbach HL. The Variable Manifestations of Multiple Enchondromatosis. *Radiology* 1971;99:377.

+ 135. Malghem J, Vande Berg B, Noel H, Maldague B. Benign Osteochondromas and Exostotic Chondrosarcomas: Evaluation of Cartilage Cap Thickness by Ultrasound. *Skeletal Radiol* 1992;21:33.

+ 136. Mandell GA, Harcke HT, Scott CI, et al. Protrusio Acetabuli in Neurofibromatosis: Nondysplastic and Dysplastic Forms. *Neurosurgery* 1992;30:552.

137. Mankin HJ. Rickets, Osteomalacia, and Renal Osteodystrophy: An Update. *Orthop Clin North Am* 1990;21:81.

138. Mankin HJ. Metabolic Bone Disease. *Instr Course Lect* 1995;44:3.

139. Marini JC, Gerber NL. Osteogenesis Imperfecta: Rehabilitation and Prospects for Gene Therapy [Clinical Conference]. *JAMA* 1997;277:746.

+ 140. Martich V, Ben-Ami T, Yousefzadeh DK, Roizen NJ. Hypoplastic Posterior Arch of C-1 in Children with Down Syndrome: A Double Jeopardy. *Radiology* 1992;183:125.

+ 141. Mathoulin C, Gilbert A, Azze RG. Congenital Pseudarthrosis of the Forearm: Treatment of Six Cases with Vascularized Fibular Graft and a Review of the Literature. *Microsurgery* 1993;14:252.

142. Mautner VF, Tatagiba M, Guthoff R, et al. Neurofibromatosis 2 in the Pediatric Age Group. *Neurosurgery* 1993;33:92.

+ 143. McAllion SJ, Paterson CR. Causes of Death in Osteogenesis Imperfecta. *J Clin Pathol* 1996;49:627.

+ 144. Menelaus MB. Talectomy for Equinovarus Deformity in Arthrogryposis and Spina Bifida. *J Bone Joint Surg* 1971;53B:468.

* 145. Menezes AH, Ryken TC. Craniovertebral Abnormalities in Down's Syndrome. *Pediatr Neurosurg* 1992;18:24.

! 146. Minamitani K, Minagawa M, Yasuda T, Niimi H. Early Detection of Infants with Hypophosphatemic Vitamin D Resistant Rickets (HDRR). *Endocr J* 1996;43:339.

+ 147. Morton RE, Khan MA, Murray-Leslie C, Elliot S. Atlantoaxial Instability in Down's Syndrome: A Five Year Follow Up Study. *Arch Dis Child* 1995;72:115.

+ 148. Msall ME, Reese ME, Di Gaudio K, et al. Symptomatic Atlantoaxial Instability Associated with Medical and Rehabilitative Procedures in Children with Down Syndrome. *Pediatrics* 1990;85:447.

+ 149. Murray C, Fixsen JA. Management of Knee Deformity in Classical Arthrogryposis Multiplex Congenita (Amyoplasia Congenita). *J Pediatr Orthop B* 1997;6:186.

+ 150. Nabarro MN, Giblin PE. Monostotic Fibrous Dysplasia of the Thoracic Spine. *Spine* 1994;19:463.

+ 151. Nawata K, Teshima R, Minamizaki T, Yamamoto K. Knee Deformities in Multiple Hereditary Exostoses: A Longitudinal Radiographic Study. *Clin Orthop* 1995; 313:194.

+ 152. Nelson J, Thomas PS. Clinical Findings in 12 Patients with MPS IV A (Morquio's Disease): Further Evidence for Heterogeneity. Part III: Odontoid Dysplasia. *Clin Genet* 1988;33:126.

+ 153. Nguyen BD, Lugo-Olivieri CH, McCarthy EF, et al. Fibrous Dysplasia with Secondary Aneurysmal Bone Cyst. *Skeletal Radiol* 1996;25:88.

+ 154. Nicholas RW, James P. Telescoping Intramedullary Stabilization of the Lower Extremities for Severe Osteogenesis Imperfecta. *J Pediatr Orthop* 1990;10:219.

+ 155. Niki H, Staheli LT, Mosca VS. Management of Clubfoot Deformity in Amyoplasia. *J Pediatr Orthop* 1997; 17:803.

+ 156. Nishi Y, Kajiyama M, Miyagawa S, et al. Growth Hormone Therapy in Achondroplasia. *Acta Endocrinol* 1993;128:394.

+ 157. O'Brien MF, Bridwell KH, Lenke LG, Schoenecker PL. Intracanalicular Osteochondroma Producing Spinal Cord Compression in Hereditary Multiple Exostoses. *J Spinal Disord* 1994;7:236.

+ 158. Olmastroni M, Seracini D, Lavoratti G, et al. Magnetic Resonance Imaging of Renal Osteodystrophy in Children. *Pediatr Radiol* 1997;27:865.

! 159. Olsen CL, Cross PK, Gensburg LJ, Hughes JP. The Effects of Prenatal Diagnosis, Population Ageing, and Changing Fertility Rates on the Live Birth Prevalence of Down Syndrome in New York State, 1983–1992. *Prenat Diagn* 1996;16:991.

+ 160. Oppenheim WL, Fischer SR, Salusky IB. Surgical Correction of Angular Deformity of the Knee in Children with Renal Osteodystrophy. *J Pediatr Orthop* 1997; 17:41.

+ 161. Oppenheim WL, Shayestehfar S, Salusky IB. Tibial Physeal Changes in Renal Osteodystrophy: Lateral Blount's Disease. *J Pediatr Orthop* 1992;12:774.

* 162. Parfenchuck TA, Bertrand SL, Powers MJ, et al. Posterior Occipitoatlantal Hypermobility in Down Syndrome: An Analysis of 199 Patients. *J Pediatr Orthop* 1994;14:304.

163. Parfitt AM. Renal Osteodystrophy. *Orthop Clin North Am* 1972;3:681.

+ 164. Patel L, Clayton PE, Brain C, et al. Acute Biochemical Effects of Growth Hormone Treatment Compared with Conventional Treatment in Familial Hypophosphataemic Rickets. *Clin Endocrinol* 1996;44:687.

+ 165. Patel MD, Filly RA. Homozygous Achondroplasia: US Distinction Between Homozygous, Heterozygous, and Unaffected Fetuses in the Second Trimester. *Radiology* 1995;196:541.

166. Paterson D. Congenital Pseudarthrosis of the Tibia: An Overview. *Clin Orthop* 1989;247:44.

+ 167. Pauli RM, Horton VK, Glinski LP, Reiser CA. Prospective Assessment of Risks for Cervicomedullary-junction Compression in Infants with Achondroplasia. *Am J Hum Genet* 1995;56:732.

+ 168. Pauli RM, Breed AM, Horton VK, et al. Prevention of Fixed Angular Kyphosis in Achondroplasia. *J Pediatr Orthop* 1997;17:726.

169. Peterson HA. Multiple Hereditary Osteochondromata. *Clin Orthop* 1989;239:222.

+ 170. Peterson HA. Deformities and Problems of the Forearm in Children with Multiple Hereditary Osteochondromata. *J Pediatr Orthop* 1994;14:92.

* 171. Ponseti IV. Skeletal Growth in Achondroplasia. *J Bone Joint Surg* 1970;52A:701.

+ 172. Porsborg P, Astrup G, Bendixen D, et al. Osteogenesis Imperfecta and Malignant Hyperthermia. Is There a Relationship? *Anaesthesia* 1996;51:863.

173. Poussa M, Merikanto J, Ryoppy S, et al. The Spine in Diastrophic Dysplasia. *Spine* 1991;16:881.

+ 174. Przybylski GJ, Pollack IF, Ward WT. Monostotic Fibrous Dysplasia of the Thoracic Spine: A Case Report. *Spine* 1996;21:860.

+ 175. Pueschel SM, Moon AC, Scola FH. Computerized Tomography in Persons with Down Syndrome and Atlantoaxial Instability. *Spine* 1992;17:735.

176. Pueschel SM, Scola FH, Tupper TB, Pezzullo JC. Skeletal Anomalies of the Upper Cervical Spine in Children with Down Syndrome. *J Pediatr Orthop* 1990;10:607.

+ 177. Pueschel SM, Scola FH, Pezzullo JC. A Longitudinal Study of Atlanto-dens Relationships in Asymptomatic Individuals with Down Syndrome. *Pediatrics* 1992;89: 1194.

+ 178. Quinn CM, Wigglesworth JS, Heckmatt J. Lethal Arthrogryposis Multiplex Congenita: A Pathological Study of 21 Cases. *Histopathology* 1991;19:155.

+ 179. Raupp P, Kemperdick H. Neonatal Radiological Aspect of Enchondromatosis (Ollier's Disease). *Pediatr Radiol* 1990;20:337.

+ 180. Richards BS. Atlanto-axial Instability in Diastrophic Dysplasia: A Case Report. *J Bone Joint Surg* 1991;73A: 614.

+ 181. Rizzolo S, Lemos MJ, Mason DE. Posterior Spinal Arthrodesis for Atlantoaxial Instability in Down Syndrome. *J Pediatr Orthop* 1995;15:543.

+ 182. Rosenbloom AL, Smith DW. The Natural History of Metaphyseal Dysostosis. *J Pediatr* 1965;66:857.

! 183. Rousseau F, Bonaventure J, Legeai-Mallet L, et al. Mutations in the Gene Encoding Fibroblast Growth Factor Receptor-3 in Achondroplasia. *Nature* 1994;371:252.

! 184. Rowe PS, Goulding J, Francis F, et al. The Gene for X-linked Hypophosphataemic Rickets Maps to a 200-300 kb Region in Xp22.1 and Is Located on a Single YAC Containing a Putative Vitamin D Response Element (VDRE). *Hum Genet* 1996;97:345.

! 185. Rowe PS, Goulding J, Read A, et al. Refining the Genetic Map for the Region Flanking the X-linked Hypophosphataemic Rickets Locus (Xp22.1-22.2). *Hum Genet* 1994;93:291.

+ 186. Roy M, Baxter M, Roy A. Atlantoaxial Instability in Down Syndrome—Guidelines for Screening and Detection. *J R Soc Med* 1990;83:433.

+ 187. Rubinovitch M, Said SE, Glorieux FH, et al. Principles and Results of Corrective Lower Limb Osteotomies for Patients with Vitamin D–Resistant Hypophosphatemic Rickets. *Clin Orthop* 1988;237:264.

+ 188. Rudolf MK, Arulanantham K, Greenstein RM. Unsuspected Nutritional Rickets. *Pediatrics* 1980;66:72.

+ 189. Ruggieri P, Sim FH, Bond JR, Unni KK. Malignancies in Fibrous Dysplasia. *Cancer* 1994;73:1411.

+ 190. Ryoppy S, Poussa M, Merikanto J, et al. Foot Deformities in Diastrophic Dysplasia: An Analysis of 102 Patients. *J Bone Joint Surg* 1992;74B:441.

! 191. Saggese G, Baroncelli GI, Bertelloni S, Perri G. Long-term Growth Hormone Treatment in Children with Renal Hypophosphatemic Rickets: Effects on Growth, Mineral Metabolism, and Bone Density. *J Pediatr* 1995;127:395.

+ 192. Sanchez CP, Salusky IB. The Renal Bone Diseases in Children Treated with Dialysis. *Adv Ren Replace Ther* 1996;3:14.

! 193. Sanguinetti C, Greco F, De Palma L, et al. Morphological Changes in Growth-plate Cartilage in Osteogenesis Imperfecta. *J Bone Joint Surg* 1990;72B:475.

194. Scarborough MT, Moreau G. Benign Cartilage Tumors. *Orthop Clin North Am* 1996;27:583.

+ 195. Schajowicz F, Santini-Araujo E. Adamantinoma of the Tibia Masked by Fibrous Dysplasia: Report of Three Cases. *Clin Orthop* 1989;238:294.

* 196. Schenk EA, Haggerty J. Morquio's Disease: A Radiologic and Morphologic Study. *Pediatrics* 1964;34:839.

! 197. Schipani E, Langman CB, Parfitt AM, et al. Constitutively Activated Receptors for Parathyroid Hormone and Parathyroid hormone–related Peptide in Jansen's Metaphyseal Chondrodysplasia. *N Engl J Med* 1996;335:708.

+ 198. Schorry EK, Crawford AH, Egelhoff JC, et al. Thoracic Tumors in Children with Neurofibromatosis-1. *Am J Med Genet* 1997;74:533.

* 199. Schwartz HS, Zimmerman NB, Simon MA, et al. The Malignant Potential of Enchondromatosis. *J Bone Joint Surg* 1987;69A:269.

* 200. Segal LS, Drummond DS, Zanotti RM, et al. Complications of Posterior Arthrodesis of the Cervical Spine in Patients Who Have Down Syndrome. *J Bone Joint Surg* 1991;73A:1547.

+ 201. Sells JM, Jaffe KM, Hall JG. Amyoplasia, the Most Common Type of Arthrogryposis: The Potential for Good Outcome. *Pediatrics* 1996;97:225.

+ 202. Shaw ED, Beals RK. The Hip Joint in Down's Syndrome: A Study of Its Structure and Associated Disease. *Clin Orthop* 1992;278:101.

+ 203. Shea D, Mankin HJ. Slipped Capital Femoral Epiphysis in Renal Rickets: Report of Three Cases. *J Bone Joint Surg* 1966;48A:349.

+ 204. Shearer P, Parham D, Kovnar E, et al. Neurofibromatosis Type I and Malignancy: Review of 32 Pediatric

Cases Treated at a Single Institution. *Med Pediatr Oncol* 1994;22:78.

+ 205. Sheffield EG. Double-layered Patella in Multiple Epiphyseal Dysplasia: A Valuable Clue in the Diagnosis. *J Pediatr Orthop* 1998;18:123.

! 206. Shen MH, Harper PS, Upadhyaya M. Molecular Genetics of Neurofibromatosis Type 1 (NF1). *J Med Genet* 1996;33:2.

! 207. Shohat M, Lotan R, Magal N, et al. A Gene for Arthrogryposis Multiplex Congenita Neuropathic Type is Linked to D5S394 on Chromosome 5qter. *Am J Hum Genet* 1997;61:1139.

* 208. Sillence D. Osteogenesis Imperfecta: An Expanding Panorama of Variants. *Clin Orthop* 1981;159:11.

+ 209. Sillence D, Butler B, Latham M, Barlow K. Natural History of Blue Sclerae in Osteogenesis Imperfecta. *Am J Med Genet* 1993;45:183.

! 210. Sillence DO. Craniocervical Abnormalities in Osteogenous Imperfecta: Genetic and Molecular Correlation. *Pediatr Radiol* 1994;24:427.

+ 211. Simonis RB, Shirali HR, Mayou B. Free Vascularized Fibular Grafts for Congenital Pseudarthrosis of the Tibia. *J Bone Joint Surg* 1991;73B:211.

+ 212. Sirois JLD, Drennan JC. Dystrophic Spinal Deformity in Neurofibromatosis. *J Pediatr Orthop* 1990;10:522.

+ 213. Smith MD, Phillips WA, Hensinger RN. Fusion of the Upper Cervical Spine in Children and Adolescents: An Analysis of 17 Patients. *Spine* 1991;16:695.

+ 214. Snearly WN, Peterson HA. Management of Ankle Deformities in Multiple Hereditary Osteochondromata. *J Pediatr Orthop* 1989;9:427.

+ 215. Sodergard J, Ryoppy S. The Knee in Arthrogryposis Multiplex Congenita. *J Pediatr Orthop* 1990;10:177.

+ 216. Sodergard J, Ryoppy S. Foot Deformities in Arthrogryposis Multiplex Congenita. *J Pediatr Orthop* 1994;14:768.

+ 217. Sodergard J, Hakamies-Blomqvist L, Sainio K, et al. Arthrogryposis Multiplex Congenita: Perinatal and Electromyographic Findings, Disability, and Psychosocial Outcome. *J Pediatr Orthop B* 1997;6:167.

* 218. Sofield HA, Miller EA. Fragmentation, Realignment and Intramedullary Rod Fixation of Deformities of the Long Bones in Children: A Ten-year Appraisal. *J Bone Joint Surg* 1959;41A:1371.

+ 219. Sperry K. Fatal Intraoperative Hemorrhage during Spinal Fusion Surgery for Osteogenesis Imperfecta. *Am J Forensic Med Pathol* 1989;10:54.

* 220. Staheli LT, Chew De, Elliot JS, Mosca VS. Management of Hip Dislocations in Children with Arthrogryposis. *J Pediatr Orthop* 1987;7:681.

+ 221. Stanescu V, Stanescu R, Maroteaux P. Pathogenic Mechanisms in Osteochondrodysplasias. *J Bone Joint Surg* 1984;66A:817.

+ 222. Stanton RP, Hansen MO. Function of the Upper Extremities in Hereditary Multiple Exostoses. *J Bone Joint Surg* 1996;78A:568.

+ 223. Steinbach HL, Kolb FO, Gilfillan R. Mechanism of Production of Pseudofractures in Osteomalacia (Milkman's Syndrome). *Radiology* 1954;62:388.

! 224. Steiner RD, Pepin M, Byers PH. Studies of Collagen

Synthesis and Structure in the Differentiation of Child Abuse from Osteogenesis Imperfecta. *J Pediatr* 1996; 128:542.

+ 225. Stephenson RB, London MD, Hankin FM, Kaufer H. Fibrous Dysplasia: An Analysis of Options for Treatment. *J Bone Joint Surg* 1987;69A:400.

+ 226. Stevens JM, Kendall BE, Crockard HA, Ransford A. The Odontoid Process in Morquio-Brailsford's Disease: The Effects of Occipitocervical Fusion. *J Bone Joint Surg* 1991;73B:851.

+ 227. Stickler GB, Morgenstern BZ. Hypophosphataemic Rickets: Final Height and Clinical Symptoms in Adults. *Lancet* 1989;2:902.

+ 228. Stockley I, Bell MJ, Sharrard WJ. The Role of Expanding Intramedullary Rods in Osteogenesis Imperfecta. *J Bone Joint Surg* 1989;71B:422.

! 229. Stoilov I, Kilpatrick MW, Tsipouras P. A Common FGFR3 Gene Mutation Is Present in Achondroplasia but Not in Hypochondroplasia. *Am J Med Genet* 1995; 55:127.

! 230. Superti-Furga A, Rossi A, Steinmann B, Gitzelmann R. A Chondrodysplasia Family Produced by Mutations in the Diastrophic Dysplasia Sulfate Transporter Gene: Genotype/phenotype Correlations. *Am J Med Genet* 1996;63:144.

+ 231. Swierstra BA, Diepstraten AF, vd Heyden BJ. Distal Femoral Physiolysis in Renal Osteodystrophy: Successful Nonoperative Treatment of 3 Cases Followed for 5 years. *Acta Orthop Scand* 1993;64:382.

+ 232. Szoke G, Staheli LT, Jaffe K, Hall JG. Medial-approach Open Reduction of Hip Dislocation in Amyoplasia-type Arthrogryposis. *J Pediatr Orthop* 1996;16:127.

! 233. Takeyama K, Kitanaka S, Sato T, et al. 25-Hydroxyvitamin D3 1 Alpha-hydroxylase and Vitamin D Synthesis. *Science* 1997;277:1827.

+ 234. Thomas B, Schopler S, Wood W, Oppenheim WL. The Knee in Arthrogryposis. *Clin Orthop* 1985;194:87.

+ 235. Thompson EM. Non-invasive Prenatal Diagnosis of Osteogenesis Imperfecta. *Am J Med Genet* 1993;45:201.

! 236. Timperlake RW, Cook SD, Thomas KA, et al. Effects of Anticonvulsant Drug Therapy on Bone Mineral Density in a Pediatric Population. *J Pediatr Orthop* 1988; 8:467.

237. Tolo VT. Spinal Deformity in Short-stature Syndromes. *Instr Course Lect* 1990;39:399.

+ 238. Treble NJ, Jensen FO, Bankier A, et al. Development of the Hip in Multiple Epiphyseal Dysplasia: Natural History and Susceptibility to Premature Osteoarthritis. *J Bone Joint Surg* 1990;72B:1061.

* 239. Tredwell SJ, Newman DE, Lockitch G. Instability of the Upper Cervical Spine in Down Syndrome. *J Pediatr Orthop* 1990;10:602.

+ 240. Trumble ER. Myseros JS, Smoker WR, et al. Atlantooccipital Subluxation in a Neonate with Down's Syndrome: Case Report and Review of the Literature. *Pediatr Neurosurg* 1994;21:55.

+ 241. Tuncay IC, Johnston CE, Birch JG. Spontaneous Resolution of Congenital Anterolateral Bowing of the Tibia. *J Pediatr Orthop* 1994;14:599.

+ 242. Uchida Y, Kojima T, Sugioka Y. Vascularised Fibular Graft for Congenital Pseudarthrosis of the Tibia: Long-term Results. *J Bone Joint Surg* 1991;73B:846.

+ 243. Uno K, Kataoka O, Shiba R. Occipitoatlantal and Occipitoaxial Hypermobility in Down Syndrome. *Spine* 1996;21:1430.

+ 244. Vaara P, Peltonen J, Poussa M, et al. Development of the Hip in Diastrophic Dwarfism. *J Bone Joint Surg* 1998;80B:315.

245. van der Burgt I, Haraldsson A, Oosterwijk JC, et al. Cartilage Hair Hypoplasia, Metaphyseal Chondrodysplasia Type McKusick: Description of Seven Patients and Review of the Literature. *Am J Med Genet* 1991; 41:371.

+ 246. van Mourik J, Weerdenburg H. Radiographic Anthropometry in Patients with Multiple Epiphyseal Dysplasia. *AJR Am J Roentgenol* 1997;169:1105.

* 247. Verge CF, Lam A, Simpson JM, et al. Effects of Therapy in X-linked Hypophosphatemic Rickets. *N Engl J Med* 1991;325:1843.

! 248. von Deimling A, Krone W, Menon AG. Neurofibromatosis Type 1: Pathology, Clinical Features and Molecular Genetics. *Brain Pathol* 1995;5:153.

249. Walker BA, Scott CI, Hall JG, et al. Diastrophic Dwarfism. *Medicine* 1972;51:41.

! 250. Wallis GA, Rash B, Sykes B, et al. Mutations within the Gene Encoding the Alpha 1 (X) Chain of Type X Collagen (COL10A1) Cause Metaphyseal Chondrodysplasia Type Schmid but Not Several Other Forms of Metaphyseal Chondrodysplasia. *J Med Genet* 1996; 33:450.

251. Walton J. Familial Hypophosphatemic Rickets: A Delineation of Its Subdivisions and Pathogenesis. *Clin Pediatr* 1976;15:1007.

+ 252. Ward BA, Harkey HL, Parent AD, et al. Severe Cervical Kyphotic Deformities in Patients with Plexiform Neurofibromas: Case Report. *Neurosurgery* 1994;35:960.

! 253. Warman ML, Abbott M, Apte SS, et al. A Type X Collagen Mutation Causes Schmid Metaphyseal Chondrodysplasia. *Nat Genet* 1993;5:79.

254. Waters KA, Everett F, Sillence D, et al. Breathing Abnormalities in Sleep in Achondroplasia. *Arch Dis Child* 1993;69:191.

+ 255. Waters KA, Everett F, Sillence DO, et al. Treatment of Obstructive Sleep Apnea in Achondroplasia: Evaluation of Sleep, Breathing, and Somatosensory-evoked Potentials. *Am J Med Genet* 1995;59:460.

+ 256. Waters PM, Van Heest AE, Emans J. Acute Forearm Lengthenings. *J Pediatr Orthop* 1997;17:444.

+ 257. Weber G, Prinster C, Meneghel M, et al. Human Growth Hormone Treatment in Prepubertal Children with Achondroplasia. *Am J Med Genet* 1996;61:396.

+ 258. Weiland AJ, Weiss AP, Moore JR, Tolo VT. Vascularized Fibular Grafts in the Treatment of Congenital Pseudarthrosis of the Tibia. *J Bone Joint Surg* 1990; 72A:654.

! 259. White KS, Ball WS, Prenger EC, et al. Evaluation of the Craniocervical Junction in Down Syndrome: Correlation of Measurements Obtained with Radiography and MR Imaging. *Radiology* 1993;186:377.

+ 260. Wicklund CL, Pauli RM, Johnston D, Hecht JT. Natural History Study of Hereditary Multiple Exostoses. *Am J Med Genet* 1995;55:43.

+ 261. Wilde PH, Upadhyay SS, Leong JC. Deterioration of Operative Correction in Dystrophic Spinal Neurofibromatosis. *Spine* 1994;19:1264.

+ 262. Wilson DM, Lee PD, Morris AH, et al. Growth Hormone Therapy in Hypophosphatemic Rickets. *Am J Dis Child* 1991;145:1165.

* 263. Winter RB, Moe JH, Bradford DS, et al. Spine Deformity in Neurofibromatosis: A Review of One Hundred and Two Patients. *J Bone Joint Surg* 1979;61A:677.

+ 264. Wirganowicz PZ, Watts HG. Surgical Risk for Elective Excision of Benign Exostoses. *J Pediatr Orthop* 1997;17:455.

+ 265. Yamada Y, Ito H, Otsubo Y, Sekido K. Surgical Management of Cervicomedullary Compression in Achondroplasia. *Childs Nerv Syst* 1996;12:737.

+ 266. Yamate T, Kanzaki S, Tanaka H, et al. Growth Hormone (GH) Treatment in Achondroplasia. *J Pediatr Endocrinol* 1993;6:45.

+ 267. Yasui N, Kawabata H, Kojimoto H, et al. Lengthening of the Lower Limbs in Patients with Achondroplasia and Hypochondroplasia. *Clin Orthop* 1997;344:298.

+ 268. Yong-Hing K, MacEwen GD. Scoliosis Associated with Osteogenesis Imperfecta. *J Bone Joint Surg* 1982;64B:36.

+ 269. Yundt KD, Park TS, Tantuwaya VS, Kaufman BA. Posterior Fossa Decompression without Duraplasty in Infants and Young Children for Treatment of Chiari Malformation and Achondroplasia. *Pediatr Neurosurg* 1996;25:221.

+ 270. Zionts LE, Ebramzadeh E, Stott NS. Complications in the Use of the Bailey-Dubow Extensible Nail. *Clin Orthop* 1998;348:186.

! 271. Zionts LE, Nash JP, Rude R, et al. Bone Mineral Density in Children with Mild Osteogenesis Imperfecta. *J Bone Joint Surg* 1995;77B:143.

+ 272. Zucconi M, Weber G, Castronovo V, et al. Sleep and Upper Airway Obstruction in Children with Achondroplasia. *J Pediatr* 1996;129:743.

Index

Note: Page numbers followed by f indicate illustrations; those followed by t indicate tables.

1

Myelomeningocele. *See* Spina bifida
Myelopathy
  cervical spondylotic, 3749, 3750
    clinical manifestations of, 3751
    evaluation of, 3751
    operative treatment for,
      3756–3757
  in rheumatoid arthritis, of cervical
    spine, 3890
Myocutaneous flap
  complications of, 175–179
  design of, 174–175
Myofascial pain, trigger point injection
  for, 150
Myofibroblasts, in Dupuytren's disease,
  1735
Myotonic dystrophy, 4522–4524
  adult, 4523–4524
  congenital, 4522–4523, 4523f
Myotonic syndromes, 4522–4524,
  4523f

N

Nafcillin, 319t, 3518t, 3520, 3522t
  for hand infections, 1991t, 1992t
  for osteomyelitis, 3534–3535, 3535t
  for septic arthritis, 3569
Naftifine, 3530
Nail. *See* Fingernail
Nail bed
  anatomy of, 1257–1258, 1258f
  avulsion of, 1259–1260, 1260f,
    1261f
    lateral deviation and, 1262, 1262f
  infection of, 2003–2004
  injury of, 1257–1263
    classification of, 1259
    etiology of, 1258, 1258t
    initial treatment of, 1258–1259
  repair of, 1259, 1259t
  shortening of, 1263
Nail flap, 1263
Nails. *See also* Implant; Intramedullary
    nailing; Rod
  Alta, 359, 360f, 361, 362, 363f,
    364f
  AO, 359
  Brooker-Wills, 361, 362f
  care of, in diabetics, 3078
  Ender, 360, 362f
  gamma, 363, 365f
  Grosse-Kempf, 359, 360f, 361
  Hansen-Street, 359–360
  Harris, 361f
  interlocking, 371
  Klemm, 359, 361
  Küntscher, 359, 360f
  locking, 361–362, 362f
  Lottes tibial, 360, 361f, 794–796
  malposition of, 373
  nonreamed, 359–361, 360f
  normal flora of, 3508
  reamed, 359, 360f
  reaming for, 369–370

removal of, 374, 375
  in nonunion, 864
Russell-Taylor, 359, 362, 363f
Sage, 360, 363
Sampson, 359, 360
Schneider, 359–360, 361f
Seidel, 361
size of, 370–371
specialized, 362–365
Uniflex, 359
Zickel, 362–363
Nanocolloid, for bone scan, 67. *See
  also* Bone scan
Narcotics
  abuse of, perioperative management
    of, 82t, 82–83
    in failed back surgery syndrome,
      3880
  intrathecal, implantable pump for,
    152
Navicular
  accessory, 3143–3145, 3144f
  tarsal
    fracture of
      avulsion, 2988–2990, 2992
      in Chopart's joint fracture-
        dislocation, 2987–2992
      isolated, 2992–2994
    osteonecrosis, 3302
Naviculocalcaneal coalition, 3142,
  3142f, 3143
Naviculocapitate syndrome,
  1370–1371
Nd:YAG laser, 2539
Neck pain
  differential diagnosis of, 3750
  in disc disease, 3749, 3750–3751,
    3752
Necrotizing fasciitis, 3507
  in hand, 1994–1995
Needle biopsy. *See also* Biopsy
  of cervical tumors, 3917
  muscle, pediatric, 4509
  of soft-tissue tumors, 3454
  of spinal tumors, 3937, 3937f
Needle holders, for arterial injury, of
  upper extremity, 1116
Needle sticks, infection from, 110–111
Neer classification, of proximal
  humeral fracture, 453, 454f
Neer II proximal humerus, 2630,
  2630f, 2631f
Neonatal rickets, 4588
Nerve, repair of
  anatomic basis of, 1537–1538
  epineurial, 1539
  fascicular, 1539–1540, 1540f
  free tissue transfer and, 1176–1177
  newer techniques for, 1541–1542
  postoperative care after, 1541
  principles of, 1533–1542
  rehabilitation after, 1541
  replantation and, 1158–1159
  surgical indications for, 1537–1541,
    1538f, 1540f
Nerve biopsy, in children, 4509

Nerve block
  in deep peroneal nerve entrapment
    diagnosis, 3050
  peripheral, 140, 141t. *See also*
    Anesthesia
  regional, 95–96, 140–143, 141t. *See
    also* Anesthesia
  sympathetic, 150
    replantation and, 1162
Nerve conduction studies
  in cervical disc disease, 3752
  in compression neuropathy, 1547f,
    1547–1548
  pediatric, 4508
  in pronator syndrome, 1562–1563
Nerve disorders, pediatric, evaluation
  of, 4506–4509
Nerve grafting, 1539, 1540–1541
  for brachial plexus injury, 1713,
    1713t
  for neuroma, 1612
Nerve injury, 1533–1534. *See also
  specific nerve*
  in bone grafting, 210
  classification of, 1534, 1534t
  vs. compartment syndrome,
    398–399, 399t
  compression, from casts, 284
  contusion, 1533
  in femoral shaft fracture, 695
  in intramedullary nailing, 374
  intraoperative, 178–179
    in hip osteotomy, 2761
    in revision hip arthroplasty, 2740
    in spinal surgery, 3836–3837
    in total hip arthroplasty, 2787
  knee surgery and, 2438
  laceration, 1533
  natural history of, 1534–1535
  in pelvic trauma, 535–536, 536t,
    581–582
  peripheral, clinical assessment of,
    1535t, 1535–1537, 1536f
  in spinal stenosis correction,
    3836–3837
  in tibial fracture, 804
Nerve root compression
  in cervical spine instability, in
    rheumatoid arthritis, 3990f,
    3990–3992
  in spondylolisthesis, 4147
Nerve root injury, in spinal surgery,
  3836–3837
Nerve transfer, for brachial plexus
  injury, 1713–1717,
  1714f–1716f
Neuralgia, intercostobrachial, thoracic
  outlet surgery and, 1732
Neural tube defects. *See* Spina bifida
Neurapraxia, 1534
Neurectomy
  simple excisional, 1613f,
    1613–1614, 1614f
  ulnar motor, 1756–1757, 1846
Neurilemmoma, 3464
  of hand, 2026